third edition

REHABILITATION
for the Postsurgical Orthopedic Patient

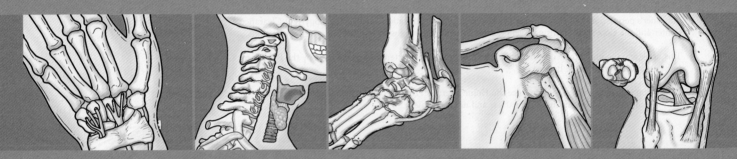

LISA MAXEY, PT
California Hand and Physical Therapy
Oxnard, California

JIM MAGNUSSON, PT, ATC
Owner
Performance Therapy Center, Inc.
Oxnard and Camarillo, California;
Team Physical Therapist
Oxnard College and Pacifica High School
Oxnard, California;
Wellness/Fitness Coordinator
Oxnard/Ventura Fire Departments
Oxnard and Ventura, California

ELSEVIER

3251 Riverport Lane
St. Louis, Missouri 63043

Rehabilitation for the Postsurgical Orthopedic Patient, Third Edition   978-0-323-07747-7

Notices

Knowledge and best practice in this field are constantly changing. As new research and experience broaden our understanding, changes in research methods, professional practices, or medical treatment may become necessary.

Practitioners and researchers must always rely on their own experience and knowledge in evaluating and using any information, methods, compounds, or experiments described herein. In using such information or methods they should be mindful of their own safety and the safety of others, including parties for whom they have a professional responsibility.

With respect to any drug or pharmaceutical products identified, readers are advised to check the most current information provided (i) on procedures featured or (ii) by the manufacturer of each product to be administered, to verify the recommended dose or formula, the method and duration of administration, and contraindications. It is the responsibility of practitioners, relying on their own experience and knowledge of their patients, to make diagnoses, to determine dosages and the best treatment for each individual patient, and to take all appropriate safety precautions.

To the fullest extent of the law, neither the Publisher nor the authors, contributors, or editors, assume any liability for any injury and/or damage to persons or property as a matter of products liability, negligence or otherwise, or from any use or operation of any methods, products, instructions, or ideas contained in the material herein.

Previous editions copyrighted 2007, 2001

Library of Congress Cataloging-in-Publication Data

Rehabilitation for the postsurgical orthopedic patient / [edited by] Lisa Maxey, Jim Magnusson.—3rd ed.
    p. ; cm.
    Includes bibliographical references and index.
    ISBN 978-0-323-07747-7 (hardcover: alk. paper)
    I. Maxey, Lisa.   II. Magnusson, Jim.
    [DNLM: 1. Physical Therapy Modalities.   2. Postoperative Care–rehabilitation.   3. Orthopedic
Procedures–rehabilitation.   WB 460]
    617.4′706–dc23
                                                                              2012031888

Vice President: Linda Duncan
Content Manager: Jolynn Gower
Senior Content Development Specialist: Christie M. Hart
Publishing Services Manager: Pat Joiner-Myers
Project Manager: Prathibha Mehta
Design Direction: Karen Pauls

Printed in China

Last digit is the print number: 9   8   7   6   5   4   3   2   1

In thanksgiving for all His blessings.
Lisa Maxey

To my two children, Nicholas and Michelle.
Jim Magnusson

CONTRIBUTORS

Mayra Saborio Amiran, PT
Owner
California Hand and Physical Therapy
Newbury Park and Oxnard, California

James R. Andrews, MD
Clinical Professor of Surgery
Division of Orthopaedic Surgery
University of Alabama at Birmingham School of Medicine
Birmingham, Alabama;
Clinical Professor of Orthopaedics & Sports Medicine
University of Virginia Medical School
Charlottesville, Virginia;
Clinical Professor
Department of Orthopaedic Surgery
University of Kentucky Medical Center
Lexington, Kentucky;
Senior Orthopaedic Consultant
Washington Redskins Professional Football Team
Washington, DC;
Medical Director
Tampa Bay Devil Rays Professional Baseball Team
Tampa Bay, Florida;
Co-Medical Director
Intercollegiate Sports at Auburn University
Auburn, Alabama;
Orthopaedic Surgeon
Alabama Sports Medicine & Orthopaedic Center
Birmingham, Alabama

Danny Arora, MD
Resident
Department of Surgery
Queen's University
Kingston, Ontario, Canada

Babak Barcohana, MD
Southern California Orthopedic Institute
Van Nuys, California

Mark T. Bastan, DPT, CSCS
Coordinator of Clinical Research and Development
Elite Physical Therapy
Warwick, Rhode Island

Clive E. Brewster, COO
Kerlan-Jobe Orthopaedic Clinic;
Administrator
Kerlan-Jobe Surgery Center
Los Angeles, California

Andrew A. Brooks, MD, FACS
Attending Orthopedic Surgeon
Southern California Orthopedic Institute
Van Nuys, California;
Attending Orthopedic Surgeon
Encino Hospital
Encino, California;
Attending Orthopedic Surgeon
Motion Picture and Television Hospital
Woodland Hills, California;
Attending Orthopedic Surgeon
Specialty Surgical Center
Encino and Beverly Hills, California

Tom Burton, PT
Director
The Center for Rehabilitation Medicine
Van Nuys, California

Adam Cabalo, MD
Orthopedic Surgeon
Kaiser Permanente Maui
Maui, Hawaii

James H. Calandruccio, MD
Associate Professor
Department of Orthopaedic Surgery
University of Tennessee
Memphis, Tennessee;
Physician, Hand and Upper Extremity
Campbell Clinic Orthopaedics
Germantown, Tennessee

Robert Cantu, PT, MMSc, MTC
Clinic Director, Physiotherapy Associates
Woodstock, Georgia;
Continuing Education Instructor
University of St. Augustine for Health Sciences
St. Augustine, Florida;
Adjunct Instructor
School of Occupational Therapy
University of Indianapolis
Indianapolis, Indiana

Erin Carr, PT, DPT
Adjunct Faculty
Department of Physical Therapy
Mount St. Mary's College
Los Angeles, California;
Staff Physical Therapist
Knight Physical Therapy, Inc
Garden Grove, California

Diane Coker, PT, DPT, CHT
Associate Instructor
Loma Linda University
Riverside, California;
Director, Hand Therapy Services
South County Hand Center
Laguna Woods, California

Kyle Coker, MD
Medical Director
South County Hand Center
Laguna Woods, California

Steven L. Cole, MEd, ATC
Athletic Trainer
College of William and Mary
Williamsburg, Virginia

Benjamin Cornell, PT, OCS
Adjunct Professor
Department of Physical Therapy
Mount St. Mary's College
Los Angeles, California;
Physical Therapist
Department of Physical Therapy
HealthCare Partner's Medical Group
Torrance, California

Curtis A. Crimmins, MD
Hand Surgery, Ltd.
Milwaukee, Wisconsin

Linda de Haas, PT, MPT, OCS, CHT
Professional Physical Therapy Associates
Whittier, California

Rick B. Delamarter, MD
Director
The Spine Institute
St. John's Medical Center
Santa Monica, California

Robert Donatelli, PhD, PTOCS
National Director
Sports Specific Rehabilitation and Performance Enhancement
Physiotherapy Associates
Las Vegas, Nevada

Daniel A. Farwell, PT, DPT
Adjunct Professor of Clinical Physical Therapy
Department of Biokinesiology and Physical Therapy
University of Southern California
Los Angeles, California;
Owner/Director
Private Practice
Body Rx Physical Therapy
Glendale, California

Richard D. Ferkel, MD
Assistant Clinical Professor
Department of Orthopedic Surgery
University of California, Los Angeles
Los Angeles, California;
Sports Medicine Fellowship Director
Southern California Orthopedic Institute
Van Nuys, California

Morgan L. Fones, PT, DPT, OCS, ATC
Head Physical Therapist
Mt. Tam Physical Therapy
Larkspur, California

Jonathan E. Fow, MD
Board Certified
Orthopaedic Surgery & Sports Medicine
Arroyo Grande, California

Freddie H. Fu, MD
Professor and Chairman
Department of Orthopaedic Surgery
School of Medicine
University of Pittsburgh
Pittsburgh, Pennsylvania

Ralph A. Gambardella, MD
Kerlan Jobe Orthopedic Clinic
Los Angeles, California

Joshua Gerbert, DPM, FACFAS
Professor Emeritus
Department of Podiatric Surgery
California School of Podiatric Medicine at Samuel Merritt
   University
Oakland, California;
Past Chairman
Department of Podiatric Surgery
St. Mary's Medical Center
San Francisco, California

Mark Ghilarducci, MD
Department of Orthopedic Surgery
St. John's Regional Medical Center;
Department of Sports Medicine
Ventura Orthopedic Medical Group
Oxnard, California;
Ventura Orthopedics
Ventura, California

Eric Giza, MD
Central Maine Orthopedics Group
Auburn, Maine

Patricia A. Gray, MS, PT
Physical Therapist
Rehabilitation/Health At Home
San Francisco General Hospital
San Francisco, California

Jane Gruber, PT, DPT, OCS
Department of Rehabilitation Services
Newton Wellesley Hospital
Newton, Massachusetts

Carlos A. Guanche, MD
Adjunct Clinical Professor
University of Southern California;
Teaching Faculty
Southern California Orthopedic Institute
Van Nuys, California

Will Hall, PT, DPT, OCS
Regional Vice President—Southeast
Physiotherapy Associates
Cumming, Georgia

Karen Hambly, PhD, MCSP
Senior Lecturer
School of Sport and Exercise Sciences
University of Kent
Kent, United Kingdom

Timothy Hartshorn, MD
Resident
Orthopaedic Surgery
University of Southern California
Los Angeles, California

George F. Rick Hatch III, MD
Assistant Professor of Orthopaedic Surgery
University of Southern California
Keck School of Medicine
Los Angeles, California

Eric S. Honbo, PT, DPT, OCS
Co-Owner
Advanced Physical Therapy & Sports Medicine
Thousand Oaks, California

Chris Izu, MPT, DPT, OCS
Adjunct Professor
Department of Physical Therapy
Mount St. Mary's College
Los Angeles, California;
Physical Therapist
Human Performance Center
Santa Barbara, California

Reza Jazayeri, MD
Department of Orthopaedic Surgery
Sports Medicine
Southern California Permanente Medical Group
Woodland Hills, California

Richard Joreitz, PT, DPT, SCS, ATC
Senior Physical Therapist
UPMC Centers for Rehab Services;
Adjunct Clinical Instructor
Department of Physical Therapy
University of Pittsburgh;
Physical Therapist
Pittsburgh Penguins Team
Pittsburgh, Pennsylvania

Kelly Akin Kaye, PT, CHT
Physical Therapist PRN
Campbell Clinic Orthopedics
Germantown, Tennessee

Paul D. Kim, MD
Orthopedic Surgery
Spine Institute
San Diego, California

Linda J. Klein, OTR, CHT
Hand Surgery, Ltd.
Milwaukee, Wisconsin

Graham Linck, PT
Physiotherapy Associated
Las Vegas, Nevada

Kristen G. Lowrance, OTR/L, CHT
Occupational Therapist
Clinical Manager
Campbell Clinic
Germantown, Tennessee

Jim Magnusson PT, ATC
Owner, Performance Therapy Center, Inc.
Oxnard and Camarillo, California;
Team Physical Therapist
Oxnard College and Pacifica High School
Oxnard, California;
Wellness/Fitness Coordinator
Oxnard/Ventura Fire Departments
Oxnard and Ventura, California

Bert R. Mandelbaum, MD
Assistant Professor
Division of Orthopedic Surgery
Department of Surgery
University of California, Los Angeles
Los Angeles, California;
Chief Surgeon
Medical Plaza Orthopedic Surgery Center;
Chief of Orthopedics
Department of Orthopedic Surgery
St. John's Hospital and Health Center
Santa Monica, California

Joel M. Matta, MD
Associate Professor of Clinical Orthopaedics
University of Southern California School of Medicine;
John C. Wilson Jr. Chair of Orthopaedic Surgery
Good Samaritan Hospital
Santa Monica, California

Lisa Maxey, PT
California Hand and Physical Therapy
Oxnard, California

Neil McKenna, DPT, FAAOMPT, OCS, CSCS
Physical Therapist
Solana Beach, California

Kai Mithoefer, MD
Department of Orthopedics
Harvard Vanguard Medical Associates
Harvard Medical School
Boston, Massachusetts

Erica V. Pablo, PT, DPT, OCS
Clinical Director
Knight Physical Therapy, Inc
Garden Grove, California

David Pakozdi, PT, OCS
Director
Kinetic Orthopaedic Physical Therapy
Santa Monica, California

Mark R. Phillips, MD
Clinical Assistant Professor
Department of Orthopedic Surgery
University of Illinois College of Medicine at Peoria;
Department of Orthopedic Surgery
Methodist Medical Center;
Department of Orthopedic Surgery
Proctor Hospital;
Orthopaedic Surgeon
Great Plains Orthopaedics
Peoria, Illinois

Haideh V. Plock, PT, DPT, OCS, ATC, FAAOMPT
Manager
Department of Physical Therapy
Palo Alto Medical Foundation
Palo Alto, California

Luga Podesta, MD, FAAPMR
Clinical Assistant Professor
Department of Physical Medicine and Rehabilitation
Western University of Health Sciences
Pomona, California;
Medical Director
Podesta Orthopedic and Sports Medicine Institute
Thousand Oaks, California;
Kerlan-Jobe Orthopedic Clinic;
Team Physician
Los Angeles Angels of Anaheim
Los Angeles, California;
Performance Medicine Consultant
Cirque du Soleil–IRIS

Ben B. Pradhan, MD
Spine Surgeon
Director of Clinical Research
Los Angeles, California;
The Spine Institute
Santa Monica, California

Edward Pratt, MD
Memphis Spine Center
Germantown, Tennessee

Christine Prelaz, DPT, MS, OCS, CSCS
HealthPath Physical Therapy & Wellness
Denver, Colorado

Brian E. Prell, MSPT, RRT
Rehabilitation and Performance Center
Greensboro, Georgia

Michael M. Reinold, PT, DPT, SCS, ATC, CSCS
Head Physical Therapist
Boston Red Sox Baseball Club
Boston, Massachusetts

Michael D. Ries, MD
Professor of Orthopaedic Surgery
University of California, San Francisco
San Francisco, California

Diane R. Schwab, MS, RPT
San Diego, California

Jessie Scott, PT, MBA
California Pacific Medical Center
San Francisco, California

Chris A Sebelski, PT, DPT, OCS, CSCS
Assistant Professor
Department of Physical Therapy & Athletic Training
Doisy College of Health Sciences
Saint Louis University
St. Louis, Missouri

Holly J. Silvers, MPT
Director of Research/Physical Therapist
US Soccer Federation Medical Team / CD Chivas USA /
    LA Galaxy
Santa Monica, California

Paul Slosar, MD
Spine Care Medical Group
Daly City, California

Renee Songer, DPT, OCS, FAAOMPT
Agile Physical Therapy
Palo Alto, California

Jason A. Steffe, DPT, OCS, MTC
Group Director
Physiotherapy Associates
Atlanta, Georgia

Derrick G. Sueki, PT, DPT, GCPT, OCS, FAAOMPT
Adjunct Faculty
Department of Physical Therapy
Mount St. Mary's College
Los Angeles, California;
President
Knight Physical Therapy, Inc
Garden Grove, California

Steven R. Tippett, PT, PhD, SCS
Professor
Department of Physical Therapy and Health Science
Bradley University
Peoria, Illinois

Timothy F. Tyler MS, PT, ATC
Clinical Research Associate
NISMAT at Lenox Hill Hospital
New York, New York

Kevin E. Wilk, PT, OPT
Adjunct Assistant Professor
Physical Therapy Department
Marquette University
Milwaukee, Wisconsin;
Clinical Director
Champion Sports Medicine;
Vice President of Education
Benchmark Medical, Inc.
Birmingham, Alabama

Julie Wong, PT, CLT
Director/Owner
Julie Wong's Proactive Clinic
San Francisco, California

James Zachazewski, PT, DPT, SCS, ATC
Clinical Director
Department of Physical and Occupational Therapy
Massachusetts General Hospital
Boston, Massachusetts;
Adjunct Assistant Clinical Professor
Programs in Physical Therapy
MGH Institute of Health Professions
Charlestown, Massachusetts

Boris A. Zelle, MD
Assistant Professor
University of Texas Health Science Center at San Antonio
Division of Orthopaedic Traumatology
Department of Orthopaedic Surgery
San Antonio, Texas

Craig Zeman, MD
Department of Orthopedics
St. Johns Hospital
Oxnard, California

PREFACE

We initially set out on this project to help bring knowledge that was lacking in the field regarding postoperative rehabilitation for the orthopedic outpatient population. We knew that it was a subject that would continue to grow, as in the previous editions, as new surgical and rehabilitative techniques were enhanced and/or refined. Our purpose remains the same with this third edition, adding new chapters and updating prior ones. We are confident that this book provides the clinician with the most comprehensive evidence-based view of postoperative rehabilitation.

In this third edition, we are excited about the addition of a home exercise component (Exercise Pro online) to accompany the Suggested Home Maintenance Program. We also have included new chapters, Clinical Applications for Platelet Rich Plasma Therapy (Chapter 10), Lumbar Spine Disc Replacement (Chapter 17), Autologous Chondrocyte Implantation (Chapter 25), and Bunionectomies (Chapter 32). In keeping in line with returning our clients to their prior level of function, we have included Transitioning the Patient Back to Running (Chapter 34) to augment the guidelines in Transitioning the Jumping Athlete Back to the Court (Chapter 33) and Transitioning the Throwing Athlete Back to the Field (Chapter 13).

The third edition begins with an overview regarding the principles of soft tissue healing and treatment presented by experts in their field. Clinicians must remember the biology of the healing process and the many factors that influence it. Some of the concepts touched on are controversial and experimental, but others that were once thought of as experimental are being performed with increasing regularity (e.g., platelet rich plasma therapy). The descriptions are meant to give the clinician visualization of the healing process from a cellular level.

The practice of physical therapy continues to undergo transformations. Over the past 60 years it has evolved into a science that is continually being scrutinized by third-party payers challenging us to prove that what we do is effective and efficient. We are at a crucial point in our profession in which we need to justify how many treatments are necessary to manage a condition or ICD-9 code; at times, this practice ignores the person we are treating. This book is not a "cookbook" for success but rather a compass from which the clinician can find guidance. This text is our effort to provide a resource that the clinician can reference as a guideline in the rehabilitation of the postsurgical patient.

We feel that this third edition will, like the previous two editions, be an invaluable resource for every clinician practicing in an orthopedic setting. We have brought together over 70 authors from throughout the United States and England. Many of the authors are widely published, and some are just excellent clinicians who have agreed to share their experiential philosophy. We wanted the clinician to be able to visualize the common surgical approaches to each case (through the physicians' portion) and then follow the therapists' guidelines to establish an efficient treatment plan. When we first began this journey in 2001, the prototype of this text had not been explored, to our knowledge, in this much depth (and with this many contributors). We believe it is a unique text, since we have continued to develop the content by going beyond the clinical setting and transitioning the client back to his or her prior activity level.

HOW TO USE THIS BOOK

This third edition has evolved and expanded, as has our knowledge base over the last 5 years. We have added five new chapters, as mentioned previously. We have made the table guidelines and Home Maintenance Programs easier to follow and added more vignettes to assist the clinician in problem-solving and clinical reasoning. We have also added Exercise Pro so that therapists can easily make custom home exercise programs to hand to their patients. We believe that these additions to the book make it an invaluable tool for every clinician treating postoperative orthopedic patients.

This book gives the therapist a clear understanding of the surgical procedures required for various injuries and conditions so that a rehabilitation program can be fashioned appropriately. Each chapter presents the indications and considerations for surgery; a detailed look at the surgical procedure, including the surgeon's perspective regarding rehabilitation concerns; and therapy guidelines to use in designing the rehabilitation program. During rehabilitation, areas that might prove troublesome are noted with appropriate ways to address the problems.

The indications and considerations for surgery and a description of the surgery itself are described by an outstanding surgeon specializing in each area. All of the information presented should be valuable in understanding the mechanics of the injury and the repair process.

The therapy guidelines section is divided into three parts:

- Evaluation
- Phases of rehabilitation
- Suggested home maintenance

Every rehabilitation program begins with a thorough evaluation at the initial physical therapy visit, which provides pertinent information for formulating the treatment program. As the patient progresses through the program, assessment continues. Activities too stressful for healing tissues at one point are delayed and then reassessed when the tissue is ready for the stress. Treatment measures are outlined in tabular format for easy reference.

The phases each patient faces in rehabilitation are clearly indicated, both as a way to break the program into manageable segments and as a way to provide reassurance to the patient that rehabilitation will proceed in an orderly fashion. The time span covered by each phase and the goals of the rehabilitation process during that phase are noted. The exercises are carefully explained, and photographs are provided for assistance.

Home maintenance for the postsurgical patient is an essential component of the rehabilitation program. Even when the therapist is able to follow the patient routinely in the clinic, the patient is still on his or her own for most of the day. The patient must understand the importance of compliance with the home program to maximize postoperative results. In the successful home maintenance program, the patient is the primary force in rehabilitation, with the therapist acting as an informed and effective communicator, an efficient coordinator, and a motivator. When the therapist successfully fulfills these obligations and the patient is motivated and compliant, the home maintenance program can be especially rewarding.

When the patient is not motivated or not compliant or possesses less-than-adequate pain tolerance, a no-nonsense and forthright dialogue with the surgeon, referring physician, rehabilitation nurse, or any other professional involved is essential. Timely, accurate, and straightforward documentation also is significant in the case of the "problem" patient. Emphasizing active patient involvement in an exercise program at home is even more imperative in light of the prescriptive nature of current managed care dictums.

The keys to an effective home maintenance program are structure, individuality, prioritization, and conciseness. The term *structure* refers to exercises that are well defined in terms of sets, repetitions, frequency, resistance, and technique. The patient must know what to do and how to do it. Home programs with photographs or video demonstrations are helpful in assisting the patient to visualize what is intended. Some computer-generated home exercise programs also offer adequate visual descriptions of the desired exercises. Stick figures and drawings that the physical therapist makes are often unclear and confusing to the patient.

Individuality, in the clearest sense, involves prescribing exercises that address the specific needs of a patient at a specific point in time. It includes being flexible enough to allow the patient to work the home program into the daily schedule as opposed to following only an "ideal" treatment schedule. Other components inherent in the concept of individuality include assistance available to the patient at home, financial implications, geographical concerns that influence follow-up, and the patient's cognitive abilities.

Prioritization and conciseness involve maximizing the use of the patient's time to perform the exercises at home. If the patient is being seen in the clinic, home exercises should stress activities not routinely performed in the clinic. If the patient is constrained for time, the therapist can identify the most beneficial exercises and prescribe them. It is best not to prescribe too many exercises to be done at home. Ideally, the patient should have to concentrate on no more than five or six at a time. To help keep the number of exercises manageable, the therapist should discontinue less taxing exercises as new exercises are added to the program.

Lisa Maxey
Jim Magnusson

ACKNOWLEDGMENTS

Once again I would like to thank Jim Magnusson, Clive Brewster, and all the contributing authors for their hard work and dedication to their profession. I am continually amazed the people I've met in the health care profession and their dedication to serving others. And I am grateful to be a part of the physical therapy profession. I have truly been blessed through the professionals I work with and the patients I've treated. And I am especially grateful to my family: Albert and Yvonne Liddicoat, Albert Jr. Liddicoat, Brent Liddicoat, Jim Maxey, Paul Maxey, Rebecca Maxey, Jessica Maxey, Stephen Maxey, and Christine Maxey.

Lisa Maxey

I would like to acknowledge my wife, Tracy, who continues to amaze me with her patience and understanding. My parents, Nancy and Chuck, who gave me the foundations of respect, honesty, and love. My brothers, Bill and Bob, who remind me of the values of having faith, being humble, challenging ourselves, and never giving up on your dreams, and my favorite—James 3:13.

My grandfather, Dr. James Logie, who helped me understand the dedication of those who aspire to become the best in their profession. I studied some of his own hand drawings of the human anatomy when he was in school and have seen how, through his dedication to serving his patients, his life has been blessed. He has taught me the importance of patience and showed me the art of fly fishing.

In the course of a lifetime, we meet people who have made impressions on us. Good or bad, they change us and shape our vision of who we want to become. In my experience (25 years) working in the field of physical therapy, I also have worked with individuals who, not only through clinical work but also through life experience, have taught me the value of compassion, dedication, empathy, and respect. Although a number of physical therapists have individually helped, the ones I've singled out also have positively influenced countless other therapists: Dee Lilly, Rick Katz, Gary Souza, and Charles Magistro.

I continue to thank God (and Dee) for helping me find that special person in my wife, partner in life, and peer— Tracy Magnusson, PT.

Jim Magnusson

CONTENTS

ENHANCE YOUR LEARNING AND PRACTICE EXPERIENCE

The image to the right is a QR code. The code will take you to the companion site where you will find links to selected Exercise Pro home exercise programs you can print and deliver to patients, suggested home maintenance programs you can print and/or edit as needed, and more. All can be accessed on your mobile device for quick reference in a lab or clinical setting.

For fast and easy access, right from your mobile device, follow these instructions. You can also find them at http://booksite.elsevier.com/Maxey_rehab3e/.

What You Need

- A mobile device, such as a smart phone or tablet, equipped with a camera and Internet access
- A QR code reader application (If you do not already have a reader installed on your mobile device, look for free versions in your app store.)

How It Works

- Open the QR code reader application on your mobile device.
- Point the device's camera at the code and scan.
- The codes take you to a main page where you can link to specific chapters for instant viewing of the references where you can further access the website content—no log-on required.

Main Page Code.

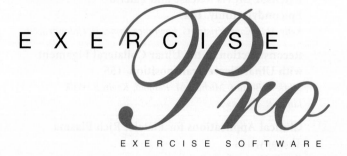

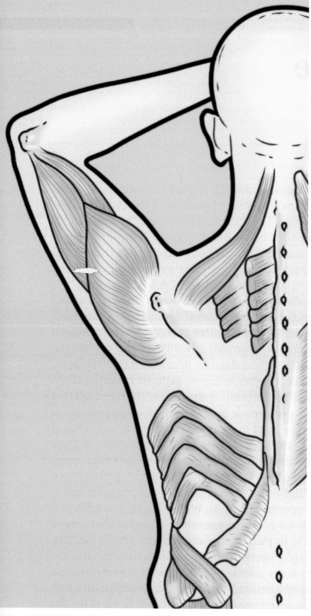

PART 1

Introduction

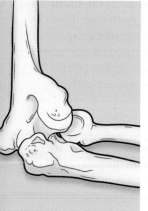

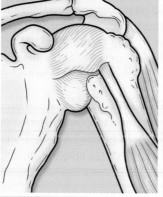

CHAPTER 1

Pathogenesis of Soft Tissue and Bone Repair

Boris A. Zelle, Freddie H. Fu

Musculoskeletal injuries usually result from supraphysiologic stresses that overwhelm the intrinsic stability of the musculoskeletal apparatus. The consequence is injury to the bone, tendon, muscle, ligaments, or a combination of these structures. The physiologic healing response varies among these tissues and is influenced by various intrinsic and extrinsic factors. Among these are the degree and anatomic location of the injury, the patient's physiology, and the mode of treatment rendered. The aim of this chapter is to review the concept of soft tissue and bone healing and to describe the factors that influence the healing response.

INCISION AND WOUND HEALING

With regard to epithelial tissue, the surgical incision is considered to be a "controlled trauma." Incision and wound healing begins immediately after surgery and progresses through four distinct phases: (1) the coagulation phase (Fig. 1-1), (2) the inflammatory phase, (3) the granulation phase (Fig. 1-2), and (4) the scar formation and maturation phase. Table 1-1 gives an approximate time frame for each of these phases with hallmarks of what each phase accomplishes. Wound healing requires a clean environment, good circulation, appropriate approximation of wound edges, and a balance of the cellular mechanisms that ensure a proper immune response in the wound environment. Wound healing occurs through scar formation. Many intrinsic factors (e.g., age, metabolic and circulatory disorders, patient physiology, and comorbidities) and extrinsic factors (e.g., nutrition, hydration, smoking, wound exposure, and wound management) will influence the healing response and formation of the scar.

LIGAMENT INJURIES AND HEALING

Ligament Anatomy and Function

Ligaments are anatomic structures of dense, fibrous connective tissue. They can be divided into two major subgroups: (1) ligaments connecting the elements of the bony skeleton (skeletal subgroup) and (2) ligaments connecting other organs, such as suspensory ligaments in the abdomen (visceral subgroup). The skeletal ligaments are the focus of this chapter. The nomenclature of the ligaments usually relates to their anatomic location and bony attachments (i.e., medial collateral, posterior talofibular), as well as their shape and function (i.e., triangular, cruciate, or deltoid ligament).

Structurally, ligaments contain rows of fibroblasts within parallel bundles of collagen fibers. Approximately two thirds of the wet weight of a ligament is water, whereas collagen fibers account for approximately 70% of the dry weight. More than 90% of the collagen in ligaments is type I collagen. Trace amounts of other collagens exist, such as type III, V, X, XII, and XIV.[1] The primary structure of the type I collagen consists of a polypeptide chain with high concentrations of glycine, proline, and hydroxyproline. Almost two thirds of the primary structure of type I collagen consists of these three amino acids. Intermolecular forces cause three polypeptide chains to combine into a triple helical collagen molecule. This ropelike configuration imparts great tensile strength properties (Fig. 1-3). Within the ligament, the collagen fibrils are usually organized in a longitudinal pattern and are held in place by the extracellular matrix (see Fig. 1-1).[2] Collagen fibers in the extracellular matrix are surrounded by water-soluble molecules, such as proteoglycans, glycosaminoglycans, and structural glycoproteins. Although these molecules represent only approximately 1% of the dry weight of ligaments, they are important for proper ligament formation and organization of the ligament meshwork. Their hydrophilic properties are crucial for the viscoelastic capacity of ligament tissue and ensure adequate tissue lubrication and proper gliding of the fibers. Moreover, proteoglycans couple adjacent collagen fibrils together and support the mechanical integrity of the ligaments.[3]

Ligament Injury

From the clinical standpoint, ligamentous injuries are classified into three grades.[4] Grade I injuries include mild sprains. The structural integrity of the ligament is intact,

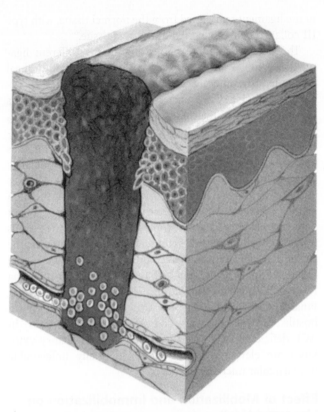

Fig. 1-1 Coagulation phase of wound healing; wound gap is filled with a blood clot. (From Browner BD, et al: Skeletal trauma—basic science, management, and reconstruction, ed 3, Philadelphia, 2003, Saunders.)

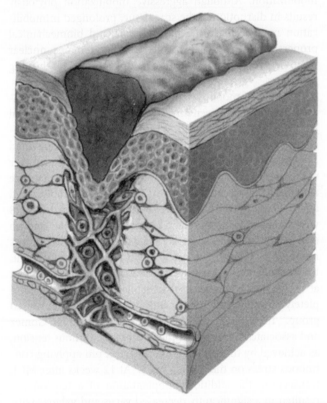

Fig. 1-2 Granulation phase of wound healing, fibroplasias, angiogenesis, epithelialization, and wound contraction. (From Browner BD, et al: Skeletal trauma—basic science, management, and reconstruction, ed 3, Philadelphia, 2003, Saunders.)

TABLE 1-1 Epithelial Tissue Healing

Coagulation Phase (see Fig. 1-1)	Vasoconstriction, platelet aggregation, clot formation	Begins immediately and lasts minutes
Inflammatory Phase	Vasodilation, polymorphonuclear (PMN) leukocytes, phagocytes	At the edges of wounds, epidermis immediately begins thickening; within the first 48 hours entire wound is epithelialized; lasts hours
Granulation Phase	Fibroplasia, epithelialization, wound contraction	Fibroblasts appear in 2-3 days and are dominant cell by day 10
Scar Formation/ Maturation Phase (see Fig. 1-2)	Collagen synthesis; rarely regain full elasticity and strength	Lasts weeks to months and even up to 1 year

Adapted from Browner BD, et al: Skeletal trauma—basic science, management, and reconstruction, ed 3, Philadelphia, 2003, Saunders.

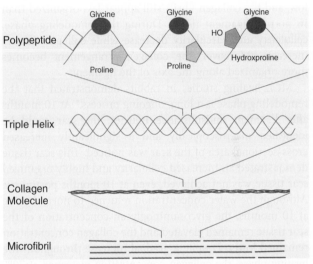

Fig. 1-3 Schematic drawing of the collagen structure. A linear polypeptide with a high percentage of proline, glycine, and hydroxyproline is folded into an α-helix. Three polypeptide chains form a triple helix. The collagen molecules are packed to form the microfibrils. (Adapted from Gamble JC, Edward C, Max S: Enzymatic adaptation of ligaments during immobilization. Am J Sports Med 12:221-228, 1984.)

although edema, swelling, and punctate ligament bleeding may be present. In grade II injuries, individual fibrils are torn, but the overall continuity of the ligament is maintained. Significant edema and bleeding is usually noted, and ligament stability is reduced. Grade III injuries are characterized by complete disruption of the ligament substance. Most ligamentous injuries can be diagnosed through a clinical examination and joint stability tests. Magnetic resonance imaging (MRI) represents the most commonly performed imaging study for diagnosing ligamentous injuries.

Multiple healing studies involving the medial collateral ligament (MCL) of the knee have been performed and have contributed to our knowledge of ligament healing. The healing phases of ligaments are traditionally divided by their morphologic appearance into an inflammatory phase (first days postinjury), a proliferative phase (1 to 6 weeks postinjury), and a remodeling phase (beginning at 7 weeks postinjury) (Table 1-2).[5] It is important to appreciate that these three phases represent a continuum rather than distinct phases. The predominant cell types in the inflammatory phase are inflammatory cells and erythrocytes. As the ligament ruptures, its torn ends retract and have a ragged, "mopend" appearance. The gap between these torn ends is filled with hematoma from ruptured capillaries. Histologically, the inflammatory reaction is characterized by increased vasodilation, capillary permeability, and migration of leukocytes. During the inflammatory phase, water and glycosaminoglycans are increased in the injured tissue. During the proliferative phase, a highly cellular scar develops, with fibroblasts as the dominating cell type. New collagen fibrils can be identified as early as 4 days after the injury. After approximately 2 weeks, the newly formed collagen fibrils bridge the gap between the torn ligament ends. However, the water content of the scar remains elevated, the collagen density remains low, and the collagen fibrils still appear less organized than in normal ligament tissue. During the remodeling phase, cellularity and vascularity decrease while collagen density increases. Moreover, the collagen arrangement becomes more organized along the axis of the ligament.

MCL healing studies in rabbits demonstrated that the remodeling phase is a long, ongoing process.[6] At 10 months after ligament midsubstance injuries, the scar could be identified macroscopically and a significantly increased cross-sectional area of the scar was noticed. This scar tissue demonstrated an increased cellularity and highly organized scar tissue was not achieved, even at 10 months postinjury. Although the water concentration returned to normal value at 10 months, the glycosaminoglycan concentration of the scar tissue remained elevated and the collagen concentration remained lower. Despite a gradual increase throughout the healing phase, the collagen concentration plateaued at 70% of uninjured ligament tissue. In addition, the collagen types in the ligament scar varied from the normal tissue, with type III collagen being increased in the scar tissue.[6]

The healing response varies among the different ligaments. While MCL injuries have the potential to heal spontaneously, other ligament injuries, such as anterior cruciate ligament (ACL) injuries, rarely show a spontaneous healing response. Recent experimental studies in rabbits have demonstrated an increased expression of myofibroblasts and growth factor receptors in the injured MCL as compared with the injured ACL.[7] Various reasons may account for the superior healing response of the MCL as compared with the ACL. It must be assumed that the high stress carried by the ACL prevents the ruptured ligament ends from having sufficient contact. In addition, the ACL is not embedded in a strong soft tissue envelope. Moreover, the ACL is an intraarticular structure; when it ruptures, the blood is diluted by the synovial fluid, preventing hematoma formation and hence initiation of the healing mechanism. Finally, it has been suggested that the synovial fluid is a hostile environment for soft tissue healing. Thus in ACL-deficient knees, the levels of proinflammatory cytokines are elevated, leading to a potentially unfavorable intraarticular microenvironment.[8]

Effect of Mobilization and Immobilization on Ligament Healing

An important aspect of the rehabilitation of patients with ligament injuries represents the timing of postinjury mobilization. Although aggressive mobilization obviously results in disruption of the scar tissue, prolonged immobilization may decrease the morphologic and biomechanical properties of the newly formed scar. It remains unclear what degree of immobilization is appropriate for healing ligaments.

The role of mobilization versus immobilization on ligament healing has been investigated in numerous animal studies.[9-11] In an MCL healing study in rats, Vailas and associates[11] compared the healing properties of the transected MCL across the following four groups: (1) surgical repair with 2 weeks of immobilization and 6 weeks of normal cage activity; (2) surgical repair with 2 weeks of immobilization and 6 weeks of treadmill exercise; (3) surgical repair with 8 weeks of immobilization; and (4) no surgical repair and no exercise. All animals were sacrificed at 8 weeks. The authors reported that the wet ligament weight, dry ligament weight, total collagen content of the ligament, and the ultimate load at failure of the ligament substance was lowest in the completely immobilized group and highest in the exercised group.[11] In an MCL transsection model in the rabbit, Gomez and associates[9] investigated the effect of continuous tension, as achieved by the implantation of a steel pin applying continuous stress on the healing MCL. At 12 weeks after MCL transection, the additional implantation of a tension pin resulted in a significantly decreased varus and valgus laxity, decreased cellularity of the scar tissue, and a more longitudinal alignment of the collagen fibers. These authors concluded that the application of controlled stress helped to

TABLE 1-2 Ligament Healing

Inflammatory Phase	Vasodilation, fibrin clot formation, increased capillary permeability, and migration of leukocytes	Begins immediately and lasts minutes to hours
Proliferative Phase	Fibroblasts are the dominate cell type, collagen fibrils (as early as 4 days postinjury)	1-6 wk postinjury
Remodeling Phase	Collagen synthesis and increased density; rarely regain full elasticity and strength	7 wk up to 1 yr

augment the biochemical, morphologic, and biomechanical properties of the healing MCL.[9] In a more recent study, Provenzano and associates[10] investigated the effect of hind limb immobilization on the healing response of transected MCLs in a rat model. The authors reported significantly superior biomechanical ligament properties in the mobilized group. Microscopic analysis revealed abnormal scar formation and cell distribution in the immobilized group, as suggested by disoriented fiber bundles and discontinuities in the extracellular ligament matrix.[10]

These experimental data clearly emphasize the importance of stress and motion for the functional recovery of healing ligaments. However, the ideal amount of mobilization and immobilization during ligament healing is difficult to determine by animal studies, because animal studies are limited by the differing physiology and joint kinematics of animals. In addition, the amount of mobilization is difficult to control, and an exact titration of the stress cannot be performed with current in vivo models. Future clinical trials are necessary to determine the optimal amount of applied stress for the various ligament injuries.

TENDON INJURIES AND HEALING

Tendon Anatomy and Function

Tendons are bands of dense, fibrous connective tissue interposed between muscles and bones. They transmit the forces created in the muscles to the bone, making joint motion possible. Some tendons may also connect two muscle bellies (e.g., digastrics, omohyoid). The gross tendon structure varies considerably from tendon to tendon, ranging from cylindrical rounded cords to flattened bands, called aponeuroses. The cross-sectional area of the more rounded tendons usually correlates with the isometric strength of the muscle from which they arise. The bony insertion site of the tendon is often accompanied by a small synovial bursa (e.g., subacromial bursa, pes anserinus, retrocalcaneal bursa). The tendon bursae are usually located in those anatomic sites where a bony prominence would otherwise compress the gliding tendon.

Microscopically, tendons and ligaments are similar. The tendon tissue is a complex composite of parallel collagen fibrils embedded in a matrix; cells are relatively rare, and fibroblasts represent the predominant cell type within the tendon; and the fibroblasts are arranged in parallel rows between the collagen fibrils (Fig. 1-4, A and B). The biochemical composition of ligaments and tendons are also very similar. Water is the major constituent of the wet tendon weight, whereas type I collagen accounts for approximately 70% to 80% and elastin for approximately 1% to 2% of the dry tendon substance. As in ligaments, other collagen types exist only in small amounts. The proteoglycans and glycosaminoglycans in the extracellular matrix play an important role for the viscoelastic properties and the tensile strength of the tendon. Their hydrophilic capacity provides the tendon with lubrication and facilitates gliding of the fibrils during tensile stress.

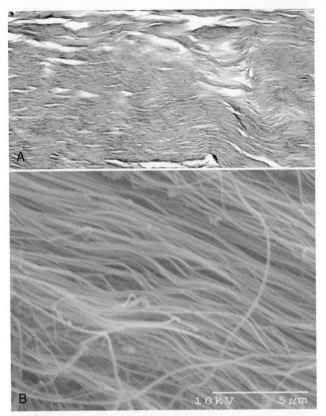

Fig. 1-4 Microscopic longitudinal sections of the patellar tendon. **A,** The hematoxylin and eosin (H&E) staining demonstrates the parallel arrangement of the collagen fibers and the fibroblasts under the light microscope. **B,** Electron microscopy demonstrates the wavy pattern of the fibers (i.e., "crimp"). (From Fu FH, Zelle BA: Ligaments and tendons: basic science and implications for rehabilitation. In Wilmarth MA, editor: Clinical applications for orthopaedic basic science: Independent study course, La Crosse, Wis, 2004, American Physical Therapy Association.)

According to their envelope, tendons can be divided into tendons within a synovial sheath (i.e., sheathed tendons) and paratenon-covered tendons. In particular, tendons in the hand and foot are often enclosed in a synovial tendon sheath. The tendon sheath directs the path of the tendon and produces a synovial fluid, which allows tendon gliding and contributes to tendon nutrition. True tendon sheaths are only found in areas with an increased friction or sharp bending of the tendons (e.g., flexor tendons of the hand). A simple membranous thickening of the surrounding soft tissue, called the paratenon, usually surrounds tendons without a true synovial tendon sheath, such as the Achilles tendon. The paratenon is composed of loose fibrillar tissue. It also functions as an elastic sleeve and permits free movement of the tendon against the surrounding tissue, although it is not as efficient as a true tendon sheath.

Just like ligaments, tendons have a limited blood supply. The vascular supply of tendons has been described by injection studies, which demonstrated that tendons are usually surrounded by a network of blood vessels.[12] Arteries supplying the tendon might come from the attached muscle, the bony insertion site, the paratenon, or the tendon sheath along the length of the tendon. However, there seems to be a difference between the nutrition of the sheathed tendons and the paratenon-covered tendons. The paratenon-covered tendons receive the majority of their blood supply from vessels in the paratenon. In sheathed tendons, the synovial sheath minimizes the vascular supply to the tendon substance, and avascular regions have been identified within the midsubstance of these tendons.[12-14] Hence the diffusion of nutrients through the synovial fluid of sheathed tendons is critical for their homeostasis. Indeed, in sheathed tendons this process may be even more important than vascular perfusion. The digital flexor tendons, for example, receive up to 90% of their nutrition by diffusion.[15] For this reason, sheathed tendons have also been referred to as avascular tendons, whereas the paratenon-covered tendons have been referred to as vascular tendons.

Tendon Injury

Tendon injuries may occur as a result of direct or indirect trauma (Fig. 1-5, *A* and *B*). Direct trauma includes contusions and lacerations, such as lacerations of the flexor tendons of the hand. Indirect tendon injuries are usually a consequence of tensile overload. Because most tendons can withstand higher tensile forces than their associated muscles or osseous insertion sites, avulsion fractures and ruptures at the myotendinous junctions are more likely than midsubstance ruptures. Midsubstance ruptures of the tendon after indirect trauma are usually associated with preexisting tendon degeneration. This has been supported by histologic investigations of ruptured Achilles tendons, which demonstrated increased tenocyte necrosis, loss of fiber structure, increased vascularity, decreased collagen content, and increased glycosaminoglycan content in previously ruptured tendons.[16-18]

Tendon Healing

The repair process in paratenon-covered tendons is also initiated by the influx of extrinsic inflammatory cells. As in ligaments, the healing of the ruptured tendon proceeds through an inflammatory phase, a proliferative phase, and a remodeling phase.[19-21] During the inflammatory phase, healing is initiated by the formation of a blood clot bridging the gap between the ruptured ends. During the first few days after the injury, the proliferative phase begins; disorganized fibroblasts are the dominating cell types, and collagen synthesis can be detected. The collagen fibers orient themselves along the axis of the tendon during the remodeling phase. The remodeling phase continues for many months. It is characterized by increased organization of the collagen fibers, an increase in the number of intermolecular bonds between the collagen fibers, subsequent reduction of scar tissue, and increased tensile strength (Table 1-3).

Although it seems well accepted that the healing response in paratenon-covered tendons is initiated by the influx of inflammatory cells, the initiation of the healing response of sheathed tendons remains controversial. Both an intrinsic mechanism and an extrinsic mechanism have been proposed. The extrinsic concept suggests that similar to

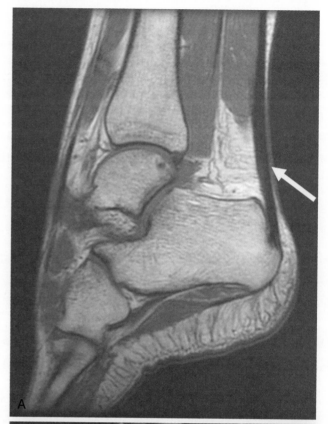

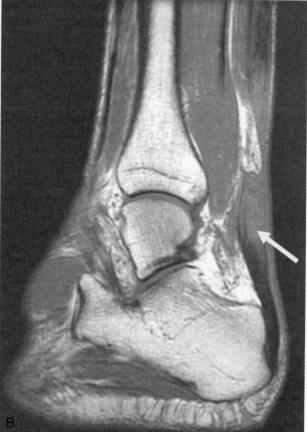

Fig. 1-5 Magnetic resonance imaging (MRI) evaluation of the Achilles tendon. The T1-weighted sagittal cuts show normal continuity of the Achilles tendon (**A**) *(arrow)* and a ruptured Achilles tendon (**B**) *(arrow)*.

TABLE 1-3 Tendon Healing

Inflammatory Phase	Vasodilation, hematoma formation to bridge the defect (or gap), increased capillary permeability, and migration of leukocytes; influx of extrinsic/ intrinsic inflammatory cells	Begins immediately and lasts minutes to hours
Proliferative Phase	Fibroblasts are the dominant cell type, collagen synthesis	1-6 wk postinjury
Remodeling Phase	Collagen synthesis and increased density	Can last for several months

paratenon-covered tendons, the healing of sheathed tendons occurs by granulation from the tendon sheath and the surrounding tissue, although the tenocytes themselves play no important role in this repair. According to the intrinsic theory, cells from within the tendon proliferate at the wound site, leading to production of collagen and extracellular matrix.[15,20] With regard to the initiation of the healing response, it appears probable that both intrinsic and extrinsic healing exist.

Effect of Mobilization and Immobilization on Tendon Healing

The ideal mobilization regimen for the various tendon injuries is beyond the scope of this discussion. Clearly, overaggressive early mobilization may result in rerupture of the tendon. **Scientific evidence suggests that motion and stress increase collagen production, accelerate remodeling, and improve the biomechanical properties of healing tendons.[22-24] However, the optimal level of stress and motion of the healing tendon must be established based on clinical evidence.**

SKELETAL MUSCLE INJURIES AND HEALING

Anatomy and Function of Skeletal Muscle

Skeletal muscle represents the largest tissue mass in the body and accounts for almost 50% of the total body weight. Skeletal muscle originates from bone and inserts into bone via tendon. The primary function of skeletal muscle is to provide mobility to the bony skeleton. This is accomplished by muscle contraction (i.e., shortening) and force transmission through the muscle-tendon-bone complex.

The basic structural element of the skeletal muscle is the muscle fiber. The muscle fiber is a syncytium of many cells fused together with multiple nuclei. The muscle fibers consist of contractile elements, the myofibrils, which give skeletal muscle a striated appearance by light microscopy. The myofibrils consist of myofilaments (actin and myosin filaments). Individual muscle fibers are organized into muscle by surrounding connective tissue (i.e., endomysium, perimysium, epimysium) that provide integrated motion among the

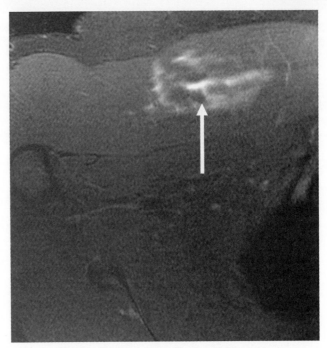

Fig. 1-6 Magnetic resonance imaging (MRI) evaluation of a partial tear of the pectoralis muscle. The T2-weighted axial cuts depict the edema formation *(arrow)* within the pectoralis muscle.

muscle fibers. The endomysium surrounds the individual muscle fibers. Groups of muscle fibers are arranged together to fascicles surrounded by the perimysium. The fascicles are grouped together by the epimysium to form the whole muscle belly.

Skeletal muscle contraction is accomplished by sliding of its filaments.[25,26] The basic contractile unit is the sarcomere. The active contractile units within the sarcomere are the actin and the myosin filaments. These myofilaments are arranged in a parallel fashion in which the larger myosin filaments interdigitate between the small actin filaments. The actin filaments actively slide along the surface of the myosin filaments through cross-bridges originating from the myosin. The coordinated sliding of actin and myosin filaments throughout the muscle translates into contraction of the entire unit, which generates force and motion.

Muscle Injuries and Healing

Skeletal muscle injuries constitute the majority of sports-related injuries.[27,28] Skeletal muscle injuries can be classified as indirect and direct injuries. Indirect injuries result from an overload that overwhelms the muscle's ability to respond normally, such as muscle strains and delayed-onset muscle soreness. Direct injuries are usually a result of external forces, such as muscle contusions and muscle lacerations. Most injuries are diagnosed clinically. MRI has been found to be highly sensitive to muscle edema and hemorrhage and is the primary imaging modality for determining the type of injury and the degree of muscle involvement (Fig. 1-6).[18,29] Large muscle injuries have a limited healing capacity, and the repair process usually results in the formation of scar tissue.

Severe muscle injuries may result in the inability to train or compete for several weeks, and they have a high tendency to recur.[30,31]

Similar to ligaments and tendons, injured skeletal muscle undergoes phases of disruption and degeneration, inflammation, proliferation, and fibrosis (Table 1-4). After trauma to the muscle, the disrupted muscle ends retract and the gap is filled by a local hematoma. Disruption of the muscle fibers leads to increased extracellular calcium levels, activation of the complement cascade, and myofiber necrosis. Inflammation is an early response to muscle tissue injury. Neutrophils rapidly invade the injury site and release inflammatory cytokines followed by an increase in macrophages that phagocytose cell debris. Structural damage of the muscle fibers usually heals with formation of scar tissue (Fig. 1-7, A to D).[29]

The most common muscle injuries include delayed-onset muscle soreness (DOMS), muscular contusion, muscular strain, and muscular laceration. Among these types of injuries, the mechanism of injury, pathologic changes, treatment, and outcome vary greatly. Therefore these issues will be discussed in detail for each of these muscle injuries.

Delayed Onset Muscle Soreness

DOMS is a consequence of extensive exercise and usually occurs approximately 12 to 48 hours after exercise. The symptoms of DOMS occur when the amount of stress applied to the muscle exceeds its ability to elongate without disrupting the structural integrity. The symptoms of DOMS are particularly intense after eccentric muscle contraction exercises, whereas repetitive submaximal muscle contractions cause less severe symptoms.[32,33] DOMS is characterized by alterations of the structural integrity, an inflammatory response, and the loss of functional capacity.[34,35] The inflammatory component is most likely a response to the damage of the structural muscle integrity and usually lasts for a few days. To reduce the inflammatory response, the treatment during the first 2 to 3 days consists of rest, ice, compression, and elevation (RICE). Stretching exercises are recommended thereafter to allow superior scar tissue remodeling and fiber alignment of the repair tissue. However, most competitive athletes resume their normal activities quickly after DOMS onset. Permanent impairment after DOMS does not occur.[32]

Muscular Contusion

Muscular contusions are caused by direct blunt trauma to the muscle resulting in damage and partial disruption of the muscle fibers. Frequently, muscle contusions are associated with capillary rupture and local hematoma formation. This is associated with an inflammatory reaction, including increased neutrophil and phagocytic activity, release of inflammatory cytokines, prostaglandin production, and local edema. Clinical signs and symptoms may include ecchymosis, superficial and deep soft tissue swelling, pain, local tenderness, and decreased or abnormal range of motion (ROM). Jackson and Feagin[36] classified the muscular contusions into three degrees, according to the clinical symptoms. A mild contusion is characterized by localized tenderness, near normal ROM, and near normal gait pattern. A moderate contusion usually includes a swollen tender muscle mass, a 50% decrease in ROM, and an antalgic gait. A severe contusion is characterized by marked tenderness and swelling, a 75% decrease in ROM, and a severe limp.[36]

The initial treatment consists of RICE to prevent further hemorrhage. This is followed by active and passive ROM exercises and eventually the use of heat, a whirlpool, and ultrasound. Functional rehabilitation includes strengthening exercises. Muscular contusions heal by formation of dense connective scar tissue with variable amounts of muscle regeneration. Early stretching exercises of the injured muscle play an important role in the functional scar tissue remodeling process and normal alignment of the newly formed collagen fibers. In contrast, it seems that prolonged immobilization is associated with an inferior recovery of muscle function.[36]

Muscular Strain

Muscular strains are tears in the muscle, which may occur as a result of excessive stress (i.e., acute strain) or constant overuse (i.e., chronic strain).[33] In particular, muscles that cross two joints, such as the hamstring muscles and the gastrocnemius, seem to be particularly susceptible to muscular strains. Chronic muscle strains usually occur as a result of repetitive overuse, causing fatigue of the muscle. Acute strains, on the other hand, are the result of an excessive force applied to the muscle. The injury usually occurs at the weakest part of the muscle, the myotendinous junction. Histologically, muscle strains are characterized by hemorrhage and an inflammatory response. However, the extent of muscle strain may vary. Mild strains occur when no appreciable structural damage exists to the muscle tissue and pathologic changes are confined to an inflammatory response with swelling and edema, causing discomfort with exercise. With moderate damage, an appreciable muscular defect occurs and the inflammatory response, edema, and discomfort are increased as compared with mild strains. Severe strains are characterized by complete rupture of the muscle belly or the myotendinous junction.

TABLE 1-4 Muscle Healing (Involving Disruption of Muscle Cell Structure)

Inflammatory Phase (Disruption and Degeneration)	Vasodilation, hematoma formation, increased capillary permeability, increased extracellular calcium, and migration of leukocytes	Begins immediately and lasts minutes to hours
Proliferative Phase	Neutrophil and macrophage migration	1-6 wk postinjury
Remodeling/ Fibrosis Phase	Collagen synthesis and increased density; scar formation	Can last for several months

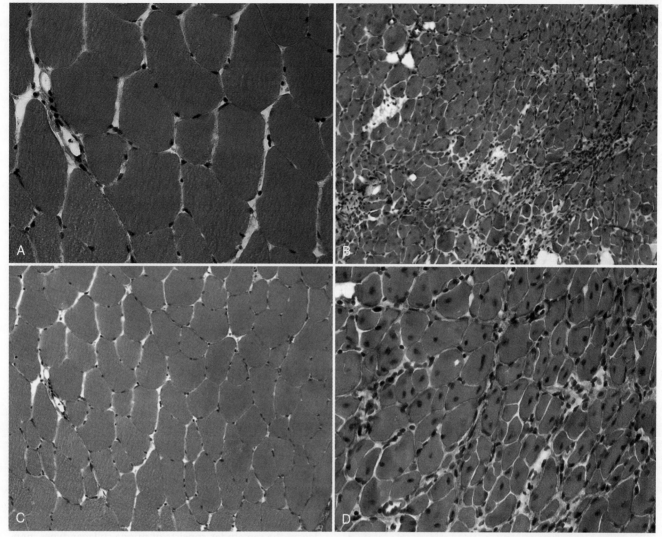

Fig. 1-7 Histologic pictures of muscle tissue from mice. **A** and **B** show normal muscle tissue. **C** and **D** show evidence of fibrosis and regenerating myofibers in the trichrome stain at 2 weeks after experimental muscle laceration.

The treatment of muscular strains is completely dependent on the grade of the injury. Although mild strains are usually treated symptomatically with RICE, severe strains may require surgical reconstruction. Muscular strains usually heal with the formation of fibrous scar tissue that can be visualized by MRI.[29]

Muscle Laceration

Muscle lacerations may be caused by penetrating trauma to the muscle and the surrounding soft tissue. Recovery of the muscle function depends on the orientation of the laceration. Lacerations perpendicular to the muscle fibers may create a denervated segment, which is associated with a poor recovery.[37,38] Suture repair of these lesions usually results in scar formation across the laceration. Thus muscle regeneration does not occur across the laceration site, and the functional continuity is usually not restored after muscle laceration.[37,38] In addition, the distal segment is often denervated, and even surgical repair of the muscle belly may not restore the innervation of this part of the muscle. Therefore the functional recovery is usually limited after muscle laceration.

Myositis Ossificans

The term myositis ossificans is used to describe ectopic bone formation within a muscle. Myositis ossificans represents a common complication after muscle injuries. Although common locations of myositis ossificans are the anterior thigh and the upper arm, it may occur in any muscle of the body. The clinical symptoms suggesting myositis ossificans include localized tenderness, swelling, and muscle weakness. Myositis ossificans can usually be detected on plain radiographs (Fig. 1-8, *A* and *B*). MRI studies may provide additional information with regard to location within the muscle and extent of the lesion. In addition, nuclear bone scans may play a role in the early detection of the lesion and may help judging the maturity and activity of the process. The pathogenesis of myositis ossificans is not completely understood. Myositis ossificans commonly occurs adjacent to the bone shaft, suggesting that bone-forming cells from the

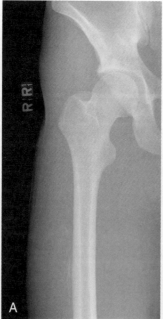

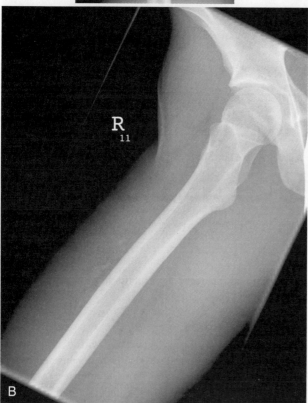

Fig. 1-8 Radiographs of the right femur with anteroposterior (**A**) and lateral view (**B**) demonstrate an ectopic bone formation lateral to the femur in the middle third of the bone.

periosteum migrate into the muscle tissue and produce bone within the injured muscle or the muscle hematoma.[39,40] In some cases, however, the ectopic calcifications occur within the muscle and are not in the close proximity of the bone. For these lesions, the pathogenesis remains unclear. One theory is that after the muscle injury, the circulation within the traumatized muscle decreases and leads to ossification.[41]

Other authors theorize that after the muscle injury, rapidly proliferating nondifferentiated connective tissue forms calcifications within the muscle.[42]

In the early stages of myositis ossificans, RICE is the preferred treatment. Ectopic calcification in the soft tissue surrounding the hip joint after total hip replacement or treatment of acetabular fractures represent a major clinical challenge. A meta-analysis of the literature demonstrated that treatment with moderate to high doses of nonsteroidal anti-inflammatory drugs (NSAIDs), such as indomethacin, at the time of surgery decreases the risk of ectopic bone formation.[43] The method by which NSAIDs prevent ectopic bone formation has not been completely understood, but early inhibition of prostaglandin-dependent osteogenic cells appears to be the likely mechanism. Early surgery is contraindicated in myositis ossificans because reossification commonly occurs. Surgical exploration and excision of heterotopic bone formations is only indicated in symptomatic patients and when bone scans and consecutive radiographs suggest low activity and mature bone formation.[40]

BONE INJURY AND HEALING

Bone Morphology

Bone is a composite of material consisting of minerals, proteins, water, cells, and other macromolecules (i.e., lipids, sugar). The composition of the bone tissue varies and depends on age, diet, and general health status. In general, minerals account for 60% to 70% of the bone tissue, water accounts for 5% to 10% of the bone tissue, and the organic bone matrix makes up the remainder. The mineral component is mainly composed of calcium hydroxyapatite $(Ca_{10}(PO4)_6(OH)_2$. Approximately 90% of the organic bone matrix is type I collagen; the remainder consists of minor collagen types, non-collagenous proteins, and other macromolecules.

The major cell types of bone tissue are osteoblasts, osteocytes, and osteoclasts. The osteoblasts represent the bone-forming cells. The osteoblasts line the surface of the bone matrix and the osteocytes are encased within the mineralized bone matrix. Both cell types are derived from the same osteoprogenitor cell type. A layer of unmineralized bone matrix (osteoid) lies between the osteoblast and the mineralized bone matrix. Once an osteoblast becomes surrounded by mineralized bone matrix, it is referred to as an osteocyte. Osteocytes are characterized by a higher nucleus-to-cytoplasm ratio and contain fewer cell organelles than osteoblasts. Osteoclasts are the major resorptive cells of bone and are characterized by their large size and multiple nuclei. Osteoclasts derive from pluripotent cells of the bone marrow, which are hematopoietic precursors that also give rise to monocytes and macrophages. They lie in regions of bone resorption in pits called Howship lacunae.

Bone Injuries and Healing

A fracture of a bone is a complete or partial break in the continuity of the bone. Fractures usually occur as a result of trauma and may arise from low energy forces that are cyclically repeated over a long time period (i.e., stress fractures) or from forces having sufficient magnitude to cause structural failure after a single impact. Most fractures can be identified on plain radiographs. In some cases, computed tomography (CT) scans or MRI may provide additional information on the fracture pattern. Fracture repair is unique in that healing occurs without scar formation, and only mature bone remains in the fracture site at the end of the repair process. This repair process consists of four stages, including inflammation, soft callus, hard callus, and remodeling (Table 1-5).

The inflammation period begins immediately after the fracture is sustained and is characterized by the presence of hemorrhage, necrotic cells, hematoma, and fibrin clots. The predominant cell types are platelets, polymorphonuclear neutrophils, monocytes, and macrophages. Shortly thereafter, fibroblasts and osteoprogenitor cells appear and blood vessels start growing into the defect. This neoangiogenesis is initiated and maintained by a tissue oxygen gradient and is enhanced by angiogenic factors.

The stage of soft callus is characterized by fibrous or cartilaginous tissue within the fracture gap and a great increase in vascularity (Fig. 1-9, *A* and *B*). The bony ends are no longer freely moveable. Clinically, subsiding pain and swelling characterize this stage.

During the stage of hard callus, the fibrous callus is replaced by immature woven bone. (Fig. 1-10, *A* and *B*). The transition of soft callus to hard callus is somewhat arbitrary,

and overlap exists between these two stages because different regions may progress at different rates. During the remodeling process, the woven bone slowly converts to lamellar bone and the trabecular structure responds to the loading conditions according to Wolff's law.[44] The remodeling process may continue for years after the fracture.

The vast majority of fractures (90% to 95%) are treated successfully.[45] However, a variety of local and systemic factors may affect fracture healing. Local factors that may impede fracture healing include extensive injury to the surrounding soft tissue envelope, decreased local blood supply, inadequate reduction, inadequate mobilization, local infection, or malignant tissue at the fracture site. Systemic factors may include endocrinologic factors (e.g., diabetes mellitus, menopause), general bone loss (e.g., osteopenia, osteoporosis), patient nutrition (smoking, insufficient vitamin or calcium uptake), and peripheral circulation (vascular disease). In many fractures that do not heal, multiple risk factors may exist. Impaired bone healing may present as delayed osseous union or osseous nonunion. Delayed union is usually defined as the failure of the fractured bone to heal within the expected time course, while maintaining the potential to heal. Nonunion is defined as a state in which all healing processes have ceased before fracture healing has occurred.

TABLE 1-5 Bone Healing for a Stable Fracture

Inflammatory Phase	Hemorrhage, necrotic cells; hematoma and fibrin clot formed to bridge the gap	Begins immediately
Soft Callus Phase	Fibrous and cartilaginous tissue forms between the fracture ends, increase in vascularity and ingrowth of capillaries into the fracture callus; increase in cellular proliferation, osteoclasts remove dead bone fragments	1-6 wk postinjury
Hard Callus Phase	Woven bone develops when the callus converts from fibrocartilaginous; osteoclasts continue removing dead bone; osteoblast activity abundant	4-6 wk postinjury
Remodeling Phase	Woven bone slowly changes to lamellar bone; medullary canal is then reconstituted; fracture diameter decreases to the original width	6 wk and up to several months or years (depends on a number of anatomic and physiologic factors)

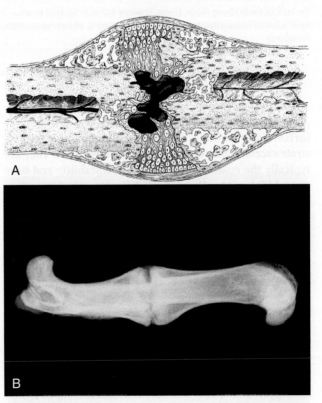

Fig. 1-9 In the second stage of structural fracture healing (i.e., soft callus), subperiosteal bone and medullary callus have formed in the adjacent region, but the central region has filled with cartilage and fibrous tissue, and the peripheral region covers them with dense fibrous tissue forming a new periosteum (**A**), which is not evident radiographically (**B**). (From Browner BD, et al: Skeletal trauma—basic science, management, and reconstruction, ed 3, Philadelphia, 2003, Saunders.)

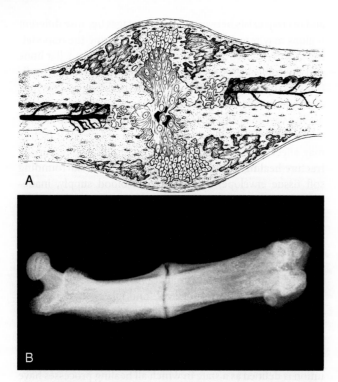

Fig. 1-10 The third stage of structural fracture healing (i.e., hard callus). **A,** Bone begins to form in the peripheral callus region supplied by vascular invasion from the surrounding soft tissue. **B,** This early bone formation may be very thin and not radiographically dense, and the central region is still the bulk of the bridging tissue. (From Browner BD et al: Skeletal trauma—basic science, management, and reconstruction, ed 3, Philadelphia, 2003, Saunders.)

Nonunions can be classified as hypertrophic and atrophic. Nonunions lack the potential to heal and require further interventions. Hypertrophic nonunions demonstrate excessive vascularity and callus formation. They are typically the result of biomechanical instability and have a good biologic healing potential. Treatment of hypertrophic nonunions requires biomechanical stabilization of the fracture site. Atrophic nonunions have a limited healing potential, decreased vascularity, and show decreased callus formation. Treatment of atrophic nonunions is challenging, and the treatment may include débridement, stabilization, and use of bone grafts or other bone stimulating agents.

BIOLOGIC TREATMENT APPROACHES

The successful treatment of musculoskeletal injuries remains challenging. Both ligaments and tendons have a poor vascular supply and a low cell turnover. Recent experimental investigations have attempted to establish novel biologic treatment methods, such as growth factor stimulation. Although most of these novel techniques have not been established in the clinical practice, we provide a brief review of the current research and discuss future perspectives in this area.

TABLE 1-6 Effects of Growth Factors on Musculoskeletal Tissues

	Muscle	Cartilage	Meniscus	Ligament/Tendon	Bone
IGF-1	+	+	+	+	+
(a, b) FGF	+	+	+	+	+
NGF	+				
PDGF (AA, AB, BB)	+		+	+	+
EGF		+	+	+	
TGF-α		+			
TGF-β		+	+	+	+
BMP-2		+	+		+
BMP-4					+
BMP-7					+
VEGF					+

BMP-2, Bone morphogenetic protein-2; *BMP-4,* bone morphogenetic protein-4; *BMP-7,* bone morphogenetic protein-7; *EGF,* endothelial growth factor; *FGF,* fibroblast growth factor; *IGF-1,* insulin-like growth factor-1; *NGF,* nerve growth factor; *PDGF,* platelet-derived growth factor; *TGF-α,* transforming growth factor-alpha; *TGF-β,* transforming growth factor-beta; *VEGF,* vascular endothelial growth factor.

Growth Factors and Gene Therapy

Growth factors are proteins that can be synthesized by both the resident cells (e.g., fibroblasts) and by immigrating cells (e.g., macrophages). Growth factors have the ability to stimulate cell proliferation, cell migration, and cell differentiation.[46] Several authors have investigated the role of growth factors in stimulating the musculoskeletal healing response. Stimulating effects of various growth factors have been demonstrated in a variety of tissue (Table 1-6).[47]

The use of most of these growth factors is limited by their short biologic half-lives, requiring repeated applications.[48,49] To overcome this problem, gene transfer techniques have been tested in experimental studies. Gene therapy is based on the modification of cellular genetic information (Fig. 1-11). Thus the genes encoding for growth factors are transferred into local cells at the injury site to modify their genetic codes so that growth factors are continuously produced. This continuous excretion of growth factors will result in an uninterrupted stimulation of the injured musculoskeletal tissue. To achieve gene expression, the DNA encoding for the growth factors must be transferred into the nucleus of the host cells. After gene transfer, the treated cells generously express the intended factor (Fig. 1-12). Usually, viral vectors are used for the gene transfer, with adenoviruses and retroviruses representing the most commonly used vectors. Two strategies are used for the transfection of the host cells: (1) the in vivo approach and (2) the ex vivo approach.[48,49] The in vivo approach includes the injection of a virus (usually an adenovirus) encoding the growth factor gene at the injury site. The ex vivo approach includes harvesting cells from the host, genetic modification in vitro (usually by a retrovirus),

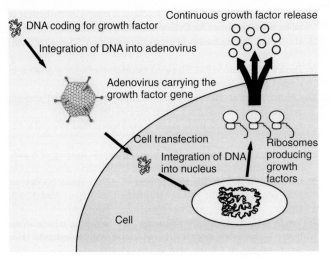

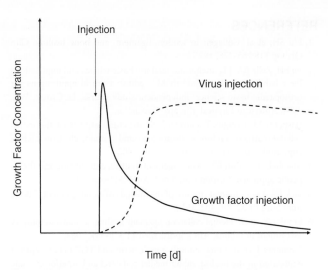

Fig. 1-11 Gene expression pathway. The DNA encoding for a growth factor is inserted into a viral vector. The viral vector is transfecting the cell, and the growth factor gene is inserted into the cell nucleus. The growth factor is then produced by the transfected cells and released into the extracellular space. (Adapted from Lattermann C, Fu FH: Gene therapy in orthopaedics. In Huard J, Fu FH, editors: Gene therapy and tissue engineering in orthopaedics and sports medicine, New York, 2000, Birkhauser Boston.)

Fig. 1-12 Growth factor concentration after injection of the pure protein versus gene therapy. After injection of the pure growth factor, the concentration reaches a maximum and returns instantly to the baseline level. Gene therapy results in a continuous growth factor concentration in the target tissue over a longer time period. (Reprinted from Fu FH, Zelle BA: Ligaments and tendons: basic science and implications for rehabilitation. In Wilmarth MA, editor: Clinical applications for orthopaedic basic science: independent study course, La Crosse, Wis, 2004, American Physical Therapy Association.)

and reinjection of the modified cells to the injury site. Although the in vivo approach appears to be technically simpler, the ex vivo approach appears to be safer because the transfection of the cells occurs under controlled conditions in vitro.

Although experimental data have demonstrated the great potential of gene therapy techniques, gene therapy has not been established as a standard treatment in patients with musculoskeletal injuries. The major concern surrounding gene therapy is the safety of this technique. Potential risk factors include uncontrolled overstimulation and overgrowth of the repair tissue, mutation of the viral vectors, development of malignancies, and immunologic reactions. Future research is required to investigate and optimize the safety of gene therapy to translate this treatment approach into clinical practice.

CLINICAL CASE REVIEW

1 What can patients do to improve wound healing?

Wound healing occurs through scar formation. Extrinsic factors (e.g., nutrition, hydration, smoking, wound exposure, and wound management) will influence the healing response and the scar formation.

2 Why can some ligaments heal, whereas others need to be repaired?

The healing response varies among the different ligaments. For this answer, let us consider the knee as an example. While MCL injuries have the potential to heal spontaneously, other ligament injuries, such as ACL injuries, rarely show a spontaneous healing response due to:

1. High stress carried by the ACL that prevents the ruptured ligament ends from having sufficient contact.
2. The ACL is not embedded in a strong soft tissue envelope and it is an intraarticular structure; when it ruptures, the blood is diluted by the synovial fluid, preventing hematoma formation and hence initiation of the healing mechanism.
3. Increased expression of myofibroblasts and growth factor receptors were found in the injured MCL as compared with the injured ACL.[7]

REFERENCES

1. Liu SH, et al: Collagen in tendon, ligament, and bone healing. Clin Orthop 318:265-278, 1995.

2. Fu FH, Zelle BA: Ligaments and tendons: basic science and implications for rehabilitation. In Wilmarth MA, editor: Clinical applications for orthopaedic basic science: independent study course, La Crosse, Wis, 2004, American Physical Therapy Association.

3. Raspanti M, Congiu T, Guizzardi S: Structural aspects of the extracellular matrix of tendon: an atomic force and scanning electron microscopy study. Arch Histol Cytol 65:37-43, 2002.

4. Marshall JL, Rubin RM: Knee ligament injuries: a diagnostic and therapeutic approach. Orthop Clin North Am 8:641-668, 1977.

5. Jack EA: Experimental rupture of the medial collateral ligament. J Bone Joint Surg Br 32:396-402, 1950.

6. Frank CB, et al: Medial collateral ligament healing: a multidisciplinary assessment in rabbits. Am J Sports Med 11:379-389, 1983.

7. Menetrey J, et al: alpha-Smooth muscle actin and TGF-beta receptor I expression in the healing rabbit medial collateral and anterior cruciate ligaments. Injury 42(:8)735-741, 2011.

8. Cameron M, et al: The natural history of the anterior cruciate ligament-deficient knee: Changes in synovial fluid cytokine and keratan sulfate concentrations. Am J Sports Med 25:751-754, 1997.

9. Gomez MA, et al: The effects of increased tension on healing medial collateral ligaments. Am J Sports Med 19:347-354, 1991.

10. Provenzano PP, et al: Hindlimb unloading alters ligament healing. J Appl Physiol 94:314-324, 2002.

11. Vailas AC, et al: Physical activity and its influence on the repair process of medial collateral ligaments. Connect Tissue Res 9:25-31, 1981.

12. Kolts I, Tillmann B, Lullmann-Rauch R: The structure and vascularization of the biceps brachii long head tendon. Ann Anat 176;75-80, 1994.

13. Hergenroeder PT, Gelberman RH, Akeson WH: The vascularity of the flexor pollicis longus tendon. Clin Orthop 162:298-303, 1982.

14. Zbrodowski A, Gajisin S, Grodecki J: Vascularization of the tendons of the extensor pollicis longus, extensor carpi radialis longus and extensor carpi radialis brevis muscles. J Anat 135:235-244, 1982.

15. Manske PR, Lesker PA: Comparative nutrient pathways to the flexor profundus tendons in zone II of various experimental animals. J Surg Res 34:83-93, 1983.

16. Cetti R, Junge J, Vyberg M: Spontaneous rupture of the Achilles tendon is preceded by widespread and bilateral tendon damage and ipsilateral inflammation: A histopathologic study of 60 patients. Acta Orthop Scand 74:78-84, 2003.

17. Maffulli N, Barrass V, Ewen SW: Light microscopic histology of Achilles tendon ruptures: A comparison with unruptured tendons. Am J Sports Med 28:857-863, 2000.

18. Steinbach LS, Fleckenstein JL, Mink JH: Magnetic resonance imaging of muscle injuries. Orthopedics 17:991-999, 1994.

19. Gelberman RH, et al: Flexor tendon repair in vitro: a comparative histologic study of the rabbit, chicken, dog, and monkey. J Orthop Res 2:39-48, 1984.

20. Manske PR, et al: Intrinsic flexor-tendon repair: A morphological study in vitro. J Bone Joint Surg Am 66:385-396, 1984.

21. Russell JE, Manske PR: Collagen synthesis during primate flexor tendon repair in vitro. J Orthop Res 8:13-20, 1990.

22. Feehan LM, Beauchene JG: Early tensile properties of healing chicken flexor tendons: Early controlled passive motion versus postoperative mobilization. J Hand Surg Am 15:63-68, 1990.

23. Kubota H, et al: Effect of motion and tension on injured flexor tendons in chickens. J Hand Surg [Am] 21:456-463, 1996.

24. Mass DP, et al: Effects of constant mechanical tension on the healing of rabbit flexor tendons. Clin Orthop 296:301-306, 1993.

25. Huxley HE: The mechanism of muscular contraction. Science 164:1356-1366, 1969.

26. Huxley AF, Simmons RM: Proposed mechanism of force generation in striated muscle. Nature 233:533-538, 1971.

27. Croisier JL, et al: Hamstring muscle strain recurrence and strength performance disorders. Am J Sports Med 30:199-203, 2002.

28. Garrett WE, Jr: Muscle strain injuries. Am J Sports Med 24(suppl 6):S2-S8, 1996.

29. Speer KP, Lohnes J, Garrett WE, Jr: Radiographic imaging of muscle strain injury. Am J Sports Med 21:89-95, 1993.

30. Orchard J, Best TM: The management of muscle strain injuries: an early return versus the risk of recurrence. Clin J Sport Med 12:3-5, 2002.

31. Verrall GM, et al: Clinical risk factors for hamstring muscle strain injury: A prospective study with correlation of injury by magnetic resonance imaging. Br J Sports Med 35:435-439, 2001.

32. Friden J, Sjostrom M, Ekblom B: Myofibrillar damage following intense eccentric exercise in man. Int J Sports Med 4:170-176, 1983.

33. Stauber WT: Eccentric action of muscles physiology, injury, and adaptation. Exerc Sport Sci Rev 17:157-185, 1989.

34. Barash IA, et al: Desmin cytoskeletal modifications after a bout of eccentric exercise in the rat. Am J Physiol Regul Integr Comp Physiol 283:958-963, 2002.

35. Lieber RL, Shah S, Friden J: Cytoskeletal disruption after eccentric contraction-induced muscle injury. Clin Orthop 403:S90-S99, 2002.

36. Jackson DW, Feagin JA: Quadriceps contusions in young athletes. J Bone Joint Surg Am 55:95-105, 1973.

37. Botte MJ, et al: Repair of severe muscle belly lacerations using tendon grafts. J Hand Surg 12A:406-412, 1987.

38. Garrett WE, et al: Recovery of skeletal muscle after laceration and repair. J Hand Surg 9A:683-692, 1984.

39. Arrington ED, Miller MD: Skeletal muscle injuries. Orthop Clin North Am 26:411-422, 1995.

40. King JB: Post-traumatic ectopic calcification in the muscles of athletes: A review. Br J Sports Med 32:287-290, 1998.

41. Hierton C: Regional blood flow in experimental myositis ossificans. Acta Orthop Scand 54:58-63, 1983.

42. Illes T, et al: Characterization of bone forming cells in post traumatic myositis ossificans by lectins. Pathol Res Pract 188:172-176, 1992.

43. Neal BC, et al: A systematic overview of 13 randomized trials of non-steroidal anti-inflammatory drugs for prevention of heterotopic bone formation after major hip surgery. Acta Orthop Scand 71:122-128, 2000.

44. Regling G, editor: Wolff's law and connective tissue regulation: Modern interdisciplinary comments on Wolff's law of connective tissue regulation and rational understanding of common clinical problems, Berlin, NY, 1992, W de Gruyter.

45. Einhorn TA: Enhancement of fracture healing. J Bone Joint Surg Am 77:940-956, 1995.

46. Zelle BA, et al: Biological considerations of tendon graft incorporation within the bone tunnel. Oper Tech Orthop 15:36-42, 2005.

47. Huard J: Gene therapy and tissue engineering for sports medicine. J Gene Med 5:93-108, 2003.

48. Evans C, Robbins PD: Possible orthopaedic applications of gene therapy. J Bone Joint Surg Am 77:1103-1114, 1995.

49. Robbins PD, Ghivizzani S: Viral vectors for gene therapy. Pharmacol Ther 80:35-47, 1998.

CHAPTER 2

Soft Tissue Healing Considerations After Surgery

Robert Cantu, Jason A. Steffe

Physical therapists work daily on a variety of connective tissue types that are dynamic and have an amazing capacity for change. Changes in these types of tissues are driven by a number of factors, including trauma, surgery, immobilization, posture, and repeated stresses. The physical therapist should have a good working knowledge of the normal histology and biomechanics of connective tissue. Additionally, the astute therapist should have a thorough understanding of the way connective tissue responds to immobilization, trauma, and remobilization. Both experienced and novice physical therapists can benefit from a good "mental picture" of how connective tissue operates as they think through, strategize, and treat postsurgical patients.

The classic view of connective tissue and its response to trauma and immobilization is that these tissues are inert and noncontractile, with muscle fibers being the only contractile element. While the body of literature documenting this view is solid and well accepted, newer studies have uncovered some exciting possibilities regarding the "contractility" of connective tissue. If fascia, ligaments, and tendons have a limited ability to behave like contractile tissue, many of the changes therapists have felt immediately after performing manual techniques can be validated and substantiated. Additionally, treatment strategies would change, or if not change, be better explained. In the context of postsurgical management, treating "inert" tissue as "contractile" could certainly change treatment perspectives.

SURGERY DEFINED

Because this text primarily considers postsurgical rehabilitation, an operational definition of surgery is in order. For the purpose of considering injury and repair of soft tissue, *surgery* may be defined as *controlled trauma produced by a trained professional to correct uncontrolled trauma.* The reason for this specific, contextual definition is

that connective tissues respond in characteristic ways to immobilization and trauma. Because surgery is itself a form of trauma that is usually followed by some form of immobilization, the physical therapist must understand the way tissues respond to both immobilization and trauma.

This chapter begins by presenting the classical view of basic histology and the biomechanics of connective tissue. Next, the histopathology and pathomechanics of connective tissue (i.e., the way connective tissues respond to immobilization, trauma, and remobilization) will be addressed. This chapter will also address some basic principles of soft tissue mobilization based on the basic science behind immobilization, trauma, and remobilization of the connective tissue. Finally, there will be a discussion of the more recent literature suggesting the limited contractility potential of connective tissue.

HISTOLOGY AND BIOMECHANICS OF CONNECTIVE TISSUE

The connective tissue system in the human body is quite extensive. Connective tissue makes up 16% of the body's weight and holds 25% of the body's water.[1] The "soft" connective tissue forms ligaments, tendons, periosteum, joint capsules, aponeuroses, nerve and muscle sheaths, blood vessel walls, and the bed and framework of the internal organs. If the bony structures were removed, then a semblance of structure would remain from the connective tissue.[1-5]

A majority of the tissue affected by mobilization are "inert" connective tissue. During joint mobilization, for example, the tissues being mobilized are the joint capsule and the surrounding ligaments and connective tissue. Arthrokinematic rules are followed, but the tissue being mobilized is classified as inert connective tissue. Therefore, background knowledge of the histology and histopathology of connective tissue is essential for the practicing physical therapist.

Normal Histology and Biomechanics of Connective Tissue Cells

Connective tissue has two components: (1) the cells and (2) the extracellular matrix. The two cells of primary importance in connective tissue are the fibroblast and the myofibroblast. The fibroblast synthesizes all the inert components of connective tissue, including collagen, elastin, reticulin, and ground substance.[1-5] The myofibroblast is a specialized cell that contains smooth muscle elements and has a capacity to contract.[6-9]

Extracellular Matrix

The extracellular matrix of connective tissue includes connective tissue fibers and ground substance. The connective tissue fibers include collagen (the most tensile), elastin, and reticulin (the most extensible). Collagen, elastin, and reticulin provide the tensile support that connective tissue offers. Extensibility or the lack of it is driven by the relative density and percentage of the connective tissue fibers. Tissues with less collagen density and a greater proportion of elastin fibers are more pliable than tissue with a greater density and proportion of collagen fibers.[1-3]

The ground substance of connective tissue plays a very different role in the connective tissue response to immobility, trauma, and remobilization. The ground substance is the viscous, gel-like substance in which the cells and connective tissue fibers lie. It acts as a lubricant for collagen fibers in conditions of normal mobility and maintains a crucial distance between collagen fibers. The ground substance also is a medium for the diffusion of nutrients and waste products and acts as a mechanical barrier for invading microorganisms. It has a much shorter half-life than collagen and, as will be discussed, is much more quickly affected by immobilization than collagen.[4,10]

Three Types of Connective Tissue

Connective tissue is classified according to fiber density and orientation. The three types of connective tissue found in the human body are (1) dense regular, (2) dense irregular, and (3) loose irregular (Table 2-1).[11,12]

Dense regular connective tissue includes ligaments and tendons (Fig. 2-1).[5] The fiber orientation is unidirectional for the purpose of attenuating unidirectional forces. The high density of collagen fibers accounts for the high degree of tensile strength and lack of extensibility in these tissue. Relatively low vascularity and water content account for the slow diffusion of nutrients and the resulting slower healing times. Dense regular connective tissue is the most tensile and least extensible of the connective tissue types.

Dense irregular connective tissue includes joint capsules, periosteum, and aponeuroses. The primary difference between dense regular and dense irregular connective tissue is that dense irregular connective tissue has a multidimensional fiber orientation (Fig. 2-2). This multidimensional orientation allows the tissue to attenuate forces in numerous directions. The density of collagen fibers is high, producing

TABLE 2-1 Classification of Connective Tissue

Tissue Type	Specific Structures	Characteristics of the Tissue
Dense regular	Ligaments, tendons	Dense, parallel arrangement of collagen fibers; proportionally less ground substance
Dense irregular	Aponeurosis, periosteum, joint capsules, dermis of skin, areas of high mechanical stress	Dense, multidirectional arrangement of collagen fibers; able to resist multidirectional stress
Loose irregular	Superficial fascial sheaths, muscle and nerve sheaths, support sheaths of internal organs	Sparse, multidirectional arrangement of collagen fibers; greater amounts of elastin present

From Cantu R, Grodin A: Myofascial manipulation: Theory and clinical application, Gaithersburg, Md, 1992, Aspen.

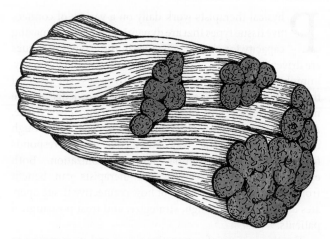

Fig. 2-1 Dense regular connective tissue. The parallel compact arrangement of the collagen fibers should be noted. (Modified from Williams P, Warwick R, editors: Gray's anatomy, ed 35, Philadelphia, 1973, Saunders.)

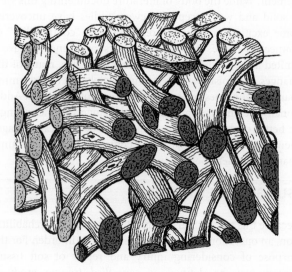

Fig. 2-2 Dense irregular connective tissue with multidimensional compact arrangement of collagen fibers. (Modified from Williams P, Warwick R, editors: Gray's anatomy, ed 35, Philadelphia, 1973, Saunders.)

a high degree of tensile strength and a low degree of extensibility. Dense irregular connective tissue also has low vascularity and water content, resulting in slow diffusion of nutrients and slower healing times.[5]

Loose irregular connective tissue includes, but is not limited to, the superficial fascial sheath of the body directly under the skin, the muscle and nerve sheaths, and the bed and framework of the internal organs. Similarly to dense irregular connective tissue, loose irregular connective tissue has a multidimensional tissue orientation. However, the density of collagen fibers is much less than that of dense irregular connective tissue. The relative vascularity and water content of loose irregular connective tissue is much greater than dense regular and dense irregular connective tissue. Therefore, it is much more pliable and extensible, and exhibits faster healing times after trauma. Loose irregular connective tissue also is the easiest to mobilize.[5]

Normal Biomechanics of Connective Tissue

Connective tissues have unique deformation characteristics that enable them to be effective shock attenuators. This is termed the viscoelastic nature of connective tissue.[1-3,13] This viscoelasticity is the very characteristic that makes connective tissue able to change based on the stresses applied to it. The ability of connective tissue to thicken or become more extensible based on outside stresses is the basic premise to be understood by the manual therapist seeking to increase mobility.

In the viscoelastic model, two components combine to give connective tissue its dynamic deformation attributes. The first is the elastic component, which represents a temporary change in the length of connective tissue subjected to stress (Fig. 2-3). A spring, which elongates when loaded and returns to its original position when unloaded, illustrates this. This elastic component is the "slack" in connective tissue.[1-3]

The viscous, or plastic, component of the model represents the permanent change in connective tissue subjected to outside forces. A hydraulic cylinder and piston illustrates this (Fig. 2-4). When a force is placed on the piston, the piston slowly moves out of the cylinder. When the force is removed, the piston does not recoil but remains at the new length, indicating permanent change. These permanent changes result from the breaking of intermolecular and intramolecular bonds between collagen molecules, fibers, and cross-links.[1-3]

The viscoelastic model combines the elastic and plastic components just described (Fig. 2-5). When subjected to a mild force in the midrange of the tissue, the tissue elongates in the elastic component and then returns to its original length. If, however, the stress pushes the tissue to the end range, then the elastic component is depleted and plastic deformation occurs. When the stress is released, some permanent deformation has occurred. It should be noted that not all the elongation (only a portion) is permanently retained.[1-3]

Clinically, this phenomenon occurs frequently. For example, a client with a frozen shoulder that has only 90° of elevation is mobilized to reach a range of motion (ROM) of 110° by the end of the treatment session. When the client returns in a few days, the ROM of that shoulder is less than 110° but more than 90°. Some degree of elongation is lost and some is retained.

This viscoelastic phenomenon can be further illustrated by the use of stress-strain curves. By definition, stress is the force applied per unit area, and strain is the percent change in the length of the tissue. When connective tissue is initially stressed or loaded, very little force is required to elongate the tissue. However, as more stress is applied and the slack or spring is taken up, more force is required and less change occurs in the tissue (Fig. 2-6). When the tissue is subjected to repeated stresses, the curve shows that after each stress the tissue elongates and then only partially returns to its original length. Some length is gained each time the tissue is taken into the plastic range. This phenomenon is seen clinically in repeated sessions of therapy. ROM is gained during a session, with some of the gain being lost between sessions.[1-3]

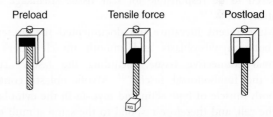

Preload   Tensile force   Postload

Fig. 2-4 The viscous, or plastic, component of connective tissue. (From Grodin A, Cantu R: Myofascial manipulation: theory and clinical management, Centerpoint, NY, 1989, Forum Medical.)

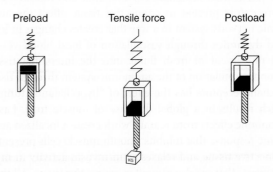

Preload   Tensile force   Postload

Fig. 2-5 The viscoelastic nature of connective tissue. (From Grodin A, Cantu R: Myofascial manipulation: Theory and clinical management, Centerpoint, NY, 1989, Forum Medical.)

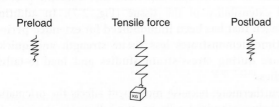

Preload   Tensile force   Postload

Fig. 2-3 The elastic component of connective tissue. (From Grodin A, Cantu R: Myofascial manipulation: Theory and clinical management, Centerpoint, NY, 1989, Forum Medical.)

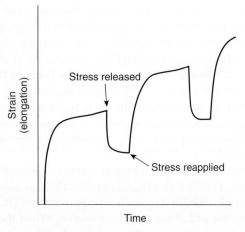

Fig. 2-6 Stress-strain curves indicating the progressive elongation of connective tissue with repeated stresses. (From Grodin A, Cantu R: Myofascial manipulation: Theory and clinical management, Centerpoint, NY, 1989, Forum Medical.)

New Developments—Connective Tissue Is Contractile and Dynamic

The older model of connective tissue does not explain completely the quick changes that can occur in connective tissue during manual therapy. Several theories have emerged to explain these quick changes. The most substantial body of literature suggests that connective tissues have a limited contractile ability resulting from the presence of myofibroblasts. Myofibroblasts are differentiated fibroblasts that not only synthesize collagen and ground substance, but also retain the ability to contract. These specialized cells were first recognized to be present in immature scar tissue, and were believed to be responsible for scar tissue shrinkage and contracture.[6,7,14-16]

More recent literature has documented the presence of both myofibroblasts and smooth muscle fibers in normal connective tissue, including the fascia cruris and the lumbodorsal fascia.[16,17] Myofibroblasts contain smooth muscle of type actin and myosin in the cytoplasm of the cell, and therefore respond to the same stimuli that affect smooth muscle.[20] Schleip and associates have described several autonomic mechanisms by which connective tissue "tone" can possibly be affected.[14,15,18,19]

First, manual stimulation of interstitial and Ruffini mechanoreceptors present in connective tissue affect the autonomic nervous system in a way that creates changes in local fluid dynamics through vasodilation of local blood vessels and movement of fresh fluids into the interstitial tissue. Second, stimulation of the autonomic system through tissue mechanoreceptors has the effect of "hypothalamic tuning," which results in a global decrease of muscle tone. Lastly, autonomic effects from manual work create a localized autonomic response that inhibits smooth muscle cells present in connective tissue and relaxes actin/myosin activity in myofibroblasts that are also present in connective tissue. All three of these basic mechanisms can better explain the relatively immediate changes that are palpable after manual therapy.

As an example, consider the patient who is referred for therapy 4 weeks after rotator cuff repair, who has developed significant capsular tightness of the shoulder, and who is reactive and guarded with passive range of motion. Gentle soft tissue work in the shoulder girdle, including the scapulathoracic area, lateral scapula, upper trapezius, and the pectoralis major and minor usually result in immediate increases in range of motion and less reactivity from the patient. Mechanical changes in the joint capsule are not likely to have occurred in such a short time to explain the increased range of motion. A more plausible explanation would be that gentle manual work around the shoulder complex created an autonomic response, which in turn relaxed the contractile elements present in the connective tissue.

EFFECTS OF IMMOBILIZATION, REMOBILIZATION, AND TRAUMA ON CONNECTIVE TISSUE

Immobilization

Immobilization and trauma significantly change the histology and normal mechanics of connective tissue. A majority of the historic studies in the area of immobilization follow the same basic experimental mode.[13,20-27] Laboratory animals are fixated internally for varying periods. The fixation is removed and the animals are then sacrificed. Histochemical and biomechanical analyses are performed to determine changes in the tissue. In some studies, the fixation is removed and the animals are allowed to move the fixated joint for a period before performance of the analysis. This is done to determine the reversibility of the effects of immobilization.[28]

Macroscopically, fibrofatty infiltrate is evident in the recesses of the immobilized tissue. With prolonged immobilization, the infiltrates develop a more fibrotic appearance, creating adhesions in the recesses. These fibrotic changes occur in the absence of trauma. Histologic and histochemical analyses show significant changes primarily in the ground substance, with no significant loss of collagen. The changes in the ground substance consist of substantial losses of glycosaminoglycans and water. Because a primary function of ground substance is binding water to assist in hydration, the loss of ground substance results in a related loss of water.

Another purpose of ground substance is to lubricate adjacent collagen fibers and maintain a crucial interfiber distance. If collagen fibers approximate too closely, then the fibers will adhere to one another. These cross-links create a series of microscopic adhesions that limit the pliability and extensibility of the tissue (Fig. 2-7). **In addition, collagen that has been immobilized for extended periods of time demonstrates less tissue strength and quicker failure during stress-strain studies and load-to-failure studies.**[10,25,27,29-33]

Furthermore, because movement affects the orientation of newly synthesized collagen, the collagen in the immobilized joints studied was laid down in a more haphazard, "haystack" arrangement. This orientation restricts tissue

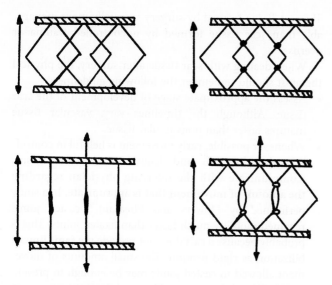

Fig. 2-7 The basket weave configuration of connective tissue. With immobilization, the distance between fibers is diminished, forming cross-link adhesions. (From Cantu R, Grodin A: Myofascial manipulation: Theory and clinical application, Gaithersburg, Md, 1992, Aspen.)

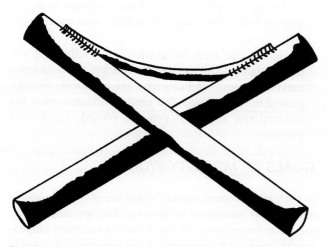

Fig. 2-8 The random haystack arrangement of immobilized scar tissue creating additional adhesions. (From Cantu R, Grodin A: Myofascial manipulation: Theory and clinical application, Gaithersburg, Md, 1992, Aspen.)

mobility further by adhering to existing collagen fibers (Fig. 2-8).

Biomechanical analysis reveals that as much as 10 times more torque is necessary to mobilize fixated joints than normal joints. After repeated mobilizations, these joints gradually return to normal. The authors of these studies implicate both fibrofatty microadhesions and increased microscopic cross-linking of collagen fibers in the decreased extensibility of connective tissue.[13,20-27]

Remobilization

The classic research seems to suggest that mobility and remobilization prevent the haystack development of collagen fibers within ligaments and tendons, as well as stimulate the production of ground substance. When connective tissue is stressed with movement, the tissue rehydrates, collagen cross-links are diminished, and new collagen is laid down in a more orderly fashion.[13,20-28,34]

Also, the collagen tends to be laid down in the direction of the forces applied and in an appropriate length. In addition, early mobilization leads to enhanced ligament and tendon strength, resistance to tensile forces, greater joint stability, and improved resistance of the ligament to avulsion.[4,9,10,25-27,29,31,34-36]

Additionally, macroadhesions formed during the immobilization period partially elongate and partially rupture during the remobilization process, increasing the overall mobility of the tissue. Both passive mobilization and active ROM produce similar results.

Trauma

The previously described studies have limited application because they involve the immobilization of normal, healthy joints. To complete this discussion, we must superimpose the effects of trauma and scar tissue on immobilization.

Scar

Scar tissue mechanics differ somewhat from normal connective tissue mechanics. Normal connective tissue is mature and stable, with limited pliability. Immature scar tissue is much more dynamic and pliable. Scar tissue formation occurs in four distinct phases. Each of these phases shows characteristic differences during phases of immobilization and mobilization.[1-3]

The first phase of scar tissue formation is the inflammatory phase. This phase occurs immediately after trauma. Blood clotting begins almost instantly and is followed by migration of macrophages and histiocytes to start débriding the area. This phase usually lasts 24 to 48 hours, and immobilization is usually important because of the potential for further damage with movement. Some exceptions to routine immobilization exist. For example, in an anterior cruciate ligament (ACL) reconstruction, in which the graft is safely fixated and damage from gentle movement is unlikely, there may be a great advantage in moving the tissue as early as the first day after surgery. Research indicates that early mobilization leads to more rapid ligament regeneration and ultimate load to failure strength in surgically repaired ACLs.[32]

The second phase of scar tissue formation is the granulation phase. This phase is characterized by an uncharacteristic increase in the relative vascularity of the tissue. Increased vascularity is essential to ensure proper nutrition to meet the metabolic needs of the healing tissue. The granulation phase varies greatly depending on the type of tissue and the extent of the damage. Generally speaking, the entire process of scar tissue formation is lengthened if the damaged tissue is less vascular in its nontraumatized state. For example, tendons and ligaments require more time for scar tissue formation than muscle or epithelial tissue. Movement is helpful in this phase, although the scar tissue can be easily damaged. The physician and therapist need to work closely to determine the extent of movement relative to the risk.

The third phase of scar tissue formation is the fibroplastic stage. In this stage the number of fibroblasts increases, as does the rate of production of collagen fibers and ground substance. Collagen is laid down at an accelerated rate and binds to itself with weak hydrostatic bonds, making tissue elongation much easier. This stage presents an excellent window of opportunity for the reshaping and molding of scar tissue without great risk of tissue reinjury. This stage lasts 3 to 8 weeks, depending on the histologic makeup and relative vascularity of the damaged tissue. Scar tissue at this phase is less likely to be injured but is still easily remodeled with stresses applied (Fig. 2-9). Additionally, myofibroblasts are the most active in the last two phases of scar tissue maturation. Myofibroblasts are believed to be responsible for the scar tissue shrinkage that occurs in this and the next phase of scar tissue healing.[1,3,6-8,37]

The final phase of scar tissue formation is the maturation phase. Collagen matures, solidifies, and shrinks during this phase. Maximal stress can be placed on the tissue without risk of tissue failure. Because collagen synthesis is still accelerated, significant remodeling can take place when appropriate mobilizations are performed. Conversely, if they are left unchecked, then the collagen fibers can cross-link and the tissue can shrink significantly. At the end of the maturation phase, tissue remodeling becomes significantly more difficult because the tissue reverts to a more mature, inactive, and nonpliable status.

Surgical Perspective

Surgery has been defined in this chapter as controlled trauma produced by a trained professional to correct uncontrolled trauma. Postsurgical cases are subject to the effects of immobilization, trauma, and scar formation. However, they have the advantage of resulting from controlled trauma.

The scar tissue formed by surgery is usually more manageable than scar tissue formed by uncontrolled trauma or overuse.

When dealing with scar tissue after surgery, the physical therapist should remember the following guidelines:

- Assess the approximate stage of development of the scar tissue. Although the timelines vary, vascular tissue matures faster than nonvascular tissue.
- Whenever possible, early movement is helpful in controlling the direction and length of the scar tissue. **Communicate with the referring physician regarding the amount of movement that is appropriate.** In a study performed by Flowers and Pheasant,[38] casted joints regained mobility much faster than fixated joints. This is probably because a cast does not provide the same immobilization as rigid fixation. The small amounts of movement allowed in casted joints may be enough to prevent some of the changes caused by rigid fixation.
- Recognize the window of opportunity to stress scar tissue, and keep in mind the associated risk of tissue injury or microtrauma (see Fig. 2-9). Although the potential to change scar tissue may be greater in earlier stages, the risk of damage is higher. The third stage appears to be the stage at which the reward of mobility work exceeds the risk.
- Recognize that even the gentlest and soothing of soft tissue mobilizations can positively affect the autonomic nervous system,[39] and can relax the contractile element present in these tissues. This gentle, autonomic effect has minimal risk and great potential reward. Touch your patients!

GOALS OF MOBILITY WORK

In 1945 John Mennell wrote, "There are only two possible effects of any movement or massage: they are reflex (autonomic) and mechanical."[36] The following summary emphasizes the goals of the mechanical and autonomic changes of mobility work:

- Mobility work allows for the hydration and rehydration of connective tissue through both mechanical and autonomic mechanisms.
- Mobility work causes the breaking and subsequent prevention of cross-links in collagen fibers.
- Mobility work allows for the breaking and prevention of macroadhesions.
- Mobility work allows for the plastic deformation and permanent elongation of connective tissue.
- Mobility work allows for the laying down of collagen fibers and scar tissue in the appropriate length and direction of the stresses applied.
- Mobility work allows for the molding and remolding of collagen fibers during the fibroplastic and maturation stages of scar tissue formation.
- Mobility work prevents scar tissue shrinkage through both mechanical and autonomic mechanisms.

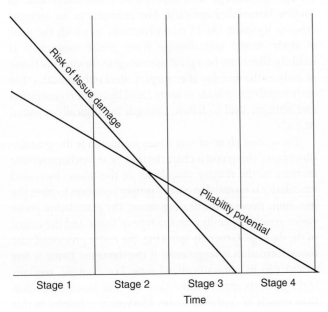

Fig. 2-9 Relationship of tissue pliability to relative risk of injury.

- Mobility work allows for the generalized autonomic effects of increased blood flow, increased venous and lymphatic return, and increased cellular metabolism.
- Mobility work allows for specific autonomic effects, which include the relaxation of smooth muscle fibers present in connective tissue and the relaxation of the actin-myosin complexes found in myofibroblasts.

PRINCIPLES FOR MOBILIZATION OF CONNECTIVE TISSUES

This section attempts to integrate the principles of basic scientific research and years of clinical experience into a series of techniques useful for the physical therapist in treating immobilized tissue.

Three-Dimensionality of Connective Tissue

Connective tissue is three-dimensional. Especially after trauma and immobilization, the scar tissue can follow lines of development not consistent with the kinesiology or arthrokinematics of the area. Therefore the ability to feel the location and direction of the restriction becomes important in the mobilization of scar tissue.

Creep

Creep is another term for the plastic deformation of connective tissue. Active scar tissue is more "creepy" than normal connective tissue (i.e., it is more easily elongated by external forces).[2] Creep occurs when all the "slack" has been let out of the tissue. It is best accomplished with low-load,

prolonged stretching but also can be accomplished with other manual techniques. Dynamic splinting is another technique used to elongate connective tissue. The tissue should be elongated along the lines of normal movement; however, at times the restrictive lesion may not follow the line of movement. The therapist must identify the direction of the restriction and mobilize directly into the restriction. The scar may be a transverse or horizontal plane. Mobilizing the scar in the direction of the restriction usually results in more movement along conventional planes.[1,3]

The Contractile Characteristic of Soft Tissues

As previously mentioned, connective tissues have a contractile element by virtue of the presence of smooth muscle cells and myofibroblasts. Instantaneous "creep" is an autonomic phenomenon.[14,15] Gentle manual work, through stimulation of mechanoreceptors, can create the autonomic effect of relaxation, resulting in increased pliability of connective tissue, increased range of motion, and decreased pain.

Principle of Short and Long

The principle of short and long is the idea that tissues mobilized in a shortened range often become more extensible when they are immediately elongated (Fig. 2-10). For example, in a lateral epicondylitis, cross-friction massage may be performed over the lateral epicondyle with the elbow passively flexed and the wrist passively extended. Immediately after the cross-friction in the shortened range, the tissue is stretched into the plastic range. In the shortened range, deeper tissue can be accessed. When tissue is taut, only the more superficial layers can be accessed. When the tissue has

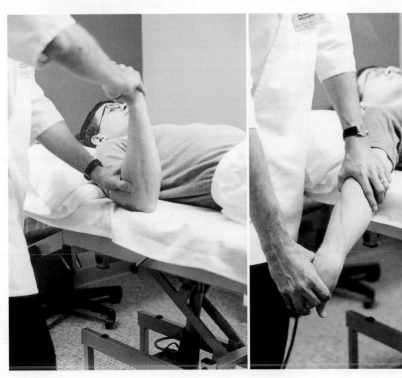

Fig. 2-10 The principle of short and long. Soft tissue immobilization is performed in a shortened range, then immediately elongated.

some slack, the deeper tissue can be accessed and prepared for stretching.[2]

The principle of short and long has neuromuscular implications as well. If a muscle is guarded, then shortening the muscle by mobilizing it has an inhibitory effect that makes immediate elongation easier.

SAMPLE TECHNIQUES FOR MOBILIZATION OF CONNECTIVE TISSUES

The following techniques and associated photographs illustrate some examples of simple manual techniques effective in mobilizing soft tissue.

Muscle Splay

Muscle splay is a term that implies a widening or separation of longitudinal fibers of muscle or connective tissue that have adhered to one another (Fig. 2-11). These adhesions limit the ability of the tissue to be lengthened passively or shortened actively. When muscle bundles or connective tissue bundles stick together, the muscle fibers become less efficient in their contractions. For example, muscle splay in the wrist flexors often produces a slightly greater grip strength immediately after soft tissue work. This is not greater strength, but greater muscle efficiency produced by increased soft tissue pliability. The muscle can contract more efficiently within its connective tissue compartments.[2]

Transverse Muscle Bending

Transverse muscle bending takes the contractile unit and mobilizes it perpendicular to the fibers (Fig. 2-12). This perpendicular bending mobilizes connective tissue in a way similar to the bending of a garden hose (Fig. 2-13). The connective tissue sheath surrounding a muscle may be likened to the hose itself, with the muscle being analogous to the water inside it. If the connective tissue sheath is stiff and rigid, then the muscle inside has difficulty contracting. The unforgiving sheath does not allow the muscle to expand transversely, creating a lack of efficiency and a low-grade "compartment syndrome." By mobilizing these muscle sheaths, overall mobility is enhanced along planes of normal movement.[2]

Additionally, muscle bending specifically stimulates the Ruffini type mechanoreceptor. Ruffini endings are particularly sensitive to lateral/transverse type stretching. This type of stretching, therefore, has the autonomic effect of decreasing sympathetic tone in the "garden hose," creating greater connective tissue pliability.[14,15]

Bony Clearing

Bony clearing is similar to muscle splay, except the mobilization is applied longitudinally along the soft tissue that borders or attaches to a bony surface (Fig. 2-14). A good example of this is longitudinal stroking of the anterior lateral border of the tibia in conditions such as shin splints. The connective tissue along the border of the tibia thickens and becomes adhered, and the therapist attempts to mobilize the tissue in this plane.[2]

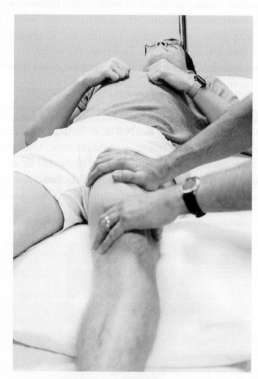

Fig. 2-12 The bending of the fascial sheath surrounding the muscles.

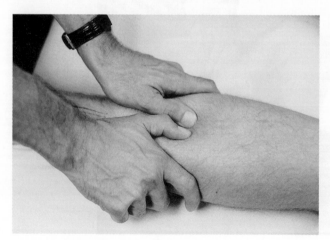

Fig. 2-11 The splaying, or longitudinal separation, of fascial planes.

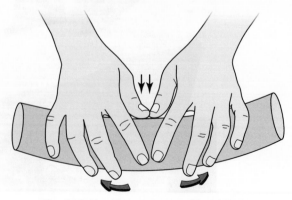

Fig. 2-13 Transverse movement of fascial planes.

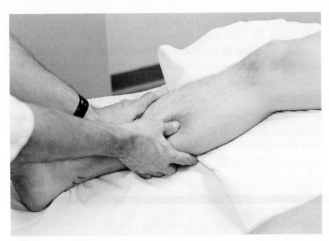

Fig. 2-14 Longitudinal stroke clearing fascia away from a bony surface.

Cross-Friction

Cross-friction massage, which was developed and advocated by the late James Cyriax, is excellent for mobilizing scar tissue and nonvascular connective tissue. It is an aggressive form of soft tissue mobilization designed to break scar tissue adhesions and temporarily increase the blood flow to nonvascular areas. Ligaments and tendons struggling to heal completely are excellent candidates for cross-friction massage. This technique can be used on scar tissue as well, and it should be performed at many different angles to access fibers in all directions.[2]

MUSCLE BALANCING

As connective tissue pliability is increasing through manual therapy and passive range of motion, attention is also given to active range of motion and strengthening. Individual muscles surrounding joints can be grouped together according to their response to dysfunction. Typically, postural muscles respond to injury, abnormal stress, and surgery by tightening or becoming facilitated. Phasic muscles tend to respond to injury, abnormal stress, and surgery by weakening or becoming inhibited.[2]

Each joint complex in the body has groups of muscles that are dedicated to functioning as stabilizers and muscles that function as prime movers. For example, it is well known that the vastus medialis oblique (VMO) at the knee functions to stabilize the patella during knee flexion and extension. It is also well known that the VMO, along with the other three quadricep muscles, responds to dysfunction by weakening, becoming inhibited, and displaying atrophy. Conversely, the hamstring muscle group responds to dysfunction by tightening.[2]

During postsurgical rehabilitation, the therapist should expect to provide manual treatment for the postural muscles that act on the involved joint and strengthen (when healing constraints permit) the phasic muscles that have invariably weakened. A prime example is the shoulder after rotator cuff surgery. Initially, during the acute and protective phases of rehab, the therapist should treat levator scapulae, trapezius,

TABLE 2-2 Classification of Postural and Phasic Muscles of the Shoulder

Classification	Muscles
Postural	Upper traps
	Levator scapulae
	Pectoralis major
	Pectoralis minor
	Subscapularis
	Teres major
Phasic	Lower traps/middle lower rhomboids
	Latissimus dorsi
	Middle traps
	Rhomboids
	Teres minor, infraspinatus, supraspinatus

From Cantu R, Grodin A: Myofascial manipulation: Theory and clinical application, Gaithersburg, Md, 1992, Aspen.

TABLE 2-3 Classification of Postural and Phasic Muscles of the Hip

Classification	Muscles
Postural	Iliopsoas
	Tensor fasciae latae
	Hip adductors
	Hip internal rotators
	Quadratus lumborum
	Piriformis
Phasic	Gluteus maximus
	Gluteus medius/minimus
	Hip external rotators
	Transverse abdominis

TABLE 2-4 Classification of Postural and Phasic Muscles of the Knee

Classification	Muscles
Postural	Hamstrings
	Gastrocnemius
Phasic	Quadriceps (vastus medialis oblique [VMO])
	Dorsiflexors

From Cantu R, Grodin A: Myofascial manipulation: Theory and clinical application, Gaithersburg, Md, 1992, Aspen.

subscapularis, teres major, and pectoralis minor (all postural muscles that act on the shoulder complex). After the patient enters into the active phase of rehab, efforts should be shifted to strengthening of the external rotators, lower traps, rhomboids, and serratus anterior (all phasic muscles that stabilize the shoulder complex).[2]

Tables 2-2 to 2-4 illustrate and summarize the groupings of postural and phasic muscles by region, and agonist-antagonist relationships.

SUMMARY

This chapter outlines the basic principles and guidelines for soft tissue management after surgery and discusses the stages of scar tissue formation. **The time frames for these stages are variable based on the vascularity of the tissue and the surgical procedure performed.** They are delineated in more detail in the following chapters.

The physical therapist must understand connective tissue responses to immobilization, trauma, remobilization, and scar remodeling to treat injured tissue effectively. Additionally, the therapist should be aware of the global and specific autonomic effects of manual therapy that affect tissue contractility. Awareness of both mechanical and autonomic principles of soft tissue management, along with good physician-client communication, ensures consistently effective management of postsurgical rehabilitation.

CLINICAL CASE REVIEW

1 What is the mechanism by which ROM is achieved during a session of manual therapy?

Stimulation of the autonomic nervous system through manual stimulation of interstitial and Ruffini mechanoreceptors has the effect of "hypothalamic tuning," which results in a global decrease of muscle tone.

2 Why is it important to be respectful of the connective tissue following immobilization?

During immobilization collagen fibers become dehydrated, and if collagen fibers approximate too closely, then the fibers will adhere to one another. These cross-links create a series of microscopic adhesions that limit the pliability and extensibility of the tissue. In addition, collagen that has been immobilized for extended periods of time demonstrates less tissue strength and quicker failure during stress-strain studies and load-to-failure studies.

3 At what point is it advisable to stress scar tissue?

There is a window of opportunity to stress scar tissue. Keep in mind the associated risk of tissue injury or microtrauma if the scar tissue is overstressed in its immature stage. Although the potential to change scar tissue may be greater in earlier stages, the risk of damage is higher. The third stage (fibroplastic) appears to be the stage at which the reward of mobility work exceeds the risk. This stage lasts 3 to 8 weeks depending on the histologic makeup and relative vascularity of the damaged tissue.

REFERENCES

1. Cummings GS, Crutchfield CA, Barnes MR: Orthopedic physical therapy series: Soft tissue changes in contractures, Atlanta, 1983, Stokesville Publishing.
2. Cantu R, Grodin A: Myofascial manipulation: Theory and clinical application, Austin, Tex, 1992, ProEd Publishers.
3. Cummings GA: Soft tissue contractures: Clinical management continuing education seminar, course notes, Atlanta, March 1989, Georgia State University.
4. Ham AW, Cormack DH: Histology, Philadelphia, 1979, JB Lippincott.
5. Warwick R, Williams PL: Gray's anatomy, ed 35, Philadelphia, 1973, Saunders.
6. Darby IA, Hewitson TD: Fibroblast differentiation in wound healing and fibrosis. Int Rev Cytol 257:143-175, 2007
7. Gabbiani G: The myofibroblast in wound healing and fibrocontractive diseases. J Pathol 200:500-503, 2003.
8. Hinz B, et al: Biological perspectives: the myofibroblast—One function, multiple origins. Am J Pathol 190(6):1807-1816, 2007.
9. Inoue M, et al: Effects of surgical treatment and immobilization on the healing of the medial collateral ligament: A long-term multidisciplinary study. Connect Tissue Res 25(1):13-26, 1990.
10. Goldstein WM, Barmada R: Early mobilization of rabbit medial ligament and collateral ligament repairs: Biomechanics and histological study. Arch Phys Med Rehab 65(5):239-242, 1984.
11. Copenhaver WM, Bunge RP, Bunge MB: Bailey's textbook of histology, Baltimore, 1971, Williams & Wilkins.
12. Sapega AA, et al: Biophysical factors in range-of-motion exercise. Phys Sportsmed 9:57-65, 1981.
13. Woo S, et al: Connective tissue response to immobility. Arthritis Rheum 18:257-264, 1975.
14. Schleip R: Fascial plasticity—a new neurobiological explanation: Part 1. J Bodywork Movement Ther 7(1):11-19, 2003.
15. Schleip R: Fascial plasticity—a new neurobiological explanation: Part 2. J Bodywork Movement Ther 7(2): 104-116, 2003
16. Yahia LH, Pigeon P, DesRosiers EA: Viscoelastic properties of the human lumbodorsal fascia. J Biomed Eng 15:425-429, 1993.
17. Stecco C, et al: A histological study of the deep fascia of the upper limb. J Anat Embryol 111(2):1-5, 2006.
18. Schleip R: Active contraction of the thoracolumbar fascia—indications of a new factor in low back pain research with implications for manual therapy, 5th Interdisciplinary World Congress on Low Back and Pelvic Pain, Melbourne, Australia, 2004.

19. Schleip R, Klinger W, Lehmann-Horn F: Active fascial contractility: Fascia may be able to contract in a smooth muscle-like manner and thereby influence musculoskeletal dynamics. Med Hypotheses 65:273-277, 2005.

20. Akeson WH, Amiel D: The connective tissue response to immobility: A study of the chondroitin 4 and 6 sulfate and dermatan sulfate changes in periarticular connective tissue of control and immobilized knees of dogs. Clin Orthop 51:190-197, 1967.

21. Akeson WH, Amiel D: Immobility effects of synovial joints: The pathomechanics of joint contracture. Biorheology 17:95, 1980.

22. Akeson WH, et al: The connective tissue response to immobility: An accelerated aging response? Exp Gerontol 3:289-301, 1968.

23. Akeson WH, et al: The connective tissue response to immobility: Biochemical changes in periarticular connective tissue of the immobilized rabbit knee. Clin Orthop 93:356, 1973.

24. Akeson WH, et al: Collagen cross-linking alterations in the joint contractures: changes in the reducible cross-links in periarticular connective tissue after 9 weeks of immobilization. Connect Tissue Res 5:15, 1977.

25. Woo S, et al: The biomechanical and morphological changes in the medial collateral ligament of the rabbit after immobilization and remobilization. J Bone Joint Surg Am 69(8):1200-1211, 1987.

26. Woo SL, et al: New experimental procedures to evaluate the biomechanical properties of healing canine medial collateral ligaments. J Orthop Res 5(3):425-432. 1987.

27. Woo SL, et al: Treatment of the medial collateral ligament injury. II: Structure and function of canine knees in response to differing treatment regimens. Am J Sports Med 15(1):22-29, 1987.

28. Evans E, et al: Experimental immobilization and mobilization of rat knee joints. J Bone Joint Surg 42A:737, 1960.

29. Gelberman RH, et al: Effects of early intermittent passive mobilization on healing canine flexor tendons. J Hand Surg Am 7(2):170-175, 1982.

30. Hart DP, Dahners LE: Healing of the medial collateral ligament in rats. The effects of repair, motion, and secondary stabilizing ligaments. J Bone Joint Surg Am 69(8):1194-1199, 1987.

31. Lechner CT, Dahners LE: Healing of the medial collateral ligament in unstable rat knees. Am J Sports Med 19(5):508-512, 1991.

32. Muneta T, et al: Effects of postoperative immobilization on the reconstructed anterior cruciate ligament: An experimental study in rabbits. Am J Sports Med 21(2):305-313, 1993.

33. Thornton GM, Shrive NG, Frank CB: Healing ligaments have decreased cyclic modulus compared to normal ligaments and immobilization further compromises healing ligament response to cyclic loading. J Orthop Res 21(4):716-722, 2003.

34. Piper TL, Whiteside LA: Early mobilization after knee ligament repair in dogs: An experimental study. Clin Orthop Relat Res 150:277-282, 1980.

35. Gomez, MA, et al: The effects of increased tension on healing medial collateral ligaments. Acta Orthop Scand 54(6):917-923. 1983.

36. Mennell JB: Physical treatment by movement, manipulation and massage, ed 5, London, 1945, Churchill Livingstone.

37. Tomasek JJ, et al: Myofibroblasts and mechano-regulation of connective tissue remodeling. Mol Cell Biol 3:349-362, 2002.

38. Flowers KR, Pheasant SD: The use of torque angle curves in the assessment of digital stiffness. J Hand Ther 1(2)69-74, 1988

39. Dicke E, Schliack H, Wolff A: A manual of reflexive therapy of the connective tissue, Scarsdale, NY, 1978, Sidney S Simon.

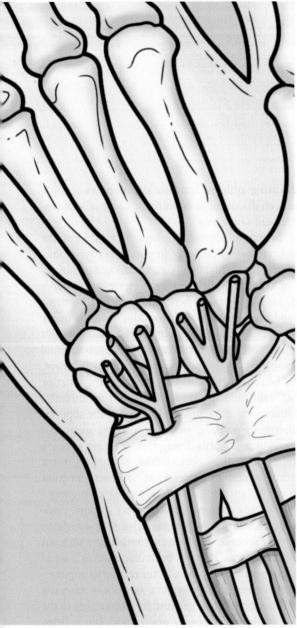

PART 2

Upper Extremity

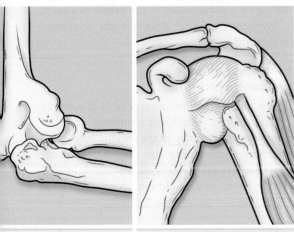

CHAPTER 3

Acromioplasty

Steven R. Tippett, Mark R. Phillips

Before the broad topic of acromioplasty is addressed, the topic of subacromial impingement syndrome must be explored. In 1972 Neer[1] described subacromial impingement as a distinct clinical entity. He correlated the anatomy of the subacromial space with the bony and soft tissue relationships and described the impingement zone. Neer[2] also described a continuum of three clinical and pathologic stages. This study provides a basis for understanding the impingement syndrome, which ranges from reversible inflammation to full-thickness rotator cuff tearing. The relationships among the anterior third of the acromion, the coracoacromial ligament, and the acromioclavicular (AC) joint and the underlying subacromial soft tissue—including the rotator cuff—remain the basis for most of the subsequent surgery-related impingement studies. Many other researchers have contributed to the current knowledge regarding the subacromial shoulder impingement syndrome. The works of Meyer,[3] Codman,[4] Armstrong,[5] Diamond,[6] and McLaughlin and Asherman[7] provide a historical perspective.

SURGICAL INDICATIONS AND CONSIDERATIONS

Anatomic Etiologic Factors

Any abnormality that disrupts the intricate relationship within the subacromial space may lead to impingement. Both intrinsic (intratendinous) and extrinsic (extratendinous) factors have been implicated as etiologies of the impingement process. The role of muscle weakness within the rotator cuff has been described as leading to tension overload, humeral head elevation, and changes in the supraspinatus tendon, which is used most often in high-demand, repetitive overhead activities.[8,9] Authors[10-12] also have described inflammation and thickening of the bursal contents and their relationship to the impingement syndrome. Jobe[13] and Jobe, Kvitne, and Giangarra[11] studied the role of microtrauma and overuse in intrinsic tendonitis and glenohumeral instability and their implications for overhead-throwing athletes. Intrinsic degenerative tenopathy also has been discussed as an intrinsic cause of subacromial impingement symptoms.[14]

Extrinsic or extratendinous etiologic factors form the second broad category of causes of impingement syndrome. Rare secondary extrinsic factors (e.g., neurologic pathology secondary to cervical radiculopathy, supraspinatus nerve entrapment) are not discussed here, but the primary extrinsic factors and their anatomic relationships are of primary surgical concern. The unique anatomy of the shoulder joint sandwiches the soft tissue structures of the subacromial space (i.e., rotator cuff tendons, coracoacromial ligament, long head of biceps, bursa) between the overlying anterior acromion, AC joint, and coracoid process and the underlying greater tuberosity of the humeral head and the superior glenoid rim. Toivonen, Tuite, and Orwin[15] have supported Bigliani, Morrison, and April's description[16] of three primary acromial types and their correlation to impingement and full-thickness rotator cuff tears. AC degenerative joint disease also can be an extrinsic primary cause of impingement disease.[1,2] Many authors support Neer's original position on the contribution of AC degenerative joint disease to the impingement process.[17,18] The os acromiale, the unfused distal acromial epiphysis, also has been discussed as a separate entity and a potential etiologic factor related to impingement.[19] Glenohumeral instability is a secondary extrinsic cause or contribution to impingement. Its relationship to the impingement syndrome is poorly understood, but it helps explain the failure of acromioplasty in the subset of young, competitive, overhead-throwing athletes with a clinical impingement syndrome.[11,20,21]

Diagnosis and Evaluation of the Impingement Syndrome

History and physical examinations are crucial in diagnosing subacromial impingement syndrome. Findings may be subtle, and symptoms may overlap in the various differential diagnoses; therefore, appreciating the impingement syndrome symptom complex may be difficult. The classic history has an insidious onset and a chronic component that develops over months, usually in a patient over 40 years old. The patient frequently describes repetitive activity during recreation, recreational sports, competitive athletics, and work. Pain is the most common symptom, especially pain with specific high-demand or repetitive away-from-the-chest and overhead shoulder activities. Night pain is seen later in impingement syndrome, after heightening of the inflammatory response. Weakness and stiffness may occur secondary to pain inhibition. If true weakness persists after the pain is eliminated, then the differential diagnoses of rotator cuff tearing or neurologic cervical entrapment type of pathologies must be addressed. If stiffness persists, then frozen shoulder–related conditions (e.g., adhesive capsulitis, inflammatory arthritis, degenerative joint disease) must be ruled out.[22] Younger athletic and throwing patients need continual assessment for glenohumeral instability.

The physical examination of a patient with impingement syndrome focuses on the shoulder and neck regions. Physical examination of the neck helps rule out cervical radiculopathy, degenerative joint disease, and other disorders of the neck contributing to referred pain complexes in the shoulder area. The shoulder evaluation includes a general inspection for muscle asymmetry or atrophy, with emphasis on the supraspinatus region. Range of motion (ROM) and muscle strength testing and generalized glenohumeral stability testing are emphasized during the evaluation. The Neer impingement sign[2] and Hawkins-Kennedy sign[23] are gold standard tests to help diagnose impingement. The impingement test, which includes subacromial injection of a Xylocaine type of compound and repeated impingement sign maneuvers, is most helpful in ascertaining the presence of an impingement syndrome. The AC joint also is addressed during the shoulder evaluation. The clinician should note AC joint pain with direct palpation and pain on horizontal adduction of the shoulder. Selective AC joint injection also may be helpful. Long head biceps tendon pathology, including ruptures, is rare but may occur in this subset of patients. Physical examination will define the tendon's contribution to the symptom complex. Instability testing, especially in the younger athletic patient, also should be performed. The clinician should assess for classic apprehension signs and perform the Jobe relocation test, recording any positive findings.

Radiographic Evaluation

Standard radiographic evaluation is carried out with special attention to anteroposterior (AP), 30° caudal tilt AP, and outlet views of the shoulder.[24,25] These plain studies are helpful in demonstrating acromial anatomy types, hypertrophic coracoacromial ligament spurring, AC joint osteoarthrosis, and calcific tendonitis. These views, in combination with an axillary view, can uncover os acromiale lesions. Magnetic resonance imaging (MRI) also is helpful in revealing relationships in impingement syndrome, especially if rotator cuff tear and other internal derangement pathologies (e.g., glenolabral or biceps tendon pathologies) are suspected.[26]

SURGICAL PROCEDURE

Subacromial impingement syndrome that has not responded to rehabilitation techniques and nonoperative means may require surgery. If proven trials of rehabilitation, activity modification, use of nonsteroidal antiinflammatory agents (NSAIDs), and judicious use of subacromial cortisone injections are unsuccessful, then acromioplasty and subacromial decompression (SAD) should be considered.

Historically, open acromioplasties produced excellent results and still have a significant role in surgical treatment.[1,19,27] Ellman[28] is credited with the first significant arthroscopic SAD techniques and studies, and many surgeons and investigators have developed techniques and arthroscopic SAD advancements for the surgical treatment of subacromial impingement syndrome.[29-34] Indications for surgery to correct subacromial impingement syndrome include persistent pain and dysfunction that have failed to respond to nonsurgical treatment, including physician- or therapist-directed physical therapy, trials of NSAIDs, subacromial cortisone or lidocaine injections, and activity modification.

The most controversial surgical indication topic concerns the amount of time that should elapse before nonoperative management is considered a failure.[19] Most surgeons and investigators recommend a trial period of approximately 6 months. However, this depends on the individual patient and pathologic condition and should be tailored to the circumstances. For example, a 42-year-old patient with a history of several months of progressive symptoms has an occupation or recreational activity that requires high-demand, repetitive overhead movement. In the absence of instability, with a hooked acromion (type III) and MRI-documented, partial-thickness tearing, this patient need not endure the 6-month trial period to meet surgical indications for the treatment of his condition. On the other hand, a noncompliant patient in a workers' compensation–related situation who has a flat acromion and equivocal, inconsistent clinical findings may never meet the surgical indications.

Procedure

Both open acromioplasty and the arthroscopic SAD procedure are discussed in the following sections. Open acromioplasty techniques have been well documented, their outcomes have been well researched, and their results have been rated as very good to excellent in numerous studies.[1,27,29,30,35] Because of these factors and the high technical demands of arthroscopic decompression, surgeons should never completely abandon this proven technique for the surgical management of persistent shoulder impingement. Surgeons also may resort to these open techniques in the event of arthroscopic procedure failure or intraoperative difficulties. Depending on surgical experience and expertise, an open procedure may be used in deference to an arthroscopic SAD procedure.

Arthroscopic SAD for the surgical treatment of impingement syndrome has a number of advantages. First, the arthroscopic technique allows evaluation of the glenohumeral joint for associated labral, rotator cuff, and biceps pathology, as well as assessment of the AC joint and surgical treatment of any condition contributing to impingement. Second, this technique produces less postoperative morbidity and is relatively noninvasive, minimizing deltoid muscle fiber detachment. However, arthroscopic SAD is a technically demanding procedure with a learning curve that can be higher than for other orthopedic procedures.

Many different arthroscopic techniques have been described, but the authors of this chapter recommend the modified technique initially described by Caspari.[36] The patient is usually anesthetized with both a general and a scalene block regional anesthetic. In most community settings this combination has been highly successful in allowing patients to have this procedure done on an outpatient basis. A scalene regional block and home patient-controlled analgesia (PCA) provide acceptable pain control and ensure a comfortable postoperative course.

After the patient has reached the appropriate depth of anesthesia, the shoulder is evaluated in relationship to the contralateral side in both a supine and a semisitting beach chair position. Any concern regarding stability testing can be further assessed at this time, taking advantage of the complete anesthesia. Then, using the standard beach chair positioning, the surgeon begins the arthroscopic procedure. An inflow pressure pump (Davol) is used to maintain appropriate tissue space distention. Epinephrine is added to the irrigation solution to a concentration of 1 mg/L, thus enhancing hemostasis.

Specific portal placement is important to eliminate technical difficulties. Carefully addressing the palpable bony topography of the shoulder and marking the acromion, clavicle, AC joint, and coracoid process greatly facilitate portal placement (Fig. 3-1). First, the sulcus is palpated directly posterior to the AC joint. From this universal landmark, appropriate orientation can be obtained and consistent

reproducible posterior, anterior, and lateral portal placement can be achieved.

Using the standard posterior portal, the surgeon inserts the arthroscope into the glenohumeral joint. In a routine and sequential fashion, the glenohumeral joint is evaluated with attention directed to the biceps tendon and the labral and rotator cuff anatomy. Any incidental pathology can be addressed arthroscopically at this point. Subacromial space arthroscopy can now be performed.

For subacromial procedures, a long diagnostic double-cannula arthroscope is recommended. The cannula with a blunt trocar is placed from the posterior portal superior to the cuff, and exits through the anterior portal.

Using this cannula as a switch stick equivalent, the surgeon places a cannula with a plastic diaphragm over the arthroscopic instrument and returns it to the subacromial space. Gently retracting the arthroscopic cannula and inserting the arthroscope allows the inflow and arthroscopic cannulas to be close together. Adequate distention and maintenance of inflow and outflow are crucial for visualization and indirect hemostasis. This technique has been successful in achieving these goals. At this point the lateral portal is fashioned, generally on the lateral aspect of the acromion just posterior and inferior to a line drawn by extending the topographic anatomy of the anterior AC complex (see Fig. 3-1). A spinal needle may assist in the accurate placement of this portal, which is crucial to instrument placement and subsequent visualization.

Starting from the posterior portal and using an aggressive synovial resector with the inflow in the anterior portal, the surgeon uses the lateral portal to perform a bursectomy and débride the soft tissue of the subacromial space. This is done in a sequential manner, working from the lateral bursal area to the anterior and medial AC regions. Spinal needles can be placed in the anterolateral and AC joint region to facilitate visualization and reveal spatial relationships. After the subacromial bursectomy and denudement of the undersurface of the acromion, the superior rotator cuff can be visualized along with the AC joint and anterior acromial anatomy is more easily defined. The surgeon must take care not to violate the coracoacromial ligament during this initial bursectomy procedure.

At this point the surgeon inserts the arthroscope in the lateral portal for visualization. Using the posterior portal and following the posterior slope of the normal acromion, the surgeon performs sequential acromioplasty with an acromionizer instrument. In the technique described by Caspari,[36] the shank of the acromionizer is directed flat against the posterior acromial slope and acromioplasty is completed from the posterior to the anterior aspect. This accomplishes two goals. First, it provides a reliable and reproducible template to convert any abnormal hooked, sloped, or curved acromion to the therapeutic goal of a flat, type I configuration. Second, it allows for the removal of the coracoacromial ligament from its bony attachment with minimal chance for coracoacromial artery bleeding, thereby maximizing arthroscopic visualization and minimizing technical

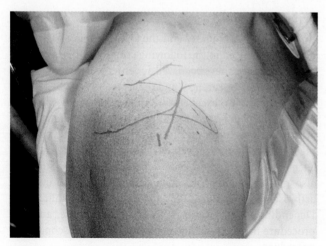

Fig. 3-1 The lateral portal is fashioned on the lateral aspect of the acromion just posterior and inferior to a line drawn by extending the topographic anatomy of the anterior acromioclavicular (AC) complex.

difficulties. At this point any further modification or "fine tuning" may be done through both the lateral and the anterior portals. Any residual coracoacromial ligament is removed from its acromial insertion while its bursal extension is excised.

The AC joint also may be assessed at this stage, and minimal inferior osteophytes may be excised. Depending on the results of the preoperative evaluation, distal clavicle procedures can be performed at this point either through directed arthroscopic techniques or, as the authors of this chapter prefer, through a small incision located over the AC joint region. If AC joint symptoms are present with horizontal adduction and direct palpation, if radiographs confirm the pathology, or if both occur, then the surgeon should proceed with a distal clavicle excision. A T-type capsular incision is located over the AC joint region, with the anterior and posterior capsular leaves elevated subperiosteally from the distal clavicle. Using small Homan retractors, the surgeon can excise the distal clavicle (usually 1.5 to 2 cm) with an oscillating saw. The distal clavicle can then be easily palpated and rasped smooth. With a simple digital confirmation, the undersurface of the acromion also can be checked and any residual osteophytes rasped through this minimal-incision technique.

The soft tissue is then closed in anatomic fashion, with essentially no deltoid detachment. A routine subcuticular skin closure is used. The patient is placed in a postoperative pouch sling, and cryotherapy is frequently suggested. The patient is discharged to continue treatment as an outpatient; if insurance or health demands require it, overnight observation is used. Physical therapy may begin immediately on the first postoperative day and should follow the standard program discussed previously.[36]

Outcomes

The surgical outcomes for arthroscopic SAD, partial acromioplasties, and distal clavicle excisions[16,32,33] have been most favorable. Many studies have compared open and closed techniques and obtained similar overall findings.[19,35,37] SAD procedures have three general goals:

1. To return the patient to a premorbid ROM and strength perimeters
2. To eliminate pain
3. To eliminate the anatomic mechanical component of the impingement syndrome

Challenges and Precautions

The most common causes of surgical failures are associated with incomplete bone resection and not addressing AC joint arthropathy. These common pitfalls can be eliminated by carefully considering surgical techniques and including (if necessary) distal clavicle excision or combined open techniques. Another common reason for failure of arthroscopic SAD surgery is inappropriate diagnosis or patient selection. Again, with careful assessment—especially regarding instability, underlying lesions, and differential diagnoses—these failures can be lessened dramatically.

Rehabilitation Concerns: The Surgeon's Perspective

Therapists spend more time with postoperative patients than most surgeons do, and their input and direction are important in achieving a successful outcome. Their understanding of the procedure, postoperative pain, patient apprehension, and general medical concerns is vital. Physical therapy–directed early diagnosis of any wound problems (evidenced by erythema) or superficial infection can eliminate potential major complications. Postoperative inflammation also can be assessed with careful observation. Stiffness in frozen shoulder syndrome, although rare, can develop postoperatively and is addressed optimally with early diagnosis and progressive physical therapy.

THERAPY GUIDELINES FOR REHABILITATION

The goal of the therapeutic exercise program after a SAD procedure is to augment the surgical decompression by increasing the subacromial space. Additional clearance for subacromial structures can be gained by strengthening the scapular upward rotators and humeral head depressors. Exercises to enhance the surgical decompression are straightforward.

 The challenge for the physical therapist is to implement the appropriate therapeutic exercise regimen without overloading healing tissue.

The postoperative rehabilitation program can be divided into three phases:

1. Phase one emphasizes a return of ROM.
2. Phase two stresses regaining muscle strength.
3. Phase three stresses endurance and functional progression.

These three phases are not distinct entities and they do overlap. Together they serve as a template on which the physical therapist can build a management protocol for the post-SAD patient. An absence of pain is the primary guideline for progressing to more strenuous activities.[38] The phases are simply guidelines and should be adapted to each patient. Patients with significant rotator cuff involvement, articular cartilage defects, significant preoperative motion or strength loss, perioperative or intraoperative complications, and glenohumeral instability require special consideration and may not progress as rapidly as indicated in the standard rehabilitation program, which assumes that no glenohumeral instability exists and that the rotator cuff tendons are intact.

Signs that therapeutic activities are too aggressive include the following:

- Increased levels of referred pain to the area of insertion of the deltoid
- Night pain
- Pain that lasts more than 2 hours after exercising[39]
- Pain that alters the performance of an activity or exercise[39]

Evaluation

Every rehabilitation program begins with a thorough evaluation at the initial physical therapy visit. This evaluation provides pertinent information for formulating a treatment program. As the patient progresses through the program, assessment is ongoing. Activities that are too stressful for healing tissue at one point are reassessed when the tissue is ready for the stress. Measures to be included in the physical therapy evaluation are provided in Box 3-1.

Phase I

TIME: First 2 to 3 weeks after surgery
GOALS: Emphasis on measures to control normal postoperative inflammation and pain, protect healing soft tissue, and minimize the effects of immobilization and activity restriction (Table 3-1)

Control of Inflammation and Pain. The surgeon may have prescribed NSAIDs to control normal postoperative inflammation and pain. These can be an adjunct to the other means the physical therapist uses to decrease inflammation (i.e., gentle therapeutic exercise, cryotherapy).

The therapist should determine whether a scalene block was performed in addition to the general anesthetic. If a block was performed, then the onset of immediate postoperative pain may be delayed; the patient should be monitored for signs of delayed motor return and prolonged or abnormal hypesthesia. If narcotics are used past the first few postoperative days, then the therapist must undertake the therapeutic exercise program cautiously.

Cryotherapy can be used to help manage postoperative pain. Crushed ice conforms nicely to the shoulder, but commercially available cryotherapy and compression units (PolarCare, Cryocuff), although tedious to use, can be less messy. Sterile postoperative liners allow the source of the cold to be placed under the initial bulky dressing. The physical therapist should be aware of reimbursement practices for these units and use them accordingly.

Protection of Healing Soft Tissues. Decreased use of the upper extremity is required to protect healing soft tissue after SAD. A sling may be prescribed depending on the surgeon's protocol and operative findings. The sling helps decrease the forces on the supraspinatus tendon by centralizing the head of the humerus in the glenoid fossa in a dependent position. Use of the sling is encouraged for the first 2 to 3 days after surgery in most cases, with the patient's level of discomfort dictating the degree of sling use.

Although the sling is used to minimize pain, it can add to the patient's discomfort. A "critical zone" of hypovascularity in the supraspinatus tendon initially described by Rathbun and McNab[40] may contribute to shoulder pain in a resting-dependent position. Some authors debate the existence of this critical zone, but recent work by Lohr and Ulthoff[41] corroborates Rathbun and McNab's initial findings. This critical

---

BOX 3-1 Components of the Physical Therapy Evaluation

Background Information
- Status of capsule
- Status of rotator cuff
- Status of articular cartilage
- Previous procedures
- Associated medical problems that can influence rehabilitation (e.g., cardiovascular concerns, diabetes mellitus)
- Work-related injury
- Insurance status
- Motivation
- Comprehension

Subjective Information
- Previous level of function
- Present level of function
- Patient's goals and expectations
- Intensity of pain
- Location of pain
- Frequency of pain
- Presence of night pain
- Assistance at home
- Access to rehabilitation facilities
- Medication (dose, effect, tolerance, compliance)

Objective Information
- Observation:
  - Muscle wasting
  - Resting posture
  - Use of sling
  - Wound status
  - Swelling
  - Color
- Range of motion (ROM) (active/passive):
  - G/H PROM with in pain tolerance
  - Upper thoracic spine
  - Scapulothoracic joint
  - Sternoclavicular joint
  - Acromioclavicular (AC) joint
  - Scapulothoracic rhythm
- Strength
- Rotator cuff
- Scapular upward rotators
- Scapular retractors
- Scapular protractors
- Deltoid
- Biceps

Note: Strength testing should be delayed until safe and appropriate. Bicep testing could be performed earlier than the deltoid strength test. Care must be taken so that the recovering tissue is not compromised and irritated.

TABLE 3-1 Acromioplasty

Rehabilitation Phase	Goals	Intervention	Rationale	Anticipated Impairments and Functional Limitations	Criteria to Progress to This Phase
Phase Ia Postoperative 1-2 days	• Decrease pain • Prevent infection • Minimize wrist and hand weakness from disuse	• Cryotherapy 20-30 minutes • Monitoring of incision site • Grip strength exercises (with arm elevated if swollen)	• Self-manage pain and manage edema • Prevent complications during healing • Minimize disuse atrophy and promote circulation	• Pain • Edema • Dependent upper extremity (usually in a sling or airplane splint depending on degree of repair)	• Postoperative
Phase Ib Postoperative 3-10 days	• Improve PROM, avoiding aggravating surgical site • Produce fair to good muscular contraction of rotators • Restore/maintain scapula mobility • Reduce pain/joint stiffness	Continue intervention as in phase Ia with addition of the following: • PROM of shoulder as indicated • Isometrics—submaximal to maximal internal and external rotation in sling or supported out of sling in neutral resting position • AROM—scapular retraction/protraction (position as with isometrics) • Joint mobilization to the SC and AC joints as indicated	• Increase PROM preparing to advance AROM exercises • Minimize reflex inhibition of rotator cuff • Minimize disuse atrophy of scapula stabilizers • Use low-grade (resistance free) mobilizations to decrease muscle guarding and progress grades as tolerated to restore arthrokinematics	• As in phase Ia	• No wound drainage or presence of infection
Phase Ic Postoperative 11-14 days	• Flexion PROM to 150° • External/internal rotation PROM to functional levels (or full ROM) • Scapulothoracic PROM to full mobility • Supine AROM flexion to 120° • Symmetric AC/SC mobility • Increase AROM tolerance in water to 100° flexion • Minimize cardiovascular deconditioning • Improve general muscular strength and endurance	Continue as in phases Ia & Ib: • AROM—External rotation (at 60°-90° abduction) • Supine flexion • AROM—Supine scapular protraction (elbow extended) "punches" side-lying (midrange) external rotation with support (towel) in axilla • Prone scapular retraction • Pool therapy (with appropriate waterproof dressing if incision site not fully closed) • Cardiovascular exercise (bike, walking program) • Depending on job activities, return to limited work duties	• Increase capsular extensibility with flexion/elevation and rotation exercises • Make rotator cuff ready for supine elevation • Initiate strengthening of scapula stabilizers (proximal stability) • Support axilla to allow for vascular supply to cuff during exercises • Encourage AC/SC accessory motions required for full shoulder mobility • Note that buoyant effects of water allow an environment where the water assists in flexion • Prescribe lower-extremity conditioning exercises to promote healing and improve cardiovascular fitness • Provide ergonomic education early to prevent future complications	• Intermittent pain • Limited upper extremity use with reaching/lifting activities • Limited ROM • Limited strength	• Comfortable out of sling • No signs of infection or night pain

AC, acromioclavicular; *AROM,* active range of motion; *PROM,* Passive range of motion; *ROM,* range of motion; *SC,* sternoclavicular.

zone corresponds to the anastomoses between osseous vessels and vessels within the supraspinatus tendon. Vessels in this critical zone fill poorly when the arm is at the side,[2] but this wringing out of the supraspinatus tendon is not observed when the arm is abducted.[42] If the patient experiences increased shoulder discomfort after prolonged periods with the arm at the side, then he or she should place a small bolster (2 to 3 inches in diameter) in the axilla (resting the arm in a supported, slightly abducted position) to help decrease the pain.

Immobilization and Restricted Activities. Although the sling protects the healing tissue around the glenohumeral joint, motion should be encouraged at proximal and distal joints. Scapular protraction, retraction, and elevation can be performed in the sling. The patient should remove the arm from the sling at least three to four times daily to perform supported elbow, wrist, and hand ROM exercises.

The patient should always perform warm-up activities. This enhances the rate of muscular relaxation, increases the mechanical efficiency of muscle by decreasing viscous resistance, allows for greater hemoglobin and myoglobin dissociation in the time spent working, decreases resistance in the vascular bed, increases nerve conduction velocity, decreases the risk for electrocardiographic abnormalities, and increases metabolism.[43]

The physical therapist should educate the patient and help him or her to understand that discomfort experienced with passive stretching into external rotation comes from the capsule and occurs because the supraspinatus muscle is slack. Patients with sedentary occupations who do not have lifting duties typically can return to work during phase one. Those returning to work should perform scapular, elbow, wrist, and hand exercises during working hours.

Phase II

TIME: From 3 to at least 6 weeks after surgery
GOALS: Emphasis on muscle strengthening, with continued work on rotator cuff musculature and scapula stabilizer strengthening (Table 3-2)

Many of the exercises used to strengthen the rotator cuff and scapular stabilizers have been assessed by electromyography (EMG).[44] EMG (both superficial and fine wire) has been used to document electrical activity in the rotator cuff and intrascapular musculature during the performance of various therapeutic exercises. Strengthening of the rotator cuff muscles can be selectively progressed from supine active exercises to upright resistive exercises.[45] Muscles of the rotator cuff (especially the supraspinatus) have relatively small cross-sectional areas and short lever arms. When working with them, the therapist should apply minimal resistance, starting at 8 oz, then increase to 1 lb, and then advance in ½ lb or 1 lb increments as tolerated. Weights seldom have to exceed 3 to 5 lb for the supraspinatus. The infraspinatus and subscapularis can be stressed to a greater degree, and weights can be progressed from 5 to 8 lb. The

therapist should emphasize scapular stabilizer efforts for proximal stability before addressing distal mobility.

Townsend, Jobe, and Pink[46] assessed the EMG output of three slips of deltoid, pectoralis major, latissimus dorsi, and the four rotator cuff muscles during 17 exercises. Findings from this study indicate that the majority of the muscles studied are most effectively recruited with the following:

- Scaption (with internal shoulder rotation)
- Flexion
- Horizontal abduction with external rotation
- Press-ups

Because the supraspinatus is the most frequently involved cuff muscle necessitating a subacromial decompression, diligent efforts to return supraspinatus strength are vital. The most effective exercise position to maximally recruit the supraspinatus has been evaluated in numerous studies with varying results. Elevation in the plane of the scapula (i.e., scaption) with the shoulder internally rotated is referred to as the empty-can position (Fig. 3-2).

To decrease the likelihood of compressing the supraspinatus between the greater tuberosity of the humerus and the subacromial structures, care should be taken never to perform the empty-can exercise past 60° to 70° of elevation.

Scaption can also be performed with the humerus externally rotated (Fig. 3-3). Another position that is very effective in recruiting the supraspinatus is prone horizontal abduction of the shoulder, with the shoulder abducted to

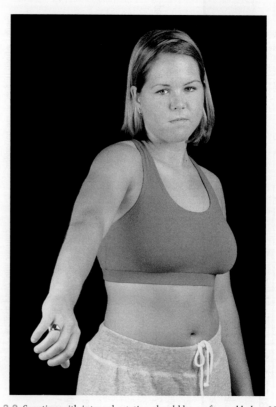

Fig. 3-2 Scaption with internal rotation should be performed below 90° to prevent impinging subacromial structures.

TABLE 3-2 Acromioplasty

Rehabilitation Phase	Goal	Intervention	Rationale	Anticipated Impairments and Functional Limitations	Criteria to Progress to This Phase
Phase IIa Postoperative 3-6 wk	• PROM full in all ranges • Symmetric AROM flexion • Symmetric accessory motions of glenohumeral and SC/AC joints • AROM flexion in standing to shoulder height without substitution from scapulothoracic region • Symmetric strength scapula stabilizers and shoulder rotators	• Continue exercises from previous phases as indicated: • PREs — elastic tubing exercises for internal rotation and scapular retraction At 3 wk, add external rotation and scapular protraction • Isotonics — side-lying external rotation (with axilla support) with ½ to 1 lb • Standing scaption with shoulder externally rotated • Standing shoulder flexion with ½ to 1 lb • Elbow and wrist PREs with appropriate weight • Assess lateral scapular slide	• Restore previous functional use and ROM of the upper extremity • Begin strengthening; internal rotators (subscapularis) usually not affected by surgery • Initiate scapular retraction as long lever arm forces are minimal (versus protraction) • Progress exercise to include external rotators and scapula protraction as tolerance to exercises improves • Recognize that supraspinatus is secondary mover for straight plane external rotation • Strengthen upper quarter musculature • Accompany gravity-resisted shoulder flexion and abduction by substitution with scapular elevation	• Limited reach and lifting abilities, especially above shoulder height • Limited strength and endurance of arm above shoulder height • Limited AROM	• AROM to 120° flexion • AROM improving trend • Gait with normal arm swing • Strength of rotators to 4/5 (manual muscle test [MMT] — 5/5 normal • Self-manage pain
Phase IIb Postoperative 6-8 wk	• Symmetric strength of supraspinatus and deltoid • Restoration of normal arm strength ratios (involved/uninvolved) • Return to previous levels of activities/sport as indicated by strength and tolerance • Prevention of poor mechanics with throwing • Preparation of upper extremity for advanced activities	• Continue with exercises from previous phases as indicated; maintain rotator cuff strength • AROM PREs — standing scaption with shoulder internal rotation (empty can); perform below 70° scaption • Prone or bent over horizontal abduction with shoulder at 100° abduction • Begin exercises unresisted, then add weight, beginning with ½ lb • Progress weight as indicated • Initiate throwing program as outlined in Chapter 13 • Begin gentle plyometrics	• Continue to restore ROM and strength of upper quarter musculature • Strengthen supraspinatus as a prime mover • Advance strength demand on the scapula stabilizers • Progress resistance on a conservative basis • Progress activity on a sequential basis	• Unable to work overhead for prolonged periods of time • Unable to participate in overhead-throwing athletics	• Gravity-resisted flexion and abduction without scapulothoracic substitution • Symmetric strength of external rotators

AC, acromioclavicular; *AROM,* active range of motion; *PREs,* progressive resistance exercises; *PROM,* Passive range of motion; *ROM,* range of motion; *SC,* sternoclavicular.

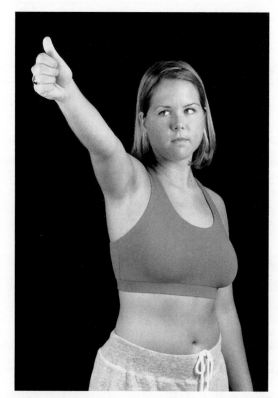

Fig. 3-3 Scaption with external rotation can safely be performed through full available range of motion (ROM).

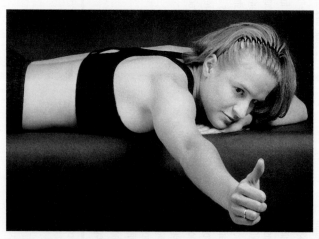

Fig. 3-4 Prone horizontal abduction with the humerus abducted to 100°. The physical therapist should take care with patients with concomitant anterior glenohumeral instability.

BOX 3-2 Supraspinatus Strengthening Exercises*	
Jobe	EC
Blackburn	HA (100° abduction) > EC
Townsend	MP > EC
Worrell	HA (100° abduction) > EC
Malanga	EC = FC
Kelly	EC = FC
Takeda	EC = FC > HA
Reinold	HA (100° abduction) > ER

*EC, Empty can; FC, full can; HA, horizontal abduction; MP, military press.

significant role in activities involving abduction (in the plane of the body and plane of the scapula) especially with combined external rotation and when greater resistance is applied.[55] The teres minor assists the infraspinatus in the above activities to a minor extent and is most effective in horizontal abduction of the humerus along with scapular retraction and glenohumeral extension.[56] Two practical and comprehensive reviews of shoulder muscle activity and function in common shoulder exercises may be of particular benefit to the reader.[57,58]

Although isolation of specific muscles is vital to ensure a comprehensive strengthening program, work with muscles contracting in synchrony about a joint also is an important consideration. Wilk[59] and Toivonen, Tuite, and Orwin[15] note that in overhead activities the subscapularis is counterbalanced by the infraspinatus and teres minor in the transverse plane, whereas the deltoid is opposed by the infraspinatus and teres minor in the coronal plane. Because overhead movements are incorporated in the rehabilitation program, the physical therapist also should address the force couple of the upper and lower trapezius for scapular upward rotation. Upper and lower trapezius recruitment may increase during glenohumeral flexion and abduction exercises when using dynamic reactive instruments as opposed to elastic or cuff weight resistance.[60] Multiplanar work can be beneficial by incorporating dynamic trunk, scapulothoracic, and glenohumeral activities simultaneously. Two activities in the standing position that recruit firing of the upper and lower trapezius before the serratus anterior include trunk extension with simultaneous unilateral scapular retraction/upward rotation combined with elbow flexion, glenohumeral extension, and external rotation (lawnmower exercise); and trunk extension with simultaneous bilateral scapular retraction/upward rotation with elbow flexion, glenohumeral extension, and external rotation (robbery exercise).[61]

When strengthening the shoulder internal rotators, do not work with the patient in a side-lying position. Lying on the involved shoulder often increases shoulder pain; therefore, internal rotation should be performed in the standing or prone position. When working on strengthening the supraspinatus and standing flexion and abduction in the same exercise session, perform the gravity-resisted elevation

100° (Fig. 3-4). In cases of secondary impingement related to glenohumeral instability, care must be taken not to position the arm to increase stress on static restraints. Inherent humeral head localization is enhanced during strengthening exercises by performing these activities in the plane of the scapula.[47]

Box 3-2 summarizes research findings relative to the most effective exercise position to recruit the supraspinatus.[48-54]

Remaining muscles of the rotator cuff cannot be neglected. The infraspinatus is most actively recruited via external rotation at zero degrees of abduction. This muscle also plays a exercises before the strengthening ones. This sequence allows a nonfatigued supraspinatus to contribute effectively to achieve an adequate force couple. Cadaveric analysis of rotator cuff composition indicates that these muscles consist of a mix of type I and type II fibers.[62] Resistance applied to the muscles should be a healthy fix of function-specific velocities and repetitions.

Exercise combinations can be used effectively to strengthen the muscles of the shoulder girdle. Wolf[63] describes a "four square" combination of tubing-resisted flexion, extension, external rotation, and internal rotation (IR) followed by stretching of the external rotators and abductors. A combination of "around the world" exercises of flexion, abduction, and horizontal abduction followed by rotator cuff stretching also can be used during phase two. The physical therapist should use care when performing flexibility exercises of the rotator cuff because horizontal adduction can reproduce or cause impingement symptoms.

Strong scapular stabilizers are required to provide a stable base for the glenohumeral joint, elevate the acromion, and provide for retraction and protraction around the thoracic wall.[64] Moseley and associates[65] studied eight scapular muscles via indwelling EMG and identified a core group of four strengthening exercises that include scaption with external rotation (i.e., full can), rowing, press-ups, and push-ups with a plus. Ludewig and associates[66] found a push-up with a plus to be effective in recruiting the serratus anterior with less activity of the trapezius musculature. Lear and Gross[67] noted increased serratus anterior activity during a push-up with a plus with the feet elevated. Decker and associates[68] noted push-ups with a plus (both traditional and on the knees), punching, scaption, and a dynamic hug all resulted in serratus anterior activity greater than 20% of a maximum voluntary contraction. Ekstrom, Donatelli, and Soderberg[69] found a seated shoulder diagonal movement of forward flexion, horizontal adduction, and external rotation to be most effective in recruiting the serratus anterior when compared with nine other open-chain exercises.

In addition to careful observation of scapulohumeral rhythm during overhead motions, scapular stabilizer efficiency can be assessed with the lateral scapular slide test. This test, which was initially described by Kibler,[64] involves observing and measuring scapular motion during abduction of the shoulder. The steps of the modified lateral scapular slide test are described in Box 3-3. The lateral scapular slide is a valid tool to assess scapular motion.[70] Kibler[64] described side-to-side differences of 1 cm as an indicator of scapulohumeral dysfunction. Other authors assessing the reliability of the lateral scapular slide, however, note that a 1 cm difference cannot be used as an indicator of dysfunction and that 1 cm can fall within intertester variability.[71]

Continue ROM efforts during phase two, especially if limited capsular extensibility detrimentally affects physiologic motion. In addition to aggressive stretching exercises and mobilization of the glenohumeral joint, self-mobilizations also may be of benefit.[72] Patients with glenohumeral laxity also require special consideration as ROM and strengthening

---

BOX 3-3 Modified Kibler's Lateral Scapular Slide Test*

1. Patient stands with the arms resting against the sides.
2. Therapist palpates the spinous process immediately between the inferior angles of the scapula (usually T-7).
3. Therapist measures and records the distance from the spinous process to each scapular inferior angle.
4. Patient abducts the arms to 90°.
5. Patient internally rotates the shoulders so that the thumbs point to the floor.
6. Therapist measures and records the distance from the spinous processes to each scapular inferior angle.

*Normal test is symmetry between right and left sides.

---

exercises progress. For patients with anterior instability, exercises should not stress extremes of horizontal abduction and external rotation. Posterior glenohumeral instability requires care with horizontal adduction and IR. Strengthening programs for patients with glenohumeral instability are best performed in the plane of the scapula.

Phase III

TIME: Weeks 9 to 12

GOALS: Emphasis on enhancing kinesthesia and joint position sense, building endurance, strengthening the scapular stabilizer, and performing work-specific and sport-specific tasks (Table 3-3)

After the patient has progressed through the first two phases, the obvious deficits resulting from surgery (i.e., pain, limited motion, decreased strength) have essentially been eliminated. Deficits in endurance and proprioception are not as readily apparent. Violation of the capsule, decreased use of the shoulder, and abnormal or restricted movement of the shoulder may decrease endurance and proprioception. One study[73] has demonstrated decreased proprioception in lax shoulders, with patients able to sense external rotation movements with greater ease than IR, especially at end range. Exercises to improve both passive detection of shoulder movement and active joint repositioning may help enhance kinesthesia and joint position sense, respectively. Voight and associates[74] noted decreased glenohumeral joint proprioception with muscle fatigue of the rotator cuff.

Decreasing the weight used with strengthening exercises and increasing the repetitions address endurance training. Scapular stabilizer strengthening has been performed in sets of 30 repetitions to this point, and repetitions can be increased as required. Work- and sport-specific tasks should be used as guidelines to the number of prescribed repetitions. The supraspinatus tendon is the one most frequently involved in the injury, so it should be strengthened last.

TABLE 3-3 Acromioplasty

Rehabilitation Phase	Goals	Intervention	Rationale	Anticipated Impairments and Functional Limitations	Criteria to Progress to This Phase
Phase III Postoperative 9-12 wk	• Unrestricted overhead work and sporting activity	• Formal return to throwing and overhead activities	• Create a specific training principle to return the patient to the desired activity	• Decreased work or sport-specific endurance	• Symmetric range of motion and strength of upper quarter

The physical therapist also can address proprioception by having the patient perform functional tasks and emphasizing the timing of muscle contraction and movement without substitution. When rehabilitating overhead-throwing athletes, Pappas, Zawacki, and McCarthy[75] suggest timing muscle recruitment to correlate with the throwing sequence of active abduction, horizontal extension, and external rotation. Appropriate timing of muscle contraction also can be addressed using proprioceptive neuromuscular facilitation techniques.[76] Although the majority of upper extremity function in daily, work, or sport activities occur in the open kinetic chain, closed kinetic chain activities provide stimulation to the glenohumeral joint to enhance joint awareness and kinesthesia (important in secondary impingement). Activities in the closed chain should progress from low ground reaction forces (as a percent of body weight) to higher forces that have been shown to recruit greater shoulder girdle musculature as evidenced by the percentage of maximum volitional isometric contraction.[77]

A functional progression program can be used to enhance the return of proprioception and endurance. Functional progression involves a series of sport- or work-specific basic movement patterns graduated according to the difficulty of the skill and the patient's tolerance. Providing a comprehensive functional progression program for every job or sport that a patient is involved in is impossible. Programs to return the patient to throwing, swimming, and tennis activities can be found in other sources.[78,79] Plyometric activities help restore endurance, proprioception, and muscle power.[80,81]

SUGGESTED HOME MAINTENANCE FOR THE POSTSURGICAL PATIENT

Box 3-4 outlines the shoulder rehabilitation the patient is to follow. The physical therapist can use it in customizing a patient-specific program.

Unlike more complex arthroscopic procedures or sophisticated open operative procedures, the need for structured clinic-based rehabilitation of the SAD patient should be the exception rather than the rule. Most of the rehabilitation for the patient after an uneventful SAD procedure can take place through a comprehensive home exercise program. Special cases may warrant a more formal and structured treatment program after the SAD procedure to detect problems. These

special situations typically involve patients with the following conditions:

- Inadequate preoperative ROM
- Full-thickness rotator cuff pathology
- Biceps tendon or labral pathology
- Articular cartilage involvement
- Secondary "impingement"
- Tendency for excessive scarring
- History of regional complex pain syndrome or reflex sympathetic dystrophy (RSD)

TROUBLESHOOTING

1. Scapulothoracic concerns. If the patient cannot perform gravity-resisted flexion or abduction without substituting with scapular elevation, then keep all efforts within the substitution-free ROM. Monitor scapular dynamic stability with the lateral scapular slide test. Because breakdown of the normal scapulothoracic muscle is more obvious with slow, controlled arm lowering, pay special attention to the eccentric component of gravity-resisted flexion and abduction.
2. Appropriate exercise dose. Dye[82] has described the envelope of function, which is defined as the range of load that can be applied across a joint in a given period without overloading it. The challenge is to stress the healing tissue to maximize functional collagen cross-linking without exceeding the envelope of function. As functional levels are increased, alter the therapeutic exercise dose. In cases of significant scapulothoracic dysfunction (long thoracic nerve neuropathy), scapulothoracic taping or figure-eight strapping may be used for additional stability.[83]
3. Monitoring for complications. Postoperative complications after SAD are rare, but the therapist must guard against RSD. Pain disproportionate to the patient's condition should be construed as RSD until proven otherwise. Institute aggressive ROM and pain control efforts daily. Prolonged (i.e., more than 3 weeks after surgery) loss of accessory joint motions may predispose the patient to adhesive capsulitis. Give treatments three times a week for mobilization and aggressive ROM.
4. Loading contractile tissue. Progressively load contractile tissue. Stress healing tissue initially as a secondary mover (receiving assistance from other muscles) before using the tissue in its role as a prime mover.

Suggested Home Maintenance for the Postsurgical Patient

Week 1

GOAL FOR THE WEEK: Control pain and swelling, and begin regaining range of motion (ROM) for joints.

Days 0 to 2: Perform grip strength exercises. Elevate your arm if it is swollen.

Days 3 to 7:

1. Do pendulum exercises for 2 minutes, 3 to 4 times each day.
2. Go through the active ROM for your elbow, wrist, and hand. Do three sets of 15 repetitions in all directions, 3 to 4 times each day.
3. Do internal and external rotation isometrics for 10 seconds each, with 10 repetitions 10 times each day.
4. Apply ice after you exercise.

Week 2

GOAL FOR THE WEEK: Prevent disuse atrophy.

Days 8 to 10: Continue your program from days 3 to 7 and add these exercises:

1. Active assisted supine flexion to tolerance. Do three sets of 15 repetitions, twice a day.
2. Supine scapular protraction at 90° of flexion. Do three sets of 30 repetitions, twice a day.
3. Side-lying unresisted outward rotation to parallel with the floor. Do three sets of 15 repetitions twice a day.

Days 11 to 14: Discontinue the exercises you did on days 3 to 7 and only do the ones listed for days 8 to 10. Continue to apply ice after you exercise.

Week 3 (Only One Visit Required)

GOAL FOR THE WEEK: Prevent adhesive capsulitis and minimize disuse atrophy.

1. If passive ROM is not within normal limits and symmetrical, then institute organized outpatient treatment for mobilization. Schedule three times per week.
2. Begin tubing- or Theraband-resisted IR. Do three sets of 15 repetitions each twice a day.
3. Begin tubing- or Theraband-resisted scapular retraction exercises. Do three sets of 30 repetitions each twice a day.
4. Begin side-lying external rotation (support under arms) using 8 oz to 1 lb weights. Do three sets of 15 repetitions each twice a day.
5. Begin progressive resistance exercises (PREs) for elbow flexion and extension.
6. Assess lateral scapular slide.

Weeks 3-6 (Only One or Two Visits Required Over 3-Week Period)

GOAL FOR THE PERIOD: Supply added resistance for greater demand on scapular stabilizers.

1. Add tubing- or Theraband-resisted external rotation. Do three sets of 15 repetitions twice each day.
2. Do full ROM unresisted exercises for standing forward flexion and abduction. Begin PREs using 8 oz or 1 lb weights.
3. Continue IR as previously, but decrease to daily; then every other day.
4. Add gravity-resisted scaption with the shoulder externally rotated and unresisted. Do three sets of 15 repetitions twice each day.
5. Add tubing- or Theraband-resisted scapular protraction exercises. Do three sets of 30 repetitions twice each day.
6. Continue scapular retraction exercises as previously described.
7. Expand cardiovascular activities to include upper extremity use (e.g., using stair-climbing machine, rowing machine, upper body ergometer [UBE]).

Weeks 7-8

GOALS FOR THE PERIOD: Return to normal work or sports (with restricted activities as needed) and normal dominant-to-nondominant muscle strength ratios.

1. Add scaption with the shoulder internally rotated (use an empty can) at no greater than 70° of abduction. Begin with unresisted exercises; then add weight beginning with 8 oz and progressing in 8 oz to 1 lb increments. Do three sets of 15 repetitions twice each day.
2. Add prone and bent over horizontal abduction with the shoulder at 100° of abduction. Begin unresisted exercises in the middle range. Do three sets of 15 repetitions twice each day.
3. Begin return to throwing program (Appendix A).
4. Begin gentle plyometrics.

Weeks 9-12 (Only One or Two Visits Required Over 4 Weeks)

GOALS FOR THE PERIOD: Obtain ROM and muscle strength sufficient to reintroduce more aggressive occupational or sports demands.

1. Make formal return to throwing and overhead activities.

---

5. Prevention. As the old adage goes, an ounce of prevention is worth a pound of cure. Preventing early primary impingement symptoms from becoming chronic may eliminate the need for surgery. Nirschl[8] notes the following factors as keys in preventing chronic impingement syndrome: relief of inflammation, strengthening (especially the external rotators, abductors, and scapular stabilizers), flexibility (especially shoulder internal rotators and adductors), general fitness, education, and proper equipment.

SUMMARY

This chapter discusses the surgical procedure of SAD along with principles that govern postoperative rehabilitation. A surgeon with sound diagnostic, management, and surgical skills, along with a physical therapist with the expertise to advance the patient through the postoperative phase, typically produces a favorable result. Of even greater importance is the rapport established between surgeon and therapist, and the relationship between the health care providers and the patient.

CLINICAL CASE REVIEW

1 Carl arrives for therapy 5 weeks after a shoulder acromioplasty. He is having difficulty performing shoulder flexion and scaption exercises correctly. He occasionally demonstrates a mild shoulder hike with arm elevation exercises above 70° of elevation. How can the therapist sequence his exercises to maximize his ability to elevate his arm above shoulder height?

If the patient is going to be strengthening the supraspinatus and performing shoulder elevation exercises (i.e., shoulder flexion, abduction, or scaption exercises), he should perform the gravity-resisted elevation exercises first. The supraspinatus works more efficiently, without fatigue, to achieve an adequate force couple, thereby helping Carl to execute the elevation exercises correctly.

2 Drew is a 55-year-old plumber. He has a history of shoulder pain over the past 2 years and has a slouched posture. He had an acromioplasty performed 8 weeks ago. He still has minimal deficits with average range of motion (AROM) for reaching overhead objects and cannot reach into his back pocket. On evaluation, Drew demonstrates near full passive range of motion (PROM) for shoulder flexion. PROM for IR and a combined movement of IR with shoulder extension is limited. What are some essential points to address and treatment techniques to use during Drew's treatment?

After correction of Drew's posture he was able to reach higher above his head. His slouched posture had previously restricted full active shoulder flexion. The shoulder capsule needs to be assessed immediately for restrictions. Emphasizing capsular mobilization of a restricted capsule allows for better joint arthrokinematics and increased ROM. The anterior, posterior, and inferior capsule were all restricted. General mobilizations were performed for all areas of the capsule, and specific mobilizations were performed for the anterior capsule. Drew then performed ROM and stretching to the shoulder, including stretches with the hand behind the back. A considerable increase in PROM and AROM for the hand behind the back was noted after this treatment.

3 Kelly had an acromioplasty on her right shoulder 6 weeks ago. She complains of a pinching pain when reaching above her head, through the last 20° of shoulder flexion and abduction. She also has a pinching pain when actively reaching across her body in horizontal adduction. With PROM for horizontal adduction, shoulder flexion, and abduction, she has pain near the end of the ranges. What type of treatment may be helpful during her next session?

Kelly was treated with joint mobilizations to the glenohumeral joint as usual to increase shoulder flexion and shoulder abduction. AC mobilizations have been performed in the past, with the arm in anatomic position while the patient was supine. However, today AC mobilizations were performed with the shoulder in horizontal adduction and again with the shoulder in flexion above 140°. An assistant was required to hold the extremity of the patient in place while the therapist performed the mobilizations. AROM for shoulder flexion, abduction, and horizontal adduction increased by 10° of pain-free motion. In addition, the complaints of pain intensity were less when experienced. After one more visit for the same treatment, the patient exhibited full ROM.

4 Cynthia had an acromioplasty on her right shoulder 5 days ago. She complains of moderate to severe pain intermittently throughout the day. She also has difficulty sleeping secondary to shoulder pain. She is a mother of young children. Patient uses arm for light activities of daily living (ADLs) when possible. ROM is limited in all directions. Strength is not tested secondary to healing tissue and pain levels. How did the therapist advise her and treat her for pain management?

The therapist encouraged her to use a sling for a couple of days to prevent overuse of the healing extremity. She was told to use the sling when she was up and about for protection and for rest. Children as well as others would be less likely to bump or grab her arm. She was also encouraged to use cryotherapy intermittently throughout the day. The therapist advised her to try sleeping in a recliner chair or a semireclined position with her shoulder supported in a loose packed position. Treatment consisted of assessing the cervical area. Gentle mobilizations were done in the cervical area along with massage to the cervical and scapular musculature to decrease muscle guarding and spasms. The patient's pain level decreased slightly after the treatment. Pain began subsiding over the next couple of days.

5 Mike had an acromioplasty on his right shoulder 4 weeks ago. He notes aching in the shoulder after early functional progression consisting of a short toss program. This discomfort is in the posterior aspect of the shoulder. The discomfort is most pronounced during the follow though in the throwing motion. He has no night pain but has minimal discomfort with daily overhead activities. His rotator cuff strength is excellent, and he has a normal scapulohumeral rhythm. What additional concerns should be addressed?

As Mike is a throwing athlete, the cause of his rotator cuff issues may have been due to secondary impingement as a result of anterior glenohumeral instability. Subtle anterior instability may be increased due to a tight posterior capsule. Since this is where Mike's symptoms are present, stretching of the posterior capsule may be indicated. Manual techniques the therapist can employ include horizontal adduction without stabilization of the axillary border of the scapula progressing to stabilizing the scapula and focusing on glenohumeral motion. The sleeper stretch (side-lying on the involved shoulder with the arm forward flexed while passively pushing the forearm toward the floor) may be helpful, but should be done carefully with the arm flexed to no more than 70°.

6 Tim is employed as a truck driver who has responsibilities for overhead lifting and stacking. His SAD was done 5 weeks ago and he is readying to return to work. His rehab has gone well, with the only difficulty being the last 5° to 8° of flexion needed to get to the upper shelves in his delivery truck. The restriction is not painful but is accompanied by stiffness. His motion preoperatively was also slightly restricted due to pain and stiffness. In addition to passive ROM of the shoulder what other areas may be of concern?

The last few degrees of elevation can be troublesome. Many issues can contribute to decreased mobility at the cervical-thoracic junction and throughout the midthoracic spine. Assessment of joint play in these regions may reveal one or more hypomobile segments. Restoring normal accessory motions in these areas may assist in regaining full shoulder elevation.

7 John has been referred to you from a surgeon from out of state. He states that he had a shoulder decompression 6 weeks ago and did not have postoperative physical therapy. He found a rotator cuff strengthening program online and has been doing those exercises daily and is using "3 or 4 lb." In addition to significant rotator cuff weakness, your evaluation demonstrates scapular malposition, inferior medial border prominence, pain at the coracoids, and an abnormal scapulohumeral rhythm. How will you modify John's program?

Excessive loads can be placed on the rotator cuff with insufficient proximal stability afforded at the scapulothoracic joint. In addition, muscles of the rotator cuff (especially the supraspinatus) may not tolerate excessive external resistance due to short lever arms and a relatively small physiologic cross-sectional area. John should not be performing progressive resistive exercises for the cuff at this juncture. You should emphasize anterior chest muscle flexibility and strengthening of the scapular stabilizers.

8 Ann works in a data entry position and has had right shoulder pain off and on for 3 years with occasional complaints of "carpal tunnel." She had a SAD performed 3 weeks ago and has yet to start rehabilitation because of poorly localized postoperative pain. Two days after your initial evaluation, Ann returned for a follow-up visit with complaints of increased shoulder pain and occasional numbness and tingling down the right arm and into the hand. Is it safe to proceed with rehabilitation?

You should counsel Ann that any increase in activity may result in discomfort. Ann may be experiencing delayed onset muscle soreness and/or her level of activity may be in excess of what she is ready for. You can certainly trouble shoot Ann's level of activities and exercise. You can also determine if discomfort is delayed-onset muscle soreness in nature or from joint and healing tissue. The issue of occasional numbness and tingling is not a contraindication for exercise, but it also cannot be ignored. If you have not yet done so, Ann's cervical spine should be cleared, nerves cleared for adverse neural tension/compression, and peripheral nerve entrapments.

REFERENCES

1. Neer CS II: Anterior acromioplasty for the chronic impingement syndrome in the shoulder: A preliminary report. J Bone Joint Surg Am 54-A:41-50, 1972.
2. Neer CS II: Impingement lesions. Clin Orthop 173:70, 1983.
3. Meyer AW: The minute anatomy of attrition lesions. J Bone Joint Surg Am 13:341-360, 1931.
4. Codman EA: Rupture of the supraspinatus tendon and other lesions in or about the subacromial bursa. In Codman EA, editor: The shoulder, Boston, 1934, Thomas Todd.
5. Armstrong JR: Excision of the acromion in treatment of the supraspinatus syndrome: Report of ninety-five excisions. J Bone Joint Surg Am 31-B(3):436-442, 1949.
6. Diamond B: The obstructing acromion: Underlying diseases, clinical development and surgery, Springfield, Ill, 1964, Charles C Thomas.
7. McLaughlin HL, Asherman EG: Lesions of the musculotendinous cuff of the shoulder. IV. Some observations based upon the results of surgical repair. J Bone Joint Surg Am 33-A:76-86, 1951.
8. Nirschl RP: Rotator cuff tendinitis: Basic concepts of patho-etiology. In The American Academy of Orthopedic Surgeons, editor: Instructional course lectures, vol 38, Park Ridge, Ill, 1989, The American Academy of Orthopedic Surgeons.
9. Nirschl RP: Rotator cuff tendinitis: Basic concepts of patho-etiology. In Nicholas JA, Hershman EB, editors: The upper extremity in sports medicine, St Louis, 1990, Mosby.
10. Ark JW, et al: Arthroscopic treatment of calcific tendinitis of the shoulder. Arthroscopy 8:183-188, 1992.
11. Jobe FW, Kvitne RS, Giangarra CE: Shoulder pain in the overhand or throwing athlete: The relationship of anterior instability and rotator cuff impingement. Orthop Rev 18:963-975, 1989.
12. Uhthoff HK, et al: The role of the coracoacromial ligament in the impingement syndrome: A clinical, radiological and histological study. Int Orthop 12:97-104, 1988.
13. Jobe FW: Impingement problems in the athlete. In Nicholas JA, Hershmann EB, editors: The upper extremity in sports medicine, St Louis, 1990, Mosby.
14. Ogata S, Uhthoff HK: Acromial enthesopathy and rotator cuff tear: A radiologic and histologic postmortem investigation of the coracoacromial arch. Clin Orthop 254:39-48, 1990.
15. Toivonen DA, Tuite MJ, Orwin JF: Acromial structure and tears of the rotator cuff. J Shoulder Elbow Surg 4:376-383, 1995.
16. Bigliani LU, Morrison DS, April EW: The morphology of the acromion and its relationship to rotator cuff tears. Orthop Trans 10:228, 1986.
17. Kessel L, Watson M: The painful arc syndrome. Clinical classification as a guide to management. J Bone Joint Surg Am 59-B(2):166-172, 1977.
18. Watson M: The refractory painful arc syndrome. J Bone Joint Surg 60-B(4):544-546, 1978.
19. Bigliani LU, Levine WN: Current concepts review: Subacromial impingement syndrome. J Bone Joint Surg Am 79-A(12):1854-1868, 1997.
20. Fu FH, Harner CD, Klein AH: Shoulder impingement syndrome: A critical review. Clin Orthop 269:162-173, 1991.
21. Glousman RE: Instability versus impingement syndrome in the throwing athlete. Orthop Clin North Am 24:89-99, 1993.
22. Nevaiser RJ, Nevaiser TJ: Observations on impingement. Clin Orthop 254:60-63, 1990.
23. Hawkins RJ, Kennedy JC: Impingement syndrome in athletes. Am J Sports Med 8:151-158, 1980.
24. Gold RH, Seeger LL, Yao L: Imaging shoulder impingement. Skeletal Radiol 22:555-561, 1993.
25. Ono K, Yamamuro T, Rockwood CA: Use of a thirty-degree caudal tilt radiograph in the shoulder impingement syndrome. J Shoulder Elbow Surg 1:546-552, 1992.
26. Beltran J: The use of magnetic resonance imaging about the shoulder. J Shoulder Elbow Surg 1:321-332, 1992.
27. Rockwood CA Jr, Lyons FR: Shoulder impingement syndrome: Diagnosis, radiographic evaluation, and treatment with a modified Neer acromioplasty. J Bone Joint Surg Am 75-A:409-424, 1993.
28. Ellman H: Arthroscopic subacromial decompression: Analysis of one-to three-year results. Arthroscopy 3:173-181, 1987.
29. Altchek DW, et al: Arthroscopic acromioplasty: technique and results. J Bone Joint Surg Am 72-A:1198-1207, 1990.
30. Esch JC, et al: Arthroscopic subacromial decompression: Results according to the degree of rotator cuff tear. Arthroscopy 4:241-249, 1988.
31. Johnson LL: Diagnostic and surgical arthroscopy of the shoulder, St Louis, 1993, Mosby.
32. Kuhn JE, Hawkins RJ: Arthroscopically assisted techniques in diagnosis and treatment of rotator cuff tendonopathy. Sports Med Arthrosc 3:60, 1995.
33. Paulos LE, Franklin JC: Arthroscopic S.A.D. Development and application: A 5 year experience. Am J Sports Med 18:235-244, 1990.
34. Snyder SJ: A complete system for arthroscopy and bursoscopy of the shoulder. Surg Rounds Orthop, pp 57-65, July 1989.
35. Basamania CJ, Wirth MA, Rockwood CA Jr: Treatment of rotator cuff tendonopathy by open techniques. Sports Med Arthroscopy Rev 3(1):68, 1995.
36. Caspari R: A technique for arthroscopic S.A.D. Arthroscopy 8(1):23-30, 1992.
37. Gartsman GM, et al: Arthroscopic subacromial decompression: An anatomical study. Am J Sports Med 16:48-50, 1988.
38. Buuck DA, Davidson MR: Rehabilitation of the athlete after shoulder arthroscopy. Clin Sports Med 15(4):655, 1996.
39. O'Connor FG, Sobel JR, Nirschl RP: Five-step treatment for overuse injuries. Phys Sportsmed 20(10):128-142, 1992.
40. Rathbun JB, McNab I: The microvascular pattern of the rotator cuff. J Bone Joint Surg Am 52B:540, 1970.
41. Lohr JF, Ultoff HK: The microvascular pattern of the supraspinatus tendon. Clin Orthop 254:35-38, 1990.
42. Chansky HA, Ianotti JP: The vascularity of the rotator cuff. Clin Sports Med 10(4):807-822, 1991.
43. Wenger HA, McFayeden R: Physiological principles of conditioning. In Zachazewski JE, Magee DJ, Quillen WS, editors: Athletic injuries and rehabilitation, Philadelphia, 1996, Saunders.
44. Bradley JP, Tibone JE: Electromyographic analysis of muscle action about the shoulder. Clin Sports Med 15(4):789-805, 1991.
45. McCann PD, Wooten ME, Kadaba MP: A kinematic and electromyographic study of shoulder rehabilitation exercises. Clin Orthop 288:179-188, 1993.
46. Townsend H, Jobe FW, Pink M: Electromyographic analysis of the glenohumeral muscles during a baseball rehabilitation program. Am J Sports Med 19(3):264-272, 1991.
47. Graichen H, et al: Glenohumeral translation during active and passive elevation of the shoulder: A 3D open-MRI study. J Biomech 33:609-613, 2000.
48. Blackburn TA, et al: EMG analysis of posterior rotator cuff exercises. J Athl Train 25(1):40-45, 1980.
49. Jobe FW, Moynes DR: Delineation of diagnostic criteria and a rehabilitation program for rotator cuff injuries. Am J Sports Med 10:336-339, 1982.
50. Kelly BT, Kadrmas WR, Speer KP: The manual muscle examination for rotator cuff strength: An electromyographic investigation. Am J Sports Med 24:581-588, 1996.
51. Malanga GA, et al: EMG analysis of shoulder positioning in testing and strengthening of the supraspinatus. Med Sci Sports Exerc 28:661, 1996.
52. Reinold MM, et al: Electromyographic analysis of the rotator cuff and deltoid musculature during common shoulder external rotation exercises. J Orthop Sports Phys Ther 34(7):385-394, 2004.
53. Takeda Y, et al: The most effective exercise for strengthening the supraspinatus muscle: Evaluation by magnetic resonance imaging. Am J Sports Med 30(3):374-381, 2002.

54. Worrell TW, Corey BJ, York SL: An analysis of supraspinatus EMG activity and shoulder isometric force development. Med Sci Sports Exerc 24(7):744-748, 1992.

55. Alpert SW, et al: Electromyographic analysis of deltoid and rotator cuff function under varying loads and speeds. J Shoulder Elbow Surg 9(1):47-58, 2000.

56. Meyers JB, et al: On the field resistance-tubing exercises for throwers: An electromyographic analysis. J Athl Train 40(1):15-22, 2005.

57. Escamilla RA, et al: Shoulder muscle activation and function in common shoulder rehabilitation exercises. Sports Med 39(8):663-685, 2009.

58. Reinold ML, Escamilla R, Wilk KE: Current concepts in the scientific and clinical rationale behind exercises for glenohumeral and scapulothoracic musculature. J Orthop Sports Phys Ther 39(2):105-115, 2009.

59. Wilk KE: The shoulder. In Malone TR, McPoil T, Nitz AJ, editors: Orthopaedic and sports physical therapy, ed 3, St Louis, 1997, Mosby.

60. Lister JL, et al: Scapular stabilizer activity during Bodyblade®, Cuff Weights, and Theraband® use. J Sport Rehabil 16:50-67, 2007.

61. Kibler WB, et al: Electromyographic analysis of specific exercises for scapular control in early phases of shoulder rehabilitation. Am J Sports Med 36(9):1789-1798, 2008.

62. Lovering RM, Russ DW: Fiber type composition of cadaveris human rotator cuff muscles. J Orthop Sports Phys Ther 38(11):674-680, 2008.

63. Wolf WB: Shoulder tendinoses. Clin Sports Med 11(4):871-890, 1992.

64. Kibler WB: The role of the scapula in the overhead throwing motion. Contemp Orthop 22(5):525-532, 1991.

65. Moseley JB, et al: EMG analysis of the scapular muscles during a shoulder rehabilitation program. Am J Sports Med 20(2):128-134, 1992.

66. Ludewig PM, et al: Relative balance of serratus anterior and upper trapezius muscle activity during push-up exercises. Am J Sports Med 32(2):484-493, 2004.

67. Lear LJ, Gross MT: An electromyographical study of the scapular stabilizing synergists during a push-up progression. J Orthop Sports Phys Ther 28(3):146-157, 1998.

68. Decker MJ, et al: Serratus anterior muscle activity during selected rehabilitation exercises. Am J Sports Med 27(6):784-791, 1999.

69. Ekstrom RA, Donatelli RA, Soderberg GL: Surface electromyographic analysis of exercises for the trapezius and serratus anterior muscles. J Orthop Sports Phys Ther 33(5):247-258, 2003.

70. Tippett SR, Kleiner DM: Objectivity and validity of the lateral scapular slide test. J Athl Train 31(2):S40, 1996.

71. Odom CJ, Hurd CE, Denegar CR: Intratester and intertester reliability of the lateral scapular slide test and its ability to predict shoulder pathology. J Athl Train 30(2):S9, 1995.

72. Hertling D, Kessler RM: The shoulder and shoulder girdle. In Hertling D, Kessler RM, editors: Management of common musculoskeletal disorders: Physical therapy principles and methods, ed 3, Philadelphia, 1996, Lippincott.

73. Blasier RB, Carpenter JE, Huston LJ: Shoulder proprioception: effect of joint laxity, joint position, and direction of motion. Orthop Rev 23(1):45-50, 1994.

74. Voight ML, et al: The effects of muscle fatigue and the relationship of arm dominance to shoulder proprioception. J Orthop Sports Phys Ther 23(6):348-352, 1996.

75. Pappas AM, Zawacki RM, McCarthy CF: Rehabilitation of the pitching shoulder. Am J Sports Med 13(4):223-235, 1985.

76. Lephart SM, Kocher MS: The role of exercise in the prevention of shoulder disorders. In Matsen FA, Fu FH, Hawkins RJ, editors: The shoulder: A balance of mobility and stability, Rosemont, Ill, 1992, American Academy of Orthopaedic Surgeons.

77. Uhl TL, Carver TJ, Mattacola CG: Shoulder muscular activation during upper extremity weight-bearing exercise. J Orthop Sports Phys Ther 33(3):109-117, 2003.

78. Andrews JR, Whiteside JA, Wilk KE: Rehabilitation of throwing and racquet sport injuries. In Buschbachler RM, Braddom RL, editors: Sports medicine and rehabilitation: A sport-specific approach, Philadelphia, 1994, Hanley & Belfus.

79. Tippett SR, Voight ML: Functional progressions for sport rehabilitation, Champaign, Ill, 1995, Human Kinetics.

80. Goldstein TS: Functional rehabilitation in orthopaedics, Gaithersburg, Md, 1995, Aspen.

81. Voight ML, Draovitch P, Tippett SR: Plyometrics. In Albert M, editor: Eccentric muscle training in sports and orthopaedics, ed 2, New York, 1995, Churchill Livingstone.

82. Dye SF: The knee as a biologic transmission with an envelope of function: a theory. Clin Orthop 323:10-18, 1996.

83. Host HH: Scapular taping in the treatment of anterior shoulder impingement. Phys Ther 75(9):803-812, 1995.

CHAPTER 4

Anterior Capsular Reconstruction

Renee Songer, Reza Jazayeri, Diane R. Schwab, Ralph A. Gambardella, Clive E. Brewster

INTRODUCTION

Anterior shoulder instability is one of the most commonly diagnosed and treated conditions of the shoulder in athletes. This encompasses a wide spectrum of pathology, and similarly various surgical approaches have been used to address the specific pathoanatomy involved. Treatment of anterior shoulder instability has evolved due to advances in arthroscopic techniques along with an improved understanding of shoulder anatomy and its complex biomechanics. Although the treatment of anterior glenohumeral instability has been a topic of debate over the last couple of decades, a consensus exists regarding the necessity of an individualized treatment plan based on the patients' functional demands and their associated type and degree of instability. Treating anterior shoulder instability requires an accurate diagnosis, a detailed operative plan, experience with advanced arthroscopic and open procedures, and individualized rehabilitation programs.

ETIOLOGY/EVALUATION

Shoulder instability is often not an isolated diagnosis, but rather one point of a continuum of pathology (Fig. 4-1). This is particularly evident in overhead-throwing athletes who place a tremendous amount of force on the shoulder joint and surrounding soft tissue structures. Repetitive microtrauma and stresses placed on the shoulder can lead to injury of the glenohumeral joint and various supporting structures including the rotator cuff, glenohumeral ligaments, and labrum.

Shoulder instability is often associated with internal impingement, a process where the posterosuperior labrum and the articular undersurface of the rotator cuff tendons impinge and become injured. The cause of internal impingement is multifactorial in throwing athletes. Poor mechanics such as hyperangulation of the arm during the cocking phase and poor endurance can lead to pathologic stretching of the anterior shoulder structures. This is often exacerbated by underlying weak periscapular stabilizers and deficits in internal rotation. The combination of these factors and the repetitive nature of throwing sports can lead to internal impingement with damage to the surrounding structures.

Many patients cannot be simply placed into categories represented by the eponyms TUBS and AMBRI. TUBS stands for traumatic instability, unidirectional, Bankart lesion, treated with surgery. AMBRI stands for atraumatic instability, multidirectional, bilateral, with treatment being initially rehabilitation; if nonoperative treatment fails, then surgical treatment is an inferior capsular shift. Shoulder instability may be better addressed when classified into one of four groups as shown in Box 4-1.

Clinical examination of group 1 patients with anterior shoulder instability commonly demonstrate glenohumeral internal rotation deficit (GIRD), with positive apprehension and relocation signs. Associated posterior capsular tightness contributes to anterior and superior shifting of the humeral head, leading to posterior impingement and labral pathology. If left untreated, this instability can lead to internal impingement with rotator cuff and labral tearing (group 2).

Some patients also have signs of external impingement or a diagnosis of rotator cuff tendinitis, bursitis, or bicipital tendinitis. Generally, this group is older than those who experience internal impingement. This group often has persistent symptoms despite both nonoperative treatment and surgical subacromial decompression.

Young patients with generalized ligamentous laxity (group 3) are another group of patients that can have shoulder instability, as well as a positive relocation test and internal impingement. Lastly, (group 4) a traumatic episode can lead to anterior instability as a result of a Bankart lesion. These patients, however, show no evidence of impingement.

The majority of patients will respond to conservative treatment if the diagnosis of anterior shoulder instability is made early during the pathologic course. As many as 95% of patients can return to their previous level of competition. The focus of these exercises is on posterior capsular stretching, strengthening the periscapular muscles, and emphasis of proper throwing mechanics. Activity modification and rest from throwing combined with a supervised therapy

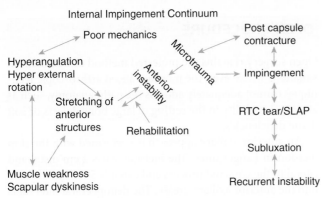

Fig. 4-1 Instability continuum.

program are instrumental in protecting the anterior shoulder structures. Persistence and attention to detail are both essential to a successful outcome: the elimination of pain and return to full activity without surgical intervention.

Patients who do not respond to 3 to 6 months of appropriate nonoperative management are possible candidates for anterior capsulolabral reconstruction (ACLR) for recurrent instability or repair of their Bankart lesion for traumatic instability.

SURGICAL CONSIDERATIONS

It is imperative to determine the correct etiology of instability by a thorough history, physical examination, and imaging studies for selection of the appropriate procedure. A surgical approach that combines careful preoperative and intraoperative evaluation maximizes the possibility of good and excellent outcomes. Both open and arthroscopic surgical repairs have a role in the management of anterior shoulder instability. While arthroscopic capsulolabral repair has recently become the standard of care for the treatment of anterior shoulder instability, open approaches remain a reliable, time-tested option and in certain cases continue to be the gold standard.

All patients are examined under anesthesia. Subtle instabilities, which were not apparent previously, are often better appreciated with the patient asleep. Regardless of surgical approach, a thorough diagnostic arthroscopy is performed. The patient is placed in the lateral position, and the shoulder is distracted with 10 lb using an overhead traction

suspension unit. The arthroscope is introduced into the shoulder via the posterior portal. The glenohumeral joint is evaluated for subtle changes—such as attenuation or absence of the inferior glenohumeral ligament, a loose redundant capsule—with a positive "push-through" test. Often an internal impingement between the undersurface of the supraspinatus tendon and the posterior labrum is evident with fraying or a partial articular supraspinatus tendon avulsion (PASTA) lesion in more advanced cases.

In cases of traumatic anterior shoulder instability, a Bankart lesion, and occasionally a Hill-Sachs deformity can be seen. The subacromial space usually appears normal in the younger overhead-thrower who has an anterior instability without the inflamed, thickened bursa and decreased space that is characteristically found with external impingement.

Based on the preoperative workup, evaluation under anesthesia and diagnostic arthroscopy, the surgical approach that will best address the patient's issues is elected.

ARTHROSCOPIC PROCEDURE

Arthroscopic surgical stabilization is currently the preferred method of treatment for most patients with anterior instability. Surgical goals remain similar to open approaches, including addressing any Bankart/anterior labral periosteal sleeve avulsion (ALPSA) lesion back to its anatomic position on the glenoid, eliminating any capsular hyperlaxity, and repairing any clinically significant rotator interval laxity. Furthermore, an arthroscopic approach allows better identification and treatment of associated pathologic conditions including superior labral anterior-posterior (SLAP) lesions, release of posterior capsular tightness, and any possible subacromial impingement.

Traditionally, open stabilization has been the gold standard. However, more recent arthroscopic suture anchor techniques have recurrence rates equal to open techniques, even in high-demand contact athletes. Recent reports documented 92% to 97% good to excellent results, with 91% of high-demand contact athletes with traumatic anterior instability returning to sports. Multidirectional instability also may be treated by arthroscopic stabilization with predictably good results.

Arthroscopy is minimally invasive; avoiding open surgical dissection decreases morbidity and facilitates an outpatient approach. Maintaining subscapularis integrity improves postoperative muscle function and facilitates rehabilitation, particularly in the overhead athlete.

Initially, a diagnostic arthroscopy is performed through a standard posterior portal. An anterior superior portal is created just anterior to the biceps tendon. This portal is used for mobilization of the capsulolabral complex and for subsequent suture management. An anterior inferior portal is placed just above the superior edge of the subscapularis and is used for inferior placement of suture anchors on the lower aspect of the glenoid neck. Assessment of the mobility of the capsuloligamentous complex is crucial in determining whether the soft tissues have been displaced or are scarred in a medial position on the neck of the glenoid as in an ALPSA lesion. Adequate inferior soft tissue mobilization to the 6 o'clock position on the glenoid face is carried out using a combination of probes, rasps, motorized shavers, and periosteal elevators.

The anterior glenoid is rasped and decorticated in preparation for suture anchor insertion. The anchors are then placed on the edge of the articular surface in the 2 o'clock, 3 o'clock, and 5 o'clock positions. A suture lasso* or similar device is used to shift the labroligamentous complex superiorly and medially as needed. The suture is passed through the tissue, and arthroscopic knots are then used to securely fix the soft tissue to the glenoid. After all suture anchors are tied, the repair is evaluated for stable fixation and restoration of an anterior "buttress" to inhibit instability.

Adjunctive procedures may need to be performed to completely correct all pathology associated with the instability, such as rotator interval (RI) incompetence and capsular laxity. Arthroscopic findings consistent with RI tears are capsular redundancy between the supraspinatus and subscapularis, biceps tendon fraying, superior glenohumeral ligament (SGHL) tear, and the superior border of the subscapularis fraying. Arthroscopic closure of the deep layer of the SGHL to the middle glenohumeral ligament (MGHL) imbricates the anterosuperior capsule and can address RI capsular incompetence.

Contraindications to arthroscopic treatment include large Hill-Sachs lesions (25% to 35% of the humeral arc), Hill-Sachs lesions that engage the anterior glenoid rim in abduction-external rotation, or a loss of more than 20% to 25% of the anteroinferior glenoid.

Multiple dislocations can lead to attenuated capsulolabral tissue. This remaining poor quality tissue is often difficult to mobilize and repair arthroscopically, and an open stabilization may be preferred in these patients. Other relative indications for open stabilization include recurrent instability after failed arthroscopic stabilizations and avulsion of the capsulolabral tissue from the humerus (the humeral avulsion of the glenohumeral ligaments [HAGL] lesion).

Recent stabilization techniques have also expanded the arthroscopic scope of treating anterior shoulder instability. The "Remplissage" procedure (French for "to fill") described by Wolf consists of an arthroscopic capsulotenodesis of the posterior capsule and infraspinatus tendon to fill the Hill-Sachs lesion.[†] Although others have also demonstrated satisfactory results with this technique,[‡] alterations in biomechanics of the shoulder remain a valid concern.[§]

---

*Arthrex, Naples, Fla.

[†]Hill-Sachs "remplissage": an arthroscopic solution for engaging the Hill-Sachs lesion.

[‡]Arthroscopic double-pulley remplissage technique for engaging Hill-Sachs lesions in anterior shoulder instability repairs.

[§]Decreased range of motion following arthroscopic remplissage.

OPEN PROCEDURE

Open surgery remains the preferred method of treatment in situations where even the most advanced arthroscopic techniques cannot adequately address the pathoanatomy, such as anterior instability in the setting of large bone defects or soft tissue deficiencies.

An anterior axillary approach is performed with the skin incision in Langer lines. The incision starts 2 cm distal and lateral to the coracoid process and extends 5 to 7 cm distally into the anterior axillary crease. The deltopectoral interval is identified, and the cephalic vein is retracted laterally with the deltoid. The conjoined tendon is identified and retracted medially. With the shoulder in external rotation, the subscapularis tendon is split transversely in line with its fibers at the junction of the upper two thirds and lower one third.

The subscapularis muscle is dissected free from the underlying capsule, starting medially in the muscular portion of the subscapularis and extending laterally. Retractors are positioned to maintain the subscapularis interval, allowing a horizontal anterior capsulotomy to be made in line with the split of the subscapularis tendon. Tag sutures are placed on either side of the capsular flaps just lateral to the labrum exposing the glenoid.

If a Bankart lesion is noted, it is repaired using suture anchors back to its anatomic location on the anterior-inferior glenoid neck. The capsule is assessed for its volume, quality, and ability to buttress the anterior inferior margin. The degree of capsular shift is tailored to the degree of laxity. If the capsule is deemed lax or incompetent, it is overlapped to obliterate the redundancy. The inferior leaf of the capsule and accompanying inferior glenohumeral ligament are advanced proximally. The superior portion of the capsule is brought over the inferior portion and labrum, resting along the anterior scapular neck. The inferior and superior leaflets are overlapped using a vest-over-pants technique with nonabsorbable sutures. If the labrum is intact and does not require repair, a capsular imbrication alone is adequate to reduce the volume of the joint.

After capsular closure, the arm is taken through a ROM, noting the extent of motion which places tension on the repair. This will mark the limitation of motion that the patient is permitted postoperatively. The surgeon must clearly communicate with the therapist to ensure that this safe zone is observed.

After determining a safe postoperative motion, the surgeon reapproximates the subscapularis and closes the deltopectoral interval, followed by subcuticular closure of the skin with the addition of adhesive strips. The arm is splinted in abduction and external rotation.

DISCUSSION

The management of anterior shoulder instability continues to evolve as advances in arthroscopy provide an effective alternative to traditional open surgery. Furthermore, arthroscopic procedures allow improved evaluation and treatment of associated pathologies, including SLAP lesions, partial rotator cuff tears, subacromial impingement, RI, and capsular laxity while avoiding the common morbidities associated with open procedures.

Open surgical stabilization, however, continues to play an important role in certain injury patterns that cannot be adequately addressed arthroscopically. Decision-making regarding surgery for instability is influenced by the relevant pathologic findings and the surgeon's experience.

Careful patient selection and a thorough understanding of the involved pathoanatomy are paramount in maximizing patient outcome. Regardless of the surgical approach chosen, our success should be based on retaining range of motion, decreasing recovery time, maintaining proprioceptive control, and ultimately returning patients to their prior level of activity.

THERAPY GUIDELINES FOR REHABILITATION

Because no muscles are cut during the surgical reconstruction, rehabilitation proceeds promptly with two familiar goals: restore structural flexibility and strengthen dynamic glenohumeral and scapulothoracic stabilizers. This chapter includes exercises and manual interventions to restore the trinity of normalcy: range of motion, strength, and endurance. The key to success is restoring all three components concurrently rather than addressing each component sequentially. The best plan is an integrated one: do not wait for full range of motion to return before initiating strengthening, and address muscular endurance as gross strength improves. The likelihood of an optimal postoperative outcome increases dramatically when the physical therapist monitors postoperative exercises carefully to ensure correct execution. Be cautious and avoid pushing for full ROM too early and disrupting the healing tissue.

Phase IA

TIME: Day 1 to 2 weeks (Table 4-1)
GOALS: Manage pain and protect the surgical wounds from infection
Protect the anterior capsule from excessive stress
Activate scapular stabilizers and encourage proper scapular positioning
Initiate passive and active assisted ROM with a goal of 135° in the flexion plane
Maintain functional ROM at the elbow and wrist

For 2 to 4 weeks, the arm will be in an abduction sling. Protection of the surgically repaired tissue is essential for a successful long-term outcome. Many of these patients have some joint laxity and rarely have difficulty regaining motion with a normal course of rehabilitation. The inflammatory and initial fibroblastic/granulation stages of physiologic healing occur during the first 2 weeks following surgery.[1-3]

Taking care not to extend the inflammatory phase with overly aggressive treatments will allow maximal collagen fiber deposition with minimal disruption leading to better healing in the end. **Avoid stressing the anterior capsule with your interventions.**

On the first visit, remove the sling and measure passive range of motion (PROM) in flexion and abduction in the scapular plane (scaption). Do not move into external rotation past zero degrees at this time to prevent excessive stress to the anterior capsule. Measure internal rotation to the limits permitted by pain tolerance because there is no concern about disrupting healing tissue in this direction. Assess wrist and elbow motion at the first visit as well. Early mobilization has been shown to improve tissue healing following surgery.[4,5] Without mobilization the patient is less likely to regain full motion; therefore, it is important to begin ranging the shoulder within the limits of discomfort immediately. Because pain typically prevents independent active range of motion (AROM) in the first few days after surgery, perform passive or manual active-assisted range of motion (AAROM). Independent AAROM can be safely initiated using wand exercises, table slides, and wall walks into flexion and scaption. When the postoperative pain subsides, measure active elevation in the scapular plane.

Assess scapular positioning and active scapular mobility immediately and begin scapular positioning exercises. Emphasis should be placed on activation of the serratus anterios and the middle and lower trapezius muscles to promote retraction and upward rotation of the scapula.[6] Exercises may include (1) proprioceptive neuromuscular facilitation (PNF) interventions for scapular positioning, which are very effective and safe immediately postoperatively[7]; and (2) prone or standing scapular retraction. Avoid excessive activation of upper trapezius or latissimus dorsi, which leads to improper scapular elevation or depression, respectively.[6]

A home exercise program should begin immediately (Box 4-2). Remove the sling three to four times per day to perform exercises for 15 minutes including: scapular retraction, AROM elbow flexion/extension, pronation/supination, wrist flexion, extension, radial and ulnar deviation, and squeezing a gripper ball. Follow this routine with ice and return to the sling. Codman's pendulum exercises are also appropriate at home if the patient has no contraindications due to extreme laxity.[8]

Pain management modalities, such as electrical stimulation and cryotherapy, may be used as needed throughout the course of therapy. If the patient is having an excessive amount of pain, assessment and treatment of the cervical spine may be appropriate. Preoperative compensations, intraoperative positioning, and postoperative guarding can lead to joint and soft tissue dysfunction in the neck. Comparable objective findings locally at cervical levels 3, 4, and 5 may explain excessive pain, muscle inhibition, or excessive tightness in the shoulder and the therapist should intervene appropriately.[9]

TABLE 4-1 Anterior Capsular Reconstruction

Rehabilitation Phase	Criteria to Progress to This Phase	Anticipated Impairments and Functional Limitations	Intervention	Goal	Rationale
Phase 1A Postoperative 1 day–2 wk • Postoperative protection	• Postoperative	• Postoperative pain • Postoperative edema • UE in abduction sling • Limited ROM • Limited strength • Limited ADLs	• **Modalities:** • Cryotherapy • Electrical stimulation • **PROM:** • All directions as needed if patient is unable to perform AAROM because of pain • **AAROM:** Wand exercises, table slides, and wall walks • Shoulder—flexion, internal rotation, and abduction, avoiding stress on the anterior capsule • **AROM:** • Elbow—Flexion, extension, pronation, supination • Wrist—Flexion, extension, radial and ulnar deviation • **Submaximal Isometrics:** • Shoulder—All movements in a neutral position • Scapular stabilization • **Manual Intervention:** • Grade I, II GH mobilization • PNF patterns • **Scapular Positioning Exercises:** • PNF for scapular positioning • Prone and standing scapular retraction • **Core strengthening when able**	• **Modalities:** • Manage pain and edema • **PROM:** • Produce 135° of flexion in the scapular plane • **AAROM:** • Produce 135° of flexion in the scapular plane • ER limited to 0° • **AROM:** • Maintain full ROM of elbow and wrist • **Isometrics:** • Produce good-quality contraction of shoulder girdle musculature • **Manual Intervention:** • **Function:** • Allow ADLs below shoulder height to tolerance	• **Modalities:** • Minimize edema to minimize discomfort and inhibitory effects on local musculature • **PROM:** • Maintain ROM if patient is unable to perform exercises independently due to pain • **AAROM:** • Minimize ROM loss while protecting the anterior capsule • **AROM:** • Minimize loss at secondary joints • **Isometrics:** • Activate rotator cuff and scapular stabilizers to minimize atrophy • **Manual Intervention:** • Minimize adhesions and manage pain • Facilitate muscle activation and scapular positioning • **Function:** • Maximize functional use within the limits of protecting the surgical repair

AAROM, active-assisted range of motion; *ADLs,* activities of daily living; *AROM,* active range of motion; *ER,* external rotation; *GH,* glenohumeral; *PNF,* proprioceptive neuromuscular facilitation; *PROM,* passive range of motion; *ROM,* range of motion; *UE,* Upper extremity.

Begin core strengthening exercises immediately. Abdominals, lumbar extensor muscles, and gluteals are all critical components in the kinetic chain for athletes and physical laborers alike. Core and lower body strengthening are safe and easy to incorporate into the training program. Once the patient is safe and independent, transition these exercises into a home exercise program to allow more time for close supervision of the shoulder exercises during therapy sessions.

Phase IB

TIME: 2 weeks to 4 weeks (Table 4-2)
GOALS:
• Progress from PROM to AAROM to AROM while protecting the anterior joint capsule
• Progress scapular stabilization exercises

• Initiate rotator cuff exercises while protecting the anterior joint capsule

Typically, the arm comes out of the sling during this phase. Physiologic healing is progressing from the granulation stage into the proliferative/fibroblastic stage.[1-3] Due to the deposition of collagen fibrils, the healing tissues are developing some internal integrity enabling them to tolerate gentle stresses. The skin wounds should be healing and pain should be minimal.

Measure active range of motion to the onset of discomfort including: flexion, scaption, and internal rotation. Measure external rotation to 45° or onset of discomfort, whichever comes first. Assess scapular mobility and quality of motion during AROM looking for abnormalities in scapular winging, scapulothoracic or scapulohumeral rhythm, and quality of

BOX 4-2 Suggested Home Exercise Program for the Postsurgical Patient

Phase IA: 0-2 Weeks

15 minutes 2 to 4 times per day as discomfort permits
ROM
Codman's pendulum exercises
Elbow: flexion, extension
Forearm: pronation, supination
Wrist: flexion, extension, radial and ulnar deviation
Scapular stability
Scapular retraction: in sling and out of sling
Grip/squeeze ball
Ice as needed for discomfort throughout day/night

Phase IB: 2-4 Weeks

ROM:
AAROM:
Wand: flexion, full can, ER to 45°, hand behind back
Wall walks: flexion, full can
Stretching if indicated:
Cross-body posterior capsule
Scapular stability
Static hold "Row"
Static hold serratus press
Rotator cuff strengthening
Isometrics with elbow at side: flexion, extension,
    abduction, internal and external rotation
Variable load isometrics (once scapular control is
    achieved and therapist is confident the patient can
    correctly perform exercises)
Ice as needed for discomfort throughout day
PRECAUTION: Do not force external rotation at this time.
    Limit the patient to 45° to prevent excessive stretching
    while unsupervised at home.

Phase II: 4-8 Weeks

ROM:
AAROM/AROM:
Wand, progressing to full ROM in flexion, scaption,
    external rotation, hand behind back
Stretching if indicated:
Sleeper stretch
Scapular stability:
Scapular protraction:
Serratus press progression:
Wall: two arms > one arm
Table height: two arms > one arm
Plank: knees > full

Dynamic hug below 90° elevation
Scapular retraction:
Prone row, extension
Rotator cuff strengthening:
Side-lying external rotation, abduction, and horizontal
    flexion
Standing internal and external rotation with resistance
    bands
OKC flexion, full can

Phase III: 2-3 Months

ROM: expected to be normalized at this time. Continue
    with ROM as indicated in any restricted directions
Stretching: continue as indicated
Scapular stability:
Scapular protraction/upward rotation:
Serratus anterior:
Wall slides into forward elevation above shoulder/head
    height
Hug at 120° elevation
Scapular retraction:
Prone full can
Prone row with external rotation
Rotator cuff strengthening:
Supraspinatus mid-range overhead punch
Supine internal and external rotation at 45° to 90°
    abduction with resistance bands
General Strength:
Biceps, triceps, latissimus, pectorals, trapezius strength
    using traditional exercises as appropriate based on
    scapular stability, overall strength, and safety.

Phase IV: 3-4 Months

Scapular Stability:
Planks, walkouts pike press
Endurance: ball bounce in overhead position for 30-90
    seconds
Rotator cuff strengthening:
External rotations eccentric strengthening with
    resistance bands
General strengthening:
Becoming more sport specific as appropriate

Phase V: 4-6 Months

Sport-specific training progresses
Full range of motion push-ups

muscle contraction. Gentle strength assessment of the rotator cuff in all planes from a neutral position is also appropriate as pain tolerance allows. The goal is to assess muscle activation rather than to perform break testing, which would require maximal force production and potentially damage the surgically repaired tissue and cause pain.

Active-assisted ROM exercises can include wand flexion and abduction in the scapular plane, external rotation to 45°, and hand behind the back. The patient should move into the ROM until he or she begins to feel an initial stretch. Make certain the patient understands that the goal of therapy in this phase is to initiate range of motion without stressing the

TABLE 4-2 Anterior Capsular Reconstruction

Rehabilitation Phase	Criteria to Progress to This Phase	Anticipated Impairments and Functional Limitations	Intervention	Goal	Rationale

Phase 1B
Postoperative 2-4 wk
• Postoperative protection
• ROM initiation and muscle activation
	• No signs of infection
	• Pain controlled with medication or modalities
	• No loss of ROM from initial assessment
		• Patient comes out of sling
		• Limited ROM
		• Limited strength
		• Minimal functional use of arm for self-care and ADLs due to weakness and discomfort
		• Full elbow and wrist AROM
			• **Modalities:**
			  • Continue modalities as needed by pain and edema
			• **AAROM:** as needed
			• **AROM:**
			  • Shoulder—Flexion, scaption, and internal rotation to tolerance; external rotation to 45°
			  • Avoid stress on the anterior capsule
			  • Continue with elbow and wrist as needed
			• **Isometrics:**
			  • Shoulder—Progressive load isometrics
			• **Isotonics:**
			  • Scapular stabilization exercises standing and prone
			  • Prone extension
			  • Side-lying series
			  • Static serratus press
			  • Static hold "row"
			• **Manual Intervention:**
			  • Soft tissue mobilization
			  • GH and scapulothoracic mobilization
				• **Modalities:**
				  • Manage pain and edema
				• **AAROM/AROM:**
				  • Shoulder—Flexion, scaption, and internal rotation 70% of uninvolved side for functional requirements
				  • External rotation limited to 45° to avoid stress on the anterior capsule
				  • Continue with elbow and wrist as needed
				• **Isometrics:**
				  • Strong, tonic contraction of rotator cuff without pain
				• **Isotonics:**
				  • Good scapular control in standing and prone exercises without cues
				  • Prone and side-lying series: good form maintained through 3×10 repetitions
				• **Manual Intervention:**
				  • Maximize ROM
				  • Maximize mechanical alignment
				• **Function:**
				  • Independent for self-care and ADLs below shoulder height
				  • Participation in core and lower body strengthening
					• **Modalities:**
					  • Minimize edema to minimize discomfort and inhibitory effects on local musculature
					• **AAROM/AROM:**
					  • Shoulder—Progress with ROM quickly but safely
					  • Avoid stress on the anterior capsule
					• **Isometrics:**
					  • Once good muscle activation is achieved, quickly progress into more advanced exercises if able
					• **Isotonics:**
					  • Scapular control is required to advance into more challenging rotator cuff exercises
					  • Through range motions in safe positions to build strength and endurance
					• **Manual Intervention:**
					  • Decrease mechanical barriers preventing normal ROM and strength
					• **Function:**
					  • Minimize dependency for functional activities
					  • Maintain fitness to minimize losses

AAROM, active-assisted range of motion; *ADLs,* activities of daily living; *AROM,* active range of motion; *ROM,* range of motion; *GH,* glenohumeral; *UE,* Upper extremity.

anterior capsule. These exercises can be incorporated into a home program.

During this phase the patient must learn to actively control the position of the scapula without cues. The goal is to maximize scapular stability and minimize scapular winging. Proper control of scapular position is required to progress with rotator cuff exercises. Three key muscles to activate are the middle trapezius, lower trapezius, and serratus anterior. Progress prone or standing scapular retractions to a static row using an exercise band. The patient

grasps an exercise band with two hands, and performs a scapular retraction creating tension in the band, while the elbows remain bent to 90° and in the plane of the body. The patient then walks slowly backward to increase tension in the band while maintaining a scapular retraction to load the posterior scapular stabilizers. Static rows can be performed with an isometric hold in the loaded position or simply by moving repeatedly through the motion to load and relax the muscles. Early activation of the serratus anterior can be achieved with a static hold serratus press in a modified push-up position at the wall (Fig. 4-2, *A*). This position is similar to the "plus" position of the traditional "push-up plus," which demonstrates high EMG activity in the serratus anterior.[10,11] The patient places the hands on the wall at shoulder height, with the head and spine in neutral alignment. Instruct the patient to press the hands into the wall and the body away from the hands using a scapular protraction motion to achieve the "plus" position. Progress into a more challenging position by lowering the hands to the height of a table, thereby increasing gravitational forces and increasing the workload on the serratus (Fig. 4-2, *B*). These are safe exercises to add to the patient's home program because there is no active motion being performed at the glenohumeral joint (see Box 4-2).

Once scapular positioning can be achieved and maintained by the patient, slowly progress rotator cuff strengthening as tolerance, strength, and proper form allow. *Caution the patient that the elbow should never be behind the plane of the body to avoid stressing the anterior capsule.* To begin, submaximal isometric strengthening exercises can be performed in a neutral position into shoulder flexion, extension, internal and external rotation, and abduction (Fig. 4-3). Progression of these initial rotator cuff exercises includes variable load isometrics using resistance bands. The patient stands holding the band as if to perform classic isotonic internal and external rotation exercises. Yet rather than move the arm, the patient holds the arm still while stepping away from the anchor point of the band, thereby increasing resistance and loading the rotator cuff muscles in a safe manner. Another technique for safe early strengthening is performing active motion from the prone position with a stable scapula. Prone extension is an excellent exercise for initiating dynamic scapular stabilization and activation of the middle trapezius (cools) (Fig. 4-4, *A*). The elbow should remain in full extension and the motion ends at the plane of the body to protect the anterior capsule.

Posterior shoulder soft tissue restriction or posterior capsule tightness can accompany anterior shoulder instability. If restriction is present, as determined by the Tyler test[12] and available horizontal adduction ROM,[13] it may lead to

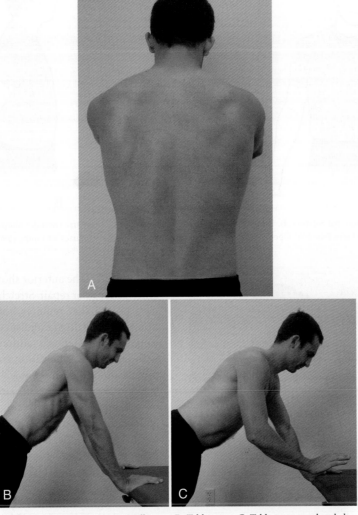

Fig. 4-2 Serratus press: **A,** Wall press. **B,** Table press. **C,** Table press one-handed.

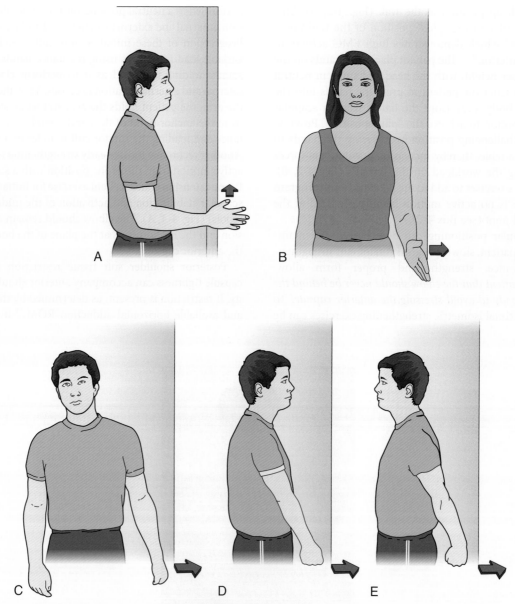

Fig. 4-3 **A,** Isometric shoulder internal rotation. **B,** Isometric shoulder external rotation. **C,** Isometric shoulder abduction. **D,** Isometric shoulder flexion. **E,** Isometric shoulder extension. (From Jobe FW: Operative techniques in upper extremity sports injuries, St Louis, 1996, Mosby.)

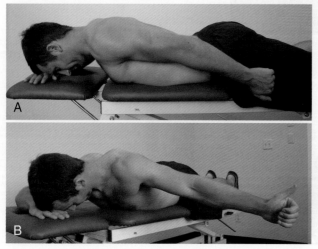

Fig. 4-4 Prone: **A,** Extension. **B,** Horizontal abduction.

aggravation of the anterior shoulder structures and stress the anterior capsular repair. Stretching the posterior capsule may be a project that requires both manual interventions and home self-stretching exercises over the course of many weeks to normalize. Manually address posterior capsule tightness with soft tissue mobilization and anterior-posterior GH joint mobilizations.[14,15] The physical therapist should take care to avoid excessive compression forces on the anterior shoulder with hand-holds because this can be very painful for the patient. Cross-body stretching of the posterior capsule can be included in the home program if appropriate for the patient (Fig. 4-5).[16,17]

Grade II manual GH mobilizations in the anterior-posterior and cephalad/caudad directions can be used for pain management[18] and to prevent excessive adhesion formation during this phase.[14]

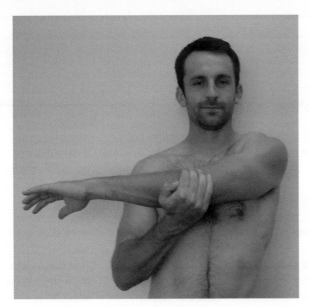

Fig. 4-5 Cross-body stretch.

Nighttime discomfort may continue to be a problem and the therapist can advise the patient regarding sleeping positions. Pillow support under the elbow maintains the shoulder in the scapular plane while sleeping and reduces stress on the anterior capsule. Pillows should not be placed under the shoulder directly because this forces the scapula into a more protracted and anteriorly tipped position.

Phase II

TIME: 4 weeks to 8 weeks (Table 4-3)
GOALS:

- Full ROM is expected by 8 weeks.
- Progress dynamic scapular stabilization and rotator cuff strengthening exercises.
- Return to ADLs and functional activities that do not stress the anterior capsule.

Physiologically, the healing tissue is well advanced into the proliferative/fibroblastic stage during this phase.[1-3] There is an abundance of collagen fibers in the region and the surgical repair has fair integrity. At a cellular level, the goal of physical therapy is to align these collagen fibers in the proper orientation along lines of normal stress.[15] This phase is the optimal time period for elongating tissue with a progressively lessening amount of risk for damage. Moving the arm through a large pain-free range of motion will allow appropriate stresses to the healing tissue, resulting in an optimal outcome.

Typical manual muscle testing and active range of motion assessment in all directions are appropriate at this time. Include strength testing of the rotator cuff and scapular stabilizers to be certain all aspects of the kinetic chain are progressing as required. **Do not force motion into extension, external rotation, or horizontal abduction to avoid stretching the anterior capsule.**

Functional mobility begins to return during this phase. Overhead reaching into flexion typically is the most comfortable direction and most easily regained after surgery. Often, patients continue to complain of pain with functional activities involving extension and external rotation, such as putting on a jacket. The patient should have full PROM and nearly full AROM by two months following surgery with the exception of external rotation, which may lack approximately 10°.[20] Slowly begin exercises that gently stretch the anterior capsule through the active range rather than forcing a stretch by passive manual interventions, for example, wand scaption or external rotation. If by 6 weeks postsurgery a deficit in external rotation of 25° or larger remains, incorporate more aggressive manual techniques or self-stretching exercises to regain full motion. It is the authors' opinion that a 5° to 10° loss of external rotation in a neutral position and at 90° of abduction at 8 weeks postoperative is not uncommon and not detrimental to the final outcome. The surgical reconstruction will continue to stretch over the next 2 to 4 months. Keep in mind that the goal of the surgery was to decrease pathologic laxity. Aggressively stretching the repair site can put the patient back into their preoperative state of excessive laxity and should be avoided during this phase. The patient should continue with ROM exercises at home as needed (see Box 4-2).

During this phase, emphasis must be on proper dynamic scapulothoracic and scapulohumeral rhythm. Allowing excessive motion at the glenohumeral joint as a compensation for improper scapulothoracic motion can overstress the anterior capsule and the repair. It is best to observe scapulothoracic and scapulohumeral rhythm with the patient shirtless to ensure proper mechanics are present before advancing the program. The scapular slide test,[21] although inconsistently validated in the literature, can be used as an assessment tool early in the rehabilitation process to quantify gross differences in scapular motion. The physical therapist measures the distance from the inferior angle of the scapula to the midline of the thoracic spine at the level of the inferior angle of the scapula. The measurements should be symmetrical for the involved and uninvolved shoulders at zero degrees hands at sides, 45° hands on hips, and 90° of abduction with internal rotation. Assess the quality of the motion in addition to the quantity of motion. The goal is to have a smooth contraction and appropriate firing patterns on both the concentric and eccentric phases of motion. A jerky pattern with visible muscle fasciculations would be considered abnormal and needs to be addressed before progressing into more difficult exercises.

Proper function of the serratus anterior muscle is critical to normal shoulder function and is essential if the patient is to avoid an external impingement problem. Progress the serratus press exercise into one-handed stabilization at table height (see Fig. 4-2, *C*). Further progression moves to the floor in a kneeling plank position (Fig. 4-6, *A*), and finally a full plank position on the floor (Fig. 4-6, *B*). The serratus dynamic hug below 90° of elevation is an excellent progression into functional through range serratus activation[10] (Fig. 4-7).

TABLE 4-3 Anterior Capsular Reconstruction

Rehabilitation Phase	Criteria to Progress to This Phase	Anticipated Impairments and Functional Limitations	Intervention	Goal	Rationale
Phase II Postoperative 4-8 wk • Cautious ROM and initial strengthening	• Strong, tonic isometric muscle activation • Independent with scapular positioning and stability for initial prone and side-lying exercises • Pain controlled with medication or modalities • No loss of ROM	• Limited ROM • Limited strength • Limited tolerance of UE for reach, lift, and carry activities	• **Modalities:** • Continue modalities as needed by pain and edema • **AAROM:** As needed • **AROM:** • Continue phase I as needed • Shoulder—Flexion, scaption, ER and IR to tolerance • **Isotonics:** • Continue phase I as needed • Scapular stabilization: serratus press progression on wall>table>floor>(4-4c) one handed • Plank: knees>full (4-8A, 4-8B) • Scapular retraction—prone row extension • Scapular protraction/upward rotation • Dynamic hug below 90° • 4 wk: prone extension and row; through range ER/IR • 6 wk: prone horizontal abduction; OKC in side-lying ER, IR, abduction, horizontal flexion • 8 wk: OKC flexion, scaption; resistance bands for ER and IR • UBE, initiate with involved arm being passive • **Manual Intervention:** • Soft tissue mobilization • GH and ST mobilization • PNF patterns in diagonals and functional positions	• **Modalities:** • Manage pain and edema • **AAROM/AROM:** • Full shoulder AROM by 8 wk • Possible limitation of 10° in external rotation is expected • **Isotonics:** • Good scapular control in standing and prone and closed chain positions • Prone, side-lying, and standing exercises: good form maintained through 3×20 repetitions • Standing OKC: good form maintained through 3×10 repetitions • **Manual Intervention:** • Maximize ROM • Maximize mechanical alignment • **Function:** • Independent for self-care and ADLs at and above head height without pain • Strength 60%-70% • Lift 5 lb • Participation in core, lower body strengthening, and cardio program	• **Modalities:** • Minimize edema to minimize discomfort and inhibitory effects on local musculature • **AAROM/AROM:** • Shoulder—Progress with ROM quickly but safely • Avoid excessive stress on the anterior capsule as indicated by discomfort • **Isotonics:** • Scapular control is required to advance into more challenging rotator cuff and functional exercises • Progressively challenge the scapular stabilizers, rotator cuff, and prime movers to build strength and endurance • **Manual Intervention:** • Decrease mechanical barriers preventing normal ROM and strength • **Function:** • Minimize dependency for functional activities • Maintain fitness to minimize losses

AAROM, active-assisted range of motion; *ADLs,* activities of daily living; *AROM,* active range of motion; *ER,* external rotation; *GH,* glenohumeral; *OKC,* open kinetic chain; *PNF,* propioceptive neuromuscular facilitation; *ROM,* range of motion; *ST,* scapulothoracic; *UBE,* upper body ergometer; *UE,* Upper extremity.

Prone horizontal abduction (see Fig. 4-4, *B*) and prone row (Fig. 4-8) target the middle and lower trapezius muscles[22] and posterior rotator cuff.[23] Begin with AROM only to retrain proper scapular control and progress to light weight to increase the demand on the muscle. Because the patient is retrained in a manner minimizing risk to the anterior shoulder, these are excellent exercises for building muscle endurance.

Once dynamic scapular control is achieved, advance with more specific rotator cuff muscle-strengthening exercises. Side-lying external rotation,[23] abduction, and horizontal forward flexion,[24] all limited to body plane range of motion, require more dynamic scapular stability while maintaining a safe range of motion for the shoulder. Watch carefully to ensure excessive scapular adduction and trunk rotation do not substitute for proper stabilization by the middle and lower trapezius.

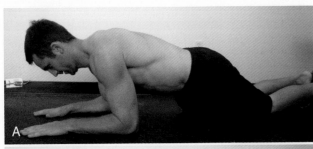

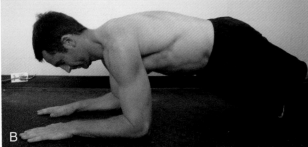

Fig. 4-6 Plank: **A,** Kneeling half plank. **B,** Full plank.

Progress to through-range external and internal rotation with resistance bands, emphasizing scapular stability to ensure proper rotator cuff activation.[25,26] Use an axillary towel roll to reinforce proper positioning, increase muscle activation, and to improve synergistic function of the adductors and external rotators.[23]

Begin open kinetic chain exercises in standing, including shoulder scaption in a full can position,[23] flexion, and abduction using gravity as resistance. These exercises can be used to train proper scapulohumeral rhythm through AROM and are less effective for specific muscle strengthening. Add light-weight or resistance bands as movement patterns, scapular stability, and overall strength increase. Poor eccentric control and scapular winging tend to be limiting factors in progression with added resistance.

The upper body ergometer (UBE) may be incorporated early in rehab. Initially the involved arm is passive to focus on mobility, with the uninvolved arm doing the majority of the work. An easy five-minute program alternates forward and backward revolutions at a comfortable pace. With repeated use, the involved arm may begin to participate more as tolerance allows, progressively increasing the effort until the patient is predominantly using the involved arm by 2 months postoperation.

If anterior shoulder pain, a protracted scapula,[27] or an anteriorly translated humeral head are noted, reassess for possible restriction in the posterior shoulder. If capsular or muscular restriction is present, incorporate more aggressive manual interventions and home exercises. Grade IV+ posterior mobilizations in varying angles of humeral flexion and rotation may be indicated to redress this dysfunction and normalize mechanics.[14] The sleeper stretch (Fig. 4-9) is a good home exercise to improve the extensibility of the posterior capsule.[17,28] Additionally, the excursion and pliability of the subscapularis muscle often becomes restricted

following surgery and prevents the patient from regaining full range of motion. Gentle soft tissue mobilization can ease this restriction, allowing the patient to actively move into increased range.

Phase III

TIME: 2 to 3 months (Table 4-4)
GOALS:
- Full range of motion in all directions
- Progressive strengthening with resistance in all planes of motion
- Normal functional tasks without limitations with the exception of sports

Physiologically, the capsular tissue is progressing out of the proliferative/fibroblastic stage and into the remodeling/maturation stage.[1-3] As the collagen tissue matures, it becomes more resilient to stress, therefore more stress can be placed on the capsule without risk of damage. Because of this increasing tissue strength, the window of opportunity to increase ROM is closing during this phase. Be certain you have achieved the desired ROM, otherwise it may be very hard to regain later.

The primary goal of the third postoperative month of physical therapy is strengthening throughout the full active range of motion. The patient may add resistance to an exercise when (1) the motion can be performed with proper scapulohumeral and scapulothoracic motion patterns; (2) he or she can demonstrate good eccentric control through the range of motion; and (3) such motion is pain-free.

It is necessary to perform break testing in all planes of motion, including end range, to assess functional strength. Performing manual muscle tests only in neutral positions is not a sufficient assessment to ensure adequate functional strength and endurance in athletes. If weakness is present in overhead positions, many overhead athletes will be unable to regain all necessary function.

Adequate strength of the serratus anterior is critical to maintain scapular protraction and to prevent scapular winging throughout open and closed kinetic chain activities.[6] Concentric and eccentric control must be evaluated during all exercises. A modified minirange push-up plus with a narrow grip and elbows hugged tightly to the body can be the next step in strengthening.[11] Begin these on the wall and progress to table height, then the floor. Do not jeopardize the anterior capsule by progressing too quickly. **Patients should not be performing normal full range push-ups at this time, as the tensile strength of the healing tissue is inadequate. Many athletes view a push-up as a gold-standard of functional strength and will strive to return to push-ups too quickly, leading to pain or damage in the shoulder.** The serratus also functions to upwardly rotate and posteriorly tip the scapula when the arm is overhead.[29] Use wall slides to train overhead motion, with the emphasis on pushing the hands into the wall and the body away from the wall (Fig. 4-10).[30] Once the motor pattern is learned, progress into a serratus punch at a 120° elevation

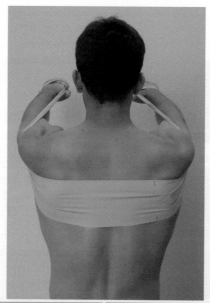

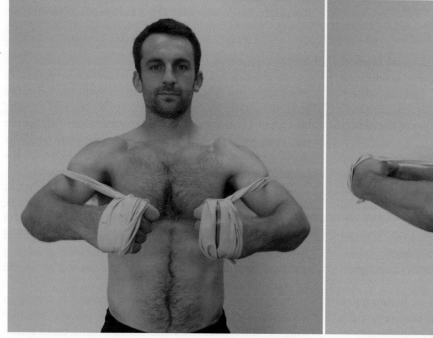
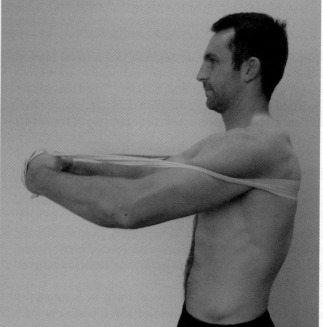

Fig. 4-7 Serratus dynamic hug below 90° elevation.

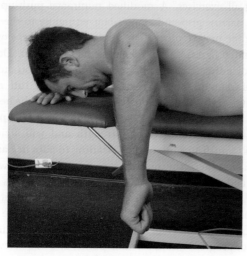

Fig. 4-8 Prone row.

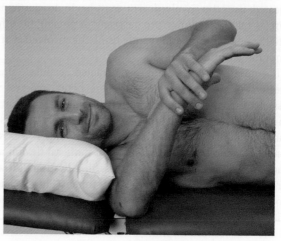

Fig. 4-9 Sleeper stretch.

TABLE 4-4 Anterior Capsular Reconstruction

Rehabilitation Phase	Criteria to Progress to This Phase	Anticipated Impairments and Functional Limitations	Intervention	Goal	Rationale
Phase III Postoperative 2-3 months • Progressive strengthening	• Maintain full ROM in all planes with possible exception of 10° loss of ER • Independent with proper scapular positioning and stability for initial prone, side-lying, and standing exercises • Execute 3×20 repetitions of prone and side-lying exercises and 3×10 repetitions of standing OKC exercises with proper form	• Limited strength for overhead activities • Limited strength for lift and carry activities • Not participating in UE sports	• **Modalities:** • Continue modalities as needed • **AROM:** • Continue phase II as needed for ER loss if present • **Isotonics:** • Continue phase II • Advance scapular stabilization with closed chain exercises: narrow push-up, wall slides, serratus punch at 120° • 8 wk: prone full can • 10 wk: supraspinatus punch; prone row with ER • 12 wk: resisted eccentric ER, IR • UBE: progress into one arm • Initiate strengthening of bicep, tricep, latissimus, deltoid, and pectoral muscles when scapular stability allows • **Manual Intervention:** • Soft tissue and GH mobilization as needed • PNF patterns in diagonals and functional positions with increased speed and resistance	• **Modalities:** • Manage pain • **AROM:** • Full shoulder AROM all directions by 12 wk • **Isotonics:** • Good scapular control and proper form for all prone, side-lying, and standing exercises: 3×20 repetitions • **Manual Intervention:** • Maximize ROM • Maximize mechanical alignment • **Function:** • Independent with ADLs above head height without pain • Strength 80% • Carry 5 lb • Participation in core, lower body strengthening, and cardio program	• **Modalities:** • Minimize discomfort • **AROM:** • Normalized capsular excursion in all planes • **Isotonics:** Add resistance to an exercise when: —Demonstrate proper SH and ST motion pattern —Demonstrate good eccentric control —Exercise is pain free at current level • Scapular control in CKC and overhead positions is critical for normal athletic participation and to avoid impingement • Progressively challenge the scapular stabilizers, rotator cuff, and prime movers to build strength and endurance • **Manual Intervention:** • Normalize GH and ST mechanics • Window for gaining capsular excursion closes during this phase • Increase tolerance of anterior shoulder muscles to movement • **Function:** • Maximize functional activities in an effort to return patient to previous level of function

ADLs, activities of daily living; *AROM,* active range of motion; *CKC,* closed kinetic chain; *ER,* external rotation; *GH,* glenohumeral; *IR,* internal rotation; *OKC,* open kinetic chain; *PNF,* propioceptive neuromuscular facilitation; *ROM,* range of motion; *SH,* scapulohumeral; *ST,* scapulothoracic; *UBE,* upper-body ergometer; *UE,* Upper extremity.

(Fig. 4-11) which demonstrates high EMG activity through a functional overhead motion.[10]

Lower and middle trapezius muscle strength and endurance are progressed by moving the arm into different planes of motion. Prone full can (Fig. 4-12) emphasizes the lower trapezius while a prone row emphasizes the middle trapezius.[22] Prone rows can be progressed by adding external rotation into the 90°/90° position (Fig. 4-13) when strength and eccentric control of the scapular stabilizers and rotator cuff

are adequate. *Avoid pain at end range external rotation because this is a position that stresses the anterior capsule.*

Progress rotator cuff exercises described above by increasing either resistance or repetitions. Given their role as dynamic glenohumeral stabilizers[31,32] we must consider the rotator cuff muscles as muscles of endurance rather than power and focus on lighter weight with more repetition. This is a more appropriate training strategy than using heavier weight and fewer repetitions. The supraspinatus punch in

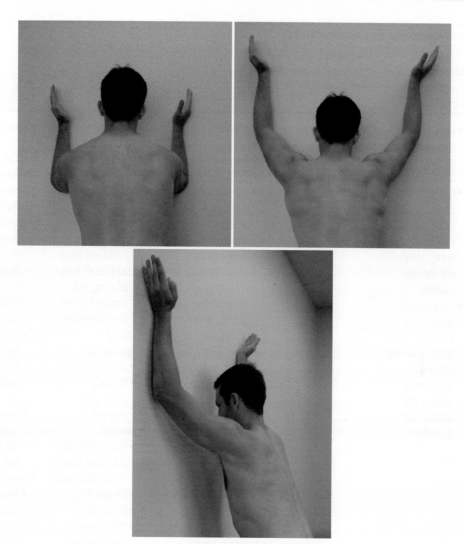

Fig. 4-10 Wall slide overhead.

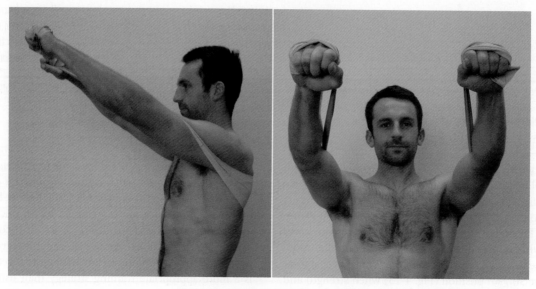

Fig. 4-11 Serratus punch at 120° elevation.

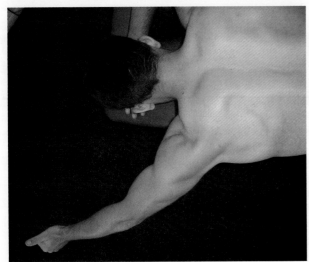

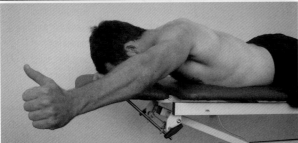

Fig. 4-12 Prone full can.

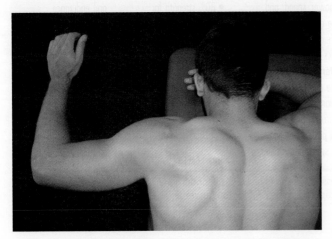

Fig. 4-13 Prone row with external rotation into 90°/90° position.

Strengthening of the biceps, triceps, latissimus dorsi, deltoid, and pectoral muscles becomes more important once the therapist is certain there is adequate strength and endurance of the rotator cuff muscles and scapular stabilizers. Athletes often push toward lifting heavy weights for these larger muscle groups, yet progressing with light to medium weights is more appropriate. Remember that it has been several months since the last true training session was possible and the rotator cuff and scapular muscles must provide the necessary stability to the shoulder complex. Allowing a patient to return to 45 lb bicep curls on the first attempt simply because that is "what I was lifting before surgery" will cause shoulder discomfort.

Progress the UBE to using only the involved arm with emphasis on endurance training and increased speed.

Phase IV

TIME: 3 to 4 months (Table 4-5)
GOALS:

- Continue with progressive strengthening exercises into functional range of motion based on anticipated sports or work demands
- Initiate a return to an overhead sports training program at approximately 4 months postoperatively

While tissue remodeling continues, we can be confident the surgical repair is strong and can tolerate increasing stresses. We become less and less concerned about damaging the surgical repair as time goes on. Full range of motion is expected at this time. Functionally, the patient should feel normal with the exception of overall gross power for heavier lifting and endurance for longer duration activities. Overhead sports and work specific activities likely remain challenging from a strength and endurance perspective.

Consider sport-specific activities and positional requirements to identify ongoing impairments that need continued attention. Have the patient move through patterns of motion similar to their sport, without speed or load. If the patient is a pitcher, assess objective ability and subjective tolerance to the cocking position of the arm, then with the full body pitching motion before allowing him or her to throw a ball. If the patient is a volleyball player, mimic the serving and blocking motions starting with just the arm and progressing into slow, purposeful full body motion. Look for the ability to control the concentric and eccentric phases of motion. Question the patient about any pain, restriction, or weakness with the action. Use this information to guide the next several weeks of treatment ensuring that the patient is ready to transition to sport-specific training at 4 months postoperation.

Advance serratus anterior strength with planks or walkouts on an exercise ball (Fig. 4-14), and continue to emphasize scapular protraction and upward rotation throughout the exercise. Pressing from a plank into a pike position (Fig. 4-15) on the floor will train closed chain overhead serratus control. Pikes can be performed using a stability ball (Fig. 4-16) and are a very challenging high-level exercise,

midrange in the scapular plane is a good method of initiating overhead strengthening.[10] Supine internal and external rotation with the arm positioned in 45° to 90° of abduction using resistance bands allows for a safe progression of range by moving the arm into more functional positions.

PNF continues to be a valuable manual tool in this patient population. The therapist can use PNF patterns to strengthen muscles in terminal ranges of motion, as well as for gross motor patterning throughout the range of motion.[7] Minimal resistance is applied to focus the effort on proper muscle firing patterns more than gross power or speed.

TABLE 4-5 Anterior Capsular Reconstruction

Rehabilitation Phase	Criteria to Progress to This Phase	Anticipated Impairments and Functional Limitations	Intervention	Goal	Rationale

Phase IV Postoperative 3-4 months
 • Functional and eccentric strengthening
	• Full shoulder AROM all directions by 12 wk
	 • Good scapular control and proper form for all prone, side-lying, and standing exercises: 3×20 repetitions
	 • Independent with ADLs above head height without pain
	 • Strength 80%
	 • Carry 5 lb
		• Limited strength and endurance of UE
		 • Unable to perform sustained or repetitive reaching and overhead activities
		 • Limited tolerance to carrying objects
			• **Modalities:**
			   • As needed after exercise
			 • **AROM:**
			   • Maintenance stretching
			 • **Isotonics:**
			   • Continue phase III
			   • Advance scapular stabilization exercises: floor/ball plank, floor/ball pike, table height push-up plus
			   • Overhead OKC for eccentric control
			   • Sustained overhead endurance work
			   • Eccentric strengthening rotator cuff in functional positions
			   • Advance power training of prime movers of the shoulder girdle
			 • **Sport-Specific Strengthening:**
			   • Strengthening in related positions
			   • Address power, speed, and endurance components of specific training
			   • Plyometrics
			 • **Manual Intervention:**
			   • Soft tissue and GH mobilization as needed
			   • PNF patterns in diagonals and functional positions with increased speed and resistance
				• **Modalities:**
				   • Manage pain
				 • **AROM:**
				   • No deficits
				 • **Isotonics:**
				   • Good scapular control and proper form for all prone, side-lying, and standing exercises: 3×20 repetitions
				   • 90% strength throughout shoulder complex and core
				 • **Manual Intervention:**
				   • Maximize ROM
				   • Maximize mechanical alignment
				 • **Function:**
				   • Gross strength 90%
				   • 80% strength for overhead lifting
				   • 90% strength for carrying below shoulder height
				   • Initiate return to sport programs
					• **Modalities:**
					   • Minimize discomfort
					 • **AROM:**
					   • Normalized capsular excursion in all planes
					 • **Isotonics:** Add resistance to an exercise when:
					   —Demonstrate proper SH and ST motion pattern
					   —Demonstrate good eccentric control
					   —Exercise is pain free at current level
					   • Scapular control in CKC and overhead positions is critical for normal athletic participation and to avoid impingement
					   • Progressively challenge the scapular stabilizers, rotator cuff and prime movers to build strength and endurance
					 • **Manual Intervention:**
					   • Maintenance of ROM as needed as patient returns to sports
					 • **Function:**
					   • Maximize functional activities in an effort to return patient to previous level of function

ADLs, activities of daily living; *AROM,* active range of motion; *CKC,* closed kinetic chain; *GH,* glenohumeral; *OKC,* open kinetic chain; *PNF,* propioceptive neuromuscular facilitation; *ROM,* range of motion; *SH,* scapulohumeral; *ST,* scapulothors acic; *UE,* Upper extremity.

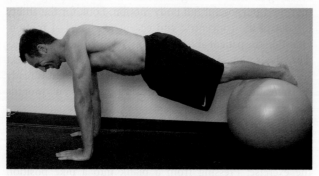

Fig. 4-14 Stability ball walk-out.

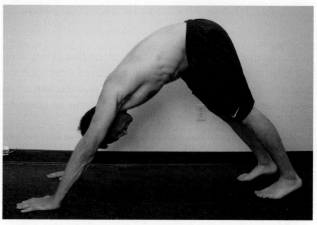

Fig. 4-15 Pike press on the floor.

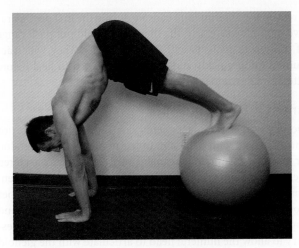

Fig. 4-16 Pike press on stability ball.

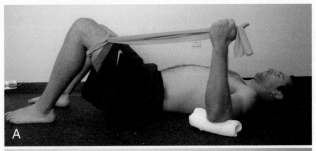

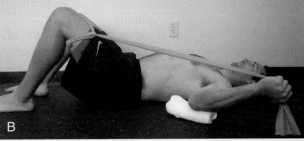

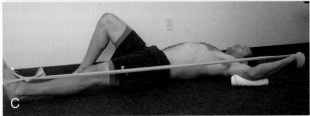

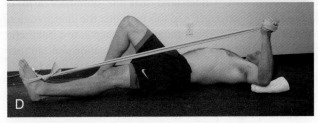

Fig. 4-17 Eccentric external rotation. **A,** Start. **B,** Loading into 90°/90° position. **C,** Loading with lower extremity extension. **D,** Eccentric control to return to start position.

which may be appropriate for only the strongest individuals near the end of this phase of rehab. Full-range, overhead, open kinetic chain exercises, such as forward flexion, full can, and supraspinatus press, can be used to train eccentric control of the scapula as the arm is lowered to the side. This is more of a neuromuscular retraining exercise than a true strength building exercise. Again, assess the quality of motion, not simply the quantity of motion or weight lifted.

If the patient is an overhead athlete or worker, endurance for maintaining the arms overhead can be critical to returning to these activities. Bounce a light ball, gym ball, or medicine ball overhead for 30 to 60 seconds, focusing on scapular stability in a retracted, posteriorly tipped, and upwardly rotated position.

It is essential to achieve good eccentric control of the rotator cuff muscles before returning to sports activity. This is particularly important when working with overhead athletes since the posterior rotator cuff is responsible for the eccentric deceleration of the arm in activities such as throwing, serving, or hitting.[33,34] Therapist-assisted prone external rotation can be used for eccentric strengthening of the posterior rotator cuff. A heavier but controllable weight is selected, and the therapist helps the patient preposition the arm into the 90°/90° position, then releases the weight, forcing the patient to control the weight in the negative direction. To eccentrically strengthen internal rotation, have the patient lie supine and perform the same therapist-assisted 90°/90° exercise. A home exercise for eccentric posterior rotator cuff strengthening is performed with resistance bands. The patient lies supine with a resistance band tied to the foot and the band wrapped around the hand (Fig. 4-17, *A*). The arm is positioned at 90° abduction in neutral rotation. With the band slack, the arm is externally rotated into the 90°/90° position, the thumb pointing toward the floor (Fig. 4-17, *B*). The leg is extended tensioning the band, while maintaining the arm in the 90°/90° position (Fig. 4-17, *C*). Slowly, the arm is returned to the neutral starting position in a controlled manner creating eccentric loading of the posterior cuff (Fig. 4-17, *D*).

Increase the speed and resistance applied when performing PNF patterns.[7] Speed work into internal and external rotation in multiple planes in both the concentric and eccentric directions is effective training for overhead activities. Sports such as volleyball, tennis, swimming, water polo, and throwing sports can benefit greatly from D1/D2 patterning into end ranges of motion. These exercises can also be performed with resistance bands and transitioned into sport-specific warm-up drills as the patient progresses toward independence.

Power training for the deltoids, biceps, triceps, latissimus dorsi, and pectoral muscles becomes more important in this last phase of therapy before returning to sports activity. Whereas the rotator cuff and scapular stabilizers are control and endurance muscles, the prime movers of the arm are the power muscles.[33-35] Incorporate lat pull-downs, bicep curls, tricep extensions, and rows into the program with heavier weight and fewer repetitions.

Phase V

TIME: 4 to 6 months (Table 4-6)
GOALS:
- Return to sports or work
- Avoid recurrence of shoulder pain

At this time, many patients have returned to normal activities including sports played below shoulder height or sports demanding very little of the upper extremity. Overhead athletes must have adequate strength and endurance to transition into sport-specific training.

Plyometrics are a critical part of rehabilitation for athletes. Ball toss to a trampoline while in tall kneel, half kneel, or standing can mimic required motions for sports. Playing catch with a light medicine ball allows concentric and eccentric training of the throwing motion. While lying prone the patient catches the ball in the 90°/90° position, eccentrically lowering the ball to 90° abduction with neutral rotation, then tosses the ball back to the therapist by externally rotating the arm back to the 90°/90° position. For larger motion patterns, throw a 5 to 10 lb medicine ball against a wall in a chest pass, side pass, or overhead toss. There is no limit to the options for ball related plyometrics that can be very sport-specific.

Isokinetic strength measurement is an excellent way to determine overall power and endurance compared with the uninvolved arm. Understand that the dominant arm is expected to be stronger, and this may alter the interpretation of strength testing. The authors of this chapter test isokinetic strength at 120° per second for internal rotation and 240° per second for external rotation. **Sport-specific training begins when the involved arm demonstrates 70% to 80% strength of the uninvolved arm.**

Sport-specific programs are indicated in Boxes 4-3 through 4-6.

TROUBLESHOOTING

Misapprehending Tissue Quality

Patients with "normal" or tight connective tissue must work early and diligently to reacquire motion, while avoiding stress on the anterior joint capsule during the first postoperative month. Conversely, the therapist should not push range of motion in patients with hyperelasticity. They will reacquire motion quickly and should be allowed to heal before attempting extremes of motion.

Anterior Shoulder Pain

Despite surgery, some patients continue to have anterior shoulder pain with palpation of the proximal biceps tendon or transverse humeral ligament. This may be considered "leftover inflammation." Although the structural problem has been rectified surgically, the residual inflammation does not disappear overnight. Assess the posterior cuff and capsule for adequate tissue length. Stretching may be necessary to allow the humeral head to articulate with the glenoid at its normal contact point, which will eliminate stress on the anterior structures and allow the irritation to resolve. The therapist can use modalities to reduce discomfort at the clinic and the patient should follow through at home with a cryotherapy routine.

Posterior Shoulder Pain

Many patients note pain in the posterior shoulder, especially with activity that requires elevation above 120° and motion that requires horizontal abduction posterior to the frontal plane. Another potentially difficult motion is hyperextension posterior to the plane of the body. Occasionally, patients develop a tendinopathy of the rotator cuff external rotators, specifically the teres minor, which may be treated symptomatically. The therapist may note pain on palpation of the posterior cuff insertion, the posterior capsule, or the proximal third of the axillary border of the scapula, as well as decreased extensibility of the posterior structures, which may affect the alignment of the humeral head in the glenoid. Treat accordingly with modalities, stretching, and progressive strengthening.

Insufficient Range of Motion

If too much time elapses after surgery before the patient regains normal motion, capsular adhesion may

Rehabilitation Phase	Criteria to Progress to This Phase	Anticipated Impairments and Functional Limitations	Intervention	Goal	Rationale
Phase V Postoperative 4 months and beyond • Return to sport	• Good concentric and eccentric control for all isotonic exercises • 90% strength throughout shoulder complex and core • Gross strength 90% • Strength for carrying below shoulder height 90% • Strength for overhead lifting 80%	• Decreased endurance for sport-specific activities	• Continue phase IV as needed • Push-up on floor • Isokinetics for internal and external rotation at 200 degree/sec • Sport-specific drills when strength is 80%-90% (see Chapter 13)	• Return to sports	• Strengthen and improve endurance of shoulder muscles using high-speed resistance training • Return to sport or activity safely and without injury

TABLE 4-6 Anterior Capsular Reconstruction

BOX 4-3 Rehabilitation Throwing Program for Pitchers*

Step 1: Toss the ball (no windup) against a wall on alternate days. Start with 25 to 30 throws, build up to 70 throws, and gradually increase the throwing distance.

Number of Throws	Distance (ft)
20	20 (warm-up)
25-40	30-40
10	20 (cool down)

Step 2: Toss the ball (playing catch with easy windup) on alternate days.

Number of Throws	Distance (ft)
10	20 (warm-up)
10	30-40
30-40	50
10	20-30 (cool down)

Step 3: Continue increasing the throwing distance while still tossing the ball with an easy windup.

Number of Throws	Distance (ft)
10	20 (warm-up)
10	30-40
30-40	50-60
10	30 (cool down)

Step 4: Increase throwing distance to a maximum of 60 feet. Continue tossing the ball with an occasional throw at no more than one half speed.

Number of Throws	Distance (ft)
10	30 (warm-up)
10	40-45
30-40	60-70
10	30 (cool down)

Step 5: During this step, gradually increase the distance to 150 feet maximum.

Phase 5-1

Number of Throws	Distance (ft)
10	40 (warm-up)
10	50-60
15-20	70-80
10	50-60
10	40 (cool down)

Phase 5-2

Number of Throws	Distance (ft)
10	40 (warm-up)
10	50-60
20-30	80-90
20	50-60
10	40 (cool down)

Phase 5-3

Number of Throws	Distance (ft)
10	40 (warm-up)
10	60
15-20	100-110
20	60
10	40 (cool down)

Phase 5-4

Number of Throws	Distance (ft)
10	40 (warm-up)
10	60
15-20	120-150
20	60
10	40 (cool down)

Step 6: Progress to throwing off the mound at one half to three fourths speed. Try to use proper body mechanics, especially when throwing off the mound:
- Stay on top of the ball.
- Keep the elbow up.
- Throw over the top.
- Follow through with the arm and trunk.
- Use the legs to push.

Phase 6-1

Number of Throws	Distance (ft)
10	60 (warm-up)
10	120-150 (lobbing)
30	45 (off the mound)
10	60 (off the mound)
10	40 (cool down)

Phase 6-2

Number of Throws	Distance (ft)
10	50 (warm-up)
10	120-150 (lobbing)
20	45 (off the mound)
20	60 (off the mound)
10	40 (cool down)

Continued

BOX 4-3 Rehabilitation Throwing Program for Pitchers—cont'd

Phase 6-3

Number of Throws	Distance (ft)
10	50 (warm-up)
10	60
10	120-150 (lobbing)
10	45 (off the mound)
30	60 (off the mound)
10	40 (cool down)

Phase 6-4

Number of Throws	Distance (ft)
10	50 (warm-up)
10	120-150 (lobbing)
10	45 (off the mound)
40-50	60 (off the mound)
10	40 (cool down)

At this time, if the pitcher has successfully completed phase 6-4 without pain or discomfort and is throwing approximately three fourths speed, then the pitching coach and trainer may allow the pitcher to proceed to step 7: up-down bullpens. Up-down bullpens is used to simulate a game. The pitcher rests between a series of pitches to reproduce the rest period between innings.

Step 7: Up-down bullpens: (one half to three fourths speed)

Day 1

Number of Throws	Distance (ft)
10 warm-up throws	120-150 (lobbing)
10 warm-up throws	60 (off the mound)
40 pitches	60 (off the mound)
Rest 10 minutes	
20 pitches	60 (off the mound)

Day 2

Off

Day 3

Number of Throws	Distance (ft)
10 warm-up throws	120-150 (lobbing)
10 warm-up throws	60 (off the mound)
30 pitches	60 (off the mound)
Rest 10 minutes	
10 warm-up throws	60 (off the mound)
20 pitches	60 (off the mound)
Rest 10 minutes	
10 warm-up throws	60 (off the mound)
20 pitches	60 (off the mound)

Day 4

Off

Day 5

Number of Throws	Distance (ft)
10 warm-up throws	120-150 (lobbing)
10 warm-up throws	60 (off the mound)
30 pitches	60 (off the mound)
Rest 8 minutes	
20 pitches	60 (off the mound)
Rest 8 minutes	
20 pitches	60 (off the mound)
Rest 8 minutes	
20 pitches	60 (off the mound)

At this point the pitcher is ready to begin a normal routine, from throwing batting practice to pitching in the bullpen. This program can and should be adjusted as needed by the trainer or physical therapist. Each step may take more or less time than listed, and the trainer, physical therapist, and physician should monitor the program. The pitcher should remember that it is necessary to work hard but not overdo it.

---

*Patients start at the step that is appropriate for them. Postsurgical patients begin at step 1. Patients progress depending on the maintenance of their pain-free status and their strength and endurance.
From Jobe FW: Operative techniques in upper extremity sports injuries, St Louis, 1996, Mosby.

develop, permanently limiting the total motion available in the shoulder. The best defense for this problem is a good offense: the physical therapist should know the patient's tissue type and encourage motion early if appropriate. As noted earlier, normal ROM differs for different patients and a very carefully planned stretching program should be implemented based on the patient's tissue type and functional requirements. This plan should include manual stretching by the therapist and stretching independently by the patient with a goal of returning the patient to functional

ROM requirements without excessive motion. For example, a baseball pitcher may require 130° of external rotation for function, while most other populations have more modest requirements. **While an athlete does need this amount of external rotation, too much external rotation can lead to instability.** A very narrow margin exists between being able to perform and having a problem. Precisely correct mechanics is crucial to prevent recurrence.

If the patient is having difficulty gaining the last few degrees of shoulder flexion because of pain or stiffness and

BOX 4-4 Rehabilitation Program for Catchers, Infielders, and Outfielders

- Note: Perform each step three times.
- All throws should have an arc or "hump."
- The maximum distance thrown by infielders and catchers is 120 feet.
- The maximum distance thrown by outfielders is 200 feet.

Step 1: Toss the ball with no windup. Stand with your feet shoulder-width apart and face the player to whom you are throwing. Concentrate on rotating and staying on top of the ball.

Number of Throws	Distance (ft)
5	20 (warm-up)
10	30
5	20 (cool down)

Step 2: Stand sideways to the person to whom you are throwing. Feet are shoulder-width apart. Close up and pivot onto your back foot as you throw.

Number of Throws	Distance (ft)
5	30 (warm-up)
5	40
10	50
5	30 (cool down)

Step 3: Repeat the position in step 2. Step toward the target with your front leg and follow through with your back leg.

Number of Throws	Distance (ft)
5	50 (warm-up)
5	60
10	70
5	50 (cool down)

Step 4: Assume the pitcher's stance. Lift and stride with your lead leg. Follow through with your back leg.

Number of Throws	Distance (ft)
5	60 (warm-up)
5	70
10	80
5	60 (cool down)

Step 5: Outfielders: Lead with your glove-side foot forward. Take one step, crow hop, and throw the ball.

Infielders: Lead with your glove-side foot forward. Take a shuffle step and throw the ball. Throw the last five throws in a straight line.

Number of Throws	Distance (ft)
5	70 (warm-up)
5	90
10	100
5	80 (cool down)

Step 6: Use the throwing technique used in step 5. Assume your playing position. Infielders and catchers, do not throw farther than 120 feet. Outfielders, do not throw farther than 150 feet (midoutfield).

Number of Throws	Infielders' and Catchers' Distance (ft)	Outfielders' Distance (ft)
5	80 (warm-up)	80 (warm-up)
5	80-90	90-100
5	90-100	110-125
5	110-120	130-150
5	80 (cool down)	80 (cool down)

Step 7: Infielders, catchers, and outfielders all may assume their playing positions.

Number of Throws	Infielders' and Catchers' Distance (ft)	Outfielders' Distance (ft)
5	80 (warm-up)	80-90 (warm-up)
5	80-90	110-130
5	90-100	150-175
5	110-120	180-200
5	80 (cool down)	90 (cool down)

Step 8: Repeat step 7. Use a fungo bat to hit to the infielders and outfielders while in their normal playing positions.

From Jobe FW: Operative techniques in upper extremity sports injuries, St Louis, 1996, Mosby.

BOX 4-5 Rehabilitation Program for Tennis Players

The following tennis protocol is designed to be performed every other day. Each session should begin with the warm-up exercises below. Continue with your strengthening, flexibility, and conditioning exercises on the days you are not following the tennis protocol.

Warm-Up

Lower extremity:
- Jog four laps around the tennis court.
- Stretches:
- Gastrocnemius
- Achilles tendon
- Hamstring
- Quadriceps
  Upper extremity:
- Shoulder stretches:
- Posterior cuff
- Inferior capsule
- Rhomboid
- Forearm/wrist stretches
- Wrist flexors
- Wrist extensors
  Trunk:
- Side bends
- Extension
- Rotation
  Forehand ground strokes:
- Hit toward the fence on the opposite side of the court.
- Do not worry about getting the ball in the court.
  During all of the strokes listed previously, remember these key steps:
- Bend your knees.
- Turn your body.
- Step toward the ball.
- Hit the ball when it is out in front of you.

Avoid hitting with an open stance because this places undue stress on your shoulder. This is especially more stressful during the forehand stroke if you have had anterior instability or impingement problems. This is also true during the backhand if you have had problems of posterior instability.

On the very first day of these sport-specific drills, start with bouncing the ball and hitting it. Try to bounce the ball yourself and hit it at waist level. This will allow for consistency in the following:
- How the ball comes to you
- Approximating your timing between hits
- Hitting toward a target to ensure follow-through and full extension
- Using the proper mechanics, thereby placing less stress on the anterior shoulder

Week 1

Day 1:
- 25 forehand strokes
- 25 backhand strokes

Day 2:
- If no problems occur after the first-day workout, increase the number of forehand and backhand strokes.
- 50 forehand strokes
- 50 backhand strokes

Day 3:
- 50 forehand strokes (waist level)
- 50 backhand strokes (waist level)
- 25 high forehand strokes
- 25 high backhand strokes

Week 2

Progress to having the ball tossed to you in a timely manner, giving you enough time to recover from your deliberate follow-through (i.e., wait until the ball bounces on the other side of the court before tossing another ball). Always aim the ball at a target or at a spot on the court.

If you are working on basic ground strokes, have someone bounce the ball to you consistently at waist height.

If you are working on high forehands, have the ball bounced to you at shoulder height or higher.

Day 1:
- 25 high forehand strokes
- 50 waist-height forehand strokes
- 50 waist-height backhand strokes
- 25 high backhand strokes

Day 2:
- 25 high forehand strokes
- 50 waist-height forehand strokes
- 50 waist-height backhand strokes
- 25 high backhand strokes

Day 3:
- Alternate hitting the ball crosscourt and down the line, using waist-high and high forehand and backhand strokes.
- 25 high forehand strokes
- 50 waist-height forehand strokes
- 50 waist-height backhand strokes
- 25 high backhand strokes

Week 3

Continue the three-times-per-week schedule. Add regular and high forehand and backhand volleys. At this point you

BOX 4-5 Rehabilitation Program for Tennis Players—cont'd

may begin having someone hit tennis balls to you from a basket of balls. This will allow you to get the feel of the ball as it comes off another tennis racket. Your partner should wait until the ball that you hit has bounced on the other side of the court before hitting another ball to you. This will give you time to emphasize your follow-through and not hurry to return for the next shot. As always, emphasis is placed on proper body mechanics.

Day 1:
- 25 high forehand strokes
- 50 waist-height forehand strokes
- 50 waist-height backhand strokes
- 25 high backhand strokes
- 25 low backhand and forehand volleys
- 25 high backhand and forehand volleys

Day 2:
- Same as day 1, week 3

Day 3:
Same as day 2, week 3, with emphasis on direction (i.e., down the line and crosscourt). Remember, good body mechanics is still a must:
- Keep knees bent.
- Hit the ball on the rise.
- Hit the ball in front of you.
- Turn your body.
- Do not hit the ball with an open stance.
- Stay on the balls of your feet.

Week 4

Day 1:
Continue having your partner hit tennis balls to you from out of a basket. Alternate hitting forehand and backhand strokes with lateral movement along the baseline. Again, emphasis is on good mechanics as described previously.

Alternate hitting the ball down the line and crosscourt. This drill should be done with a full basket of tennis balls (100 to 150 tennis balls).

Follow this drill with high and low volleys using half a basket of tennis balls (50 to 75 balls). This drill also is performed with lateral movement and returning to the middle of the court after the ball is hit.

Your partner should continue allowing enough time for you to return to the middle of the court before hitting the next ball. This is to avoid your rushing the stroke and using faulty mechanics.

Day 2:
Same drill as day 1, week 4

Day 3:
Same drills as day 2, week 4

Week 5

Day 1:
Find a partner able to hit consistent ground strokes (able to hit the ball to the same area consistently [e.g., to your forehand with the ball bouncing about waist height]).

Begin hitting ground strokes with this partner alternating hitting the ball to your backhand and to your forehand. Rally for about 15 minutes, then add volleys with your partner hitting to you from the baseline. Alternate between backhand and forehand volleys and high and low volleys. Continue volleying another 15 minutes. You will have rallied for a total of 30 to 40 minutes.

At the end of the session, practice a few serves while standing along the baseline. First, warm up by shadowing for 1 to 3 minutes. Hold the tennis racquet loosely and swing across your body in a figure eight. Do not swing the racquet hard. When you are ready to practice your serves using a ball, be sure to keep your toss out in front of you, get your racquet up and behind you, bend your knees, and hit up on the ball. Forget about how much power you are generating, and forget about hitting the ball between the service lines. Try hitting the ball as if you are hitting it toward the back fence.

Hit approximately 10 serves from each side of the court. Remember, this is the first time you are serving, so do not try to hit at 100% of your effort.

Day 2:
Same as day 1, week 5, but now increase the number of times you practice your serve. After working on your ground strokes and volleys, return to the baseline and work on your second serve hit up on the ball, bend your knees, follow through, and keep the toss in front of you. This time hit 20 balls from each side of the court (i.e., 20 into the deuce court and 20 into the ad court).

Day 3:
Same as day 2, week 5, with ground strokes, volleys, and serves. Do not add to the serves. Concentrate on the following:
- Bending your knees
- Preparing the racket
- Using footwork
- Hitting the ball out in front of you
- Keeping your eyes on the ball
- Following through
- Getting in position for the next shot
- Keeping the toss in front of you during the serve

The workout should be the same as day 2, but if you emphasize the proper mechanics listed previously, then you should feel as though you had a harder workout than in day 2.

Continued

BOX 4-5 Rehabilitation Program for Tennis Players—cont'd

Week 6

Day 1:

After the usual warm-up program, start with specific ground stroke drills, with you hitting the ball down the line and your partner on the other side hitting the ball crosscourt. This will force you to move quickly on the court. Emphasize good mechanics as mentioned previously.

Perform this drill for 10 to 15 minutes before reversing the direction of your strokes. Now have your partner hit down the line while you hit crosscourt.

Proceed to the next drill with your partner hitting the ball to you. Return balls using a forehand, then a backhand, then a put-away volley. Repeat this sequence for 10 to 15 minutes. End this session by serving 50 balls to the ad court and 50 balls to the deuce court.

Day 2:

Day 2 should be the same as day 1, week 6, plus returning serves from each side of the court (deuce and ad court). End with practicing serves, 50 to each court.

Day 3:

Perform the following sequence: warm-up; crosscourt and down-the-line drills; backhand, forehand, and volley drills; return of serves; and practice serves.

Week 7

Day 1:

Perform the warm-up program. Perform drills as before and practice return of serves. Before practicing serving, work on hitting 10 to 15 overhead shots. Continue emphasizing good mechanics. Add the approach shot to your drills.

Day 2:

Same as day 1, week 7, except double the number of overhead shots (25 to 30 overheads).

Day 3:

Perform warm-up exercises and crosscourt drills. Add the overhead shot to the backhand, forehand, and volley drill, making it the backhand, forehand, volley, and overhead drill.

If you are a serious tennis player, you will want to work on other strokes or other parts of your game. Feel free to gradually add them to your practice and workout sessions. Just as in other strokes, the proper mechanics should be applied to drop volley, slice, heavy topspin, drop shots, and lobs (offensive and defensive).

Week 8

Day 1:

Warm up and play a simulated one-set match. Be sure to take rest periods after every third game. Remember, you will have to concentrate harder on using good mechanics.

Day 2:

Perform another simulated game but with a two-set match.

Day 3:

Perform another simulated game, this time a best-of-three match.

If all goes well, you may make plans to return to your regular workout and game schedule. You also may practice or play if your condition allows it.

From Jobe FW: Operative techniques in upper extremity sports injuries, St Louis, 1996, Mosby.

---

the physical therapist determines the glenohumeral and scapular mobility are normal, the problem may be in the spine. Assess the lower cervical and upper thoracic spine for hypomobility.[36,37] The cervicothoracic junction is required to move into extension during end range shoulder flexion. At times, this region of the spine can become restricted and actually limits functional end range shoulder flexion. Mobilizing the spine into extension restores normal scapulothoracic and cervicothoracic motion and allows terminal functional flexion to be achieved.

Strength and Endurance

Often rehabilitation programs concentrate on increasing strength. However, for most patients, including overhead throwers, endurance is probably much more important to overall function than gross strength. Endurance training is equally important for patients who are hurt on the job. With inadequate endurance, the patient will develop muscle substitution patterns to enable them to continue to perform an activity, which will lead to altered mechanics for a given task

or sport. Such substitutions and alterations are often the forerunners of tissue breakdown. The therapist should prescribe focused strengthening exercises for specific muscle groups based on their functional use for shoulder motion. The scapular upward rotators and the rotator cuff require more endurance training, while the larger prime mover muscles of the shoulder, such as the shoulder flexors, extensors, and abductors, tend to require more power training.

One specific and often overlooked area of concern is scapular anterior tipping and winging with active motion. Often this is a result of weakness or poor endurance in the serratus anterior. It is easily observed during the eccentric phase in open kinetic chain arm motions or in dynamic closed kinetic chain activities such as stability ball walk-outs. This lack of dynamic scapular control leads to excessive stresses throughout the shoulder and may contribute to a recurrence of the original presurgery symptoms. If adequate strength and endurance are present, the patient should be able to raise and lower the arm through a full range of motion while maintaining the scapula flat against the thoracic wall.

BOX 4-6 Rehabilitation Program for Golfers

This sport-specific protocol is designed to be performed every other day. Each session should begin with the warm-up exercises outlined here. Continue the strengthening, flexibility, and conditioning exercises on the days you are not playing or practicing golf. Advance one stage every 2 to 4 weeks, depending on the severity of the shoulder problem, as each stage becomes pain-free in execution.

Warm-Up

Lower extremities: jog or walk briskly around the practice green area three or four times; stretch the hamstrings, quadriceps, and Achilles tendon.

Upper extremities: stretch the shoulder (i.e., posterior cuff, inferior cuff, rhomboid) and wrist flexors and extensors.

Trunk: do side bends, extension, and rotation stretching exercises.

Stage 1

Putt	50	3 times/week
Medium long	0	0 times/week
Long	0	0 times/week

Stage 2

Putt	50	3 times/week
Medium long	20	2 times/week
Long	0	0 times/week

Stage 3

Putt	50	3 times/week
Medium long	40	3 times/week
Long	0	0 times/week
Not more than one third best distance		

Stage 4

Putt	50	3 times/week
Medium long	50	3 times/week
Long	10	2 times/week
Up to one half best distance		

Stage 5

Putt	50	3 times/week
Medium long	50	3 times/week
Long	10	3 times/week

Stage 6

Putt	50	3 times/week
Medium long	50	3 times/week
Long	20	3 times/week
Play a round of golf in lieu of one practice session per week.		

From Jobe FW: Operative techniques in upper extremity sports injuries, St Louis, 1996, Mosby.

For closed chain assessment, demonstrating dynamic control under load, the athletic patient should be able to perform 10 walk-outs on a stability ball while maintaining the scapula flush with the thoracic wall in a protracted position. Lastly, functional strength and endurance of the serratus must be observed during the actual motion pattern the patient requires. For example, the physical therapist must observe a pitcher mimicking the pitching motion repeatedly, at normal speeds, to ensure the scapular control is adequate to allow a safe return to pitching. The physical therapist must ensure there is adequate dynamic control of the serratus anterior before allowing high-level functional activities.

Stretching Considerations

Patients with anterior instability may have a tight posterior capsule. Despite surgical correction, the posterior tightness may remain and, if left untreated, lead to a recurrence of the original complaint. Two excellent self-stretching techniques for the posterior capsule are the cross body stretch with scapular stabilization (see Fig. 4-5) and the sleeper stretch (see Fig. 4-9).

Periscapular muscles that tend to be restricted include the pectoralis minor and levator scapula. Both of these muscles will contribute to an anteriorly tipped and downwardly rotated scapula, thus preventing normal rotation of the scapula and therefore contributing to shoulder impingement. The therapist should be suspicious if the patient has rounded shoulders and a protracted scapula. Stretching of both muscles can be performed manually or independently. Soft tissue mobilization can be very effective in treating these restrictions as well. Remember to protect the anterior capsule from being overstretched when addressing these issues.

The therapist must not stretch the anterior shoulder structures of any throwing athlete unless he or she is certain that tightness exists. By and large, all these patients can demonstrate anterior laxity in the dominant shoulder. Assess ROM carefully and consider all factors of the patient and physical demands before proceeding with any stretching of the anterior shoulder.

Mechanics

Even though the patient may have good ROM, strength, and endurance in the shoulder itself, important work remains to be done. Poor body mechanics may be one of the reasons the patient was injured in the first place. Understanding the mechanics of the sport the patient is resuming is essential. For example, in the throwing athlete, the physical therapist must ensure the full kinetic chain is functioning properly, including the front foot pointing toward the plate, appropriate stride length, adequate balance, and that the front foot does not hit the ground before the arm is in the fully cocked position. An awareness of the mechanics of tennis, volleyball, swimming, and golf is critically important when working with these athletes. Without incorporating a review of proper mechanics and a "tune up" when necessary, it is likely that the player will return to old habits formed before the shoulder surgery, possibly leading to reaggravation and injury.

CLINICAL CASE REVIEW

1 John is a 35-year-old surfer. He had several episodes of shoulder dislocation while paddling his surfboard. He also complained of anterior shoulder pain. Conservative treatment failed, so he underwent an anterior capsular reconstruction 11 weeks ago. Passive range of motion (PROM) and AROM are good. John's main complaint is continuing anterior shoulder pain. The pain can be elicited by palpation over the biceps tendon and transverse humeral ligament. This symptom has delayed progress with strengthening. How was the patient treated?

John was treated for biceps tendonitis, or inflammatory symptoms occurring in the area of the proximal biceps tendon and transverse humeral ligament. Despite the structural corrections, these tissues may remain irritable. Because the posterior capsule also was slightly restricted, posterior capsular mobilizations were performed to allow the humeral head to articulate with the glenoid at its normal contact point, eliminating this as a source of continuing aggravation for these anterior structures.

2 Peter is a 20-year-old pitcher for a baseball team. He had right-shoulder laxity and a painful shoulder secondary to impingement problems. He underwent capsular reconstruction on his right shoulder 10 weeks ago. His shoulder flexion and abduction with PROM is still limited by 15° for flexion and 20° for abduction. PROM for internal rotation also is limited by 20°. At this time, should decreased ROM be a concern? If yes, what techniques were used to improve ROM?

On further investigation a tight posterior capsule was noted. The therapist used posterior capsular mobilizations in the next treatment to increase shoulder flexion and internal rotation. The patient gained 10° to 15° more for flexion and internal rotation and 5° to 10° more for abduction. After mobilization and PROM were performed, the patient executed AROM exercises for shoulder flexion, abduction, and internal rotation.

3 Caroline is an 18-year-old high school volleyball player who experienced recurrent anterior subluxations during play. At 16 weeks postoperation, she notes a clicking with mild pain in the anterior shoulder while performing overhead motions mimicking a volleyball serve. Her involved shoulder motion and strength are considered normal. However the uninvolved side had 30° more internal rotation than the involved shoulder. What structures are possibly at fault?

Recheck her shoulder internal rotation at 90° and above. Despite her internal rotation being normal for the average population, she is still lacking 30° compared with her uninvolved side. By aggressively mobilizing the soft tissue in the posterior cuff, she is able to regain what is normal mobility for her and the pain and clicking has resolved.

4 Lucy is a 13-year-old middle school competitive swimmer who experienced anterior shoulder pain and impingement signs primarily with backstroke. She is 3 weeks since the operation and has full PROM in external rotation without resistance or pain. How do you proceed?

Educate Lucy and her parents regarding the physiology and goal of the surgery and the concern you have about her arm moving too far into external rotation. Explain that you would like her to limit this motion as much as possible to allow physiologic healing to occur. Do not give her any stretching exercises involving external rotation at this time.

5 Steve is a 29-year-old computer programmer who is 4 weeks postoperation. His anterior shoulder pain is not resolving as expected. Progress with ROM is hampered by pain more than stiffness and the end feel is empty in all directions. He is also having difficulty sleeping at night because of pain. What steps should you take?

Assess the cervical spine. Include ROM, palpation, and cervical strength testing. Often times there is segmental cervical dysfunction, which can contribute to referred shoulder pain and restriction. This is different than a cervical radiculopathy because there are no hard neurologic findings such as myotomal weakness, altered reflexes, or sensation.

6 Kari is a 40-year-old mother who plays recreational volleyball and runs. She noted nondominant shoulder subluxations with basic reaching activities of increasing frequency over the past 2 years. She had to stop playing volleyball because of the shoulder instability. Kari is 6 weeks postoperation and notes minimal pain. She is able to gain ROM during therapy sessions but is unable to maintain the range between sessions. What can be addressed to help her maintain her range?

After the patient/therapist is done stretching the shoulder, PNF patterns can be useful to initiate muscle contraction into the newly gained ROM. PNF D1 and D2 patterns with minimal resistance performed in a pain-free range can facilitate the rotator cuff and scapular muscles to help Kari maintain these gains. At home, the exercises can be performed with no resistance or light band resistance to reinforce the active end range control.

7 Marc is a 42-year-old recreational basketball player who is 5 months postoperation. He has full ROM in all directions but continues to have anterior shoulder pain at end range flexion in his initial attempts to return to play. Every time he reaches for a lay up, the shoulder pain is sharp but settles quickly. What would you expect to find with your palpation examination?

Likely Marc has tightness in muscles of the posterior rotator cuff and tenderness over the proximal bicep tendon. When he reaches with speed and force into full flexion, impingement of the bicep tendon under the acromion may occur if the force couple of the rotator cuff musculature is not functioning properly.

8 Angela is a competitive gymnast who underwent ACR surgery 2 weeks ago. She presents to you at her physical therapy evaluation with empty end feels for external rotation at 30°, flexion at 150° with minimal pain, and abduction at 90°. She notes minimal postoperative pain

at this time and is wearing the sling "only because my doctor told me to." What is your treatment on day one?

At a physiologic level, collagen fibers must be deposited and bond together to limit the extensibility of the capsular tissue. If you work to increase ROM at this time, you may be hampering the healing of the newly restricted capsule by excessively elongating the new fibers. Focus on AAROM exercises within the guidelines of restricted ROM despite her ability to move beyond the suggested precautions. When more time has elapsed, progress ROM according to the doctors recommended limitations.

9 Two muscles are particularly critical to create proper scapulohumeral rhythm. What are they?

Levator scapula and serratus anterior. If the levator scapula is restricted and lacks the normal extensibility, it will prevent the scapula from moving into upward rotation as the arm moves into elevation. If the serratus anterior is weak, it will not properly guide the scapula into upward rotation as the arm moves into elevation. If either of these muscles is not performing properly, the scapula becomes dysfunctional and will lead to secondary impingement. Be certain to assess and reassess the function of these two muscles throughout the course of rehabilitation.

REFERENCES

1. Frank CB: Ligament structure, physiology and function. J Musculoskelet Neuronal Interact 4(2):199-201, 2004.
2. Hardy MA: The biology of scar formation. Phys Ther 69(12):22-32, 1989.
3. Woo SL, Apreleva M, Hoher J: Tissue biomechanics of ligaments and tendons. In Kumar S, editor: Biomechanics in ergonomics, Philadelphia, 1999, CRC Press.
4. Burroughs P, Dahners LE: The effect of enforced exercise on the healing of ligament injuries. Am J Sports Med 18:376-378, 1990.
5. Lechner CT, Dahners LE: Healing of the medial collateral ligament in unstable rat knees. Am J Sports Med 19:508-512, 1991.
6. Mottram SL: Dynamic stability of the scapula. Manual Ther 2(3):123-131, 1997.
7. Saliba V, Johnson GS, Wardlaw C: Proprioceptive neuromuscular facilitation. In Basmajian JV, Nyberg RE, editors. Rational manual therapies, Baltimore, 1992, Williams & Wilkins.
8. Long JL, et al: Activation of the shoulder musculature during pendulum exercises and light activities. J Orthop Sports Phys Ther 40(4):230-237, 2010.
9. Dwyer A, Aprill C, Bogduk N: Cervical zygapophyseal joint pain patterns: A study in normal volunteers. Spine 15(6):453-457, 1990.
10. Decker MJ, et al: Serratus anterior muscle activity during selected rehabilitation exercises. Am J Sports Med 27(6):784-791, 1999.
11. Moseley JB Jr, et al: EMG analysis of the scapular muscles during a shoulder rehabilitation program. Am J Sports Med 20:128-134, 1992.
12. Tyler TF, et al: Reliability and validity of a new method of measuring posterior shoulder tightness. J Orthop Sports Phys Ther 29(5):262-269, 1999.

13. Laudner KG, Stanek JM, Meister K: Assessing posterior shoulder contracture: The reliability and validity of measuring glenohumeral joint horizontal adduction. J Athl Train 41:375-380, 2006.
14. Hengeveld E, Banks K, editors: Maitland's peripheral manipulation, ed 4, Philadelphia, 2005, Butterworth-Heinemann.
15. Threlkeld A: Effects of manual therapy on connective tissue. Phys Ther 72(12):893-902, 1992.
16. Warner JJP, et al: Patterns of flexibility, laxity, and strength in normal shoulders and shoulders with instability and impingement. Am J Sports Med 18:366-375, 1990
17. McClure P, et al: A randomized controlled comparison of stretching procedures for poster shoulder tightness. J Orthop Sports Phys Ther 37(3)108-114, 2007.
18. Conroy DE, Hayes KW: The effect of joint mobilization as a component of comprehensive treatment for primary shoulder impingement syndrome. J Orthop Sports Phys Ther 28(1):3-14, 1998.
19. Reference 19 deleted in proof.
20. Ellenbecker TS, Mattalino AJ: Glenohumeral joint range of motion and rotator cuff strength following arthroscopic anterior stabilization with thermal capsulorraphy. J Orthop Sports Phys Ther 29(3):160-167, 1999.
21. Kibler WB: The role of the scapula in athletic shoulder function. Am J Sports Med 36(9):1789-1798, 1998.
22. Ekstrom RA, Donatelli RA, Soderberg GL: Surface electromyography analysis of exercises for the trapezius and serratus anterior muscles. J Orthop Sports Phys Ther 33(45):247-258, 2003.
23. Reinold MM, et al: Electromyographic analysis of the rotator cuff and deltoid musculature during common shoulder external rotation exercises. J Orthop Sports Phys Ther 34:385-394, 2004.

24. Cools AM, et al: Rehabilitation of scapular muscle balance: Which exercises to prescribe? Am J Sports Med 35(10):1744-1751, 2007.

25. Myers JB, et al: On-the-field resistance-tubing exercises for throwers: an electromyographic analysis. J Athl Train 40:15-22, 2005.

26. Hintersmeister RA, et al: Electromyographic activity and applied load during shoulder rehabilitation exercises using elastic resistance. Am J Sports Med 26(2):210-220, 1998.

27. Laudner KG, Moline MT, Meister K: The relationship between forward scapular posture and posterior shoulder tightness among baseball players. Am J Sports Med 38(10):2106-2112, 2010.

28. Laudner KG, Sipes RC, Wilson JT: The acute effects of sleeper stretches on shoulder range of motion. J Athl Train 43(4):359-363, 2008.

29. Ludewig PM, Cook TM, Nawoczenski DA: Three-dimensional scapular orientation and muscle activity at selected positions of humeral elevation. J Orthop Sports Phys Ther 24:57-65, 1996.

30. Hardwick DH, et al: A comparison of serratus anterior muscle activation during a wall slide exercise and other traditional exercises. J Orthop Sports Phys Ther 36(12):903-910, 2006.

31. Escamilla RF, et al: Shoulder muscle activity and function in common shoulder rehabilitation exercises. Sports Med 39(8):663-685, 2009.

32. Lee SB, et al: Dynamic glenohumeral stability provided by the rotator cuff muscles in the mid-range and end-range of motion: A study in cadavera. J Bone Joint Surg Am 82:849-857, 2000.

33. Jobe FW, et al: An EMG analysis of the shoulder in throwing and pitching: A preliminary report. Am J Sports Med 11(1):3-5, 1983.

34. Jobe FW, et al: An EMG analysis of the shoulder in pitching: A second report. Am J Sports Med 12(3):218-220, 1984.

35. Jobe FW, Pink M: Classification and treatment of shoulder dysfunction in the overhead athlete. J Orthop Sports Phys Ther 18(2):427-432, 1993.

36. Crosbie J, et al: Scapulohumeral rhythm and associated spinal motion. Clin Biomech 23(2):184-192, 2008.

37. Boyles RE, et al: The short-term effects of thoracic spine thrust manipulation on patients with shoulder impingement syndrome. Manual Ther 14(4):375-380, 2009.

CHAPTER 5

Rotator Cuff Repair and Rehabilitation

Lisa Maxey, Mark Ghilarducci

ETIOLOGY

Rotator cuff disorders are generally thought to have a multifactorial cause, including trauma, glenohumeral (GH) instability, scapulothoracic dysfunction, congenital abnormalities, and degenerative changes of the rotator cuff. Intrinsic factors of primary tendon degeneration and extrinsic mechanical factors have been described extensively and are felt to be the primary contributors of rotator cuff pathology. Intrinsic tendon degeneration has been described. In 1931, Codman and Akerson[1] suggested that degenerative changes in the rotator cuff lead to tears. Microvascular studies of the vascular pattern of the rotator cuff have demonstrated a hypovascular zone in the supraspinatus adjacent to the supraspinatus insertion into the humerus.[2-4] Relative ischemia in this hypovascular zone is believed to lead with aging to decreased tendon cellularity and the eventual disruption of the rotator cuff attachment to bone.

Compression of the rotator cuff between the acromion and the humeral head may subject the cuff to wear as the supraspinatus passes under the coracoacromial arch. Neer[5,6] postulated that 95% of rotator cuff tears are caused by impingement of the rotator cuff under the acromion. Neer[5] classified three stages of impingement as a continuum that eventually led to cuff tears. Stage I is characterized by subacromial edema and hemorrhage of the rotator cuff and usually occurs in patients younger than 25 years old. Stage II includes fibrosis and tendinosis of the rotator cuff and occurs more commonly in patients 25 to 40 years old. Stage III is a continued progression characterized by partial or complete tendon tears and bone changes. Typically, this involves patients older than 40 years old.[5] Bigliani, Morrison, and April[7] described three types of acromion shapes: (1) type I is flat, (2) type II is curved, and (3) type III is hooked. An increased incidence of rotator cuff tears is associated with a curved (type II) or a hooked (type III) acromion. Other sources of extrinsic impingement postulated include acromioclavicular (AC) osteophytes, the coracoid process, and the posterosuperior aspect of the glenoid.[8]

A rotator cuff tear may occur spontaneously after a sudden movement or a traumatic event.[9] Ruptures of the rotator cuff have been estimated to occur in up to 80% of persons older than 60 years of age with GH dislocations.[10] Cuff tears usually occur late in the shoulder deterioration process (after secondary impingement) and in older adults.

In athletes who participate in repetitive overhead activities (e.g., throwers, swimmers, tennis players), small rotator cuff tears may appear late in the deterioration process from secondary impingement. Secondary impingement is caused by instability of the GH joint or by functional scapulothoracic instability.[11] The primary underlying GH instability may progress along a continuum from anterior subluxation to impingement to rotator cuff tearing. Treatment must be directed to the primary instability problem.[12]

The throwing athlete also may have secondary impingement caused by functional scapular instability. Fatigue of the scapular stabilizers from repetitive throwing leads to abnormal positioning of the scapula. As a result, humeral and scapular elevation lose synchronization and the acromion is not elevated enough to allow free rotator cuff movement.[11] The rotator cuff abuts the acromion, causing microtrauma and impingement. A tear may gradually or spontaneously occur.

In summary, rotator cuff disease has a multifactorial cause. Vascular factors, impingement, degenerative processes, and developmental factors all contribute to the overall evolution and progression of rotator cuff disorders (Box 5-1).

Clinical Evaluation

History

The majority of patients with rotator cuff dysfunction have pain. They may complain of fatigue, functional catching, stiffness, weakness, and symptoms of instability. An acute or macrotraumatic presentation is important to distinguish from an overuse or microtrauma presentation. Most patients report a gradual onset of pain with no history of trauma. A gradual onset of weakness is usually associated with a chronic tear and an acute onset of weakness after years of shoulder pain is suggestive of an acute on chronic tear.

> **BOX 5-1** Rotator Cuff Deterioration Process
>
> ### In Older Persons or Laborers
> Osteophyte develops
> Decreased subacromial space (more accentuated with a slouched posture)
> Continuous microtrauma from impingement leads to degenerative cuff changes
> Gradual partial tear or complete tear develops
>
> ### In Athletes Secondary to Glenohumeral (GH) Instability
> Overused biceps tendon and rotator cuff become weak and fatigued
> Passive restraints are overloaded
> Cuff laxity
> Anterosuperior GH instability
> Humeral head migrates superiorly and impinges the rotator cuff
> Continuous microtrauma from recurrent impingement leads to degenerative cuff changes
> Gradual or sudden rotator cuff tear occurs
>
> ### Secondary to Functional Scapular Instability
> Weak scapulothoracic muscles
> Abnormal scapular positioning
> Humeral head elevation is not synchronized with scapular elevation and upward rotation (disrupted scapulohumeral rhythm)
> Acromion requires more elevation to allow unrestricted movement of the rotator cuff
> Rotator cuff impinged under the coracoacromial arch
> Continuous microtrauma from a recurrent impingement leads to degenerative cuff changes
> Gradual partial tear or a complete tear develops

Pain is typically localized in the upper arm in the region of the deltoid tuberosity and anterior lateral acromion. Pain is usually worse at night. Overhead activities often induce the patient's symptoms. Typical findings are a loss of endurance during activities, catching, crepitus, weakness, and stiffness.

Physical Examination

A thorough examination of the shoulder should include evaluation of the cervical spine and an upper extremity neurologic examination. The opposite shoulder must also be examined for comparison. Inspection, palpation for tenderness, and range of motion (ROM) tests should be completed. Palpation should include the AC joint, sternoclavicular (SC) joint, subacromial space, biceps tendon, trapezius muscle, and cervical spine. Impingement sign tests as described by Hawkins, Misamore, and Hobeika[13] (i.e., forward flexion to 90° and internal rotation) and by Neer and Welch[14] (forward

elevation and internal rotation) are performed to elicit pain. If these tests produce pain, then they are considered positive signs of impingement and suggest rotator cuff dysfunction. The rotator cuff muscles are tested for strength. Subscapularis muscle strength tests include the lift-off test and the belly-press test. The lift-off test places the arm behind the back and up the spine. The patient is then asked to lift the hand off the back against restriction. The belly-press test places the arms onto the elbows bent to 90°, and the elbows are then lifted anteriorly against resistance. Examination for instability is performed. Apprehension sign, a positive-relocation test, or inferior sulcus sign are all indicative of instability. Stability testing should be performed in different positions (i.e., seated, supine) to eliminate instability as the cause of secondary impingement. Evidence of rotator cuff pathology includes painful impingement signs or weakness and a painful arc of motion.[5]

Diagnostic Testing

Diagnostic testing includes injections, radiographs, arthrogram, or magnetic resonance imaging (MRI) or ultrasonography. An impingement test (subacromial space injection with at least 10 mL of 1% lidocaine) is invaluable in evaluating the origin of shoulder pain. Physical examination several minutes after the injection, including for ROM, impingement signs, strength, and instability should be completed. Resolution of the shoulder symptoms without instability indicates primary rotator cuff pathology or impingement. Relief of pain with evidence of instability indicates possible primary instability with secondary rotator cuff changes because of altered shoulder mechanics.

Convention radiography is an important tool in the evaluation of rotator cuff tear pathology and is used to rule out arthritis and fractures, assess the morphology of the acromion, and look for calcifications about the shoulder. Arthrography is no longer the gold standard for identification of rotator cuff tears. Although reliable for the diagnosis of complete rotator cuff tears, it is less reliable for the evaluation of partial-thickness rotator cuff tears. MRI has evolved to provide an excellent noninvasive tool in the diagnosis of rotator cuff pathology and the shoulder labrum and is the modality of choice for the evaluation of cuff tear pathology, followed by ultrasonography. MRI provides information not available by other diagnostic testing, including muscle atrophy, amount of rotator cuff retraction in full-thickness tears, bursal swelling, the status of the AC joint, and the shoulder articular cartilage. The combination of intraarticular contrast (gadolinium) and MRI (magnetic resonance arthrography) has been developed to better delineate abnormalities of the rotator cuff and labrum including partial surface rotator cuff tears.[15,16] Ultrasonography of the shoulder has increased in popularity, and as technical advances continue to improve, it has become an increasingly useful tool in the diagnosis of cuff pathology. Ultrasonography has several advantages. These include a relatively low cost, the lack of the contraindications as with MRI, and its use in the examination of the patient both statically and dynamically. Unfortunately, the accuracy of ultrasonography is operator dependent and typically requires a long learning curve.

Treatment

Symptoms of rotator cuff dysfunction are usually treated initially in a nonoperative fashion (tendonitis, partial- or full-thickness rotator cuff tears). Nonsteroidal antiinflammatory drugs (NSAIDs), heat, ice, relative rest, cortisone injection, and rehabilitation programs are used in the treatment. The initial goal of treatment is restoration of normal ROM. This is followed by a rotator cuff strengthening program. Stretch cords for resistance are initiated and are followed by free weights as tolerated. To avoid aggravation of the rotator cuff, all strength training initially should be below shoulder level. External rotation strengthening with the arm at the side may minimize subacromial pressure and pain while increasing the cuff's ability to act as a humeral head depressor.

Nonoperative treatment programs usually continue for 3 to 6 months. Success varies from 50% to 90%.[17-21] Approximately 50% of patients with complete symptomatic rotator cuff tears have satisfactory results with nonoperative measures, but these results may deteriorate with time.[22] This wide range of outcomes is likely the result of lack of uniformity in classification, indications, and treatment. Some individuals have rotator cuff tears with no pain and normal function, whereas others may have debilitating pain. This demonstrates a need for better understanding of the factors that lead to symptoms.

Indications for Surgery

Indications for rotator cuff surgery include failure of 3 to 6 months of conservative care or an acute full-thickness tear in an active patient younger than 50 years. Failure of treatment can be determined before an entire rehabilitation course is completed. Indications for earlier surgical treatment can include return to full strength with persistent symptoms, failure to tolerate therapy because of pain, or plateau of initial improvement with persistent symptoms. Early surgical intervention is also indicated for patients sustaining acute trauma with full-thickness tears associated with significant rotator cuff weakness and posterior cuff involvement, particularly in young patients with higher functional demands. In addition, patients with acute tears or extension of chronic cuff tears may benefit from early surgery.[23]

In general, the duration of nonoperative treatment must be individualized based on pathology involved, the patient's response to treatment, and individual functional demands and expectations.

Surgical Goals

The primary goal of rotator cuff surgery is decreased pain, including rest pain, night pain, and pain with activities of daily living (ADLs). Arrest of the progression of rotator cuff pathology and improved shoulder function are additional surgical goals.

SURGICAL PROCEDURES

Tendonitis and Partial Rotator Cuff Tear

Surgical management for impingement syndrome generally involves open anterior acromioplasty as described by Neer[63] or arthroscopic subacromial decompression (SAD) with release or partial release of the coracoacromial ligament. The coracoacromial ligament is released from the undersurface of the anterior and lateral acromion. An acromioplasty is performed using a burr to achieve a flat acromion. If osteophytes are present on the inferior surface of the AC joint, they are removed from the distal clavicle. Partial thickness cuff tears may be bursal or articular sided. Partial thickness cuff tears may be treated with débridement alone, débridement and acromioplasty, or rotator cuff repair. A subacromial decompression/acromioplasty is generally indicated if the partial tear is bursal sided or there are signs of mechanical impingement. Partial rotator cuff tears greater than 50% of the width of the tendon generally are treated with arthroscopic repair insitu or transtendineus repair, or may be treated with takedown and repair of the rotator cuff either miniopen or arthroscopic.[24] Repair of partial-thickness tears improves results compared with débridement alone in this patient group. The overhead throwing athletes with rotator cuff disease have different requirements. Acromioplasty is rarely necessary in the throwing athlete.

Results of surgical treatment of low-grade (<50%) partial-thickness rotator cuff tears after débridement with and without acromioplasty have reported 75% to 88% satisfactory outcome on short-term follow-up.[18,25-27] Repair of a high-grade (>50%) partial-thickness tear has had similar outcome to débridement of a low-grade partial-thickness tear or repair of a small full-thickness cuff tear.[28]

Full-Thickness Tears

The mainstay of treatment for full-thickness tears is surgical repair. The type, pattern, and size of the tear, as well as the surgeon's preference, dictate whether the repair is a full-arthroscopic, miniopen, or a completely open procedure.

Small- or moderate-sized (3 cm or less) partial- or full-thickness supraspinatus or infraspinatus tears may be repaired fully with an arthroscopic or miniopen technique. Large width (3 to 5 cm) tears may also be repaired miniopen or arthroscopic if the cuff is mobile enough to allow anatomic repair.

Large, immobile cuff tears involving the subscapularis or teres minor, as well as tears of the musculotendinosis junction, may require an open approach. Massive chronic atrophic cuff tears should be considered for arthroscopic débridement for pain control.

SURGICAL TECHNIQUE

All operative procedures discussed in recent literature for primary repair of rotator cuff tears include use of an anterioinferior acromioplasty to decompress the subacromial space.

The author presently performs GH arthroscopy and subacromial bursoscopy on all patients undergoing surgery for cuff pathology.

Shoulder arthroscopy and decompression is performed as previously described. After acromioplasty, the bursal surface of the rotator cuff is evaluated. With shoulder rotation, the cuff can be completely visualized. Mobile tears may be treated with a miniopen technique or with arthroscopic repair.

Arthroscopic Rotator Cuff Repair

In the past decade as arthroscopic repair of rotator cuff tears has become more widespread, there have been significant advances in arthroscopic surgical techniques and instrumentation. Arthroscopic repair involves the same general steps as miniopen or open rotator cuff repair. Bony landmarks are outlined and marked with a sterile pen. Multiple arthroscopic portals are made. Posterior, anterior, and lateral portals are made for all arthroscopic repairs. Additional portals are made depending on the rotator cuff tear configuration and include posterior lateral, anterior lateral, and lateral acromial portals. These allow access to various rotator cuff configurations and for suture anchor placement. The GH joint is completely and systematically evaluated followed by subacromial bursoscopy. The subacromial bursa is excised, and the anterior acromion is flattened with a burr. If symptomatic, then the AC joint is excised arthroscopically. The rotator cuff is visualized. The quality and the integrity of the rotator cuff are evaluated. The mobility of the cuff is evaluated. Adhesions on the bursal and articular sides of the tear are released. The goal is a mobile cuff which can be repaired to the normal footprint on the greater tuberosity with minimal tension. A three dimensional understanding of the cuff tear configuration is developed. Margin convergence repair principles are used for U-shaped tears or L- or reverse L-shaped tears. Sutures are placed in a side-to-side fashion through the anterior and posterior leafs of the tear. This convergences the edges of the tear and minimizes the tension on the tendon to bone repair. The result may be an arthroscopic repair of an otherwise irreparable tear. The greater tuberosity of the humerus is lightly decorticated with a burr. The tendon is then repaired to bone with suture anchors. The number of suture anchors used is predicated on the size of the tear and its configuration. In general, one suture anchor is used for each one centimeter of cuff tear.

Miniopen Rotator Cuff Repair

In the miniopen procedure, the lateral subacromial portal incision is extended either longitudinally or transversely to expose the deltoid fascia. The deltoid fascia is then split in line with its fibers directly over the tear. The anterior deltoid insertion of the anterior acromion is preserved. The deltoid fibers should not be split more than 4 cm lateral to the lateral acromion to avoid axillary nerve injury (Fig. 5-1). Rotation of the arm provides access to the tear. Digital palpation can be used to assess the adequacy of the acromioplasty. A bony trough is prepared in the greater tuberosity of the humerus. The rotator cuff may then be repaired through a bony bridge

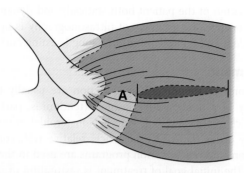

Fig. 5-1 Line of incision for partially open repair. The deltoid split begins at the lateral edge of the acromion *(A)* and should not extend more than 4 cm lateral to the acromion to avoid injury to the axillary nerve.

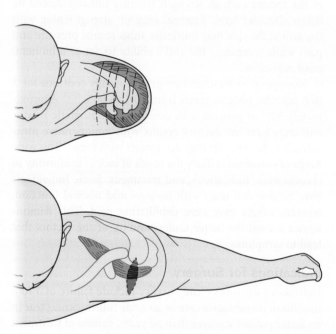

Fig. 5-2 Incision placed in Langer lines produces the best cosmesis.

or with suture anchors. The permanent sutures are tied, pulling the rotator cuff down into its trough on the humerus.

Open Rotator Cuff Repair

Tears that are fixed, retracted, but reparable, may be repaired open using principles developed by Neer.[5,6] An oblique incision in Lagers line from the anterior edge of the acromion to a point about 2 cm lateral to the coracoid process is made. The anterior deltoid is released from the anterior aspect of the acromion and splitting the deltoid no more than 4 cm lateral to the acromion (Fig. 5-2). The deltoid origin over the acromion is elevated subperiosteally. The coracoacromial ligament is released.

The anterior acromion is osteotomized. The acromion anterior to the anterior aspect of the clavicle is removed, and the undersurface of the acromion is flattened from anterior to posterior. The AC joint may be removed if arthritic and symptomatic. The distal clavicle is excised parallel to the AC joint so that no contact occurs with adduction of the arm.

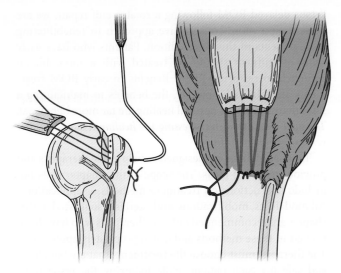

Fig. 5-3 Transosseous repair of rotator cuff tendon. A trough is created in the proximal humerus just lateral to the articular surface. Sutures are tied over the bone bridge in the greater tuberosity.

The cuff tear is visualized and mobilized. A bony trough 0.5 cm in width parallel to the junction of the humeral articular cartilage and greater tuberosity of the humerus is made. The rotator cuff tear is repaired to bone with suture anchors or through a bony bridge in the greater tuberosity using permanent sutures (Fig. 5-3). The goal is to repair the cuff with minimal tension with the arm at the side.

Watertight repairs are not necessary for good functional outcome. Excellent and good results have been shown in patients with residual cuff holes.[29,30] The anterior deltoid is repaired back to the acromion by preserved periosteum or through drill holes with permanent sutures. Routine skin closure is performed.

Postoperative management of cuff repairs must be individualized to incorporate tear size, tissue quality, difficulty of repair, and patient goals. Passive motion is initiated immediately. In general, supine active-assisted motion is started on the first postoperative day. Waist-level use of the hand can usually be started after surgery. Active ROM and isotonic strengthening are started 6 to 8 weeks after surgery. Progress of strengthening is individualized with full rehabilitation taking from 6 to 12 months. Function can continue to improve for 1 year after surgery.

MANAGEMENT OF MASSIVE TENDON DEFECTS

The management of massive irreparable tendon defects remains controversial. Options include SAD and débridement of nonviable cuff tissue without attempt at repair, use of autogenous or allograft tendon grafts, and use of active tendon transfers. Operations that require tendon transfer to nonanatomic sites to cover rotator cuff defects are likely to alter mechanics of the shoulder unfavorably.[31] Débridement may be pursued (either open or arthroscopic).

RESULTS OF TREATMENT OF FULL-THICKNESS ROTATOR CUFF TEARS

Satisfactory results after rotator cuff repair for pain relief occur 85% to 95% of the time[5,13,32,33] and appear to correlate with the adequacy of the acromioplasty and SAD. Functional outcomes correlate with integrity of the cuff repair, preoperative size of the cuff tear, and quality of the tendon issue. Poor outcomes are also associated with deltoid detachment or denervation.[34]

Arthroscopic-assisted miniopen rotator cuff repair provides favorable clinical results. Results comparable with open cuff repair have been reported for small- and moderate-sized rotator cuff repair (less than 3 cm.).[35-37] These studies have shown the most important factor affecting outcome was cuff tear size. Tears of small or moderate size had better results. Blevins and associates,[38] in a retrospective study, have shown 83% good or excellent results regardless of cuff size. Most studies have shown more rapid return to full activities with miniopen repair.

Fully arthroscopic repair studies have shown outcomes approaching the results of open rotator cuff repair or miniopen rotator cuff repair.[39-47]

A surgical technique that initially includes arthroscopy has the advantage of providing identification and treatment of intraarticular pathology (articular cartilage, labrum, biceps tendon). Additional advantages of arthroscopic rotator cuff repair include decreased soft tissue dissection, improved cosmesis, preservation of the deltoid attachment, decreased postoperative pain, and earlier return of normal ROM.

Unfortunately, rehabilitation cannot be accelerated for arthroscopic or miniopen cuff repairs because the limiting factor, tendon-to-bone healing, is not changed by the surgical technique.

No ideal surgical technique exists. Each surgeon must individualize treatment based on the type of lesion present, as well as the expertise of the physician. As has been noted over the past decade with the widespread use of shoulder arthroscopy and improved surgical technique and instrumentation, arthroscopic rotator cuff surgery will continue to increase in frequency and open or miniopen cuff repairs will continue to decrease in frequency. All these methods have a role in the treatment of rotator cuff tears.

THERAPY GUIDELINES FOR REHABILITATION

The general guidelines that follow are for the rehabilitation of a type 2 rotator cuff tear (a medium-to-large rotator cuff tear that is larger than 1 cm and smaller than 5 cm). We have also included a table of guidelines to follow for large tears. The protocol is designed for active patients (i.e., recreational athletes, laborers). Older, more sedentary individuals progress through the stages more slowly. These patients are not appropriate candidates for the more aggressive exercises.

Recent studies suggest that longer periods of immobilization and a more conservative approach to restoring ROM early on leads to more successful outcomes in terms of fewer repeat tears following surgery or insufficient healing of the rotator cuff. Even if the tear is not completely healed, the patient can be satisfied with the results. However, they are happier if the cuff is healed. Therefore, the goal is for a healed rotator cuff repair. Too many ROM exercises or too much stress on the repaired tissues early on may create an increase in scar tissue. This tissue has a poorer quality of intracellular tissue. Studies have also shown that after 1 year there is no difference in the ROM of patients in different groups following surgery.[48] Groups that received early ROM treatment versus groups that received delayed ROM treatments had the same ROM at 1 year. The group that delayed ROM treatments actually had a higher rate of healing versus the group who received passive range of motion (PROM) early in the rehabilitation process.[48]

Many factors contribute to the healing rates of these repairs: retraction of the tissue, age, early repair versus late repair, surgical technique, patient selection, and postoperative rehabilitation. Poorer outcomes have been noted with patients over 65 years of age, manual laborers, those with poor bone stock, tears greater than 5 cm, workers' compensation cases, or active litigation clients. Better outcomes have been noted with younger patients, smaller tears, and early surgical repair. In light of the recent discussion of early versus delayed ROM following a rotator cuff repair, we are presenting a more conservative approach to rehabilitating these patients in this third edition. Patients who have early signs of stiffness should be treated with a more liberal approach to restoring ROM. Benefits to early ROM treatments are minimal; however, the benefits to maintaining a safe environment for optimal healing are far more beneficial. *The goal is to avoid overstressing the healing tissues and preventing shoulder stiffness.*

These guidelines are designed to help guide therapists and provide treatment ideas. The scope of this chapter does not include instructions on treatment methods or applications. All modalities, mobilizations, and exercises suggested in this chapter are recommended only for therapists who have been trained in these methods and can appropriately apply them. The therapist must choose the treatments that are beneficial and safe for each patient while following the restrictions outlined by the operating surgeon.

Phase I

TIME: 1 to 4 weeks after surgery
GOALS: Comfort, maintain integrity of repair, increasing ROM as tolerated without progressing to full range, decreased pain and inflammation, minimal cervical spine stiffness, protection of the surgical site, maintenance of full elbow and wrist ROM (Table 5-1)

TABLE 5-1 Rotator Cuff Repair for Moderate-Sized Tears

Rehabilitation Phase	Criteria to Progress to this Phase	Anticipated Impairments and Functional Limitations	Intervention	Goal	Rationale
Phase I Postoperative 1-4 wk	• Postoperative	• Limited ROM • Limited strength • Pain • Initial restriction to PROM of shoulder • Dependent upper extremity immobilized in sling or airplane splint	• Cryotherapy • Electrical stimulation • PROM: Pendulum exercises at 2-3 wk; initiate PROM for shoulder flexion, ER, and abduction in scapular plane • AROM: Elbow flexion and extension • PREs: Hand gripping, exercises with putty • Joint mobilization resistance free to shoulder • Rx of C/S mobilizations as needed • Rx of soft tissue msg. to C/S and upper back musculature as needed • Instruct in AROM and appropriate stretches to C/S area	• Decrease pain • Manage edema • Improve PROM and tolerance to movement • Increase quality of muscle recruitment • Maintain and improve ROM of joints proximal and distal to surgical site • Maintain and improve distal muscle strength • Control pain	• Pain control • Edema management • Prevention of joint stiffness • Promotion of healthy articular surface and collagen synthesis and organization • Prevention of further atrophy of upper-extremity musculature • Elimination of neuromuscular inhibition • Prevention of associated weakness, stiffness, and dysfunction of neighboring joints • Gaiting of pain and preparation for stretches into resistance • decreases muscle guarding, stiffness, and pain to shoulder and cervical area • allows for improved ROM at shoulder

AROM, active range of motion; *C/S,* cervical spine; *ER,* external rotation; *PREs,* progressive resistance exercises; *PROM,* passive range of motion; *ROM,* Range of motion; *Rx,* treatment.

Refer to Box 5-2 for a shoulder evaluation following a rotator cuff repair. The therapist must maintain the protection of the patient and the surgical repair while obtaining an evaluation; therefore, some tests will need to be deferred until later in the treatment process.

To reduce pain and swelling, use cryotherapy. Electrical stimulation may also be used for pain reduction. Instruct the patient in posturing for comfort. Encourage the patient to experiment with different positions. Usually a loose packed GH position (shoulder in some flexion, abduction, and internal rotation) with the arm supported by pillows while supine or sitting is more comfortable. Usually patients cannot sleep much after surgery in the supine position. Therefore suggest sleeping semireclined in a recliner chair with the upper extremity supported in the loose packed position. The patient may also try the supine position in bed, with the arm supported by pillows in a loose packed position.

Gentle mobilizations using grades I and II oscillations, and distractions may help reduce pain, muscle guarding, and spasms. These mobilizations also help maintain nutrient exchange and therefore prevent the painful and degenerating effects that long periods of immobilization produce (i.e., a swollen and painful joint).[18] Occasionally, some people produce increased levels of scar tissue and tighten up quickly. For these cases, passive exercises provide nourishment to the articular cartilage and assist in collagen tissue synthesis and organization.[49-51] The organization of collagen may then follow stress patterns, and adverse collagen tissue formation may be minimized. Limited periods of PROM and pendulum exercises are initiated during this initial stage. For large to massive tears, consider withholding PROM exercises until 4 weeks postsurgery. Recently, it has been suggested that early ROM or excessive ROM treatment of the GH joint may delay tissues from healing. Therefore, when conducting PROM treatments, be careful to protect healing tissues from too much stress from ROM exercises. PROM exercises are done in protected planes. PROM exercises for shoulder flexion are initiated in the scapular plane with the elbow flexed 90°, and external rotation is done with the palm facing the patient and beginning at 45° of abduction.[52] Performing PROM exercises in the scapular plane is beneficial because of decreased tension on the capsuloligament-tendon complex.[52] "Rotation exercises should be initiated at 45° of abduction to minimize tension across the repair."[52]

Remember to avoid horizontal adduction, extension, and internal rotation during this phase. Also advise

---

BOX 5-2 Components of the Physical Therapy Evaluation

Background Information
- Status of the capsule
- Status of rotator cuff
- Status of articular cartilage
- Previous procedures
- Associated medical problems that can influence rehabilitation (e.g., cardiovascular concerns, diabetes mellitus)
- Work-related injury
- Insurance status
- Comprehension

Subjective Information
- Previous level of function
- Present level of function
- Patient's goals and expectations
- Intensity of pain
- Location of pain
- Frequency of pain
- Irritability of symptoms
- Presence of night pain
- Amount of hours able to sleep at night
- Assistance at home
- Access to rehabilitative facilities
- Medication (i.e., dose, effect, tolerance, compliance)

Objective Information
Observations
- Muscle wasting
- Muscle spasms

- Resting posture
- Use of sling
- Wound status
- Swelling
- Color

Passive Range of Motion (PROM) of Shoulder
- Shoulder flexion within the limits of tolerance
- Shoulder abduction within the limits of tolerance
- Shoulder external rotation
- Scapulothoracic joint

Palpation
- Biceps tendon (when tenderness and swelling near the surgical site have decreased)
- Trapezius muscle
- Cervical musculature
- Upper thoracic spine
- SC joint
- Acromioclavicular (AC) joint (2 weeks status after surgery)

Modified Cervical Spine Evaluation
Delay active range of motion (AROM) testing of the shoulder until 7 to 8 weeks post surgery

Delay strength testing until tissues have appropriately healed and testing can be done without irritating the shoulder. Avoid strength testing directly on the rotator cuff until approved by surgeon.

patients to avoid leaning on the elbow, sleeping on the affected side, sudden movements, pushing/pulling, lifting, and carrying for 12 weeks.[53]

A general guideline to use in judging the force being applied is slight discomfort with a slight increase in motion after several repetitions. Remain sensitive and aware of the feedback the patient's body is exhibiting during ROM or mobilization techniques. The patient's response will dictate the amount of force applied or the plane of movement chosen. If muscle guarding continues to increase after several repetitions, the force being applied should be reduced or the plane of movement chosen needs to be slightly altered or decreased (or both need to be done) to avoid pinching sensations or increased pain. The therapist usually can find a groove (i.e., line of movement that can be progressed more easily) or line of motion with less muscle guarding. Therefore, constantly assess treatment application while treating the patient with manual PROM. Vary the treatment application as the patient's feedback dictates (i.e., exact plane of movement, force, and repetitions). An increase in ROM will often accompany a decrease in pain if executed with a sensitive hand. However, general treatment soreness may be expected. Treatment soreness is usually more pronounced when progressing the patient from PROM to active range of motion (AROM) and then again when progressing

to resisted ROM exercises. *Remember during this stage we do not want full ROM. The superseding goal is to provide an environment where the tissues can heal while preventing stiffness.*

Patients usually exhibit protective muscle guarding from the necessary insult of the surgery and the preceding shoulder pathology. Muscle guarding is present in the cervical region and the shoulder musculature. Therefore patients perform cervical AROM exercises and stretches. Appropriate cervical spine mobilization techniques may be valuable for decreasing cervical joint stiffness and muscle guarding, allowing more unrestricted movement of the shoulder complex.

Phase II

TIME: 5 to 8 weeks after surgery

GOALS: Protection of surgical site, improvement of ROM, increase in active strength, decrease in pain and inflammation, maintenance of elbow and wrist ROM, and minimizing of cervical stiffness (Table 5-2)

During the second phase, the therapist should avoid overstretching muscles into positions that could compromise the repaired tissues (e.g., horizontal adduction, internal rotation beyond 70°, shoulder extension).

TABLE 5-2   Rotator Cuff Repair for Moderate-Sized Tears

Rehabilitation Phase	Criteria to Progress to this Phase	Anticipated Impairments and Functional Limitations	Intervention	Goal	Rationale
Phase II Postoperative 5-8 wk	• Incision area well healed • Decreased pain to minimum levels • Improved ROM • Improved sleep patterns	• Limited tolerance to ROM • Limited strength • Relatively dependent upper extremity	• Continue phase I exercises • Initiate A/AROM (supine) at 6 wk, progressing toward AROM • Initiate A/AROM at 6 wk for upper-extremity (PNF) D1 and D2 patterns using elbow and wrist movements in supine and progress to AROM • A/AROM for shoulder flexion, ER, abduction, and scaption • Soft tissue mobilization as needed after incision has healed • Cardiovascular conditioning (e.g., bicycling, walking program) • Initiate wand exercises for shoulder flexion, ER, and abduction	• PROM shoulder flexion/abduction 150° to 180° ER 70°, internal rotation 55° • A/AROM reach above head height • Prevent increase of pain • Improve scar mobility; decrease pain • Improve fitness level	• Continuation of phase I exercises to minimize stiffness of adjacent joints • Mimicking and strengthening of functional movements • Improvement of ROM and strength • Improvement of tolerance to movement and preparation for AROM • Performance of exercises to ease subacromial pressures • Normalization of skin mobility and desensitization of scar • Provision of a good healing environment and normalization of arm swing with gait • Allow for ROM exercises at home

A/AROM, Active/assisted range of motion; *AROM,* active range of motion; *ER,* external rotation; *PNF,* proprioceptive neuromuscular facilitation; *PROM,* passive range of motion; *ROM,* Range of motion.

Strength should begin to improve, with the patient progressing from PROM to active assistive range of motion (A/AROM) to AROM movements against gravity. A/AROM can begin at 6 weeks, and AROM can be initiated as able after 7 to 8 weeks. Submaximal isometrics can be initiated to eliminate neuromuscular inhibition, reiterate muscle firing, and retard muscle atrophy. The therapist can incorporate active assistive proprioceptive neuromuscular facilitation (PNF) D1 and D2 patterns to mimic functional movements and strengthen the areas in functional planes.15 In the D1 pattern, the shoulder moves into flexion-abduction-external rotation. With the D2 pattern, the shoulder moves into extension-adduction-internal rotation.[21,41] Initiate these exercises in the supine position with the assistance of the therapist using PROM. Then progress to A/AROM in D1 and D2 patterns. Near the end of this phase, use independent performance of the PNF patterns in the supine position, advancing to a standing position when able. Eventually, active shoulder flexion, external rotation, and scaption exercises (Fig. 5-4) are performed after 7 weeks. Active shoulder flexion and scaption are usually initiated between zero and 70° (with the elbow bent at 90°) and progress according to the patient's ability to execute these exercises correctly. Incorrect performance of shoulder elevation exercises can lead to impingement problems. Again evaluate for cervical spine (C/S) and thoracic spine (T/S) issues that may be causing secondary issues of pain and muscle tightness. Address joint or soft tissue issues.

Precautions at this stage include no resisted exercises for 8 weeks. Between 6 and 12 weeks, advise patient to only perform waist level activities and no heavy lifting for 4 to 6 months. *Marked increases in swelling, pain, or wound drainage (or the presence of red, streaking marks) must be reported immediately, and exercises should be discontinued.*

Phase III

TIME: 8 to 13 weeks after surgery
GOALS: Expansion of ROM, avoidance of impingement problems, gaining of near full ROM, increased strength, alleviation of pain, increased function, and decreased soft tissue restrictions and scarring (Table 5-3)

To advance to this phase, the patient should have minimal pain, near full ROM, and greater than three over five for strength generally throughout the shoulder movements. Often when progressing a patient to a new level of exercises (i.e., going from A/AROM to AROM) muscle soreness will be more pronounced initially. The patient will usually adapt to the new demands of the program within the first week.

During the period from 9 to 12 weeks after surgery, the patient should progress to full ROM. By 12 weeks the repaired tissues are now strong enough to tolerate stretching within the patient's tolerance level. Passive stretching of the internal and external rotators is important. Tightness in these areas could promote abnormal shoulder mechanics, particularly in the throwing athlete. Tight external rotators lead to anterior translation and superior migration of the humeral head, which can produce impingement problems.[54] ROM will normally progress without much difficulty.

AC joint pain is common in many patients who have undergone rotator cuff repair. The symptoms may result from a previous trauma, be caused by primary generalized osteoarthritis (OA), or follow abnormalities in the GH joint, such as degeneration and rupture of the rotator cuff.[17] The

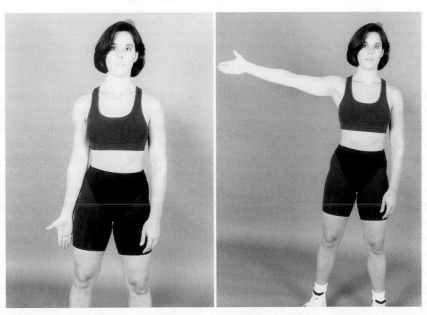

Fig. 5-4 Isotonic scaption exercises. These are elevation exercises done in the scapular plane. The patient holds the arm with the thumb up and the elbow straight and lifts the arm at a 45° angle to shoulder level. Patient progresses to full elevation and then gradually adds weight.

TABLE 5-3 Rotator Cuff Repair for Moderate-Sized Tears

Rehabilitation Phase	Criteria to Progress to this Phase	Anticipated Impairments and Functional Limitation	Intervention	Goal	Rationale

Phase III Postoperative 8-12 wk	• Steady improvement in ROM and strength (tolerance to movement)
	 • Pain controlled with therapy and medication
	 • Strength > 3/5 generally
		• Limited AROM
		 • Limited tolerance to use of upper extremity
		 • Limited reaching
		 • Limited lifting
			• Continue exercises from phases I and II as indicated.
			 • AROM: Wand exercises (i.e., flexion, extension, abduction) progress to independent use of wand
			 • AROM progressing to isotonics
			 • Begin shoulder ER with light weights and axillary roll then progress to using Thera-Band near end of phase
			 • Isotonics: Shoulder flexion and abduction in scapular plane after 10 wk
			 • Scapular exercises
			   • reverse rows
			   • horizontal abduction (see Fig. 5-8); prone at 90° abduction then ER without weight
			   • Scaption performed initially without weight
			   • Prone shoulder extension
			   • Standing push-ups against the wall
			 • Initiate low-level Body Blade exercises then progress as appropriate
			 • Manual resistance added to PNF patterns
			   • rhythmic stabilization and slow reversal holds
				• Increase exercises that patient can perform at home
				 • Full PROM
				 • Strength of shoulder generally >55%
				 • Minimal pain associated with overhead activity
				 • Able to perform self-care activities using involved upper extremity
					• Promotion of self-management
					 • Transition to AROM program with emphasis as appropriate on PROM
					 • Strengthening of shoulder and upper quarter musculature with a variety of resistance devices and positions
					 • Scapular exercises to promote proximal stability for distal mobility
					 • Progression from AROM to PREs as tolerance to activity improves
					 • Performance of cuff-stabilization exercises with pain-free ranges

AROM, Active range of motion; *ER,* external rotation; *PNF,* proprioceptive neuromuscular facilitation; *PREs,* progressive resistance exercises; *PROM,* passive range of motion; *ROM,* Range of motion.

AC joint will especially be tender if an acromioplasty was performed. When the AC joint is hypomobile and symptomatic, mobilization can help alleviate a portion of the symptoms and allow greater mobility (Fig. 5-5).

After the incision is healed and closed, the therapist can apply soft tissue mobilization over the incision areas and instruct the patient in massaging the scarred area. Early movement minimizes tightness from scarring. Normal skin mobility allows normal movement to occur.[9]

Resistance exercises are initiated around 10 weeks. Patients should demonstrate correct active movements before resistance is added in a particular range. The patient must perform the resisted exercises correctly or the movement needs to be altered. Isotonic exercises are important for strengthening and promoting dynamic shoulder stabilization. The humeral head stabilizers are used during this phase.

The supraspinatus, infraspinatus, teres minor, and subscapularis muscles pull the humeral head securely into the glenoid and control humeral rotation so that the humeral head stays in good alignment with the glenoid.[49] In addition, it should be noted that the primary depressors of the humeral head during shoulder elevation are the infraspinatus, teres minor, and subscapularis muscles. Because the infraspinatus is involved in two critical force couples about the GH joint, the quality of shoulder motion is directly related to its function.[52]

When resisted exercises are initiated, begin external rotation with hand-held weights with the patient in a side-lying position on the unaffected side. The elbow is maintained in 90° of flexion, and the patient starts with the shoulder in internal rotation, then moves into external rotation (Fig. 5-6, *A* and *B*). Eventually the patient can be progressed to concentric-eccentric movements using a Thera-Band for external rotation and internal rotation. An axillary roll can be placed under the shoulder to avoid a fully adducted position, which can cause a vascular stress on the supraspinatus and biceps tendon.[10,26] Resisted elbow flexion exercises can be done with exercise tubing for the biceps. The long head of the biceps brachialis has been revealed as a strong humeral head depressor and acts to steer.[52] Baylis and Wolf[55] described a "four square" combination of tubing-resisted exercises for shoulder flexion, shoulder extension, internal rotation, and external rotation (see Fig. 5-6), followed by stretching of the external rotators and abductors.

Remember that proximal stability is essential for controlling distal mobility.[41] Moseley and associates[56] reported that four exercises appeared to significantly enhance recruitment of the scapular muscles. These exercises included shoulder elevation in the scapular plane, upright rowing, a press-up, and a push-up with a "plus."[52] Shoulder flexion and abduction exercises in the scapular plane (instead of the straight planes) are more functional and less problematic to the rotator cuff. Prone rowing can also be done (Fig. 5-7).

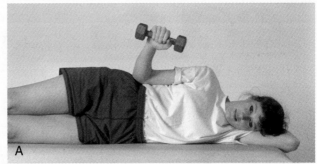

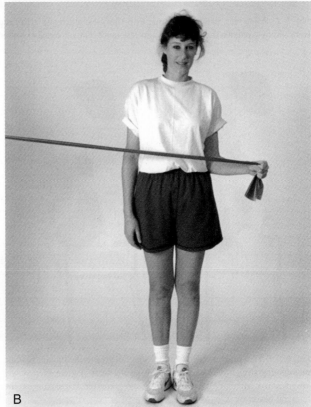

Fig. 5-6 **A,** Patient lies on the unaffected side, in the side-lying position. Patient maintains a 90° bend in the elbow while holding a hand-held weight and moving the arm into external rotation. **B,** Again, the patient maintains the elbow in 90° of flexion while externally rotating the shoulder against resistance of the band.

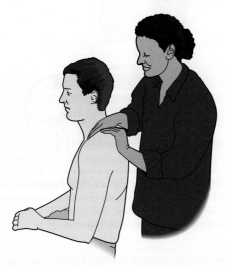

Fig. 5-5 Acromioclavicular (AC) mobilization through posteroanterior (PA) movement. The therapist stabilizes the midclavicle while applying PA pressure through the spine of the scapula.

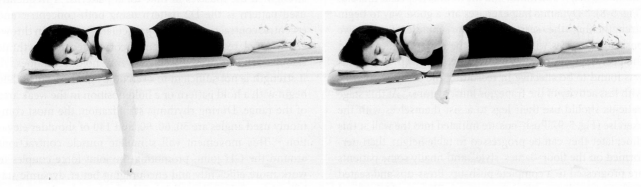

Fig. 5-7 Prone rowing. Patient hangs arm over edge of table, pulls hand upward while bending the elbow and tightening the scapular muscles, and slowly releases.

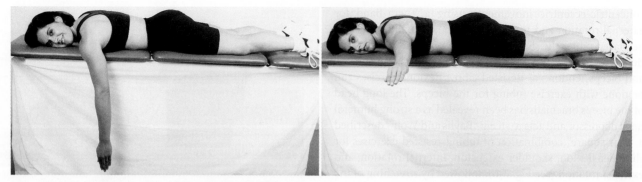

Fig. 5-8 Prone flies. Patient lies prone with elbow extended and arm hanging down. Therapist instructs patient to abduct the arm horizontally. Patient can start without weights, then gradually add resistance. Patient can also perform this with the shoulder in 135° of abduction.

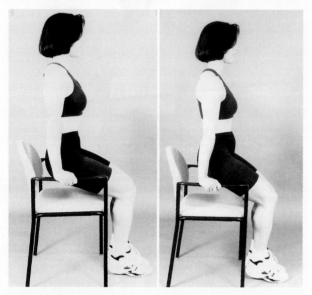

Fig. 5-9 Seated push-ups with a plus. Patient depresses the shoulders while maintaining straight elbows, thereby lifting the torso. Patient then slowly lowers torso, attempting to avoid excessive superior translation of the humeral head.

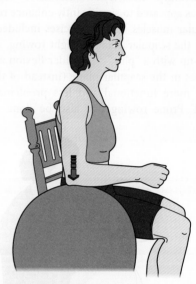

Fig. 5-10 Shoulder girdle depressions using a Swiss ball. Patient sits next to Swiss ball and places elbow on the ball. Patient maintains a 90° bend in the elbow while depressing the scapula to push the elbow down into the ball. This exercise is good for those who cannot or should not perform seated push-ups with a plus (e.g., older patients).

Rowing is excellent for all portions of the trapezius, levator scapula, and rhomboids. These muscles help maintain the scapula in good alignment during shoulder movements. The higher and the lower trapezius musculature stabilizes the scapula for overhead activities. In addition, prone horizontal abduction can be incorporated to strengthen the rhomboid major and minor and the middle trapezius muscles (Fig. 5-8).[56] Dynamic hug exercises are a good way to begin strengthening the serratus anterior muscle. Progressive push-up exercises will strengthen the serratus anterior and the pectoralis minor muscles. A seated push-up with a plus was found to be effective in recruiting the serratus anterior with less activity of the trapezius musculature.[56] At this stage patients should use their legs to assist themselves with the exercise (Fig. 5-9). Push-ups are initiated into the wall at this time; later they can be progressed to table height, then performed on the floor "ladies' style," and finally some patients are progressed to a complete push-up. Press-ups and seated push-ups are done with active patients. They can be initiated with support from the lower extremities and eventually

progressed to only balance assisted by the lower extremities. These exercises help strengthen the serratus anterior muscle, which encourages humeral head depression with shoulder elevation. Older, more sedentary patients can strengthen their serratus anterior muscle using a Swiss ball (Fig. 5-10).

Resisted exercises also are performed in PNF patterns to strengthen the muscles in functional patterns. A frequently used pattern is the D2 pattern using both concentric and eccentric contractions. This is particularly effective in throwers. Manual resistance is again incorporated for rhythmic stabilization exercises and slow reversal hold techniques.[21,41] If strength is not sufficient to overcome light resistance then begin with a hold pattern or a hold position in the weak area of the range. During rhythmic stabilization, the most commonly used angles are 30, 60, 90, and 140 of shoulder elevation.[52] This movement will stimulate muscle contractions around the GH joint, promoting the joint force couples to work more efficiently and encouraging better dynamic stabilization of the humeral head.[52] Good angles to work on with rhythmic stabilization are areas of increased weakness;

therefore one can specifically strengthen at the weakest point, allowing improvement for the entire movement.

Strengthening begins with normalizing AROM while initiating light resistance into an appropriate arc of motion. AROM for shoulder elevation begins with the elbow flexed. The patient can add light resistance when he or she performs active elevation correctly with the elbow extended. Resistance may be added for elevation up to 70° of motion and progressed as the patient is able to perform AROM correctly through 80° and progressing to 150° of elevation. The patient must also demonstrate good scapular humeral mechanism without pain and perform 20 repetitions. This must be executed correctly before resistance is added.[53] If challenged by 10 repetitions but able to do 20, then maintain the level of resistance. Do not train for power. The patient needs good muscle endurance over time, therefore do 30 repetitions before gradually increasing the load.[53] When using resistance, begin abduction movement to 45°. Shoulder flexion can be performed between 70° and 80°. External rotation can be initiated in a supported position, then advanced to unsupported. When using a Thera-Band, have the patient begin with yellow and do 10 repetitions. If challenged and eager to rest, then go to another exercise. If easy then do 10 more repetitions. If still easy then do another set of 10 repetitions and move on. If the patient executes 30 repetitions well, the therapist may gradually increase resistance.[53] Even today, the low intensity resistance, high repetitions technique may be the best regimen for athletes with injuries of insidious onset and during early rehabilitation phases.[57] By 20 weeks, the athlete can advance to heavier weight lifting.[48]

In my experience, the Body Blade has been helpful for active patients. Exercises with the Body Blade are initiated with the shoulder and upper arm against the trunk. Eventually patients progress to operating the Body Blade with the arm extended away from the body and elevated. In even more advanced stages, patterns of motion can be followed while maintaining the oscillations of the blade and proper body mechanics. These exercises enhance contractions around a joint, increase strength, a increase proprioception, as well as improve coordination and increase endurance. The Body Blade has also been shown to produce greater scapular activity than traditional resistance techniques.[58]

Often times, older patients with fair tissue status and massive tears have difficulty progressing to active shoulder flexion against gravity. Eccentric shoulder flexion exercises without weights help provide these patients with a transition to active shoulder flexion. Help patients lift their arms in the scapular plane above their heads; then instruct them to lower their arms without allowing them to fall. These patients also need to emphasize strengthening of their humeral head depressors. Finally, have them exercise in front of a mirror so that they can readily correct the tendency to hike their shoulder.

Strengthening of the trunk and legs is important for athletes. Numerous studies indicate that the trunk and legs are responsible for more than 50% of the kinetic energy expended during throwing (see Chapter 13). Endurance training also

begins during this phase. Patients begin on the upper body ergometer with short-duration and low-intensity bouts, and then they advance to longer durations and higher intensity bouts. Modalities are minimally used during this stage. Pain is generally minimal but will increase with moderate to dramatic changes in activity levels.

Precautions are necessary when initiating isotonic shoulder elevation exercises. All exercises should be performed with little or no joint pain. Complaints of muscle discomfort are acceptable and even desirable.[19] **However, if the patient complains of sharp pain through particular ranges, then the therapist needs to modify the exercises to avoid a painful arc.**

Phase IV

TIME: 13 to 16 weeks after surgery
GOALS: Maintenance of full ROM, increased strength and endurance, improved function (Table 5-4)

The patient should have full ROM by 13 to 16 weeks. If this is not the case, then progressing with ROM needs to be the primary focus during treatments until this has been achieved. The therapist can emphasize more aggressive mobilization using grades +3 and +4 on the GH capsule to stretch the specific areas of capsular restrictions, thereby normalizing arthrokinematics at the GH joint. These mobilizations also can be performed near the physiologic end ROM, and they can be performed near end of ranges in conjunction with combined movements (refer to the question-and-answer scenario for an application example). Adequate capsule laxity is necessary to allow normal rolling and gliding between the bony surfaces of a joint. Patients should continue the necessary stretches to gain and maintain ROM in restricted areas (Figs. 5-11 through 5-13 illustrate some of the suggested stretches).

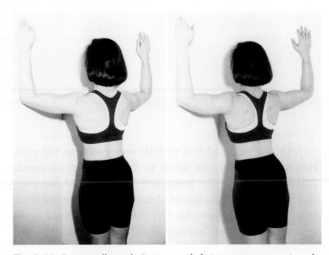

Fig. 5-11 Corner wall stretch. Patient stands facing a corner approximately one stride length away. The patient then places the forearms on the wall, keeping the elbows at shoulder height. The therapist instructs the patient to lean into the corner until he or she feels a stretch on the anterior portion of the shoulders.

TABLE 5-4 Rotator Cuff Repair for Moderate-Sized Tears

Rehabilitation Phase	Criteria to Progress to this Phase	Anticipated Impairments and Functional Limitations	Intervention	Goals	Rationale
Phase IV Postoperative 13-16 wk	• Full ROM or near-full ROM • Pain controlled and self-managed • No loss of strength with addition of phase III exercises • No increase in night pain	• Limited tolerance to overhead activities • Pain with activities involving prolonged use of upper extremity • Limited strength of rotator cuff	• Exercises for phase III continued and progressed as appropriate • Stretches: Corner wall stretch if necessary (see Fig. 5-11); posterior capsule stretch if restricted (see Fig. 5-12); hand-behind-back stretch (see Fig. 5-13) • PREs progressed • Prone horizontal abduction at 90 degrees and ER of the shoulder for higher-level patients • Closed-chain exercises; wall push-ups plus progressing to table push-ups then floor push-ups if able; seated push-ups plus for active patients (see Fig. 5-9); shoulder girdle depressions using a Swiss ball for sedentary patients (see Fig. 5-10) • May initiate plyometrics near end of phase • Movement patterns to simulate work or sport activity • Progress with Body Blade exercises • Trunk- and leg-strengthening exercises for return to previous level of functioning • Stretching/mobilization to cervical and thoracic spine as needed	• Self-management of home exercises • Full AROM • Strength > 70% (dependent on extent of tear) • Self-management of pain associated with overhead activity • Reach in front and to side for light-weight objects • Carry light weight for short periods (i.e., grocery bags)	• Preparation of patient for discharge and continued self-management • Improvement of capsular mobility • Restoration of end-range joint arthrokinematics • Strengthening of upper quarter, especially scapula stabilizers, in stable but challenging environment • Co-contraction exercises to enhance dynamic joint stability • Preparation of patient for activity-specific demands • Maintenance and improvement of cardiovascular fitness, incorporating upper extremities • Restoration of end-range joint arthrokinematics

AROM, Active range of motion; *ER,* external rotation; *PREs,* progressive resistance exercises; *ROM,* range of motion.

It should be noted that with throwing athletes the anterior capsule does not need to be stretched as much. Patients with anterior instability issues should not exercise near extreme ranges of abduction and external rotation. Those with posterior GH instabilities should avoid extreme ranges of horizontal adduction and internal rotation.

If the patient cannot elevate the arm without shoulder hiking (i.e., scapulothoracic substitution), then continue to focus on the humeral head–stabilizing exercises and exercise the humeral head depressors. Remember the primary function of the rotator cuff is to provide good humeral head alignment with the glenoid fossa; this must be mastered before any complex movements are initiated. The efficiency of the GH force couples is vital for success. The primary couples of the GH joint are the subscapularis counterbalanced by the infraspinatus and teres minor and the anterior deltoid and supraspinatus counterbalanced by the infraspinatus and teres minor.

Strengthening exercises are progressed with progressive resistance exercises (PREs) progressing to 3 to 5 lb or the green Thera-Band if able. See Fig. 5-16 for exercises using

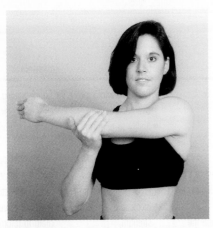

Fig. 5-12 Posterior capsular stretch. Patient horizontally adducts arm across body and then uses the other hand to pull the affected arm into further horizontal adduction.

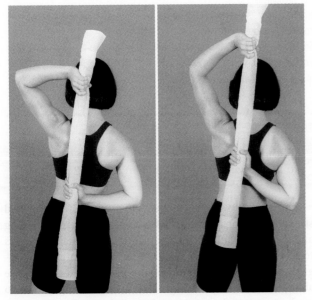

Fig. 5-13 Hand-behind-back stretch. Patient stands with towel in both hands and places the involved arm behind the buttock or low back. Patient places the uninvolved arm behind the head and slowly pulls with the superior hand up the back until he or she feels a stretch.

the Thera-Band. The supraspinatus and infraspinatus muscles (also known as decelerators) produce slow, controlled movements. These muscles are subjected to larger stresses and also are injured more frequently in overhead sporting activities.[59] Through the use of electromyographic studies, Blackburn found that the best isolation for the infraspinatus and teres minor muscles occurs during prone exercises incorporating horizontal abduction and external rotation. An optimal exercise for athletes who need GH congruity and stability is prone external rotation with the shoulder at 90° abduction and the elbow flexed to 90°.[60] These exercises should be performed at a functional speed starting without weight then adding resistance.[61] Resisted external rotation with abduction is another good strengthening exercise for athletes.

Continue with push-ups while leaning into a wall and progress to ladies' style push-ups if able. More active patients

or athletes can progress to the standard push-ups on the floor, as previously mentioned. Closed-chain exercises help promote cocontractions and enhance dynamic joint stability.[62]

Therapists must also consider the neuromuscular system that provides joint stability through proprioceptive awareness, because proprioceptive training of the shoulder can lead to improved neuromuscular control, which can improve the overall dynamic stability of the GH joint.[63] Appropriate shoulder exercises using the Body Blade provide proprioceptive training, dynamic-stabilization training, and endurance training. Eventually (during the later stages of rehabilitation) the patient can be progressed using the Body Blade through a vast range of shoulder movements, allowing athletes and workers to train and exercise in specific patterns or postures. These movements mimic a pattern of movement or a position used during a sport or work activity. In a later phase, resistance can be added to these movement patterns with the use of a Thera-Band (see Fig. 5-17). Caution must be used while progressing the patient from 10 to 18 weeks because pain is usually absent.

Phase V

TIME: 17 to 21 weeks after surgery
GOALS: Maintenance of full ROM, increased strength and endurance, improvement of neuromuscular control, return to functional activities, initiation of sport-specific activities (Table 5-5)

The therapist can continue the stretching program and instruct the patient in self-mobilization techniques if indicated. The patient can maintain a shoulder-strengthening program and continue PREs with increasing hand weights. Isokinetic training can also be beneficial. These exercises can be performed throughout the range because of the accommodation factor in isokinetic training. If a patient cannot move through the resistance at a particular arc of motion, he or she still can train with resistance throughout the whole range.

Athletes and other appropriate patients can begin plyometric exercises, which involve a stretch-shortening cycle of the muscle. Plyometrics can be performed two times a week. All sporting movements involve this explosive stretch-shortening cycle (e.g., jumping, throwing, running, swimming).[45] Progressive plyometric exercises are done with appropriate patients who exhibit correct execution of the exercises. Recreational and competitive athletes perform exercises at higher speeds, using more eccentric muscle contractions and higher level progressions. These exercises are excellent intermediate steps between traditional strengthening exercises and training activities before initiating throwing drills.[63]

Resisted exercises using tubing with concentric-eccentric contractions, isokinetics, and scapulothoracic strengthening can be done. Athletes or workers required to do continuous overhead activities can perform exercises with a Thera-Band for external rotation, starting with an axillary pillow between

TABLE 5-5 Rotator Cuff Repair for Moderate-Sized Tears

Rehabilitation Phase	Criteria to Progress to this Phase	Anticipated Impairments and Functional Limitations	Intervention	Goal	Rationale
Phase V Postoperative 17-26 wk	• Progression through phase IV without loss of strength or increase in pain • Potential to return to high level functional use of the upper extremity (i.e., competitive athletics)	• Limited strength and endurance of rotator cuff muscles • Continued manageable pain with overhead activities	• Continuation of phase IV exercises as indicated • Joint mobilization as appropriate • PREs progressed • Prone shoulder abduction in various ranges with light weights • Thera-Band for ER with the shoulder abducted to 90° and the elbow at 90° (athletes only) • Initiation of strengthening in sport-specific activity • Initiate isokinetic exercises • Plyometrics • Initiation of throwing program when appropriate (see Chapter 13)	• Pain free with overhead activity • Ability to perform ADLs without increased pain • Return to previous level of functioning • Increase in strength, endurance, and neuromuscular control	• Strengthening of rotator cuff in specific ranges (overhead and reaching to the side) • Provision of optimal ROM for client to perform associated activity • Provision of vehicle for client to return at or close to previous level of functioning

ADLs, Activities of daily living; *ER*, external rotation; *PREs*, progressive resistance exercises; *ROM*, range of motion.

the trunk and arm, then to the scapular plane position, and then to the 90°/90° position if able. D2 diagonal patterns can be executed with tubing. Latissimus strengthening and scapular retraction exercises can be performed using a Thera-Band.[64] Athletes and higher level patients can perform these exercises at a faster and higher speed while maintaining control over the movement. They can also perform at a slower and more deliberate pace. Specific applications of eccentric training to the posterior cuff using a Thera-Band and/or isokinetics are essential to pitchers and ball players.

Later, when the patient is ready, initiate sport-specific drills for athletes along with an interval sports program (see Chapter 13). Throwing techniques need to be evaluated. **If the patient is using bad body mechanics, using improper techniques while throwing, or both, then tissues may be overstressed, eventually causing rotator cuff problems once again.** Older, sedentary patients should work on specific ADLs. As appropriate, patients may progress to more difficult tasks.

In general golfers can usually start putting at 14 to 16 weeks and then progress as able. At 20 to 22 weeks tennis players can begin hitting their forehand and backhand strokes and progress to serving. And swimming can be initiated between 20 and 26 weeks. By 7 to 9 months the athlete may be able to reengage in sports activities competitively.

Phase VI

TIME: 22 and more weeks after surgery
GOAL: Return to normal activities, maintenance of full ROM, continued strengthening and endurance,

gradual return to full activities. Athletes can return to their sports usually between 6 and 12 months

During weeks 22 to 26 patients maintain a stretching and strengthening program. Athletes continue on strengthening and on a sports interval program. Others gradually progress to recreational activities. Older individuals continue to progress with PREs and work on more advanced ADLs. The ability to return to more high-level activities ranges from 26 weeks to more than 1 year after surgery. After 26 weeks, patients continue with their stretching and strengthening program as long as they anticipate using the shoulder aggressively in ADLs or sports. The patient can maintain a shoulder-strengthening program and continue PREs with increasing hand weights up to 6 to 10 lb for athletes or 1 to 5 lb for more sedentary people. Isokinetic exercises may be initiated with athletes when they are able to lift 5 to 10 lb in external rotation and 15 to 20 lb in internal rotation without pain or significant edema.[38] The patient should begin strength and endurance training at 200°/second.[38,72]

TROUBLESHOOTING

Considering influential factors outside the GH joint during treatment will aid the therapist in helping the patient progress more efficiently. General suggestions are given; however, it is beyond the scope of this book to instruct therapists in the use and application of techniques. The following areas are addressed:

- Cervical spine
- Thoracic spine
- Adverse neural tension (ANT)
- AC joint
- SC joint
- Scapulothoracic joint

Cervical Spine

Evaluation of the cervical spine may prove vital in addressing cervical issues that may be inhibiting progress. Although the cervical spine is not the primary cause of shoulder dysfunction when dealing with rotator cuff repairs, it may be a contributory factor. Often cervical spine disorders occur in conjunction with a traumatic shoulder injury (e.g., falling onto the upper extremity may cause injury to the shoulder and the cervical spine). Furthermore, prolonged muscle guarding secondary to the shoulder injury or pathology affects the cervical area. Muscles in spasm originating or inserting along the cervical spine can lead to cervical symptoms. Thus a patient may have a combination of cervical and shoulder signs and symptoms. Treatment to the appropriate cervical joints can alleviate a portion of the symptoms and signs, thereby decreasing the complaints of pain and potentially allowing more GH movement and function. Clinicians may notice that after treating cervical spine dysfunctions, treatment of the shoulder is more effective.

Common patterns in cervical pathology are addressed to assist clinicians with differentiating shoulder and cervical symptoms because they frequently occur together. Spinal disorders may cause referred pain (Fig. 5-14). Joint movement disorders may cause joint pain and be associated with an altered range of cervical spine joint movement or shoulder movement. Therefore the cervical spine should be assessed for additional joint disorders that may be causing local pain or pain that is referred into the shoulder and arm region.[32] (Suggested readings for treatment of the cervical spine are Practical Orthopedic Medicine by Corrigan and Maitland[32] and Vertebral Manipulation by Maitland.[36])

Thoracic Spine

Thoracic mobility affects shoulder mobility. During unilateral shoulder flexion, contralateral side flexion of the spine occurs; bilateral shoulder flexion produces spinal extension.[22] Therefore decreased thoracic extensibility or increased thoracic kyphosis can inhibit shoulder ROM.[65]

Postural education is important, especially with patients who can voluntarily correct and maintain good posture. Maintaining an erect posture while performing upper extremity activities allows greater ROM at the shoulders. Better posture decreases the amount of impingement, which a patient can see in the following maneuver:

1. Have the patient flex the shoulder through its available ROM while in a seated slouched position.
2. Ask the patient to flex the shoulder while seated with good posture.

The patient will be able to lift the arm higher when maintaining a more upright posture. A slouched position causes

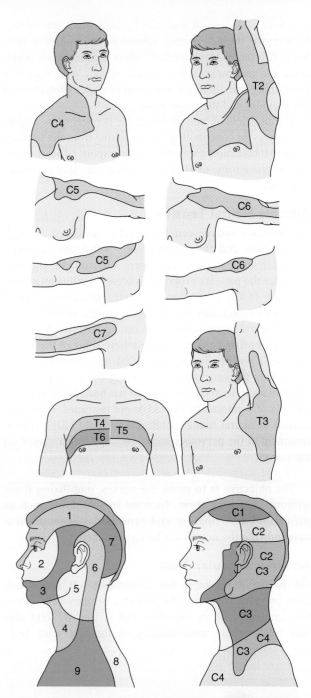

Fig. 5-14 Dermatomal pattern of the upper extremity. (From Maxey L: Cervical spine. In Magee DJ, editor: Orthopedic physical therapy assessment, ed 3, Philadelphia, 1997, Saunders.)

depressed forward-displaced shoulders and GH internal rotation. The potential for shoulder impingement increases with this type of posture.[65]

Evaluation and treatment of the thoracic spine may prove helpful for patients having difficulty progressing in ROM in the latter stages. Addressing issues of hypomobility and decreased ROM of the thoracic spine and treating them appropriately allows for better progress. Mobilization of a hypomobile thoracic spine and ROM exercises to increase thoracic extension (e.g., supine on a Swiss ball) can be beneficial. A foam roll also may be used when appropriate to increase thoracic spinal extension and mobility (Fig. 5-15). (Vertebral Manipulation[36] offers instruction on evaluation and treatment of the thoracic spine.) With regard to positioning, the therapist also must consider protection of the shoulder and the surgery site.

If complaints of pain persist in the cervical spine region, then assess for contributing factors arising from the thoracic spine. Mobilization to a stiff thoracic spine (if warranted) may alleviate some or all of the cervical pain that continues to persist.[66]

Adverse Neural Tension

The nervous system can be directly mobilized through tension tests and their derivatives.[40] Adhesions in neural tissue can affect shoulder movement and strength, and may influence the patient's progress. However, the therapist must be aware of any precautions or contraindications. A good evaluation is necessary for addressing adverse neural tension issues. Neural tissue mobilization can be effective when used with appropriate patients to help relieve some of the symptoms and potentially improve ROM and strength. These issues may be better addressed during the latter phases of rehabilitation when the tissue repair has healed and shoulder ROM is only minimally limited or not restricted. Clinicians trained in neural tissue mobilization should only perform treatment to the nervous system. Avoid placing a stretch on the nerves.

The objective is to move the nerves, mobilizing them without stretching them. Increase in symptoms such as pain, numbness, tingling, and paresthesias down the arm may indicate the nerves are being stretched.[73]

Acromioclavicular Joint

OA in the AC joint is not uncommon.[67] It may result from previous trauma or be part of a primary generalized OA, impingement, or capsulitis. OA in the AC joint also may follow other abnormalities in the GH joint (e.g.,

degeneration and rupture of the rotator cuff) that allow the head of the humerus to sublux upward.[32] In our experience, many patients with repaired and unrepaired rotator cuff tears have some symptoms arising from the AC joint.

Because the movement of all of the joints affects the shoulder complex, it is essential to evaluate and treat the entire shoulder complex to improve upper extremity function.[68] Table 5-6 shows some of the joint movements that occur within the shoulder complex. Restrictions in one area will affect other areas of the shoulder complex.

Complaints of AC joint pain are usually localized over the joint. An active movement that may best implicate this joint as a source of pain is horizontal adduction of the arm across the chest. The therapist may determine whether the AC joint is hypomobile or hypermobile by passive accessory movement tests of the joint.[69] If the AC joint is stiff and tender, then its mobilization often relieves a portion of the symptoms and promotes better shoulder ROM. The AC joint may also be tender from an acromion osteotomy if performed with the rotator cuff. Eventually gentle movements of the AC joint may be beneficial when the patient can tolerate the treatment. If the AC joint has been removed because it is arthritic or symptomatic then do not attempt to mobilize the area.

Accessory movements can be applied to the clavicle or acromion. When applied to the clavicle, they affect only the AC joint; however, when applied to the acromion, they affect both the AC and GH joint.[6] Accessory AC joint movements should be used within the limits of pain. To increase motion at the AC joint, the therapist can use an anterior glide to the acromion through the posterior spine of the scapula while stabilizing the midclavicle. This allows mobilization of the AC joint without direct manual pressure over the joint or inflamed tissues.

As the available shoulder ROM progresses, this same technique can be applied with the shoulder in some degree of available flexion or in horizontal adduction (see Fig. 5-5).

Corrigan and Maitland[32] describe a similar technique for the AC joint. In this method an anterior-posterior movement is produced by applying pressure over the anterior

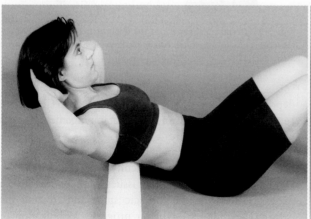
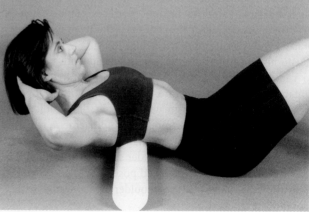

Fig. 5-15 Thoracic extension on foam roll or using tennis balls. Patient lies supine with both knees bent and places roll or balls at the middle thoracic spine levels. Patient then places hands under head and slowly leans back (taking care not to arch over the roll or balls) until a stretch is felt.

TABLE 5-6 Shoulder Complex—Range and Axis of Motion*

Joint Motion	Range (Degrees)	Axis of Motion
Sternoclavicular rotation (counterclockwise)	0-50	Longitudinal axis of clavicle
Glenohumeral (GH) flexion	0-180	Coronal through
Abduction	0-180	Sagittal through
Horizontal adduction	0-145	GH joint Vertical through GH joint
Internal rotation	0-90	Vertical axis through
External rotation	0-90	Shaft of humerus
Acromioclavicular (AC) winging of scapula	0-50	Vertical axis through AC joint
Abduction of scapula	0-30	Anteroposterior axis
Inferior angle of scapula tilts away	0-30	Coronal axis from chest wall
Scapulothoracic		
Upward rotation	0-60	From 0-30° near vertebral border on spine of scapula; from 30-60° near acromial end of spine of scapula

*When conflicting information occurred, the most frequently cited numbers were used.

Data from Codman EA, Akerson IB: The pathology associated with rupture of the supraspinatus tendon. Am Surg 93:348, 1931; Akeson WH, Woo SLY, Amiel D: The connective tissue response to immobility: biomechanical changes in periarticular connective tissue of the immobilized rabbit knee. Clin Orthop 93:356, 1973; Andrews JR, Kupferman SP, Dillman CJ: Labral tears in throwing and racquet sports. Clin Sports Med 10(4):901, 1991; Abrams JS: Special shoulder problems in the throwing athlete: Pathology, diagnosis and nonoperative management. Clin Sports Med 10:839, 1991; Bigliani LU et al: Operative management of failed rotator cuff repairs. Orthop Trans 12:674, 1988; Bross R, et al: Optimal number of exercise bouts per week for isokinetic eccentric training of the rotator cuff musculature. Wisc Phys Ther Assoc Newsl 21(5):18, 1991 (abstract); Butler DS: Mobilization of the nervous system, New York, 1991, Churchill Livingstone.

surface of the outer third of the clavicle with counter pressure along the spine of the scapula.

Sternoclavicular Joint

Degenerative changes are not found as commonly in the SC joint as in the AC joint but may occur as the result of trauma or overuse of the shoulder.[70] Movements such as shoulder abduction or flexion may increase pain originating from this joint because of rotation of the inner end of the clavicle. SC joint pain is usually localized to the SC area, but it may radiate to other areas. Signs that implicate the SC joint as a contributing factor include reproduction of pain with horizontal flexion and passive accessory movements of the SC joint. The capsule and surrounding ligaments are likely to be thickened and tender.[69]

Treatment of the SC area includes rest, modalities, and mobilization, depending on the condition of the joint.[32] A hypomobile SC joint may be correctly mobilized in several ways depending on its restrictions. To increase shoulder elevation, a caudal glide to the proximal clavicle can be used.[32,37]

Scapulothoracic Joint

Scapular muscles have been included in the rotator cuff repair protocol. However, some patients require more intense conditioning of these muscles. The scapula moves with concentric-eccentric motions. Patients with poor eccentric control of the scapular stabilizers demonstrate scapula winging on the return from full shoulder flexion. The serratus anterior is essential for stabilizing the medial border and inferior angle of the scapula, preventing scapula internal rotation (winging) and anterior tilt.[60] These same patients may have full ROM and normal movement during flexion. If muscle weakness is apparent, then ensuring normal muscle strength around the scapulothoracic and GH joints is the goal. If the scapular muscles are weak and overstretched, then scapular motion during arm elevation may result in excessive lateral gliding of the scapula. Abnormal scapular muscle firing patterns, weakness, fatigue, or injury causes the shoulder to function less efficiently and the risk of injury increases.[60]

The therapist can use various PNF techniques, such as scapular slow reversal holds, rhythmic stabilization, and timing for emphasis, to intensify the dynamic control and kinesthesia of the scapulothoracic joint. Other recommended exercises are scapular protraction, retraction, elevation, and depression against manual resistance.[71]

Exercises are encouraged that enhance dynamic control of the scapulothoracic musculature.[71] These should be directed to the scapular rotator muscles (i.e., the serratus anterior, rhomboid, trapezius, levator scapula) to position the glenoid and coracoid appropriately for the humerus. Exercises that mimic the rowing motion and shoulder horizontal abduction are both excellent for all portions of the trapezius and for the levator scapulae and rhomboid muscles. Flexion and scaption (i.e., scapular plane elevation) exercises are valuable for most of the scapular muscles (see Fig. 5-4). In addition, shoulder shrugs and press-ups with a plus are essential exercises for the levator scapula, upper trapezius, serratus anterior, and pectoralis minor muscles. Also refer to the "Prone Program Plus" for more exercise ideas.

SUMMARY

The general guidelines described in this chapter help guide therapists and provide treatment ideas. Rotator cuff repairs vary in size from small to massive. The condition of the torn tissue and the joints (i.e., AC, GH) varies. Along with these differences, therapists must consider the patient's unique history, profile, and abilities. They must consider each case and choose the treatment ideas that will work best, constantly assessing the patient's responses. Therapists must always address the individual when deciding on a treatment plan.

Suggested Home Maintenance for the Postsurgical Patient

The following is the suggested home maintenance for the postsurgical patient with minimal and moderate tears. Improvise to accommodate for massive tears.

This home maintenance box outlines ideas for rehabilitation the patient can follow after rotator cuff repair. The physical therapist can use it in customizing a patient-specific program. Patients require a program that suits their needs and abilities. Some exercises may be appropriate for certain patients but not for others. Some patients progress slower than others. The therapist must take into account the patient's age, the condition of the repaired tissues, the size of the tear, the cause of the tear, the rate of healing, and the patient's abilities and previous level of function.

Older, more sedentary patients will progress more slowly than younger, more active patients. Some of the exercises suggested may be inappropriate for the older patient. The therapist can alter the home exercise prescription according to the individual's abilities, status, and needs. Improvise this program to accommodate for rotator cuff repair (RCR) for large tears.

Weeks 1-4
GOALS FOR THE PERIOD: Achieve control of pain and inflammation; increase ROM as tolerated, and promote firing of muscles.
1. Do active cervical spine rotations.
2. Do upper trapezius (UT) stretches.
3. Do pendulum exercises.
4. Begin wand exercises or pulley exercises (for passive range of motion [PROM]) after 2 to 3 weeks. Do 3 sets of 10 repititions 2x/day for flexion, scapular plane abduction, and external rotation.
5. Apply a cold or ice pack intermittently throughout the day for pain control and inflammation.
6. Instruct the patient in the use of pillows to maintain the shoulder in a more loose packed position when supine, sitting, semireclined, or side-lying.

Weeks 5-8
GOALS FOR THE PERIOD: Continue to increase ROM, decrease pain and inflammation, and increase muscle activity.
1. Use cold or ice packs as needed.
2. Continue with previous exercises.
3. Initiate wand exercises for A/AROM at 6 weeks. Do 4 sets of 10 repititions 3x/day.
4. Add active shoulder flexion in supine position when cleared by the surgeon (usually 6 to 8 weeks postsurgery). Initiate this exercise with elbow bent to 90°.

5. Massage the scar area when the incision has appropriately healed.

Weeks 8-12
GOALS FOR THE PERIOD: Increase range of motion (ROM) to full, and continue to increase strength. Use upper extremity for light activities of daily living (ADLs).
1. Continue with wand exercises for ROM.
2. Continue with active cervical ROM and UT stretches as needed.
3. Instruct the patient in self-mobilization of the T/S using tennis balls or foam roll if needed (may not be appropriate for older or kyphotic patients).
4. Perform active shoulder flexion and abduction in the functional plane while facing a mirror; be sure to maintain voluntary humeral head depression (keeping the shoulder from hiking). Initially perform with elbow flexed to 90°. Do 3 sets of 10 repititions, 3x/day.
5. Resisted elbow flexion with arm at side
6. At 11 weeks, initiate isotonic exercises within a controlled ROM using light weights (without substitution patterns). Do 3 sets of 10 repititions for the following exercises 3x/day:
   a. Deltoid (initiate at 10 to 12 weeks depending on size of tear) (Fig. 5-16, C and D)
   b. Supraspinatus (initiate at 10 to 12 weeks depending on size of tear)
   c. Scaption exercises (initiate at 10 to 12 weeks depending on size of tear)
7. Use tubing or Thera-Band for internal rotation at 8 weeks, then add external rotation (use axillary roll) and abduction at 11 to 12 weeks (see Fig. 5-16).
8. Do standing reverse rows using tubing or Thera-Band.
9. Do push-ups with a plus while standing and using a wall.
10. If necessary, add shoulder depression exercises using a Swiss ball for resistance (see Fig. 5-10).
11. Athletes can initiate prone horizontal abduction in neutral position without weights at 10 or 11 weeks if able. Also may perform same exercise at 135° of abduction (see Fig. 5-9).

Weeks 13-16
GOALS FOR THE PERIOD: Increase ROM, strength, and endurance, and begin transitioning into higher activity levels.
1. Continue with the wand exercises.
2. Continue with active ROM of the cervical spine, UT stretches, and T/S mobilizations.
3. Perform a corner wall stretch for pectoralis muscles and the anterior capsule if needed.

4. Use a horizontal adduction stretch for the posterior capsule.
5. Place a hand behind the back and stretch, using a towel for assistance.
6. Continue and progress with isotonic exercises for endurance and strength training.
Do 10-15 repititions for 3 sets.
7. Continue and progress resistance with tubing and Thera-Band exercises (see Fig. 5-16).
8. Consider seated push-ups with a plus if patient is more active (see Fig. 5-9).
9. Perform prone horizontal abduction exercises without weights and then a light dumbbell if able.

Weeks 17-21

1. Continue with previous stretches as needed.

2. Continue with progressive resistance exercises (PREs) (i.e., isotonics).
3. Continue to progress with tubing and Thera-Band exercises for reverse rows.
4. Complete proprioceptive neuromuscular facilitation (PNF) patterns using a Thera-Band for resistance (Fig. 5-17).
5. Begin an interval sports program, refer to throwing program in Chapter 13.

Weeks 22-26

1. Continue stretches.
2. Continue PREs.
3. Progress with interval sports program.

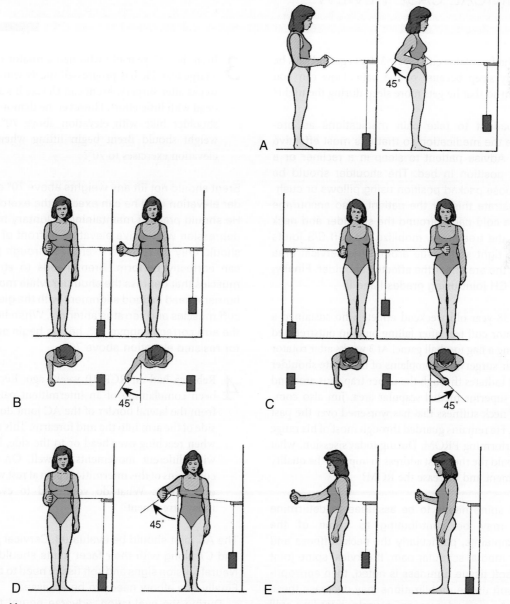

Fig. 5-16 **A,** Shoulder extension. **B,** External rotation. **C,** Internal rotation. **D,** Shoulder abduction. **E,** Shoulder flexion with elbow extension. (From Wirth MA, Basamania C, Rockwood CA Jr: Nonoperative management of full-thickness tears of the rotator cuff. Orthop Clin North Am 28:59-67, 1997.)

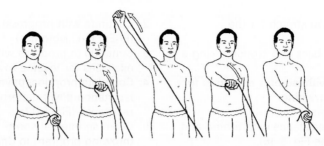

Fig. 5-17 Diagonal proprioceptive neuromuscular facilitation patterns using Thera-Band for resistance. (From Trumble TE, Cornwall R, Budoff J: Core knowledge in hand, elbow and shoulder, Philadelphia, 2006, Mosby.)

CLINICAL CASE REVIEW

1 Paul just had a rotator cuff repair 3 days ago and says he can hardly sleep because of the pain. How can you advise him so that he gets more sleep during the night?

Encourage patient to take pain medications as prescribed. Time the medication so that it is most effective at bed time. Advise patient to sleep in a recliner or a semireclined position in bed. The shoulder should be placed in a loose packed position using pillows or cushions. Demonstrate this for the patient. Also encourage patient to use cold packs around the shoulder and neck area. During the treatment, mobilize the stiff C/S joints and mobilize tight soft tissue around the cervical area emphasizing the area near the affected shoulder. Finally, mobilize the GH joint using grades I and II.

2 Jim is a 38-year-old weekend athlete who sustained a large rotator cuff tear after falling onto an outstretched arm during a flag football game. At 3 weeks after rotator cuff repair surgery, he complains of moderate shoulder pain that radiates through the upper trapezius area and into the superior medial scapular area. Jim also complains of neck stiffness that has worsened over the past few days. He remains guarded through most of his range when performing PROM. During today's session, what areas should the therapist address to improve the quality of movement and increase the ROM?

The cervical spine needs to be assessed to determine whether it may be contributing to some of the patient's complaints, particularly the neck stiffness and the superior medial scapular pain. If cervical spine joint stiffness or soft tissue tightness is noted, then appropriate joint or soft tissue mobilizations may decrease these symptoms. As pain decreases, muscle guarding will lessen, allowing the shoulder to move more freely.

3 Brent is a 27-year-old who had a rotator cuff repair for a large tear. He has progressed nicely with PROM. At 9 weeks after surgery, Brent can elevate his arm above his head with little effort. However, he demonstrates a mild shoulder hike with elevation above 70°. How much weight should Brent begin lifting when performing elevation exercises to 70°?

Brent should not lift any weights above 70° during shoulder elevation until he can execute the exercise correctly. He should practice maintaining voluntary humeral head depression with active elevation in front of a mirror. He should only do resisted exercises through the range he can correctly perform. Brent needs to strengthen the muscles that depress the shoulder while maintaining the humeral head in good alignment with the glenoid (rotator cuff muscles and serratus anterior). When he can elevate the arm correctly above 70°, he can begin adding weight for resisted elevation above 70°.

4 Rebecca had an RCR 10 weeks ago. Recently she has been complaining of an intermittent pain that travels from the lateral border of the AC joint down the lateral side of the arm into the mid forearm. This usually occurs when reaching over head or to the side, but will occur with different movements as well. On occasion she complains of this intermittent pain at rest with a decrease of intensity. What do you need to evaluate during today's treatment?

The AC joint should be evaluated. Cervical joints C5, C6, and C7 along with their facet joints should be checked. Neural tension signs and soft tissue need to be addressed. Finally, the elbow needs to be assessed.

During the evaluation, adverse neural tension signs were positive and reproduced pain in the area of complaint. Neural mobilization techniques were performed and the intensity and frequency of symptoms dramatically decreased.

5 Barbara is a 68-year-old woman who had a massive rotator cuff repair 12 weeks ago. Her favorite hobby is making jewelry. To work with the jewelry she needed to make a sawing motion with her affected (right dominant) arm. At this point the patient had −3/5 strength for flexion and abduction. She exhibited +3/5 for external rotation and −4/5 for internal rotation. The patient did not have the strength to make this sawing motion against much resistance throughout the range. She was weak, and her endurance was low. Tissue status was fair. How should the therapist exercise this patient?

Patient had full PROM throughout the affected shoulder. The therapist mostly performed manual assisted and resisted exercises with this patient to maximize strengthening at her weakest points in the range. The therapist performed PNF patterns for the upper extremity and the scapular muscles. Manual resisted exercises for serratus anterior strengthening and rotation strengthening. Resisted shoulder depression exercises were also done. In addition, rhythmic stabilization was used. Shoulder eccentric lowering was done for shoulder flexion strengthening because she could not perform AROM shoulder flexion against gravity (AROM shoulder flexion to 30° before initiating a shoulder hike). Manual exercises with light resistance were done (and progressed) to mimic the sawing motion used with making jewelry. Surprisingly the patient did return to making jewelry after 5 to 6 weeks of exercising in physical therapy, along with home exercises. This patient was motivated and compliant.

6 Ruth is a 65-year-old sedentary female who had an RCR 10 weeks ago. She continues to demonstrate a moderate shoulder hike with elevation above 70°. What exercises need to be emphasized to eliminate this movement dysfunction?

Exercising the muscles that promote shoulder depression with elevation is critical. These muscles would include the rotator cuff, especially the infraspinatus muscle. The serratus anterior also keeps the humeral head depressed with elevation and the biceps help to keep the humeral head in place. Because Ruth is an older sedentary woman, she would have more success initially with the "shoulder girdle depression exercises using a Swiss ball." Other exercises are mentioned in the chapter. Having her elevate her arm in front of a mirror while she concentrates on maintaining a depressed shoulder is also very helpful. Exercising the shoulder flexors in eccentric contractions also proved helpful.

7 Christine is a young mother who had a rotator cuff repair 6 months ago. She is returning to therapy because of stiffness issues in her shoulder. Her main complaints are reaching behind to grasp objects. Particularly difficult to reach toward the back seat of the car, which she needs to do frequently (small children in the back seat). She also would like to clasp her bra from the back. Upon evaluation she exhibited minimal restrictions for shoulder flexion and shoulder abduction near the end of the ranges. Shoulder internal rotation and extension were also limited, but the combined movement of internal rotation and extension with hand-behind-the-back movements was the most restricted. The patient's thumb actively reached to T11 behind the back. What types of mobilization techniques would be particularly helpful?

Mobilizations were performed in various areas of the capsule to improve all functional ranges. Mobilizations were also done near end ranges with combined movements using grades 3 and +4 to improve her hand-behind-the-back motions. The patient used her unaffected upper extremity to hold her other hand behind her back while the therapist applied a posterior-anterior force to the superior humerus. This was done to stretch the anterior capsule of the GH joint near its end range of combined movement. This was followed by the hand-behind-the-back stretch using a towel as shown in Fig. 5-13. The patient's range improved dramatically after two treatments with the execution of home exercises that reinforced the hand-behind-the-back movements.

8 Yvonne is a 55-year-old female who had an RCR for a 5 cm tear. She had surgery 4 weeks ago and has been immobilized in a sling since surgery. She is coming to you for her first visit. Her physician wants her to use the sling for another week to 2 weeks. Should this be a concern regarding her rehabilitation program?

If the patient demonstrates greater than 120° with shoulder flexion without a leathery or hard end feel then she should progress normally with ROM in therapy while using the sling for another 2 weeks. However, if she has a history of shoulder capsulitis, or stiff joints after surgery or injuries, or the ROM is limited to less than 120° of elevation with PROM, then the therapist may want to make the physician aware of these concerns.

9 James is a weekend athlete who had an RCR 6 weeks ago. His shoulder had been getting progressively worse for many years. The surgery went well and he's been progressing nicely with PROM to his shoulder. After PROM has been done to his shoulder then shoulder flexion is 0 to 160. He complains of a moderate pain on the superior aspect of his shoulder near the end ranges of shoulder flexion and abduction. Pain at end of range is slowing progress with ROM. Slight tenderness with deep pressure is noted over the AC joint. No complaints are made about cervical pain when asked.

AROM for cervical rotation and lateral side bending are within functional limits; however, it is slightly diminished with right rotation and, left and right side bending. What needs to be investigated?

With further evaluation, the therapist noted tenderness with right unilateral posterior anterior pressures over C3-4 and C4-5. There was minimal tenderness with palpation over the biceps tendon. Cervical musculature on the right C/S area was tighter than on the left. The therapist performed grade III mobilization techniques on the right C3-4 and C4-5 facet joints. The therapist then retested the ROM for shoulder flexion. The therapist noted a 5° to 10° increase with shoulder flexion and slight decrease in pain. The therapist then continued with another bout of grade III right unilateral posterior anterior pressures followed by some stretching to the right UT and right cervical musculature. Again ROM slightly increased and c/o pain diminished to a minimal level at end of range. After another treatment, ROM was within normal limits for the right shoulder in all directions.

10 Silvia is a 45-year-old woman who fell onto her outstretched arm and obtained a rotator cuff tear. She had a repair 14 weeks ago. She has been progressing but continues to have pain around the anterior, lateral, and superior area of the shoulder. She has full ROM. Resisted shoulder flexion and abduction with light weights increases the pain. The patient can perform resisted shoulder extension, resisted elbow flexion, resisted elbow extension, and resisted internal rotation and external rotation without much discomfort. No complaints are made of pain when carrying light objects close to her body. However, carrying objects or lifting objects away from her

body causes pain. What are your thoughts, given only the above information?

Most likely the biceps tendon is inflamed. This may have happened during the initial fall. The biceps are one of the primary humeral head depressors during shoulder movement and the biceps are used for shoulder elevation. The biceps tendon can get over used, especially if already strained. And if the rotator cuff is not functioning at its full capacity, there is an increased demand on the biceps.

The patient had pain during AROM with flexion and abduction. Manual muscle testing elbow flexion and forearm supination was pain free despite the irritation at the tendon. Resisted shoulder flexion and abduction are painful. Tenderness with palpation was noted over the biceps tendon. Therefore the biceps tendon was treated for tendonitis.

11 David is a 22-year-old athlete. He had a 5-cm RCR 8 weeks ago. He has been progressing with therapy and has full ROM for all directions. He is feeling good. What key issue needs to be addressed during this next stage?

Educate the patient regarding the importance of allowing the repair to heal. Active young men especially need to hear this warning. More healing needs to occur at this point before much stress is applied. The patient needs to avoid any substantial lifting or use of the affected arm and avoid overhead activities. The patient can perform light activities with the hand at waist level or below. Light resisted exercises will begin after 10 to 12 weeks. David feels great and is eager to try new things. The therapist needs to explain that he will jeopardize the repair if he puts too much stress on the repair. He needs to know that he will feel great but that is no indication that the repair is strong.

REFERENCES

1. Codman EA, Akerson IB: The pathology associated with rupture of the supraspinatus tendon. Am Surg 93:348, 1931.
2. Moseley HF, Goldie I: The arterial pattern of the rotator cuff of the shoulder. J Bone Joint Surg Br 45:780, 1963.
3. Rathburn JB, Macnab I: The microvascular pattern of the rotator cuff. J Bone Joint Surg Br 45:540, 1970.
4. Rothman RM, Parke WW: The vascular anatomy of the rotator cuff. Clin Orthop 41:176, 1965.
5. Neer CS: Anterior acromioplasty for the chronic impingement syndrome in the shoulder: A preliminary report. J Bone Joint Surg Am 54:41, 1972.
6. Neer CS: Impingement lesions. Clin Orthop 173:70, 1983.
7. Bigliani LU, Morrison DS, April EW: The morphology of the acromion and its relationship to rotator cuff tears. Orthop Trans 10:216, 1986.
8. Gerber C, Terrier F, Fane R: The role of the coracoid process in the chronic impingement syndrome. J Bone Joint Surg Am 67B:703, 1985.
9. Craven WM: Traumatic avulsion tears of the rotator cuff. In Andrews JR, Wilk KE, editors: The athlete's shoulder, New York, 1994, Churchill Livingstone.
10. Neviaser RJ, Neviaser TJ, Neviaser JS: Concurrent rupture of the rotator cuff and anterior dislocation of the shoulder in the older patient. J Bone Joint Surg Am 70:1308, 1988.
11. Brotzman BS: Clinical orthopaedic rehabilitation, St Louis, 1996, Mosby.
12. Kvitne RS, Jobe FW: The diagnosis and treatment of anterior instability in the throwing athlete. Clin Orthop 291:107, 1993.
13. Hawkins RJ, Misamore GW, Hobeika PE: Surgery for full-thickness rotator cuff tears. J Bone Joint Surg Am 67A:139, 1985.
14. Neer CS, Welsh RP: The shoulder in sports. Orthop Clin North Am 8:583, 1977.
15. Nelson MC, et al: Evaluation of the painful shoulder. J Bone Joint Surg Am 73(5):707-716, 1991.
16. Roger B, et al: Imaging findings in the dominant shoulder of throwing athletes: Comparison of radiography, arthrography, CT arthrography, and MR arthrography with arthroscopic correlation. AJR Am J Roentgenol 172:1371-1380, 1999.
17. Caspari RB, Thal R: A technique for arthroscopic subacromial decompression. Arthroscopy 8:23, 1992.
18. Gartsman GM, Milne JC: Articular surface partial-thickness rotator cuff tears. J Shoulder Elbow Surg 4(6):409-415, 1995.

19. Roye KP, Grana WA, Yates CK: Arthroscopic subacromial decompression: Two to seven year follow up. Arthroscopy 11:301, 1995.

20. Ryu RK: Arthroscopic subacromial decompression: A clinical review. Arthroscopy 8:141, 1992.

21. Seitz WH, Froimson AI, Shapiro JD: Chronic impingement syndrome: the role of ultrasonography and arthroscopic anterior acromioplasty. Orthop Rev 18:364, 1989.

22. Itoi E, Tabata S: Conservative treatment of rotator cuff tear. Clin Orthop 275:165, 1992.

23. Iannotti JP, et al: Prospective evaluation of rotator cuff repair. J Shoulder Elbow Surg 2:69, 1993.

24. Weber SC: Arthroscopic debridement and acromioplasty versus mini-open repair in the treatment of significant partial-thickness rotator cuff tear. Arthroscopy 15:126-131, 1999.

25. Patel V, et al: Arthroscopic subacromial decompression: Results and factors affecting outcome. J Shoulder Elbow Surg 8:231, 1999.

26. Payne L, et al: Arthroscopic treatment of partial rotator cuff tears in young athletes: A preliminary report. Am J Sports Med 25:299, 1997.

27. Synder S, et al: Partial thickness rotator cuff tears: Results of arthroscopic treatment. Arthroscopy 7:1, 1991

28. Wright S, et al: Management of partial-thickness rotator cuff tears. J Shoulder Elbow Surg 5:458, 1996.

29. Calvert PT, Packer NP, Staker DJ: Arthrography of the shoulder after operative repair of the torn rotator cuff. J Bone Joint Surg Br 68:147, 1986.

30. Lui SH: Arthroscopically-assisted rotator cuff repair. J Bone Joint Surg Br 76:592, 1994.

31. Burkhart S: Reconciling the paradox of rotator cuff repair versus debridement: A unified biomechanical rationale for treatment of rotator cuff tears. Arthroscopy 10(1):4, 1994.

32. Cofield R, et al: Surgical repair of chronic rotator cuff tears. J Bone Joint Surg Am 83A:71, 2005.

33. Harryman DT II, et al: Repairs of the rotator cuff: Correlation of functional results with integrity of the cuff. J Bone Joint Surg Am 73:982, 1991.

34. Bigliani LU, et al: Operative treatment of failed repairs of the rotator cuff. J Bone Joint Surg Am 74A:1505, 1992.

35. Baker CL, Liu SH: Comparison of open and arthroscopically assisted rotator cuff repairs. Am J Sports Med 23:99, 1995.

36. Lui SH, Baker CL: Arthroscopically-assisted rotator cuff repair: Correlation of functional results with integrity of the cuff. Arthroscopy 10:54, 1991.

37. MacConaill MA, Basmajian JV: Muscles and movements: A basis for human kinesiology, Baltimore, 1969, Williams and Wilkins.

38. Blevins FT, et al: Arthroscopic assisted rotator cuff repair: Results using a mini-open deltoid splitting approach. Arthroscopy 12:50, 1996.

39. Bishop J, et al: Cuff integrity after arthroscopic versus open rotator cuff repair: A prospective study. J Shoulder Elbow Surg 15:290, 2006.

40. Burkhart SS, Danaaceau SM, Pearce CE Jr: Arthroscopic rotator cuff repair: Analysis of results by tear size and by repair technique margin convergence versus direct tendon to bone repair. Arthroscopy 17:905, 2001.

41. Kim S, et al: Arthroscopic versus mini-open salvage repair of rotator cuff tear. Arthroscopy 19(7):746, 2003.

42. Murray T, et al: Arthroscopic repair of medium to large full-thickness rotator cuff tears: Outcome at 2- to 6-year follow-up. J Shoulder Elbow Surg 11(1):19-24, 2002.

43. Sauerbrey A, et al: Arthroscopic versus mini open rotator cuff repair: A comparison of clinical outcome. Arthroscopy 21:1415, 2005.

44. Severud E, et al: All-arthroscopic versus mini-open rotator cuff repair: A long-term retrospective outcome comparison. Arthroscopy 19(3):234, 2003.

45. Verma N, et al: All-arthroscopic versus mini-open rotator cuff repair: A retrospective review with a minimum 2-year follow-up. Arthroscopy 22:587, 2006.

46. Warner J, et al: Arthroscopic versus mini-open rotator cuff repair: A cohost comparison study. Arthroscopy 21(3):328, 2005.

47. Youm T, et al: Arthroscopic versus mini-open rotator cuff repair: A comparison of clinical outcomes and patient satisfaction. J Shoulder Elbow Surg 14:455, 2005.

48. Wilcox R: Controversies in rehabilitation progression following rotator cuff repair: An evidenced-based consensus guideline, 2010; Williams G: Am PT Association's 2nd combined sections meeting CSM 2010, Resourceful Recordings 2010

49. Akeson WH, Woo SLY, Amiel D: The connective tissue response to immobility: Biomechanical changes in periarticular connective tissue of the immobilized rabbit knee. Clin Orthop 93:356, 1973.

50. Davies GJ, Dickoff-Hoffman S: Neuromuscular testing and rehabilitation of the shoulder complex. J Orthop Sports Phys Ther 18(2):449, 1993.

51. De Palma AF, Cooke AJ, Prabhakar M: The role of the subscapularis in recurrent anterior dislocations of the shoulder. Clin Orthop 54:35, 1967.

52. Jenp NY, et al: Activation of the rotator cuff in generating isometric shoulder rotation torque. Am J Sports Med 24(4):477, 1996.

53. Leggon B: Controversies in rehabilitation progression following rotator cuff repair: An evidenced-based consensus guideline, 2010; Williams G: Am PT Association's 2nd Combined Sections Meeting CSM 2010, Resourceful Recordings 2010.

54. Brewster C, Moynes-Schwab D: Rehabilitation of the shoulder following rotator cuff injury or surgery. J Orthop Sports Phys Ther 18(2):422, 1993.

55. Baylis RW, Wolf EM: Arthroscopic rotator cuff repair: clinical and arthroscopic second-look assessment. Paper presented at annual meeting of the Arthroscopy Association of North America, San Francisco, May 1995.

56. Maitland GD: Peripheral joint manipulation, ed 3, Newton, Mass, 1991, Butterworth.

57. Andrews JR, Harrelson GL, Wilk KE: Physical rehabilitation of the injured athlete, ed 3, Philadelphia, 2004, Saunders.

58. Lister JL, et al: Scapular stabilizer activity during Bodyblade, cuff weights, and Thera-Band use. J Sports Rehabil 16(1):50-67, 2007.

59. Andrews JR, Kupferman SP, Dillman CJ: Labral tears in throwing and racquet sports. Clin Sports Med 10(4):901, 1991.

60. Escamilla RF, et al: Shoulder muscle activity and function in common shoulder rehabilitation exercises. Sports Med 39(8):663-685, 2009.

61. Cyriax J: Textbook of orthopaedic medicine: diagnosis of soft tissue lesions, vol 1, Baltimore, 1975, Williams and Wilkins.

62. Kelly M, Clark W: Orthopedic therapy of the shoulder, Philadelphia, 1995, Lippincott.

63. Trott PH: Differential mechanical diagnosis of shoulder pain. Proceedings of the Manipulative Therapists Association of Australia, 1985.

64. Escamilla RF, Andrews JR: Shoulder muscle recruitment patterns and related biomechanics during upper extremity sports. Sports Med 39(7):569-590, 2009

65. Ayoub E: Posture and the upper quarter. In Donatelli R, editor: Physical therapy of the shoulder, New York, 1987, Churchill Livingstone.

66. Walser RF, Meserve BB, Boucher TR: The effectiveness of thoracic spine manipulation for the management of musculoskeletal conditions: A systematic review and meta-analysis of randomized clinical trials. J Man Manip Ther 17(4):237-246, 2009

67. Dehne E, Tory R: Treatment of joint injuries by immediate mobilization, based upon the spinal adaptation concept. Clin Orthop 77(218): 1971.

68. Lazarus MD, et al: Comparison of open and arthroscopic subacromial decompression. J Shoulder Elbow Surg 3:1, 1994.

69. Smith RH, Brunolti J: Shoulder kinesthesia after anterior glenohumeral joint dislocation. Phys Ther 69:106, 1989.

70. De Palma AF: Degenerative changes in the sternoclavicular and acromioclavicular joints in various decades, Springfield, Ill, 1957, Thomas.

71. Tibone JE, et al: Shoulder impingement syndrome in athletes treated by anterior acromioplasty. Clin Orthop 134:140, 1985.

72. Bross R, et al: Optimal number of exercise bouts per week for isokinetic eccentric training of the rotator cuff musculature. Wis Phys Ther Assoc Newsl 21(5):18, 1991 (abstract).

73. Butler DS: Mobilization of the nervous system, New York, 1991, Churchill Livingstone.

CHAPTER 6

Superior Labral Anterior Posterior Repair

Timothy F. Tyler, Craig Zeman

INTRODUCTION

Superior labral anterior posterior (SLAP) lesions were not realized until the advent of shoulder arthroscopy. Andrews, Carson, and McLeod[1] were the first to describe labral tears of the biceps anchor, but it was Synder[2] who was the first to classify them, outline their treatment, and describe four basic types of lesions: I to IV (Fig. 6-1). Since then, several other variants have been described. So as to not get caught up in the subtleties of the classifications, SLAP lesions can best be understood by how they are treated and by the patient's concurrent diagnosis. The two major ways that a SLAP lesion can be treated are by débridement and repair. SLAP lesions are seen in patients who either have instability or impingement, and the kind of rehabilitation patients receive is determined by which factors they have.

Overall, nonoperative management has proven unsuccessful for a large number of patients with unstable SLAP lesions,[1,3,4] but Edwards feels that a course of nonoperative conservative management of nonsteroidal antiinflammatory drugs (NSAIDs) and physical therapy should be tried. A 50% failure rate was observed in their study.[5] In many studies, patients underwent diagnostic arthroscopy at an average of 12 to 30 months from their initial symptoms. In one study, patients had an extended trial of activity modification and rehabilitation exercises.[6] Most patients had been treated with rest, physical therapy, steroid injections, and NSAIDs without relief of their symptoms before diagnostic arthroscopy. Arthroscopic tools, anchors, and sutures have continued to advance making the surgical treatment more effective and easier to perform.[7-16] Treatment of these lesions is directed according to their type.* In general, type I and III lesions are débrided, whereas type II and many type IV lesions are repaired.[4,17-19] After all SLAP repairs, rehabilitation plays an integral part in the patient's outcome.[20]

---

*Tables detailing the rehabilitation guidelines for SLAP repair can be found on the CD.

SURGICAL INDICATIONS AND CONSIDERATIONS

Cause

The superior labral is part of the attachment of the long head of the biceps.[3,9,11,21] The role of the long head of the biceps is to be a humeral head depressor and an anterior stabilizer.[7,10] The SLAP area is in continuity with the anterior and posterior labrum. Therefore a tear in the superior labrum can affect the entire labrum, and conversely a tear in the anterior or posterior labrum can disrupt the superior labrum. The classic mechanism to develop a SLAP lesion is force, which either pushes the humeral head over or pulls the humeral head away from the superior labrum.[8,22] The humeral head will pull on the superior labrum and the biceps anchor tearing them away from the glenoid.[23,24] In addition, a tear of the anterior or posterior labrum from a dislocation can extend into the superior labrum. Repetitive overhead lifting, which can pinch the superior labrum and pull on it in a downward fashion, can also cause degenerative SLAP tears. In the deceleration phase of pitching, the biceps fires to stop the elbow from hyperextending, which causes a force to be placed across the superior labrum. It is this repetitive action that is felt to cause SLAP lesions in pitchers.[25]

Clinical Evaluation

The therapist should look in the patient's history for an injury that placed an upward shear force across the shoulder—a fall on an outstretched arm that was overhead or that placed a traction force across the arm, a sudden grab and pull on something, having the arm pulled forcefully (e.g., the shoulder getting pulled on while waterskiing)—as well as mild instability in the shoulder with the repetitive throwing motion.[26-28] Some patients can develop SLAP lesions with no apparent cause. In questioning for cause, it is important to ask about repetitive overhead lifting and throwing activities. Patient complaints can range from instability to a vague ache in the shoulder. Many patients can show signs of impingement, and some have symptoms of locking, popping, and catching. No classic symptom

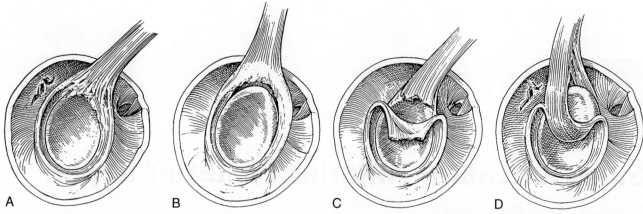

Fig. 6-1 SLAP lesions classifications. **A,** Type I. **B,** Type II. **C,** Type III. **D,** Type IV. (From Snyder SJ, et al: SLAP lesions of the shoulder. Arthroscopy 6[4]: 274-279, 1990.)

pinpoints a SLAP lesion. Many physical examination tests have been described to help diagnose a SLAP lesion.[4,17,20,29] The two most common are the Speeds test and O'Brien test, which are modified supraspinatus isolation tests and therefore can be positive if the patient has impingement.[30] The problem with diagnosing a SLAP lesion is that it is usually found in combination with either impingement or instability. Overall it appears that the primary authors of these tests report overall good sensitivity and specificity but other authors are unable to repeat their results when tested.[31-39] The clinician needs to be aware of other problems that can be associated with SLAP lesions such as ganglion cyst, rotator cuff tears, posterior instability, and acromioclavicular (AC) joint arthritis.[40-46]

Diagnostic Testing

Plain radiographs are of little use in evaluating a SLAP lesion. Magnetic resonance imaging (MRI) with gadolinium is probably the best way to see a SLAP lesion.[47-56] An MRI without gadolinium has been reported to have had some success.[57] The problem with an MRI is that it can be too sensitive and tends to "overread" the lesion. A computerized tomography (CT) scan with contrast and three-dimensional (3-D) reconstruction can also be used to see labral tears, but once again it can be too sensitive. A glenolabral cyst can be seen on both MRI and CT scan and can be commonly caused by a SLAP lesion.[58]

SURGICAL PROCEDURE

The treatment of SLAP lesions is an arthroscopic procedure. It is very difficult if not impossible to treat a SLAP lesion open. Most SLAP lesions are found on diagnostic arthroscopy; therefore the surgeon must be prepared to treat a SLAP lesion at the time of surgery.

Type I

These lesions are simply the fraying of the superior labrum without any significant detachment of the labrum from the superior glenoid (Figs. 6-1, *A*, and 6-2). The frayed area

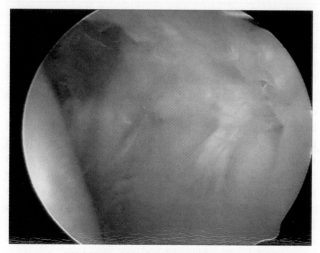

Fig. 6-2 SLAP type I lesion. Fraying of the superior labrum.

usually covers a portion of the superior glenoid; however, no gross instability of the labral tissue exists. This lesion is commonly seen in patients with impingement or rotator cuff tears. It is not usually seen in patients with instability and it does not seem to cause capsular laxity. These lesions are simply débrided down to the attached base of the superior labrum with an arthroscopic shaver (Fig. 6-3).[59]

Type II

These lesions have an unstable attachment of the superior labrum. The base of the labrum is pulled away from the superior glenoid and is highly mobile (Figs. 6-1, *B*, and 6-4, *A*). If the labrum pulls away from the superior glenoid more than 3 to 4 mm when traction is applied to the biceps tendon, the tear is considered unstable.[60-63] When the labrum is reduced, one will usually see a reduction in the capsular volume and a change in the position of the anterior and posterior labrum to a more upright position (Fig. 6-4, *B*). A type II lesion needs to be surgically reduced (Fig. 6-5, *A* and *B*). It is done through three portals: one posterior and two anterior. Some type of anchor with suture attached will be used to repair the tear. The detached labrum will be reattached to its anatomic position on the glenoid.

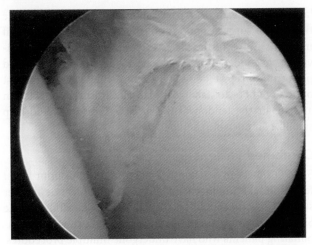

Fig. 6-3 SLAP type I lesion after débridement.

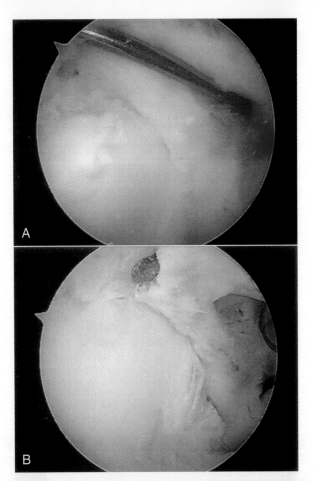

Fig. 6-5 **A,** SLAP type II lesion (repeat of tear probe picture RS). **B,** SLAP type II lesion (repaired).

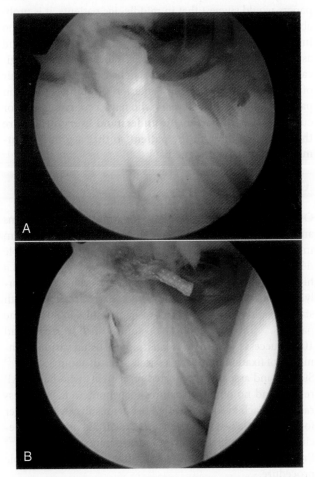

Fig. 6-4 **A,** SLAP type II lesion. Base of labrum pulled away from the glenoid. **B,** SLAP type II lesion (repaired).

Once the portals have been established, a burr is used to débride the bone of the superior glenoid under the torn labrum. This exposes a bleeding bed of bone that will aid in the healing process. Any loose or frayed ends of the labrum are débrided down to a stable base, and an anchor is placed into the prepared bone through the superior portal. The next task is to pull the two suture ends through the torn labral tissue. This can be done in a multitude of ways; the general concept is as follows: A device with a loop on the end is passed through the torn labral tissue. One end of the suture is then placed into this loop, which is then pulled back through the labral tissue pulling the suture through the labrum. This process is repeated again so that both ends of the suture are passed through the labrum. Using arthroscopic tying techniques, the torn labrum is firmly reattached back down to the bone of the glenoid (Fig. 6-6). Depending on the size of the tear, more anchors may need to be used to get a secure repair.

Type III

A type III SLAP can be thought of as a bucket handle tear of the labrum (Figs. 6-1, *C*, and 6-7, *A* and *B*). The unstable handle portion floats around inside the glenohumeral (GH) joint, getting caught between the humeral head and the glenoid during shoulder range of motion (ROM). This pulls on the labral and capsular tissue, producing pain in the shoulder. The portion of the labrum not involved in the tear is normally firmly attached to the glenoid; therefore the symptomatic part is the bucket handle tear, which can simply be débrided down to a stable base such as a meniscus tear in the knee.

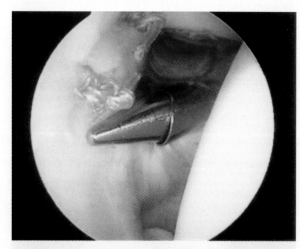

Fig. 6-6 SLAP type II lesion (repaired using sutures).

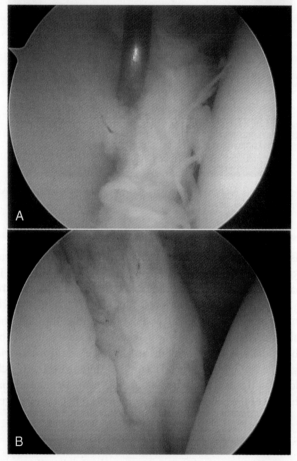

Fig. 6-7 **A,** SLAP type III tear (unstable bucket handle tear). **B,** SLAP type III tear débrided much like resolving a bucket handle tear in the knee meniscus.

Type IV

This lesion involves a bucket handle tear of the labrum, which extends into the biceps tendon (Figs 6-1, *D,* and 6-8, *A-C*). Treatment of these lesions depends on the extent of the tear and the age and activity level of the patient. If at least 30% of the biceps remains and the remaining portion of the

labrum is stable, the torn part can be débrided down to stable tissue. The surgical options are much more complicated if more than 30% of the biceps is torn. In a less active individual, a good option would be to débride the tear and perform a biceps tenodesis. In a throwing athlete, the best option might be to stabilize the labral tear like a type II lesion and repair the tendon of the biceps. A repair would help stabilize an unstable shoulder.

Combined Lesions

SLAP lesions can be seen with anterior and posterior labral tears and with impingement and rotator cuff tears. All other surgical lesions should be treated at the same time as the SLAP repair. More times than not, the therapist will be rehabilitating patients who have undergone multiple procedures. There has been controversy over whether during a rotator cuff repair a SLAP repair should be done. A review of these papers would suggest that in middle-age patients, it is probably best not to repair the SLAP because this can lead to increased stiffness after the surgery.[64-66] In contrast, Levy and associates[67] demonstrated that predictable short-term surgical results and return to activity can be expected after repair of type II superior labrum anterior posterior lesions in patients younger than 50 years who have a coexistent rotator cuff tear. **It is important to understand every procedure that has been done to the patient so that a proper treatment plan can be designed.**

OUTCOMES

Overall mixed results of operative treatment of SLAP lesions and nonoperative care have been reported.[68-71] Short-term improvement can be seen in patients with just simple débridement, but at long-term follow-up, the patients had a high failure rate.[72] This failure is probably because the underlying instability was not addressed. Early treatment with staple fixation yields good to excellent results in 80% of the patients.[68] The first reports of suture anchor repair had 100% success.[29] A review of later reports using various techniques of fixation have seen a success rate of about 85%.[17,20,73] Stetson and associates[4] reported on patients who had SLAP repairs and no other procedures for whom an 82% success rate was achieved. Recently, better results with longer follow-up have been reported after type II SLAP repair, especially in those athletes with traumatic injury and repair.[73,74] Properly performed treatment of SLAP lesions is a reliable procedure.

THERAPY GUIDELINES FOR REHABILITATION

Postoperatively, the shoulder is placed in a sling without a swathe for 2 to 4 weeks to minimize biceps muscular activity and protect any additional structures addressed during the surgical procedure. The position of the arm is in internal rotation (IR) slightly anterior to the frontal plane. Because the early labral tensile strength is weak, the early rehabilita-

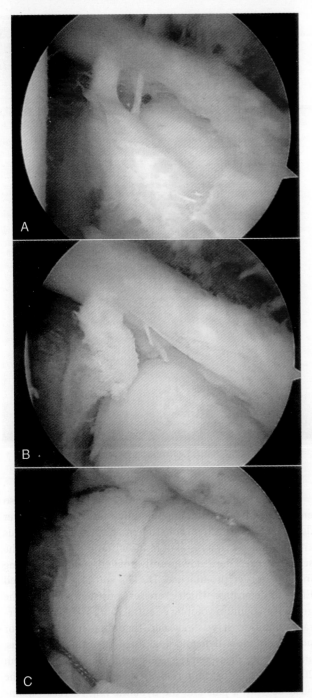

Fig. 6-8 **A,** SLAP type IV bucket handle tear that extends into the biceps tendon. **B,** SLAP type IV bucket handle tear, débrided and prepared for suturing. **C,** SLAP type IV repaired using sutures.

tion program is more conservative than other open-stabilization procedures.[29,47,68]

The main focus of the early protective postoperative period (up to 4 weeks) is to maintain proximal and distal strength and mobility, provide pain relief, and prevent selective hypomobility of sections of the capsule as a result of iatrogenic change from the surgery. During this period, elbow ROM and gripping exercises are encouraged. The authors have found that instructing patients to sleep with a

pillow under their elbow to support the shoulder may take stress off the labrum and reduce discomfort. Modalities can be useful tools in providing pain relief. The level of pain, postoperative swelling, and type of SLAP tear that was surgically addressed will determine progression of the patient.[48,49] As the treating clinician, good communication with the surgeon is essential to proper care.[48] Understanding the specific procedure, concomitant injuries, and tissue quality may also affect the level of progression.

The rehabilitation process will focus on four keys to success:

1. Regaining ROM
2. Providing scapular stabilization
3. Restoring posterior shoulder extensibility
4. Returning rotator cuff strength

Phase I (Early Protective Phase)

TIME: Day 1 to 4 weeks after surgery
GOALS: Protect surgical procedure, educate patient on procedure and therapeutic progression, regulate pain and control inflammation, initiate ROM and dynamic stabilization, neuromuscular reeducation of external rotators and scapulothoracic muscles

Initial Postoperative Examination

Outpatient physical therapy can begin as early as 3 days after SLAP repair. At this time the mobility of the sternoclavicular (SC) joint, AC joint, and scapulothoracic joint are addressed and mobilized if indicated. Initial evaluation documentation should include the observation of the portal sites, atrophy, swelling, posture, and functional difficulties. Observation and documentation of ROM and general willingness to move the shoulder and neurovascular measurements should be documented. **Care should be taken to avoid contracting the biceps (active elbow flexion) until week 2. Tests to assess shoulder instability or labral pathology at this point would be inappropriate.**

Early Protective Postoperative Rehabilitation

Once the milestone of mobility of the proximal joints is obtained, manual scapular stabilization is initiated. In the side-lying position, manual resistance can be given to the scapula to resist elevation, depression, protraction, and retraction (Fig. 6-9). Pain can be a limiting factor for starting scapular stabilization and rotator cuff isometrics; however, submaximal pain-free alternating isometrics for IR and external rotation (ER) may begin as early as 7 days after surgery (Fig. 6-10). Because the rotator cuff muscles are not violated, this exercise can begin with the arm at the side. Early mobilization exercises such as the pendulums are recommended for pain relief and could prevent adhesions from forming. Pendulums have been shown to produce very little muscular activity and are considered to be a safe exercise during this period for most shoulder surgeries.[58]

However, some surgeons feel the arm hanging in a dependent position may put unwanted stress on the

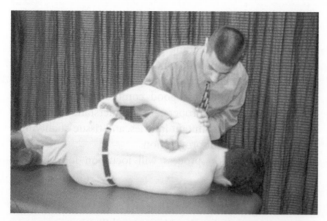

Fig. 6-9 Mobilization and rhythmic stabilization position for the scapula.

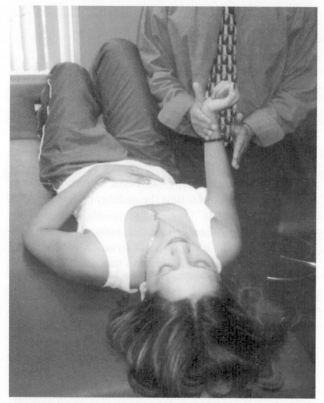

Fig. 6-10 Rhythmic stabilization exercise for internal rotation (IR) and external rotation (ER) in 0° of abduction.

repaired labral. Initiation of active assistive range of motion (A/AROM) using a pulley for sagittal plane flexion and scapular plane elevation is advised. In addition, a cane, golf club, or umbrella can be used to assist with regaining flexion, abduction, adduction, and ER at 0° and 30° of abduction (or where the surgeon sets the shoulder during surgery). Gentle mobilization (grades I and II) consisting of posterior glides can be performed at this time for pain relief.

Contraindications
- No ER past the set point for 3 weeks
- No ER in the 90°/90° position for 6 weeks to avoid the peel-back mechanism
- No active biceps contraction for 4 weeks

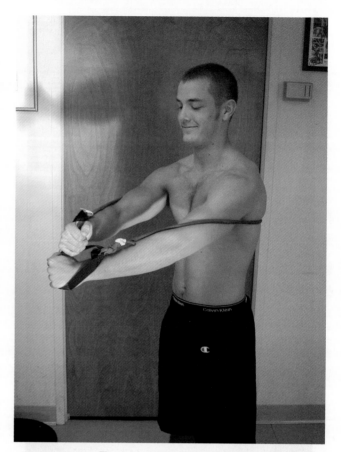

Fig. 6-11 Dynamic hug exercise.

Early strengthening of the serratus anterior muscle is also encouraged if it is maintained slightly below 90° of shoulder flexion and is pain free. Subsequent atrophy of the serratus anterior muscle, as a result of immobilization, may allow the scapula to rest in a downwardly rotated position, causing inferior border prominence. Decker and associates[75] used EMG to determine which exercises consistently elicited the greatest maximum voluntary contraction (MVC) of the serratus anterior. It was revealed that the serratus anterior punch, scaption, dynamic hug, knee push-up with a plus, and push-up plus exercises consistently elicited more than 20% of MVC. Most importantly, it was determined that the push-up with a plus and the dynamic hug exercises maintained the greatest MVC, as well as maintained the scapula in an upwardly rotated position (Fig. 6-11). Although it would be too early in the rehabilitation process to perform these later exercises, Decker and associates[75] highlighted the serratus anterior punch as a valuable exercise. Performed in a controlled, supervised setting, this is an excellent choice to initiate early serratus anterior strengthening. Transition to the more challenging serratus anterior exercises should occur after 8 weeks and be based on logical exercise progression.

A fine line exists between pushing patients too hard and progressing them as planned. Often patients may feel better than expected during this early protective phase, so therapists must always respect the laws of tissue healing.

Three milestones to achieve for progression to the next phase of rehabilitation are (1) to educate the patient on the procedure he or she had and what to expect during the rehabilitation, (2) to provide some pain relief so that the patient is able to tolerate submaximal isometrics of the rotator cuff muscles at 0° abduction, and (3) to attain symmetrical mobility of the SC, AC, and scapulothoracic joints, as well as the ability to protract, retract, elevate, and depress the scapula against submaximal manual resistance. A/AROM goals include achieving flexion to 110° to 130°, abduction to 70°, scapula plane IR to 60°, and scapula plane ER to set point.

Phase II (Intermediate Phase)

TIME: 5 to 8 weeks after surgery
GOALS: Normalize arthrokinematics, gains in neuromuscular control, normalization of posterior shoulder flexibility

During weeks 5 to 8, three visits per week should focus on the return of scapular stability and GH ROM. Later in this period, rotator cuff isotonic strengthening is initiated. During this period, the patient removes the sling, and more aggressive A/AROM exercises are initiated. These exercises may include the use of a pulley or cane to assist in forward elevation in the plane of the scapula and IR. Initially, ER stretching is performed in the guarded neutral position with the arm at the side, and then it is progressed into the scapular plane. While progressing through rehabilitation, the therapist should always consider patients' morphology, understanding if they are hypermobile by nature and returning motion quickly and easily; if so, they do not need to be pushed.

Patients with excessive joint laxity or generalized joint hypermobility must be progressed under a watchful eye.[76] Excessively stretching ER in the 90°/90° position in these patients too early during their postoperative care may jeopardize the end result. Burkhart and Morgan[77] discovered the peel-back mechanism, which can occur during rehabilitation when ER is forced passively in the 90°/90° position before healing has occurred. Kuhn and associates[78] demonstrated failure of the biceps superior labral complex in 9 of 10 cadaveric shoulders when the biceps was tensioned in the cocking position. The peel-back phenomenon occurs when the biceps-labral complex is abducted and externally rotated causing a posterior biceps vector, and shearing the biceps anchor repair off its origin.

One therapeutic intervention that can assist in decreasing tension in the biceps-labral complex is restoring posterior extensibility. By restoring posterior capsule extensibility, it allows the humeral head to centralize in the glenoid fossa and not be forced anterior. A tight posterior capsule forces the humeral head anterior, creating unwanted tension in the biceps-labral complex as the phenomenon occurs. Stretching and mobilization of the posterior capsule should be emphasized because tightness of the posterior shoulder structures has been linked to a loss of IR ROM.[79] Loss of mobility can potentially limit progress, considering a tight posterior capsule is thought to cause anterior-superior migration of the humeral head with forward elevation of the shoulder, possibly contributing to a SLAP tear.[80] If posterior shoulder tightness and a decrease in IR ROM are observed, careful assessment must be undertaken. The Tyler test for posterior shoulder tightness can be performed to determine if posterior shoulder tightness is present (Fig. 6-12).[79,81] Recently Mullaney and associates[82] have made the measurement easier and shown its reproducibility using a digital level. To further determine if the loss of IR is due to capsular contracture, a posterior glide must be performed (Fig. 6-13). An effective method of stretching this area is to stabilize the patient's scapula at the inferior angle manually while the patient provides a cross-chest adduction force in the supine position (Fig. 6-14). Further stretch may be felt by having

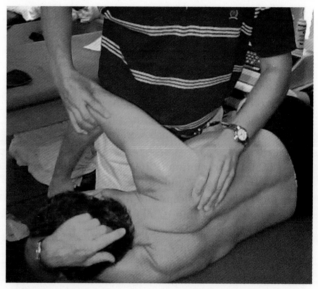

Fig. 6-12 The Tyler test for posterior shoulder tightness.

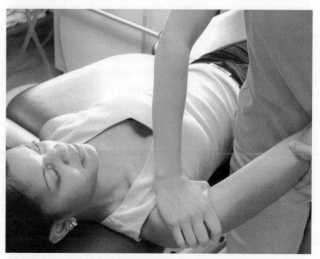

Fig. 6-13 A posterior glide in the plane of the scapula to distinguish posterior capsule tightness.

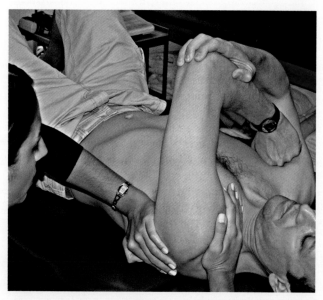

Fig. 6-14 Supine scapula stabilized assisted posterior shoulder stretch.

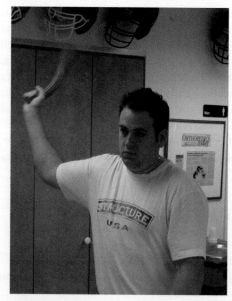

Fig. 6-15 Shoulder oscillation in the plane of the scapula keeping the wrist, elbow, and shoulder steady.

the patient add slight pressure into IR by pressing inferiorly on the dorsal aspect of the hand or wrist. This posterior shoulder protocol has been shown to be effective in the correction of posterior shoulder tightness in patients with internal impingement, six of which were more than 6 months after SLAP repair.[83]

Passive range of motion (PROM) of ER and abduction should be limited to 65° and 70°, respectively, as to not put stress on the healing biceps-labral complex. Initial ROM goals are to achieve within 10° of full IR and 150° to 165° of passive flexion in the plane of the scapular. The goal is to maintain available mobility and prevent excessive scarring. Similar to Burkhart and Morgan[84] and Burkhart, Morgan, and Kibler,[85] isotonic strengthening exercises are initiated for abduction, scaption, IR, and ER in the scapular plane.[86] In addition, rhythmic stabilization at the end ROM can be performed at this time. To have normal scapulohumeral rhythm, dynamic scapula stability of this joint needs to be restored. Scapula exercises are encouraged in this phase of rehabilitation to counteract scapulohumeral dissociation and provide a stable base of support for active range of motion (AROM) to be performed.[87] Recently, the authors of this chapter reported on the importance of scapula stability in generating shoulder rotation torque in microinstability patients. The results of the authors' study demonstrated patients with microinstability exhibited a significant decrease in peak shoulder ER and IR torque after exercise-induced fatigue of the scapular stabilizer.[88] Many authors have examined the EMG activity during scapular strengthening exercises; however, when choosing the appropriate exercise, the clinician must keep the activity pain free and protect the surgical repair.[89-92] Three relatively low-level exercises the authors like to use after SLAP repair are (1) elastic resistance rows (not to brake the frontal plane with the involved elbow); (2) standing scapular retraction against elastic resistance

with straight arms just below 90° of shoulder flexion; and (3) shoulder oscillation in the plane of the scapula, keeping the wrist, elbow, and shoulder steady (Fig. 6-15). Finally, in the later phases of rehabilitation, the patient can progress to more demanding open and closed kinetic chain scapular strengthening exercises.

Strengthening exercises should progress to resistance training with elastic bands for IR, ER, abduction, and extension. Maintaining the GH joint in the scapular plane (30° to 45° anterior to the frontal plane) will minimize the tensile stress placed on the labral repair.[93]

The authors have found that giving verbal feedback to lift the chest up and pinch the shoulders back can facilitate scapular stabilization while training the external rotators. Hintermeister and associates[94] found shoulder elastic resistance training to have a low load on the shoulder and therefore to be safe for postoperative patients.

It is our opinion that the use of free weights with the arm in a dependent position should be used accordingly during this period to minimize the potential for detrimental humeral head translation. Side-lying ER is typically initiated during the later portion of this phase (Fig. 6-16). Proper technique, weight, and ROM are important to execute this safely. Stabilizing the humerus to the thorax and not allowing the elbow to drift past the frontal plane of the body will place minimal winding on the labral repair.

At this phase, minimal weight should be used within the comfortable ROM to prevent ill-advised stress to the healing biceps-labral complex. It may also be recommended that the patient wait until the end of the intermediate postoperative period to initiate jogging or running for this same reason (the humeral head may be forcibly thrusted anteriorly). It is imperative that the therapist maintain supervision of the ROM progression during this period to protect the healing tissue.[86] Clinical milestones to progress to the next

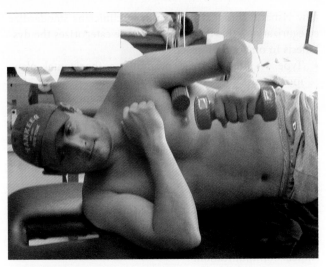

Fig. 6-16 External rotation strengthening in the side-lying position with a free weight.

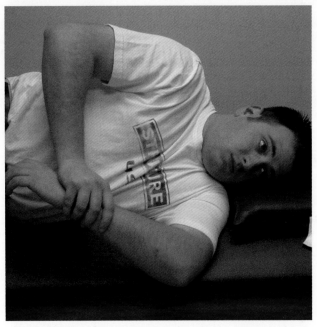

Fig. 6-17 Sleeper stretch for gaining internal rotation.

phase of rehabilitation include (1) achieving 160° of flexion in the scapular plane, (2) scapular plane ER to 65°, (3) ER at 90° abduction to 45°, (4) near full IR in the scapular plane, (5) IR at 90° abduction to 45°, (6) 150° of abduction, (7) symmetrical posterior shoulder flexibility, and (8) improved isotonic internal and external strength in available ROM.

Phase III (Strengthening Postoperative Phase)

TIME: 9 to 14 weeks after surgery
GOALS: Normalize ROM, progression of strength, normalize scapulothoracic motion and strength, overhead activities without pain

During weeks 9 to 14 (usually two to three treatment sessions per week), rehabilitation continues to work toward full GH ROM and dynamic stability of the humeral head in the glenoid fossa. Gaining or maintaining full AROM within 10° of flexion in the sagittal plane and ER are to be achieved later during this time phase. At this time, regaining ER, abduction, and flexion does not seem to be a limiting factor for recovery. Once the patient has achieved the milestone of 70° to 80° ER in the plane of the scapula, he or she will begin to acquire ER ROM at 90° of abduction. Although in the past it has been expected that the patient will have full AROM 8 weeks after SLAP repair, most patients do not achieve this at 8 weeks. In our experience, ER and IR ROM measured in the supine position with the GH joint abducted 90° typically does not achieve full ROM until 10 to 12 weeks or longer, depending upon the patient.

It is at this point that a sleeper stretch may safely be given to a patient to regain passive IR ROM (Fig. 6-17). This is in agreement with other authors who demonstrated a lack of full return of ROM in patients 12 weeks after SLAP repair.[84,85,95,96] In our opinion, the key to a successful rehabilitation of these patients, at this phase, is finding the balance point between stretching ER and letting them naturally regain their ROM.

An arm upper body ergometer (UBE) using light resistance can be beneficial at this time to facilitate ROM and initiate active muscular control of the shoulder.

The axis of rotation of the UBE should remain below the level of the shoulder joint so as not to force forward flexion above 80°. To avoid stress to the biceps-labral complex, the patient should be positioned at a distance from the axis of rotation that does not allow the elbow to move posterior to the frontal plane when performing ergometer revolutions. This exercise is not initiated earlier because the amount of stress placed on the biceps-labral complex during the use of an UBE is unknown.

When designing the strengthening program, it is important to match patients' needs with their limitations and goals. A properly designed strengthening program will address their needs by attempting to get the most benefit from each exercise prescription. Previous EMG studies have set forth which shoulder exercises activate particular muscles, and these should be considered as the clinician prescribes a program.[58,75,76,90,91] We have combined many of these programs to address generalized specific weaknesses. From these studies, we have developed the "prone program plus" to address scapular stability and generalized weakness. The prone program plus can be started in this phase of the rehabilitation if the exercises are pain free. The prone program plus includes prone GH horizontal abduction with GH IR (thumb down), prone scapula adduction with GH ER (thumb up), prone rows, prone shoulder flexion in the scapular plane, prone 90°/90° ER, push-ups with a plus (therapist initiates exercise in quadruped), and ball press downs. Patients can easily get into poor habits or begin performing these exercises with improper form. It is recommended that clinicians educate their patients on these exercises and allow ample time for them to develop proper form before prescribing these as part of a home program.

Proprioceptive neuromuscular facilitation (PNF) can be described as movements that combine rotation and diagonal components that closely resemble the movement patterns required for sport and work activities. PNF acts to enhance the proprioceptive input and neuromuscular responses while stressing motor relearning in the postoperative phases of rehabilitation. PNF patterns are initiated with the scapula because scapular stability is essential for total function of the shoulder. Scapular patterns are generally performed in the side-lying position, with the head and neck in neutral alignment. The coupled patterns of anterior elevation–posterior depression and anterior depression–posterior elevation are used, respectively. Trunk rotation should eventually be combined with scapular and extremity PNF patterns to maximize combined muscular movement patterns. Techniques such as hold-relax, slow reversals, and contract-relax are used specifically to improve motion, whereas rhythmic stabilization, repeated contractions, and combination isotonics are used to enhance concentric and eccentric muscle action. Specifically, the D2-flexion pattern combines flexion, abduction, and ER, emphasizing the posterior rotator cuff and posterior deltoid (Fig. 6-18). These neuromuscular control exercises strive to reestablish scapular positioning and stability of the humeral head in the glenoid.[87]

As the patient progresses through the program, periodical reevaluation of the scapular dyskinesis is highly recommended. The authors stress this, especially as the patient gains full ROM and may no longer be inhibited by tight soft tissue structures. The term scapular dyskinesis, although indicating that an alteration exists, is a qualitative collective term that does not differentiate between types of scapular positions or motions.[97] Therefore scapular evaluation and categorization is challenging. The most common techniques for objective quantification include visual evaluation, the lateral scapular slide test (LSST), and 3-D techniques. Kibler and associates[97] have recently introduced a

new visual technique that may help clinicians standardize categorization. This dynamic technique categorizes the dyskinesis in one of four groups:

- Type I—inferior angle prominence (horizontal plane movement)
- Type II—medial border prominence dorsally (frontal plane movement)
- Type III—shoulder shrug motion without winging (sagittal plane movement)
- Type IV—bilaterally symmetrical movement (normal movement)

Like all scapular categorization techniques, the therapist must be concerned with combined movements, a learning curve, and patient experience; however, it does present clinicians with a valuable tool that, with practice, may enhance clinical communication.

The authors also believe that exercises directed toward facilitation of functional muscular firing patterns in both the open and closed chain may provide useful input for return to function after SLAP repair. Lear and Gross[93] demonstrated scapular muscle activity increases with a wall push-up progression. **However, the strain on the biceps-labral complex is unknown and may be too great for patients after SLAP repair. This exercise should be gradually built up to and proceeded to with caution.** Clinicians should hold this exercise until the advanced strengthening postoperative phase to protect the healing tissue.

Isotonic exercises emphasizing light resistance and increased repetitions are used for isolated and combined movement patterns of the shoulder. The authors use a progression from three sets of 10, to two sets of 15, and on to one set of 30 repetitions. If the patient can perform one set of 30 repetitions with good form and no substitution, he or she can be progressed to 1- to 2-lb weights and back down to three sets of 10 to repeat the cycle. This rationale is based on lending objectivity to the progression and the tonic nature of the rotator cuff muscles and the scapular stabilizers. Isolated exercises are used to enhance or increase the strength of a particular muscle. Combining isotonic exercises in functional-movement patterns are performed with PNF patterns using elastic resistance or the cable column to enhance coordinated movement. In the case of a swimmer, the D1 pattern with elastic resistance will lead to a carryover to his athletic function. Initiation of isokinetic strengthening at this phase may enhance the shoulder's ability to strengthen in a pain-free ROM. It is encouraged that slower speeds be used when strengthening patients with shoulder instability. Isokinetic principles suggest that faster isokinetic speeds create greater translational forces, whereas slower speeds create stronger compressive forces (which stabilize the shoulder). Milestones that should be met to move to the next rehabilitation phase include (1) within 10° of full AROM in flexion, abduction, IR, and ER in the plane of the scapula; (2) normalized scapulothoracic motion and strength; (3) moderate overhead activities without pain; and (4) isometric internal and external strength should be at least 50% that of the uninjured side.

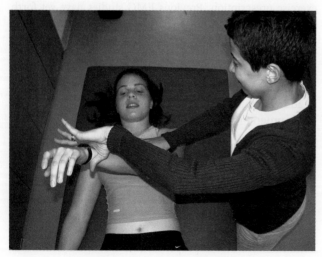

Fig. 6-18 D2 flexion with manual resistance.

Phase IV (Advanced Strengthening Phase)

TIME: 15 to 24 weeks after surgery
GOALS: Pain-free full ROM, improve muscular endurance, improve dynamic stability

After 15 weeks the patient is in the final phase of rehabilitation. Full AROM should be attained at this time. The only restriction on ROM is that ER should not be stretched beyond 90°. It may be preferable to allow the athlete to regain additional degrees of ER over time rather than stress the biceps-labral complex, potentially stretching the repair.

Posterior capsule stretching is appropriate if full IR has not been obtained yet. Performing the side-lying sleeper stretch encourages ROM for IR (see Fig. 6-17). At the onset of this phase, a thorough strength assessment is needed to evaluate the direction of strengthening needed for the particular patient. This assessment may include manual muscle testing, hand-held dynamometry, and isokinetic strengthening (or a combination of these techniques). Assessment should include the primary shoulder movers, shoulder rotators, and scapula stabilizers. Results of this assessment should be addressed with a well-rounded strengthening program to include isotonic, concentric, and eccentric loading exercises. When designing these programs, consider the everyday demands of each patient. For an overhead-throwing athlete, strengthening in the throwing position is imperative (Fig. 6-19). Once this phase of rehabilitation is reached, treatment should begin to streamline toward the functional demands of the patient.[98]

Initiation of a properly designed plyometric training program is often the missing link to discharging a high-level patient. Plyometric training for the upper extremity is used to generate rapid and powerful muscular contractions in response to a dynamic stretch–inducing load to a muscle or group of muscles. It is suggested that plyometrics train the entire neuromuscular system, using the principles of stored elastic energy to use strength as quickly and forcefully as possible. The myotatic stretch reflex develops stored elastic potential. If the exercise movement is slow, such as in weight lifting, the energy is dissipated and nonproductive. However, with rapid movement, this stored elastic energy can be used to generate a force greater than that of the concentric contraction of the muscle alone. Plyometrics use the principles of progressive loading with the ultimate goal of power development. Using a trampoline will increase the EMG activity and elevate the level of eccentric loading of the shoulder rotators.[99] Therefore a progression from two-handed, side-to-side throws to overhead throws to one-handed overhead throws is encouraged to maximize the power development of the overhead athlete. A well-rounded program will address both the internal and external rotators of the shoulder, together with the core muscles of the trunk. Externally challenging the patient, by permitting stability from a naturally unstable surface, such as a ball, will challenge the entire kinetic chain. Advanced exercises, such as the Physioball "walk outs," exemplify this concept (Fig. 6-20). As the patient walks out from the ball with the hands, core stabilizers, as well as GH stabilizers, are challenged. Milestones to progress to the final phase of rehabilitation include (1) pain-free full ROM, (2) less than 20% strength deficits for IR and ER at 90°/second, and (3) 20% strength deficits in all positions.

Phase V (Return-to-Activity-and-Sport Phase)

TIME: 4 to 6 months after surgery
GOALS: Pain-free full ROM, normalized strength, return to sport or activity program

This is the phase of rehabilitation at which very few therapists have the opportunity to discharge patients.

All too often patients lose interest, exhaust insurance coverage, or just neglect the importance of fine-tuning their shoulders before fully returning to their lifestyle. This stage is designed to prepare patients to return, without hesitation, to full participation in all activities. Milestones to successfully complete this phase include (1) total confidence in the shoulder, (2) pain-free full ROM, and (3) an isokinetic or hand-held dynamometry with less than 10% deficit in all positions.[100]

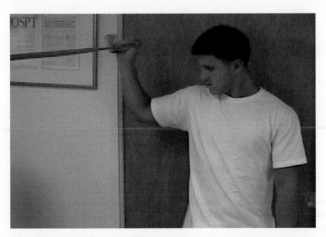

Fig. 6-19 External rotation strengthening in the 90°/90° position with elastic resistance.

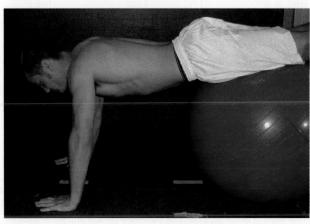

Fig. 6-20 Physioball wall walkouts.

Exercises in this phase continue to emphasize functional positions, including the plyometric program (isokinetic strengthening at 90° of abduction). A gradual return to sport is permitted once the patient is pain free, has nearly full ROM in all planes, confidence in the shoulder, and 85% to 90% of the strength of the opposite side on isokinetic testing at 90°, 180°, and 300°/second for IR and ER motions.

Confidence is achieved with the ability to perform pain-free functional movement in the patient's sport. Our experience has demonstrated that the throwing athlete requires an additional 1 to 2 months to allow the shoulder to adjust to the motion. Patients also report that it takes up to 1 year before the shoulder feels "normal" after SLAP repair. We currently are using the American Shoulder and Elbow Surgeons Shoulder Evaluation Form to standardize the documentation of pain, motion, strength, stability, and function. Although it remains difficult to gather enough data to determine a criterion score for return to sports, once 6 months have passed and clinical milestones have been met, the athlete is cleared for full throwing. This time frame is in agreement with other authors' findings[101] (Table 6-1).

SUMMARY

Considerations must be given if additional procedures are performed for reattachment of the labrum, ligaments, or the biceps tendon. However, stronger fixation techniques have allowed the rehabilitation to progress more rapidly with these procedures. These guidelines are a continuum of rehabilitation phases based on the effect the surgery has on the tissue and the surrounding structures. Scientific rationale is applied whenever possible; however, as surgical procedures evolve, so must the rehabilitation. These guidelines are by no means set in stone, and all exercises are not distinct to particular phases. The goals and exercises need to be modified

based on the performer, the pathology, and the performance demands. Exercise prescriptions should not be viewed as protocol but as guidelines upon which to base rehabilitation. These rehabilitation guidelines are outlined in Box 6-1.

TROUBLESHOOTING

Hypomobility and Hypermobility of the Glenohumeral Joint

In the process of rehab after a SLAP repair, it is not uncommon to have difficulty restoring a patient's normal ROM. With these hypomobile patients, it is necessary to begin early mobilization and stretching to regain normal arthrokinematic and osteokinematic motion. Using grade III and IV mobilizations can help to increase capsular pliability, especially in the posterior and inferior directions.

The therapist should avoid stretching patients into the apprehension position without applying a posterior "relocation" force because this may cause impingement internally.

After SLAP repair, some patients will experience a hypermobility issue. Often times this is due to generalized ligament laxity that affects all joints. This is tested by thumb-to-forearm, metacarpophalangeal and distal interphalangeal extension, as well as elbow and knee recurvatum. These patients will regain normal ROM on their own as they progress to doing functional movements of the shoulder. Therefore it is necessary for the therapist to mobilize and stretch the GH complex. It is important to progress these patients more slowly and allow them to regain the motion on their own.

Poor Scapular Stabilization

Scapular dyskinesis, or poor scapulohumeral rhythm, is often a problem that patients and therapists face after SLAP repair surgery. Poor scapular stability may have been a

TABLE 6-1 Time to Return to Sports After SLAP Surgery

Study	Year	Surgery	Type of SLAP	Population	Return to Sports*	Full Throwing
Yoneda, et al[68]	1991	Repair	Type II	Athletes	ND	ND
Resch, et al[102]	1993	Repair	Type II	Not specified	6 months	ND
Cordasco, et al[72]	1993	Débridement	Type II	Not specified	ND	ND
Pagnani, et al[6]	1995	Repair	Types II & IV	Not specified	4 months	6 months (not specified)
Field & Savoie[29]	1993	Repair	Types II & IV	Not specified	ND	ND
Berg & Ciullo[103]	1997	Repair	Types II & IV	Not specified	ND	ND
Segmuller, et al[104]	1997	Repair	Types II & IV	Not specified	6 months	ND
Morgan, et al[105]	1998	Repair	Type II	Athletes & nonathletes	4 months	7 months
Samani, et al[106]	2001	Repair	Type II	Athletes & nonathletes	ND	ND
O'Brien, et al[30]	2002	PAL, repair	Type II	Athletes & nonathletes	ND	ND
Jazrawi, et al[107]	2003	Repair with ATCS	Type II	Athletes	3-4 months	11.2 months

ATCS, Arthroscopic thermal capsular shift; *ND*, not documented; *PAL*, partial anterolateral acromioplasty.
*In most papers, time to return refers to the initial return, not to full return.
Data from O'Brien SJ, et al: The trans-rotator cuff approach to SLAP lesions: Technical aspects for repair and a clinical follow-up of 31 patients at a minimum of 2 years. Arthroscopy 18(4):372-377, 2002.

BOX 6-1 Rehabilitation Guidelines for SLAP Repair

I. Early Protective Phase (0 to 4 Weeks)

A. Goals:

- Protect surgical procedure
- Educate patient on procedure and therapeutic progression
- Regulate pain and control inflammation
- Initiate ROM and dynamic stabilization
- Neuromuscular reeducation of external rotators and scapulothoracic muscles

B. Treatment Plan (0 to 2 Weeks):

- Sling immobilization for 2 to 4 weeks
- Gripping exercises
- Elbow, wrist, and hand ROM
- Pendulum exercises
- Shoulder PROM F/ABD/IR/ER Do not go beyond the position set at time of surgery for ER (progress flexion to A/AROM)
- IR and ER proprioception training (controlled range)
- Initiate gentle alternating isometrics for IR and ER in 0° abduction to scapular plane
- Initiate passive forward flexion to 90°
- Initiate scapular mobility

C. Treatment Plan (2 to 4 Weeks):

- ROM progression
  - Forward flexion to 110° to 130°
  - ER in scapular plane to 35° (position set at time of surgery)
  - IR in scapular plane to 60°
- Progress submaximal alternating isometrics for IR and ER in scapular plane
- Initiate scapular strengthening
  - Manual scapula retraction
  - Resisted band retraction

(Note: No shoulder extension past trunk)

- Deltoid isometrics in all directions
- Biceps-triceps strengthening
- Initiate light band work for IR and ER

D. Milestones For Progression:

- Forward flexion to 90°
- Abduction to 70°
- ER in scapular plane to 30°
- IR in scapular plane to 20°
- Tolerance of submaximal isometrics
- Knowledge of home care and contraindications
- Normalize mobility of related joints (AC, SC, ST)

II. Intermediate Phase (5 to 8 Weeks)

A. Goals:

- Normalize arthrokinematics
- Gains in neuromuscular control

- Normalization of posterior shoulder flexibility
- Limit PROM of ER/ABD to 65° to 70° to protect the healing biceps/labral complex

B. Treatment plan:

- ROM progression
  - Flexion in the scapula plane passively 150° to 165°
  - ER in the scapula plane to 65°
  - IR in the scapula plane, full or to within 10°
- Initiate joint mobilizations as necessary
- Initiate posterior capsular stretching
- Progress strengthening
  - IR/ER (with GH in the scapula plane) with elastic band
  - Side-lying ER
  - Scaption full can (no weight if substitution patterns)
  - Clockwise/counterclockwise ball against wall
  - Body Blade at neutral or rhythmic stabilization

C. Milestones for progression:

- Forward flexion to 160°
- ER in scapular plane to 65°
- Full IR in scapular plane
- Symmetrical posterior capsule mobility
- Progressing isotonic strength with IR and ER in available range

III. Strengthening Phase (9 to 14 Weeks)

A. Goals:

- Normalize ROM
- Progression of strength
- Normalize scapulothoracic motion and strength
- Overhead activities without pain

B. Treatment plan:

- ROM progression; stretching ER at 90° of GH abduction
  - Within 10° of full AROM in all plans
- Progression of scapular retractors and stabilizers
  - Prone program; LT, MT, rhomboid
  - LT; scapular depression
  - Progress strengthening
  - Challenging rhythmic stabilization
  - Upper body ergometer
  - Initiate isokinetic IR and ER in scapular plan
  - Initiate IR and ER at 90° of GH abduction
  - Isotonic strengthening; flex, abduction
  - Closed kinetic chain exercise

C. Milestones for progression:

- Within 10° of full active range in scapular plane
- Isometric strength IR and ER less than 50% deficit
- Less than 30% strength deficits; primary shoulder muscles and scapular stabilizers

Continued

BOX 6-1 Rehabilitation Guidelines for SLAP Repair—cont'd

IV. Advanced Strengthening Phase (15 to 24 Weeks)

A. Goals:

- Pain-free full ROM
- Improve muscular endurance
- Improve dynamic stability

B. Treatment plan:

- Maintain flexibility
- Progress strengthening
- Advanced closed kinetic chain exercise
- Wall push-ups; with and without ball
- Continue with overhead strengthening
- Continue with isokinetic IR and ER strengthening; 90° of GH abduction
- Advance isotonic strengthening
- Advance rhythmic stabilization training in various ranges and positions
- Initiate plyometric strengthening
  - Chest passes
  - Trunk twists
  - Overhead passes
  - 90°/90° position single-arm plyometrics

C. Milestones for progression:

- Pain-free full ROM
- Strength deficits less than 20% for IR and ER at 90° of GH abduction
- Less than 20% strength deficits throughout

V. Return-to-Activity and Sport Phase (4 to 6 Months)

A. Goals:

- Pain-free full ROM
- Normalized strength
- Return to sport or activity program

B. Treatment plan:

- Continue isokinetic training
- Continue with stability training
- Advance plyometric training
- Continue with closed kinetic chain exercise

C. Milestones for activity:

- Confidence in shoulder
- Strength deficits less than 10% throughout
- Pain-free full ROM
- Completion of return to sport or activity program

A/AROM, active assistive range of motion; *AC*, acromioclavicular; *AROM*, active range of motion; *ER*, external rotation; *GH*, glenohumeral; *IR*, internal rotation; *LT*, lower trapezius; *MT*, middle trapezius; *PROM*, Passive range of motion; *SC*, sternoclavicular; *ST*, scapulothoracic; *UBE*, upper body ergometer.

---

precursor that helped lead to the SLAP tear, or it may be a direct result of the disuse after surgery and wearing a sling. In these cases it is necessary to establish a stable base by working the rhomboids, middle and lower trapezius, and the serratus muscles in an endurance fashion. Because normal motion requires these muscles to be tonically active, it is necessary to work them to fatigue. Failing to establish this stable base will lead to the peal-back mechanism occurring when the arm is in the 90°/90° position. Winging of the scapula causes an increased anterior force on the humeral head that will increase the traction force on the long head of the biceps as the arm moves up into the throwing motion. It is important to avoid rotator cuff strengthening in the 90°/90° position until scapulohumeral motion has been normalized.

Posterior Shoulder Extensibility

The throwing athlete has been known to have an increase in ER ROM and a decreased/limited IR ROM. Not maintaining total ROM with a severe loss of IR ROM may lead to a SLAP tear. The cause of the IR ROM loss may be a tight posterior capsule and musculature. If the therapist is lucky enough to see the patient before surgery, this can be addressed. In fact, the surgeon may do a posterior capsule release during the SLAP repair.

More often the posterior shoulder tightness needs to be treated after the surgery by the physical therapist. Focus-ing on the posterior shoulder will ensure recovery of total ROM.

Impingement Symptoms During Return-to-Activity Phase

Sometimes after SLAP repair, a patient will report back to the physical therapist with shoulder pain after returning to activity. It is not uncommon for an athlete to forget about the home exercise program or fail to complete rehabilitation. The athlete commonly complains of mechanical shoulder impingement symptoms. If this is the case, it is helpful to closely examine ER strength in the 90°/90° position, poste-rior shoulder strength, and scapulohumeral rhythm. It is more than likely that one or all of these parameters have not been normalized before the patient returned.

Suggested Home Maintenance for the Postsurgical Patient

Because the patient spends only an estimated 2 to 3 hours per week with the physical therapist, it is what the patient does on his or her own that influences the eventual outcome. Physical therapists are teachers; they intervene manually when necessary but direct the rehabilitation based on the basic science of healing tissue. Adherence to a home exercise program is crucial for a successful outcome after SLAP repair. The home program for any patient must be individualized based on the patient's postoperative condition, age, nutritional status, limitations, and individual needs. Frequency, sets, and repetitions are determined based on the therapist's professional opinion of the expected outcome.

1. Early (0 to 4 Weeks)
- Shoulder and elbow A/AROM flexion
- Pendulums
- No active biceps activity
- Isometric ER at 0° abduction
- Scapula pinches, gripping exercises

2. Intermediate (5 to 8 Weeks)
- Isotonic ER at 45° of abduction with Thera-Band
- Rows with Thera-Band (not to break the frontal plane with the involved elbow)
- Wall crawls
- Side-lying ER with soup can
- Golf club ER stretch at 45° (limit ROM of ER/ABD to 65° to 70°)
- Scaption
- Biceps curls, elbow supported (no support later, 6 to 8 weeks)
- Ball proprioception

3. Dynamic Strengthening (9 to 14 Weeks)
- ER at 90° abduction with Thera-Band
- Sleeper stretch
- UE stabilization in quadriplegic
- Door stretch
- Thrower's ten
- Eccentric biceps curls, shoulder unsupported with supination
- PNF D1, D2 pattern with Thera-Band
- Mirroring exercise—Stand in front of mirror, flex good arm to 45°, copy motion with bad arm and eyes closed

4. Return to Sports
ER 90°/90° position with Thera-Band, three sets to fatigue
- Definitions of fatigue
  - Failure to complete full ROM (0° to 90°)
  - Upper arm breaking the frontal plane
  - Dropping of elbow
- Maintain full IR at 90°/90° position
- Sleeper stretch
- Push-ups with a plus
- Rows
- Horizontal ABD, front raises, lateral raises, posterior raises
- Completion of interval throwing program

A/AROM, Active assistive range of motion; *ABD*, abduction; *ER*, external rotation; *PNF*, proprioceptive neuromuscular facilitation; *UE*, upper extremity.

CLINICAL CASE REVIEW

1 Aimee just felt a pop in her shoulder 4 hours ago while throwing a softball from center field to home plate. She has iced her arm and now arrives at your clinic to determine the possible source of pain. What special test might you perform during your physical examination to evaluate for a SLAP tear?

The Speeds test and O'Brien test are commonly used tests.

2 Tom is continuing to have pain after his nonoperative rehabilitation of his type I SLAP tear. His MRI is not showing any increased pathology to the biceps complex. What associated injury could be causing pain in his shoulder?

Other problems that can be associated with SLAP lesions include ganglion cysts, rotator cuff tears, posterior instability, and AC joint arthritis.

3 Sally is a 42-year-old female who arrives at the clinic 4 days after a SLAP repair. In passing, she tells the therapist that she has not been feeling well since surgery; she reports feeling "rundown" with a low-grade fever and fatigue the last few days. She is also complaining of severe aching around the shoulder joint. She notes her pain as 10 out of 10, and nothing she can do will make it better. "It even hurts when I don't move, and it often wakes me up." Upon inspection the therapist notices that the entire area around the shoulder is red, swollen, and has moderate wound seepage. The area surrounding the incision is hot to the touch, and the skin is very firm. What is the most likely cause of the patient's pain and discomfort?

Sally is exhibiting signs of a postoperative sepsis infection. A feeling of general malaise and low-grade fever are signs of systematic infection. Sally should be referred back to her physician immediately.

4 Tom is a 52-year-old male who arrives at the clinic 4 weeks after a SLAP repair. By recommendation of his physician, Tom has worn a sling religiously for the past 4 weeks. Upon the therapist's initial evaluation, it is noted that Tom has painful and severely restricted motion in all planes. What is the most likely cause of Tom's ROM deficit, and how would this deficit be treated most successfully?

Tom most likely has some iatrogenic GH adhesive capsulitis (i.e., frozen shoulder). Because he is still in the tissue-healing phase of his rehabilitation, the therapist cannot use grade III or IV mobilizations to normalize arthrokinematic motion because it may disrupt the repair. Tom's treatment should be with PROM and A/AROM to decrease and prevent further loss of ROM secondary to adhesive capsulitis. He should be encouraged to remove his sling several times a day and perform pendulum exercises to provide distraction and gentle ROM.

5 Dwight, who is 6 weeks postoperation for SLAP repair of the right shoulder, presents for his initial evaluation complaining of aching pain on the top of the shoulder laterally and posteriorly, with a feeling of shoulder tightness. You notice that he holds his shoulder in a protective, hiked position. While observing him performing therapeutic exercises, you notice he "shrugs" his shoulders bilaterally with performance of rows and on the right side with scaption AROM. What do you think is the culprit of his complaints, what should be evaluated, and what should your treatment plan consist of?

Based on his subjective complaints, he is likely experiencing upper trapezius muscle tightness with pain being referred to the distal insertion site of the muscle. Based on objective observation, Dwight is overusing the upper trapezius muscle both at rest and with execution of exercises and is using substitution patterns secondary to abnormal scapulohumeral rhythm. Scapulothoracic joint mobility should be assessed, as well as posterior shoulder musculature tightness and posterior capsule mobility.

Treatment should consist of soft tissue mobilization/massage to the upper trapezius muscle, scapulothoracic mobilizations, and joint mobilization to surrounding joints as appropriate, including the GH and sternoclavicular joints. Special attention should be paid to execution of exercises. Because he tends to activate the upper trapezius muscles when performing shoulder movements, visual and tactile cues to keep the shoulders "down and back" should be used, as well as visual or EMG biofeedback for upper trapezius muscle inhibition. Scapular stabilization exercises to strengthen the serratus anterior and other parts of the trapezius should also be added to assist in scapular upward rotation.

6 Shannon is a 47-year-old college professor who had a SLAP repair 12 weeks ago on her dominant arm. She is compliant with physical therapy and postsurgical precautions. She comes to the clinic complaining of increased pain and discomfort when writing on the chalkboard and reaching for things. Upon assessment, the therapist finds poor scapulohumeral rhythm, a winging scapular, and the following postmanual muscle testing (MMT) grades: serratus anterior 3/5, rhomboids/midtrapezius 3/5, and lower trapezius 2/5. Based on the clinical findings, what therapeutic exercise should be added to Shannon's program to resolve her complaints?

The following therapeutic exercises should be added to Shannon's program: dynamic hugs, push-ups with a plus, serratus punches, scaption, and manual scapula rhythmic stabilization.

7 At 12 weeks after SLAP repair, Lily has 45° of GH IR PROM and 40° of AROM. She has been doing the sleeper stretch but has not made any gains in ROM in the last 4 weeks. How does the therapist determine if the limitation in IR ROM is capsular or muscular to ensure that the correct therapeutic exercises are prescribed?

The therapist should perform a Tyler test and a posterior glide looking for side-to-side restriction. If the Tyler test is positive but the posterior glide is negative, the therapist can determine that the lack of IR is caused by muscle tightness and not capsular tightness.

8 Demetrius is 20 weeks s/p type II SLAP repair when he begins to get anxious about returning to his recreational baseball team in time for the playoffs, which start in 2 weeks. How should the therapist determine when he is ready to return to sports and at what level of competition?

A patient must first meet the return to activity/sport goals which include pain-free full ROM, normalized strength (i.e., <15% measured contralaterally), and the confidence necessary for the specific sport. Once these goals are met, the patient must then complete a return to activity program (e.g., return to throwing program). The American Shoulder and Elbow Surgeons Shoulder Evaluation Form can be used for documentation and comparison purposes. The literature has generally demonstrated a return to sports between 4 to 6 months for an athlete with a type II SLAP repair.

9 Steve is a 22-year-old collegiate baseball pitcher who the therapist has been treating for the last 23 weeks after right-sided SLAP repair (throwing arm). Steve began a throwing program that the therapist designed 3 weeks earlier, and he has been throwing without problems. However, now that the number of pitches has increased in his throwing program, he has been complaining of anterior shoulder pain that bothers him most during the "ball release" and "follow-through" phases of his pitching mechanics. Ruling out a possible compromise of the SLAP repair, what else could possibly be causing Steve's pain during the late period of his throw?

Because the biceps acts as an elbow flexor and a forearm supinator, its functions in the late phases of throwing are to decelerate the arm and extend the elbow. Overuse of the biceps if it has not been properly strengthened can lead to bicipital tendonitis. The therapist should have Steve back off the throwing program and begin eccentric strengthening of the biceps once the inflammation of the tendonitis has subsided. In addition, Steve's rotator cuff strength should be checked because the biceps will often be overused as a humeral head depressor if the rotator cuff is weak and not functioning properly.

10 Mariano arrives at the clinic after completion of an interval throwing program after 24 weeks of SLAP rehabilitation. He states his shoulder hurts after he is done throwing. After taking a history, the therapist feels that he is having some mechanical impingement. What are three likely causes of this impingement?

Three likely causes of this impingement are (1) poor scapular stability, (2) tight posterior shoulder structure, and (3) weak external rotator.

11 Jon is a 16-year-old male, s/p SLAP repair with a small Hill Sachs lesion and is 26 weeks postoperation. His primary complaint is an inability to make the throw from third base to first base, stating he has no velocity. His MMT is 4/5 in all shoulder motions; ER ROM is within normal limits; slight glenohumeral IR deficit of 15°. What should Jon's continued treatment consist of?

Jon should respond well to continued stretching of his shoulder via sleeper stretch, and posterior shoulder stretches. Included with stretching was continued strengthening with the "Throwers 10" exercises, and continued work with a return to throw interval program.

REFERENCES

1. Andrews JR, Carson WG Jr, McLeod WD: Glenoid labrum tears related to the long head of the biceps. Am J Sports Med 13:337-341, 1985.
2. Snyder SJ, et al: SLAP lesions of the shoulder. Arthroscopy 6(4):274-279, 1990.
3. Prodromos CC, et al: Histological studies of the glenoid labrum from fetal life to old age. J Bone Joint Surg Am 72:1344-1348, 1990.
4. Stetson WB, et al: Long term clinical follow-up of isolated SLAP lesions of the shoulder. Paper presented at the 65th Annual Meeting of the American Academy of Orthopaedic Surgeons, New Orleans, March 23, 1998.
5. Edwards SL, et al: Nonoperative treatment of superior labrum anterior posterior tears: Improvements in pain, function, and quality of life. Am J Sports Med 38:1456-1461, 2010.
6. Pagnani MJ, et al: Arthroscopic fixation of superior labral lesions using a biodegradable implant: A preliminary report. Arthroscopy 11(2):194-198, 1995.
7. Itoi E, et al: Stabilizing function of the biceps in stable and unstable shoulders. J Bone Joint Surg Br 75:546-550, 1993.
8. Maffet MW, Gartsman GM, Moseley B: Superior labrum-biceps tendon complex lesions of the shoulder. Am J Sports Med 23:93-98, 1995.
9. Pal GP, Bhatt RH, Patel VS: Relationship between the tendon of the long head of biceps brachii and the glenoidal labrum in humans. Anat Rec 229:278-280, 1991.
10. Rodosky MW, Harner CD, Fu FH: The role of the long head of the biceps muscle and superior glenoid labrum in anterior stability of the shoulder. Am J Sports Med 22:121-130, 1994.
11. Vangsness CT Jr, et al: The origin of the long head of the biceps from the scapula and glenoid labrum: Anatomical study of 100 shoulders. J Bone Joint Surg Br 76:951-954, 1994.
12. Gartsman GM, Hasan SS: What's new in shoulder surgery. J Bone Joint Surg Am 83:45, 2001.
13. Rhee YG, Lee DH, Lim CT: Unstable isolated SLAP lesion: Clinical presentation and outcome of arthroscopic fixation. Arthroscopy 21(9):1099, 2005.
14. Wilk KE, et al: Current concepts in the recognition and treatment of superior labral (SLAP) lesions. J Orthop Sports Phys Ther 35(5):273-291, 2005.
15. Ide J, Maeda S, Takagi K: Sports activity after arthroscopic superior labral repair using suture anchors in overhead-throwing athletes. Am J Sports Med 33:507-514, 2005.
16. Boileau P, et al: Arthroscopic treatment of isolated type II slap lesions: Biceps tenodesis as an alternative to reinsertion. Am J Sports Med 37:929-936, 2009.
17. Resch H, et al: Arthroscopic repair of superior glenoid labral detachment (the SLAP lesion). J Shoulder Elbow Surg 2:147-155, 1993.
18. Brockmeier SF, et al: Outcomes after arthroscopic repair of type-II SLAP lesions. J Bone Joint Surg Am 91:1595-1603, 2009.

19. Fleega BA: Overlap endoscopic SLAP lesion repair. Arthroscopy 15(7):796-798, 1999.

20. Snyder SJ, Banas MP, Karzel RP: An analysis of 140 injuries to the superior glenoid labrum. J Shoulder Elbow Surg 4:243-248, 1995.

21. Cooper DE, et al: Anatomy, histology, and vascularity of the glenoid labrum: An anatomical study. J Bone Joint Surg Am 74:46-52, 1992.

22. Morgan CD, et al: Type II SLAP lesions: Three subtypes and their relationships to superior instability and rotator cuff tears. Arthroscopy 14(6):553-565, 1998.

23. Seneviratne A, et al: Quantifying the extent of a type II SLAP lesion required to cause peel-back of the glenoid labrum–a cadaveric study. Arthroscopy 22(11):1163,e1-6, 2006.

24. McMahon PJ, et al: Glenohumeral translations are increased after a type II superior labrum anterior-posterior lesion: A cadaveric study of severity of passive stabilizer injury. J Shoulder Elbow Surg 13(1):39-44, 2004.

25. Burkhart SS, Morgan CD, Kibler WB: Shoulder injuries in overhead athletes: The "dead arm" revisited. Clin Sports Med 19(1):125-158, 2000.

26. Oh JH, et al: The evaluation of various physical examinations for the diagnosis of type II superior labrum anterior and posterior lesion. Am J Sports Med 36:353-359, 2008.

27. D'Alessandro DF, Fleischli JE, Connor PM: Superior labral lesions: Diagnosis and management. J Athl Train 35(3):286-292, 2000.

28. Kim TK, et al: Clinical features of the different types of slap lesions: an analysis of one hundred and thirty-nine cases. J Bone Joint Surg Am 85:66-71, 2003.

29. Field LD, Savoie FH III: Arthroscopic suture repair of superior labral detachment lesions of the shoulder. Am J Sports Med 21:783-790, 1993.

30. O'Brien SJ, et al: A new and effective test for diagnosing labral tears and AC joint pathology. J Shoulder Elbow Surg 6:175, 1997 (abstract).

31. Mimori K, et al: A new pain provocation test for superior labral tears of the shoulder. Am J Sports Med 27:137-142, 1999.

32. Kim SH, Ha KI, Han KY: Biceps load test: A clinical test for superior labrum anterior and posterior lesions in shoulders with recurrent anterior dislocations. Am J Sports Med 27:300-303, 1999.

33. Berg EE, Ciullo JV: A clinical test for superior glenoid labral or "SLAP" lesions. Clin J Sports Med 8(2):121-123, 1998.

34. Holtby R, Razmjou H: Accuracy of the Speed's and Yergason's tests in detecting biceps pathology and SLAP lesions: comparison with arthroscopic findings. Arthroscopy 20(3):231-236, 2004.

35. Kim SH, et al: Biceps load test II: A clinical test for SLAP lesions of the shoulder. Arthroscopy 17(2):160-164, 2001.

36. Guanche CA, Jones DC: Clinical testing for tears of the glenoid labrum. Arthroscopy 19(5):517-523, 2003.

37. Myers TH, Zemanovic JR, Andrews JR: The resisted supination external rotation test: A new test for the diagnosis of superior labral anterior posterior lesions. Am J Sports Med 33:1315-1320, 2005.

38. Parentis MA, et al: An evaluation of the provocative tests for superior labral anterior posterior lesions. Am J Sports Med 34:265-268, 2006.

39. Ebinger N, et al: A new SLAP test: The supine flexion resistance test. Arthroscopy 24(5):500-505, 2008.

40. Lichtenberg S, Magosch P, Habermeyer P: Compression of the suprascapular nerve by a ganglion cyst of the spinoglenoid notch: The arthroscopic solution. Knee Surg Sports Traumatol Arthrosc 12(1):72-79, 2004.

41. Baums MH, et al: Treatment option in a SLAP-related ganglion cyst resulting in suprascapular nerve entrapment. Arch Orthop Trauma Surg 126(9):621-623, 2006.

42. Hosseini H, et al: Arthroscopic release of the superior transverse ligament and SLAP refixation in a case of suprascapular nerve entrapment. Arthroscopy 23(10):1134.e1-4, 2007.

43. Berg EE, Ciullo JV: The SLAP lesion: A cause of failure after distal clavicle resection. Arthroscopy 13(1):85-89, 1997.

44. Chochole MH, et al: Glenoid-labral cyst entrapping the suprascapular nerve: Dissolution after arthroscopic debridement of an extended SLAP lesion. Arthroscopy 13(6):753-755, 1997.

45. Forsythe B, et al: Concomitant arthroscopic SLAP and rotator cuff repair. J Bone Joint Surg Am 92:1362-1369, 2010.

46. Kessler MA, et al: SLAP lesions as a cause of posterior instability. Orthopade 32(7):642-646, 2003.

47. Chandnani VP, et al: Glenoid labral tears: Prospective evaluation with MR imaging, MR arthrography, and CT arthrography. AJR Am J Roentgenol 161:1229-1235, 1993.

48. Karzel RP, Snyder SJ: Magnetic resonance arthrography of the shoulder: A new technique of shoulder imaging. Clin Sports Med 12:123-136, 1993.

49. Tirman PFJ, et al: Magnetic resonance arthrography of the shoulder. Magn Reson Imaging Clin N Am 1:125-142, 1993.

50. Tirman PF, et al: The Buford complex–a variation of normal shoulder anatomy: MR arthrographic imaging features. AJR Am J Roentgenol 166:869-873, 1996.

51. Jee WH, et al: Superior labral anterior posterior (slap) lesions of the glenoid labrum: Reliability and accuracy of mr arthrography for diagnosis. Radiology 218:127-132, 2001.

52. Liu SH, et al: Diagnosis of glenoid labral tears: A comparison between magnetic resonance imaging and clinical examinations. Am J Sports Med 24:149-154, 1996.

53. Stetson WB, Templin K: The Crank test, the O'Brien test, and routine magnetic resonance imaging scans in the diagnosis of labral tears. Am J Sports Med 30:806-809, 2002.

54. Bencardino JT, et al: Superior labrum anterior-posterior lesions: Diagnosis with MR arthrography of the shoulder. radiology 214:267-271, 2000.

55. De Maeseneer M, et al: CT and MR arthrography of the normal and pathologic anterosuperior labrum and labral-bicipital complex. Radiographics 20:S67-S81, 2000.

56. Tuite MJ, et al: Superior labrum anterior-posterior (SLAP) tears: Evaluation of three MR signs on T2-weighted images. Radiology 215:841-845, 2000.

57. Connell DA, et al: Noncontrast magnetic resonance imaging of superior labral lesions: 102 cases confirmed at arthroscopic surgery. Am J Sports Med 27:208-213, 1999.

58. Ellsworth AA, et al: Electromyography of selected shoulder musculature during unweighted and weighted pendulum exercises. Proceedings of the American Physical Therapy Association Combined Sections Meeting, Nashville Tenn, February 17, 2004.

59. Waldherr P, Snyder SJ: SLAP-lesions of the shoulder. Orthopade 32(7):632-636, 2003.

60. Snyder SJ: Shoulder arthroscopy, New York, 1994, McGraw-Hill.

61. Davidson PA, Rivenburgh DW: Mobile superior glenoid labrum: A normal variant or pathologic condition? Am J Sports Med 32:962-966, 2004.

62. Choi NH, Kim SJ: Avulsion of the superior labrum. Arthroscopy 20(8):872-874, 2004.

63. Mihata T, et al: Type II SLAP lesions: a new scoring system–the sulcus score. J Shoulder Elbow Surg 14(1 suppl S):19S-23S, 2005.

64. Franceschi F, et al: No advantages in repairing a type II superior labrum anterior and posterior (SLAP) lesion when associated with rotator cuff repair in patients over age 50: A randomized controlled trial. Am J Sports Med 36:247-253, 2008.

65. Abbot AE, Li X, Busconi BD: Arthroscopic treatment of concomitant superior labral anterior posterior (SLAP) lesions and rotator cuff tears in patients over the age of 45 years. Am J Sports Med 37:1358-1362, 2009.

66. Oh JH, et al: Results of concomitant rotator cuff and SLAP repair are not affected by unhealed SLAP lesion. J Shoulder Elbow Surg 20(1):138-145, 2010.

67. Levy HJ, et al: The effect of rotator cuff tears on surgical outcomes after type II superior labrum anterior posterior tears in patients younger than 50 years. Am J Sports Med 38(2):318-322, 2010.

68. Yoneda M, et al: Arthroscopic stapling for detached superior glenoid labrum. J Bone Joint Surg Br 73:746-750, 1991.

69. Katz LM, et al: Poor outcomes after SLAP repair: descriptive analysis and prognosis. Arthroscopy 2009 25(8):849-855.

70. Gorantla K, Gill C, Wright RW: The outcome of type II SLAP repair: a systematic review. Arthroscopy 26(4):537-545, 2010.

71. Kim SH, et al: Results of arthroscopic treatment of superior labral lesions. J Bone Joint Surg Am 84:981-985, Jun 2002.

72. Cordasco FA, et al: Arthroscopic treatment of glenoid labral tears. Am J Sports Med 21:425-431, 1993.

73. Brockmeier SF, et al: Outcomes after arthroscopic repair of type-II SLAP lesions. J Bone Joint Surg Am 91(7):1595-1603, 2009.

74. Friel NA, et al: Outcomes of type II superior labrum, anterior to posterior (SLAP) repair: Prospective evaluation at a minimum two-year follow-up. J Shoulder Elbow Surg 19(6):859-867, 2010.

75. Decker MJ, et al: Serratus anterior muscle activity during selected rehabilitation exercises. Am J Sports Med 27:784-791, 1999.

76. Tyler TF, et al: Electrothermally assisted capsulorrhaphy (ETAC): A new surgical method for glenohumeral instability and its rehabilitation considerations. J Orthop Sports Phys Ther 30(7):390-400, 2000.

77. Burkhart SS, Morgan C: The peel-back mechanism: Its role in producing and extending posterior type II SLAP lesions and its effect on SLAP repair rehabilitation. Arthroscopy 14(6):637-640, 1998.

78. Kuhn JE, et al: Failure of the biceps superior labral complex: a cadaveric biomechanical investigation comparing the late cocking and early deceleration positions of throwing. Arthroscopy 19(4):373-379, 2003.

79. Tyler TF, et al: Reliability and validity of a new method of measuring posterior shoulder tightness. J Orthop Sports Phys Ther 29:262-274, 1999.

80. Harryman D, et al: Translation of the humeral head on the glenoid with passive glenohumeral motion. J Bone Joint Surg 72A(9):1334-1343, 1990.

81. Tyler TF, et al: Quantification of posterior capsule tightness and motion loss in patients with shoulder impingement. Am J Sports Med 28(5):668-673, 2000.

82. Mullaney MJ, et al: Reliability of shoulder range of motion comparing a goniometer to a digital level. Physiother Theory Pract 26(5):327-333, 2010.

83. Tyler TF, et al: Correction of posterior shoulder tightness is associated with symptom resolution in patients with internal impingement. Am J Sports Med 38(1):114-119, 2010.

84. Burkhart SS, Morgan C: SLAP lesions in the overhead athlete. Orthop Clin North Am 32(3):431-441, 2001.

85. Burkhart SS, Morgan CD, Kibler WB: The disabled throwing shoulder: Spectrum of pathology. II. Evaluation and treatment of SLAP lesions in throwers. Arthroscopy 19(5):531-539, 2003.

86. Diederichs S, Harndorf M, Stempfle J: Follow-up treatment with physiotherapy after arthroscopic reconstruction in SLAP lesions. Orthopade 32(7):647-653, 2003.

87. Kibler WB: Shoulder rehabilitation: principles and practice. Med Sci Sports Exerc 4S:40-50, 1998.

88. Tyler TF et al: Effect of scapular stabilizer fatigue on shoulder external and internal rotation strength in patients with microinstability of the shoulder. Paper presented at the AOSSM Annual Meeting, Keystone, Colo, 2005.

89. McCann P, et al: A kinematic and electromyographic study of shoulder rehabilitation exercises. Clin Orthop Relat Res 288:179-187, 1993.

90. McMahon PJ, et al: Comparative electromyographic analysis of shoulder muscles during planar motions: anterior glenohumeral instability versus normal. J Shoulder Elbow Surg 2:118-123, 1996.

91. Moseley JB, et al: ECG analysis of scapular muscles during a shoulder rehabilitation program. Am J Sports Med 20:128-134, 1994.

92. Schachter AK, et al: Electromyographic activity of selected scapular stabilizers during glenohumeral internal and external rotation contractions. J Shoulder Elbow Surg 19(6):884-890, 2010.

93. Lear LJ, Gross MT: An electromyographical analysis of the scapular stabilizing synergists during a push-up progression. J Orthop Sports Phys Ther 28(3):146-157, 1998.

94. Hintermeister RA, et al: Electromyographic activity and applied load during shoulder rehabilitation exercises using elastic resistance. Am J Sports Med 26(2):210-232, 1998.

95. Cordasco FA, et al: Arthroscopic treatment of glenoid labral tears. Am J Sports Med 21(3):425-430, 1993.

96. Warner JJ, Kann S, Marks P: Arthroscopic repair of combined Bankart and superior labral detachment anterior and posterior lesions: Technique and preliminary results. Arthroscopy 10(4):383-391, 1994.

97. Kibler WB, et al: Qualitative clinical evaluation of scapular dysfunction: A reliability study. J Shoulder Elbow Surg 11(6):550-556, 2002.

98. Burkhart SS, Morgan CD, Kibler WB: Shoulder injuries in overhead athletes: The "dead arm" revisited. Clin Sports Med 19(1):125-158, 2000.

99. Cordasco FA, et al: An electromyographic analysis of the shoulder during a medicine ball rehabilitation program. Am J Sports Med 24(3):386-392, 1994.

100. McFarland EG, et al: Results of repair of SLAP lesion. Orthopade 32(7):637-641, 2003.

101. Park HB, et al: Return to play for rotator cuff injuries and superior labrum anterior posterior (SLAP) lesions. Clin Sports Med 23(3):321-334, 2004.

102. Resch H, et al: Arthroscopic repair of superior glenoid detachment (the SLAP lesion). J Shoulder Elbow Surg 2:147-155, 1993.

103. Berg EE, Ciullo JV: The SLAP lesion: A cause of failure after distal clavicle resection. Arthroscopy 13(1):85-89, 1997.

104. Segmuller HE, Hayes MG, Saies AD: Arthroscopic repair of glenolabral injuries with an absorbable fixation device. J Shoulder Elbow Surg 6(4):383-392, 1997.

105. Morgan CD, et al: Type II SLAP lesions: three subtypes and their relationships to superior instability and rotator cuff tears. Arthroscopy 14(6):553-565, 1998.

106. Samani JE, Marston SB, Buss DD: Arthroscopic stabilization of type II SLAP lesions using an absorbable tack. Arthroscopy 17(1):19-24, 2001.

107. Jazrawi LM, McCluskey GM III, Andrews JR: Superior labral anterior and posterior lesions and internal impingement in the overhead athlete. Instr Course Lect 52:43-63, 2003.

CHAPTER 7

Total Shoulder Arthroplasty

Chris A. Sebelski, Carlos A. Guanche

CLINICAL EVALUATION

History

The most common complaint in patients with advanced osteoarthritis (OA) of the shoulder is pain—more specifically, night pain. Most often, the pain is insidious in its onset, although an occasional patient will report acute symptomatology only to discover severe osteoarthritic changes in the glenohumeral (GH) joint. In many cases night pain is a major problem; specifically, difficulty with lying on the affected side is a common complaint.[1]

A careful history should be taken with respect to prior injuries and prior surgical procedures. For a total shoulder replacement to be viable and functional, an intact rotator cuff is necessary. In certain patients with long-standing rotator cuff disruption, the initial clinical signs are progressive pain that comes with the developing secondary arthropathy.[2]

Another area of concern is whether the patient has undergone any prior stabilization procedures. The reason this is important to remember is that preferential wear of certain parts of the glenoid can occur in long-standing cases that have undergone excessive capsular-tightening procedures.[3] Most commonly, this is posterior wear. In addition, in certain types of stabilization procedures, a variety of bony transfer procedures are performed, including a lateralization of the lesser tuberosity and a transfer of the coracoid transfer. As a result, the surgical exposure in these cases can be difficult because of the distorted anatomy.

Physical Examination

The most important predictor of the outcome of a total shoulder replacement is the preoperative range of motion (ROM).[4,5] **It is therefore incumbent on the physician to document all directions of the patient's motion and to discuss the implications of lack of mobility on the overall outcome.** Another important aspect is the integrity of the rotator cuff; a successful standard replacement depends very heavily on the presence of an intact cuff. The supraspinatus, infraspinatus, teres minor, and the subscapularis should all be carefully examined. If any doubt exists as to the function of the cuff, magnetic resonance imaging (MRI) is indicated. In cases in which a rotator cuff disruption coexists with severe OA, a determination should be made as to the possibility of repairing the cuff. In those cases in which significant chronicity of the cuff is noted, either by history or MRI examination, a simple hemiarthroplasty or a reverse total shoulder replacement (in cases in which pseudoparalysis of the arm exists) should be considered.[6]

SURGICAL INDICATIONS AND CONSIDERATIONS

Those patients with refractory pain and limitation of motion that do not respond to conservative methods of treatment (i.e., a trial of physical therapy, antiinflammatory medications, activity modification, avoidance of inciting factors, and intraarticular corticosteroid injections) are candidates for shoulder replacement. Ideally, the patient's age should also fit within the acceptable parameters for a joint replacement. Although the ideal patient should be over the age of 65 and have a relatively limited activity level, the reality is that many patients do not fit such criteria.

In cases in which the patient's age is significantly under 65 years or the activity level is not commensurate with their age, avoiding the surgery should be considered (in some of these patients, a case can be made for fusion of the joint). In addition, a spectrum of replacement procedures can be used, including a partial humeral replacement (classically termed a hemiarthroplasty), a hemiarthroplasty with a biologic resurfacing of the joint, and a standard total shoulder replacement; in more severe cases of patients with concurrent unrepairable rotator cuff tears, a reverse total shoulder can be used.

SURGICAL PROCEDURE

The choice of anesthesia depends on the clinical experience of the surgeon and anesthesiologist. Ideally, the anesthesia would include an interscalene block, either by itself or as a supplement to a general anesthetic. The use of such blocks has been shown to significantly affect the patient's postoperative course in a very positive manner.[7] In cases in which interscalene anesthesia is not used, the preemptive administration of a long-acting anesthetic (Marcaine) is also well-founded in the literature and has been shown to positively affect recovery.[8]

The standard approach to a shoulder replacement operation includes positioning the patient in a semirecumbent (beach chair) position, with a small bolster under the scapula to effectively stabilize the glenoid for exposure. In addition, the operative shoulder should be examined under anesthesia with all of the directions of motion measured and documented. Finally, it is important to ensure that the operative arm can be extended and rotated appropriately for delivery of the humeral head and subsequent resection during the surgical procedure (Fig. 7-1). This is called the ability to shotgun the arm into this position.

The standard incision is a deltopectoral approach that is typically centered immediately lateral to the coracoid process of the scapula and extends down the proximal arm, avoiding the axilla (Fig. 7-2). It is important to allow for distal

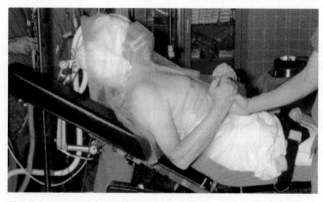

Fig. 7-1 Position for total shoulder arthroplasty (TSA), ensuring that the arm can be positioned for the insertion of the humeral device.

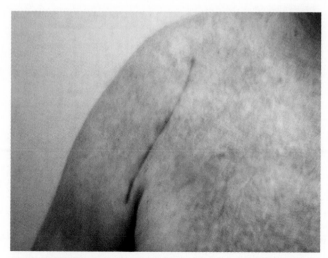

Fig. 7-2 Standard incision along the anterior aspect of the shoulder. The typical incision is about 4 inches long.

exposure of the wound should the need arise for a more complex humeral approach, such as in complications associated with humeral shaft fractures on prosthetic insertion.

The exposure includes identification of the deltopectoral interval with identification of the cephalic vein and subsequent medial retraction. The pectoralis tendon is identified laterally and, in severe cases, released for a distance of 1 to 2 cm for improved GH joint exposure. In addition, the deltopectoral interval is exposed in its entirety from the leading edge of the clavicle to the lower end of the pectoralis muscle. Commonly, significant subdeltoid adhesions need to be released for proper delivery of the humeral head out of the wound.

After complete exposure of the deltopectoral interval, the conjoint tendon is identified and released at its proximal portion for a distance of 1 cm, and the medial retractor is placed behind the tendon. Care should be taken to protect the musculocutaneous nerve when performing this maneuver.

The subscapularis tendon is now identified and released from superior to inferior, beginning at its lateral corner. The tendon is released directly off the lesser tuberosity and retracted medially. The release continues inferiorly, cauterizing the vascular leash consisting of the anterior inferior humeral circumflex vessels and proceeding along the inferior humeral head, while externally rotating the humerus (Fig. 7-3). The extent of the release is variable. However, the requirement is that the entire humeral head can be delivered for resection and that adequate exposure of the glenoid is possible if resurfacing of that portion is being performed.

Once the exposure is complete, a variety of humeral resection techniques can be used, depending on the manufacturer's individual surgical protocol. The design the author of this chapter uses involves resection of the humeral head at its anatomic base. Before completing this cut, the head must be exposed and all peripheral osteophytes should be removed to appropriately resect the head in an anatomic fashion (Fig. 7-4).

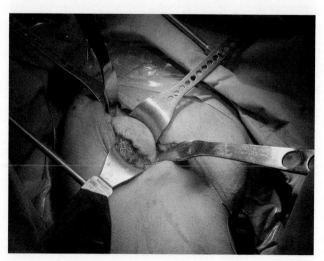

Fig. 7-3 Right humeral head exposed through the wound. The complete absence of normal cartilage on the surface and the peripheral osteophytes around the articular margin should be noted.

After resection of the head, the humeral canal is prepared for the prosthetic device being implanted. A series of reamers are inserted down the medullary canal, stopping when the appropriate-sized device is used. The size is typically judged from templates that measure the size of the medullary canal based on their radiographic dimension. However, ultimately the choice is made intraoperatively, based on the surgeon's experience as he or she advances the device into the shaft.

The humeral metaphysis is then prepared with a series of broaches that contour the proximal humerus for insertion of the actual component. The type of implant varies, with two major types being available: (1) cemented and (2) cementless. A cementless device uses the body's ability to grow bone into some of its surfaces; these surfaces are often prepared with a sintered metal (Fig. 7-5). In a cemented device, the prosthesis is implanted using polymethylmethacrylate cement for immediate fixation of the device. The theoretic

advantages of one device over another are beyond the scope of this chapter; the reader is directed to the appropriate references.[9-11]

Attention is now directed to the glenoid. It is important to be able to access the entire area of the glenoid from anterior to posterior and superior to inferior to effectively prepare the bony surface for the implant. The capsule of the joint is excised, beginning with the most anterior, superior portion and extending inferiorly and posteriorly as far as necessary to allow for adequate exposure (Fig. 7-6). Once the exposure is gained, the central point of the glenoid is identified; then the surface is prepared for accepting the actual component. Finally, the device is cemented into position using polymethylmethacrylate cement.

The final decisions that need to be made include choosing the appropriately sized humeral head component to allow a relatively normal passive range of motion (PROM) with minimal to no instability before closure of the subscapularis muscle tendon (Fig. 7-7). Once the appropriate head is chosen and implanted, the subscapularis muscle tendon is reapproximated to the lesser tuberosity with the use of sutures that have been prepositioned through the bone before implantation of the humeral component (Figs. 7-8 and 7-9). The repair of the subscapularis is the critical element that needs attention during the first 6 weeks because of the importance of the subscapularis for component stability and overall shoulder girdle strength. Moreover, a disruption of the repair is notoriously difficult to diagnose in the early phases and extremely difficult to salvage when a chronic diagnosis is made.

The closure is done in layers, with a subcuticular skin closure protected by Steri-Strips being the final step. In some cases a drain may be exteriorized via a separate stab wound incision. This is typically removed on the first postoperative day. The final and perhaps most important part of the surgical procedure occurs at this time. The surgeon takes the arm through a PROM to assess the overall total motion possible without joint instability of disruption of the subscapularis

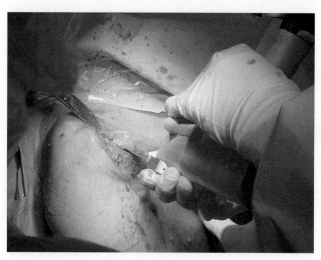

Fig. 7-4 Resection of the humeral head after removal of the peripheral osteophytes and the normal anatomic reference is found.

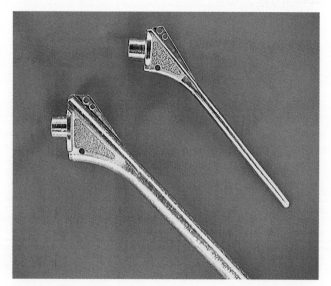

Fig. 7-5 Typical shoulder (humeral) components. These are standard components with a porous metal interface at that proximal portion to promote bony ingrowth.

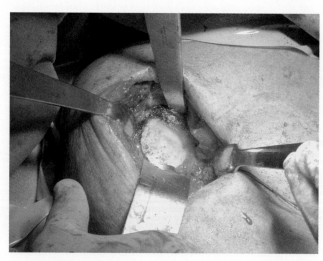

Fig. 7-6 Glenoid exposure after soft tissue resection circumferentially around the joint.

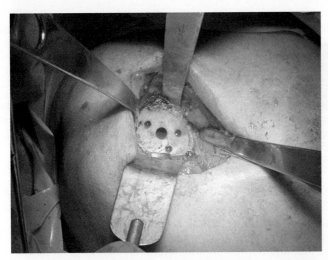

Fig. 7-7 Prepared glenoid face after drilling of central canal and preparation of face.

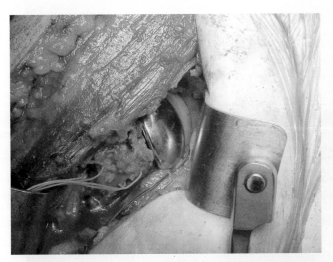

Fig. 7-8 Final view of humeral and glenoid implants before closure of the subscapularis tendon.

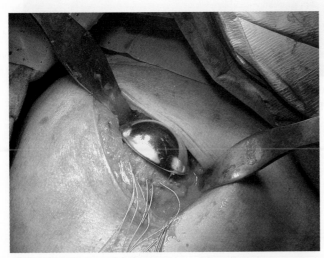

Fig. 7-9 Prepared proximal humerus with sutures through the lesser tuberosity in preparation for reattachment of the subscapularis tendon.

tendon repair. This ROM will be used to guide the limits that will be allowed in the first phases of rehabilitation. Final radiographs are typically obtained immediately postoperatively to ensure an appropriate position of all the components and also to ascertain that no intraoperative complications such as a humeral shaft fracture have occurred (Fig. 7-10).

THERAPY GUIDELINES FOR REHABILITATION

Total shoulder arthroplasty is performed less frequently than hip or knee total joint replacements in the United States.[8] There is evidence that a decreased hospital stay and a higher likelihood of discharge to home may be associated with those patients treated in surgical centers with a higher volume of total shoulder arthroplasties.[12,13] No attempts to correlate the patient's functional limitations and impairments on discharge have been found with length of stay or "successful discharge." The clinician must use physiologic healing principles to assist in gaining functional return of shoulder ROM following surgical intervention.

Successful rehabilitation of a total shoulder arthroplasty (TSA) depends in large part on the collegial communication between the surgeon and the therapist. Appropriate rehabilitation needs to recognize and address the preoperative history and impairments, the surgical technique, prosthetic type, and the surgeon's assessment of the tissue status upon finalization of the repair.

The majority of these issues dictate the postoperative precautions and guidelines that are placed upon the rehabilitation timeline to ensure that protection of the position of the prosthesis and the appropriate healing of the subscapularis occurs (Box 7-1).

The patient and therapist must be aware that the primary goal for nontraumatic TSA is pain relief. It appears that the achievement of functional ROM goals are more achievable today than 5 years ago; however, the improvement of ROM is not as well substantiated in the literature as the successful achievement of decreased pain.[14] The preoperative diagnosis also impacts the postoperative outcome. Completion of a TSA because of primary OA is more likely to result in functional use of the upper extremity than those completed as a result of trauma, rheumatoid arthritis of the GH joint,

---

BOX 7-1 Potential Preoperative Impairments for Primary TSA Because of OA[14]

Pain with attempted activities
Loss of elevation range of motion
Loss of external rotation range of motion
Inability to complete activities overhead
Inability to complete activities of daily living
Interrupted sleep patterns because of pain

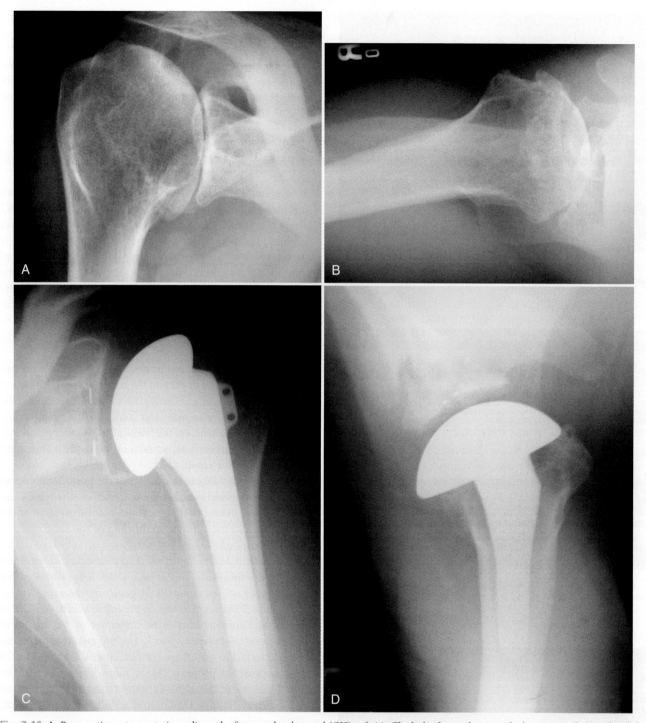

Fig. 7-10 A, Preoperative anteroposterior radiograph of severe glenohumeral (GH) arthritis. The lack of space between the humerus and glenoid and the peripheral osteophytes should be noted. **B,** Axillary view showing GH relationship with no joint space. **C,** Final anteroposterior radiograph of total shoulder replacement. **D,** Final axillary view of the total shoulder arthroplasty.

capsulorrhaphy, arthropathy, or rotator cuff arthropathy (Box 7-2).[15]

To prognosticate functional outcomes, including achievement of active ROM against gravity, the clinician should examine the patient's prior surgical history, duration of impairments before surgery, presence and severity of a preoperative rotator cuff tear,[15] the underlying cause for the surgical technique, and finally, the postoperative ROM at the

shoulder while under anesthesia. These factors can help the clinician predict the maximal outcome that may be achieved. Both the patient's status before surgery and the underlying causative factors leading to surgery can be obtained via patient interview. It is rare that the treating physical therapist would have the opportunity to perform a physical examination to potentially address postural deficits preoperatively. The surgical information including comments on ROM and

BOX 7-2 Preoperative Factors for Better Outcomes Following TSA

Better Outcomes

No previous surgery
Higher level of preoperative function[54,56]
Minimal rotator cuff pathology[56]
Overall well-being of the patient before surgery[43]
Surgery because of primary osteoarthritis

Worse Outcomes

Surgery because of rheumatoid arthritis or trauma
Severe loss of passive range of motion
Increased number of comorbidities[56]
Radiographic evidence of humeral head subluxation
Loss of posterior glenoid bone
Significant rotator cuff pathology
Increased fatty degeneration of the infraspinatus, subscapularis[50]

Data from Hettrich CM, et al: Preoperative factors associated with improvements in shoulder function after humeral hemiarthroplasty. J Bone Joint Surg Am 86-A(7):1446-1451, 2004; Iannotti JP, Norris TR: Influence of preoperative factors on outcome of shoulder arthroplasty for glenohumeral osteoarthritis. J Bone Joint Surg Am 85-A(2):251-258, 2003; Matsen FA III, et al: Correlates with comfort and function after total shoulder arthroplasty for degenerative joint disease. J Shoulder Elbow Surg 9(6):465-469, 2000; Edwards TB, et al: The influence of rotator cuff disease on the results of shoulder arthroplasty for primary osteoarthritis: Results of a multicenter study. J Bone Joint Surg Am 84-A(12):2240-2248, 2002; Franklin JL, et al: Glenoid loosening in total shoulder arthroplasty. Association with rotator cuff deficiency. J Arthroplasty 3(1):39-46, 1988; Rozencwaig R, et al: The correlation of comorbidity with function of the shoulder and health status of patients who have glenohumeral degenerative joint disease. J Bone Joint Surg Am 80(8):1146-1153, 1998.

BOX 7-3 Common Postsurgical Precautions

Passive range of motion for up to 6 weeks
Abduction pillow for up to 8 weeks
External rotation limited to 30° with humerus at 0° of adduction
Sling to be worn for comfort

The periodization of the rehabilitation program for a TSA must balance protection of the healing tissues, structures with the need for ROM gain to prevent overall stiffness of the shoulder. There are indications that an increased immobilization period increases the risk of a contracture of the deltoid and the rotator cuff. This soft tissue imbalance is theorized to be one of the reasons for revision surgery of a TSA. Other reasons for surgical revision include glenoid loosening, rotator cuff tear, humeral head subluxation, proximal humeral head migration, and GH instability.[1,14,20,55] **The following guidelines should not supersede the communications from the surgeon nor should they override sound clinical judgment to create an independent plan of care based on your patient's comorbidities, physical health, and functional needs.**

Initial Postoperative Examination

Patient examination following surgery typically occurs on day 0 (day of surgery) or on postoperative day 1. The therapist will note IV lines for postsurgical fluid intake, sanguineous drains, postoperative dressing, and the upper extremity in a sling for comfort. Physical examination should include cognitive testing for orientation to name, time, place, and reason and vital sign assessment on the noninvolved extremity in supine, sitting, and standing. Testing specific to the involved upper extremity should adhere to the postoperative restrictions according to the patient's chart (Box 7-3).

Neural screening should be completed as allowed within the postsurgical restrictions, including myotome, dermatome, and deep tendon reflex (DTR) testing. Active range of motion (AROM) of the cervical spine, thoracic spine, and elbow, wrist, and fingers should be assessed. PROM of the shoulder should be assessed with the patient in supine, understanding that some limitation in mobility may be contributable to the dressing or IV lines. Girth measurements should be noted at the elbow and at the wrist for comparison with the uninvolved extremity. Additionally, the anterior and posterior chest wall should be monitored for ecchymosis.

Functional mobility assessment should be initiated with instructions cautioning against direct pushing or pulling of the involved upper extremity during transferring. Patients must be assessed for independent mobility from supine to sit to stand and vice versa. Once standing is achieved, balance must be assessed for single limb support without loss of balance. Frequently, postoperative day 0 or day 1 will require the patient to use a temporary single upper extremity support (IV pole or single point cane) because of anxiety and a deconditioned state. Monitoring of vitals and

the condition of the repaired tissue may be obtained from communications with the surgeon including the surgical report.

Rehabilitation progression may further be guided by precautions and recommendations directly from the surgeon. In some instances formal physical therapy may not be used depending on the surgeon's experiences.[16] Typically, the patient will present in an abduction pillow or at the very least a shoulder sling. Additional positioning options or passive ROM (PROM) restrictions may be in place for a patient with a history of rheumatoid arthritis. A long history of rotator cuff pathology may require positioning that decreases the mechanical stresses placed on the healing structures. **An external rotation restriction of less than 30° to 40° is typical for protection of the healing subscapularis muscle and the anterior capsule, which is disrupted during placement of the prosthetic. This restriction may last up to 6 weeks.**[17-19]

orientation during the transfer and gait assessment is necessary due to risk of hypotensive episodes. The clinician should encourage the use of coughing and incentive spirometry throughout the hospital stay because of the greater level of inactivity following surgery intervention.

Phase I: Hospital Phase of Rehabilitation

TIME: 2 to 6 days after surgery[13]
GOALS: Protection of healing structures, pain control, independent functional mobility for transfers, dressing and ambulation, education, and the institution of a home exercise program within the surgical restrictions (Table 7-1)

Treatment during the hospital phase of rehabilitation focuses on the achievement of appropriate pain control, independent functional mobility for transfers, dressing and ambulation, education, and the institution of a home exercise program within the surgical restrictions. Length of hospital stay depends on multiple factors including the volume and experience of the hospital and the surgeon experienced in the total shoulder procedure. Home support, comorbidities, and demographic features play a smaller role. Unlike the total knee arthroplasty where a certain objective measure of knee flexion is often one of the impairment goals for discharge, common discharge goals regarding functional level, pain control, and impairment objective measurements for total shoulder procedures have not been established in the literature.[12,13]

Typically, PROM is initiated on day 0 or 1, with a progression to self-assisted ROM exercises including pendulum or table top activities.

The home exercise program should be completed multiple times per day for short durations of 5 minutes maximum per bout of exercise.[18] **If there is a strict passive ROM restriction in place, then this will require the education of a caregiver or family member to assist with the execution of the home program.** This caregiver must understand all postsurgical restrictions that limit ROM. Self-assisted ROM exercises can be based on patient comfort or surgeon preference.

Pendulum exercises involve a static position of forward flexion of the trunk with movement of the hips and trunk to drive the dangling upper extremity into multiple planes of motion (Fig. 7-11). The benefits of this activity for this patient population includes the addition of traction to the joint, stretching of the capsule, and **avoidance of active muscular contraction at the shoulder joint.**[21] Overall, the goal is prevention of soft tissue contracture and possible modulation of pain via the rhythmic movement of the upper extremity through a PROM.[17,22] *There are several challenges with the correct performance of this exercise as it applies to the patient with a recent TSA.* Frequently, the patient demonstrates inappropriate performance by recruiting excessive muscular action at the deltoid and pectoralis major muscles. The recommended posture for pendulum exercises emphasizes poor mechanical alignment of the scapula on the thorax with promotion of scapular abduction. And lastly, the excessive and unopposed stretching of the recently repaired musculature and tissues from the surgical procedure may actually generate greater pain response.

The Neer protocol for TSA[23] placed wall slides in the same phase as pendulum activities with literary evidence of low muscular activity about the healing structures.[21] Modification of this position to a lower gravitational demanding position would be self-assisted ROM using a table top. This table top modification is frequently used before wall slides during this early intervention phase. The patient stands at a table top with bilateral upper extremities resting at a comfortable placement. The hands maintain a static position and then ROM is attained by the lower extremity stepping into the various planes of motion.[17] There are several benefits to this type of exercise prescription. The position of weight bearing promotes ROM gains through planar lower extremity

TABLE 7-1 Total Shoulder Replacement

Rehabilitation Phase	Criteria to Progress to This Phase	Anticipated Impairments and Functional Limitations	Intervention	Goal	Rationale
Phase I (Hospital phase) Postoperative 2-6 days	Things to watch out for: • Hypotension • Neurologic deficits	• Edema • Pain • Inadequate ROM	• ROM of proximal and distal joints to surgical site • Balance activities of trunk • Development of home exercise program: closed kinetic chain versus open kinetic chain discussion	• Modified independent bed-to-sitting transfers • Modified independent sit-to-stand transfers • Instruction on sleeping positions • Independent with home exercise program • Controlled pain	• Maintain ROM of proximal and distal joints to surgical site • For trunk activation • Continue to progress with home exercises

ROM, Range of motion.

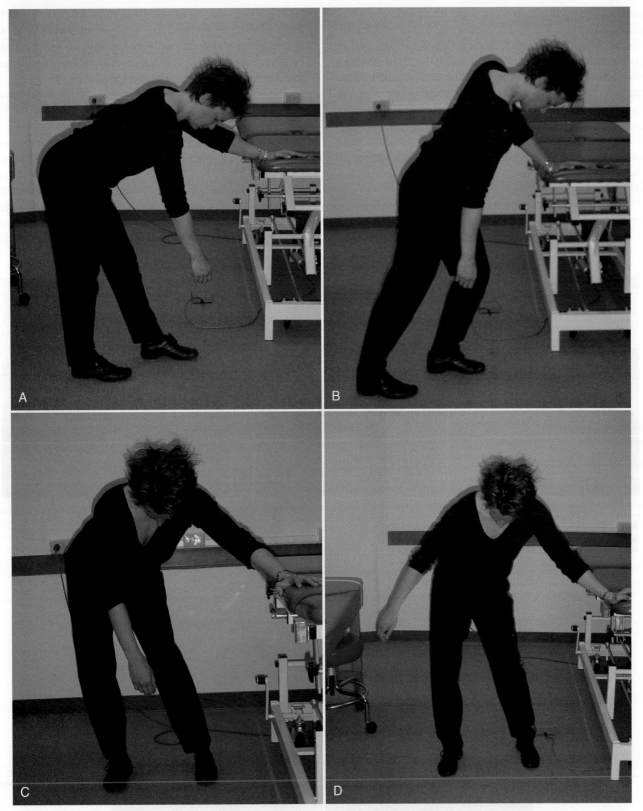

Fig. 7-11 Pendulum. **A** and **B,** Sagittal plane. **C** and **D,** Frontal plane.

motion. The trunk is moving underneath the scapula, which promotes interaction of the scapula and thorax in preparation for later stages of rehabilitation (Fig. 7-12). The patient is able to control the excursion of the ROM of the shoulder via decreasing the step size. The supported position of the shoulder via the hand decreases the unopposed stress on the healing tissue that may be achieved in the open kinetic chain position of the pendulum. Finally, closed kinetic chain activities at the shoulder reap similar benefits as stated for other extremities including: muscular cocontraction, decrease of shear forces, increased joint compression, and increased stability about the joint.[3,24]

The home exercise program should require AROM of the cervical and thoracic spines through the cardinal planes and active movement of the elbow, wrist, and hand. **If the patient is supine then flexion of the elbow should occur only with the humerus supported by a towel underneath it to decrease the strain on the biceps tendon at its insertion.** Frequent bouts of exercise for short durations are recommended for the earlier stages of rehabilitation.

The home exercise program contains education for passive and/or self-assisted ROM at the shoulder, active ROM for proximal and distal structures, and education on sleeping postures. This should include positional support via the use of pillows or an immobilizer to support the healing structures during the night. The encouragement of experimentation to attain the best possible sleeping posture should be discussed. *Anecdotally, patients following shoulder surgery feel better sleeping in a semireclined posture with the involved upper extremity supported by pillows or bolsters (Fig. 7-13).*

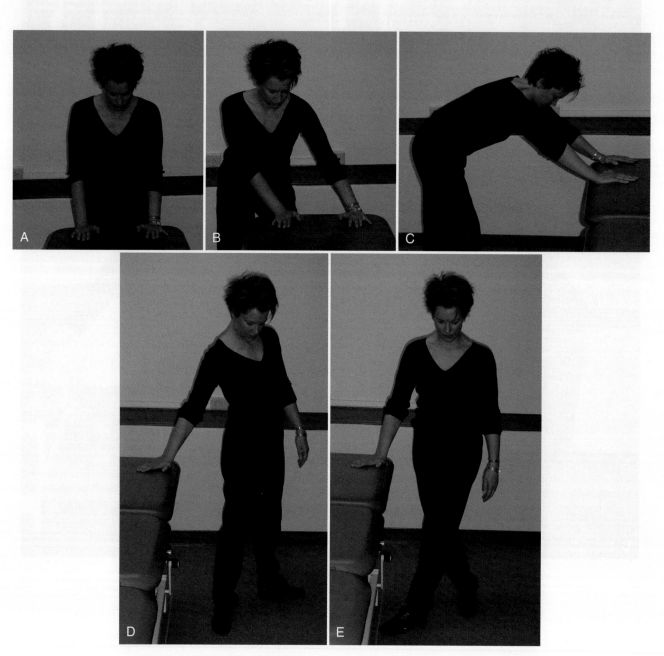

Fig. 7-12 Table top position. **A,** Starting position. **B,** Abduction. **C,** Flexion. **D,** External rotation. **E,** Internal rotation.

Phase II: Outpatient Rehabilitation–Early Range of Motion 0 to 6 Weeks

TIME: 0 to 6 weeks
GOALS: Protection of healing structures, pain control, uninterrupted sleep pattern, normalized circumference measurements between upper extremities, mobilization of scar, ability to

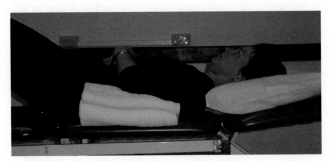
Fig. 7-13 Supine elbow support position.

demonstrate normalized posture, and increased ROM (Table 7-2)

Outpatient rehabilitation begins as a progression of the home exercise program given during the hospital stay. It is recommended to incorporate the use of a self-reported outcome measure tool, such as the simple shoulder test (SST) or the disability assessment of shoulder and hand (DASH) to monitor functional changes through rehabilitation.[7] *It is important to remind the patient that their rehabilitation will continue past discharge from formal physical therapy as functional return may proceed for 1 to 2 years after surgical intervention.*[25]

The focus of the first 6 weeks of rehabilitation is twofold: protection of the healing structures and progression of ROM for prevention of muscular contracture and joint capsule stiffness. A limited amount of literature is available to support the variety of intervention plans employed during this phase.[18,26-28] *Adherence to postsurgical precautions is paramount. Treatment of the postsurgical impairments of pain, edema, and scar*

TABLE 7-2 Total Shoulder Replacement

Rehabilitation Phase	Criteria to Progress to This Phase	Anticipated Impairments and Functional Limitations	Intervention	Goal	Rationale

Phase II (ROM) Postoperative 0-6 wk	• Progression to next stage, physician clearance of tissue healing
	• Things to watch for:
	  • Quick achievement of ROM before 8-12 wk
	  • Excessive ER with UE at side
	  • Sustained edema in the distal UE greater than 4 wk
		• Edema
		• Pain
		• Inadequate ROM
			• ROM of proximal and distal joints to surgical site
			• Balance activities
			• Soft tissue mobilization when adequate healing has occurred (subscapularis, posterior cuff, biceps tendon)
			• PROM (performed in functional planes of movement and respecting postsurgical limitations)—Shoulder flexion, shoulder abduction, and ER (no greater than 30°)
			• ROM activities of the involved extremity
			• Wand versus Codman exercises
			• Closed kinetic chain
			• Modalities—Ice, ES for pain control
			• Lymphatic massage
			• Scapular mobility
			• MWM, PNF patterns versus cat-camel (many patients will require scapular adduction, upward rotation, and elevation because of typical postural dysfunction of scapular abduction and downward rotation secondary to sling posture)
				• Protection of healing structures
				• Pain control
				• Uninterrupted sleep pattern
				• Normalized circumference measurements between UEs
				• Mobilization of scar when appropriate
				• Ability to demonstrate normalized posture
				• Increased shoulder ROM—Flexion = 0°-140°
				0°-30°, ER
				0°-70°, IR
				0°-110°, abduction
					• Maintain ROM of proximal and distal joints
					• Activation for trunk
					• Realignment of scar tissue and collagen (to allow more unrestricted ROM)
					• Prevent joint contractures (pain modulation)
					• Joint traction (stretching to capsule, pain modulation)
					• Proprioception training (proximal segment over distal segment promotes scapula and thorax interaction, cocontractions around a joint increase stability of the joint)
					• Modalities for pain control
					• Lymphatic massage for lymphatic drainage
					• Prepares connective tissue around the scapula for future ROM

ER, External rotation; *ES*, electric stimulation, *IR*, internal rotation; *MWM*, mobilizations with movement; *PNF*, proprioceptive neuromuscular facilitation; *PROM*, passive range of motion; *ROM*, range of motion; *UE*, upper extremity.

mobility will naturally lead to increased ROM in the shoulder.

Pain control should be assisted via the adherence to medications prescribed by the surgeon and alleviating positions. Use of the sling should be gradually removed as the patient progresses through this phase. Control of pain will also be gained via the interventions to address the postsurgical inflammation and edema, and those interventions to improve the limited functional use of the upper extremity. Edema may be present in the distal upper extremity and ecchymosis may be present in the thorax from the overload of the lymphatic system following surgery. Modality use including ice, elevation, and electric stimulation are appropriate for edema management.[29] Diaphragmatic breathing followed by localized lymphatic massage techniques beginning at the proximal segments of the thorax and ipsilateral axilla and progressing distally in sequential order may also be employed for effective management.

Sleeping postures should be recommended to include positional support of the humerus via the use of pillows or a bolster. As mentioned, patients following shoulder surgery may prefer sleeping in a semireclined posture; the therapist should encourage the patient to experiment.

Progression of ROM may be elicited via soft tissue mobilization. Soft tissue mobilization, a form of massage, has the support of an animal model for potential cellular changes.[30] Initiation of soft tissue mobilization techniques at the posterior cuff and the deltoid will promote appropriate muscular length. Because of the probable postsurgical hypersensitivity, care should be taken at or near the surgical scar. For each of these techniques, the upper extremity position should be adjusted to ensure the muscle or area of skin being addressed is relaxed and in a protected posture. Initial positioning should address the targeted muscle in a position of a passively shortened length. This will decrease sensitivity and spasm at the introduction of this type of intervention.

The external rotation limitation is in place to promote soft tissue healing and protection of those structures injured during the surgical procedure, specifically the subscapularis muscle. As outlined previously, the subscapularis is taken down and reattached during the arthroplasty procedure. **Direct passive ROM to "stretch" this tissue is contraindicated during the early phases of rehabilitation and soft tissue mobilization is an appropriate intervention to address the inflammatory condition of this muscle and prevent adhesion development.** The technique of soft tissue mobilization promotes change to the myofascia via proposed realignment of the scar tissue and collagen. Slow, deep strokes to the myofascia of the subscapularis will assist in improvement of external rotation ROM, pain control, and eventual overhead reach.[31] The best patient position for improvements to the subscapularis length is approximately 45° of humeral abduction with a neutral rotation of the humerus.

Consideration of the other joints of the shoulder complex should be initiated during this phase. During the hospital stay, the patient had been instructed in cervical and thoracic AROM. Distally, the elbow and hand should be used during daily functional activities, thereby limiting the extent of distal disuse atrophy. Realization of the influence of the scapulothoracic juncture on GH motion can assist with restoration of this motion early in rehabilitation.

Protective posturing from the postsurgical sling typically places the scapula in an abducted and down rotated position. Lack of humeral motion in all of the planes through the initial weeks of rehabilitation leads to further disuse of the scapula and its contribution to shoulder ROM. Scapular mobilization on a stable thorax with the GH joint in its resting position for greatest volume prepares the scapula and its connecting tissue for future shoulder ROM (Fig. 7-14). Because of the typical postural dysfunction of scapular abduction and down rotation, many patients will require facilitation of adduction, upward rotation, and elevation. The lack of a true joint capsule about the scapula places this type of intervention into a mobilization of the myofascial connections. The clinician should recall the scapulohumeral rhythm and carefully monitor the position of the humerus when facilitating positions of the scapula (Box 7-4). For example, *scapular mobilizations into upward rotation should only occur with the humerus passively flexed greater than 60° or abducted greater than 30°, as these are the ranges at which the scapula and humerus begin a more associated phase of motion.*[32]

PROM via a family member in a gravity-eliminated position of supine or self-assisted ROM during table top weight

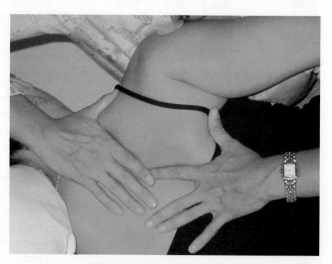

Fig. 7-14 Scapular mobilization.

BOX 7-4 A Review of Scapulohumeral Rhythm for Movement Analysis[32]
Initial phase: 0° to 60° primarily humeral motion Mid phase: 60° to 140° (ratio is inconsistent throughout motion with primarily humeral motion initially then mainly scapular motion) Ending phase: 140° to 180° with the majority of motion occurring at other joints

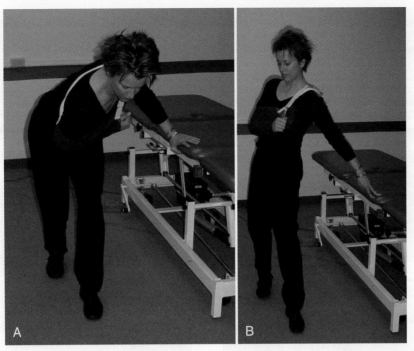

Fig. 7-15 **A,** Sling with internal rotation. **B,** Sling with external rotation.

bearing will be the primary method to promote ROM during this time frame (see Fig. 7-12). Progression should be dictated by the report of pain. **PROM performed by the therapist, patient, or caregiver should not exceed any precautions or restrictions given by the surgeon.** A tip for improved pain tolerance for motion of the upper extremity is to bias toward the plane of the scapula instead of true sagittal plane flexion.[33] A recommendation for moving into passive external rotation is the alignment of the humerus perpendicular to the center of the glenoid. This occurs at approximately 30° of abduction and ensures that the capsular structures will relax, achieving a better outcome.[18]

Self-assisted activities for ROM can be varied by direction, surface, and patient position. These types of exercise promote the mobility of the proximal segments over the involved upper extremity in a stable position. The trunk may move away from the upper extremity in various directions to promote the cardinal planes.[26] For example, in the early stages when the patient may still be most comfortable in the sling or supported position, relative external rotation and facilitation of scapular control may be achieved via contralateral trunk rotation and a return to neutral.[34] In an advanced stage of self-assisted exercises, the involved upper extremity may rest on a stability ball and the patient rolls the stool away from the stability ball in the frontal plane, promoting self-assisted abduction of the involved extremity. Or the patient may progress to gravity-dependent positions using the wall as the support and the trunk moving under the body to facilitate various planes of motions (Fig. 7-15).

Other self-assisted activities that have been recommended during this time include wand activities and pulley stretches.[18,26-28] Examination of pulley and wand activities compared to therapist-assisted exercises[35] indicate that

---

BOX 7-5 Goal of Passive Range of Motion Expected for Phase II (Supine)[34]

Flexion: 140 °
External rotation: 30° to 45°
Internal rotation: >70°
Abduction: 110°

---

therapist activities elicit less muscular activity of the supraspinatus, infraspinatus, anterior deltoid, and trapezius muscles. Therefore, *therapist-assisted activities should be used initially during this phase with a progression to wand or pulley activities as pain or surgical restrictions allow (Figs. 7-16, 7-17, and 7-18).*[18,26-28]

Progression from the initial outpatient phase (phase II) to the late ROM phase (phase III) is listed in Box 7-5. **The most significant requirement is physician clearance for AROM, especially into external rotation.** Many patients' restrictions will be lifted between weeks 2 and 6, thereby blurring the activities of phase II and phase III. The therapist should monitor the patient's ROM to assist with "staging" the patient's rehabilitation. This is one of the most challenging components of the transition from phase II to phase III. As noted, the passive motion goal of phase II is 40° while the patient will have achieved full PROM at the end of phase III. Additionally at the end of phase III, the patient should have active external rotation ROM of 45°. This ROM measure is the key to successful overhead motion.

Recall that optimal GH and scapular mechanics require near normal ROM of external rotation of the GH joint to complete functional tasks, such as touching the back of the head, reaching overhead, and donning/doffing shirts.[36] If the

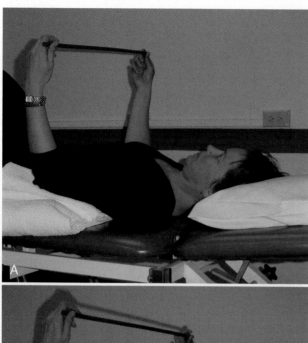

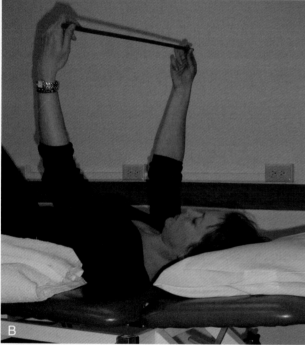

Fig. 7-16 **A,** Starting wand position. **B,** Scaption plane with wand.

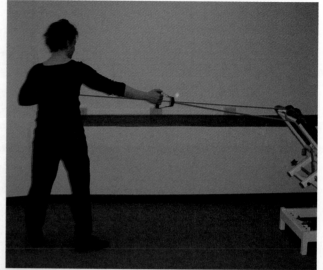

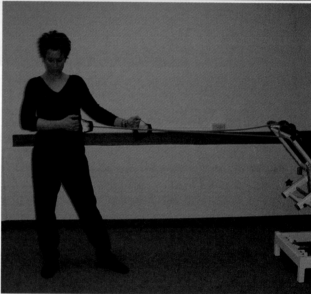

Fig. 7-17 Horizontal pulley.

GH joint ROM into external restriction is restricted to 45°, then a significant loss of function occurs, dramatically impacting a patient's quality of life. *As the patient will not have near normal external rotation ROM at the end of phase II, it is ill-advised to focus on repetitive or strengthening activities that are overhead because the mechanics will be less than optimal.* To prevent complications of overuse or tissue irritation, exercises and activities should be performed with the correct mechanics and without symptoms before progression to the next phase.

Complications

There are several signs and symptoms that should alert the therapist for possible complications (Box 7-6). Each must be examined with close consideration to the context and

---

BOX 7-6 Cautionary Signs and Symptoms During Early Range of Motion

Sustained edema in the distal upper extremity greater than 4 weeks
Excessive humeral external rotation (>30°) with upper extremity at side
Quick achievement of range of motion before 8 to 12 weeks
Biceps tendonitis
Progressively increasing pain

---

associated or corroborating signs and symptoms. Sustained edema in the distal upper extremity may be indicative of a systemic issue, such as infection. Excessive external rotation or quick achievement of ROM may indicate compromised muscular integrity. Biceps tendonitis indicates an overuse of the biceps for shoulder motion or stabilization. The biceps has an active role as a humeral depressor and with postsurgical muscular inhibition of the rotator cuff, successful accomplishment of shoulder flexion may rely on the biceps as the primary humeral depressor.[37] As a patient successfully progresses through the different stages of rehabilitation, pain is expected to plateau, decrease, or alter to more muscular fatigue or muscular soreness. Progressively increasing pain is often thought of as an indicator of serious pathology.

Phase III: Outpatient Rehabilitation—Late ROM and Early Strengthening

TIME: Approximately 6 to 12 weeks
GOALS: Return to everyday activities below 90° of shoulder flexion, increased ROM, improved muscle flexibility, improved neuromuscular control, increased strength, protection of healing structures (Table 7-3)

As the patient's ROM progresses, the patient will enter a mixed phase that consists of stretching to gain motion and strengthening to use the range gained. Exercise selection should place the protection of the healing structures as the primary concern. **This may include protection of the anterior joint capsule and the subscapularis via limit of external rotation when the humerus is in 0° of abduction and a limitation of hyperextension of the humerus when in the supine position for resting or exercise positioning.**[18,26] Communication with the surgeon will assist with determining which restrictions need to be maintained.

The emphasis of this phase is use of ROM and progression to muscle strengthening. Interventions to address muscular flexibility of the rotator cuff, deltoid, and scapular stabilizers should be continued from the previous phase. Pain has been found to inhibit muscular strength and therefore can be a limitation for achievement of active ROM.[6] Consideration that the source of pain may be from structures other than the traumatized muscle tissue will provide options for other interventions. Gentle joint mobilizations (grade I to II oscillatory) to the GH joint may be used to decrease possible capsular adhesions and to alter nociceptive input.[18,26]

There can be considerable discussion on the most appropriate exercises to initiate strengthening activities following a TSA. The clinician should always consider *how* mobility is achieved and what movement patterns may be adopted during this time period. *As the body transitions from limited mobility and muscular inhibition, the patient is at risk of developing faulty movement patterns that may later impede the ability to achieve active ROM in gravity-resisted positions.* It is strongly encouraged to instruct the patient in activities that promote the correct scapulohumeral rhythm for overhead activities. Application of this movement reasoning includes activities that emphasize the separation of scapular and the humeral motion during the initial phases and late phases of flexion and abduction and then emphasize coordination of the motion of the scapula and the humerus during the mid phases of motion.

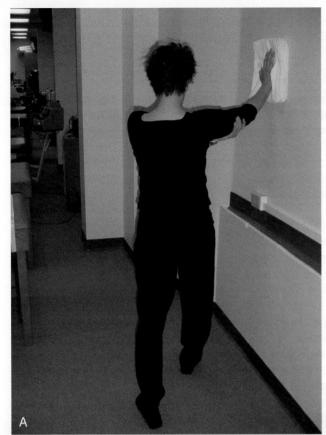
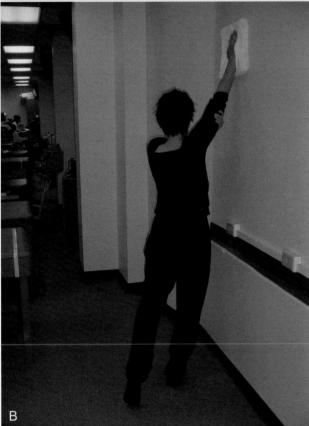

Fig. 7-18 **A,** Wall slides starting position. **B,** Finish position.

TABLE 7-3 Total Shoulder Replacement

Rehabilitation Phase	Criteria to Progress to This Phase	Anticipated Impairments and Functional Limitations	Intervention	Goal	Rationale
Phase III (Late ROM to strengthening) Postoperative 6-12 wk	• No signs of infection • No increase in pain or loss of ROM and physician clearance to progress	• Movement dysfunction—Early/unopposed shoulder elevation • Inadequate strength • Inadequate ROM	• Continue STM • Joint mobility at GH joint if painful (greater than I-II) • NMES—Rotator cuff and deltoid • Isometric exercises (initially submaximal) progress to walk aways • Progression of table dusting to wall washing • Progression of CKC from weight bearing at table to wall to floor • Pseudo CKC to OKC with UE supported but moving through ROM (angled table position) • Eccentric shoulder strengthening for flexion, abduction, and functional planes (assisted elevation of arm to shoulder height, then have patient slowly lower arm)	• Return to activities below 90° of shoulder flexion • Increased AROM of the shoulder in supine: flexion 0°-140°, abduction 0°-120°, ER 0°-40°; with shoulder abducted to 90°, then ER 0°-40° • AROM sitting flexion 0°-120° • Improved muscle flexibility • Improved neuromuscular control • Increase in strength • Protection of healing structures	• Realignment of scar tissue and collagen (to allow more ROM with less soft tissue restrictions) • Decrease possible capsular adhesions • Decrease nociceptor input • Targeting for specific muscles • Promote muscle contractions • Benefits of CKC exercises as stated before • Progression for antigravity strengthening • Eccentric strengthening • Progression to next stage

AROM, Active range of motion; *CKC,* closed kinetic chain; *GH,* glenohumeral; *NMES,* neuromuscular electric stimulation; *OKC,* open kinetic chain; *ROM,* range of motion; *STM,* soft tissue massage; *UE,* upper extremity; *ER,* external rotation.

Isometric training is supported for early strength training, especially in the cases where muscular contraction is desired yet the patient lacks sufficient strength for mobility through ROM.[26] **The clinician should be aware that significant muscular contraction can be elicited during isometric contraction exercises and therefore these exercises may be inappropriate during a healing phase where maximum tissue protection is required.**[21] Initiation of isometric training of the deltoids with a contraction of the rotator cuff establishes a muscular cocontraction or force couple that is required for motion (Figs. 7-19 and 7-20).

Isometric training of the scapular stabilizers with an eccentric contraction of the deltoid and rotator cuff from a prone position is an option for the introduction of strength training below 90° of shoulder flexion. A slow lowering toward the floor after a passive preposition into horizontal abduction at 90° will activate each of these key muscles. Introduction of concentric flexion and abduction may be introduced by progressively tilting supine positioning toward upright with and without weights (Figs. 7-21 and 7-22).[19]

If the patient is demonstrating significant difficulty performing an active contraction of targeted muscles in the absence of a neurologic injury, neuromuscular electric stimulation (NMES) may be used. Though specific parameters are outside the scope of this chapter, dual channel stimulation to provide for the deltoid activation and the

> **BOX 7-7** Goals of Active Range of Motion Expected for Phase III
>
> Full passive range of motion in supine
> Active range of motion (AROM) humeral flexion in supine: 140°
> AROM humeral abduction in supine: 120°
> AROM humeral external rotation in supine with humerus positioned at 0° of abduction: 45°
> AROM humeral external rotation in supine with humerus positioned at 90° of humeral abduction: 45°
> Active humeral flexion in a sitting/standing posture: 120°

scapular rotation necessary to achieve shoulder motion greater than 90° is recommended. Scapular rotation may be stimulated via the lateral rotator cuff muscles on the scapula or by stabilizing the scapula by stimulating the muscles with attachments to the medial border of the scapula. Electrode size and placement are key points for effective use of NMES.[29]

Progression to the final phase requires an improvement in passive and active ROM. The patient must be able to perform all home exercises with the correct form and minimal correction by the therapist (Box 7-7).

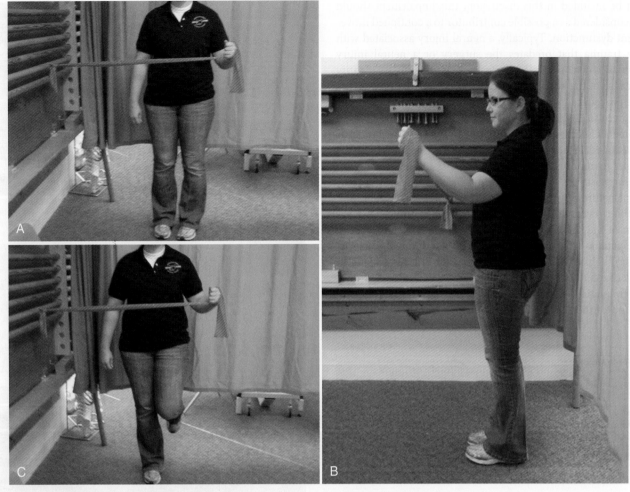

Fig. 7-19 Isometric holds. **A,** Front view. **B,** Sagittal view. **C,** Progression.

Phase IV: Outpatient Rehabilitation—Late Phase Strengthening

TIME: 12 weeks and more postsurgery
GOALS: Return to normal activities including overhead, increased ROM, improved neuromuscular control and strength. Full potential of function achieved between 6 and 12 months (Table 7-4).[7]

The goal of this phase of rehabilitation is strengthening of targeted muscles for use of the AROM gained and to establish a home exercise program that promotes continued strengthening upon discontinuation of therapy. Interventions addressing pain control and edema should be progressively phased out as they are no longer needed. Mobility of the scapula should occur with the humerus positioned into greater ranges of motion into shoulder flexion or abduction or completed in a mobilization with a movement model, with the patient performing the motion and the clinician providing overpressure to engage scapular motion at the appropriate time. The intention of mobilizations to the GH joint should change from addressing pain relief to the residual capsular stiffness or asymmetry through oscillation grades III and IV. Strengthening activities should address the dynamic stabilization system of the shoulder that is necessary for overhead movement.

Several underlying impairments may be responsible for the continued limited ability of the patient to demonstrate appropriate sequential motion when attempting to raise the arm above shoulder height. A number of factors may create barriers to successful progression. These include appropriate and timely surgical intervention, a rehabilitation course that has minimal medical complications, and/or appropriate motivation by the patient. If no barriers are apparent to progress, the primary impairment for limited overhead motion is due to inadequate motor performance of the force couples of the shoulder. The force couple *between the deltoid muscles and the rotator cuff musculature is the primary focus.*[17,27] If the AROM demonstrated in the supine position is approaching the ROM goals for therapy—yet the patient is unable to demonstrate similar range in sitting—then this type of motor control and/or pattern of weakness should be considered (Box 7-8).

Though specific rehabilitation parameters for those patients exhibiting weakness because of neural injury will not be included in this discussion, this impairment should be considered as a possible contributor to a continued movement dysfunction. Typically, a neural injury associated with the trauma that predates the surgery or a neural injury from a recent surgical intervention is difficult to identify because of the amount of surgically induced trauma during the procedure. Neural injury may be identified via atrophic changes to the muscle, inability of the patient to elicit an isometric contraction of the muscle with the humerus positioned in neutral, and possible sensory changes in the upper extremity. Isolated neural injuries following shoulder arthroplasty are considered a low risk because of the transient nature of the injuries and the tendency for resolution without eventual operative intervention.[38] When denervation of the shoulder musculature is present before surgery, the patient will most likely be placed in a limited goals category.[23] This category and the goals will be discussed later in this chapter.

Evaluation of weakness in patients with adequate innervation of the shoulder musculature should include manual

---

BOX 7-8 Cautionary Signs and Symptoms During Later Stages of Rehabilitation[57]

Loss of shoulder range of motion
Progressively increasing pain
"Clunk" felt during passive or active range of motion

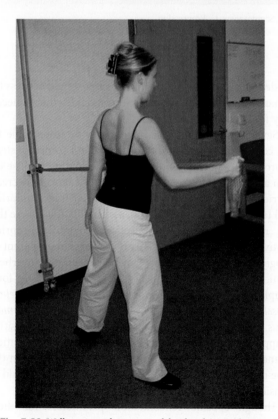

Fig. 7-20 Walk aways with isometric deltoid and external rotation.

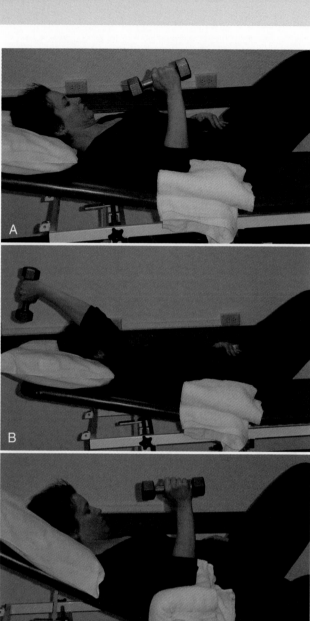

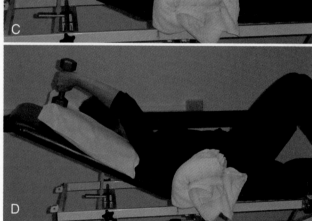

Fig. 7-21 **A,** Supine progressive tilt starting position. **B,** Finish. **C,** Supine greater angle progressive tilt starting position. **D,** Finish.

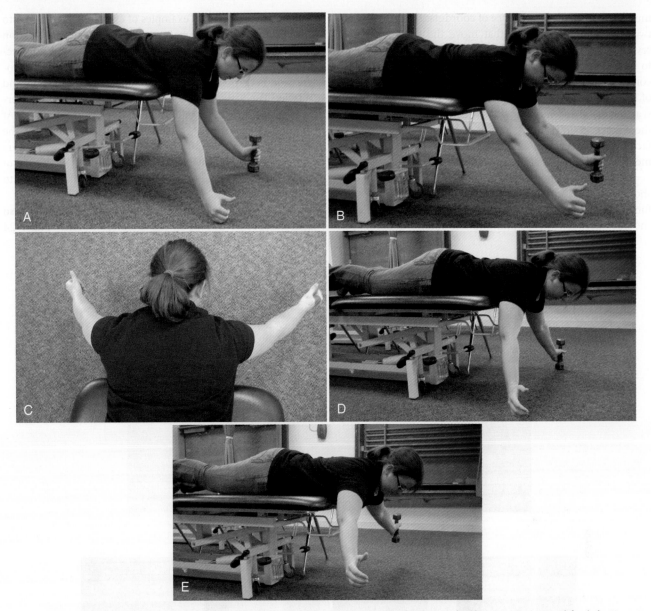

Fig. 7-22 Prone positions. **A,** Start and finish for Y-position exercise. **B,** Midposition. **C,** Overhead view of midposition. **D,** Start and finish for T-position exercise. **E,** Midposition.

TABLE 7-4 Total Shoulder Replacement

Rehabilitation Phase	Criteria to Progress to This Phase	Anticipated Impairments and Functional Limitations	Intervention	Goal	Rationale

Phase IV (Late phase strengthening) Postoperative 12 wk after surgery to discharge from therapy	• No increase in pain or loss of ROM and physician clearance to progress
	• Things to watch for:
	  • Excessive external rotation with UE at side
	  • Sustained edema in the distal upper extremity
		• Movement dysfunction—Early/unopposed shoulder elevation
		• Inadequate strength
		• Inadequate ROM
			• Continue STM
			• Joint mobility strengthening continues (both OKC and CKC)
			• Progression to terminal end ROM and home exercise program
				• Return to activities including overhead
				• Increased ROM
				• Improved strength
				• Improved neuromuscular control
					• Realignment of scar tissue and collagen (to allow more ROM with less soft tissue restrictions)
					• Decrease possible capsular adhesions
					• Decrease nociceptor input
					• Increase strength
					• Increase endurance
					• Improve function
					• Progression to discharge

CKC, Closed kinetic chain; *OKC,* open kinetic chain; *ROM,* range of motion; *STM,* soft tissue massage; *UE,* upper extremity.

muscle testing and the presence of coordination between the two primary force couples that move the shoulder. As a review, there is a delicate balance that must be maintained to move the shoulder through its full ROM. The muscular contribution to this coordinated effort is via the force couple of the deltoid muscles and the rotator cuff muscles, and the scapular stabilizer muscles with the deltoid muscles. Both of these force couples must have a balanced contraction to facilitate shoulder flexion and abduction without impingement of the humerus at the subacromial arch.[39]

Strengthening should respect the force couples of the shoulder while addressing both the concentric and eccentric functions of the targeted muscles. The force couple of the shoulder between the deltoid and the rotator cuff can be progressed from earlier examples of exercise (Fig. 7-23) into a standing exercise that maintains humeral external rotation through an isometric contraction and a concentric contraction of the deltoid. An example of an eccentric exercise progression is demonstrated through an alteration of the wand activity. The patient can complete a sitting or standing overhead wand activity initially shown in supine in Fig. 7-24. At the highest point of the wand lift, the patient releases the involved upper extremity from the wand and slowly lowers the involved extremity back toward the waist.[40] This type of training can also be initiated for strengthening into abduction.

As a final example, consider that strengthening must also address specific deficits in the targeted muscles. Fig. 7-24

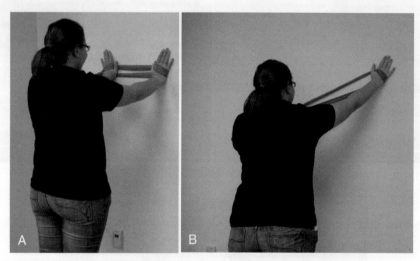

Fig. 7-23 Clock reach. **A,** Start position. **B,** Finish position.

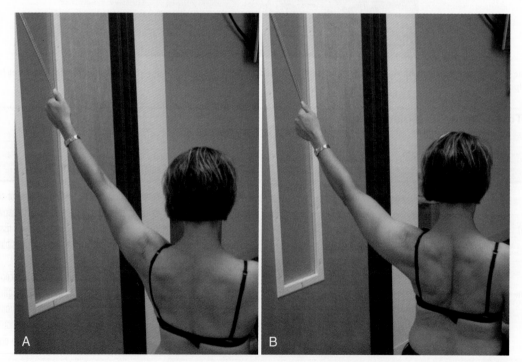

Fig. 7-24 Sitting low trapezius. **A,** Start position. **B,** Finish position.

demonstrates an exercise targeting the function of the low trapezius. The exercise emphasizes an isometric contraction of the upward rotation and a concentric action of the low trapezius as a scapular depressor. A movement dysfunction at greater than 120° in either flexion or abduction or inadequate strength as noted in a manual muscle testing would assist in determining the necessity of this exercise.

Return to recreational activities should have been a goal from the initial evaluation. Closer scrutiny to the movements necessary for the patient's chosen recreation will be strong consideration for formulation of the home program and strengthening program during this final phase. *Successful return to recreation has been noted especially with the sports of swimming, tennis, and golf.* Though the timeframe of return will vary, successful return has been noted as early as 6 months.[4]

CAUTION FOR STRENGTH TRAINING

Strength training does impart increased loads upon the healing shoulder that the clinician should monitor as the patient progresses through this phase. **Heavier loading of the shoulder or the introduction of activities with increased shear forces is discouraged until significant bone healing is evident, typically around 12 weeks.** Changes in the GH translations and loading mechanics can also be attributed to an imbalance of muscular forces either from length or strength impairments and the mobility of the joint capsule.[41] The surgical procedure also plays a role in the ability of a patient to participate in heavy loading of the shoulder either for recreation or work demands. With poor methods or inappropriate prosthetic placement in addition to increased loads, the patient may be at risk for uneven wear of the glenoid or loading of the glenoid rim, which may lead to instability or component loosening.[17,42]

It is the therapist's responsibility to ensure that there is appropriate resolution of joint mobility, optimal extremity alignment, and muscular balance. Additionally, the functional tool, the simple shoulder test, can provide guidelines on how much to load the shoulder during the rehabilitation period. It includes the ability to lift 1 lb to shoulder height, ability to lift 8 lb to shoulder level, and carrying an item weighing 20 lb.[25,43]

Additional assistance for decision-making may be found considering studies of external moments of the shoulder during activities of daily living. The average external moments to reflect loading of the shoulder during several activities of daily living, including picking up a 5-kg box, moving a 10-kg suitcase, and transferring from sit to stand, have been evaluated. The performance of these activities has been found to represent a large proportion of the upper extremity strength in normal men and women.[44] Patients who receive a TSA must be considered to possess less than normal strength especially during the rehabilitation process. **Therefore, current caution for heavy loading of the shoulder for strength training demonstrates appropriate concern by the therapist for the external moments created by these lifts thereby protecting the prosthetic and its design. Limiting the intensity prescribed to the patient for strength training exercises should be examined. Discussion with the referring surgeon may give the therapist more specific guidelines for possible lifting restrictions.**

Resolution of functional limitation in activities of daily living and ROM goals should guide the determination of timely discharge. Active ROM goals are listed in Table 7-5. **The therapist should not prognosticate attainment of full ROM following TSA. This has been demonstrated in several studies on total shoulder procedures regardless of the presence or the lack of underlying pathologies or comorbidities.**[45-50] *Additionally, both patient and therapist should be aware that function improvements continue beyond the discharge of therapy up to approximately 1 year after surgery.*[17]

TABLE 7-5 Range of Motion Goals to Advance to the Next Phase of Rehabilitation

Shoulder Motion	In Hospital[25]	Early Rehabilitation[40]	Late Rehabilitation	Phase IV[45]
Flexion	PROM supine 140°	PROM supine 140°	Full PROM in supine AROM supine 140° sitting 120°	Full PROM in supine AROM sitting 145°-150°[11]
Abduction	n/a	PROM supine 110°	AROM supine 120°	n/a
ER with humerus positioned at 0° of humeral abduction	PROM supine 40°	PROM supine 30°-45°	AROM supine 45°	AROM sitting 45°-60°[47]
ER with humerus positioned at 90° of humeral abduction	n/a	n/a	AROM supine 45°	n/a
IR with humerus positioned at 0° of humeral abduction	n/a	PROM supine >70°	AROM supine >70°	AROM supine >70°
IR with humerus positioned at 90° of humeral abduction	n/a	PROM supine >30°	AROM supine >70°	AROM supine >70°

AROM, Active range of motion; *ER,* External rotation; *IR,* internal rotation; *n/a,* not available; *PROM,* passive range of motion.
Data from Goldberg BA, et al: The magnitude and durability of functional improvement after total shoulder arthroplasty for degenerative joint disease. J Shoulder Elbow Surg 10(5):464-469, 2001; Brems J: Rehabilitation following shoulder arthroplasty. In Friedman R, editor: Athroplasty of the shoulder, New York, 1994, Thieme; Godeneche A, et al: Prosthetic replacement in the treatment of osteoarthritis of the shoulder: early results of 268 cases. J Shoulder Elbow Surg 11(1):11-18, 2002; Gartsman GM, Roddey TS, Hammerman SM: Shoulder arthroplasty with or without resurfacing of the glenoid in patients who have osteoarthritis. J Bone Joint Surg Am 82(1):26-34, 2000.

LIMITED GOALS CATEGORY FOR TOTAL SHOULDER ARTHROPLASTY

The limited goals category following TSA was first mentioned by Neer in 1982.[23] Criteria for inclusion into the limited goals category included the status of the rotator cuff and the stability of the implant. Patients were placed into a limited goals category if the rotator cuff was detached and not capable of recovery secondary to denervation or irreversible contracture or if the stability of the implant was problematic as evaluated by the surgeon during the procedure (Boxes 7-9 and 7-10). Specific diagnoses typically associated in this category include: rheumatoid arthritis, massive rotator tear, component position failure, septic arthritis, or neurovascular injury.[51]

Specific ROM goals are seldom mentioned when preparing a patient for a TSA. This is true whether a patient is placed in the standard goals category or the limited goals category. The primary focus for those patients in the limited goals category is pain relief with a decreased emphasis on ROM gains. This group will achieve less than satisfactory gains in functional ROM.[51]

Total Shoulder Secondary to Trauma

The goals for a patient with a TSA secondary to trauma are the same as that for a patient with a TSA secondary to degeneration: pain relief and resumption of daily function in both patient populations. The most important preoperative factors that influence postrehabilitation function are the timing of the surgery in relation to the injury and the skill of the surgeon. The outcome worsens the longer the delay is between the date of the trauma and the initiation of surgery. The skill of the surgeon directly relates to the ability to align the humeral tuberosities. Finally, there are improved outcomes with larger surgery centers and higher volume surgeons.[52]

For patients with a traumatic reason for their total shoulder surgery, rehabilitation may be a longer period of immobilization with passive ROM only. This is to ensure appropriate boney healing. Additional time with significant precautions may exist up to 6 weeks, further delaying the potential resumption of ROM.[52] *The most common complication following a TSA procedure for a traumatic injury is superior migration of the humeral head, which the clinician may observe as unopposed scapular elevation or "shoulder hike" as described in the next section or in Box 7-11.* There are several reasons why this may occur: failure of the rotator cuff muscles, muscular imbalance with inappropriate muscular force couple production at the shoulder, or loosening of the glenoid component.[55]

TROUBLESHOOTING

Shoulder Hike

The most common observable movement dysfunction is unopposed scapular elevation and/or inadequate separation of scapular and humeral motion, or in layman's language: "a shoulder hike." This is seen with attempts to raise the arm overhead in either a frontal or sagittal plane of motion. Weakness is only one of the impairments that may contribute to shoulder hiking. Additional impairments contributing to this movement dysfunction include inadequate transverse plane ROM, inadequate length of the scapulohumeral musculature, inadequate mobility of the glenohumeral (GH) joint capsule, and inadequate mobility of the scapula on the thorax. Determination of the primary impairment limiting this motion will guide the plan of care to eliminate the unopposed scapular elevation. For example, if the movement analysis of the patient's shoulder noted inadequate separation of scapular and humeral motion during the first 30° of shoulder abduction, then the physical examination measures would focus on inadequate GH inferior glide, inadequate strength, or neuromuscular control of the scapular muscles that provide a stabilizing force into scapular down rotation, adduction, or scapular depression or the inadequate length of the scapulohumeral muscles.

BOX 7-9 Limited Goals Category[23,26]

For Patients With Tissue Insufficiency, Rheumatoid Arthritis

Goal is joint stability
Initiation of motion delayed
Joint mobilizations are delayed
Active range of motion delayed until after 8 weeks

BOX 7-10 Limited Goals Category Range of Motion Achievement

Shoulder flexion: 75° to 90°
Shoulder abduction: 70° to 80°
External rotation: 30°
Functional internal rotation: hand behind back to L5

Data from Sojbjerg JO, et al: Late results of total shoulder replacement in patients with rheumatoid arthritis. Clin Orthop Relat Res (366):39-45, 1999; Orfaly RM, et al: A prospective functional outcome study of shoulder arthroplasty for osteoarthritis with an intact rotator cuff. J Shoulder Elbow Surg 12(3):214-221, 2003.

BOX 7-11 Possible Complications Following TSA[57]

Glenoid loosening
Glenohumeral joint instability
Infection
Neurologic injury
Recurrent cuff tear
Periprosthetic fracture

Stiffness

Stiffness of the GH joint following TSA presents a complex problem with the origin of the stiffness including: inadequate intraoperative tissue release, an intense postsurgical inflammatory response, or slow progress in rehabilitation. Communication with the referring surgeon and the history of the ROM impairment of the patient before surgical intervention may assist the therapist's decision-making to decrease the risk of stiffness. Initiating therapy with good pain control immediately postoperatively may prevent the development of pathologic stiffness. Presentation of stiffness later in the rehabilitation process must be evaluated for the primary contributing impairments. Consideration should be given to the GH joint capsule, flexibility of the scapulohumeral muscles, and the separation of scapular motion from humeral motion.

Infection

A patient who has decreasing ROM in conjunction with pain or increasing pain should alert the clinician to possible infection.[9] Infection may present in up to 15% of all total shoulder cases[53] and may occur more than 1 year following the surgical procedure.[5] Though pain and loss of ROM may be the most objective signs during therapy, the therapist should be alert for drainage, warmth at the site, erythema, and effusion. Interviewing questions regarding the presence of night sweats, fever (as noted by taking body temperature), chills, remote sites of infection, or any recent invasive procedures should be asked.[10] *Early intervention in the acute phase of the infection yields the best result, therefore the therapist should recommend an urgent return visit to the physician for blood laboratory testing.*[9]

Biceps Tendon Tendonitis

Biceps tendon tendonitis is a preventable complication during the rehabilitation process. The biceps has a role in shoulder flexion and is a primary humeral depressor.[37] **Following total shoulder surgery, the rotator cuff typically demonstrates muscular inhibition, thus increasing the demand on the biceps as the primary humeral depressor during shoulder motion.** Presentation of biceps tendon tendonitis indicates continued overuse of this muscle, therefore implicating inadequate contribution from the rotator cuff muscles. Beyond regional treatment for the inflammation of the biceps tendon such as modalities, active rest, and taping, the rotator cuff muscles should be evaluated for length, neuromuscular control, and strength. The patient will have pain during active ROM, especially with shoulder flexion and shoulder abduction. Limited shoulder extension may be noted secondary to irritation as the biceps tendon is placed at a lengthened position or required to activate eccentrically. Manual muscle testing of the biceps activates this muscle for its role as an elbow flexor and forearm supinator, therefore it may be pain free and strong despite the irritation at the tendon. Attempts at special tests for tendonitis may be inconclusive because of the surgical trauma to the area and the inability of the patient to attain the necessary positions for testing.

Suggested Home Maintenance for the Postsurgical Patient

Early Phase: 0 to 6 Weeks

GOALS FOR THE PERIOD: Aware of sleeping positions, independent with home exercise program, control pain, maintain range of motion (ROM) of proximal and distal joints, protect healing structures

Exercises:

1. Instruct the patient on sleeping positions and encourage experimentation (usually semireclined with upper extremities supported by pillows or bolster).
2. When appropriate, initiate passive range of motion (PROM) or self-assisted ROM at the shoulder (avoid external rotation beyond 40°).
3. Wear a sling for comfort.
4. Have the patient perform active range of motion (AROM) of the wrist and hand, elbow flexion only with humerus supported to decrease strain on biceps tendon, and AROM of cervical spine and thoracic spine through the cardinal planes.

Mid Phases: 6 to 12 Weeks

GOALS FOR THE PERIOD: Increase shoulder ROM, initiate strengthening, increase functional activities

Exercises:

1. Continue previously mentioned ROM exercises.
2. Initiate submaximal isometrics (being careful not to irritate the healing subscapularis muscle).
3. Perform active assistive range of motion (A/AROM) exercises in supine, then progress to AROM in supine, and finally AROM in sitting as able (the patient must perform exercise correctly).

Late Phases: 13 Weeks to Discharge

GOALS FOR THE PERIOD: Return to activities (including overhead activities), increase ROM, improve strength, improve neuromuscular control

Exercises:

1. Continue with previously mentioned exercises as needed.
2. Use AROM for concentric and eccentric strengthening at the shoulder.
3. Perform rotator cuff strengthening (elevation exercises must be performed correctly).

CLINICAL CASE REVIEW

1 SW is a 72-year-old female who slipped and fell 7 days ago sustaining a four-part humerus fracture. Surgical intervention resulted in TSA. She is currently 1 day postoperation and presents in the hospital room with a compression dressing over the surgical site. The surgical team has requested that she be cleared for discharge by this evening if possible. What functional assessments must be completed to ensure a safe discharge home?

Because of her history of falls, the patient's mobility from bed to chair, sit to stand, and ambulation must be assessed for safety. Following TSA, patients typically self-limit weight bearing through the shoulder. The patient must be assessed for independent mobility with limited use of the involved upper extremity. It would be of great benefit to the patient to integrate the treatment of potential contributing impairments to lesson her fall risk.

2 RP is a 68-year-old male who underwent a right TSA 18 weeks ago. His course has been uncomplicated thus far; however, during observation of shoulder flexion, RP demonstrates a "shoulder hike." Continued assessment for what impairments needs to occur to alter the treatment plan?

Determination of the primary impairment contributing to this movement dysfunction will guide the plan of care to eliminate the "shoulder hike." To be most efficient, the clinician must note during which phase of the shoulder motion the "shoulder hike" does occur. For example, if the shoulder hike occurs during the last phase of scapulohumeral rhythm, then there should be a separation of humeral and scapular motion. The resources necessary for this separation to occur must be evaluated for probable impairments. Potential impairments include inadequate GH joint mobility, inadequate humeral depression, inadequate length of the rotator cuff muscles, and inadequate stabilization of the scapula by the lower trapezius.

3 It is 6 weeks after surgery for JK, who had a left TSA secondary to progressive degeneration. Today there is increased swelling noted and you have concerns of a possible infection. What signs and symptoms should you look for? What special questions should you ask?

Loss of ROM with pain or increasing pain would be associated with a potential infection following TSA. Corroborating signs may be drainage and warmth at the surgical site, erythema, effusion, and systemic signs of infection such as fever. Early intervention is necessary, therefore an urgent return to the surgeon should be recommended. Infection risk may extend to 1 year after the operation.

4 AB is a 68-year-old male who is participating in rehabilitation for a total shoulder. His pain complaints have recently moved to the anterior proximal biceps area especially with attempts to move his shoulder into flexion. What may be one of the structures contributing to this pain?

The most likely structure is the proximal biceps brachii tendon. The clinical presentation may also include: contractile pain with a midline resisted test of the shoulder flexors, pain-free contraction for midline resisted tests at the elbow, increased sensitivity to placing the biceps tendon in a lengthened position, and limited or painful shoulder abduction. Presentation of tendonitis indicates overuse of the biceps brachii as a shoulder flexor and humeral depressor, thereby implicating inadequate contribution from the rotator cuff muscles. Beyond the modality intervention for the inflammation of the biceps tendon, evaluation of the function of the rotator cuff should be considered.

5 ML recently underwent a total shoulder surgery. Surgical indications included a significant loss of motion, interrupted sleep, and pain secondary to rheumatoid arthritis of the GH joint. He has many questions regarding his expected ROM. What role does his history play in your discussion of prognosticated ROM?

Because of his medical history of rheumatoid arthritis, ML would have a higher chance of being placed in the limited goals category. A conversation with the surgeon on what ROM was accomplished during the surgical procedure would be necessary to determine the impact of his significant presurgical loss of ROM. A limited goals category means that expected ROM at the shoulder is conservatively estimated to reach: flexion: 75° to 90°, abduction: 70° to 80°, external rotation: 30°, and internal rotation: hand behind back to L5.

6 GR is 3 weeks after surgery on the right. His precautions include PROM for another week. Your treatment plan includes scapular mobilizations to prepare for appropriate scapulohumeral rhythm upon discharge of his PROM precautions. Name three key considerations for this intervention.

Scapular mobilizations are introduced to ensure appropriate mobility of the scapula on the thorax for the scapulohumeral rhythm during active ROM. The rhythm consists of phases when there is movement only by the humerus and not at the scapula and a phase where the scapula and the humerus are both in motion. Therefore, the clinician must consider length and mobility issues that will affect these relationships; namely, the mobility of the scapula and those structures that attach from the glenoid to the humerus (the GH joint capsule and the rotator cuff muscles). The patient should be positioned in a manner that allows the humerus to be passively positioned at greater than 30° of humeral abduction or 60° of humeral flexion before initiating scapular mobility. The length of the rotator cuff muscles must be addressed. Glenohumeral joint mobility must be assessed and treatment initiated if hypomobility is present.

7 MJ's ROM precautions have been discharged and you wish to introduce him to active overhead activities. What is the primary impairment that must be addressed before initiating independent overhead activities?

Shoulder overhead motion is a complex motion that requires a significant amount of humeral external rotation ROM. This humeral motion is necessary to avoid impingement of the greater tuberosity of the humerus and the undersurface of the acromial arch as the humerus approaches 90° of shoulder motion. As this is the typical osteokinematic motion that is restricted within postsurgical precautions, many patients do not exhibit adequate external ROM to immediately begin overhead motion following discharge of precautions. To avoid the risk of subacromial impingement, external rotation ROM should be achieved first.

8 TA is 65-year-old male retired construction worker. You are reviewing his home program before discharge. He comments that the pendulum exercise increases his pain. What should you do?

It is not uncommon for the pendulum exercise to be misinterpreted or performed incorrectly. It was designed to be a passive motion of the involved upper extremity generated by trunk and pelvis motion. You have two immediate choices: reeducate TA on the proper performance of the pendulum exercise and/or instruct him in the alternate of table top exercises. Table top exercises emphasize an active trunk and pelvis over a supported upper extremity thereby mimicking the pendulum exercise without the gravitational traction. The dosage is dependent on the goal of prescribing the exercise. For pain relief, multiple sessions per day with 60 seconds of performance is appropriate. If the goal is to generate ROM, then a numeric prescription is more appropriate such as 3 sets of 15 repetitions each.

9 JJ is a 69-year-old male presenting to you 6 days after a TSA on the right shoulder. He states that he feels better every day but is curious about the discoloration on his chest. During the physical examination, you note large patches of bruising along the right thorax and into the axilla. The wound appears dry and clean with some dried blood along the incision. What are your concerns?

It is not uncommon following total shoulder surgery for bruising to appear and extend into the thorax, trunk, and axilla. Two competing issues would be the presence of petechiae or potential signs of infection. Petechiae are minute hemorrhagic spots that may be present on the chest and are related to injury to the long bone of the humerus. Corroborating signs and symptoms of shortness of breath, increased pain, and traumatic injury would lead to suspicions of fat embolism. For signs of infection, the integumentary integrity of the wound should be checked including drainage, warmth, redness, and/or excessive edema into the axilla or the distal arm. Following major surgery, all patients should be monitored for signs and symptoms of infection including the taking of body temperature. JJ should be educated on these signs and symptoms.

10 MP is a 71-year-old female who is 10 weeks postsurgery. Her chief concern is difficulty with overhead motion. AROM of shoulder flexion is135°. PROM of shoulder flexion is 168°. During your movement analysis, you note inadequate scapular upward rotation during the mid phase of motion (60° to 160°) of shoulder flexion. What are the hypotheses of possible contributing impairments?

Inadequate scapular upward rotation could be a result of weakness of the upper trapezius, lower trapezius, and the serratus anterior because all are upward rotators of the scapula. Other hypotheses include inadequate mobility of the scapula on the thorax because of adaptive shortening of the downward rotators or inadequate motor planning of the force couples of the serratus anterior and trapezius muscles.

11 AB is progressing in therapy and wishes to begin overhead repetitive activities. As a clinician you would stage him as between phases II and III. What is a key measurement in shoulder ROM that assists with recommending overhead motion activities?

External rotation of the shoulder at 0° of humeral abduction and at 90° of humeral abduction should be closely monitored if the patient has had surgical restrictions to avoid external rotation. The end of phase II recommends the patient have 40° of PROM into external rotation. Although 45° of AROM and full PROM into external rotation demonstrate the end of phase III, the clinician must not overemphasize overhead activities until the patient has achieved an adequate amount of external rotation for the movement to be completed without multiple compensations and risk of tissue irritation.

12 YM is nearing discharge. He is 14 weeks after surgery. Though he has been walking in the pool and using various flotation devices, he has not progressed to full, unassisted freestyle swimming. What are the key criteria for successful return to this activity?

YM's timeline for integumentary healing and bone healing is appropriate. The therapist should be knowledgeable of the stroke mechanics for freestyle swimming, especially the necessary ROM and muscle actions. If the active ROM is appropriate, then the home program will have to emphasize not only traditional strength training parameters but also a timed repetitive component to more aptly mimic the muscle activities during swimming.

REFERENCES

1. Sojbjerg JO, et al: Late results of total shoulder replacement in patients with rheumatoid arthritis. Clin Orthop Relat Res (366):39-45, 1999.
2. Visotsky JL, et al: Cuff tear arthropathy: pathogenesis, classification and algorithm for treatment. J Bone Joint Surg 86A:35-40, 2004.
3. Yack HJ, Collins CE, Whieldon TJ: Comparison of closed and open kinetic chain exercise in the anterior cruciate ligament-deficient knee. Am J Sports Med 21(1):49-54, 1993.
4. McCarty EC, et al: Sports participation after shoulder replacement surgery. Am J Sports Med 36(8):1577-1581, 2008.
5. Sperling JW, et al: Infection after shoulder arthroplasty. Clin Orthop Relat Res (382):206-216, 2001.
6. Itoi E, et al: Isokinetic strength after tears of the supraspinatus tendon. J Bone Joint Surg Br 79(1):77-82, 1997.
7. Roy JS, et al: The simple shoulder test is responsive in assessing change following shoulder arthroplasty. J Orthop Sports Phys Ther 40(7): 413-421, 2010.
8. Smith KL, Matsen FA III: Total shoulder arthroplasty versus hemiarthroplasty: Current trends. Orthop Clin North Am 29(3):491-506, 1998.
9. Coste JS, et al: The management of infection in arthroplasty of the shoulder. J Bone Joint Surg Br 86(1):65-69, 2004.
10. Bishop J, Flatow E: The failed arthroplasty: options for revision. In Warner JJP, Iannotti JP, Flatow EL, editors. Complex and revision problems in shoulder surgery, ed 2, Philadelphia, 2005, Lippincott Williams & Wilkins.
11. Orfaly RM, et al: A prospective functional outcome study of shoulder arthroplasty for osteoarthritis with an intact rotator cuff. J Shoulder Elbow Surg 12(3):214-221, 2003.
12. Hammond JW, et al: Surgeon experience and clinical and economic outcomes for shoulder arthroplasty. J Bone Joint Surg Am 85-A (12):2318-2324, 2003.
13. Jain N, et al: The relationship between surgeon and hospital volume and outcomes for shoulder arthroplasty. J Bone Joint Surg Am 86-A(3): 496-505, 2004.
14. Norris TR, Iannotti JP: Functional outcome after shoulder arthroplasty for primary osteoarthritis: a multicenter study. J Shoulder Elbow Surg 11(2):130-135, 2002.
15. Hettrich CM, et al: Preoperative factors associated with improvements in shoulder function after humeral hemiarthroplasty. J Bone Joint Surg Am 86-A(7):1446-1451, 2004.
16. Mulieri PJ, et al: Is a formal physical therapy program necessary after total shoulder arthroplasty for osteoarthritis? J Shoulder Elbow Surg 19(4):570-579, 2010.
17. Iannotti JP, Williams GR: Disorders of the shoulder: Diagnosis and management, Philadelphia, 1999, Lippincott Williams & Wilkins.
18. Brems JJ: Rehabilitation following total shoulder arthroplasty. Clin Orthop Relat Res (307):70-85, 1994.
19. Jackins S: Postoperative shoulder rehabilitation. Phys Med Rehabil Clin N Am 15(3):vi, 643-682, 2004.
20. Iannotti JP, Norris TR: Influence of preoperative factors on outcome of shoulder arthroplasty for glenohumeral osteoarthritis. J Bone Joint Surg Am 85-A(2):251-258, 2003.
21. McCann PD, et al: A kinematic and electromyographic study of shoulder rehabilitation exercises. Clin Orthop Relat Res (288):179-188, 1993.
22. Cailliet R: Shoulder pain, ed 3, Philadelphia, 1991, FA Davis.
23. Neer CS II, Watson KC, Stanton FJ: Recent experience in total shoulder replacement. J Bone Joint Surg Am 64(3):319-337, 1982.
24. Beynnon BD, et al: Anterior cruciate ligament strain behavior during rehabilitation exercises in vivo. Am J Sports Med 23(1):24-34, 1995.
25. Goldberg BA, et al: The magnitude and durability of functional improvement after total shoulder arthroplasty for degenerative joint disease. J Shoulder Elbow Surg 10(5):464-469, 2001.
26. Brown DD, Friedman RJ: Postoperative rehabilitation following total shoulder arthroplasty. Orthop Clin North Am 29(3):535-547, 1998.
27. Boardman ND III, et al: Rehabilitation after total shoulder arthroplasty. J Arthroplasty 16(4):483-486, 2001.
28. Hughes M, Neer CS II: Glenohumeral joint replacement and postoperative rehabilitation. Phys Ther 55(8):850-858, 1975.
29. Baker L, et al: Neuromuscular electrical stimulation: A practical guide, ed 4, Downey, 2000, Los Amigos Research & Education Institute, Inc.
30. Langevin HM, et al: Dynamic fibroblast cytoskeletal response to subcutaneous tissue stretch ex vivo and in vivo. Am J Physiol Cell Physiol 288(3):C747-C756, 2005.
31. Godges JJ, et al: The immediate effects of soft tissue mobilization with proprioceptive neuromuscular facilitation on glenohumeral external rotation and overhead reach. J Orthop Sports Phys Ther 33(12):713-718, 2003.
32. Inman VT, Saunders JB, Abbott LC: Observations of the function of the shoulder joint. 1944. Clin Orthop Relat Res (330):3-12, 1996.
33. Duralde X: Total shoulder replacements. In Donatelli RA, editor: Physical therapy of the shoulder ed 4, Philadelphia, 2004, Churchill Livingstone.
34. Kibler WB, McMullen J, Uhl T: Shoulder rehabilitation strategies, guidelines, and practice. Orthop Clin North Am 32(3):527-538, 2001.
35. Dockery ML, Wright TW, LaStayo PC: Electromyography of the shoulder: an analysis of passive modes of exercise. Orthopedics 21(11):1181-1184, 1998.
36. Lovern B, et al: Motion analysis of the glenohumeral joint during activities of daily living. Comput Methods Biomech Biomed Engin 13(6):803-809, 2010.
37. Kido T, et al: The depressor function of biceps on the head of the humerus in shoulders with tears of the rotator cuff. J Bone Joint Surg Br 82(3):416-419, 2000.
38. Boardman ND III, Cofield RH: Neurologic complications of shoulder surgery. Clin Orthop Relat Res (368):44-53, 1999.
39. Oatis CE: Mechanics and pathomechanics of muscle activity at the shoulder complex. In Oatis CE, editor: In Kinesiology: the mechanics & pathomechanics of human movement, Philadelphia, 2004, Lippincott, Williams & Wilkins.

40. Brems J: Rehabilitation following shoulder arthroplasty. In Friedman R, editor: Athroplasty of the shoulder, New York, 1994, Thieme.

41. Dayanidhi S, et al: Scapular kinematics during humeral elevation in adults and children. Clin Biomech (Bristol, Avon) 20(6):600-606, 2005.

42. Parsons IMT, Millett PJ, Warner JJ: Glenoid wear after shoulder hemi-arthroplasty: quantitative radiographic analysis. Clin Orthop Relat Res (421):120-125, 2004.

43. Matsen FA III, et al: Correlates with comfort and function after total shoulder arthroplasty for degenerative joint disease. J Shoulder Elbow Surg 9(6):465-469, 2000.

44. Anglin C, Wyss UP: Arm motion and load analysis of sit-to-stand, stand-to-sit, cane walking and lifting. Clin Biomech (Bristol, Avon) 15(6):441-448, 2000.

45. Godeneche A, et al: Prosthetic replacement in the treatment of osteoarthritis of the shoulder: early results of 268 cases. J Shoulder Elbow Surg 11(1):11-18, 2002.

46. Antuna SA, et al: Shoulder arthroplasty for proximal humeral malunions: Long-term results. J Shoulder Elbow Surg 11(2):122-129, 2002.

47. Gartsman GM, Roddey TS, Hammerman SM: Shoulder arthroplasty with or without resurfacing of the glenoid in patients who have osteoarthritis. J Bone Joint Surg Am 82(1):26-34, 2000.

48. Edwards TB, et al: A comparison of hemiarthroplasty and total shoulder arthroplasty in the treatment of primary glenohumeral osteoarthritis: Results of a multicenter study. J Shoulder Elbow Surg 12(3):207-213, 2003.

49. Arntz CT, Jackins S, Matsen FA III: Prosthetic replacement of the shoulder for the treatment of defects in the rotator cuff and the surface of the glenohumeral joint. J Bone Joint Surg Am 75(4):485-491, 1993.

50. Edwards TB, et al: The influence of rotator cuff disease on the results of shoulder arthroplasty for primary osteoarthritis: Results of a multicenter study. J Bone Joint Surg Am 84-A(12):2240-2248, 2002.

51. Kelley M, Leggin B: Rehabilitation. In Williams GR, et al, editors. Shoulder and elbow arthroplasty. Philadelphia, 2005, Lippincott Williams & Wilkins.

52. Mighell MA, et al: Outcomes of hemiarthroplasty for fractures of the proximal humerus. J Shoulder Elbow Surg 12(6):569-577, 2003.

53. Cofield RH, Edgerton BC: Total shoulder arthroplasty: complications and revision surgery. Instr Course Lect 39:449-462, 1990.

54. Fehringer EV, et al: Characterizing the functional improvement after total shoulder arthroplasty for osteoarthritis. J Bone Joint Surg Am 84-A(8):1349-1353, 2002.

55. Franklin JL, et al: Glenoid loosening in total shoulder arthroplasty. Association with rotator cuff deficiency. J Arthroplasty 3(1):39-46, 1988.

56. Rozencwaig R, et al: The correlation of comorbidity with function of the shoulder and health status of patients who have glenohumeral degenerative joint disease. J Bone Joint Surg Am 80(8):1146-1153, 1998.

57. Gill TJ, et al: Complications of shoulder surgery. Instr Course Lect 48:359-374, 1999.

CHAPTER 8

Extensor Brevis Release and Lateral Epicondylectomy

Kelly Akin Kaye, Kristen G. Lowrance, James H. Calandruccio

The pathologic condition of the elbow commonly termed *lateral epicondylitis* or simply *tennis elbow* refers to pathologic alterations in the extensor tendon origin(s), which often are solely alterations in the extensor carpi radialis brevis (ECRB) tendon. However, this syndrome of lateral elbow pain is rarely accompanied by acute inflammatory cells and hence is now termed *lateral epicondylosis*. Moreover, many patients who have focal tenderness just distal and anterior to the lateral epicondyle and localized pain in the same region with wrist extension do not play tennis nor related to athletic activity.[1]

SURGICAL INDICATION AND CONSIDERATIONS

Etiology

Injury to the extensor tendons at the elbow often can be attributed to repetitive trauma or overuse, leading to mechanical fatigue or biomechanical overload. Some literature reports the possibility of exostosis in the area of the extensor tendons or a degenerative process that causes pain at the lateral epicondyle.[2] Symptoms may be described as an ache at the elbow with sharp pain that infrequently radiates to the dorsal forearm and occasionally to the middle and ring fingers with attendant loss of grip.[3]

The most frequently involved tendon is that originating from the extensor carpi radialis brevis (ECRB). It is responsible for static and dynamic wrist extension required for certain tasks and stabilizes the wrist while grasping. Lesions can occur at the extensor digitorum communis, extensor carpi ulnaris, extensor digiti minimi, and supinator tendon. According to the current literature, microtraumatic ECRB tendon tears may propagate to include the common extensors.[1] Plancher and associates[1] report that gross tendon

rupture is noted in a large number of patients at the time of surgical intervention.

Microtears can result from repeated sprains, repetitive forceful wrist extension and gripping, and suboptimal mechanics in hitting. Inadequate racquet size or improper tool grip size also can predispose to injury. Other factors that may influence the onset of symptoms are inadequate strength, endurance, and flexibility of the forearm musculature; changes in regular activity; increasing age; and hormonal imbalance in women.[3] The incidence is equal in men and women during the fourth and fifth decades, with 75% of all cases involving the dominant arm.[1] Among the older population, the insult can possibly be work-related, in contrast to the sports-related injuries seen in the younger population.

Lateral epicondylitis can be successfully managed non-surgically in 90% of patients with a combination of activity modification, nonsteroidal antiinflammatory medication, functional and counterforce bracing, various therapeutic modalities, and injection therapy. A small percentage of patients with persistent and disabling symptoms require surgical intervention.[4] Lesions caused by overuse during job-related activities are more likely to require surgical intervention secondary to an inability to stop the aggravating activity.

Indications for surgery are individualized according to patient demands and activity level. The period of disability and previous conservative management must be considered before surgical management is chosen. There are no absolute indications for surgical intervention to treat lateral epicondylitis, and the clinician must exercise caution in cases in which secondary gain may be important.

The most important factors in considering surgical intervention are the intensity, frequency, and duration of disability caused by pain. The Nirschl classification system indicating the severity phase of pain, its relation to activity

TABLE 8-1 Nirschl Tendinosis Pain Phases

- **Phase 1:** Mild pain after exercise activity, resolves within 24 hours
- **Phase 2:** Pain after exercise activity, exceeds 48 hours, resolves with warm-up
- **Phase 3:** Pain with exercise activity that does not alter activity
- **Phase 4:** Pain with exercise activity that alters activity
- **Phase 5:** Pain caused by heavy activities of daily living
- **Phase 6:** Intermittent pain at rest that does not disturb sleep, and pain caused by light activities of daily living
- **Phase 7:** Constant rest pain (dull aching) and pain that disturbs sleep

and exercise, and symptom resolution following these activities may have some impact on the therapeutic intervention (Table 8-1). Constant and unrelenting focal lateral elbow discomfort is not tolerated well by active individuals and pain that accompanies exercise and activity (phase 4) may indicate pathologic tendon architectural alteration. Most patients treated surgically have symptoms for 1 year, but special consideration may be given to patients in whom other therapies have failed after 6 months of compliance with a well-tailored therapeutic regimen. Calcification around the lateral aspect of the elbow may portend a less favorable outcome to conservative measures. When symptoms are present for more than 12 months, they will rarely respond to further therapeutic management. Although cortisone injections have been the historical standard for acute pain relief in significant cases of tennis elbow, the high recurrence rate has prompted autologous whole blood, platelet rich plasma, sclerosing agents, botulinum toxin, and periarticular hyaluronate injections to provide more long-lasting results. At this time, despite some compelling reports, no consensus exists regarding the ideal injection for a given patient in a particular phase of their lateral epicondylosis malady.

Similarly, less invasive surgical interventions are being investigated by some authors for a quicker return to activity and exercise. Arthroscopic treatment when compared with open management may provide athletes a shorter time period to functional recovery. In contrast to percutaneous release, arthroscopic release appears to achieve outcomes more quickly and provide a clearer visualization of the pathology. Nonetheless, the benchmark procedure for this condition is an open release for which various modifications have been proposed. Regardless of the open method chosen, these procedures are technically simple and provide predictable and long-lasting results and rely on readily available instrumentation. No single technique has been or will be adopted by all surgeons.

SURGICAL PROCEDURE (MODIFIED NIRSCHL METHOD)

The common denominator for most lateral epicondylosis procedures, however, is the débridement of the diseased tendinous tissue, most notably the ECRB origin. Hypervascular granulation tissue is characteristically found on the undersurface of the ECRB attachment to the lateral epicondyle and appears on gross inspection as dull, tan-gray, and sometimes gritty degenerative regions. A limited approach commonly incorporated into surgical techniques consists of resection of the diseased section of the tendon and lateral epicondylectomy.

A skin pen is used to outline the intended surgical incision which is 4 to 5 cm long, gently curved, and centered over the lateral epicondyle along the lateral supracondylar ridge proximally and along a line from the lateral epicondyle center toward the Lister tubercle. The skin incision is made under tourniquet control and the skin edges are retracted. Gentle spreading of the subcutaneous tissue is done to protect any cutaneous nerves, often passing through a very superficial bursa over the lateral epicondyle. The extensor fascia is identified through this opening (Fig. 8-1, *A*). The anterior edge of the ECRB tendon origin is clearly developed by elevating the posterior border of the extensor carpi radialis longus, which at this level is muscular and partially overrides the ECRB origin. The extensor digitorum communis origin may partially obscure the deeper portion of the ECRB (Fig. 8-1, *B*). The ECRB portion of the conjoined tendon is elevated at the midportion of the lateral epicondyle, distally in line with the forearm axis toward the radiocapitellar joint. The abnormal-appearing ECRB tendon is sharply dissected from the normal-appearing Sharpey fibers. The diseased tissue may appear fibrillated and discolored, and can contain calcium deposits.

Occasionally the disease process also involves the extensor digitorum communis origin. Entrance into the radiocapitellar joint may not be routinely indicated; however, an intraarticular process such as loose bodies, degenerative joint disease, effusion, and synovial thickening on preoperative examination may require a larger incision and arthrotomy for joint exploration.

The lateral 0.5 cm of the lateral epicondyle is decorticated with a rongeur or osteotome, with the surgeon taking care not to damage the articular cartilage or destabilize the joint (Fig. 8-1, *C*). The ECRB is intimately associated with the annular ligament just proximal to the radial head, thereby limiting distal migration of the ECRB tendon. However, the remaining normal ECRB tendon may be sutured to the fascia or periosteum or attached with nonabsorbable sutures through drill holes in the epicondyle.

The extensor tendon interval is closed with absorbable sutures, with the elbow in full extension to reduce the possibility of an elbow flexion contracture. The skin incision is closed (often with absorbable subcuticular suture material reinforced with adhesive strips) and a soft dressing applied. An arm sling is given for comfort and home range of motion exercises are encouraged before the first office visit in 10 to 14 days postoperative.

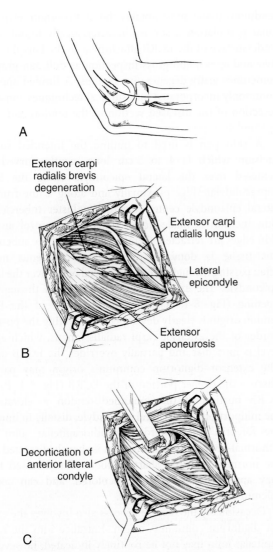

A

Extensor carpi
radialis brevis
degeneration

Extensor carpi
radialis longus

Lateral
epicondyle

Extensor
aponeurosis

B

Decortication of
anterior lateral
condyle

C

Fig. 8-1 Surgical technique for correction of tennis elbow. **A,** Skin incision. **B,** Identification of the origins of the extensor carpi radialis longus and extensor digitorum communis. **C,** Osteotome decortication. (Redrawn from Nirschl RP, Pettrone F: The surgical treatment of lateral epicondylitis. J Bone Joint Surg 61A:832-839, 1972.)

Surgical Outcomes

According to Nirschl,[5,6] 85% of patients were able to return to all previous activities without pain. Pain that occurred during aggressive activities was noted in 12% of the cases observed, and no improvement was apparent in 3% of the cases. When both medial and lateral releases are performed, a high level of patient satisfaction was achieved in a group of 53 patients followed an average of 11.7 years, and 96% of patients returned to their sports activity. Reasons for failure include misdiagnosis or the concomitant diagnosis of entrapment of the posterior interosseous nerve, intraarticular disorders, or lateral elbow instability. Poor prognostic factors include poor initial response to cortisone injections, numerous previous cortisone injections, bilateral lateral epicondylitis, other concomitant associated disorders, and smoking.

THERAPY GUIDELINES FOR REHABILITATION

Phase I

TIME: 1 to 14 days after surgery
GOALS: Achieve full range of motion (ROM) of adjacent joints, promote wound healing, control edema and pain, and increase active range of motion (AROM) of the elbow (Table 8-2)

After surgery, the therapist instructs the patient concerning the need to elevate the site to avoid edema and initiates gentle AROM exercises for the hand and shoulder. The patient is to remain immobilized in the postoperative splint with the elbow positioned at 90°. On the fifth day after surgery, the postsurgical dressing and splint are removed and therapy is initiated to the elbow.

The initial postoperative examination is conducted by a physical or occupational therapist. Upon removal of the postsurgical dressing, the examination conducted should measure and address ROM, edema, pain, functional ability, and wound healing. ROM of the hand, wrist, elbow, and shoulder along with girth measurements of the hand, forearm, elbow, and upper arm are taken. Pain levels can be monitored using a 0 to 10 VAS (Visual Analog Scale). It is recommended to have patients use this during therapy sessions and with the home exercise program for optimum accuracy. Functional ability can be monitored using the DASH (disabilities of the arm, shoulder, and hand) or PRTEE (patient-rated tennis elbow evaluation) questionnaire. The above recorded data should be taken at subsequent visits for comparison and assessment of the patient's progress.

In this phase the patient's wounds are kept clean and dry until the sutures are removed 10 to 14 days after surgery. After the operative site has been exposed, other forms of edema control can be used, including ice, pneumatic intermittent compression (performed at a 3:1 on/off ratio at a pressure of 50 mm Hg), and high-voltage galvanic stimulation (HVGS). The recommended settings for the use of HVGS to prevent edema are negative polarity with continuous modulation at 100 intrapulse microseconds and intensity to the sensory level.[7] The patient also can be fitted with a light elastic compression wrap or stockinette (such as Coban or Tubigrip) to wear intermittently throughout the day and at night for continued edema control at home (Fig. 8-2). AROM exercises also are initiated for the elbow, forearm, and wrist after the postoperative dressing is removed.[8] **Passive ROM (PROM) and joint mobilization of the elbow and forearm are contraindicated at this time.**

Some surgeons prefer to keep the elbow immobilized in a removable posterior elbow splint until the second week after surgery. This splint is typically fabricated from a low-temperature plastic with the elbow positioned at 90°; it is worn between exercise sessions and at night (Fig. 8-3).

TABLE 8-2 Extensor Brevis Release and Lateral Epicondylectomy

Rehabilitation Phase	Criteria to Progress to This Phase	Anticipated Impairments and Functional Limitations	Intervention	Goal	Rationale
Phase I Postoperative 1-14 days	Postoperative	• Postoperative pain • Postoperative edema • Limited upper extremity mobility • Unable to grasp and reach	• Monitoring of incision site • Instruction of client in activity modification • Cryotherapy • Pneumatic intermittent compression • HVGS • Elastic compression wrap or stockinette • Fabrication of removable splint • PROM-AROM — Shoulder (all ranges, maintaining elbow in neutral position) • AROM Hand (finger flexion/extension) Wrist — flexion/extension Elbow (initiate after operative dressing is removed) — Flexion/extension pronation/supination	• Prevent infection • Decrease stress on surgical site • Decrease pain • Control and decrease edema • Protect surgical site • Maintain ROM of joints proximal and distal to the surgical site • Full AROM of neighboring joints • Elbow ROM to 60% (extension will be more limited)	• Prevention of postoperative complications • Decrease stress on the common extensor tendons • Pain control • Edema management • Prevent associated joint stiffness and dysfunction of neighboring joints and muscles • AROM to assist with pain control and promote edema management • Improve ROM of elbow (sutures are usually removed at 10-14 days)

AROM, Active range of motion; *HVGS,* high-voltage galvanic stimulation; *PROM,* passive range of motion; *ROM,* range of motion.

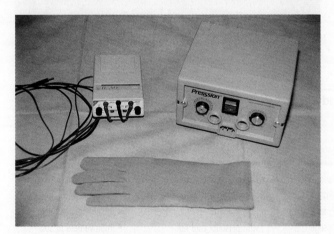

Fig. 8-2 Edema control. Portable HVGS unit, portable intermittent compression unit, and compressive garment (Isotoner glove).

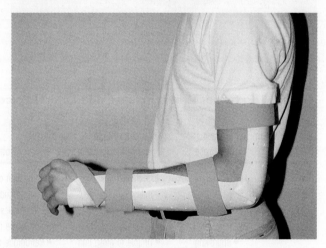

Fig. 8-3 Posterior elbow splint.

Pain can be managed using HVGS at the same settings as those used for edema control; the physician also may prescribe oral medications.

The first postoperative visit is a good time to begin patient education regarding activity modification and proper mechanics during work- and sports-related activities. **Patients should be educated to avoid forceful static grip, repetitive and static wrist extension, and resistive supination, which are commonly seen with use of hand tools such as screwdrivers, and pliers, and with keyboarding. Patients should also be advised to avoid the overhanded lifting technique.**

The primary mode of lifting should be a bilateral underhanded or neutral forearm approach (Fig. 8-4).

During this initial phase, the therapist should closely monitor the patient's reports of pain and tolerance to ROM exercises, noting any sympathetic changes that may lead to a complex pain syndrome. Signs and symptoms to be noted are as follows:

- Pain out of proportion to the stimulus
- Excessive edema
- Temperature and color changes
- Excessive joint stiffness

Phase II

TIME: 15 days to 4 to 5 weeks after surgery
GOALS: Control edema and pain, achieve full elbow PROM, maintain full ROM of adjacent joints, and promote mobility of the scar tissue (Table 8-3)

After the immobilization phase, the therapist should initiate gentle AROM exercises for the patient's elbow three to four times each day.[9] During the first ROM phase, the therapist should emphasize the importance of complying with the home exercise program and attending the regular therapy sessions.

ROM exercises to be included are as follows:

- Elbow extension and flexion
- Wrist extension and flexion
- Forearm supination and pronation

The patient should avoid positions that place maximal stress on the common extensor tendons such as elbow extension with extreme wrist flexion (Fig. 8-5).[3] To prevent reinjury, progressive resistive exercises also should be avoided at this time. Sports-related activities to avoid

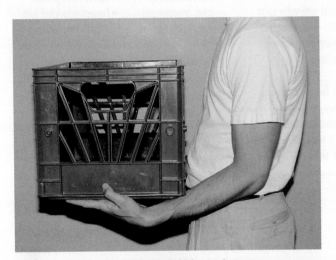

Fig. 8-4 Underhanded lifting technique.

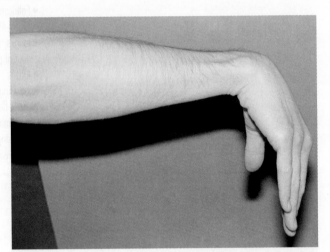

Fig. 8-5 Extreme wrist flexion with elbow extension.

TABLE 8-3 Extensor Brevis Release and Lateral Epicondylectomy

Rehabilitation Phase	Criteria to Progress to This Phase	Anticipated Impairments and Functional Limitations	Intervention	Goal	Rationale
Phase II Postoperative 3-5 wk	• Incision well healed with no signs of infection • Improving PROM of elbow • No increase in pain or edema	• Continued pain and mild edema • Limited upper extremity mobility • Unable to grasp and reach for functional use	Continuation of edema and pain management techniques as in phase I • Soft tissue massage • Retrograde massage with elevation • Scar desensitization after sutures are removed and incision is healed • Silicon gel sheet for scar pad • PROM—Elbow flexion/extension (within pain tolerance) • Isometrics (with wrist in neutral position, between 30° flexion/extension) Wrist flexion/extension	• Intermittent pain with 0/10 pain at rest • Pain rating of less than 4 of 10 with personal care ADL • Edema within 2 cm of uninvolved side • Encourage limited activities of daily living performance • Promote scar mobility and proper remodeling • Full elbow, forearm, and wrist PROM at 5 wk postoperation • 1 repetition dynamometer testing of minimum of 10 lb of surgical extremity • Encourage quality muscle contraction	• Management of edema and pain with progression to self-management • Improvement of soft tissue mobility • Use of compression to remodel scar • Promotion of normal joint arthrokinematics • Preparation of muscles for further resistive training • Encourage quality muscle contraction

ADL, Activities of daily living; *PROM,* passive range of motion.

include tennis, golf, lacrosse, or forceful throwing of a ball.

Stanley and Tribuzi[3] recommend isometric exercises with the wrist in a neutral position or at no more than 30° of extension or flexion in preparation for further resistive training. **Exercises should be performed three to four times daily with 15 to 20 repetitions being sufficient. Isometrics should be performed with submaximal effort only.**

As ROM progresses, the therapist should carefully monitor the patient's edema. The management of edema is specific to the patient and only one technique may be required. The following technique can be used for mild edema:

1. Ice and elevation for 10 minutes at the end of treatment
2. Compression wraps and stockinette
3. HVGS for 15 minutes

Moderate edema is treated with the following:

1. Retrograde massage
2. Intermittent pneumatic compression with elevation
3. HVGS with elevation and ice for 20 to 30 minutes

After the sutures are removed and the incision has healed appropriately, scar management is needed.

This includes both desensitization and scar remodeling. Because hypersensitivity can limit functional use, desensitization should begin during the patient's first therapy session after suture removal.[9] Scar remodeling consists of using massage (when appropriate) to help maintain mobility of the scar by freeing restrictive fibrous bands, increasing circulation, and allowing the pressure to flatten and smooth the scar site (Fig. 8-6).[9] The therapist also may consider using a silicone gel sheet or other silicone-based putty mix as a pad over the scar to assist in remodeling.

The therapist should instruct the patient to rub the sensitive area for 2 to 5 minutes three to four times daily with textures such as fur, yarn, rice, Styrofoam, or corn. Other useful textures include towels, clothing, dry beans, and rice.[9]

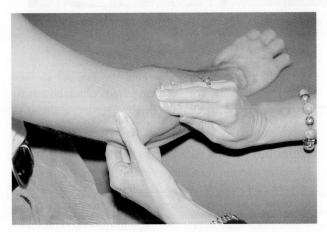

Fig. 8-6 Scar remodeling by manual massage technique.

Patients will be limited to lifting no more than 10 lb after surgery. On grip strength testing, patients typically demonstrate a 50% deficit when the operative hand is compared with the nonoperative one.

Phase III

TIME: Between 4 to 6 weeks to 6 months after surgery
GOALS: Control pain, maintain full elbow and forearm ROM, strengthen upper extremity, and regain normal forearm flexibility (Table 8-4)

Between 4 to 6 weeks after surgery, the therapist should initiate a progressive strengthening program.[9] At this point in the rehabilitative process the patient should have full ROM of the hand, wrist, and elbow, and the focus should be on building strength and training for endurance with the goal of returning the patient to work or sports.

The goal of the strengthening program is to promote conditioning of the entire upper extremity, particularly the forearm, to prevent reinjury caused by overstretching or overloading. To ensure that maximal strengthening is achieved, eccentric exercises are recommended for the extrinsic forearm muscles.[3] At this time it is appropriate to initiate extrinsic forearm stretching.

Each patient's conditioning program is formulated according to activity tolerance, previous activity level, and requirements for return to work or sports. If the patient can perform active exercises without pain, he or she is well enough to begin resistive and light work or sports-related activities using free weights and a work stimulator such as Baltimore Therapeutic Equipment (BTE) or Lido (Fig. 8-7). The key is to continue educating the patient and training her or him to lift with the forearm in a neutral position and avoid postures that stress the extensor muscles.

The components of the program are as follows:

- Hand (grip and pinch) strengthening
- Forearm strengthening
- Upper arm strengthening
- Shoulder strengthening
- Endurance training

Normally a return to activity can be anticipated by the fourth month after surgery.[8]

TROUBLESHOOTING

Problems encountered after a lateral epicondylectomy include pain, recurrence of symptoms, edema, inadequate ROM or stiffness, and scar expansion.

Increase in Pain Level or Recurrence of Symptoms

The therapist should carefully monitor the patient's pain level throughout the rehabilitation process. The Magill pain questionnaire can aid in monitoring changes in levels or characteristics of pain. Exercise progression should occur based on

TABLE 8-4 Extensor Brevis Release and Lateral Epicondylectomy

Rehabilitation Phase	Criteria to Progress to This Phase	Anticipated Impairments and Functional Limitations	Intervention	Goal	Rationale
Phase III Postoperative 6-24 wk	• PROM full and AROM near full • Pain and edema controlled and self-managed • No decrease in strength since last phase	• Minimal, intermittent pain and edema • Minimal mobility limitations in elbow • Unable to grasp and reach for functional use	Continue pain and edema management as indicated • Patient education regarding activity modification and performance of activities with good mechanics • Progressive resistance exercises—Putty exercises, finger pinch and grip • Isotonics Shoulder (see Chapter 3) Elbow—flexion, extension, pronation, and supination Wrist—flexion, extension, radial and ulnar deviation • Work simulator (12-16 wk) • Return to sports program (refer to Chapter 13) (12-16 wk)	• Self-manage pain • Prevent flare-up with progression of functional activities • Grip strength to 85% of uninvolved side • Symmetric strength of shoulder and scapula region • Wrist strength to within 80% • Return to previous activity/work level	• Avoidance of postures that place stress on the extensor musculature • Promotion of return to functional activities without flare of symptoms • Increased strength and endurance for return to work or sports • Strengthening of upper quarter to ensure optimal functional use of upper extremity • Monitoring of wrist isotonics to ensure safe, maximal strengthening • Simulation of work/sports loads in the clinic to train muscles to allow safe return to sports or work

AROM, Active range of motion; *PROM,* passive range of motion.

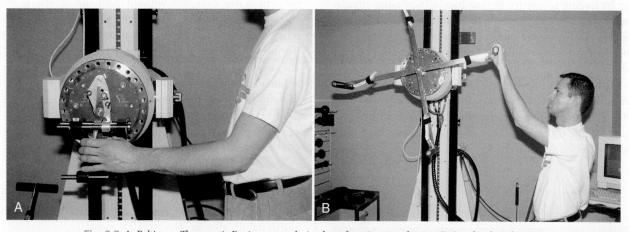

Fig. 8-7 **A,** Baltimore Therapeutic Equipment work simulator for grip strengthening. **B,** Simulated work activity.

the patient's reports of pain. In some cases of severe pain, the physician may prescribe a transcutaneous electric nerve stimulation (TENS) unit. If the pain persists or occurs at the end of the rehabilitative process, the therapist may consider the use of a counterforce brace to allow the patient to return to the previous level of activity.

Persistent Edema

Edema control involves ice, elevation, HVGS, pulsed ultra-sound, compression wraps, retrograde massage, and lymphatic massage. Continuous passive motion machines have

been used intermittently throughout the day and at night with some success to reduce edema. Decreasing the activity level or suspending the use of resistive exercises also may be necessary.

Inadequate ROM or Stiffness in Adjacent Areas

The most common mobility problem involves loss of full elbow extension. By 6 to 8 weeks after surgery, the therapist can talk to the surgeon about using static progressive or dynamic splints to improve extension. Static splinting is achieved by using custom-made, low-temperature plastic

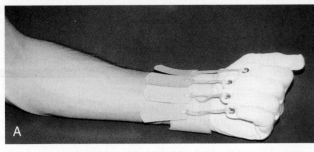
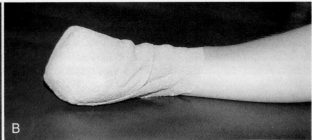

Fig. 8-8 **A,** Commercially available finger flexion glove for hand stiffness. **B,** Composite finger flexion using Coban.

material molded to the patient at the end ROM and adjusted weekly. Dynamic splints are available commercially. For hand and finger stiffness, use of a flexion glove or composite flexion stretching with a Coban or elastic (Ace) wrap is usually successful (Fig. 8-8).

Painful Scar

If the scar management techniques detailed earlier do not produce the desired result, additional methods include the following:

- Ultrasound
- Mechanical vibration
- Compressive dressings or garments to prevent scar adherence

Circumferential desensitization using fluidotherapy also may be considered.

Home Exercise Program

This program gives some general ideas for initiating and following a home exercise program. However, consideration of the patient's age, needs, and capabilities will ultimately guide the rate of progression, intensity, and type of treatment provided.

Phase 1 (1 to 2 Weeks)
1. Active range of motion 3 to 4 times daily. Begin with 1 to 2 sets of 10 repetitions progressing to 3 sets of 15 as tolerated.
2. Exercises include: elbow flexion/extension, forearm supination/pronation, wrist flexion/extension/radial deviation/ulnar deviation, finger flexion/extension/abduction/adduction, and shoulder flex/abduction/adduction/internal rotation/external rotation.
3. Edema control by using elevation and compressive stockinette. Ice packs to elbow 10 minutes three to four times daily.

Phase 2 (3 to 5 Weeks)
1. The previous exercises add passive range of motion to the elbow for flexion and extension if not achieving this actively.
2. Hold stretch for 20 to 30 seconds for 5 to 10 repetitions 3 to 4 times daily. Use unaffected

hand to passively stretch surgical elbow. Patient can use moist heat for 10 minutes before stretches if edema is under control.

Phase 3 (6 to 12 Weeks)*
1. Discontinue AROM exercises if full motion has been achieved.
2. Begin grip strengthening using light resistance putty for 5 minutes two to three times daily.
3. Begin light shoulder, arm, and forearm strengthening to include shoulder flexion/adduction/abduction/internal rotation/external rotation, biceps/triceps curls, wrist flexion/extension/radial deviation/ulnar deviation, and forearm supination/pronation. Progress from 1 lb up to 5 lb maximum for the forearm. Start light with shoulder weight, performing 1 set of 10 repetitions and progressing to 3 sets of 15. Appropriate patients may progress to 10 lb maximum.

Phase 3 Advanced (>12 Weeks)
1. Patient independently progresses exercises introduced in phase 3.

*Patients usually released back to normal activity/work or work hardening program at this time.

CLINICAL CASE REVIEW

1 Marvin is a 50-year-old diabetic who had extensor brevis release and lateral epicondylectomy 14 days ago. His sutures were removed, and he was taken out of the postoperative splint 2 days ago. He has full shoulder, forearm, and hand mobility with elbow AROM of 45° to 110°. His pain remains 3 or 4 out of 10 even at rest, and moderate edema is localized to the elbow and proximal one third of the forearm. His incision shows mild dehiscence with small amounts of exudate. What is appropriate intervention for his continued pain, edema, and suspicious wound?

The therapist should begin by ruling out infection. The patient's basal and elbow surface temperatures should be assessed, and he should be checked for redness or streaking near the elbow and forearm. If the patient shows no temperature or color change and exudate is clear, Steri-Strips should be applied to the incision and the patient's physician should be contacted. Once infection is ruled out, the following should be done: edema control using retrograde massage (avoiding the area of incision), HVGS and elevation (or both), PROM, and A/AROM to the elbow for flexion and extension. Scar remodeling should be delayed until the incision is well closed.

2 Cindy is a 60-year-old housewife who had arthroscopic release of her right tennis elbow 3 weeks ago. She is now complaining about right shoulder pain. She does not remember any injury to her elbow; she wears her arm sling for comfort during the day. On examination, her active and passive motion of the right shoulder is painful and somewhat limited. What should be added to her therapy program, and what instructions should she be given?

Cindy has developed an early adhesive capsulitis of her shoulder and should be instructed to stop wearing her arm sling. She should also be started on a shoulder program to work on her ROM. This could begin with Codman exercises and a PROM program followed by AROM and strengthening.

3 Jim is 34 years old. Approximately 7 weeks ago he had an extensor brevis release and lateral epicondylectomy performed. He is anxious to recover quickly so he can play softball on the weekends. Mild resisted exercises were initiated 1 week ago, and Jim is performing them at home. His pain level has noticeably increased over the past 4 days. However, he can control the pain with ice and antiinflammatory medication. Should Jim's exercise program be altered? If so, how should it be altered?

Jim is aggravating his symptoms with the exercises. He also may be doing the home exercises too aggressively. The primary goal should be to alleviate pain and swelling. After pain and swelling are under control, gradual strengthening can be initiated in small doses with more rest periods than before. Treatment soreness should be minimal and controllable with the administration of ice packs. The amount of exercise and resistance should be gradually increased.

4 Janet is a 35-year-old accountant. She had extensor brevis releases and a lateral epicondylectomy after various attempts at conservative treatment failed. At 7 weeks after surgery, Janet's elbow extension ROM is 15°. What type of treatment may be effective at this stage for increasing her elbow extension?

The patient should be placed in a dynamic splint or in a static progressive splint at night to gain full extension.

5 Matt is a 47-year-old business executive. He underwent an extensor brevis release with lateral epicondylectomy 4 weeks ago. Initial wound healing was good; however, he returned to frequent travel with his job. He now returns to therapy complaining of increased pain at rest reported as an 8/10, and swelling in the entire forearm and hand. He experiences shooting pains and describes a burning sensation in the involved upper extremity. Upon inspection, he has global swelling in the forearm with mottled appearance of skin and fusiform swelling around the finger joints. Range of motion has decreased in the elbow, wrist, and hand and he is unable to fully fist. Would it be appropriate to progress this patient to phase II treatment? What should your treatment consist of this treatment session?

At week 4 postoperation, a patient should have increasing range of motion and a decrease in pain. The above symptoms can indicate complex regional pain syndrome. This treatment session should consist of modalities to decrease pain and edema. No progression to the next phase in exercise regime should be made at this session. A referral back to the physician is indicated.

6 Sharon is a 45-year-old woman. She works as a computer programmer and had extensor brevis release and lateral epicondylectomy 14 weeks ago. She is performing a home exercise program of progressive resistive exercises and intrinsic stretches for the forearm and elbow four times a week and has returned to work full time. She now complains of pain at the end of the day, with

mildly noticeable swelling at the lateral elbow. She attends therapy once a week. What should the therapist evaluate at this week's appointment? What are the right recommendations?

The therapist should assess the patient's grip strength and forearm, elbow, and shoulder girdle strength as compared with the uninvolved side and previous weeks' values. Elbow mobility and edema (via palpation girth measurements) should also be checked. The patient should be asked to fill out a pain questionnaire or visual analog scale for pain. If strength values show a decrease of 10% or are less than 85% of the uninvolved side, the patient might have returned to work too early. If strength values are within desired limits but the patient shows significant edema and increased pain, she should be encouraged to decrease the weight with progressive resistive exercises and begin using ice packs for 10 to 15 minutes at the end of her work day. Stretching technique should be reviewed to make sure that the patient is not overstretching, as well as proper mechanics and activity modification while at work. The patient should be asked to wear a counterforce brace while at work (for up to 6 months after surgery).

7 Ben is a 38-year-old superintendent for a commercial construction company. He is 16 weeks past his surgery and was released from therapy 4 weeks ago with a recommendation for a functional capacity evaluation. He returns to the clinic for his 1-month reassessment. Against physician's orders, he returned to work stating that he did not do any heavy lifting with his job. He reports difficulty using his tools and soreness in the forearm when using tools with vibration. He also states that approximately midway through his day, he feels weak in the surgical hand. Upon reassessment, Ben demonstrates only 50% grip strength as compared with the nonsurgical extremity. Range of motion continues to be within normal limits. Resistive testing and palpation is negative for pain. What can be done to address his complaints?

Ben should benefit from wearing an antivibratory glove and padding tools that are used repetitively. Consultation with the surgeon regarding further rehabilitation based on his functional capacity evaluation in a work hardening setting is also indicated to increase grip and upper extremity strength and endurance required for this patient's job.

8 Madeleine is a 40-year-old veterinarian who is 4 to 5 weeks postoperation. She presents with complaints of numbness and tingling along the small and ring fingers of the affected extremity. She still has mild pain rated as 3/10 and mild edema localized to the surgical site but is tolerating passive and active range of motion and isometric exercises well since the removal of the 90° elbow

splint. She has full shoulder, forearm, and hand mobility with elbow AROM of 10° to 130°. Further questioning reveals that her preferred sleeping position is side-lying with her arms tucked under her pillow. What are the right recommendations for this patient?

Madeleine has developed an ulnar neuritis likely because of her sleeping position. She should be instructed to wear her elbow splint at night only to prevent her from sustained hyperflexion during sleep and to protect the ulnar nerve. She should progress to the phase II treatment plan as indicated.

9 Nash is a 33-year-old basketball coach who is 6 weeks postsurgery. He has full range of motion of the elbow, a mobile scar, and is tolerating self-care/activities of daily living without pain. He has not yet progressed to resistive training in his home exercise program but is doing well and seems to be ready to progress to phase III. During a therapy session, he reveals that he has been teaching/demonstrating dribbling skills to his little league team on the weekends. Should his exercise program be altered?

Nash needs to be educated regarding the time frame of the healing process after surgery. He should be reminded that at this time, full pain-free range of motion is the main goal and at this time participation in any sport or repetitive activity is prohibited. His lifting restriction continues to be 10 lb or less.

10 Ross is a 48-year-old professional race car driver. He is now 18 to 20 weeks postsurgery. He has full range of motion, equal grip strength bilaterally, and MMT of involved upper extremity of 5/5. He tolerates a 45-minute exercise session of the work simulator without residual pain. He is now ready to return to competitive driving. What guidelines would he be given for returning to racing?

Patient should be released to return to racing per physician's okay. He should be advised to allow for adequate rest periods between race practice sessions and to watch for return of symptoms, such as soreness, aching, or weakness. He can use ice to the elbow after driving as needed.

11 Tucker is a 21-year-old college football quarterback. During the off season he had a modified Nirschl procedure for lateral epicondylitis. He is now 12 weeks after surgery. He has full active and passive range of motion, is tolerating resistive strengthening exercises without reproduction of symptoms, and reports 0/10 pain at rest. He states he has only mild soreness in the elbow the day after he works out. During his leisure time he decided to go camping and presents to the clinic with a large pocket of swelling near his olecranon. What should be the next treatment?

This patient could possibly have an olecranon bursitis brought on by an infection from an insect bite. He needs to be referred back to his surgeon for possible aspiration and medication as indicated.

12 Elizabeth is a 55-year-old medical transcriptionist who had an open extensor brevis release 7 weeks ago. All goals for phase II have been met (see Table

8-3). What are appropriate guidelines for the following exercise components? Grip strength; sustained grip; forearm and wrist strength; upper arm strengthening.

Grip strengthening with light resistive putty two to three times daily for 2 minute sessions. Sustained grip with a 1-lb weight with light resistive putty for 2 minutes. Forearm and wrist PRE's with No. 1 weight, 1 to 3 sets of 10 repetitions. Upper arm strengthening varies with general health, age, sex, and lifestyle/activity level.

REFERENCES

1. Plancher KD, Halbrecht J, Lourie GM: Medial and lateral epicondylitis in the athlete. Clin Sports Med 15(2):283-305, 1996.
2. Gellman H: Tennis elbow (lateral epicondylitis). Orthop Clin North Am 23:75-82, 1992.
3. Stanley BG, Tribuzi SM: Concepts in hand rehabilitation, Philadelphia, 1992, FA Davis.
4. Canale ST: Campbell's operative orthopaedics, ed 9, St Louis, 1998, Mosby.
5. Olliveierre CO, Nirschl RP: Tennis elbow: Current concepts of treatment and rehabilitation. Sports Med 22(2):133-139, 1996.
6. Ollivierre CO, Nirschl RP, Pettroe FA: Resection and repair for medial tennis elbow: A prospective analysis. J Sports Med 23:2, 1995.
7. Hayes KW: Manual for physical agents, ed 4, Norwalk, Conn, 1993, Appleton & Lange.
8. Jobe FW, Ciccotti MG: Lateral and medial epicondylitis of the elbow. J Am Acad Orthop Surg 2(1):1-8, 1994.
9. Hunter JM, Mackin EJ, Callahan AD: Rehabilitation of the hand: Surgery and therapy, ed 4, St Louis, 1995, Mosby.

CHAPTER 9

Reconstruction of the Ulnar Collateral Ligament with Ulnar Nerve Transposition

Mark T. Bastan, Michael M. Reinold, Kevin E. Wilk, James R. Andrews

The ulnar collateral ligament (UCL) is the elbow's primary stabilizer to valgus stress within a functional range of motion (ROM). For the overhead-throwing athlete, throwing motions promote valgus stress at the elbow that exceeds the ultimate tensile strength of the UCL. Repetitive throwing motions produce cumulative microtraumatic damage and may eventually cause the ligament to overstretch and create symptomatic medial elbow instability. To correct this, both surgical intervention and a carefully coordinated rehabilitation program are required if the athlete is to return to full, pain-free function. This chapter describes the way the anatomy and biomechanics of the elbow can be applied to a scientifically based rehabilitation program for use after UCL reconstruction.

SURGICAL INDICATIONS AND CONSIDERATIONS

Bony Structures

The elbow joint has three articulations: the humeroulnar, humeroradial, and superior radioulnar joints. Collectively these joints may be classified as trochoginglymoid[1] and are enclosed by a single joint capsule.

The humeroulnar joint is a single-axis diarthrodial joint with 1° of freedom—flexion and extension. The bony structures of the joint include the distal humerus and proximal ulna (Fig. 9-1). The distal humerus flares to form the medial and lateral epicondyles, which are directly above the capitellum and trochlea, respectively. The medial epicondyle is much more prominent than the lateral epicondyle; the UCL and flexor-pronator muscle group attach to it (Fig. 9-2). The flat, irregular surface of the lateral epicondyle serves as the attachment site for the lateral collateral ligament and the supinator-extensor muscle groups. Just posterior to the medial epicondyle is the cubital tunnel, or ulnar groove, a key depression that protects and houses the ulnar nerve. Immediately above the anterior articular surface of the humerus is a bony depression called the coronoid fossa. The olecranon process of the ulna glides into this concavity during flexion. The olecranon fossa, located on the posterior aspect of the humerus, accepts the large olecranon process during extension. The proximal ulna provides the major articulation of the elbow and is responsible for its inherent stability. The trochlear ridge is a bony projection running from the olecranon posteriorly to the coronoid process anteriorly. The trochlear notch is a concave surface located on either side of the trochlear ridge; it forms a close articulation with the humeral trochlea.

The proximal radius and distal lateral aspect of the humerus articulate to form the humeroradial joint, which is also a single-axis diarthrodial joint. Similar to the humeroulnar joint, the humeroradial joint contributes to flexion and extension movements by gliding around the coronal axis. However, the humeroradial articulation also pivots around a longitudinal axis with the superior radioulnar joint to perform rotational movements. The proximal radial head is mushroom shaped,[2] with a central depression located above it. The radial head narrows distally to form the radial neck. The head and neck are not colinear, with the shaft of the radius forming an angle of approximately 15°. Further distal is the radial tuberosity, where the biceps tendon attaches. In the distal humerus the capitellum is almost spheric. A groove (the capitotrochlear groove) separates the capitellum from the trochlea. The rim of the radial head articulates with this groove throughout the arc of flexion and during pronation and supination.

The superior and inferior radioulnar joints function as single-axis diarthrodial joints that allow the elbow to pronate and supinate. Proximally, the convex medial rim of the radial head articulates with the concave radial ulnar notch. During supination and pronation, the radial head rotates within a ring formed by the annular ligament and radial ulnar notch. An interosseous membrane connects the shafts of the radius and ulna to form a syndesmosis. Distally, the ulnar head with

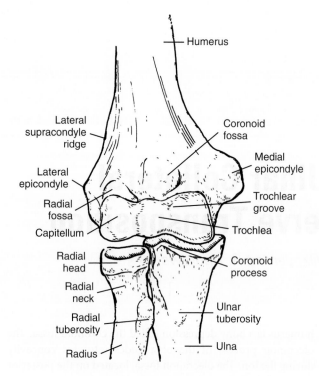

Fig. 9-1 The osseous anatomy of the elbow complex. (From Stoyan M, Wilk KE: The functional anatomy of the elbow. J Orthop Sports Phys Ther 17:279, 1993.)

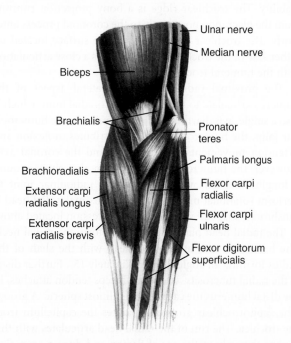

Fig. 9-2 The medial epicondyle serves as the attachment site for the ulnar collateral ligament (UCL) and flexor pronator group. (From Stoyan M, Wilk KE: The functional anatomy of the elbow. J Orthop Sports Phys Ther 17:279, 1993.)

the radial ulnar notch forms the inferior radioulnar joint articulation. This joint is L-shaped and has an articular disk between the lower ends of the radius and ulna. During supination and pronation, the ulnar notch and articular disk swing on the ulnar head.

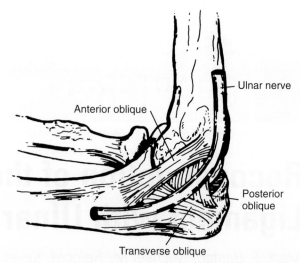

Fig. 9-3 The ulnar collateral ligament (UCL) complex of the elbow consists of three bundles: anterior, posterior, and transverse oblique. (From Stoyan M, Wilk KE: The functional anatomy of the elbow. J Orthop Sports Phys Ther 17:279, 1993.)

Ligamentous Structures

A single joint capsule surrounds the elbow joint and is lined by a synovial membrane. Specialized thickenings of the medial and lateral capsule form the collateral ligament complexes.

The UCL is traditionally described as having three portions: the anterior, posterior, and transverse bundles (Fig. 9-3).[2] The anterior bundle of the UCL is the strongest and most discrete component, coursing from the medial epicondyle to the sublime tubercle on the medial coronoid margin. The anterior bundle consists of two layers: (1) a thickening within the capsular layers and (2) an added complex superficial to the capsular layers.[3] The anatomic design of this ligament makes pathologic conditions in the central portion of the anterior bundle (as seen in a chronic, attenuated state) difficult to see during arthroscopic surgery. Functionally, the UCL is subdivided into two bands: (1) the anterior band, which is tight in extension, and (2) the posterior band, which is taut in flexion.[4]

The anterior oblique bundle of the UCL is the primary stabilizer to valgus stress at the elbow. Compromise of this structure causes gross instability in all elbow positions except full extension. The fan-shaped posterior bundle runs from the medial epicondyle to the middle margin of the trochlear notch. This band becomes especially taut in flexion beyond 60°,[5,6] but sectioning the posterior oblique ligament does not significantly affect medial elbow stability.[7] The transverse ligament (also known as the Cooper ligament) has an ulnar-to-ulnar attachment and contributes minimally to elbow stability.[5]

The anatomy of the lateral collateral ligament complex can vary significantly.[8,9] Typically four components are found: (1) the radial collateral ligament (RCL), (2) the annular ligament, (3) the lateral UCL, and (4) the accessory lateral collateral ligament (Fig. 9-4). The RCL originates

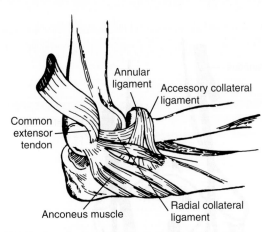

Fig. 9-4 The lateral collateral ligament complex of the elbow consists of the radial collateral ligament (RCL), annular ligament, and lateral ulnar collateral ligament (UCL). (From Stoyan M, Wilk KE: The functional anatomy of the elbow. J Orthop Sports Phys Ther 17:279, 1993.)

from the lateral epicondyle and terminates on the annular ligament. It provides varus stability by maintaining close approximation of the humeral and radial articular surfaces.[8] The annular ligament is a strong band of tissue encompassing and stabilizing the radial head in the radial ulnar notch. The anterior part of this ligament becomes taut with extreme supination and the posterior portion with extreme pronation.[10] The lateral UCL originates at the midportion of the lateral epicondyle, passes over the annular ligament, and attaches to the tubercle of the supinator. This ligament is analogous to the anterior band of the UCL and is the primary lateral stabilizer of the elbow, preventing posterolateral rotary instability.[9] Finally, the accessory lateral collateral ligament extends proximally from the inferior margin of the annular ligament and attaches distally on the tubercle of the supinator crest.

It further stabilizes the annular ligament during varus stress.[5,9-11]

Muscular Structures

The musculature surrounding the elbow joint may be divided into four main groups:
1. The elbow flexors
2. The elbow extensors
3. The flexor-pronator group
4. The extensor supinator group

The flexor group is located anteriorly and comprises the biceps brachii, brachialis, and brachioradialis muscles. The biceps brachii acts both as a major elbow flexor and as a supinator of the forearm (primarily with the elbow flexed), with a distal insertion at the radial tuberosity and bicipital aponeurosis, which attaches to the anterior capsule of the elbow. The brachioradialis originates at the proximal two thirds of the lateral supracondylar ridge of the humerus and attaches distally at the base of the styloid process of the radius, giving it the greatest mechanical advantage of the elbow flexors. The cross-sectional area of the brachialis is the largest of the elbow flexors, but this has no mechanical

advantage because it crosses so closely to the axis of rotation. As the brachialis crosses the anterior capsule, some muscle fibers insert into the capsule and help retract the capsule during flexion.

The anconeus and triceps brachii perform elbow extension and are located posteriorly. The triceps brachii has three heads (long, lateral, and medial) proximally that converge distally to form a single insertion at the posterior olecranon. The much smaller anconeus originates at the posterior aspect of the lateral epicondyle and inserts on the dorsal surface of the proximal ulna. Besides extending the elbow, the anconeus may be a lateral joint stabilizer.

The flexor-pronator muscles, which all originate completely or in part at the medial epicondyle, include the pronator teres, flexor carpi radialis, palmaris longus, flexor carpi ulnaris, and flexor digitorum superficialis. The primary role of these muscles is in hand and wrist function, but they also act as elbow flexors and dynamically stabilize the medial aspect of the elbow.

Finally, the extensor supinator muscles include the brachioradialis, extensor carpi radialis brevis and longus, supinator, extensor digitorum, extensor carpi ulnaris, and extensor digiti minimi. Each of these muscles originates near or directly onto the lateral epicondyle of the humerus and provides dynamic support over the lateral aspect of the elbow.

Neurologic Structures

The relationship of neurologic structures coursing through the elbow to their surrounding features can be crucial to function, pathologic conditions, and treatment (Fig. 9-5). The radial nerve descends anterior to the lateral epicondyle, behind the brachioradialis and brachialis muscles. At the antecubital space, the nerve divides into superficial and deep branches, with the superficial branch continuing distally in front of the lateral epicondyle and running under the brachioradialis muscle while on top of the supinator and pronator teres muscles. The deep branch pierces the supinator, travels around the posterolateral radial neck, and emerges distally 8 cm below the elbow joint to the terminal motor branches.

The median nerve follows a straight course into the medial aspect of the antecubital fossa, medial to the biceps tendon and brachial artery. From the antecubital fossa, the median nerve continues under the bicipital aponeurosis and usually passes between the two heads of the pronator teres, then travels below the flexor digitorum superficialis.

The musculocutaneous nerve innervates the major elbow flexors of the anterior brachium, then passes between the biceps and brachialis muscles to pierce the brachial fascia lateral to the biceps tendon. It continues distally to terminate as the lateral antebrachial cutaneous nerve, providing sensation over the lateral forearm.

Finally, the ulnar nerve travels anterior to posterior in the brachium through the arcade of Struthers. It then extends around the medial epicondyle and through the cubital tunnel. The cubital tunnel is the most frequent site for ulnar

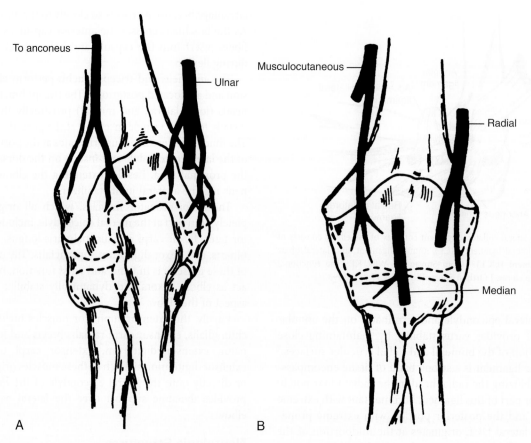

To anconeus

Ulnar

Musculocutaneous

Radial

Median

A   B

Fig. 9-5 A, Posterior view showing the ulnar nerve of the elbow ligament. **B,** Anterior view showing the neurologic innervation of the elbow. (From Stoyan M, Wilk KE: The functional anatomy of the elbow. J Orthop Sports Phys Ther 17:279, 1993.)

nerve injury; length changes in the medial ligament structures during elbow flexion can lead to significant reduction of the volume of the cubital tunnel, resulting in ulnar nerve compression.[12] This compression occurs as the cubital retinaculum, which forms a roof over the cubital tunnel, tightens with elbow flexion.[13] Absence of the cubital tunnel retinaculum has been associated with congenital ulnar nerve subluxation. After passing through the cubital tunnel, the ulnar nerve enters the forearm by traveling between the two heads of the flexor carpi ulnaris.

Cause

Injury to the UCL and resultant medial elbow instability are secondary to valgus loads that exceed the ultimate tensile strength of the ligament. Although excessive valgus loads may be secondary to trauma, as with an elbow dislocation caused by a fall or playing a sport such as football or wrestling, the most common mechanisms of injury are associated with repetitive overhead activities, such as baseball, javelin throwing, tennis, swimming, and volleyball. The single largest patient population experiencing medial elbow instability is undoubtedly overhead throwers.[14] This is secondary to the tremendous forces imparted to the elbow joint during the overhead-throwing motion.

The initiation of valgus stress occurs at the conclusion of the arm-cocking stage. The thrower's shoulder is abducted,

extended, and externally rotated about 130°, with the elbow flexed at about 90°. In transition from cocking to acceleration, the shoulder then internally rotates and the elbow flexes another 20° to 30°; this further increases the valgus load on the medial elbow. As the arm continues to accelerate, the elbow extends from about 125° to 25° of flexion at ball release.[15,16] Dillman, Smutz, and Werner[17] report that mean ultimate valgus torque measured from cadaveric testing was 33 N-m (newton-meters) (Fig. 9-6). During analysis of the dynamic demands of the pitching motion, Fleisig and associates[18] estimate that 35 N-m of valgus torque is placed on the UCL. The flexor carpi ulnaris and flexor digitorum superficialis muscles are located directly over the anterior band of the UCL and assist in combating medial joint distraction forces during the throwing motion. With any increased load transmitted to the UCL—whether with improper mechanics, warm-up, or conditioning—the structural integrity of the primary medial stabilizer of the elbow may be compromised.

Injuries to the UCL are described as either acute or chronic. An acute rupture of the UCL is frequently associated with a "pop," a feeling of pain during late acceleration or at ball release; it is often accompanied by swelling. More commonly, chronic injuries to the ligament are seen in the overhead-throwing athlete.[19] These occur from the accumulated repetitive microtrauma of overloading the ligament

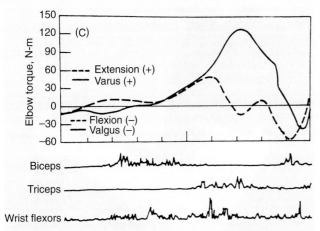

Fig. 9-6 Resting tensile strength of the ulnar collateral ligament (UCL) is measured at 33 N-m, but demands associated with pitching have been measured at 35 N-m. (From Werner SL, et al: Biomechanics of the elbow during baseball pitching. J Orthop Sports Phys Ther 17:274, 1993.)

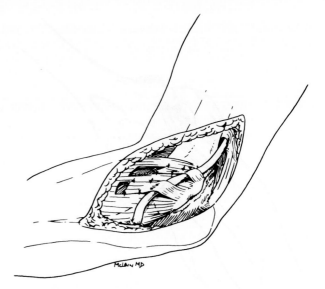

Fig. 9-7 To begin the reconstruction procedure, a medial incision is made in the elbow for ulnar collateral ligament (UCL) reconstruction and ulnar nerve transposition. (From Andrews JR, et al: Open surgical procedures for injuries to the elbow in throwers. Oper Tech Sports Med 4[2]:109, 1996.)

with throwing and can result in symptomatic medial elbow instability.[20] Accurate identification of medial instability is often difficult with clinical examination alone because laxity is only slightly increased. In addition, performing valgus laxity assessment is often difficult because of humeral rotation. Often magnetic resonance imaging (MRI) is used to confirm diagnosis. Timmerman, Schwartz, and Andrews[21] believe that use of saline-enhanced MRI improves the results when a UCL tear is suspected. The authors of this chapter have found a typical leakage of contrast fluid around the ulnar insertion of the UCL when an undersurface tear is present, which has been called the T-sign.[22]

Surgical reconstruction of the UCL is indicated in athletes who have persistent medial elbow pain, cannot throw or participate in desired sports, show documented valgus laxity, and fail a 6-month conservative course of treatment.

SURGICAL PROCEDURE

The goal of reconstruction is to restore the static stability of the anterior bundle of the UCL. The surgical procedure used at the authors' center by Dr. James Andrews is a modification of an earlier technique.

The presence or absence of the palmaris longus must be documented before surgery because it is the preferred donor tendon. If it is not present, then alternate donor sites must be evaluated, including the contralateral palmar longus, the plantaris tendon, and the extensor tendon from the fourth toe.

Surgery to correct for valgus instability is initiated with a brief arthroscopic evaluation. The procedure itself begins with arthroscopic examination to assess the integrity of the intraarticular structures and valgus instability. After that is completed, a medial incision is made with subcutaneous ulnar nerve transposition. The incision is centered over the medial epicondyle and extends about 3 cm proximally and distally (Fig. 9-7). The medial antebrachial cutaneous nerve is identified, preserved, and protected during the procedure

to avoid neuroma development. After elevating the skin flaps to expose the deep fascia covering the flexor pronator muscles, the surgeon identifies the ulnar nerve. Anterior transposition of the ulnar nerve must be performed before the medial ligament complex is explored. To do so, the cubital tunnel is first incised to mobilize the nerve. Proximally, the mobilization continues to include the arcade of Struthers, and a portion of the intermuscular septum is excised to prevent impingement of the nerve as it is transposed anteriorly. Distally, the flexor carpi ulnaris is incised along the course of the nerve. The ulnar nerve is then transposed anteriorly and preserved throughout the remainder of the procedure.

To complete visualization of the UCL, the split in the flexor carpi ulnaris is followed down to the insertion of the anterior band of the UCL on the sublime tubercle of the ulna. Starting at the insertion of the ulna, the surgeon develops the interval between the UCL and flexor muscle mass, extending proximally to the medial epicondyle. The flexor muscles are then retracted anteriorly to provide full exposure to the ligament, at which point the pathologic condition can be assessed. In a complete rupture, the joint is exposed. If the external surface appears normal, then a longitudinal incision is made in line with the fibers of the anterior bundle. This incision may reveal pathology, including tissue discoloration, fraying of the tissue, and detachment from the bony insertion on the ulna indicative of an undersurface tear, as described by Timmerman and Andrews.[23]

The remnants of the ligament are preserved and augmented with the tendon graft. After the donor tendon has been secured, muscle is stripped off the graft, the ends are trimmed, and a nonabsorbable suture is placed at each end with a locking stitch to help graft passage. Two drill holes are made at right angles just anterior and posterior to the sublime

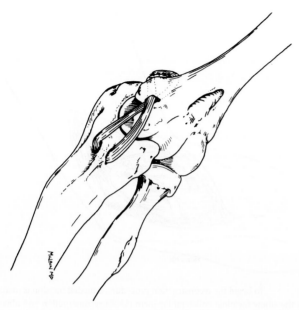

Fig. 9-8 Figure-eight reconstruction of the ulnar collateral ligament (UCL) using an autogenous graft. (From Andrews JR, et al: Open surgical procedures for injuries to the elbow in throwers. Oper Tech Sports Med 4[2]: 109, 1996.)

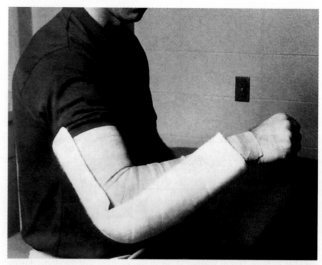

Fig. 9-9 A postoperative posterior elbow splint is used to protect healing tissues.

tubercle at the level of insertion of the anterior bundle. The drill holes are then connected with curettes and a towel clip. Proximally, two convergent tunnels are drilled to meet at the insertion of the ligament on the medial epicondyle. The graft is then passed through the ulna and crossed in a figure eight across the joint. Each end is then brought out through the two tunnels at the humerus end. If the graft is long enough, then one end is passed through a second time. The graft tension is adjusted with the elbow in 30° of flexion and by application of a varus stress. The graft is then secured with nonabsorbable 2-0 sutures over the medial epicondyle. The remaining ligament is sutured to the graft for added stability, and the flexor carpi ulnaris is loosely closed (Fig. 9-8).

Ulnar nerve transposition is now completed. An incision is made in the flexor pronator fascia, leaving attachments at the medial epicondyle; these flaps are about 3 cm long and 1 cm wide. Muscle is dissected away from the fascia, and the defect is closed to prevent herniation. The nerve is then transferred subcutaneously and anteriorly to lie under the fascial flaps. The flaps are reattached loosely to provide a sling to keep the nerve in position without compressing it. A drain is placed subcutaneously, and the skin is closed with an absorbable 3-0 subcuticular suture.

THERAPY GUIDELINES FOR REHABILITATION

Rehabilitation after UCL reconstruction should match the surgery used and meet the needs of the patient, which include additional care for the individual's specific donor site. The following guidelines are based on the procedure just described and are geared to the overhead-throwing athlete.

The complete rehabilitation program is outlined in the home maintenance box.

Phase I

TIME: 1 to 3 weeks after surgery
GOALS: Decrease pain and inflammation, retard muscle atrophy, protect healing tissues (Table 9-1)

The patient should be placed in a posterior elbow splint at 90° of flexion (Fig. 9-9), which allows initial healing of the UCL graft and soft tissue healing of the fascial slings for the transferred ulnar nerve.[24] Edema and pain are managed with frequent gripping exercises, cryotherapy, and a bulky dressing. The dressing is applied immediately after surgery and is removed between postoperative days 5 and 7.

The therapist initiates submaximal shoulder isometrics (except external rotation, which promotes a valgus stress at the elbow) and active wrist ROM to prevent neuromuscular inhibition.

The therapist evaluates ulnar nerve function postoperatively and frequently throughout the rehabilitation process. Paresthesia and impaired motor function occur at rates as high as 31% with intramuscular ulnar nerve transposition. The procedure described in this chapter uses fascial slings to complete transposition of the nerve, so the chance of postoperative neurologic complications is extremely low, usually less than 3%.

Compression wraps that are too tight and ill-fitting braces also may lead to transient ulnar nerve paresthesia and should be carefully assessed.

Early ROM and frequent assessment are vital in the early rehabilitative process. After 7 days, the posterior splint is removed and the elbow placed in a hinged brace set at 30° to 100° (Fig. 9-10). ROM is then advanced weekly by 10° of extension and 10° of flexion. Forearm supination and pronation ROM are assessed and progressed in postoperative week 2, given that these motions have no significant effect on graft

TABLE 9-1 Ulnar Nerve Transposition

Rehabilitation Phase	Criteria to Progress to This Phase	Anticipated Impairments and Functional Limitations	Intervention	Goal	Rationale
Phase I Postoperative 1-3 wk	Postoperative	• Postoperative pain • Postoperative edema • Arm immobilized in postoperative dressing • Limited elbow and wrist ROM • Limited UE strength • Limited reach, grasp, and lift capacity of UE	• Posterior splint with elbow at 90° of flexion (see Fig. 9-9) • Remove splint at 7 days after surgery and place in a hinged elbow brace set at 30° extension and 100° flexion • Brace ROM progressed by 10° of extension and 10° of flexion each week • Cryotherapy • Compression dressing (5-7 days) • Isometrics—Submaximal shoulder flexion, extension, abduction, and internal rotation (no ER) (at 2 wk, add wrist flexion/extension) At 2 wk, add wrist flexion and extension • After 2 wk, add forearm supination and pronation ROM (given that these motions have no significant strain on the graft)	• Protect surgical site • Increase elbow ROM • Improve tolerance to elbow ROM • Control pain • Manage edema • Improve UE strength and muscle contraction • Improve active ROM of wrist	• Soft tissue healing without irritating surgical site • Hinged brace to avoid valgus stress • Gradual addition of stress to surgical site, allowing ROM progression on a graduated basis • Self-management of pain and edema • Prevention of associated UE muscle atrophy without stressing UCL (avoid ER) • Nonpainful, safe strengthening of wrist musculature • Increase in available active ROM gradually as function and strength progress

ER, External rotation; *ROM,* range of motion; *UCL,* ulnar collateral ligament; *UE,* upper extremity.

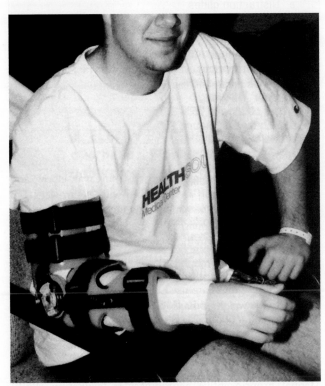

Fig. 9-10 The postoperative range of motion (ROM) brace is used to improve elbow ROM gradually while allowing soft tissue healing.

strain.[25] During the third postoperative week, active range of motion (AROM) for the wrist, elbow, and shoulder may be initiated.

Phase II

TIME: 4 to 7 weeks after surgery
GOALS: Gradually increase ROM, heal tissues, restore muscular strength (Table 9-2)

The intermediate phase begins approximately at week 4. Advancement through the rehabilitation process is adjusted based on the response of the patient to surgery, tissue healing constraints, and a criterion-based progression.

Light wrist and elbow isotonics can be initiated during week 4, as well as rotator cuff strengthening. The therapist should advance the resistance with isotonic exercises as the patient's strength improves. Typically, the patient progresses by 1 lb per week.

Training the muscles in the way they are to perform with throwing is the focus. For example, the flexor carpi ulnaris and flexor digitorum superficialis muscles are located directly over the anterior band of the UCL and may contribute to dynamic stabilization of the medial elbow. Rhythmic stabilization drills in the throwing position assist in training these muscles in a similar manner. In addition, the elbow extensors act concentrically to accelerate the arm during the

TABLE 9-2 Ulnar Nerve Transposition

Rehabilitation Phase	Criteria to Progress to This Phase	Anticipated Impairments and Functional Limitations	Intervention	Goal	Rationale
Phase II Postoperative 4-8 wk	• No sign of infection • No loss of ROM • No increase in pain	• Limited ROM • Limited UE strength • Limited reach, grasp, and lift capacity of UE • Pain	Continue exercises as in phase I as indicated • Elbow ROM 0°-135° at wk 5, discontinue brace at wk 5 • Isotonics (1-2 lb) — Wrist flexion, extension; forearm pronation, supination; elbow flexion, extension • Rotator cuff exercises (after 6 wk, see Box 9-2) After 6 wk: • Active ROM — Elbow flexion, extension • Progression of all exercises as indicated	• Elbow active ROM 0°-145° • Protect elbow from unprotected valgus force • Increase functional strength of UE • Improve tolerance to active ROM • Increase upper quarter strength • Increase lift tolerance	• Promotion of elbow ROM • Progression toward protected active ROM of elbow • Advancing of UE strength and ROM in preparation to restore previous level of functioning • Continued avoidance of valgus forces • By 6 wk, soft tissue healing should be stable enough to tolerate valgus stress • Attaining of full ROM • Objective progression of exercises

ROM, Range of motion; *UE,* upper extremity.

acceleration phase, whereas the elbow flexors act eccentrically to control the rapid rate of elbow extension during follow-through. Biasing the exercise selection appropriately for these muscle groups allows more effective strength training and provides neuromuscular training, allowing the muscles to function more efficiently when performing skilled movement patterns.

During this phase the therapist should pay careful attention to the patient's ROM. One of the most common complications after UCL reconstruction is development of an elbow flexion contracture and joint stiffness. In addition, flexion contracture is common in overhead-throwing athletes. Throwing athletes have demonstrated a 7.9° average loss of elbow extension ROM before their competitive season.[26] Therefore early intervention and progressive motion and stretching exercises are important preventatives against elbow flexion contracture (Box 9-1).[27]

ROM is gradually progressed to achieve 0° to 135° by week 5. At this time, the brace may be removed. The intimate configuration of the elbow joint is prone to develop contractures. In addition, scarring of the brachialis muscle to the capsule may further lead to loss of motion. ROM and stretching techniques are continued to ensure the prevention of motion complications. Additionally, low-load long-duration stretching may be incorporated as needed.

Phase III

TIME: 8 to 13 weeks after surgery
GOALS: Increase strength, power, and endurance, maintain full ROM, gradually add sports activities (Table 9-3)

BOX 9-1 Stretching Program to Improve Elbow Motion

1. Passive warm-up (warm whirlpool) (7 to 10 minutes)
2. Active warm-up (upper body ergometer) (10 minutes)
3. Joint mobilization
   a. Distraction glides
   b. Posterior ulnar glide for upward elbow extension
   c. Mobilization of radial head
4. Low-load, long-duration stretching (12 to 15 minutes)
5. Manual proprioceptive neuromuscular facilitation stretches using contract-relax technique
6. Passive stretching
7. Repeat process twice

During this phase aggressive wrist, forearm, elbow, and shoulder strengthening are advanced with a Thrower's Ten Program (Box 9-2). The patient may begin light plyometric exercise during this phase. Plyometrics are initiated with two-hand drills, close to the body, such as a chest pass. These exercises are progressed away from the body to include side-to-side and overhead throws and, finally, one-hand drills at week 12. These drills are used to develop power and explosiveness with weighted balls, often incorporating the functional throwing position (Fig. 9-11). Forearm plyometrics should also be introduced in this phase (Fig. 9-12). Exercises such as wrist flips and snaps will incorporate wrist flexors while extension grips will address wrist extension strength. Manual proprioceptive neuromuscular facilitation (PNF) drills integrate elbow flexion and extension with respective supination and pronation, helping to improve joint stability

TABLE 9-3 Ulnar Nerve Transposition

Rehabilitation Phase	Criteria to Progress to This Phase	Anticipated Impairments and Functional Limitations	Intervention	Goal	Rationale

Phase III Postoperative 9-13 wk	• No increase in pain
	• No loss of ROM
	• Steady progression of elbow and wrist ROM
		• Limited UE strength
		• Limited tolerance to reach, grasp, and lift activities
			Continue exercises as in phases I and II
			• Initiate plyometric exercises
			  ○ Wrist flips and snaps (see Fig. 9-12)
			  ○ Elbow flexion and extension with supination and pronation (see Fig. 9-13)
			• Isotonics—Progress wrist, elbow, and shoulder exercises
			• Initiate eccentric elbow flexion and extension exercises
			• Plyometrics—Incorporate functional throwing position (see Fig. 9-11)
			• Rhythmic stabilization
			• Proprioceptive neuromuscular facilitation patterns (see Fig. 9-14)
			• Proprioceptive neuromuscular facilitation patterns (see Fig. 9-14)
			• Light sporting activities (golf, swimming)
			• Initiate Thrower's Ten Program (see Box 9-2)
				• Increase strength of UE
				• Increase muscular control of UE
				• Prepare for return to previous activities
				• Improve recruitment of UE musculature
				• Allow client to become pain free or self-manage with gradual return to activities
				• Strengthen UE with sport-specific activities
					• Continuation of strengthening UE and progressing resistance
					• Training of muscles in movement patterns similar to overhead activities
					• Preparation of UE for accelerating and decelerating activities
					• Use of neuromuscular patterns to enhance functional strength and dynamic joint stabilization
					• Use of cross-training to vary stresses on UE
					• Specificity of training principle

ROM, Range of motion; *UE,* upper extremity.

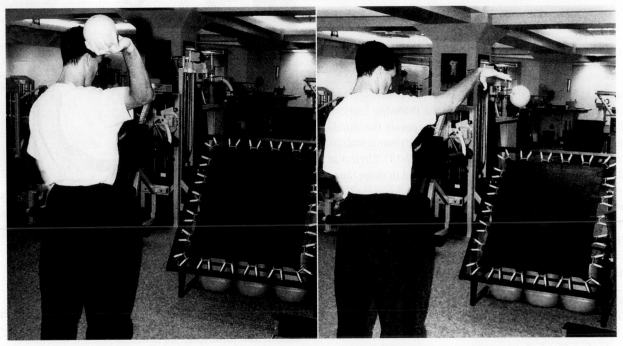

Fig. 9-11 Plyometric exercise drills develop power and explosiveness. The one-handed baseball throw to simulate throwing mechanics is shown.

BOX 9-2 Thrower's Ten Program

1. Diagonal pattern D2 flexion and extension
2. External rotation (ER) and internal rotation tubing
3. Shoulder abduction
4. Full can
5. Side-lying ER
6. Prone: horizontal abduction, horizontal abduction at 100°, row, and row into ER
7. Press-ups
8. Push-ups starting from the wall in standing
9. Elbow flexion and extension
10. Wrist extension and flexion, pronation, and supination

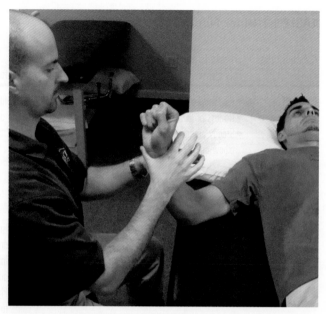

Fig. 9-13 Manual resistance proprioceptive neuromuscular facilitation (PNF) at the elbow helps promote strength and dynamic joint stability through a functional movement pattern.

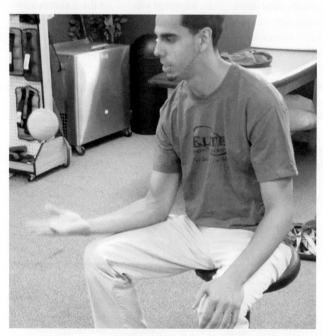

Fig. 9-12 Forearm plyometric exercises such as wrist flips help increase functional strength of the wrist flexors.

(Fig. 9-13). Emphasis should be placed on the concentric and eccentric roles of each muscle during the throwing motion. D2 flexion and extension PNF drills incorporate the shoulder, thus further encouraging strength and dynamic stabilization in functional movement patterns (Fig. 9-14). Rhythmic stabilization drills should also be incorporated in more functional throwing positions to establish control through the core stabilizers as well. Stability deficits throughout the kinetic chain will place added stress on the repaired UCL (Fig 9-15).

Phase IV

TIME: 14 to 26 weeks after surgery

GOALS: Increase strength, power, and endurance of upper extremity muscles, gradually return to sports activities (Table 9-4)

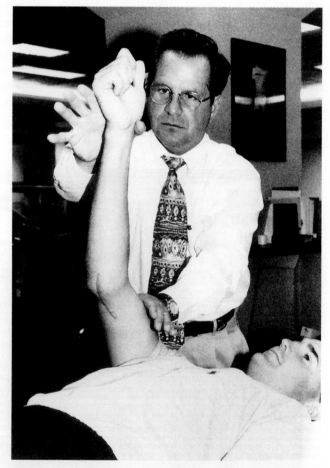

Fig. 9-14 Manual resistance proprioceptive neuromuscular facilitation (PNF) promotes strengthening in functional movement patterns and dynamic joint stabilization. This movement pattern is referred to as a D2 flexion and extension upper extremity pattern.

In this final phase, the physical therapist should take care to return the patient to sports activities gradually; an interval sports program may help ensure that goal (Boxes 9-3 and 9-4). Other throwing programs are described in Chapters 3 and 13. An interval throwing program may be initiated for an overhead thrower at 16 weeks after surgery, with throwing off the mound usually occurring around 5 to 6 months after surgery.[27] Return to competition typically occurs between 9 and 12 months. The competitive overhead athlete should participate in a year-round conditioning program that consists of isotonic strengthening, plyometric and neuromuscular training, and a sport-specific training program. Wrist,

elbow, and forearm strength should continue to improve. Professional throwing athletes have significantly greater forearm pronation and wrist flexion strength on the dominant arm.[28] In addition, the athlete should continue flexibility exercises for the elbow, wrist, and hand. The interval throwing program emphasizes a proper warm-up, correct throwing mechanics, and a gradual progression of intensity. The therapist also must teach the athlete to "listen" to the arm: if pain is present, then the patient should not advance the program prematurely.

SUGGESTED HOME MAINTENANCE FOR THE POSTSURGICAL PATIENT

The home maintenance box, as well as Box 9-2, reviews exercises that are commonly prescribed for the patient to perform at home. The exercises are progressed gradually to allow the tissue proper healing time, with the ultimate goal of full restoration of strength and ROM. The exercises are to be performed at home in conjunction with treatment sessions in the rehabilitation setting.

TROUBLESHOOTING

As already noted, the most common complication after UCL reconstruction is a flexion contracture or stiff joint. Factors that predispose the elbow joint to this loss of ROM include the following:

1. The intimate congruency of the elbow joint complex, especially the humeroulnar joint
2. The tightness of the elbow joint capsule
3. The tendency of the anterior capsule to scar and become adhesive[29]

Box 9-1 outlines a program found to be effective in combating flexion contractures of the elbow. It includes both passive and active warm-up, joint mobilizations, and manual stretching techniques. One of the most effective components to the stretching regimen is the low-load, long-duration

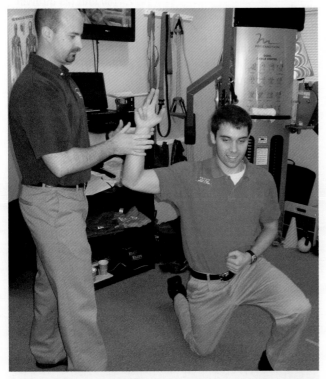

Fig. 9-15 Rhythmic stabilization in functional throwing positions helps recruit core stabilizers and prepare for the balanced transfer of force through the kinetic chain upon return to throwing.

TABLE 9-4 Ulnar Nerve Transposition

Rehabilitation Phase	Criteria to Progress to This Phase	Anticipated Impairments and Functional Limitations	Intervention	Goal	Rationale
Phase IV Postoperative 14-26 wk	• No increase in pain • No loss of range of motion • No loss of strength	• Limited tolerance to repetitive overhead activities • Limited strength	• Initiate interval throwing program (see Boxes 9-3 and Box 9-4) • Continue strengthening as in phases I through III	• Symmetric UE strength • Gradual return to unrestricted sport activity	• Normalization of UE strength to avoid reinjury with return-to-sport activities • Gradual progression to sport

UE, Upper extremity.

BOX 9-3 Interval Throwing Program Phase I

45-Foot Phase

Step 1
1. Warm-up throwing
2. 45 feet (25 throws)
3. Rest 15 minutes
4. Warm-up throwing
5. 45 feet (25 throws)

Step 2
1. Warm-up throwing
2. 45 feet (25 throws)
3. Rest 10 minutes
4. Warm-up throwing
5. 45 feet (25 throws)
6. Rest 10 minutes
7. Warm-up throwing
8. 45 feet (25 throws)

60-Foot Phase

Step 3
1. Warm-up throwing
2. 60 feet (25 throws)
3. Rest 15 minutes
4. Warm-up throwing
5. 60 feet (25 throws)

Step 4
1. Warm-up throwing
2. 60 feet (25 throws)
3. Rest 10 minutes
4. Warm-up throwing
5. 60 feet (25 throws)
6. Rest 10 minutes
7. Warm-up throwing
8. 60 feet (25 throws)

90-Foot Phase

Step 5
1. Warm-up throwing
2. 90 feet (25 throws)
3. Rest 15 minutes
4. Warm-up throwing
5. 90 feet (25 throws)

Step 6
1. Warm-up throwing
2. 90 feet (25 throws)
3. Rest 10 minutes
4. Warm-up throwing
5. 90 feet (25 throws)
6. Rest 10 minutes
7. Warm-up throwing
8. 90 feet (25 throws)

120-Foot Phase

Step 7
1. Warm-up throwing
2. 120 feet (25 throws)
3. Rest 15 minutes
4. Warm-up throwing
5. 120 feet (25 throws)

Step 8
1. Warm-up throwing
2. 120 feet (25 throws)
3. Rest 10 minutes
4. Warm-up throwing
5. 120 feet (25 throws)
6. 120 feet (25 throws)
7. Rest 10 minutes
8. Warm-up throwing

150-Foot Phase

Step 9
1. Warm-up throwing
2. 150 feet (25 throws)
3. Rest 15 minutes
4. Warm-up throwing
5. 150 feet (25 throws)

Step 10
1. Warm-up throwing
2. 150 feet (25 throws)
3. Rest 10 minutes
4. Warm-up throwing
5. 150 feet (25 throws)
6. Rest 10 minutes
7. Warm-up throwing
8. 150 feet (25 throws)

180-Foot Phase

Step 11
1. Warm-up throwing
2. 180 feet (25 throws)
3. Rest 15 minutes
4. Warm-up throwing
5. 180 feet (25 throws)

Step 12
1. Warm-up throwing
2. 180 feet (25 throws)
3. Rest 10 minutes
4. Warm-up throwing
5. 180 feet (25 throws)
6. Rest 10 minutes
7. Warm-up throwing
8. 180 feet (25 throws)

Step 13
1. Warm-up throwing
2. 180 feet (25 throws)
3. Rest 10 minutes
4. Warm-up throwing
5. 180 feet (25 throws)
6. Rest 10 minutes
7. Warm-up throwing
8. 180 feet (25 throws)

stretching technique. The three most important components of this technique are (1) duration of stretch (10 to 15 minutes), (2) intensity of stretch (low to moderate), and (3) frequency of stretch (5 to 6 times daily) (Fig. 9-16).

This stretching technique may be enhanced by the use of other modalities such as moist hot packs or ultrasound. The rationale for the success of this technique is its ability to produce a plastic response within the collagen tissue, resulting in permanent elongation.[7,30-32]

If ROM complications persist, the therapist may want to prescribe a splint to be worn both day and night. A static splint holds the joint in a constant position, whereas a dynamic splint uses a spring to exert force and create a progressive stretch. Patients are encouraged to remove the splint daily for strengthening and stretching exercises.

During the aggressive stretching program the patient often experiences increased elbow soreness or pain. Pain control using cryotherapy, high-voltage galvanic stimulation (HVGS), transcutaneous electric nerve stimulation (TENS), and interferential current is highly effective.

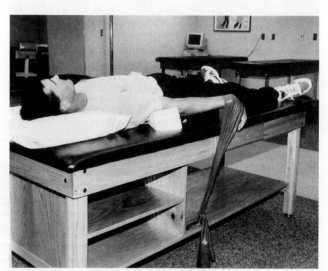

Fig. 9-16 A low-load, long-duration stretch is performed to improve elbow extension. A Thera-Band is secured at one end and wrapped around the patient's distal forearm.

BOX 9-4 Interval Throwing Program Phase II

Stage 1: Fastball Only

Step 1:
Interval throwing
15 throws off mound at 50%

Step 2:
Interval throwing
30 throws off mound at 50%

Step 3:
Interval throwing
45 throws off mound at 50%

Step 4:
Interval throwing
60 throws off mound at 50%

Step 5:
Interval throwing
30 throws off mound at 75%

Step 6:
30 throws off mound at 75%
45 throws off mound at 50%

Step 7:
45 throws off mound at 75%
15 throws off mound at 50%

Step 8:
60 throws off mound at 75%

Stage 2: Fastball Only

Step 9:
45 throws off mound at 75%
15 throws in batting practice

Step 10:
45 throws off mound at 75%
30 throws in batting practice

Step 11:
45 throws off mound at 75%
45 throws in batting practice

Stage 3

Step 12:
30 throws off mound at 75% during warm-up
15 throws off mound; 50% breaking balls
45-60 throws in batting practice (fastball only)

Step 13:
30 throws off mound at 75%
30 breaking balls at 75%
30 throws in batting practice

Step 14:
30 throws off mound at 75%
60-90 throws in batting practice; 25% breaking balls

Step 15:
Simulated game, progressing by 15 throws per workout (use interval throwing to phase 12, No. 8 in Box 9-3 as warm-up). All throwing off the mound should be done in the presence of the pitching coach to stress proper throwing mechanics. Use speed gun to aid in effort control.

Other complications include hand and grip weakness, ulnar neuropathy, rotator cuff tendonitis, and UCL failure. Intrinsic weakness of the hand may be avoided by initiating gripping exercises immediately after surgery and increasing intensity as rehabilitation progresses. Ulnar neuropathy generally develops immediately after surgery. Transposition of the ulnar nerve may cause sensory changes of the little finger and ulnar half of the ring finger. Motor deficits may include the inability to adduct the thumb, weakness of the finger abductor and adductors, adduction of the little finger, and weakness of the flexor carpi ulnaris. The most frequent patient complaint is paresthesia through the ulnar nerve sensory distribution, but this is usually transient and should resolve within 7 days.

Inactivity can lead to rapid deterioration of rotator cuff strength and a subsequent inability to stabilize the glenohumeral (GH) joint during the throwing motion. Integrating a Thrower's Ten Program with the emphasis on rotator cuff strengthening several weeks before throwing greatly reduces the chances of developing tendonitis.

UCL failure is the most serious of all postoperative complications. Graft failure or poor bone quality with inadequate graft stabilization necessitates subsequent surgery or the cessation of overhead activities. Fortunately, with advanced surgical and rehabilitation techniques, successful outcomes are much more likely than failures. Andrews and Timmerman[33] found 78% of professional baseball players returning to their previous level of play after UCL reconstruction. Additionally, Cain and associates[34] found that 83% of overhead athletes returned to their previous level or higher upon 2-year follow-up. Major complications occurred with only 4%.

Suggested Home Maintenance for the Postsurgical Patient

Weeks 1 to 3:
GOALS FOR THE PERIOD: Protect healing tissues, decrease pain and inflammation, and limit muscle atrophy
Week 1:
1. Posterior splint at 90° elbow flexion
2. Wrist assisted range of motion (AROM) extension and flexion
3. Elbow compression dressing (5 to 7 days)
4. Gripping exercises, wrist range of motion (ROM), shoulder isometrics (except shoulder external rotation [ER]), biceps isometrics, others as indicated
5. Cryotherapy
Week 2:
1. Application of functional brace 30° to 100°
2. Initiation of wrist isometrics
3. Initiation of elbow flexion and extension isometrics
4. Continuation of all exercises listed previously
Week 3:
Advance brace (gradually increase ROM; 10° of extension and 10° of flexion per week)

Weeks 4 to 7:
GOALS FOR THE PERIOD: Gradually increase ROM, healing tissues, and regain and improve muscle strength
Week 4:
1. Begin light resistance exercises for arm (1 lb), wrist curls, extensions, pronation, and supination, and elbow extension and flexion
2. Progress shoulder program, emphasizing rotator cuff strengthening
Week 5:
Continue as for week 4, discharge brace, full passive range of motion (PROM) week 5

Weeks 6 to 7:
1. ROM 0° to 145°
2. Progress elbow-strengthening exercises
3. Initiate shoulder ER strengthening
4. Progress shoulder program

Weeks 8 to 13:
GOALS FOR THE PERIOD: Increase strength, power, and endurance; maintain full elbow ROM; gradually begin sports activities
Week 8:
1. Initiate eccentric elbow flexion and extension
2. Continue isotonic program for forearm and wrist
3. Continue shoulder program (Thrower's Ten Program)
4. Begin manual resistance diagonal patterns
5. Begin two-hand plyometrics
Weeks 9 to 11:
Continue as for week 8, progress strength
Weeks 12 to 13:
1. Continue as for week 11
2. Begin one-hand plyometrics
3. Begin light sports activities (e.g., golf, swimming)

Weeks 14 to 26:
GOALS FOR THE PERIOD: Continue to increase strength, power, and endurance of upper extremity muscles; gradually return to sports activities
Week 14:
1. Continue strengthening program
2. Emphasize elbow and wrist strengthening and flexibility exercises
Weeks 15 to 21:
Continue with program
Week 16:
Begin phase I interval throwing program
Weeks 22 to 26:
Return to competitive sports as appropriate

CLINICAL CASE REVIEW

1 The patient is a 16-year-old female tennis player who had UCL reconstruction 16 weeks ago. She has full ROM and has been progressing with her isotonic strengthening program. She expresses that she is ready to start playing. What types of intervention still need to be incorporated in her program before she can begin sporting activities, and what is the rationale for doing so?

Before any overhead sporting activity such as hitting a tennis ball, it is important that the patient has progressed through a proper rehabilitation program, including isotonics, dynamic stabilization drills, a plyometric program, and an interval sport program. These exercises are essential to enhancing functional strength and dynamic joint stability, as well as preparing the upper extremity for the acceleration and deceleration forces required of her sport-specific activity.

2 The patient is a college baseball pitcher that had UCL surgery with ulnar nerve transposition 7 weeks ago. He is now performing some light isotonic exercises. What two muscles should the therapist target to enhance the dynamic stabilization of the medial elbow during a throwing motion?

The focus should be on training the muscles in the way they are to perform during throwing. The flexor carpi ulnaris and the flexor digitorum superficialis muscles are located directly over the anterior band of the UCL and may contribute to dynamic stabilization of the medial elbow.

3 The patient is a 20-year-old male pitcher who had UCL reconstruction 6 weeks ago. He arrives from another clinic with a 15° flexion contracture. What course of action should the therapist take to address this ROM deficit immediately?

The patient is behind with his ROM. The elbow joint is prone to develop a flexion contracture as the result of the intimate joint congruency. In the instance of a flexion contracture, the therapist should introduce treatments designed to create a plastic response in the collagen tissue. These include a passive warm-up, followed by active warm-up, joint mobilizations (including distraction and posterior ulnar glides), low-load, long duration, as well as contract-relax and passive stretching.

4 A patient who had UCL surgery 16 weeks ago wants to begin throwing. Is this appropriate?

Provided the patient has full ROM, good strength, and is pain free, an interval throwing program is initiated at week 16. Each stage is to be performed twice, with a day of rest in between, before moving to the next stage. Should the patient report pain or excessive soreness, he or she should move back a stage and continue from there.

5 A patient who had UCL surgery 8 months ago is beginning to throw on the mound near full effort and begins to report medial elbow pain. What should the therapist do?

The therapist should tell the patient to step back to a partial effort for a week and treat the pain symptoms. If the patient continues to feel pain when progressing, then he or she may need to see a physician and potentially stop throwing to allow time to heal while continuing with exercises.

6 A patient had UCL surgery 3 days ago and has been unable to adduct his thumb, abduct or adduct his fingers, and has weakness in the flexor carpi ulnaris. He also reports numbness in the fifth digit. What is the assessment? Is this cause for concern?

These signs and symptoms are consistent with an ulnar neuropathy, which is common after ulnar nerve transposition. The therapist can check for tight-fitting wraps or ill-fitting braces, but typically these complications resolve within 7 days after surgery.

7 Patient is a 19-year-old hockey player who had UCL reconstruction following an acute UCL tear as a result of a fall and subsequent elbow dislocation. How might the acute mechanism of injury affect progression of this patient's postoperative ROM?

Early postoperative PROM can be progressed more quickly following reconstruction of acute tears. Full PROM should be expected by week 5. Chronic tears will progress more gradually, attaining full PROM closer to postoperative weeks 6 through 8.

8 A 23-year-old pitcher is 6 weeks out of surgery following an acute UCL tear. He is having trouble achieving full extension. How aggressive should manual techniques be when trying to restore full ROM?

There are a few factors to consider when trying to determine if aggressive mobilization and stretching is indicated. Consider the end feel and what type of tissue is constraining the ROM. An empty end feel with pain or swelling should be a sign to use a more gradual, less aggressive approach. Yet, a hard, bony end feel should present as a situation where more aggressive mobilization techniques would be indicated.

9 A 32-year-old NFL quarterback is postoperative week 2 following UCL reconstruction with ulnar nerve transposition. His posterior splint has been removed and early elbow flexion/extension ROM has been initiated. Is forearm pronation/supination ROM permitted during this phase?

Pronation and supination of the forearm place no strain on the UCL graft. Therefore, PROM in these directions can be initiated during week 2. Pronation and supination isometrics also have no effect on the strain in the UCL, allowing for their addition during this phase. Initiate pronation/supination isotonics during week 4, as you would for the wrist and elbow.

10 A professional baseball pitcher has met all of the criteria to progress to phase IV of his rehabilitation and is ready to begin an interval throwing program. He is leaving our care to gradually return to sports activities with his team's training staff. What are some important things to stress to the trainers during their progression through this phase?

It is important to advance through an interval throwing program step by step, including timely progression to throwing off the mound. The overhead athlete should also participate in a year round conditioning program that includes isotonic strengthening, and plyometric and neuromuscular training. Forearm and elbow strength should continue to increase to greater than the nondominant side. Professional throwing athletes have greater wrist flexion and forearm pronation strength on their dominant arm, as well as greater strength on elbow flexion and extension.

11 Following UCL reconstruction, a patient asks why a hamstring graft was used despite the presence of palmaris longus. Are there situations where

hamstring grafts might be preferable to palmaris longus grafts?

This type of questioning should always be referred to the referring physician. However, generally speaking, use of the contralateral gracilis muscle may be indicated when there is boney involvement of the UCL. The presence of bone within the UCL represents a chronic ligamentous deficiency, which requires use of a larger graft. Data suggest use of the contralateral hamstring graft is reliable, reproducible, and may provide improved results with return to play.[35]

REFERENCES

1. Steindler A: Kinesiology of the human body, Springfield, Ill, 1955, Charles C Thomas.
2. Guerra JJ, Timmerman LA: Clinical anatomy, histology, and pathomechanics of the elbow in sports. Sports Med Arthrosc Rev 3(3):160, 1995.
3. Timmerman LA, Andrews JR: Histology and arthroscopic anatomy of the ulnar collateral ligament of the elbow. Am J Sports Med 22(5):667, 1994.
4. Andrews JR: Ulnar collateral ligament injuries of the elbow in throwers. Paper presented at the Injuries in Baseball Course, Birmingham, Ala, Jan 28, 1990.
5. Morrey BF, An RN: Articular and ligamentous contributions to the stability of the elbow joint. Am J Sports Med 11:315, 1983.
6. Warwick R, Williams PL: Gray's anatomy: Descriptive and applied, ed 35, Philadelphia, 1980, Saunders.
7. Schums GH, et al: Biomechanics of elbow stability: Role of the medial collateral ligament. Clin Orthop 146:42, 1980.
8. Morrey BF: Anatomy of the elbow joint. In Morrey BF, editor: The elbow and its disorders, Philadelphia, 1993, Saunders.
9. O'Driscoll SW, Bell DF, Morrey BF: Posterolateral rotary instability of the elbow. J Bone Joint Surg Am 73:440, 1991.
10. Martin BJ: The annular ligament of the superior radioulnar joint. J Anat 52:473, 1958.
11. Martin BJ: The oblique of the forearm. J Anat 52:609, 1958.
12. Jobe FW, Fanton GS: Nerve injuries. In Morrey BF, editor: The elbow and its disorders, Philadelphia, 1985, Saunders.
13. Morrey BF: Anatomy and kinematics of the elbow. In Tullos HS, editor: American Academy of Orthopaedic Surgeons instructional course lectures 40, St Louis, 1991, Mosby.
14. Wilk KE, Azar FM, Andrews JR: Conservative and operative rehabilitation of the elbow in sports. Sports Med Arthrosc Rev 3:237, 1995.
15. Pappas A, Zawack RM, Sullivan TJ: Biomechanics of baseball pitching: A preliminary report. Am J Sports Med 13(4):216, 1985.
16. Werner SL, Fleisig GS, Dillman CJ: Biomechanics of the elbow during baseball pitching. J Orthop Sports Phys Ther 17:274, 1993.
17. Dillman C, Smutz P, Werner S: Valgus extension overload in baseball pitching. Med Sci Sports Exerc 23:S135, 1991.
18. Fleisig GS, et al: Kinetics of baseball pitching with implications about injury mechanisms. Am J Sports Med 23(2):233, 1995.
19. Hyman J, Breazeale NM, Altchek DW: Valgus instability of the elbow in athletes. Clin Sports Med 20(1):25-45, 2001.
20. Conway JE, et al: Medial instability of the elbow in throwing athletes. J Bone Joint Surg Am 74:67, 1992.
21. Timmerman LA, Schwartz ML, Andrews JR: Preoperative evaluation of the ulnar collateral ligament by magnetic resonance imaging and computed tomography arthrography. Am J Sports Med 22(1):26, 1994.
22. Safran MR: Ulnar collateral ligament injury in the overhead athlete: Diagnosis and treatment. Clin Sports Med 23(4):643-663, 2004.
23. Timmerman LA, Andrews JR: Undersurface tear of the ulnar collateral ligament in baseball players: A newly recognized lesion. Am J Sports Med 22(1):33, 1994.
24. Wilk KE, Arrigo CA, Andrews JR: Rehabilitation of the elbow in the throwing athlete. J Orthop Sports Phys Ther 17:305, 1993.
25. Bernas G, et al: Defining safe rehabilitation for ulnar collateral ligament reconstruction of the elbow: A biomechanical study. Am J Sports Med 37(12):2392, 2009.
26. Wright RW, et al: Elbow range of motion in professional baseball pitchers. Am J Sports Med 34(2):190, 2006.
27. Wilk KE, et al: Rehabilitation following elbow surgery in the throwing athlete. Oper Tech Sports Med 4(2):69, 1996.
28. Ellenbecker TS, Mattalino AJ: The elbow in sport. Champaign, Ill, 1997, Human Kinetics.
29. Reinold MM, et al: Interval sports programs: Guidelines for baseball, tennis and golf. J Orthop Sports Phys Ther 32(6):293-298, 2002.
30. Kottke FJ, Pauley DL, Ptak RA: The rationale for prolonged stretching for correction of shortening of connective tissue. Arch Phys Med Rehabil 47:345, 1968.
31. Warren CB, Lehman JF, Koblanski JN: Elongation of cat-tail tendon: Effect of load and temperature. Arch Phys Med Rehabil 52:465, 1971.
32. Warren CG, Lehman JF, Koblanski JN: Heat and stretch procedures: An evaluation using cat-tail tendon. Arch Phys Med Rehabil 57:122, 1976.
33. Andrews JR, Timmerman LA: Outcome of elbow surgery in professional baseball players. Am J Sports Med 23(4):407, 1995.
34. Cain EL, et al: Outcome of ulnar collateral ligament reconstruction of the elbow in 1281 athletes: Results in 743 athletes with minimum 2-year follow-up. Am J Sports Med 38(12):2426, 2010.
35. Dugas JR, et al: Clinical results of UCL reconstructions done with boney involvement of ligament using gracilis tendon autograft. Unpublished data. Presented at 28th Annual Injuries in Baseball Course. Birmingham, Ala, ASMI (2010).

CHAPTER 10

Clinical Applications for Platelet Rich Plasma Therapy

Eric S. Honbo, Luga Podesta

Over the past several years, there has been significant interest in the use of biologic treatment of muscle, tendon, ligament, and bone injuries in orthopedic and sports medicine. The use of orthobiologic tissue grafts, such as platelet rich plasma (PRP) to stimulate and promote tissue healing and regeneration, has received increasing notoriety since first being reported in the February 2009 article "A Promising Treatment for Athletes, in Blood" in the *New York Times*. This article increased the public's awareness of PRP to treat the NFL's Pittsburgh Steelers football player Hines Ward before the 2009 Super Bowl.

The use of PRP to promote healing has been studied since the 1970s in both the veterinary and human literature. Ferrari and associates first reported using PRP in 1987 during cardiac surgery as an autologous transfusion component after open heart surgery to avoid homologous blood product transfusion.[1] PRP has successfully been used in various specialties, such as maxillofacial surgery, cosmetic surgery, orthopedics, and podiatry, and for general wound healing.[2-9] In humans, the higher concentrations of autologous growth factors and the secretory proteins found in PRP preparations are attributed to its ability to promote tissue healing and regeneration when applied to a variety of tissue.

DEFINITION OF PRP

Platelets are small, nonnucleated cell fragments in the peripheral blood known primarily for their role in homeostasis. The normal platelet count ranges from 150,000 μL to 400,000 μL. Platelets contain numerous proteins (growth factors), cytokines, and bioactive factors that initiate and regulate tissue healing.[10] The fluid portion of blood—plasma—also contains clotting factors, proteins, and ions. PRP is the result of concentrating the platelet count to at least 1 million platelets per microliter in 5 mL of plasma.[10,11]

PLATELET FUNCTION IN TISSUE HEALING

Platelets contain two unique types of granules—alpha granules and dense granules. Alpha granules in platelets function as storage units containing a variety of hemostatic proteins, inactive growth factors, cytokines, and other proteins such as adhesion proteins. Dense granules store and release bioactive factors that promote platelet aggregation, tissue modulation, and regeneration including adenosine diphosphate (ADP), adenosine triphosphate (ATP), calcium, serotonin, histamine, and dopamine.[12,13]

Growth factors found in these granules include platelet derived growth factor (PDGF), transforming growth factor-β_1 (TGF-β_1), vascular endothelial growth factor (VEGF), basic fibroblastic growth factor (bFGF), insulin-like growth factor (IGF-I, IGF-II), endothelial cell growth factor (ECGF), and epidermal growth factor (EGF).[4,6,10,14-16] Platelet activation is required for discharge of granule content (B5) (Table 10-1). Upon clotting, platelets are activated, resulting in degranulation and release of their growth factors from the alpha granules. Approximately 70% of the stored growth factors are released within the first 10 minutes. The majority of growth factor release occurs within the first hour after degranulation. Continued growth factor release has been shown to occur throughout the period of platelet viability, approximately 7 days.[4,8,10]

PRP is a mechanism to deliver a physiologically natural balance/ratio of growth factors, cytokines, and other bioactive proteins in supraphysiologic concentrations directly into an injured tissue to potentially optimize healing while maintaining the body's homeostatic environment.[4,17-19] Using PRP to treat a variety of soft tissue pathologies is appealing to the clinician because of its simplicity of acquisition and administration, relatively low cost when compared with surgical treatments, and absence of significant adverse effects. Since PRP is an autologous tissue graft, the risk of tissue rejection, immune response, or disease transmission is eliminated.

TABLE 10-1 Growth Factors in Platelet Rich Plasma

Growth Factor	Function	Target Cell and Tissue
Platelet-derived growth factor (PDGF)	• Stimulates the mitogenesis of mesenchymal cells • Stimulates fibroblast chemotaxis and mitogenesis • Stimulates satellite cell proliferation	Fibroblasts, smooth muscle cells, chondrocytes, osteoblasts, mesenchymal stem cells
Transforming growth factor-β (TGF-β₁)	• Stimulates mesenchymal cell proliferation • Regulates endothelial cells and fibroblast mitogenesis • Stimulates endothelial chemotaxis and angiogenesis • Inhibits macrophage and lymphocyte proliferation • Inhibits satellite cell proliferation and differentiation	Blood vessel tissue, outer skin cells Fibroblasts, monocytes Osteoblasts
Vascular endothelial growth factor (VEGF)		Blood vessel cells
Basic fibroblastic growth factor (bFGF)	• Promotes growth and differentiation of chondrocytes and osteoblasts • Mitogenetic for mesenchymal cells, chondrocytes, and osteoblasts	Blood vessels, smooth muscle, skin Fibroblasts, other cell types
Insulin-like growth factor (IGF-I, IGF-II)	• Promotes the mitogenesis of mesenchymal cells • Promotes collagen synthesis • Stimulates fibroblast chemotaxis and mitogenesis • Stimulates the proliferation and fusion of myoblasts • Inhibits myoblast apoptosis	Bone, blood vessel, skin, other tissue
Endothelial cell growth factor (ECGF)	• Cell growth, migration, new blood vessel growth • Antiapoptosis	Blood vessel cells
Epidermal growth factor (EGF)	• Stimulates endothelial chemotaxis and angiogenesis • Regulates extracellular matrix turnover • Stimulates fibroblast migration and proliferation	Blood vessel cells, outer skin cells Fibroblasts and many other cell types

TISSUE HEALING

The healing process is defined as a complex and dynamic biologic progression that results in the restoration of anatomic structure and function. Tissue healing is a process characterized by a predictable cascade of biologic tissue response triggered by the injury itself. Physiologic healing progresses through three overlapping stages: stage 1, the acute inflammatory phase; stage 2, the proliferative or repair phase; and stage 3, the remodeling phase.

The inflammatory phase, stage 1 begins with a tissue injury. Platelets are stimulated to provide hemostasis by forming a clot. Platelets in the clot then degranulate and secrete several growth factors, hemostatic factors, and cytokines from alpha granules that are necessary in the early stages of the clotting cascade. Histamine and serotonin are released from the dense granules and function to increase capillary permeability, activate macrophages, and allow inflammatory cells greater access to the injury site.[10,20,21] The inflammatory phase can last up to 72 hours and is characterized by localized pain, swelling, erythema, and increased local tissue temperature. The proliferative phase (stage 2) begins when polymorphonuclear leukocytes migrate to the inflamed tissue. During the ensuing 48 hours to 6 weeks, anatomic structures begin to be restored while tissue generation occurs. Fibroblasts begin to synthesize scar tissue and capillary neoformation begins to reestablish nutrients to the injured tissue. Stage 2 ends with the beginning of wound contraction. Stage 3 is characterized by collagen remodeling. The process of tissue remodeling can last from 3 weeks to 12 months.[14]

FORMATION OF PRP

PRP can only be derived from anticoagulated whole blood. Since platelets form part of the clot in coagulated blood and are activated triggering degranulation—thereby releasing their bioactive proteins, growth factors, and cytokines—clotted blood is not an appropriate source of blood to obtain PRP. PRP preparation begins by adding citrate to whole blood. Citrate binds to ionized calcium inhibiting the clotting cascade. The anticoagulated blood then undergoes a centrifugation process to first separate red and white blood cells from plasma and platelets, and then a second centrifugation cycle further separating the platelet rich from the platelet poor plasma. There are a number of commercially available devices on the market that produce PRP (Fig. 10-1). Current systems available to generate PRP differ in the amount of whole blood needed for processing, the anticoagulant used, the speed of the centrifuge, and the time necessary to spin the blood. Systems also differ in the final volume

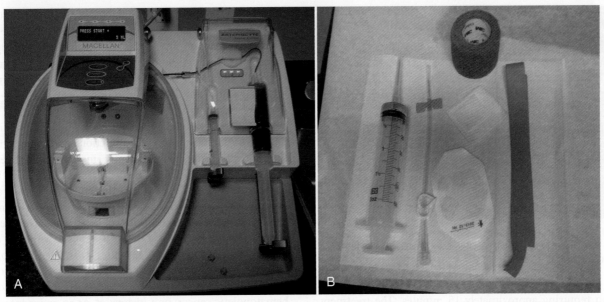

Fig. 10-1 **A,** Magellan Autologous Platelet Separator System (Arteriocyte Medical Systems). **B,** Platelet rich plasma blood collection kit (Magellan Arteriocyte Medical Systems.)

of PRP produced and the total number of platelets present in the concentrated product. As defined by the American Red Cross, PRP has 5.5×10^{10} platelets or greater per 50 mL of concentrate equaling a 2 to 7 times increase compared with whole blood. Normal platelet counts can vary between individuals. Platelet concentrations can vary greatly ranging from 2.5 to 8.0 times the concentration found in whole blood depending on the commercial system used.[4,22] Literature suggests that clinical benefits of platelet concentrations occur with the greatest predictability when a fourfold increase is achieved.[4,23] Unfortunately, evidence is lacking with regard to the appropriate and most clinically beneficial concentration of platelets.

Leukocyte concentration in PRP has become a topic of debate. Leukocyte concentrations can vary depending on the PRP system used. There is concern that the release of acid hydrolases and proinflammatory proteases from leukocytes may act as cytotoxic agents causing secondary damage to cells.[14,24]

PROCEDURAL TECHNIQUE FOR PRP DELIVERY

Treatment begins with the identification of the tissue (muscle, tendon, or ligament) and anatomic structures to be treated—after proper informed consent has been obtained and the procedure has been explained to the patient. Before treatment, pain medication is prescribed for the immediate postinjection period (3 to 5 days) and we instruct patients that nonsteroidal antiinflammatory medication cannot be used 2 to 3 weeks before and 6 to 8 weeks after the PRP treatment has been completed. Postinjection pain is common after PRP treatment. The duration and severity varies from patient to patient and with the specific tissue being treated. Before treatment, pre-PRP and post-PRP treatment

> **BOX 10-1** Pre-PRP and Post-PRP Treatment Instructions
>
> **Before PRP Treatment:**
> 1. Stop all nonsteroidal antiinflammatory drugs (NSAIDs) (e.g., Advil, Motrin, Aleve, Naproxen, Celebrex) 2 to 3 weeks before the procedure.
> 2. Apply heat packs to the painful areas 15 minutes every 2 to 3 hours as needed for pain.
> 3. Tylenol for pain as needed.
>
> **After PRP Treatment:**
> 1. Do not take NSAIDs after the procedure until told to resume use by your physician.
> 2. Apply heat packs to the painful areas 15 minutes every 2 to 3 hours as needed for pain. Use Tylenol or prescribed pain medications for pain as needed.
> 3. Perform range-of-motion exercises as tolerated after the procedure.
> 4. Increased pain and inflammation is expected in the treated tissue after the procedure.
> 5. Continue to use any braces, splints, or crutches as recommended by your physician after the treatment.

instructions are discussed with patients and all questions are answered. The patient is advised that it is normal to experience an increase in pain at the injection site after the PRP treatment, which may last for several days (Box 10-1).

The treatment area is cleaned with an alcohol/Betadine prep solution or Hibeclens solution before injection. Blood is drawn using a large bore fenestrated needle. The amount of blood drawn is dependent on the amount of PRP required for treatment. On average, 60 mL whole blood (to obtain 5 mL PRP) is drawn from the patient. The whole blood is placed into the centrifuge and the separation process is

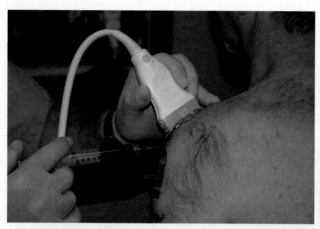

Fig. 10-2 The platelet rich plasma concentrate is delivered into the injured tissue through a 22-gauge needle under direct musculoskeletal ultrasound guidance.

begun requiring approximately 15 minutes. The treatment site is then anesthetized, first with an ethyl chloride spray followed by a local anesthetic injection of lidocaine.

When the separation process has been completed, the PRP concentrate is then delivered into the injured tissue through a 22-gauge needle under direct musculoskeletal ultrasound (US) guidance (Fig. 10-2). The precise placement of the PRP preparation is extremely important for overall outcome and efficacy of the procedure. The exact technique of delivery is dependent on the location of the tissue treated myotendinous, teno-osseous, or ligamentous. A "peppering" technique is used when treating tendons and ligaments. It is also important to touch bone at the osseous interface. Layering the PRP graft throughout the entire injury site in muscle, tendon, and ligamentous injuries will also help ensure complete coverage with the PRP preparation.

When treatment is completed, a sterile Band-Aid is applied. Protective splinting or bracing may be recommended after treating large weight-bearing tendons, such as the Achilles tendon, or areas where an extensive percutaneous tenotomy "peppering" has been performed. Application of heat after the procedure for 15 minutes every 2 to 3 hours is often recommended for postinjection pain management.

Strenuous activity for the first 7 days posttreatment is discouraged. Establishing normal range of motion after the procedure and performing activities of daily living (ADL) are encouraged as soon as possible posttreatment. At 4 to 6 weeks, the patient is reassessed. If pain persists at the treatment site a second PRP treatment might be considered at that time.

RISKS AND CONTRAINDICATION FOR PRP TREATMENT

PRP therapy is a safe and potentially very effective treatment modality for a variety of musculoskeletal soft tissue pathologies. Unfortunately, there is a paucity of randomized, placebo-controlled studies regarding treatment with PRP and its possible adverse effects. Although inherent risk is minimal, the same risks are present as with any percutaneous needle technique, including infection or puncturing a hollow

organ. When treatment is conducted with standard sterile technique, the risk of transmitting an infection or developing an allergic reaction after treatment with these autologous tissue preparations is effectively eliminated. The most common complaint from patients after PRP treatments is localized pain from the PRP injection itself.

There are a number of conditions in which treatment with PRP is contraindicated. Absolute contraindications for the use of PRP include: platelet dysfunction syndromes, critical thrombocytopenia, hemodynamic instability, septicemia, and hypofibrinogenemia. PRP treatments are relatively contraindicated in those patients that consistently used anti-inflammatory medications and systemic corticosteroid medications. It is also contraindicated in those who have received a corticosteroid injection at the treatment site within 14 days before treatment, have HGB levels less than 10 g/dL or platelet counts less than 105/µL, or have had recent fevers or illness, a rash at the donor or receptor site, bone cancer or hematopoietic cancer, or a history of, or an active infection with, *Enterococcus, Pseudomonas,* or *Klebsiella*.[12,25]

CLINICAL APPLICATION OF PRP

Despite the surge of interest in orthobiologic treatment modalities—and there recent widespread use for the treatment of a wide variety of soft tissue and boney injuries involving muscle, tendon, ligament, and articular cartilage—there remains a lack of animal and clinical studies demonstrating the efficacy of PRP. Although many studies report excellent outcomes, many of these studies unfortunately are limited case reports at best. Many of the current published studies are difficult to interpret because of the lack of standardization of PRP dosing, platelet acquisition and preparation, platelet concentration, growth factor quantity, number of treatments given, small patient sample sizes, and lack of control groups. Table 10-2 summarizes some of the recent published clinical studies regarding PRP.

REGULATION OF PRP IN SPORTS MEDICINE

The use of PRP in amateur and professional athletes remains controversial. In the United States, the use of PRP in professional sports, including the NFL, Major League Baseball, National Basketball Association, National Hockey League, Major League Soccer, National League Lacrosse, and Major League Lacrosse, is not regulated or prohibited. In addition, the National Collegiate Athletic Association currently does not regulate or prohibit the use of PRP in its participating institutions. Initially, the World Anti-Doping Agency (WADA) prohibited the use of platelet-derived preparations (PRP blood spinning) administered through an intramuscular route. Both the WADA and the U.S. Anti-doping Agency originally prohibited the injections of any growth factors affecting muscle, tendon, or ligament protein synthesis or degradation, vascularization, regenerative capacity, fiber type switching, or energy use.[14] Athletes required a therapeutic use exemption if this mode of treatment is

TABLE 10-2 Human Clinical Treatment Trials Using Platelet Rich Plasma[4,10]

Tissue	Author	Design	Level of Evidence	Study Results	Study Critique
Chronic elbow tendinosis	Mishra et al[46] 2006	Cohort, treated 15 patients with PRP	Level 2, only 5 controls	PRP patients had 93% pain reduction	Underpowered, randomized, not blinded, 3 of 5 controls left study at 8 wk
Rotator cuff	Randelli et al[47] 2008	14 patients	Level 4, case series	PRP safe and effective in treatment of rotator cuff	Small sample size
Achilles tendon	Sanchez et al[48] 2007	Case study, 6 Achilles repairs with PRP	Level 3, 6 matched retrospective controls	Plasma rich growth factor may be a new option for enhanced healing and functional recovery	Underpowered, small sample size, not randomized
Achilles tendon	de Vos et al[49] 2010	Double-blind, randomized, 54 patients	Level 1, randomized control	Improvement between groups nonsignificant	Underpowered, small sample size,
Patella tendinosis	Kon et al[50] 2009	Pilot study, 3 PRP injections, 20 patients with physical therapy	Level 4, case study	Function and pain improvement after treatment with PRP	Not controlled
Lateral epicondylitis	Peerblooms et al[51] 2010	Double-blind randomized, 100 patients, PRP vs. cortisone	Level 1, randomized controlled	Increased function exceeding the effect of corticosteroid	All patients had failed prior conservative treatment
Anterior cruciate ligament	Silva et al[52] 2009	Prospective study, 40 patients	Level 3, cohort controlled	PRP or thrombin did not appear to accelerate tendon healing	
Bone healing in nonunions	Sanchez et al[53] 2009	Retrospective, case study	Level 4, no control group	84% healed after surgical treatment; affects of PRGF unclear	Underpowered, randomized, retrospective, small sample size

PRP, Platelet rich plasma.

deemed necessary and recommended by a physician. Both organizations recently have changed their stance on PRP, since this is an autologous treatment of the patient's own blood products that have not been treated with any nonautologous growth factors.

THERAPY GUIDELINES FOR REHABILITATION

Rehabilitation progression following PRP injection is based on several individual factors: the combination of time since injection, the physiologic healing mechanism, patient's health and age, severity of injury, tissue integrity, response to physical therapy treatment dosage, and adherence to appropriate home programs. The goal of rehabilitation following PRP injections is to progressively and therapeutically place appropriate amounts of physical stress to the injured tissue to help facilitate healing. General guidelines following physiology are listed in Box 10-2. Physical stress to the tissue (muscle tendon, ligament, and bone) may include tension, torsion, compression, and shear. The stress or loading is imparted via manual therapy techniques, dosed medical exercise therapy progressions, functional strengthening, and return to play phase exercises. There is limited evidence in the literature defining specific protocols following PRP injection and limited documentation regarding tissue healing time frames following PRP injection. There is no absolute progression or transition between phases and there can be variability between patients pending each individual case.

The goal following PRP injection is to promote adequate tissue healing such that the tissue is able to once again maximally withstand the physiologic stresses and forces placed upon it with daily functional demands or sporting activities. Collagen fibers run in parallel alignment, which affords the tissue to withstand tensile forces and unilateral stress placed upon it.[26] The following information is based on clinical experience with patients who have undergone PRP injections to different tissues including muscle, tendon, bone, and ligament.

Phase I (Inflammatory Phase) (Table 10-3)

TIME: 0 to 7 days
GOALS: To allow the PRP to absorb at the injected tissue, to avoid cross-link disruption, and to facilitate integrity of cross link-formation

Phase I consists of early mobilization, gentle self-stretching, and weight-bearing functional activities to prevent the deleterious effects of immobilization and to promote tissue healing. Because of the elevated inflammatory response, the patient commonly feels an increase in pain for the next 1 to 3 days following the injection. Following PRP injection, the majority of the growth factors are released within the first hour of injection but continued release occurs up until about 7 days following injection.[24] Thus, the home program for the first 7 days following PRP injection is aimed at avoiding disruption of this physiologic mechanism and includes: rest, gentle active elbow motion, submaximal isometric holds in all pain-free planes and ranges to help fiber alignment, and heat to control symptoms. Functional outcome tools, such as the Kerlan-Jobe orthopedic score, shoulder pain and disability index and patellofemoral index

BOX 10-2 Four-Stage Rehabilitation Overview Following PRP Injection

Phase I: Postinjection—Inflammatory Phase (0 to 7 Days)

Pain peak and inflammatory response spikes and healing process commenced

- Patient response: Day 1 to 2: painful in the tissue/ joint; day 3 to 6: diminishing pain, improving significantly; day 7: sometimes no pain at all, improved quality of ROM
- Allow the PRP to absorb at the location
- Cross-link initiation and homeostasis occurring as PRP activating to prepare for cross-bridging
- Complete functional index tool (KJOC score, SCOR, SPADI) to establish baseline score
- Initiate home exercise program (HEP)—rest, gentle motion, isometric submaximal holds on all pain-free planes and ranges, heat to control symptoms

Phase II: Protection and Early Motion—Inflammatory Phase (7 to 21 Days):

Avoid homeostasis and cross-link disruption

- Maintain integrity of cross-link
- Continue active range of motion (ROM) and avoid overstretching; 90% full active ROM without stretching by end of week 2
- No ligament stressing or excessive muscle/tendon tension
- Light tissue mobilization to aid tissue fiber healing in line of stress and fiber line
- *2- to 4-week delay/slower progression with ligament injections because of decreased vascularization*

Phase III: High Repetition Loading and Light Activity— Reparative Phase (3 to 6 Weeks)

Pain threshold significantly reduced

- Adjust exercise progression based on type of tissue and severity of injury (ligaments longer to heal/ proliferate)
- Gap is filling in and matrix integrity improving
- Collagen synthesis, aligns in the longitudinal axis, tissue beginning to withstand tensile forces and loads
- Tissue stress testing/clinical examination to establish baseline

- Light deep transverse friction mobilizations, active release techniques, myofacial release
- Use of modalities to aid tissue proliferation (recommend pulsed ultrasound, laser, electrical stimulation)
- Begin-high repetition loading and concentrics (recommend 3 sets of 25 repetitions to improve tissue endurance and aid vascularization)
- Begin functional activities to mimic activities of daily living with focus on mechanics and correctness of movements. Progress with patient tolerance
- Include functional exercise in HEP
- Increased loading in the healing tissue in the direction of its fibers
- Active stretching: static and dynamic
- *Avoid ligament stress for 4 weeks with activities of daily living and exercise*

Progress to eccentrics in weeks 4 to 6

Phase IV: Eccentric Loading, Plyometric Training, Return to Sport/Activity—Remodeling Phase (6 to 12 Weeks*)

- Increased tensile strength of repaired tissue
- Improved ability to produce force and withstand tensile stretching and increased elasticity
- Continue tissue remodeling facilitation with deep transverse friction and soft tissue mobilizations
- *Eccentric loading*
- Progress to plyometrics, ballistics, explosive sport-specific activities, and exercises at approximately week 8 to 10, depending on patient status
- *Diagnostic ultrasound (approximately 8 weeks) may be repeated to determine extent of healing*
- Initiate interval sport programs (throwing, running, on field drills) pending results of diagnostic ultrasound
- Resume full functional or sporting activity at 10 to 12 weeks, depending on progress with postinjection program
- *Overlap of timelines is based on the patient's condition and severity of injury*
- *No antiinflammatory medications at home. No iontophoresis or phonophoresis in any of postinjection phases*

*Depending on individual sport and postinjection status; variable from patient to patient.

(SCOR), are commonly used to establish the patient's baseline subjective functional status.

Phase II (Inflammatory Phase) (Table 10-4)

TIME: 7 to 21 days
GOALS: To avoid disruption of collagen cross-link bridging and formation, and initiate early motion and high repetition loading exercises. Obtain 90% of full range of motion (ROM).

Phase II consists of continued gentle active elbow motion and increased activity at home. The patient should obtain greater than 90% of full ROM by the end of week 2. Light soft tissue mobilizations should commence to the ulnar collateral ligament (UCL) and common flexor origin and pronator teres at this time. **However, to avoid disruption of collagen cross-link bridging and formation, deeper soft tissue techniques (transverse friction, etc.) are not implemented until the third week following injection.** Gentle early motion of the elbow facilitates the physiologic tissue

TABLE 10-3 Platelet Rich Plasma Injection of the UCL (Inflammatory Phase)

Rehabilitation Phase	Criteria to Progress to this Phase	Anticipated Impairments and Functional Limitations	Intervention	Goal	Rationale
Phase I postinjection (0-7 days)	• Postinjection with no signs of infection	• Edema • Day 1-2: painful in the tissue/joint • Day 3-6: diminishing pain and improving significantly • Day 7: sometimes no pain at all, improved quality of ROM	• Initiate HEP rest, gentle active motion; isometric submaximal holds all pain-free planes and ranges; heat to control symptoms • No weights or stretching	• Allow the PRP to absorb at the injected tissue to cross-link disruption • Facilitate integrity of cross-link formation • Control edema and pain • Complete functional index tool (KJOC score, SCOR, SPADI) to establish baseline score	• Minimizes stress on injection site • Allow the PRP to absorb at the location • Prepare for cross bridging

HEP, Home exercise program; *KJOC*, Kerlan-Jobe orthopedic score; *PRP*, platelet rich plasma; *ROM*, range of motion; *SCOR*, patellofemoral index; *SPADI*, shoulder pain and disability index; *UCL*, ulnar collateral ligament.

TABLE 10-4 Platelet Rich Plasma Injection of the UCL (Inflammatory Phase)

Rehabilitation Phase	Criteria to Progress to This Phase	Anticipated Impairments and Functional Limitations	Intervention	Goal	Rationale
Phase II 7-21 days	• No signs of infection 2-4 wk delay/slower progression with ligament injections because of decreased vascularization	• Pain • Limited ROM • Pain with light UCL stress tests and activities of daily living • Limited UE strength	• Continue AROM, avoid valgus stress activities and overstretching; 90% full AROM without stretching by end of wk 2 • Continue modalities for symptom control • Wk 3: initiate light tissue mobilization to aid tissue fiber healing in line of stress and fiber line	• Control edema and pain • Minimize deconditioning • Initiate high repetition loading exercises and home exercise program	• Minimizes stress on injection site • Allow the PRP to absorb at the location • Prepare for cross bridging

AROM, Active range of motion; *PRP*, platelet rich plasma; *ROM*, range of motion; *UCL*, ulnar collateral ligament; *UE*, upper extremity.

healing response following PRP injection, which proceeds through the inflammatory, reparative, and remodeling phases. Furthermore, early motion and self-stretching prevent joint adhesions, increases muscle contraction, muscle fiber size, and tension, and increases resting levels of glycogen and protein synthesis. Submaximal-maximal effort elbow isometrics performed three times per day are also initiated in an attempt to create light tension in the direction of the tendon fibers. Intermittent rest and care with resuming work and normal daily functional activities are also encouraged at home to help control postinjection symptoms and early inflammatory elevation.

Progressive full arc motion in the first two phases prevents ligament atrophy and increases ligament linear tissue stress and stiffness, particularly at the bone-ligament junction. Ligament-stressing exercises or functional activities, as well as excessive muscle or tendon tension, are avoided during this phase. There may be a 2- to 4-week delay with ligament healing because of decreased tissue vascularization. **Exercises that exert tension on the UCL (valgus stress) are not begun until later (phase III).**

Early motion restoration aids connective tissue lubrication between collagen cross-links, increases collagen mass, decreases abnormal collagen cross-links, and prevents adhesion development. Following PRP injections, articular cartilage responds to early motion, intermittent compression, and decompression loading with improved metabolic activity and increased health of the cartilage matrix. Muscle, tendon, ligament, and bone tissue all respond favorably to motion. Restoring full elbow ROM is advocated during the first 10 to 14 days following PRP injection.

Modalities used in the first two phases of PRP rehabilitation can include US, laser, and electrical stimulation. The use of modalities during this phase is aimed at further stimulating tissue healing of the UCL and increasing local perfusion and oxygen delivery to the site. Nonthermal US is commonly used to facilitate tissue repair and regeneration in damaged tissue. There is research that supports the use of therapeutic US to increase bony and muscle tissue regeneration.[27-29] However, most studies that support the use of nonthermal US and a laser to aid tissue healing are based on animal studies. It is still unclear if using a pulsed nonthermal US is more effective than a low-intensity continuous protocol in terms of proliferation and tissue healing. The use of laser treatment in patients with lateral epicondylosis was found to lower subjective overall pain levels, with reports of 90% to 100% relief in over 45% of the patients who were treated with a laser.[30] Additionally, studies have found that the use of a low energy laser improves tensile strength and stiffness in repairing the medial collateral ligament in rats at 3 and 6 weeks after injury.[31] When rehabilitating after tendon PRP, we have found positive results using Russian electrical stimulation to help increase endorphin release and minimize tissue response to loading and manual mobilizations using the following parameters: 2500 Hz frequency, 50 pps, 10/10 seconds duty cycle, and 2 seconds ramp time for 10 to 12 minutes.

Progressive loading with shoulder, elbow, and wrist exercises during phases II to IV is a critical component of the post-PRP injection treatment plan. The first two phases include use of a concentric low-load, higher repetition exercise regimen: 3 sets of 20 to 25 repetitions are recommended. Once the patient reaches 3 sets of 25 repetitions, the weight is increased by 1 lb and progresses from there. Proper postural alignment, proximal and distal joint positioning, and control throughout the range, etc., are emphasized. This submaximal intensity using higher repetition progression improves tissue vascularization, helps align collagen crosslinks, promotes tissue healing, and enables the tissue to start adapting to controlled amounts of stress. Endurance training versus strengthening has been used in the early phases with success following PRP injections. Submaximal loading exercises reduce homeostasis, tissue breakdown, and symptom exacerbation during the first 2 to 4 weeks. Studies have demonstrated that resistance exercise is more effective in inducing acute muscle anabolism than high-load, low volume or work matched resistance exercise modes (isometrics).[32]

Phase III (Reparative Phase) (Table 10-5)

TIME: 3 to 6 weeks
GOALS: Adjust exercise progression based on type of tissue and severity of injury; use of modalities to aid tissue proliferation (recommend pulsed US, laser, electrical stimulation); begin high repetition loading and concentric; begin functional activities

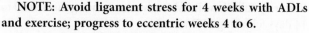

NOTE: Avoid ligament stress for 4 weeks with ADLs and exercise; progress to eccentric weeks 4 to 6.

Pain levels have typically lessened by the third week. Collagen synthesis is occurring and aligning in the longitudinal axis. At this point, the tissue is beginning to withstand tensile forces and loads. However, it is important to adjust exercise progression based on type of tissue and the severity of injury (ligament healing and proliferation take longer). Soft tissue mobilizations and progressive loading via resistance exercise are key components of the postinjection reparative and remodeling phases. The primary pathologic mechanism that leads to tendinopathy includes chronic microscopic tearing in hypovascular tendon tissue. These repetitive tears heal by

scar formation as opposed to the normal tendon healing pathways of vascularization and inflammation mechanisms.[33] Thus during the reparative and remodeling phase of muscle and tendon tissue, the use of soft tissue mobilization techniques (ASTYM, deep transverse friction mobilization, active release, Graston technique) in conjunction with appropriate exercise progressions is an important component of the healing process in order to help minimize scar formation and to promote anatomic tissue fiber healing in line of stress.

Deep transverse tissue massage (DTFM) and friction massage had been employed with positive results. As described by Cyriax,[34] DTFM is an aggressive form of soft tissue mobilization in which localized pressure or distractive manipulation of tissues is directed tangentially across the longitudinally oriented collagen component of the injured tissue. To promote normal resolution of the collagen tissue, the tissue to be treated should be in a moderate stretch position (not painful).[35] Deep transverse friction mobilizations and other soft tissue manipulation techniques have mechanical, physiologic, histologic, and neurologic effects on the tissue that facilitate the healing mechanism of PRP injections (Box 10-3). Reaction to DTFM may include rapid desensitization, latent posttreatment soreness, and moderate tissue bruising covering the area of tissue contact.[34]

Eccentric loading is initiated early in the reparative and remodeling phases at approximately weeks 4 to 6, depending on the individual patient's status. Because of its positive effect on improving tissue integrity, strength, and function, eccentric loading is the other important component of the post-PRP injection rehabilitation. Eccentric contractions function to decelerate a limb, provide shock absorption, and

---

BOX 10-3 Effects of Deep Transverse Tissue Mobilization

Mechanical
- Distortion and elongation of collagen fibers
- Increased interstitial mobility

Physiologic
- Localized hyperemia
- Stimulate white blood cell invasion and healing production
- Destruction of P substance

Histologic
- Prevents scar formation and haphazard collagen orientation
- Stimulate collagen orientation along lines of stress via "piezoelectric effect"

Neurologic
- Initial nociceptor stimulation
- Mechanoreceptor stimulation
- Pain inhibition via "central biasing mechanism"

TABLE 10-5 Platelet Rich Plasma Injection of the UCL (Reparative Phase)

Rehabilitation Phase	Criteria to Progress to This Phase	Anticipated Impairments and Functional Limitations	Intervention	Goal	Rationale
Phase III 3-6 wk	• Full ROM • No increase in pain • Pain-free moving valgus, milking stress tests and UCL stress at 0°, 30°, and 90° by end of this phase	• Limited UE strength • Limited tissue tolerance to valgus tensile loading exercises or functional activities until wk 5-6 • Pain (diminishing) • Limited tolerance with heavier lifting, pushing, pulling functional activities	• Glenohumeral stretching (HBB towel, glenohumeral flexion doorway stretching, sleeper stretch) • Shoulder strengthening program: Jobe or thrower's ten exercises, prone Hughston's progression* • Pulley concentrics 0-2 lb weight • Elbow flexion, extension (supinated grip to decrease UCL load), supination (3 sets, 15 reps) • Wrist flexion, extension, radial deviation, ulnar deviation (3 sets, 15 repetitions) • PNF and rhythmic • Stabilization exercises to shoulder only—proximal hand placement (humerus) • Scapulothoracic PNF patterns and strengthening • CKC weight shifting (elbows unlocked) **Wk 5-6:** Initiate light stretching and valgus loading of elbow (*if no pain with moving valgus, milking stress tests and UCL stress at 0°, 30°, and 90°*) • Continue deep transverse friction mobilization/massage to increase tissue vascularization and break up tissue adhesions	• Maintain glenohumeral mobility • Break up tissue adhesions • Protect from valgus loading • Increase UE function • Prepare for sport-specific interval program	• Use modalities to facilitate collagen formation and remodeling • Cross bridging occurring and matrix integrity improving • Promote full elbow ROM • Nonpainful safe elbow and wrist strengthening • Start emphasizing biceps, pronator teres, and FCU group concentrics to support medial elbow • Increase proximal joint flexibility • Cardiovascular training to improve endurance • Progress toward light valgus loading by end of phase III • UE strength gains advancing toward sport-specific retraining phase • UCL tensile strength should be strong enough to initiate valgus loading exercises

*http://www.dynoswim.com/archives/ShoulderRotatorExer.pdf.
CKC, Closed kinetic chain; *FCU*, flexor carpi ulnaris, *HBB*, hand behind back; *PNF*, proprioceptive neuromuscular facilitation; *ROM*, range of motion; *UCL*, ulnar collateral ligament; *UE*, upper extremity.

generate forces 14% to 50% greater than a maximal concentric contraction does.[36] This increased force generation improves musculotendinous integrity by inducing muscle hypertrophy and increased tensile strength, or by lengthening the musculotendinous unit.[37]

Unlike with concentric phase I to II exercises, eccentric loading has been shown to aid in stable angiogenesis in early tendon injury.[38] Daily eccentric loading was found not to have any detrimental effect on tendon vascularity or microcirculation.[38] A systematic review of tendinopathy found that eccentric exercises had the most clinical efficacy in regenerating function.[39] Other studies have found that eccentric exercise progressions are an effective treatment for chronic

tendinosis.[40,41] Eccentric tendon loading exercise progressions are thus implemented into postinjection rehabilitation by week 4, depending upon the individual patient's response through the first 2 to 4 weeks. By the end of week 6, more advanced exercise may begin (Figs. 10-3 through 10-8).

Whereas the prior table provides an overview of exercise progressions for UCL following PRP injection, examples of tendon treatment and exercise progressions are also provided (Boxes 10-4 and 10-5).

There is no clear consensus on the best nonoperative treatment for muscle injuries beyond immediate rest and antiinflammatory medications or modalities.[28] In chronic tendinosis injuries, rest has been found to be a less effective

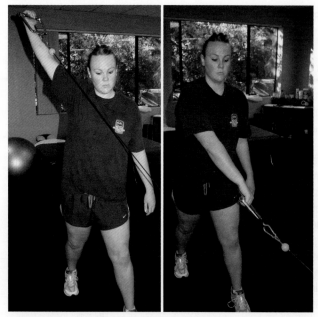

Fig. 10-3 Proprioceptive neuromuscular facilitation pulley pattern using lighter weight or speed pulley. Alter arm angle and arc of motion to simulate functional task or sport-specific plane.

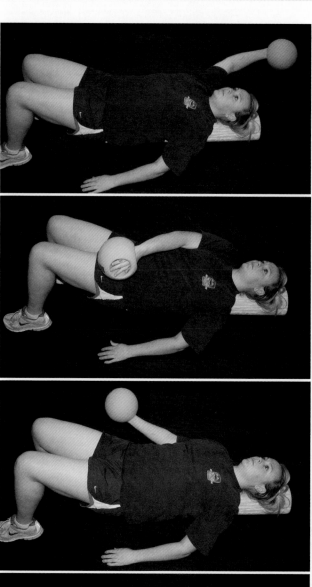

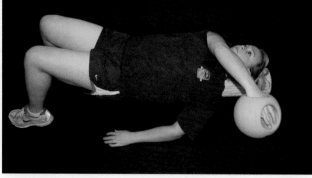

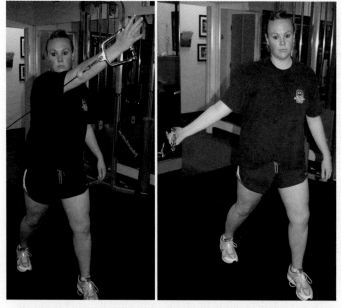

Fig. 10-4 Upper extremity pulley pattern to stress ulnar collateral ligament. Can alter plane, elbow flexion angle, and/or forearm position to alter stress through ulnar collateral ligament. Performing with hand in supinated position (underhand Frisbee toss) places further stress on ulnar collateral ligament.

Fig. 10-5 Upper extremity D1 D2 proprioceptive neuromuscular facilitation patterns using foam roller and Plyoball. Alter arm angle to challenge glenohumeral and stability or alter ulnar collateral ligament stress throughout range. Maintain core contraction keeping trunk centered on roller. Bring knees and feet together to further challenge core stability while performing the pattern.

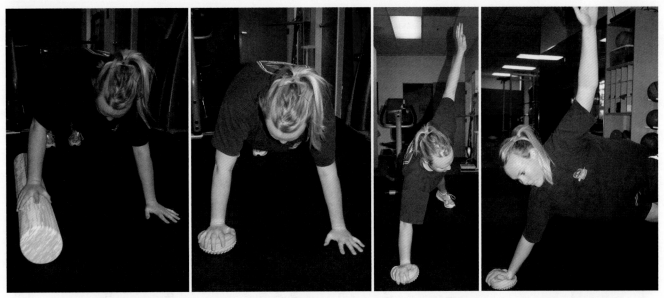

Fig. 10-6 Upper extremity D1 D2 proprioceptive neuromuscular facilitation patterns using Physioball. Maintain transverse abdominis contraction, keeping hips level and ball controlled. Bring knees closer together to challenge stability. Patient can perform at varying speeds while maintaining stability. Performing with eyes closed further challenges balance mechanism.

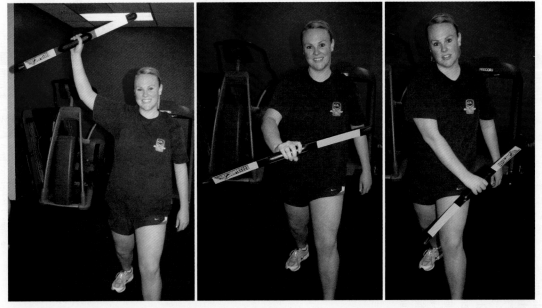

Fig. 10-7 Upper extremity patterns using Body Blade. Progress from static holds in different ranges to performing functional throwing/serving patterns. Emphasis is on endurance and longer duration holds.

treatment.[39,42] In turn, eccentric exercise and loading has been shown in many studies to be beneficial in treating patients with tendinosis.[37,38] However, the optimal dosage and frequency of eccentric loading for treating chronic tendinosis has not yet been established.[43]

Phase IV (Remodeling Phase) (Table 10-6)

TIME: 6 to 12 weeks
GOALS: Eccentric loading, plyometric training return to sport/activity; (depending upon individual sport and

postinjection status [variable from patient to patient]); continue tissue remodeling facilitation with deep transverse friction and soft tissue mobilizations

Note: Diagnostic US (at approximately 8 weeks) may be repeated to determine the extent of healing; resume full functional or sporting activity in 10 to 12 weeks depending on progress with postinjection program.

The injected tissue commonly demonstrates increased tensile strength by the remodeling phase. Tissue remodeling facilitation is continued in phase IV with the use of deep

TABLE 10-6 Platelet Rich Plasma Injection of the UCL (Reparative Phase)

Rehabilitation Phase	Criteria to Progress to This Phase	Anticipated Impairments and Functional Limitations	Intervention	Goal	Rationale
Phase IV 6-14 wk	• Objective examination results, functional testing, and subjective functional tool score indicate patient is ready to progress through phase IV to return to play status • Provocation stress test results negative (moving valgus, milking, and UCL stress tests at 30°-70°) • *Overlap of timelines is based on the patient's condition and severity of injury*	• Limited UE strength • Limited UCL tensile strength early phase IV • Altered timing and mechanics with sport-specific and functional activities	• Continue tissue remodeling and deep transverse friction mobilization • Progress Jobe exercises and add 3-4 lb • Start inner- to mid-range glenohumeral IR loading (3 sets, 15 reps) • ER progression to mid- and outer-range planes at 90/90 • Continue concentric to eccentric rotator cuff strengthening • Start upright bilateral Plyoball patterns • Light concentric resistance pulley or tubing patterns • Light resistance PNF using distal hand placements and initiating elbow and wrist motions • Light valgus loading functional pulley patterns • Early CKC exercises Wk 6-8: • Progress to fast twitch and dynamic exercises (nonthrowing medicine ball and tubing) • Increase speed and functional strengthening • Phase III-IV core strengthening • Add towel throw drills if no pain with UCL stress tests; focus on head/trunk position, balance and alignment Wk 8-10: • *Depending upon repeated US imaging findings, progress to return to play phase* • *May begin controlled overhead return to sport activities (simulated towel drills, shadow drills, controlled plyo pulley patterns, increased speed with mid- to outer-range exercises)* • Progress to two-hand throwing with lighter weight medicine ball/rebounder drills; continue CKC progression Wk 10-12: • Progress to 50%-75% of activity effort (short toss-long toss) • Begin interval return to sport program • **Start interval throwing, batting, tennis strokes, volleyball hitting programs pending repeat US imaging findings** • Outer-range cuff strengthening, ballistics, speed pulley patterns • Inner-range slide board/fitter drills for valgus loading • Rebounder tossing progressions (2 hand chest pass, overhead throw ins, shot puts, single overhed throws, eccentrics) • CKC plyometrics • Week 12: Progress from 75%-90% in controlled setting • Weeks 12-14: Gradual return to sport	• Increase UE strength • Increased muscular control • Improve UCL tensile strength • No pain with higher speed valgus loading exercises • Prepare for return to play and prior level of function • Train with sport-specific exercise progressions • Establish and transition to independent home exercise program	• Reassess functional index score to correlate with objective examination findings and determine return-to-play status • Specificity of training • Use of neuromuscular reeducation patterns to simulate functional activity, and enhance joint control and stability • Improved ability to produce force and withstand tensile loads • Increased tissue elasticity • Sport-specific interval program to enable safe return to prior functional status

CKC, Closed kinetic chain; *ER,* external rotation; *IR,* internal rotation; *PNF,* proprioceptive neuromuscular facilitation; *UCL,* ulnar collateral ligament; *UE,* upper extremity; *US,* ultrasound.

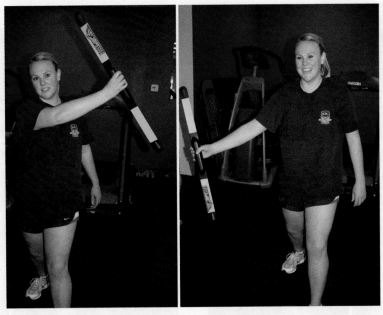

Fig. 10-8 Upper extremity patterns using Body Blade. Progress from static holds in different ranges to performing functional throwing/serving patterns. Emphasis is on endurance and longer duration holds.

transverse friction and soft tissue mobilizations. Depending on the response to the eccentric strengthening progression, the patient progresses to speed and coordination drills, plyometrics, ballistics, and more explosive, sport-specific phase IV exercises (Figs. 10-9 through 10-18).

At this point connective tissue has improved tensile strength because its fiber orientation is better aligned and suited to withstand more demanding tensile stress.[44] The functional strengthening, plyometrics, ballistics, neuromuscular power, and coordination exercises are performed at more intense levels to enable the patient to meet the demands of his or her sport or job activity. Typically, selective tissue tension tests (ligament stress tests, resistance muscle-tendon tests in lengthened position, weight-bearing and compression tests for bone) are nonprovocative. The use of follow-up functional tools is recommended to ascertain the patient's readiness to resume higher level exercises, and return to sport or work. Studies have not yet been published regarding the efficacy of using scores on subjective functional tools or questionnaires to help determine when a patient is ready to safely resume a particular activity or sport given a certain subjective score.

There is no clearly defined or objective means of determining when an athlete is able to safely return to play or a patient is able to return to a functional activity (job duty). A grading system has been used to describe tendinopathy.[45] However, the use of a detailed clinical examination together with the repeat US imaging findings, as well as the patient's subjective assertions and functional index score, are all used to assist the physician, therapist, and athletic trainer in determining when the patient is ready to resume the desired activity. Interval running programs, on field agility progressions, and interval throwing programs are initiated in phase IV. Although there are several notable documented cases in which an athlete has returned to play at an earlier time

TABLE 10-7 Timeline for Return to Activity or Interval Return Sport Phase IV

Weeks			
<1-2	<3-4	>10-12	>11-12 weeks
Rest and Therapy	Muscle Belly	Tendinosis	Ligaments

Ligament healing may be delayed 2-4 weeks; avoid varus/valgus stress for 6 weeks.

period following PRP injection, most patients have been able to resume full functional or sporting activity by 10 to 12 weeks (Table 10-7).

CONCLUSIONS

The use of orthobiologic modalities such as PRP in orthopedics and sports medicine to deliver high concentrations of naturally occurring biologically active growth factors and proteins to the site of injury is very promising. However, there remain significant clinical and basic science questions that need to be answered regarding the use of PRP in clinical practice. Questions still remain regarding the optimal concentration of PRP, how many injections are optimal, and the timing of treatments in the acute and or chronic settings. Other questions that need to be addressed include what is the optimal physiologic environment for these injections to be performed and how can PRP be optimally used in specific tissue, including muscle, tendon, ligament, or bone. Questions regarding optimal post-PRP treatment rehabilitation also need to be defined. Although PRP is widely being used in clinical practice today, a significant amount of basic science and clinical research remains to be done to define the optimal use and overall safety of PRP therapy in clinical practice.

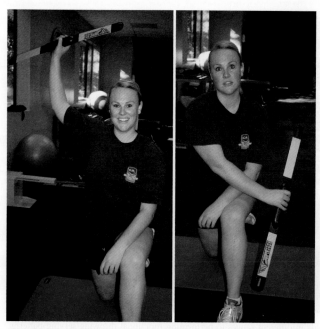

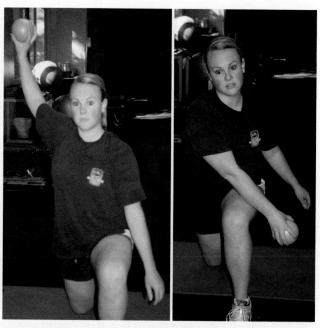

Fig. 10-9 Upper extremity strengthening in half-kneel position using Body Blade. Emphasis on scapular control, upright head/trunk position, and stability throughout pattern.

Fig. 10-10 Upper extremity strengthening in half-kneel position using Plyoball. Emphasis on scapular control, upright head/trunk position, and stability throughout pattern.

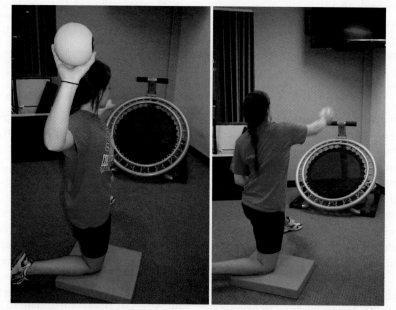

Fig. 10-11 Overhead rebounder tossing in half-kneel position. Emphasis placed on maintaining upright balance and trunk control through upper extremity strengthening pattern. Recommend using lighter weight balls (4 oz to 2 lb). Encourage and facilitate pelvis/trunk rotation and "uncoiling" mechanism for overhead athletes.

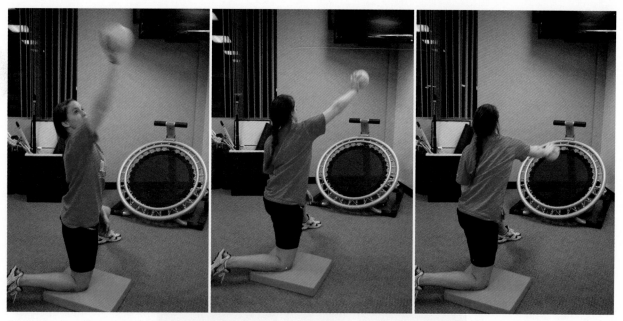

Fig. 10-12 Rotator cuff eccentrics. Patient is in half-kneel position and catches ball thrown from behind. Emphasize ball deceleration via rotator cuff and periscapular muscles by counting to 5 seconds while eccentrically lowering the ball to completion of the "follow-through" phase of the throwing arc. Emphasize a faster 2-second concentric acceleration toss back to thrower (clinician) standing behind the patient.

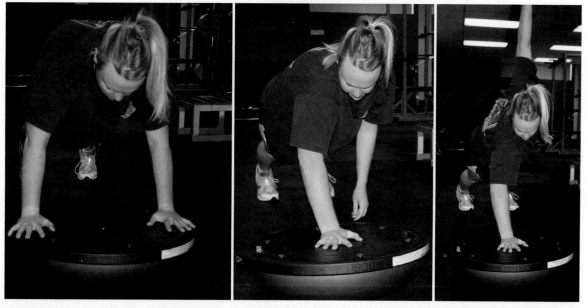

Fig. 10-13 Closed kinetic chain bilateral to single upper extremity progressions using balance disk, Bosu ball. Perform while maintaining scapula held in different retraction/protraction positions. Maintain core stability throughout.

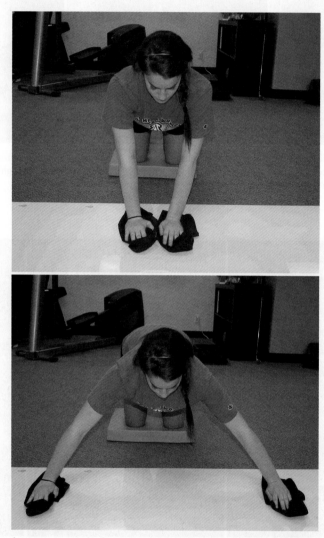

Fig. 10-14 Ulnar collateral ligament and upper extremity loading using slide board patterns. Recommend inner-range slides to assess ulnar collateral ligament tolerance to loading and progressively increase slide out distance. Can perform straight planar patterns, up/down "pluses," or diagonal angles to challenge upper extremity. Progress from performing on two knees to performing in push-up position on toes.

BOX 10-4 Post-PRP Injection Exercise Progressions—Supraspinatus/Infraspinatus Tendon Examples

Weeks 1 to 2:

No strengthening, gentle range of motion (ROM) activities only, low-grade cardiovascular training

Week 2:

Begin submaximal isometrics, progress to gravity elimi-nated strengthening or use of counterweighted pulley (3 sets of 25 reps) to increase tendon vascularization, and passive ROM and active/assisted ROM exercises within pain-free range (no stretching emphasis)

Weeks 2 to 3:

High repetition loading and submaximal to maximal isometric mid and outer ranges. Begin prone Hughston exercises (2 sets, 10 reps each); isolated supraspinatus/infraspinatus loading; Jobe or thrower's ten exercises 0- to 2-lb-weight (3 sets 15 reps); concentric mid-range internal/external rotation muscle energy technique pulley progres-sions (3 sets, 25 reps); scapulothoracic program (scapular pluses, depressions, lower/mid trapezius exercises, such as Ys, Ts, Ws over ball, scapular setting exercises) cardio-vascular training

Weeks 3 to 4:

Progress Jobe exercises and add 3 to 4 lb. Glenohumeral and scapulothoracic rhythmic stabilization (SRS) and pro-prioceptive neuromuscular facilitation (PNF) light tubing or pulley patterns (high repetition loading); Body Blade pat-terns focusing on time/endurance; outer-range rotator cuff strengthening; cardiovascular training

Weeks 4 to 5:

Progress to fast twitch, eccentrics, and dynamic exercises (nonthrowing medicine ball and tubing); PNF reversals,

higher speed pulley and Plyoball patterns; UE isokinetic strengthening; continue core strengthening and cardiovas-cular training; for throwers, integrate core strengthening and check glenohumeral internal rotation range. Integrate self-stretching (hand-behind-back towel, supine hand behind back, sleeper stretch) for cuff or capsule if appropriate

Weeks 5 to 7:

Depending upon status, may begin controlled overhead return to sport activities (simulated towel and throwing drills, shadow drills). Progress to two-hand throwing medicine/plyometric ball drills and early bilateral closed kinetic chain (CKC) girdle exercises; overhead strengthen-ing with Plyoballs, pulleys, and rebounder

Weeks 6 to 8:

Progress to 50% to 75% of activity effort. Begin interval return to sport program (short-toss, long-toss progression; 50% overhead tennis serves; free style swim strokes—all in controlled arcs and ranges). Light contact and may begin bilateral to single closed chain exercise progres-sions; progress to single overhead plyometrics, rebounder tossing

Weeks 7 to 10:

Progress from 75% to 90% in controlled setting. Return to contact.

Weeks 8 to 10:

Gradual return to sport

Overlap of timelines is based on the patient's condition and severity of injury

BOX 10-5 Post-PRP Patellar/Achilles Tendon Exercise Progression Example

Week 1:

Begin passive range of motion (ROM) for physical therapy only in the first week; towel slides in pain-free range for patellar tendon; PWB walking boot (Achilles); crutches if needed to unload tendon during gait

Week 2:

Begin low-level closed chain activity (ball sits with single-leg balance/stability/Biomechanical Ankle Platform System, standing weight shifts, standing single leg squat balance). Should get 90% of ROM without stretching by end of week 2; start submaximal isometric holds; 4-way straight leg raise; proximal joint strengthening; initiate joint mobilizations to maintain normal osteokinematics; initiate core strengthening and home exercise program; walking and light stationary bike resistance only

Weeks 3 to 4:

Begin gentle self-stretching and home exercise program; progress submaximal to maximal isometrics; start stationary bike/swimming and cardiovascular training; form run at walk pace; Thera-Band ankle foot proprioceptive neuromuscular facilitation (PNF) patterns; initiate bilateral high repetition, counterweighted, mid-range long kinetic chain (LKC) concentric strengthening (shuttle, total gym); bilateral heel raises from neutral to full plantar flexion ranges; single-leg stance (SLS) proprioception training exercises; maintain proximal joint flexibility, progress with proximal hip, and core strengthening exercises; phase II LKC proprioception retraining

Weeks 5 to 6:

Single-leg, high repetition CKC strengthening progressions; single concentric heel raises (outer-range tendon strengthening); continue cardiovascular training (stationary bike, can begin elliptical); integrate phase III SLS proprioception exercises; light trampoline weight shifts to low intensity trampoline jog intervals; start submaximal effort, higher speed isokinetics

Weeks 6 to 7:

Initiate LKC eccentrics (step up/down progressions, decline squats, heel raises (2 up, 1 down eccentric loading), Bosu ball progressions; SLS proprioception training on uneven surfaces; initiate trot or light jogging activities and 50% effort ladder drills; continue higher speed isokinetics, 75% effort

Weeks 8 to 10:

Continue longer duration cardiovascular training (elliptical, stationary bike, swimming); continue eccentric loading and isokinetic strengthening; begin bilateral counterweighted greater than body weight jump progressions on (shuttle/total gym); increase speed of agility, ladder, and controlled change of direction drills; controlled and low intensity (in place) return to sport drills, 50% to 75% effort; initiate jog, stride, and light run straight planes (no decelerations); progressive 40 to 60 yards (jog and stride). Initiation of interval programs (not long duration) depends on repeat ultrasound imaging findings, objective examination results, functional testing, and subjective functional tool scores

Weeks 10 to 12:

Continue eccentric strengthening; bilateral to single-leg jump progressions, cutting activities, sprints, and change of direction drills; progress toward single plyometrics at approximately week 10; continue functional strengthening; begin sprinting and return to sport on field activities; maximal effort isokinetic strengthening

Week >12:

Gradual return to sport

Overlap of timelines is based on the patient's condition and severity of injury

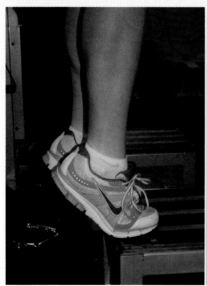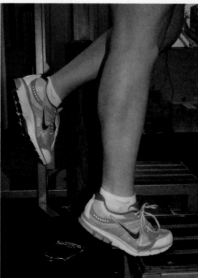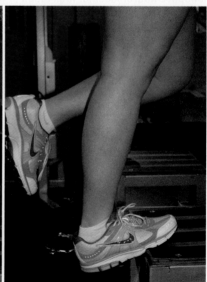

Fig. 10-15 Eccentric Achilles loading "two up, one down" decelerations. Emphasize slow controlled eccentric dorsiflexion.

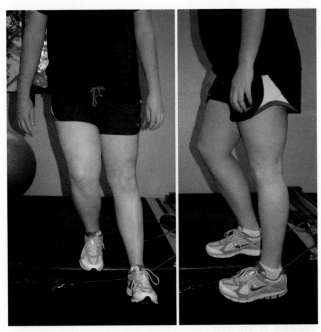

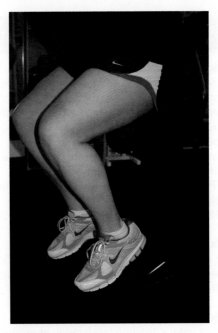

Fig. 10-16 Step down progression. Focus on sagittal plane long kinetic chain alignment, frontal plane pelvic stability, and transverse plane subtalar joint position throughout exercise. Shifting weight to metatarsal heads (maintaining heel contact on ground) on forward step down adds further tension to patellar tendon.

Fig. 10-17 Single Bosu ball squats.

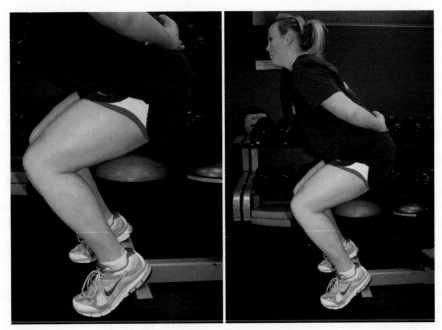

Fig. 10-18 Decline squat examples. Increased tension is placed through patellar tendon with decline squatting. Add hand weights or incorporate with closed kinetic chain isokinetic strengthening.

Suggested Home Maintenance Program Post-UCL PRP Injection

Weeks 1 to 2:

No strengthening, no activity, gentle passive range of motion (PROM) only

   Treatment: Avoid all valgus stressing activities/exercises × 4 weeks

1. Modalities (ice)
2. Isometric elbow strengthening (BID): inner- to mid-range submaximal holds
3. HEP (rest, heat, passive to light active motion, no resistance exercises or loading)
4. ROM emphasis: passive to light active ROM

Week 2:

Begin active range of motion (AROM) exercise elbow flexion, extension, and wrist; all planes within pain-free range (no weights or stretching)

Week 3:

- Avoid valgus loading (resistance shoulder internal rotation) or ligament stretching
- Maintain glenohumeral flexibility (HBB towel, glenohumeral flexion doorway stretching, sleeper stretch)
- Elbow flexion, extension (supinated grip to decrease UCL load), supination (3 sets, 20 reps)
- Wrist flexion, extension, radial deviation, ulnar deviation (3 sets, 20 reps)
- Flexion, scaption, speeds with pulleys/free weights
- Scapular mid and low rows
- Closed kinetic chain (CKC) weight shifting (elbows unlocked); upright scapular pluses against wall
  Start emphasizing biceps, pronator teres, and flexor carpi ulnaris (FCU) group concentrics to support medial elbow
  Shoulder exercises to be performed with physical therapy in the clinic to ensure proper technique

Weeks 4 to 6:

Add/begin functional diagonal and proprioceptive neuromuscular facilitation (PNF) patterns

- Initiate elbow, wrist, and hand resistance exercises. Begin with concentrics in controlled ranges, light tubing with chest press, and rows (3 sets, 15 to 20 reps)
- Add more scapular strengthening progressions (lawn mower pulls, cross hearts, depressions, Kibler scapular exercises)
- Scapular pluses and standing wall push-ups, or counterweighted (shuttle) scapular protractions
- Ball ER rolls against wall
  †Start inner- to mid-range glenohumeral IR (3 sets, 15 reps)

- ER side-lying or pulleys progress to mid- and outer-range planes @ 90/90
- Early CKC exercises (quadruped weight shifting, alternate arm/leg lifts, scapular pluses)
- Continue scapular strengthening progressions; add barrel hugs, modified push-ups on hands, knees

Weeks 6 to 8:

- Progress to fast twitch and dynamic exercises (nonthrowing medicine ball and tubing)
- Increase speed and functional strengthening phase III to IV progressions
- Continue all earlier phase exercise
- Add towel throws if no pain with UCL stress tests; focus on head/trunk position, balance and alignment

Weeks 8 to 10:

Pending follow-up US imaging findings progress to return to play phase IV exercises

- May begin controlled overhead return to sport activities (simulated towel drill, shadow drills, controlled plyometric pulley patterns, increased speed with mid- to outer-range exercises, progress to two-hand throwing with lighter weight medicine ball/rebounder drills); CKC progression including walkouts, step overs
- Isokinetic strengthening

Weeks 10 to 12:

Progress to 50% to 75% of activity effort (short toss, long toss). Begin interval return to sport/throwing program (Chapter 13). Start interval throwing, batting, tennis serve, volleyball hitting programs pending repeat US imaging findings, objective examination results, functional testing, and subjective functional tool score

- Cuff strengthening: outer ranges, ballistics, speed pulley patterns; inner range: slide board/fitter drills for valgus loading
- Rebounder progressions (two-hand chest pass, overhead throw ins, shot puts, single overhead throws, eccentrics)
- CKC plyometrics

Weeks 10 to 12:

Progress from 75% to 90% in controlled setting

Weeks 12 to 14:

Gradual return to sport

Overlap of timelines is based on the patient's condition and severity of injury

CLINICAL CASE REVIEW

1 Paul is 2 weeks post-PRP injection. He is complaining of continued medial elbow pain. Is phonophoresis/iontophoresis an appropriate choice for treatment?

No. Nonsteroidal antiinflammatory medication cannot be used 2 to 3 weeks before and 6 to 8 weeks after the PRP treatment has been completed.

2 Sam is 4 weeks post-PRP injection for a partial UCL tear. He continues to experience medial elbow pain that is limiting his progression through rehabilitation. What must be considered?

At this stage a call into the physician should be made and the potential of a second PRP injection should be considered.

3 During the initial phases of rehabilitation, what exercises should be avoided?

Any exercise that places a valgus stress on the elbow (shoulder internal rotation and proprioceptive neuromuscular facilitation [PNF] patterns with distal hand placement should be avoided)

4 Doug is 8 weeks postinjection and is making excellent progress. What must be considered before progressing to throwing activities?

Of prime concern is why the UCL was exposed and torn to begin with. Throwing mechanics should be a main concern. Doug should be performing exercises recommended in the Return to Throwing chapter, and videotaped initially and periodically thereafter to evaluate his throwing technique and progression through the throwing program.

5 What is the effectiveness of PRP injections?

The success rate for PRP injections has been reported as high as 85% in some cases. The success of the treatment depends on a number of factors, the most important being choosing the appropriate patient. I have noted a high rate of success and publication of my data is pending. However, more studies need to be done to validate the effectiveness before PRP injection can be considered a routine procedure for soft tissue injuries.

6 What is the best treatment course for an acute muscle injury?

There is no clear consensus on the best nonoperative treatment for muscle injuries beyond immediate rest and antiinflammatory medications or modalities.

7 Is rest an effective tool in managing chronic soft tissue dysfunction (tendinosis)?

In the case of chronic tendinosis injuries, rest has been found to be a less effective treatment. In turn, eccentric exercise and loading has been shown in many studies to be beneficial in treating patients with tendinosis.

REFERENCES

1. Ferrari M, et al: A new technique for hemodilution, preparation of autologous platelet-rich plasma and interoperative blood salvage in cardiac surgery. Int J Artif Org 10:47-50, 1987.

2. Gamradt SC, et al: Platelet rich plasma in rotator cuff repair. Tech Orthop 22(1):26-33, 2007.

3. Everts PA, et al: Platelet rich plasma and platelet gel: A review. J Extra Corpor Technol 38:174-187, 2006.

4. Cole BJ, et al: Platelet-rich plasma: Where are we now and where are we going? Sports Health 2(3):203-210, 2010.

5. Cervelli V, et al: Application of platelet-rich plasma in plastic surgery: Clinical and in vitro evaluation. Tissue Eng Part C Methods 15(4):625-634, 2009.

6. Kazakos K, et al: The use of autologous PRP gel as an aid in the management of acute trauma wounds. Injury 40(8):837-845, 2009.

7. Marx RE: Platelet-rich plasma: Evidence to support its use. J Oral Maxillofac Surg 62(4):489-496, 2004.

8. McCarrel T, Fontier LA: Temporal growth factor release from platelet-rich plasma trehalose lyophilized platelets and bone marrow aspirate and their effect on tendon and ligament gene expression. J Orthop Res 27(8):1033-1042, 2009.

9. Sanchez AR, Sheridan PJ, Kupp LI: Is platelet-rich plasma the perfect enhancement factor? A current review. Int J Oral Maxillofac Implants 18(1):93-103, 2003.

10. Foster, et al: Platelet-rich plasma: From basic science to clinical applications. Am J Sports Med 37(11):2258-2272, 2009.

11. Marx RE: Platelet-rich plasma (PRP): What is PRP and what is not PRP? Implant Dent 10(4):225-228, 2001.

12. Crane D, Everts P: Platelet rich plasma (PRP) matrix grafts. Pract Pain Manag 8(1):12-26, 2008.

13. Kevy SV, Jacobson MS: Comparison of methods for point of care preparation of autologous platelet gell. J Extra Corpor Technol 36:28-35, 2004.

14. Borrione P, et al: Platelet-rich plasma in muscle healing. Am J Phys Med Rehabil 89:854-861, 2010.

15. Frechette JP, Martineau I, Gagnon G: Platelet-rich plasmas: Growth factor content and roles in wound healing. J Dent Res 84(5):434-439, 2005.

16. Eppley BL, Woodell JE, Higgins J: Platelet quantification and growth factor analysis from platelet-rich plasma: implications for wound healing. Plast Reconstr Surg 114(6):1502-1508, 2004.

17. Anitua E, et al: Autologous platelets as a source of proteins for healing and tissue regeneration. Thromb Haemost 90(3):377-384, 2003.

18. Creaney L, Hamilton B: Growth factor delivery methods in the management of sports injuries: the state of play. Br J Sports Med 42(5):314-320, 2008.

19. Mishra A, Woodall JJ, Viera A: Treatment of tendon and muscle using platelet-rich plasma. Clin Sports Med 28(1):113-124, 2009.

20. Bennett NT, Schultz GS: Growth factors and wound healing: Biochemical properties of growth factors and their receptors. Am J Surg 165(6):728-737, 1993.

21. Los G, et al: Macrophage infiltration in tumors and tumor-surrounding tissue: Influence of serotonin and sensitized lymphocytes. Cancer Immunol Immunother 26(2):145-152, 1988.

22. de Mos M, et al: Can platelet-rich plasma enhance tendon repair? A cell culture study. Am J Sports Med 36(6):1171-1178, 2008.

23. Marx RE: Platelet-rich plasma (PRP): What is PRP and what is not PRP? Implant Dent 10(4):225-228, 2001.

24. Hammond JW, et al: Use of autologous platelet-rich plasma to treat muscle strain injuries. Am J Sports Med 37:1135-11342, 2009.

25. Bielecki TM, et al: Antibacterial effect of autologous platelet gel enriched with growth factors and other active substances: An in vitro study. J Bone Joint Surg 89(3):417-420, 2007.

26. Donatelli R, Owens-Burkhart A: Effects of immobilization on the extensibility of periarticular connective tissue. J Orthop Sports Phys Ther 3:67-72, 1981.

27. Byl NN, et al: Pulsed microamperage stimulation: A controlled study of healing of surgically induced wounds in Yucatan pigs. Phys Ther 74:201-213; discussion 213-218, 1994.

28. Chan YS, et al: The use of suramin, an antifibrotic agent, to improve muscle recovery after strain injury. Am J Sports Med 33:43-51, 2005.

29. Gum S, et al: Combined ultrasound, electrical stimulation, and laser promote collagen synthesis with moderate changes in tendon biomechanics. Am J Phys Med Rehabil 76:288-296, 1997.

30. Simunovic Z, Trobonjaca T: Comparison between low level laser therapy, transcutaneous electro-neural stimulation, visible incoherent polarised light and placebo in the treatment of lateral epicondylitis: A pilot clinical study on 120 patients. Lasers Surg Med (Suppl 14), 2002.

31. Fung DT, et al: Therapeutic low energy laser improves the mechanical strength of repairing medial collateral ligament. Lasers Surg Med 31:91-96, 2002.

32. Burd NA, et al: Low-load high volume resistance exercise stimulates muscle protein synthesis more than high-load low volume resistance exercise in young men. PLoS ONE 5(8):e12033, 2010. doi:10.1371/journal.pone.0012033.

33. Courville XF, Coe MP, Hecht PJ: Current concepts review: noninsertional Achilles tendinopathy. Foot Ankle Int 30(11):1132-1142, 2009.

34. Cyriax JH: Textbook of orthopaedic medicine. Volume 2: Treatment by manipulation, massage, and injection, ed 10, London, 1980, Bailliere Tindall.

35. Mattingly GE, Mackarey PJ: Optimal methods for shoulder tendon palpation: A cadaver study. Phys Ther 76(2):166-174, 1996.

36. Dean E: Physiology and therapeutic implication of negative work. Phys Ther 68:233-237, 1988.

37. Alfredson H, et al: Heavy-load eccentric calf muscle training for the treatment of chronic Achilles tendinosis. Am J Sports Med 26:360-366, 1998.

38. Nakamura K, Kitaoka K, Tomita K: Effect of eccentric exercise on the healing process of injured patellar tendon in rats. J Orthop Sci 13:371-378, 2008.

39. Magnussen RA, Dunn WR, Thompson AB: Nonoperative treatment of midportion Achilles tendinopathy: A systematic review. Clin J Sport Med 19:54-64, 2009.

40. Purdam CR, et al: A pilot study of the eccentric decline squat in the management of painful chronic patellar tendinopathy. Br J Sports Med 38:398-407, 2004.

41. Young MA, et al: Eccentric decline squat protocol offers superior results at 12 months compared with traditional eccentric protocol for patellar tendinopathy in volleyball players. Br J Sports Med 39:102-105, 2005.

42. Rompe JD, et al: Eccentric loading versus eccentric loading plus shockwave treatment for midportion Achilles tendinopathy: A randomized controlled trial. Am J Sports Med published ahead of print December 15, 2008.

43. Andres BM, Murrell GA: Molecular and clinical developments in tendinopathy: Editorial comment. Clin Orthop Rel Res 466:1519-1520, 2008.

44. Kellet J: Acute soft tissue injuries: A review of the literature. Med Sci Sports Exerc 18:489-500, 1986.

45. Blazina ME, et al: Jumper's knee. Orthop Clin North Am 4:665-678, 1973.

46. Mishra A, Pavelko T: Treatment of chronic elbow tendinosis with buffered platelet-rich plasma. Am J Sports Med 34(11):1774-1778, 2006.

47. Ranelli PS, et al: Autologous platelet rich plasma for arthroscopic rotator cuff repair: A pilot study. Disabil Rehabil 30(20-22):1584-1589, 2008.

48. Sánchez M, et al. Comparison of surgically repaired Achilles tendon tears using platelet-rich fibrin matrices. Am J Sports Med 35(2):245-251, 2007.

49. De Vos RJ, et al. Platelet-rich plasma injection for chronic Achilles tendonopathy: A randomized controlled trial. JAMA 303(2):144-149, 2010.

50. Kon E, et al: Platelet-rich plasma: new clinical application: A pilot study for treatment of jumper's knee. Injury 40(6):598-603, 2009.

51. Peerbooms JC, et al: Positive effect of autologous platelet concentrate in lateral epicondylitis in a double-blind randomized controlled trial: Platelet-rich plasma versus corticosteroid injection with a 1-year follow-up. Am J Sports Med (38):255-262, 2010.

52. Silva A, Sampaio R: Anatomic ACL reconstruction: Does the platelet rich plasma accelerate tendon healing? Knee Surg Sports Traumatol Arthrosc 17(6):676-682, 2009.

53. Sánchez M, et al. Nonunions treated with autologous preparation rich in growth factors. J Orthop Trauma 23(1):52-59, 2009.

CHAPTER 11

Surgery and Rehabilitation for Primary Flexor Tendon Repair in the Digit

Linda J. Klein, Curtis A. Crimmins

SURGICAL INDICATIONS AND CONSIDERATIONS

Flexor tendon injuries have a long history of challenging the hand surgeon and therapist. Surgical and rehabilitation techniques have evolved significantly since Bunnell[1] suggested that tendon lacerations over the proximal phalanx not be repaired, but ultimately grafted. This basic premise went unchallenged until early mobilization techniques were developed in an attempt to prevent tendon adhesions during the healing process. In the 1960s multiple investigators were able to document that primary flexor tendon repair was superior to delayed tendon grafting.[2-4]

Despite dramatic improvement in outcome over the past 25 years, research has continued with both clinical and laboratory investigations at a breakneck pace. Biomechanical studies of human cadaver tendons have been extraordinarily useful. Investigators have established how much force is applied to a tendon during rehabilitation motions and during normal hand activities.[5-8] The most recent repair techniques have greater tensile strength,[9] which has allowed early postrepair motion to advance from passive flexion to controlled active flexion. The results are fewer adhesions, with better active motion and functional outcomes.

Tendon Healing Stages

Tendon healing occurs in three general stages. The inflammatory phase lasts about 1 week and begins with a fibrin clot at the repair site. Macrophages and other inflammatory cells begin work by removing nonviable material and attracting fibroblasts. Epitenon cells bridge the repair site to restore the gliding surface. The active repair phase lasts from 1 to 2 months. Collagen bundles form and reorient to strengthen the bond between the tendon ends. The tendon begins to revascularize primarily from the intrinsic supply of the proximal stump. The remodeling phase follows until the collagen is mature along the lines of tension and the repair site strength is maximized. The maturation phase, as with all healing tissue, lasts a number of months.[10]

SURGICAL PROCEDURE

The principles of flexor tendon repair are well established and must be rigorously applied to achieve consistently good results. The first step is to educate the patient about the inherent complexity of the injury. The patient should not only understand the demanding technical nature of the injury but also the extraordinarily demanding rehabilitation. The patient must accept that a successful outcome will depend in large part on his or her commitment to and involvement in the rehabilitation protocol. If possible, the patient should be counseled by a hand therapist preoperatively to establish rapport and discuss the therapy protocol. Finally, every patient must be informed that a perfect outcome is unusual and multiple surgical procedures may be necessary.

Flexor tendon repairs should be done in the operating room by experienced hand surgeons within 1 week of the injury. Precise surgical technique is rewarded by better outcomes. Tendon ends usually retract after being cut, and an adequately large surgical incision is generally needed to locate and retrieve the tendon ends. Incisions require careful planning to allow adequate exposure without compromising the vascularity of the skin flaps. Zigzag or midaxial approaches are preferred to prevent scar contracture (Fig. 11-1).

The hallmark of successful flexor tendon repair surgery is atraumatic handling of the soft tissue, especially of the tendon itself. Flexor tendons almost always retract and must be retrieved and advanced back through the flexor sheath. This may well be the most difficult part of the operation. Great care must be exercised to avoid injury to the delicate synovial lining of the fibro-osseous sheath or the epitenon of the flexor tendon. Damage of one or the other may increase the probability of adhesion formation and a poor outcome.

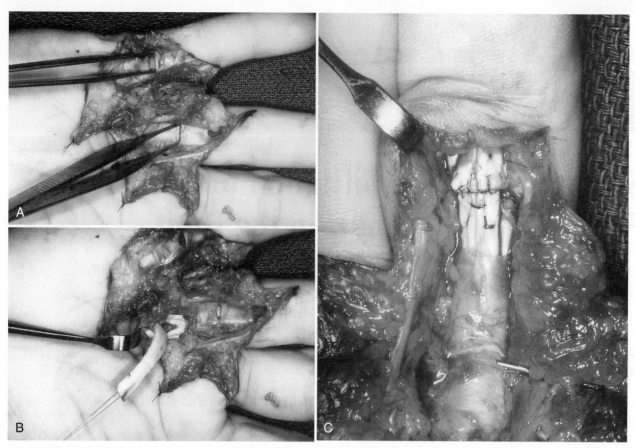

Fig. 11-1 Repair of lacerated flexor tendons in the ring and small fingers. **A,** Sheaths are empty because flexor tendons have retracted into the digit and palm. FDP and superficialis tendons are retrieved from the palm. **B,** The profundus tendon is rethreaded through the chiasm of Camper of the superficialis tendon before repair. **C,** Completed repair of flexor tendons, now placed within the sheath and pulley system, repaired between the A2 and A4 pulleys. (Courtesy Curtis Crimmins.)

Once the tendon ends have been located and threaded back through the sheath and pulleys as carefully as possible, the tendons are repaired through a window between the pulleys, while maintaining the anatomic relationship of the profundus and superficialis tendons. The flexor digitorum superficialis tendon divides into two slips over the proximal phalanx, then it merges again, creating a buttonhole type opening referred to as the chiasm of Camper, just before inserting into the middle phalanx. The flexor digitorum profundus (FDP), which lies deep to the superficialis until this point, emerges through the chiasm of Camper, continuing distally, to insert on the distal phalanx of the digit (Fig. 11-2). When both tendons are lacerated over the proximal phalanx, the surgeon must be certain to reestablish this special relationship. Furthermore, each divided slip of the superficialis has a tendency to derotate 180° as it retracts. This must also be corrected as the tendon is repaired. Only restoration of normal anatomic relationships will allow excellent return of function after repair of lacerated flexor tendons.

The actual suturing of the flexor tendons has been a major focus in the evolution of stronger repairs. The current state of the art suggests that suture repair achieve adequate strength to allow early active-flexion rehabilitation protocols. To achieve this, the repair must ensure secure knots, provide a smooth juncture of tendon ends at the repair site, prevent gapping, maintain tendon vascularity, and be relatively straightforward to perform. Biomechanical studies have definitively shown that multistrand core suture techniques can withstand forces encountered during active motion protocols. In general, at least four strands of 3-0 or 4-0 sutures are needed to cross the repair site to ensure adequate strength for an early active motion protocol. Numerous suture techniques to achieve a repair of at least four strands are described in the literature. The authors prefer a double Kessler suture to produce the four strands of suture crossing the repair site, with a running epitendinous suture[9] (Fig. 11-3).

During the process of repairing the flexor tendons, it is important to preserve as much of the flexor tendon sheath and pulley system as possible. The surgeon must attempt to preserve the A2 and A4 pulleys to prevent tendon bowstringing (Fig. 11-4).

A tendon injury at the level of either of these pulleys is technically demanding. Even repairs at other levels must be technically precise to allow gliding of the repair under preserved portions of the flexor sheath. Suture knots should be placed to minimize impingement of the flexor tendon repair as it passes through the pulley system. Current techniques

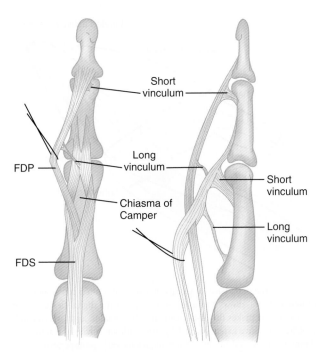

Fig. 11-2 The flexor digitorum superficialis lies volar to the FDP as the tendons enter the sheath. At the level of the proximal phalanx, the superficialis divides and the two slips pass around the profundus tendon, merging and splitting again before inserting on the middle phalanx (chiasm of Camper). (From Schneider LH: Flexor tendon injuries, Boston, 1985, Little, Brown.)

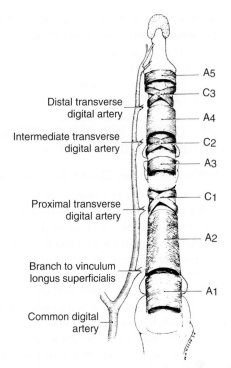

Fig. 11-4 The fibro-osseous sheath or pulley system has five annular pulleys (A1 to A5) and three cruciform pulleys (C1 to C3). The A2 and A4 pulleys must be preserved to prevent bowstringing of the flexor tendons. (From Schneider LH: Flexor tendon injuries, Boston, 1985, Little, Brown.)

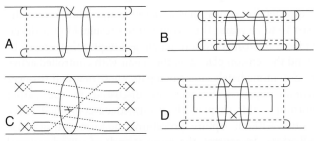

Fig. 11-3 Types of flexor tendon repairs demonstrating different amounts of suture strands crossing the repair. **A,** Modified Kessler is a two-strand repair. **B,** Double Kessler is a four-strand repair. **C,** Savage is a six-strand repair. **D,** Indiana is a four-strand repair. (From Shaieb MD, Singer DI: Tensile strengths of various suture techniques. J Hand Surg 22B[6]:765, 1997.)

THERAPY GUIDELINES FOR REHABILITATION

Flexor tendon repairs in the hand require a special rehabilitation effort. Flexor tendons will heal if positioned without tension or stress; however, adhesions to surrounding tissue will prevent tendon gliding necessary to allow active flexion once the tendon has healed. Thus the need to move a flexor tendon early in the healing process has been evident since repair of flexor tendons has begun.

After repair it takes approximately 12 weeks for a flexor tendon to regain enough tensile strength to avoid rupture with normal strong use of the hand required to grasp, hold, or lift objects during daily activities. A variety of protocols for flexor tendon rehabilitation have been developed over the past 50 years, making the choice of which protocol to use difficult. No exact method exists to determine the strength of a tendon repair during the healing process; therefore the therapist and surgeon rely on general guidelines regarding tendon healing, as well as factors that affect rate of healing to determine advancement of the patient within a flexor tendon rehabilitation protocol. The factors that are considered include the type of injury; status of the tendon, sheath, and vessels at the time of repair; injury to surrounding structures; patient health issues such as diabetes; lifestyle factors such as smoking, which decreases oxygen to the tissues; and ability to comply with the rehabilitation program. Consideration of these factors and clear

meet these requirements, and results are expectedly good, with 75% or more tendon repairs falling consistently within the excellent to good categories.

Recent and future trends in flexor tendon surgery research include investigations of the ability of substances such as platelet-derived growth factor-BB, hyaluronic acid, and 5-flourouracil to enhance tendon healing.[11-13] Polyvinyl alcohol shields and antiadhesion gels have been proposed and studied with some success to decrease adhesions.[14] As these trends continue, we must stay abreast of current developments to maximize functional outcomes for patients after flexor tendon injury.

communication with the surgeon are necessary to determine the most appropriate approach to choose for each particular patient. Before describing the variety of guidelines from which to choose for flexor tendon rehabilitation, it is important to understand how exercise concepts are modified for flexor tendon repair rehabilitation.

CONCEPTS OF HEALING AND EXERCISES FOR FLEXOR TENDON REPAIR

Role of Adhesions After Flexor Tendon Repair

Adhesions occur very early in many cases, often within 1 week after surgery, preventing gliding of the flexor tendon needed to flex the digit. The end result of dense adhesions can be a digit that does not flex any further than it did before the tendon repair was performed, but with the additional pain, discomfort, and cosmetic changes caused by extensive surgical incisions in the digit, as well as many weeks of lost use of the hand while rehabilitation is attempted. Adhesions are the most difficult to deal with in zones I and II of the hand. Zones I and II extend from the distal palmar crease of the hand to the distal phalanx, and they incorporate the area of the digit in which the flexor tendons pass under a very tight pulley system, encompassed within a tendon sheath filled with synovial fluid that allows the tendon to glide under the tight pulleys (see Fig. 11-4). When adhesions form within the sheath-pulley system in zones I and II of the digit, they are very difficult (in many cases impossible) to overcome, and the result is a digit that is limited in active flexion. Historical perspectives on tendon healing help clinicians understand the reasoning behind current approaches to flexor tendon surgery and rehabilitation. Before the 1960s, flexor tendons were allowed to heal by immobilization for the first few weeks because it was thought that the tendon could not heal without nutrition from the surrounding scar tissue.[15] This immobilization for the first few weeks resulted in dense adhesions, especially with repairs in zones I and II, with the inability to actively flex the digit. These results spurred the development of immediate passive-flexion protocols. The goal was that by passively flexing the digit and allowing partial, protected extension, the flexor tendon would glide far enough under the pulley system to prevent dense restricting adhesions and allow active motion when the tendon was adequately healed. However, in many cases, tendinous adhesions still developed. Research has shown that proximal gliding of the FDP tendon is inconsistent during passive flexion.[16] The flexor tendon, when the digit is passively flexed, is thought in some cases to kink, or bunch up, between the pulleys, rather than passively glide through the pulley system (Fig. 11-5). To ensure proximal gliding of the flexor tendon, an active contraction of the muscle is needed to pull the tendon proximally through the pulley system. Because research has shown that tendons do heal intrinsically without surrounding adhesions,[17-19] an effort to actively flex the repaired flexor tendon immediately after repair was initiated to prevent the onset of dense adhesions. To avoid rupture of the flexor tendon with active motion

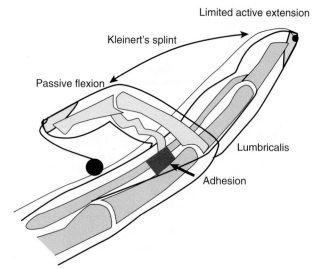

Fig. 11-5 Theoretic basis of passive flexion and limited active motion of IP joints do not always move the suture site of the digital flexor tendon. Passive flexion makes the distal segment of the tendon kink, which can be stretched by active extension of IP joints, without moving the suture site. (From Tajima T: Indication and techniques for early postoperative motion after repair of digital flexor tendon particularly in zone II. In Hunter JM, Schneider LH, Mackin EJ, editors: Tendon and nerve surgery in the hand: A third decade, St Louis, 1997, Mosby.)

immediately after surgery, however, stronger suture techniques had to be developed.

Understanding Repair Strength

Flexor tendon surgery has undergone an evolution over the past 10 to 20 years. This evolution has resulted in the development of stronger suture repair techniques that will withstand the tension placed on the repair with controlled active flexion immediately after the repair. These new and stronger tendon repair techniques, as discussed in the earlier portion of this chapter, allow immediate controlled active motion without rupture, preventing the formation of dense adhesions. In general, the more strands of suture material that cross the tendon repair, the stronger the repair (Fig. 11-6).[7-9,20,21]

Traditional surgical procedure, using a two-strand repair, will tolerate passive motion, but is not shown to be sufficiently strong enough to tolerate active motion immediately after repair.[22] A four-strand repair will tolerate gentle active motion. An eight-strand repair will certainly tolerate active motion; however, it is technically demanding and may become so bulky as to not glide under the pulleys, creating friction, possible wearing, and eventual rupture.[20] Thus a four- to six-strand repair technique is frequently chosen to apply an immediate active motion protocol.

After the traditional two-strand repair, it is safe to perform immediate passive-flexion protocols (described later in the chapter), or where necessary by patient limitation, immobilization. Immediate active-flexion protocols are generally not applied to the tendon with a traditional two-strand technique, but require a stronger four-strand technique and must be discussed with the surgeon. It is

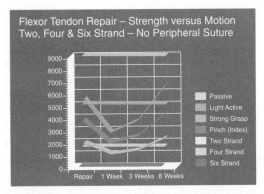

Fig. 11-6 Tensile strengths of flexor tendon repairs compared with the tension developed within the tendon with use of the hand. The comparison shows that at its weakest point after surgery, a two-strand repair is not strong enough to tolerate light gripping; however, four or more strand repairs have adequate tensile strength to tolerate light gripping. (From Strickland JW, Cannon NM: Flexor tendon repair—Indiana method. Indiana Hand Center Newsl 1:4, 1993.)

extremely important for the therapist to understand the type of suture repair that was done for a flexor tendon repair, to ensure that the protocol chosen for a particular patient stays within the tension limits of the repair.

Edema Control and Scar Management After Flexor Tendon Repair

Elevation is essential in the early phase after flexor tendon repair, because other forms of edema control are limited by the continuous splinting. Shoulder, elbow, and cervical motion exercises are performed to help with lymphatic function and circulation. In the intermediate and late phases of flexor tendon healing, use of a light compressive wrap at night is appropriate. **This should not be used during the day because compressive wraps will increase resistance to the flexor tendon during active flexion.** The therapist initiates gentle massage of the scar (for firmness) and edema massage after sutures are removed; the patient can continue this process at home when made feasible by the presence of the splint. Commercially available scar management pads may be placed or formed over the scar, applied at night only, if scars become thickened or raised. Because the splint is worn full time in the early phase of the rehabilitation programs, it is difficult for the patient to safely apply the scar management pads at night, and they are often applied beginning in the intermediate phase for this reason.

Passive-Flexion Exercises After Flexor Tendon Repair

Passive flexion of the digits is performed through all the phases of flexor tendon rehabilitation. Passive flexion of the digit after a flexor tendon repair places the repaired tendon on slack. Very little tension develops within the flexor tendon during passive flexion of the digit, as long as the patient is truly relaxed and not actively assisting the passive flexion.[5,6] After flexor tendon repair, a finger will become stiff because of swelling, incisional scarring, and pain if passive flexion is not performed within 1 week after the procedure. If passive

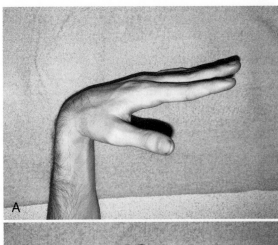

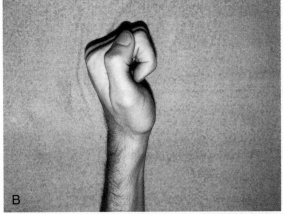

Fig. 11-7 **A,** The patient performs wrist tenodesis exercises by relaxing the wrist into flexion and extending the fingers to assist in gliding the flexor tendon distally. **B,** The wrist is then extended to 20° to 30° while the fingers are gently flexed to assist in gliding the flexor tendon proximally. (Courtesy Linda Klein.)

flexion remains limited after sutures are removed, then other therapy techniques may be used to assist in regaining passive flexion, such as heat combined with stretch into flexion before manual passive flexion within the patient's pain tolerance.

Wrist Tenodesis Exercises After Flexor Tendon Repair

Wrist tenodesis exercises use wrist motion to assist in moving the flexor tendons. The wrist is flexed to comfortable tolerance, and the fingers allowed to gently straighten at all three joints. This will give the tendon slack at the wrist and glide the tendon distally during finger extension. Next, the fingers are relaxed, the wrist is extended to 30°, and the fingers are gently flexed. The wrist extension pulls the flexors slightly proximally and gives slack to the finger extensors, allowing the flexors to glide proximally (Fig. 11-7). The wrist tenodesis exercise is started in the intermediate phase of rehabilitation after a two-strand repair, because it creates tension in the tendon. It is started within 3 days after surgery within an immediate active-flexion approach after a four (or more) strand repair unless otherwise directed by the physician.

Active Extension of the Fingers After Flexor Tendon Repair

Full extension of all three finger joints at the same time must be limited immediately after flexor tendon repair to avoid pulling the repair apart by stretch. Extension is limited in the early phase of tendon healing by positioning within the dorsal blocking splint that places the metacarpophalangeal (MP) joints in flexion. However, interphalangeal (IP) extension is very important to obtain shortly after the repair in zones I and II because the proximal interphalangeal (PIP) and distal interphalangeal (DIP) joints contract into flexion very quickly after repairs in these zones. All flexor tendon protocols emphasize attaining full IP extension immediately after surgery, unless a digital nerve has been lacerated or another injury prevents placement of the IP joints in full extension, as directed by the surgeon. When a digital nerve has been repaired in the digit, the PIP joint is generally allowed to extend to 15° less than full extension. **Composite extension of all three finger joints at the same time will place an adverse stretch effect on the flexor tendon repair in zone I or II initially after surgery, but it can be tolerated at 4 weeks after surgery with the wrist in flexion. Wrist and full finger extension are not performed at the same time until the late stage of tendon healing.**

Passive Finger Extension After Flexor Tendon Repair

Passive extension of the fingers is potentially more dangerous than active extension, because if done overaggressively, it may stretch the tendon repair apart. It is also possible for the patient to have some tension within the flexor tendon during the passive extension, resulting in resistance to the repaired tendon and possible rupture.

In the early phase of tendon healing, passive IP extension is only performed when active IP extension is limited (in the presence of PIP or DIP joint flexion contractures). When IP joint flexion contractures appear early, passive IP joint extension can be performed carefully, with the flexor tendon in a protected position and ensuring that the patient's hand is fully relaxed. The protected position for a flexor tendon is with all other joints supported in flexion while one joint is extended. For instance, to treat a PIP flexion contracture 3 weeks after repair, the therapist flexes the wrist and MP joints as far as can be tolerated, then passively extends the PIP joint by applying pressure under the middle phalanx into extension. The DIP joint is not passively extended at the same time as the PIP joint to avoid stressing the tendon across two joints in the early phase of tendon healing.

Active Finger Flexion After Flexor Tendon Repair

Active flexion introduces significantly increased tension in the repaired flexor tendon. Traditional approaches using immediate passive flexion or immobilization for the early phase of tendon healing introduce active flexion of the repaired digit in the intermediate phase of healing (4 weeks

after surgery). An assessment of flexor tendon gliding is done to determine what type of active flexion is appropriate. To assess flexor tendon gliding, passive flexion is compared with active flexion. **The initial assessment of active flexion is done cautiously, with the wrist in 20° to 30° of extension** (Fig. 11-8). When a difference exists in the repaired digit between passive and active flexion of 15° or more,[23] it indicates the presence of adhesions, limiting tendon gliding. When flexor tendon adhesions limit active more than passive flexion 3 to 4 weeks after surgery, active tendon-gliding exercises are initiated. Tendon gliding can be achieved by performing a sequence of three fists: hook fist, straight fist, and composite fist (Fig. 11-9). A hook fist is similar to a claw position, flexing the PIP and DIP joints with the MPs extended. This type of fist results in the largest differential gliding of the FDP and flexor digitorum superficialis. A straight fist results in the most excursion of the flexor digitorum superficialis. A composite fist results in the most excursion of the FDP tendon.

Active flexion is begun in the early phase of tendon healing when the patient is placed in an immediate active

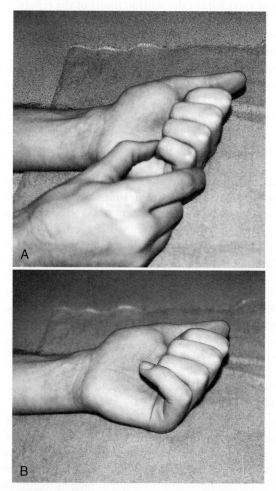

Fig. 11-8 The therapist assesses flexor tendon gliding by comparing passive flexion of the repaired digit (**A**) with active flexion (**B**). When a large difference exists between active and passive flexion, it signifies the presence of significant flexor tendon adhesions that limit active flexion. (Courtesy Linda Klein.)

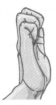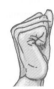

Hook fist   Straight fist   Full fist

Fig. 11-9 Active flexor tendon-gliding exercises consist of three positions: hook fist, straight fist, and full or composite fist. (From Pettengill K, van Strien G: Postoperative management of flexor tendon injuries. In Skirven TM, et al, editors: Rehabilitation of the hand and upper extremity, ed 6, Philadelphia, 2011, Mosby.)

motion flexor tendon rehabilitation approach. At the first postoperative physician or therapy visit 2 to 3 days after surgery, a controlled method of active flexion termed place-hold is begun. Place-hold flexion uses the therapist's or patient's other hand to passively place the fingers into a light fist; then the patient holds the fingers actively in the light-fist position as the other hand is removed. This requires an active muscle contraction and flexor tendon gliding in a proximal direction to keep the finger in a flexed position actively. The place-hold exercise is believed to result in less tension on the repaired tendon than if the finger were actively flexed without the assistance of the patient's opposite hand or the therapist's hand. **Within an immediate active motion approach, the three types of fists described earlier are not performed until the intermediate phase of tendon healing if flexor tendon adhesions develop in spite of early active motion attempts.**

Postoperative Guidelines

In general, three types of flexor tendon rehabilitation guidelines exist. These are (1) immobilization, (2) immediate passive flexion, and (3) immediate active-flexion approaches. The reasoning for choosing one approach over another is based on the complexity of injury, the age of the patient, patient compliance, patient health factors, and the suture repair technique. The choice of which set of guidelines within which to place a patient is best determined in conjunction with the referring surgeon, with the final decision resting with the surgeon.

Within each approach the patient progresses through three general levels or phases: early, intermediate, and late phases. The decision of when to advance a patient to the next level within each approach is determined by the amount of flexor tendon adhesion that limits the tendon gliding and the amount of time after repair. To determine the level of flexor tendon adhesion, the therapist compares passive flexion with active flexion. When a large discrepancy exists between passive and active flexion, with passive flexion 15° or more better than active flexion, it signifies the presence of flexor tendon adhesions. When adhesions limit gliding of the flexor tendon, and the time period after repair is adequate to allow increased tension on the tendon, the patient is progressed to the next level of the rehabilitation approach. **The tendon that**

does not have limiting adhesions is more at risk for rupture than the tendon with strong adhesions that surround the tendon repair site. When tendon adhesions limit active flexion more than passive flexion, the tendon can tolerate more tension before rupture, and thus can be advanced to the next level sooner than the tendon without limiting adhesions.[23] Flexor tendon adhesions are assessed on a continual basis to determine the level of the rehabilitation program that is appropriate for the patient at that time. The time after surgery, combined with the level of flexor tendon adhesion, determines the placement of the patient in the program.[23] When adhesions prevent gliding of the flexor tendon, it is appropriate to advance the patient to the next phase of rehabilitation to encourage tendon gliding, with surgeon approval. When flexor tendon gliding is adequate, the patient is kept in the current level of the program until the number of weeks after surgery dictates that the repair is strong enough to tolerate the increased tension of the next phase of the treatment protocol.

The appropriate choice of which guideline to use and advancement of the patient within the chosen guideline require in-depth knowledge of flexor tendon healing and tensile strength guidelines at various times after repair, awareness of the type of repair, and the patient's compliance level, as well as communication with the referring surgeon.

IMMOBILIZATION APPROACH

Indications for Immobilization

Immobilization is rarely used after a flexor tendon repair; however, some situations call for its application. Immobilization is used for young children, who are unable to adhere to a motion protocol with its specific precautions. Children younger than age 12 are most often placed in immobilization for the first 3 to 4 weeks, but each child should be evaluated related to his or her maturity level. Other population types that may be placed in immobilization after a flexor tendon repair would be those that have cognitive limitations (e.g., Alzheimer disease, noncompliant patients). It is sometimes difficult to know the patient's compliance ability at the first therapy session. When a patient demonstrates inability to appropriately comply with the precautions and exercises within a certain approach, it may become necessary to change the rehabilitation approach to one with less early motion, or a cast may be needed instead of a removable splint in the first 4 to 5 weeks after surgery. When a concomitant fracture or significant loss of skin requiring a skin graft occurs, a period of immobilization may be necessary to allow the bone or skin to heal adequately before beginning motion. Not all fractures require immobilization. Stable fractures or those that have had open reduction internal fixation may tolerate immediate controlled motion, as determined by the surgeon. Few sets of guidelines exist for therapy after immobilization of the repaired flexor tendon because of dense adhesion formation. The most frequently sited guideline, described as follows, encourages motion and light resistance to facilitate tendon gliding after the initial phase of tendon healing.[24,25]

Immobilization Guidelines

Phase I (Early)

TIME: 0 to 4 weeks

GOALS: Prevent joint stiffness, avoid tension on tendon repair, prevent flexion contractures, patient and family education regarding tendon protection, manage edema, full active range of motion (AROM) of upper extremity (UE) joints proximal to the wrist (Table 11-1)

Splinting. When used, the immobilization approach will place the patient's hand in a dorsal blocking cast (or in a dorsal blocking splint wrapped securely in place, with instructions not to remove the splint at home). The position of the cast or splint in the early phase of immobilization is 20° to 30° of wrist flexion, and 40° to 50° of MP flexion, with IP extension. This position keeps the flexor tendons on slack, yet prevents the most difficult joint problems (e.g., PIP flexion contractures). The cast or splint will stay in place for 3 to 4 weeks.

Exercises. Within phase I (zero to 3 or 4 weeks after surgery) the patient generally remains immobilized in the dorsal blocking splint or cast. When referred to therapy during the early phase, the therapist may perform passive flexion to prevent joint stiffness and a significant other, such as a parent, may be taught to perform passive flexion at home if he or she is reliable. Goals in the early phase of the immobilization approach include protecting the repaired flexor tendon(s) from rupture with full time splinting and patient education, obtaining passive flexion when allowed, edema control, and obtaining full active motion of the UE proximal to the wrist.

Phase II (Intermediate)

TIME: 3 or 4 weeks to 6 weeks

GOALS: Improve joint mobility (full flexion passive range of motion [PROM], partial flexion AROM, full IP extension), patient and family education, scar management, splinting to prevent tendon repair rupture between exercises (Table 11-2)

Exercises. With phase II exercises, the splint position is adjusted to bring the wrist to neutral. The splint is removed for exercises hourly. Passive flexion is initiated first, to loosen stiff joints created by immobilization, swelling, and scarring. After passive flexion, wrist tenodesis is initiated as described previously, to begin gentle tendon gliding (see Fig. 11-7). Tendon-gliding exercises are initiated, with three types of fisting exercises (i.e., straight fist, hook fist, and composite fist; see Fig. 11-9), as described previously. Assessment of flexor tendon adhesions is performed after 3 to 4 days of these exercises by comparing passive flexion with active flexion of the digit or digits. When active flexion is significantly more limited than passive flexion, blocking exercises of the PIP and DIP joints are added. Additional flexor tendon

gliding can be obtained with isolated tendon gliding exercises. The therapist can isolate the FDP tendon by blocking the MP and PIP in extension while performing active DIP flexion. The flexor digitorum superficialis (FDS) tendon is isolated with blocking of the FDP tendon by holding all other fingers in complete extension and allowing the injured finger to flex at the PIP joint. If improvement is noted in tendon gliding 1 week later, then these exercises are continued until 6 weeks after surgery.

If no improvement occurs in active flexion with blocking and tendon gliding exercises, then light resistance of gripping with very soft putty is initiated at 5 weeks after surgery. This resistance is initiated in the intermediate phase of healing only in the presence of flexor tendon adhesions that limit active flexion more than passive flexion by 15° or more.[23] Extension of the fingers is performed with the wrist flexed. When PIP flexion contractures are present, limiting the PIP joints, DIP joints, or both from full extension, they are splinted in a volar extension splint at night, beginning at 4 or 5 weeks after surgery. Goals in the intermediate phase of the immobilization approach include obtaining full passive flexion and partial active flexion, full IP extension, and protecting the repaired tendon from rupture with appropriate splinting between exercises and patient education, as well as scar management.

Phase III (Late)

TIME: 6 to 12 weeks

GOALS: Normalize PROM and AROM, improve strength to allow a light fist, patient and family education to avoid tendon repair rupture (Table 11-3)

Exercises. This phase generally lasts from 6 to 12 weeks after surgery. All protective splinting is discontinued. When passive flexion continues to be limited by joint stiffness and swelling, therapeutic techniques such as heat and PROM are continued. Active flexion, joint blocking, and tendon gliding exercises continue to attempt to bring active flexion to match the level of passive flexion. Resistance can be introduced or advanced during this phase. Light resistance can be provided with putty or light manual resistance of the therapist, and it can be advanced to light grippers in the middle of the late phase of tendon healing.

If flexor tendon adhesions are minimal, then resistance is initiated at 8 weeks after surgery, gently at first, with strong resistance restricted until after 12 weeks after surgery. Goals in the late phase of the immobilization approach include obtaining full passive and active flexion and extension of the injured finger or fingers, increasing strength to obtain a light fist, and protecting the repaired tendon from rupture with patient education.

Regardless of the goals, active motion after use of an immobilization approach is frequently limited because of adhesion formation. Limited active flexion of the repaired digit, especially the DIP joint, is frequently seen, and there may be difficulty actively flexing the adjacent digits because of the common muscle belly of the FDP to the last three

TABLE 11-1 Flexor Tendon Repair in the Digit (Immobilization Approach)

Rehabilitation Phase	Criteria to Progress to This Phase	Anticipated Impairments and Functional Limitations	Intervention	Goal	Rationale
Phase I 0-3 or 4 wk	Postoperative and cleared by physician to initiate therapy	• Edema • Pain • Limited ROM • Unable to grip, pinch, lift, or carry objects	• Postoperative splint fabrication • Inspect surgical site for drainage, erythema • Pain assessment • Edema assessment and early edema control • AROM exercises for the shoulder and elbow emphasizing avoidance of stress to the repair site • Patient/family education regarding precautions and purpose of immobilization approach as chosen by physician • Passive flexion of the MP and IP joints, in therapy only* • IP extension to limit of splint, in therapy only*	• Avoid tension on the repaired tendon • Prevent infection • Decrease pain and edema to moderate or less • Full AROM of shoulder and elbow • Patient/family to understand tendon repair precautions and purpose of immobilization • Prevent joint stiffness and flexion contractures*	• Prevent compromise of tendon repair • Promote wound healing • Manage pain and edema • Prevent proximal joint stiffness • Reduce stiffness in digits*

*In cases cleared by physician.
AROM, Active range of motion; *IP*, interphalangeal; *MP*, metacarpophalangeal; *ROM*, range of motion.

TABLE 11-2 Flexor Tendon Repair in the Digit (Immobilization Approach)

Rehabilitation Phase	Criteria to Progress to This Phase	Anticipated Impairments and Functional Limitations	Intervention	Goal	Rationale
Phase II 3/4-6 wk	• No signs of infection • No significant increase in pain • Intact tendon repair	• Edema and pain • Limited range of motion • Limited strength • Unable to grip, pinch, lift, or carry objects	• Splint adjustment to wrist neutral • Splint removed for therapy and home exercises • Modalities—heat for stiffness and pain as needed • Passive flexion of finger joints • Active IP extension • Protected passive PIP extension in the presence of contracture • Wrist tenodesis • Gentle tendon gliding and fisting exercises (Figs 11-7 and 11-9) • Gentle blocking exercises • Scar massage, scar pads at night • Edema control/light compressive wrap • Patient/family education of home exercises and tendon precautions	• Full passive flexion of finger joints • Full active IP extension • Partial active flexion • Prevent tendon rupture • Reduce tendon adhesions • Reduce scar thickness • Decrease edema • Independent home exercise program • Patient/family to understand tendon repair precautions	• Improve joint mobility • Minimize resistance to tendon gliding • Initiate tendon gliding • Manage edema, pain • Remodel tendinous adhesions • Prevent complications/rupture

IP, Interphalangeal; *PIP*, proximal interphalangeal.

TABLE 11-3 Flexor Tendon Repair in the Digit (Immobilization Approach)

Rehabilitation Phase	Criteria to Progress to This Phase	Anticipated Impairments and Functional Limitations	Intervention	Goal	Rationale
Phase III 6-12 wk	• Tolerance of A/PROM • No significant increase in pain • Intact tendon repair	• Pain • Limited range of motion • Limited strength • Limited ability to grip, pinch, lift, or carry objects	• Discontinue splint • Passive finger flexion • Passive IP extension in the presence of contractures • Composite active finger extension • Modalities—heat for stiffness and pain as needed • Progress tendon gliding, fisting, and blocking exercises • Light strengthening exercises (putty) • Light functional activities • Scar massage, scar pads at night • Edema control/light compressive wrap • Patient/family education	• Full PROM, maximize AROM of fingers • Pain-free motion • Increase strength to facilitate light use • Decrease thickness and firmness of scar • Minimal edema by 12 wk • Independent home exercises • Prevent compromise of tendon repair	• Promote restoration of full joint mobility • Pain management • Improve tendon gliding • Promote functional use of the injured hand • Prevent complications

A/PROM, Active/passive range of motion; *AROM,* active range of motion; *IP,* interphalangeal; *PROM,* passive range of motion.

digits (i.e., quadriga effect). Grip strength will be diminished secondary to loss of active flexion. It is common for flexor tendons with adhesions to require a prolonged time of therapy, with a strong emphasis on a home program of blocking exercises and resistance even longer than the 12-week healing period, to continue to facilitate tendon gliding during the long remodeling process. Further surgical procedures are available for the repaired flexor tendon with significant adhesions that limit functional use of the hand, which are most often performed between 3 and 6 months after repair.

IMMEDIATE PASSIVE-FLEXION APPROACH

Immediate passive-flexion approaches apply passive flexion to the fingers, beginning within 3 or 4 days after surgery. These guidelines are appropriate for, and have been traditionally applied to, the patient with a two-strand repair of the flexor tendon. No active contraction of the repaired flexor muscle and tendon unit occurs; therefore limited proximal gliding of the flexor tendon occurs in the early phase of tendon healing within this approach. The benefits of an immediate passive-flexion approach are that the finger does not become overly stiff, and a limited amount of gliding of the repaired tendon occurs. Results vary widely regarding results of the immediate passive-flexion approach and tendinous adhesions. Two main categories encompass all the

immediate passive-flexion guidelines. These two categories are approaches that use either elastic traction or static-positioning splints during the early phase of tendon healing. Both approaches use a dorsal blocking splint with the wrist at 20° to 30° of flexion and the MPs at 50° to 60° of flexion, with the IPs allowed full extension within the splint. The difference between the two approaches (the positioning of the fingers in either dynamic flexion or static IP extension in the early phase of healing) will be described within each guideline.

The static-positioning guideline follows the modified Duran and Houser[25-27] rehabilitation program, while the elastic traction guideline is patterned after the modified Kleinert,[3] Washington,[28] or Chow[29] rehabilitation programs. These guidelines will be generalized in the following paragraphs.

Immediate Passive Flexion With Static-Positioning Guidelines

Patients are placed into an immediate passive-flexion approach that does not use elastic traction on the fingers when it is the preference of the surgeon and therapist or when elastic traction is contraindicated. **These contraindications include questionable soft tissue tolerance to prolonged flexion, early development of IP flexion contractures, or presence of a concomitant injury such as a fracture that would not tolerate passive flexion.**

Phase I (Early)

TIME: 0 to 4 weeks

GOALS: Attain full passive flexion, full active IP extension, minimize edema, prevent rupture of flexor tendon by splinting and patient education, full AROM of UE joints proximal to the wrist (Table 11-4)

Splinting. A dorsal blocking splint is fabricated and applied within the first 5 days after surgery. The wrist is placed in 20° to 30° of flexion, the MP joints are placed in approximately 50° of flexion, and the IP joints are straight (Fig. 11-10). The patient is instructed to remain in the splint at all times for the first 4 weeks after surgery. It is removed in therapy for cleansing of the skin and splint, as well as skin assessment for pressure and fit.

Exercises. Exercises should be performed in therapy and at home, 10 repetitions every hour. Within the splint, passive PIP flexion to tolerance, passive DIP flexion to tolerance, and then composite passive flexion of MP, PIP, and DIP joints to tolerance. Duran and Houser[25,26,30] described specific passive

exercises (Fig. 11-11). Active IP extension exercises to the hood of the dorsal blocking splint are also performed.

Phase II (Intermediate)

TIME: 4 to 7 weeks

GOALS: Attain partial active flexion (at least 50%) of the injured digit, full passive flexion, full active extension, protect flexor tendon from rupture with splinting between exercises and patient education (Table 11-5)

Exercises. Exercises continue to be performed in therapy and at home, 10 repetitions every hour. Remove splint at home for exercises and bathing. Begin with wrist tenodesis exercises, and place-active hold flexion. Advance to gentle active-flexion exercises. If flexor tendon adhesions are noted (active flexion limited by 15° or more compared with passive flexion), begin blocking exercises for PIP and DIP flexion. Active finger extension is performed with wrist flexed until 6 weeks, then with the wrist neutral. Passive IP extension is begun if PIP or DIP flexion contractures exist, with the tendon in a protected position.

TABLE 11-4 Flexor Tendon Repair in the Digit (Immediate Passive-Flexion Approach)

Rehabilitation Phase	Criteria to Progress to This Phase	Anticipated Impairments and Functional Limitations	Intervention	Goal	Rationale
Phase I 0-4 wk	Postoperative and cleared by physician to initiate therapy	• Edema • Pain • Limited range of motion • Unable to grip, pinch, lift, or carry objects	• Postoperative splint fabrication • Static positioning splint* (see Fig. 11-10) • Elastic traction splint* (see Fig. 11-12) • Inspect surgical site for drainage, erythema • Pain assessment • Edema assessment and early edema control • AROM exercises for the shoulder and elbow • Passive flexion of all finger (or thumb) joints (see Fig. 11-11 in addition to composite flexion of all finger or thumb joints) • Active IP extension with MPs flexed (see Fig. 11-12, *B*, for IP extension with elastic traction approach) • Patient/family education regarding tendon precautions and home exercise program	• Protect tendon repair • Prevent infection • Decrease pain and edema to moderate or less • Full AROM of shoulder and elbow • Full passive flexion all digit joints • Full IP extension* • Patient to understand tendon repair precautions and home exercise program	• Prevent compromise of tendon repair • Promote wound healing • Manage pain and edema • Prevent proximal joint stiffness • Prevent digital joint stiffness and flexion contractures • Passively glide tendon

*Unless digital nerve is repaired, then slight flexion of the proximal interphalangeal or physician direction.
AROM, Active range of motion; *IP,* interphalangeal; *MP,* metacarpophalangeal.

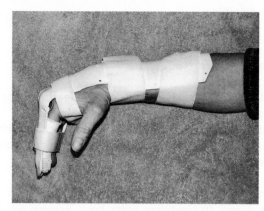

Fig. 11-10 Dorsal blocking splint with the wrist and MP joints flexed keeps slack in the repaired flexor tendon during the early healing phase. It is used for the immobilization protocol and the immediate passive-flexion protocols that do not use elastic traction. (Courtesy Linda Klein.)

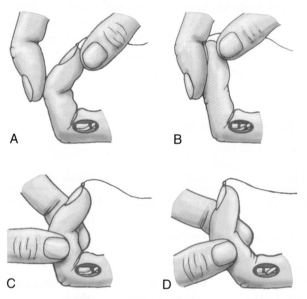

Fig. 11-11 Specific passive exercises described by Duran and Houser. With the MP and PIP joints flexed (**A**), the distal phalanx is passively extended (**B**). This moves the FDP tendon distally away from the flexor digitorum superficialis tendon. The next step is with the DIP and MP flexed (**C**), the PIP joint is passively extended (**D**). This moves both repairs distally away from the site of repair and any surrounding tissues to which they may adhere. (From Pettengill K, van Strien G: Postoperative management of flexor tendon injuries. In Skirven TM, et al, editors: Rehabilitation of the hand and upper extremity, ed 6, Philadelphia, 2011, Mosby.)

Phase III (Late)
TIME: 7 or 8 to 12 weeks
GOALS: Attain full active and passive flexion and extension of digits, light grip strength, protect repaired tendon from rupture with patient education

Discontinue use of splint. Continue with active motion exercises. If flexor tendon adhesions are present, then begin light resistive exercises. Dynamic IP extension splinting after 8 weeks is initiated if flexion contractures persist. At 12 weeks after surgery, the patient is allowed to perform normal activities (Table 11-6).

IMMEDIATE PASSIVE FLEXION WITH ELASTIC TRACTION APPROACH (refer to Tables 11-4 through 11-6 for guidelines)

Indications

Elastic traction was added to the early phase of the passive-flexion guidelines described previously in an attempt to increase proximal tendon gliding by placement of the fingers in flexion between exercises, in part by allowing more time for the tendon to be resting proximally in relation to the repair site and to the pulley system. It also decreases stiffness of the digits in the direction of flexion by applying passive flexion for a greater portion of time. **Placement in passive flexion with elastic traction to the fingers between exercises also decreases the potential for even inadvertent active flexion of the fingers in the early phase of flexor tendon healing, protecting the tendon from rupture.** The negative effect of elastic traction is the increased potential to develop IP flexion contractures, as well as the increase in complexity perceived by the patient by having a dynamic splint on the hand (as opposed to a less complicated static splint). Patients are placed into this approach by preference of the surgeon-therapist team (those patients that are not showing signs of IP flexion contracture, those that can be compliant with the rehabilitation program, and those who have no soft tissue healing complication).

Immediate Passive Flexion With Elastic Traction Guidelines

Phase I (Early)
TIME: 0 to 4 weeks
GOALS: Attain full passive flexion, full active IP extension, minimize edema, prevent rupture of flexor tendon with splinting and patient education, full AROM of UE joints proximal to the wrist

Splinting. The splint applied for this approach is the same dorsal blocking splint base as described for the static position approach, with the addition of elastic traction applied from the fingertip of the injured finger or fingers, which passes under a distal palmar pulley and is connected at the midforearm level to the proximal splint strap on the volar forearm (Fig. 11-12, *A*). The wrist is in 20° to 30° flexion, the MP joints in 50° to 60° flexion, and the IP joints straight. The elastic traction may consist of rubber bands, rubber band and monofilament line combination, or other elastic thread. It can be attached to the tip of the finger by a suture placed by the surgeon through the fingernail or an attachment such as a dress hook glued to the fingernail. Some therapists have also used self-adhesive moleskin or other fabric with a hole for the elastic traction attachment applied to the fingertip. The line is threaded through a pulley at the level of the distal palmar crease and attached at the level of the forearm, generally to the proximal splint strap, around a safety pin. The distal palmar pulley concept is important because it achieves

TABLE 11-5 Flexor Tendon Repair in the Digit (Immediate Passive-Flexion Approach)

Rehabilitation Phase	Criteria to Progress to This Phase	Anticipated Impairments and Functional Limitations	Intervention	Goal	Rationale
Phase II 4-7 or 8 wk	• No signs of infection • No significant increase in pain • Intact tendon	• Edema and pain • Limited range of motion • Limited strength • Unable to grip, pinch, lift, or carry objects	• Continue use of splint except for exercises and bathing until 6 wk after surgery. May discontinue splint at 6 wk if adhesions limit tendon gliding • May eliminate elastic traction at 4 wk postoperation in elastic traction approach • Passive digit flexion, active IP extension • Gentle passive IP extension for PIP flexion contractures with wrist flexed • Modalities—heat for stiffness and pain as needed • Initiate active digit flexion with wrist tenodesis exercises: active finger (or thumb) flexion with wrist extended; finger (or thumb) extension with wrist flexed, gradually bring wrist to neutral • Advance to blocking exercises and tendon gliding for IP flexion if adhesions limit active flexion • Edema control with light compressive wraps at night as needed • Scar massage/night pad as needed • Patient education regarding precautions	• Full passive flexion of digits • Full active extension of all digit joints with wrist flexed, advance to wrist neutral • Partial to full active digit flexion with wrist extended • Reduce peritendinous adhesions • Decrease edema • Reduce scar thickness • Independent home exercise program • Patient/family to understand tendon repair precautions • Prevent tendon rupture	• Maintain/improve joint mobility • Manage edema and pain • Minimize resistance to tendon gliding • Decrease peritendinous adhesions • Improve tendon gliding • Prevent compromise of tendon repair

IP, Interphalangeal; *PIP,* proximal interphalangeal.

passive DIP flexion. A safety pin in the strap across the palm is a simple method to obtain the distal palmar pulley. Other methods of designing a distal palmar pulley include line guides or D rings embedded in splint material that is brought across the palm.

It is important to assess IP extension on an ongoing basis because of increased potential for PIP and DIP flexion contractures (a result of the increased time in flexion during the day). Most therapists instruct the patient to remove the proximal attachment of the elastic traction at night to allow the fingers to be strapped to the dorsal hood of the splint. The splint is worn full time for the first 4 weeks. It is removed in

therapy for skin and splint cleansing and for skin assessment of pressure areas.

Exercises. Exercises should be performed in therapy and at home, 10 repetitions every hour. Passive flexion of the fingers is performed within the splint. Full passive PIP flexion, DIP flexion, and composite finger flexion are performed passively to the strap across the palm. Full active PIP and DIP extension are performed within the splint, to the dorsal hood of the splint (Fig. 11-12, *B*). It is important to maintain full IP extension, especially within this protocol, unless a digital nerve repair has been made. Goals in the

TABLE 11-6 Flexor Tendon Repair in the Digit (Immediate Passive-Flexion Approach)

Rehabilitation Phase	Criteria to Progress to This Phase	Anticipated Impairments and Functional Limitations	Intervention	Goal	Rationale
Phase III 8-12 wk	• Good progression/ tolerance of A/PROM • No significant increase in pain • Intact tendon	• Pain • Limited range of motion • Limited strength • Limited ability to grip, pinch, lift, or carry objects	• Passive finger or thumb flexion • Passive IP extension in the presence of contractures, dynamic IP extension splint with physician approval • Composite active digit extension • Full active flexion of fingers or thumb • Modalities—heat for stiffness and pain as needed • Blocking, tendon gliding if adhesions limit active motion • Gentle passive intrinsic stretch as needed • Light strengthening exercises if adhesions are present • Gradual, progressive strengthening after 12 wk • Scar massage, scar pads at night • Edema control/light compressive wrap • Patient/family education	• Full PROM, AROM of fingers or thumb • Pain-free motion • Increase strength to facilitate light use • Decrease thickness and firmness of scar • Minimal edema by 12 wk • Independent home exercises • Prevent tendon rupture • Functional use of injured hand	• Promote restoration of full joint mobility • Pain and edema management • Improve tendon gliding • Promote functional use of the injured hand • Prevent compromise of tendon repair

A/PROM, Active passive range of motion; *AROM,* active range of motion; *IP,* interphalangeal; *PROM,* passive range of motion.

early phase of the immediate passive-flexion approaches include attaining full passive flexion and active IP extension, tendon gliding as possible within these exercises, edema control, protecting the repaired flexor tendon from rupture with appropriate splinting and patient education, and attaining full UE motion proximal to the wrist.

Phase II (Intermediate)
TIME: 4 to 7 or 8 weeks
GOALS: Attain partial (at least 50%) active flexion of the injured digit, full passive flexion, full active extension, protect repaired tendon from rupture with splinting between exercises and patient education

Exercises. Exercises should continue as in phase I, and the patient can remove the splint for exercises and bathing. In therapy and at home, active flexion is initiated. Begin with wrist tenodesis exercises and gentle place-active hold in flexion exercises. Advance to active flexion and composite finger extension with the wrist flexed. At 6 weeks, discontinue protective splinting and begin active extension of the fingers with the wrist in neutral.

If flexor tendon adhesions are noted (passive flexion is better than active flexion), blocking exercises are initiated for PIP and DIP flexion. Goals in the intermediate phase of the immediate passive-flexion programs include attaining at least half range of active flexion of the injured digit, full passive flexion, full active finger extension, and protecting the repaired tendon from rupture with appropriate splinting between exercises and patient education.

Phase III (Late)
TIME: 7 or 8 to 12 weeks
GOALS: Full active and passive flexion and extension, light grip strength, protect repaired tendon from rupture with patient education

Splinting is discontinued and light active use is initiated. If flexor tendon adhesions are present, then advance to light resistive exercises at 8 weeks after surgery.

If good tendon gliding is evidenced by equal or nearly equal active and passive flexion, then delay resistance until 10 to 12 weeks after surgery and advance gradually. If IP flexion contractures are present, then passive IP extension

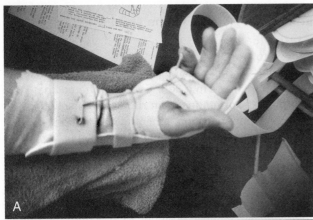

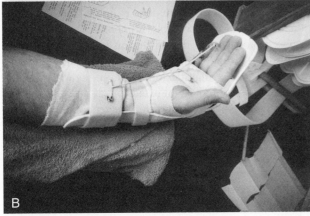

Fig. 11-12 **A,** Dorsal blocking splint with elastic traction places the MP joints and wrist in partial flexion and attaches an elastic band to the fingertip of the injured finger. **B,** Exercises are to fully passively flex the digit and to actively extend the IP joints to the hood of the splint. (Courtesy Linda Klein.)

exercises and dynamic IP extension splinting may be initiated with surgeon approval. Goals in the late phase of the immediate passive-flexion approaches include full active and passive flexion and extension, regaining light grip strength, and protecting the repaired tendon from rupture with patient education. Full grip and pinch strength can be performed as part of a home exercise program 12 weeks after surgery, at which time the repaired flexor tendon is considered to be strong enough to tolerate normal daily activities.

In general, when a digit with a repaired flexor tendon demonstrates good active flexion within the first 5 or 6 weeks after surgery, advancement to resistance is delayed because minimal additional support of adhesions to the repair site exists. When flexor tendon adhesions limit active flexion more than passive flexion, the digit can be advanced through the phases listed previously at the earlier of the times indicated because the tendon has the support of surrounding adhesions and can tolerate the additional tension applied within the advancing phases of treatment with less chance of rupture. The decision to advance a patient with a flexor tendon injury to the next phase of treatment is best done in conjunction with the referring surgeon because advancing the partially healed flexor tendon to active flexion, passive

extension, and, most significantly, resistance, creates an increase in tension at the repair site.

Full passive flexion and nearly full extension of the injured finger or fingers should be expected following use of an immediate passive-flexion approach. The amount of active flexion achieved varies, and active DIP flexion is often limited by adhesions. IP extension is occasionally limited by flexion contracture. When composite extension of the wrist and digits is limited in the late phase of tendon healing, a resting pan splint in maximum composite extension, worn at night, will help distal gliding of the tendon to allow composite extension. A finger-length splint may be used if just the IP joints are contracted in flexion. Functional deficits in motion or strength present after 12 weeks can be treated with any traditional therapy approaches, including modalities and dynamic splinting for stiffness or contractures, AROM and PROM, joint mobilization, blocking exercises, and strengthening.

IMMEDIATE ACTIVE-FLEXION APPROACH

Indications

Development of immediate active-flexion guidelines is the most recent advancement in rehabilitation after flexor tendon repairs. These guidelines have been developed after the onset of surgical advancements of stronger repair techniques described earlier in this chapter. Active-flexion approaches have been developed to minimize flexor tendon adhesions in the early phase of tendon healing and have been very successful in improving outcomes of flexor tendon repairs.[8,22,31-33] Immediate active-flexion approaches are reserved for patients who have had a strong enough surgical repair to tolerate the additional stress placed on the tendon by active flexion, as well as those who can be compliant to the splinting and exercise program. **The presence of severe edema, joint stiffness, or health factors that would slow tendon healing would prohibit placement of a patient in an active-flexion approach.** It is important to minimize the stress on the tendon, especially in the early phase of tendon healing, to prevent rupture.

Minimizing Tension on a Tendon With Immediate Active-Flexion Approaches

Because active flexion results in an increase in tension within the flexor tendon, it is important to minimize this tension in the early phase of tendon healing to prevent rupture. Edema and stiffness both present increased resistance to active flexion, thereby requiring the flexor muscles to pull harder on the tendon, increasing the work of flexion within an immediate flexion protocol. Work of flexion is a term that describes the amount of tension created within the tendon during active flexion.[34] Work of flexion increases with swelling, stiffness, or any internal friction encountered by the tendon caused by bulk of repair, tight pulleys, or swelling of the tendons, in addition to the tension normally developed during active flexion.[35] The therapist's goal is to minimize the work of flexion, thereby minimizing stress on the repaired tendon, when active motion is initiated immediately after repair. The therapist does this by minimizing edema and joint stiffness and using optimal joint positions that minimize the amount of tension developed within the tendon during active flexion.[22] Studies have shown that the wrist position that results in the least tension within the flexor tendon during active flexion is partial wrist extension and MP flexion.[36]

When the wrist is flexed, an increased amount of work is required by the flexor muscles to flex the fingers, compared with when the wrist is slightly extended. By placing the wrist in slight extension, the extensor tendons are given slack at the wrist, allowing the fingers to relax into partial flexion. It requires only a slight pull by the muscle to further flex the digits actively into a light fist. Thus most immediate active-flexion protocols use a position of wrist neutral to slightly extended during the active-flexion exercises, and avoid active digit flexion with the wrist flexed. Attaining the end ranges of active flexion also significantly increases tension within the flexor tendon, and achieving a light fist with at least 45° of DIP flexion is the main goal in the early phase of tendon healing. More than 45° of DIP flexion is allowed if attained easily by the patient, without excessive effort, when the surgeon has performed a four-strand (or more) repair. Education of the patient placed in this protocol is very important because those patients that attempt to do more than allowed are much more likely to rupture.

Immediate Active-Flexion Guidelines

Phase I (Early)

TIME: 0 to 4 or 5 weeks

GOALS: Attain full passive flexion, ability to actively hold the fingers in a light fist, minimize edema, protect flexor tendon from rupture with splinting and patient education, attain full UE motion proximal to the wrist (Table 11-7)

Splinting. A large variety of splints have been developed to apply when the patient is placed in an immediate active-flexion approach. The splint design was changed to bring the wrist into an optimal position, as described previously, during the exercises that are done at home. The wrist position in the traditional protocols (immobilization and passive-flexion protocols) was that of flexion to place slack in the repaired flexor tendon and prevent tension on the tendon at rest. During active digit flexion, however, the wrist is better placed in a position of slight extension, as described earlier, to prevent excessive tension within the tendon during active flexion. A few of the most commonly used splints will be described; however, additional options are sure to exist because splinting and guidelines are evolving constantly.

The Indiana protocol uses a wrist hinge splint that allows 30° of wrist extension and full wrist flexion, applied for exercises only (Fig. 11-13, *A* and *B*).[7,8,20,21] A static dorsal blocking splint with the wrist and MPs flexed is worn at all times

---

TABLE 11-7   Flexor Tendon Repair in the Digit (Immediate Active-Flexion Approach)

Rehabilitation Phase	Criteria to Progress to This Phase	Anticipated Impairments and Functional Limitations	Intervention	Goal	Rationale
Phase I 0-4 wk	• Repair technique of adequate strength to tolerate immediate active motion approach • Postoperative and cleared by physician to initiate therapy with immediate active motion approach	• Edema • Pain • Limited range of motion • Unable to grip, pinch, lift, or carry objects	• Postoperative splint fabrication (see text for options) • Inspect surgical site for drainage, erythema • Pain assessment • Edema assessment and early edema control • AROM exercises for the shoulder and elbow • Passive flexion all finger joints • Active IP extension with MPs flexed • Place-active hold flexion of fingers with wrist neutral or extended 20°-30° • Patient/family education regarding tendon precautions and home exercise program	• Protect tendon repair • Prevent infection • Decrease pain and edema to moderate or less • Full AROM of shoulder and elbow • Full passive flexion and IP extension • Ability to actively hold the fingers in 75° MP, 75° PIP, and 45° DIP flexion or more • Patient to understand tendon repair precautions and home exercise program	• Prevent compromise of tendon repair • Promote wound healing • Manage pain and edema • Prevent proximal joint stiffness • Prevent joint stiffness and flexion contractures • Minimize resistance to tendon gliding • Initiate active tendon gliding • Minimize tendinous adhesions

AROM, Active range of motion; *DIP,* distal interphalangeal; *IP,* interphalangeal; *MP,* metacarpophalangeal; *PIP,* proximal interphalangeal.

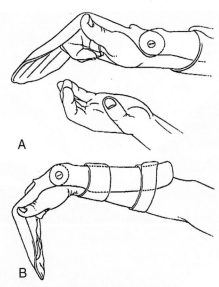

Fig. 11-13 The wrist hinge splint, designed at the Indiana Hand Center, allows 30° wrist extension while performing place-hold flexion (**A**) and wrist flexion with IP extension (**B**). (From Cannon N: Post flexor tendon repair motion protocol. Indiana Hand Center Newsl 1:13, 1993.)

between the active exercises in the early phase of tendon healing. This requires that the patient be trusted to change splints at home for exercises without inadvertent stretch applied to the tendon, or use of the hand while the splint is removed. The wrist hinge splint, worn for exercises, maximizes use of the wrist tenodesis exercises and ideal wrist position of partial extension during active flexion of the fingers.

Silfverskiold and May[32] use a cast (with the wrist neutral) that is worn at all times, for both exercises and at rest between exercises. Elastic traction is applied to all four fingers regardless of the number of injured fingers, and the elastic traction is removed or loosened for the active-flexion exercises. This concept eliminates the need for the patient to change splints at home, yet achieves the need to bring the wrist out of the flexed position for exercises. This author has used this wrist-neutral concept for both splinting and home exercises.[31] The author's preferred splint is a dorsal blocking splint with the wrist in neutral, MP joints flexed to 50°, and the IP joints allowed full extension unless a digital nerve has been repaired. The use of elastic traction with this splint is optional. If IP flexion contractures begin, the fingers may be strapped to the dorsal hood of the splint between exercises. If elastic traction is used, it is applied to all four fingers (or if the thumb flexor tendon was repaired, then elastic traction is applied to the tip of the thumb only), through a palmar pulley, attached on the proximal strap of the forearm (Fig. 11-14, *A*). The splint is not allowed to be removed at home by the patient in the early phase of tendon healing, but it is removed in therapy for splint and skin cleansing, assessment of skin for pressure areas, and exercises as follows.

Exercises. Exercises should be performed in therapy and at home, 10 repetitions every hour. The splint is worn at all times except in therapy. Passive flexion of the digits to the

palm is initiated. Active extension of the IP joints is performed fully unless a digital nerve has been repaired (Fig. 11-14, *B*). The active-flexion portion of the exercises is performed with place-active hold in flexion of the fingers. This is performed by gently, passively flexing the fingers to the palm using the patient's other hand or the therapist's hand. After placing the fingers into gentle flexion, the other hand is removed, while the patient actively holds the fingers of the injured hand in a fist (Fig. 11-14, *C* and *D*). In therapy, this is done with the wrist extended 30° to decrease tension in the extensor tendons during the place-active hold flexion. It is important to attain DIP flexion during this exercise to ensure FDP gliding. **The patient should not place pressure on the palm or squeeze the palm with any fingertips to avoid increasing tension within the tendon.** The place-active hold flexion portion of the exercise is the main difference between the immediate active and immediate passive-flexion guidelines. When the patient is successful in maintaining the actively flexed position of the digits without the repaired digit being trapped or overly supported by the adjacent digit, proximal gliding of the repaired tendon through the pulley system and the area of surgery has been achieved. This place-active hold exercise of the digits is important to obtain within the first 5 days after surgery, or flexor tendon adhesions are much more likely to limit the ability to gain full active flexion at a later time. When active flexion and passive flexion are nearly equal, it indicates good to excellent flexor tendon gliding. If good flexor tendon gliding occurs, the patient is continued in this phase longer than 6 weeks because increased tension within the well-gliding tendon is more likely to cause a rupture than in the adherent tendon (where the tendon is supported by the surrounding scar tissue). If IP flexion contractures develop, passive PIP extension may be performed with the wrist and MP supported in flexion, as described in the previous discussion of passive IP extension exercises. **Avoid passively extending the DIP joint while performing passive PIP extension in the early phase of tendon healing.** Goals in the early phase of an immediate active-flexion rehabilitation program include attaining full passive flexion, ability to actively hold in a light fist including at least 75° of PIP and 45° of DIP flexion, full PIP and DIP extension, edema control, protecting the flexor tendon from rupture with appropriate splinting and patient education, and attaining full UE motion proximal to the wrist.

Phase II (Intermediate)
TIME: 4 to 5 weeks to 8 weeks
GOALS: Attain full passive and active flexion and full finger extension, prevent intrinsic tightness, protect the repaired flexor tendon from rupture with splinting between exercises and patient education (Table 11-8)

Exercises. The splint is removed at home for bathing and exercises. If elastic traction was used in the early phase, it is discontinued at this time and the static splint is worn between

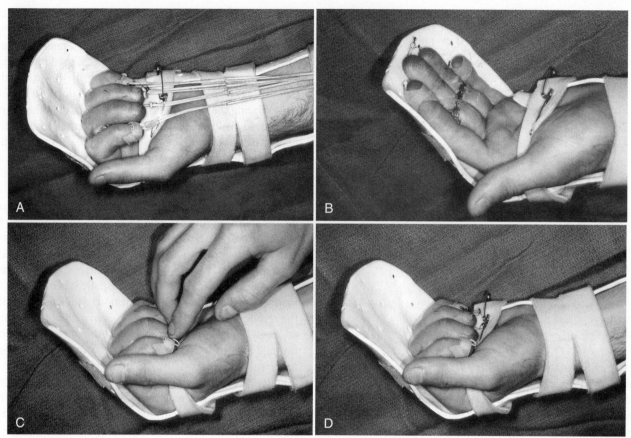

Fig. 11-14 Wrist-neutral dorsal blocking splint with elastic traction used in an immediate active-flexion protocol. Elastic traction is applied to all fingertips between exercises in this option (**A**). Exercises consist of active extension to the hood of the splint with elastic traction released (**B**) and place-active hold in flexion (**C** and **D**). The fingers are gently placed in flexion with the other hand and actively held in flexion when the supporting hand is removed. This requires proximal gliding of the flexor tendon, minimizing potential adhesions in the early phase of healing in an immediate active-flexion protocol after a four-strand or stronger repair technique. (Courtesy Linda Klein.)

TABLE 11-8 Flexor Tendon Repair in the Digit (Immediate Active-Flexion Approach)

Rehabilitation Phase	Criteria to Progress to This Phase	Anticipated Impairments and Functional Limitations	Intervention	Goal	Rationale
Phase II 4-8 wk	• No signs of infection • No significant increase in pain • Intact tendon • Compliant with splinting, home exercises, and precautions	• Edema and pain • Limited range of motion • Limited strength • Unable to grip, pinch, lift, or carry objects	• Remove splint at home for exercises and bathing • Passive flexion, active IP extension • Passive IP extension in presence of flexion contracture • Modalities—heat for stiffness and pain as needed • Wrist tenodesis exercises: active finger flexion with wrist extended; finger extension with wrist flexed • Edema control with light compressive wraps as needed • Scar massage/night pad as needed • Patient education regarding precautions and tendon healing	• Full passive flexion of all joints • Full active extension of all digit joints with wrist flexed • Functional active digit flexion with wrist extended • Reduce tendon adhesions, if present • Decrease edema • Reduce scar thickness • Independent home exercise program • Patient/family to understand tendon repair precautions • Prevent tendon rupture	• Maintain/improve joint mobility • Manage edema and pain • Minimize resistance to tendon gliding • Prevent peritendinous adhesions • Maintain/improve tendon gliding • Prevent compromise of tendon repair

IP, Interphalangeal.

exercises to protect the patient against inadvertent resistance to the well-gliding tendon. Exercises continue as in the early phase, with the addition of removing the splint to perform active motion with wrist tenodesis as described below. During this phase the patient gradually brings the wrist to neutral with the fingers extended. In therapy, gentle intrinsic stretch is performed by the therapist with the wrist flexed, MPs gently, passively extended while the IPs are held flexed.

Active finger flexion is added during this phase, but no resistance is allowed. Wrist tenodesis exercises are performed, allowing wrist extension as tolerated with the fingers in flexion and wrist flexion with the fingers extended. Some protocols discontinue the protective splint in the intermediate phase; however, with a well-gliding flexor tendon, it is possible to rupture the repaired tendon when resistance is encountered during normal daily activities. Most patients are not able to predetermine how much resistance each activity they perform with the hand will cause, and this author prefers to **continue splinting during the intermediate phase unless flexor tendon adhesions are present.** If flexor tendon adhesions limit active flexion more than passive flexion, then blocking exercises are initiated. If IP extension is limited, then passive IP extension is performed with the wrist and MPs held in flexion. Goals in the intermediate phase of the immediate active-flexion guideline include full passive and active flexion, full composite finger extension, preventing intrinsic tightness, and protecting the flexor tendon from rupture with appropriate splinting between exercises and patient education.

Phase III (Late)

TIME: 8 to 14 weeks

GOALS: Full active flexion and extension of the fingers, prevent or minimize intrinsic tightness, prevent flexor tendon from rupture with splinting during resistive activities and patient education (Table 11-9)

The splint is removed except for activities that require pinching, lifting, or strong grip. Resistance to DIP flexion (e.g., hook grasp with resistance or squeezing with the tips of the fingers) is prohibited until after 12 weeks in the case of a well-gliding flexor tendon that demonstrates flexion in the good to excellent range according to the Strickland-Glogovac formula.[27]

A small hand-based dorsal blocking splint is used to prevent the patient from performing this type of activity while at work or during heavier home management tasks. Active and passive flexion and extension of the fingers is performed with the splint off. If flexor tendon adhesions are present (active flexion more limited than passive flexion), blocking exercises continue and resistance may be added, consisting of light gripping. At 12 weeks after surgery, the patient is released to normal activities and instructed to avoid maximal resistive activities for another 2 weeks, gradually

TABLE 11-9 Flexor Tendon Repair in the Digit (Immediate Active-Flexion Approach)

Rehabilitation Phase	Criteria to Progress to This Phase	Anticipated Impairments and Functional Limitations	Intervention	Goal	Rationale
Phase III 8-14 wk	• Good progression/ tolerance of PROM and AROM • No significant increase in pain • Intact tendon • Compliance with home exercises and precautions	• Decrease in pain and edema • Minimally limited range of motion • Limited strength • Limited ability to grip, pinch, lift, or carry objects	• Adjust splint to free wrist, use at work and at night, to avoid strong use of injured hand • Passive finger or thumb flexion • Passive IP extension in the presence of contractures • Composite active digit extension • Full active flexion of fingers or thumb • Modalities—heat for stiffness and pain as needed • Blocking, tendon gliding if adhesions limit active motion • Gentle passive intrinsic stretch • Light strengthening exercises only if adhesions are present before 12 wk; gradual, progressive strengthening after 12 wk • Scar massage, scar pads at night • Edema control/light compressive wrap • Patient/family education	• Full PROM, AROM of fingers or thumb • Pain-free motion • Increase strength to facilitate light use • Decrease thickness and firmness of scar • Minimal edema by 12 wk • Independent home exercises • Prevent tendon rupture • Functional use of injured hand	• Promote restoration of full joint mobility • Pain and edema management • Maintain/improve tendon gliding • Promote functional use of the injured hand • Prevent compromise of tendon repair

AROM, Active range of motion; *IP,* interphalangeal; *PROM,* passive range of motion.

increasing tolerance to normal activities. Goals in the late phase of the immediate active motion approach include full active flexion and extension of the fingers, prevention of intrinsic tightness, and light functional use of the hand. **Prevention of flexor tendon rupture with appropriate splinting during tip pinch, strong grip and hook fist, or lifting activities, as well as patient education, is emphasized.** Regaining full grip, pinch, and full UE strength is appropriate after the 12- to 14-week flexor tendon healing process (through traditional strengthening exercises and activities).

REPAIRS IN ZONES PROXIMAL TO ZONE II

The question often arises regarding guidelines for flexor tendon repairs in other zones of the hand and distal forearm. This author uses the same guidelines described previously for all zones. Less complications of flexor tendon adhesions occur when the tendons are repaired in the midpalm, where no tight pulley system and synovial sheath is found in which to become adherent. At the wrist and distal forearm, however, there remains the problem of adhesions to the flexor retinaculum and the carpal tunnel. These areas respond more easily to efforts at regaining tendon gliding in the intermediate and late phases of tendon healing and rehabilitation than does the digit. When the repair is anywhere other than the digit itself, IP flexion contractures are much less common.

EVALUATING THE RESULTS OF A FLEXOR TENDON REPAIR

Adding flexion of the IP joints and subtracting any loss of extension is the method used to evaluate the motion of a finger in which a flexor tendon has been repaired in the hand. Although a number of formulas exist, Strickland and Glogovac's following formula[27] is commonly used.

$$\{(PIP + DIP\ flexion) - (loss\ of\ PIP\ extension + loss\ of\ DIP\ extension)\} \div 175 \times 100 = \%\ of\ normal$$

To clarify the formula, add PIP flexion + DIP flexion (measured in full-fist composite flexion). From this total, subtract any loss of extension of the PIP and DIP joints, measured in full composite extension. Divide the result by 175, and multiply by 100 to determine the percent of normal motion. The normal amount of PIP and DIP flexion is 175°, and zero is the normal loss of extension of the IP joints. Thus if the total active PIP and DIP flexion equals 175° and no loss of extension of the IP joints occurs, then the patient would have 100% of motion after the flexor tendon repair. Classification includes excellent results as 85% to 100%, good as 70% to 84%, fair as 50% to 69%, and poor as less than 50% of normal motion.

An example is a patient whose final composite motion measurements are MP 0° to 85°, PIP 10° loss of extension to 80° of flexion, and DIP 5° loss of extension to 40° of flexion. The formula applied would be as follows:

$$\{(80 + 40) - (10 + 5)\} \div 175 \times 100\%$$

which is

$$(120 - 15) \div 175 \times 100\% = 60\%$$

Sixty percent would be classified as a fair result according to this classification. MP motion is not used in this formula because it is infrequently affected by tendon repairs in zones I or II. Results in the good and excellent categories are considered functional, without need for further intervention. Fair and poor results may need further surgery or therapeutic intervention to regain function of the hand, depending on individual patient needs for ADLs and work.

SUMMARY

The amount of information available regarding flexor tendon rehabilitation is overwhelming, and the task of determining what approach to use for which patient is daunting. Patient and injury variables require the therapist to be aware of immobilization, immediate passive flexion, and immediate active-flexion guidelines for treatment of a flexor tendon repair. Within each hand treatment facility, it is typical to use one approach from the immediate passive-flexion group and one approach from the immediate active-flexion group for most patients. Then, depending on the type of surgical repair, the recommendation of the surgeon and patient compliance, placement of the patient within immediate passive- or immediate active-flexion approach is less complex. It is good, however, to be familiar with other options, because some patients will do better with elastic traction than others. Most of this author's patients are placed in the immediate active flexion with elastic traction program as described previously, because the referring surgeons are all performing four-strand repairs of the flexor tendon. If IP flexion contractures develop, the program is changed to eliminate the elastic traction or instruct the patient to intermittently strap the IPs in extension to the dorsal hood of the splint (as done at night) during the day.

For those therapists whose patients have traditional two-strand flexor tendon repairs, it is important to choose from the passive-flexion guidelines. If active flexion is performed with these patients in the early phase, then it is done very gently through partial range of flexion (and only under the supervision of the therapist).[22]

It is important to keep in mind the occasional need to place a patient in an immobilization approach, as well. Individualization of each of the guidelines is necessary. A young child may not advance as quickly as the immobilization guideline described in this chapter indicates. Discussion with the referring surgeon is necessary at each advancement point.

Understanding the concepts of flexor tendon healing in the hand and the tensile strengths of the healing tendon compared with tension demands of motion and use is important. Education of the patient regarding importance of compliance with the instructions within the guidelines and the type of activity that is likely to result in rupture is important. Study of literature and supervised experience in treating patients with this diagnosis is strongly recommended whenever possible.

CLINICAL CASE REVIEW

1 A new patient is scheduled for splint fabrication, evaluation, and treatment after repair of flexor tendons. No further information is available on the prescription. What steps should the therapist take before beginning the first session?

The therapist should contact the physician to determine the following:

- The type of repair performed (to determine whether immediate passive- or immediate active-flexion approaches should be considered)
- The surgeon's preference of elastic traction or static IP positioning in the splint

If the surgeon is not available, the therapist should begin an immediate passive-flexion approach. If passive flexion is limited, then therapy should begin with the elastic traction splint. If passive flexion is 50% or better, then the therapist may consider the static IP positioning splint.

2 A new patient is being seen for the first time in therapy after repair of both flexor tendons at the level of the proximal phalanx of a single digit. During the initial visit, the patient begins to sweat, becomes light-headed, and has significant pain with gentle passive flexion. The patient is unable to tolerate more than 30° of passive flexion at each of the IP joints of the injured finger. What can the therapist do to maximize tendon gliding and joint motion within the first week after surgery in the immediate passive- or immediate active-flexion approaches?

This patient is likely to have significant difficulty because of stiffness and adhesions unless he or she becomes more comfortable with passive motion of the digit within a few days. The patient's understanding of the cause of the pain and what to expect in the next few days is crucial at this point. A reassuring, gentle approach at the first appointment is important. The therapist should emphasize the following points:

- Most of the initial pain is related to a fresh incision, and swollen and sore joints need to be moved.
- Although the digit is very painful during the first attempts at motion, if performed to a tolerable level on a frequent basis (every $1\frac{1}{2}$ to 2 hours), then the pain usually becomes minimal within a few days.
- The finger motion may be permanently limited to the level of motion that is achieved within the first 1 or 2 weeks because adhesions develop within this time. Explaining how a tendon glides and the way in which adhesions can limit this gliding helps motivate the patient to passively flex the digit to full tolerance. If

allowed to be in an immediate active approach, then the position of active hold in flexion can only improve as passive flexion improves.

This patient may be best placed in an elastic traction approach between exercises because the elastic traction will hold the digits in flexion at a tolerable level, gradually increasing flexion as resistance of the tissue decreases. The next session should be scheduled for the next day because the patient is usually feeling better and can tolerate motion and better understand directions. If the pain level continues to significantly limit the initial exercises, then the therapist may perform slow, gentle passive flexion to demonstrate the methods to be used at home. Ongoing frequent therapy visits may be needed in the early phase of tendon healing if improvement is not seen quickly.

3 A patient had flexor tendons repaired in a digit 3 weeks ago. During active IP extension exercises, the patient is lacking 30° of PIP extension and 10° of DIP extension. What steps can be taken to improve IP extension?

In therapy, gentle PIP joint mobilization (i.e., accessory glides and gentle passive PIP extension) can be considered with the flexor tendon in the protected position of full wrist and MP flexion. The patient must be relaxed, with no tension in the flexor tendons during the passive flexion, to avoid resisting the repaired flexor tendons.

The therapist should emphasize the IP extension portion of the home exercise program. Full passive MP flexion assists IP extension. The patient should be instructed to passively flex the MP joint of the involved finger fully using the other hand while actively extending the IP joints. A dynamic IP extension splint should not be considered in this early phase of flexor tendon healing.

4 A patient had both flexor tendons repaired 5 weeks ago and has been advanced to the intermediate phase of an immediate passive approach, including gentle active motion. At this appointment, the patient shows a sudden decrease in active DIP flexion compared with the previous session, with only trace to no visible active flexion noted by the therapist. What should the therapist consider?

Whenever a sudden complete loss of flexion of the DIP joint occurs, a rupture of the FDP tendon must be considered. The therapist should have the patient make an appointment with the referring surgeon as soon as possible because some surgeons consider immediate repair. Other surgeons wait for maturation of the healing process and consider later tendon grafting if a rupture occurs. The therapist should discuss the patient's activity level to determine if he or she has used the hand actively, which would place the patient at risk for rupture. The therapist should check tendon integrity by blocking the PIP joint in extension while the patient attempts to actively flex the DIP joint. Any active DIP flexion indicates that the FDP tendon is intact.

5 A patient had flexor tendon repair 7 weeks ago. The finger has 30° active DIP flexion when the PIP is blocked in extension by the therapist but no active DIP flexion when all finger joints are flexed into a fist. What does this mean?

The FDP tendon has adhesions. When the finger is held in extension at the MP and PIP joints, it takes only a small amount of glide of the FDP tendon to result in partial DIP joint flexion. However, when the MP and PIP joints are flexed, such as in a composite fist, the FDP tendon must glide much further to pick up the slack created in the tendon by flexion of the first two joints of the finger before it can then flex the DIP joint. Adhesions limit full gliding of the tendon. The therapist should consider increasing the exercises of blocking, gradually increasing the amount of flexion at which the MP and PIP joints are blocked. The surgeon should be contacted to discuss the potential of adding ultrasound or light resistance to minimize adhesions.

6 My patient has more than the expected amount of swelling 2 weeks after surgery. Is there anything I can apply at this early stage to decrease swelling in the involved fingers?

Elevation, overhead shoulder pumping, and light edema massage proximal to the splint can be performed early after repair in all cases. In situations where there is excessive swelling, once wounds are healed, the patient can be instructed in the application of a light compressive wrap at night only, with the help of another person.

The wrist and distal strap of the splint can be opened, allowing the wrist to flex and the fingers to relax. The assisting individual may then apply the wrap to the swollen fingers lightly, not tight enough to decrease circulation. The wrap is removed during the day to avoid increasing resistance to flexion during exercises.

7 My patient has very good ability to place and actively hold the fingers in flexion. Can I advance them to the next phase of rehabilitation and initiate strengthening?

No. When a repaired flexor tendon is gliding without the restriction of adhesions, the tendon repair will be more strained by the resistance than a tendon that has the additional support of adhesions. The better the tendon excursion (better active flexion of the IP joints), the more protective the therapist is regarding advancement to resistance to avoid increasing tension across the repair, which may result in rupture. The patient should continue passive flexion, place-active hold flexion, and advance to active flexion with the splint off at the appropriate times according to the approach used, but avoid resistance until the tendon is fully healed when good active flexion is present. Resistance is used to improve tendon excursion in the presence of restricting adhesions.

8 Six weeks after surgical repair of a ring finger FDP, a patient demonstrates active flexion of 80° MP, 80° PIP, and 15° DIP. The uninjured small finger has normal passive flexion; however, active flexion is limited to 90° MP, 80° PIP, and 25° DIP flexion. Why would active flexion of an uninjured finger be limited?

This is a good example of *quadriga effect*. When the FDP tendon of one finger is not gliding proximally as in this example, the adjacent digit(s) may demonstrate limited active gliding of the FDP as well because of the common muscle belly. When one flexor tendon is tethered by a scar in the finger, the other flexor tendons are unable to be fully pulled proximally by the muscle.

REFERENCES

1. Bunnell S: Repair of tendons in the fingers and description of two new instruments, Surg Gynecol Obstet 26:103-110, 1918.
2. Kessler I, Nissim F: Primary repair without immobilization of flexor tendon division within the digital sheath: An experimental and clinical study, Acta Orthop Scand 40:587-601, 1969.
3. Kleinert HE, et al: Primary repair of lacerated flexor tendons in "no man's land," J Bone Joint Surg 49:577, 1967.
4. Verdan CE: Practical considerations for primary and secondary repair in flexor tendon injuries, Surg Clin North Am 44:951-970, 1964
5. Powell ES, Trail IA: Forces transmitted along human flexor tendons during passive and active movements of the fingers, J Hand Surg 29B:386-389, 2004.
6. Schuind F, et al: Flexor tendon forces: in vivo measurements, J Hand Surg 17A(2):291-298, 1992.
7. Strickland JW: Development of flexor tendon surgery: Twenty-five years of progress, J Hand Surg 25A:214-235, 2000.
8. Strickland JW, Cannon NM: Flexor tendon repair—Indiana method, Indiana Hand Center Newsl 1:1-12, 1993.
9. Shaieb MD, Singer DI: Tensile strengths of various suture techniques, J Hand Surg 22B(6):764-767, 1997.
10. Joyce ME, Lou J, Manske PR: Tendon healing: Molecular and cellular regulation. In Hunter JM, Schneider LH, Mackin EJ, editors: Tendon and nerve surgery in the hand: A third decade, St Louis, 1997, Mosby.
11. Moran S, et al: Effects of 5-fluorouracil on flexor tendon repair, J Hand Surg 25A(2):242-251, 2000.

12. Thomopoulos S, Das R, Silva MJ, et al: Enhanced flexor tendon healing through controlled delivery of PDGF-BB, J Orthop Res 27(9):1209-1215, 2009

13. Zhao C, Zobitz ME, et al: Surface treatment with 5-fluorouracil after flexor tendon repair in a canine in vivo model, J Bone Joint Surg Am 91(11):2673-2682, 2009.

14. Kobayashi M, Oka M, Toguchida J: Development of polyvinyl alcohol-hydroget (PV-H) shields with a high water content for tendon injury repair, J Hand Surg 26B(5):436-440, 2001.

15. Skoog T, Persson B: An experimental study of the early healing of tendons, Scand J Plast Reconstr Surg 13:384-399, 1954.

16. Silfverskiold KL, May EJ, Tornvall AH: Flexor digitorum profundus tendon excursions during controlled motion after flexor tendon repair in zone II: A prospective clinical study, J Hand Surg 17A:122-133, 1992.

17. Becker H, et al: Intrinsic tendon cell proliferation in tissue culture, J Hand Surg 6:616-619, 1981.

18. Lundborg G, Rank F: Experimental intrinsic healing of flexor tendons based upon synovial fluid nutrition, J Hand Surg 3(1)3:21-31, 1978.

19. Manske PR, Lesker PA: Biochemical evidence of flexor tendon participation in the repair process: An in vitro study, J Hand Surg 9B(2):117-120,1984.

20. Strickland JW: The scientific basis for advances in flexor tendon surgery, J Hand Ther 18(2):94-110, 2005.

21. Strickland JW: Flexor tendons: Acute injuries. In Green DP, Hotchkiss RN, Pederson WC, editors: Green's operative hand surgery, ed 4, vol 2, Philadelphia, 1999, Churchill Livingstone.

22. Evans RB, Thompson DE: The application of force to the healing tendon, J Hand Ther 6:266-284, 1993.

23. Sueoka SS, Lastayo PC: Zone II flexor tendon rehabilitation: A proposed algorithm, J Hand Ther 21(4):410-413, 2008.

24. Cifaldi Collins D, Schwarze L: Early progressive resistance following immobilization of flexor tendon repairs, J Hand Ther 4:111-116, 1991.

25. Pettengill K, van Strien G: Postoperative management of flexor tendon injuries. In Skirven TM, et al, editors: Rehabilitation of the hand and upper extremity, ed 6, Philadelphia, 2011, Mosby.

26. Duran RJ, et al: Management of flexor tendon lacerations in zone 2 using controlled passive motion postoperatively. In Hunter JM, et al, editors: Rehabilitation of the hand, ed 3, St Louis, 1990, Mosby.

27. Strickland JW, Glogovac SV: Digital function following flexor tendon repair in zone II: A comparison of immobilization and controlled passive motion techniques, J Hand Surg 5:537-543, 1980.

28. Dovelle S, Kulis Heeter P: The Washington regimen: Rehabilitation of the hand following flexor tendon injuries, Phys Ther 69:1034-1040, 1989.

29. Chow JA, et al: A splint for controlled active motion after flexor tendon repair: Design, mechanical testing and preliminary clinical results, J Hand Surg 15A:645-651, 1990.

30. Pettengill KM: The evolution of early mobilization of the repaired flexor tendon, J Hand Ther 18(2):157-168, 2005.

31. Klein L: Early active motion flexor tendon protocol using one splint, J Hand Ther 16(3):199-206, 2003.

32. Silfverskiold KL, May EJ: Flexor tendon repair in zone II with a new suture technique and an early mobilization program combining passive and active flexion, J Hand Surg 19(1):53-63, 1994.

33. Trumble TE, Vedder NB, Seiler JG, III, et al: Zone-II flexor tendon repair: A randomized prospective trial of active place-and-hold therapy compared with passive motion therapy, J Bone Joint Surg Am 92(6):1381-1389, 2010.

34. Halikis MN, et al: Effect of immobilization, immediate mobilization, and delayed mobilization on the resistance to digital flexion using a tendon injury model, J Hand Surg 22A:464-472, 1997.

35. Amadio PC: Friction of the gliding surface: Implications for tendon surgery and rehabilitation, J Hand Ther 18(2):112-127, 2005.

36. Savage R: The influence of wrist position on the minimum force required for active movement of the interphalangeal joints, J Hand Surg 13B:262-268, 1988.

CHAPTER 12

Carpal Tunnel Release

Linda de Haas, Diane Coker, Kyle Coker

Carpal tunnel syndrome (CTS) continues to be one of the most significant upper extremity (UE) injuries, with more than 500,000 procedures performed each year.[1] It results from compression of the median nerve as it crosses the wrist and is characterized by numbness, tingling, pain, and complaints of weakness in the hand. The symptoms of CTS can range from mild to severe. They may have far-reaching effects on a person's job, hobbies, and activities of daily living (ADL).[2]

CTS is also the most common entrapment neuropathy of the UE.[1] Paget described the complex of symptoms caused by median nerve entrapment at the wrist in 1854, and Moersch gave the syndrome its name in 1938. Brain, Wright, and Wilkerson published the first series of carpal tunnel releases by division of the transverse carpal ligament (TCL) in 1947. Since that time, a number of variations of this procedure have been developed, all of which involve division of the TCL.

The prevalence in the United States of self-reported CTS is approximately 1 to 3 cases per 1000 subjects per year in the adult (working and nonworking) population.[3-5] CTS affects people during their most productive years. Its prevalence peaks between the ages of 35 and 44 years for both men and women. Women are three times more likely to be affected than men.[6]

The Bureau of Labor Statistics tracks CTS under work-related musculoskeletal disorders. In 2008, 3.1% of 384,480 musculoskeletal disorders were CTS cases.[7,8] These data demonstrate the importance of clinicians fully understanding the prevention and treatment of CTS.

SURGICAL INDICATIONS AND CONSIDERATIONS

Causes

The onset of CTS can be classified into two categories: (1) acute and (2) chronic. Acute CTS is associated with a traumatic event, such as blunt trauma to the wrist, wrist fracture, infections, vascular disorders, rheumatologic disorders, hemorrhagic problems, burns, and high pressure injection injuries.[1] These traumas produce a sudden and sustained increase in interstitial pressure within the carpal tunnel, resulting in a median nerve conduction block from intra-compartmental and intraneural ischemia. This form of CTS is a medical emergency and requires immediate carpal tunnel decompression.

Chronic CTS is the result of an insidious rise of the interstitial pressure in the carpal tunnel and is classified as early, intermediate, or advanced. Patients with early CTS experience mild, intermittent symptoms that have been present less than 1 year. Intermediate CTS is characterized by more constant symptoms, including numbness and paresthesia, usually worse at night, with little or no atrophy of the thenar muscles. Surgery performed at this time uncovers a nerve that has undergone chronic changes, including epineural and intrafascicular edema. If decompression is performed at this time, then the neural changes are frequently reversible, although night symptoms may take a year to resolve. Advanced CTS is characterized by progressive paresthesia, atrophy of the thenar muscles, and pinch and grip weakness. Even after a successful surgical decompression, the chronic changes in the median nerve may be permanent.[9]

CTS can affect anyone, although females tend to have a higher incidence. Medical and ergonomic histories have been identified as independent risk factors in developing CTS, although controversy exists as to the contribution of work activities to the development of CTS.[10-12] Recent studies have looked at obesity as defined by body mass index; other biologic factors, such as genetics or structural make-up; and wrist anthropometrics as possible contributing factors.[13-18] There are some strong associations between CTS and age, gender, and female hormonal status as seen, for instance, during menopause or pregnancy.[12] Pregnancy can precipitate CTS by causing edema around the structures traversing the carpal canal. During pregnancy the symptoms of CTS tend to occur in the last trimester, secondary to fluid retention. The condition usually resolves within 6 to 12 weeks after delivery.[9]

CTS can also be associated with a number of other disease processes, including thyroid disease, rheumatoid arthritis, and diabetes, as well as with various anatomic anomalies such as a persistent median artery, median nerve variations, extramuscle bellies, and extratendinous slips.[15,18-20] Tumors and ganglions of the wrist, although rare, can precipitate CTS as the lesion occupies space within the carpal canal.[21] Wrist trauma can cause CTS because of the resulting edema and hematoma surrounding the median nerve. Variations in lumbrical origin, length, or width can increase carpal tunnel pressure as dynamic lumbrical incursion into the CT can occur during finger flexion movements.[22]

From the ergonomic side, CTS is often seen in patients who perform repetitive activities in their work or hobbies. One study of computer workers demonstrated that the angle of wrist extension (more than 20°) was associated with developing CTS.[23]

The diagnosis of CTS can usually be made based on a thorough history and careful physical examination. In cases in which the diagnosis is uncertain, electrodiagnostic studies can be helpful in either confirming or ruling out the disorder.[24]

In general, patients who are diagnosed with early stage CTS are initially treated without surgery. Nonsteroidal anti-inflammatory drugs, although often prescribed, have not been shown to be effective in any controlled study to date[25,26] In some patients with recently developed CTS (less than 1 year), local injection of steroid medication into the carpal canal or oral steroids can significantly, although temporarily, reduce the symptoms of median nerve compression (Fig. 12-1). It has not been shown that a steroid injection can actually alter the progression of the disorder.[5,27]

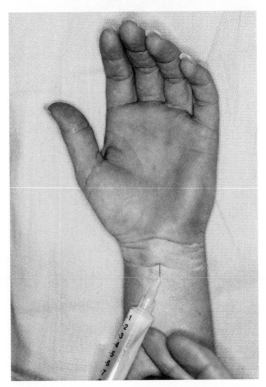

Fig. 12-1 Local injection of a corticosteroid is infiltrated into the carpal tunnel through a 25-gauge needle.

The best evidence-based conservative physical therapy treatments for CTS include splinting, deep pulsed ultrasound (US), nerve-gliding exercises, carpal bone mobilization, and yoga.[26,28] Splinting the patient's wrist can be very helpful in controlling nighttime pain symptoms.[29] The wrist is splinted in a neutral position that maximizes the carpal tunnel space[30] and minimizes the carpal tunnel pressure.[31] The splint is chosen based on the patient's needs and comfort. The metal stay of a prefabricated wrist splint is easily replaced with a custom-molded thermoplastic stay to position the wrist in neutral. A positive Berger test (the patient holds a full fist position for 30 to 40 seconds, with a positive test reproducing paresthesia) result would suggest that the metacarpal phalangeal joints should also be immobilized in the splint, as the lumbricals can descend into the carpal tunnel with active finger flexion and cause further space compromise of the carpal tunnel contents.[10,32] All patients should sleep in their splints. Patients who have constant or activity-induced paresthesia may also wear their splints during the day.[30] When such conservative measures fail to resolve symptoms, surgery is indicated.

Classic CTS symptoms include the following[5]:
1. Numbness and tingling in the median nerve distribution in the hand
2. Nocturnal paresthesia
3. Clumsiness/"weakness" of the hand
4. Weakness/atrophy in the thenar musculature (late finding)

Sensory changes are commonly the first symptoms noted. The patient typically reports paresthesia and numbness of the digits served by the sensory branches of the median nerve and in the tips of the thumb, index finger, middle finger, and radial half of the ring finger, although both sides of the ring finger can be affected. Sensory symptoms may also be restricted to a single digit, or even involve the entire hand.[1] Sensibility in the thenar eminence is usually unaffected as this area is innervated by the palmar cutaneous branch of the median nerve, which branches proximal to the carpal tunnel, entering the hand volar to the TCL.

The onset of pain is most often the primary reason a person with chronic CTS seeks medical attention. The pain associated with CTS tends to begin in the latter aspects of the early and then into the intermediate stages. The patient complains of an intermittent, vague, dull aching in the wrist or forearm. Less common is pain radiating to the elbow and even the shoulder. Night pain is a common complaint most likely caused by congestion of the venous system during sleep.[33] Neurologic muscle weakness associated with CTS occurs late in the disease process. In advanced cases, atrophy of the thenar musculature can be seen. The unlucky patient with symptoms progressed to this state is at high risk for permanent nerve damage and may require a tendon transfer to substitute for the loss of palmar abduction.

The clinician must be able to visualize the anatomic structures that make up the carpal tunnel. The carpal canal is bounded by the TCL volarly, the scaphoid tuberosity and the trapezium radially, the hook of the hamate and the pisiform ulnarly, and the volar radiocarpal ligament and volar ligamentous extensions between the carpal bones dorsally.[19,34] The carpal canal is traversed by the median nerve, the four flexor digitorum profundus tendons, the four flexor digitorum superficialis tendons, the flexor pollicis longus tendon, and the surrounding synovial membranes. Any condition that causes enlargement of the contents of the carpal canal (such as inflammation or edema) or occupies space within the canal (such as a tumor or hematoma) compresses the median nerve. This occurs because the structures that make up the carpal canal are relatively inelastic and do not expand as the contents of the canal enlarge. The resulting pressure compromises circulation within the substance of the nerve, leading to nerve ischemia, which in turn leads to the symptoms and signs seen in CTS.

SURGICAL PROCEDURE

The surgical treatment for carpal tunnel dates back to the 1940s.[35,36]

The condition could be thought of as a compartment syndrome affecting the median nerve within the carpal canal.[37] As such, the intracompartmental pressure surrounding the median nerve exceeds the local capillary pressure, thus preventing blood flow. Surgical treatment is directed at increasing the volume of the carpal canal and reducing the pressure within. Most methods rely on the release of the TCL, which forms the soft tissue roof of the carpal canal. There are three general surgical approaches to the release of the TCL.

The first surgical approach is the classic open technique in which an incision starting in the proximal third of the palm is made that extends proximally along the axis of the ring metacarpal to the wrist flexion crease (Fig. 12-2). Keeping to the ulnar side of the median nerve reduces the risk of injury to its motor branch, which will occasionally arise on the ulnar side of the nerve and cross superficially over to the thenar muscles. The incision is then continued proximally across the volar flexion creases in a zigzag fashion to avoid hypertrophic scarring. The incision is kept to the ulnar side of the palmaris longus tendon to avoid injury to the palmar cutaneous nerve. This incision gives complete exposure to the area of constriction (Figs. 12-3 and 12-4). The thick portion of the TCL between the trapezium and scaphoid tubercle radially and the hook of the hamate and pisiform on the ulnar side is divided under direct vision and extended to the superficial palmar arch distally and approximately 4 to 5 cm proximal to the volar flexion crease of the wrist. The advantage of this approach is the direct exposure to the median nerve along its entire length within the suspected area of constriction. In addition, the contents of the carpal canal can be thoroughly explored for masses, excessive synovial tissues, and bone spurs. If indicated, synovectomy or tenolysis can be performed. Disadvantages of this approach include an increased incidence of pillar pain, prolonged healing, prolonged weakness of grip because of scar

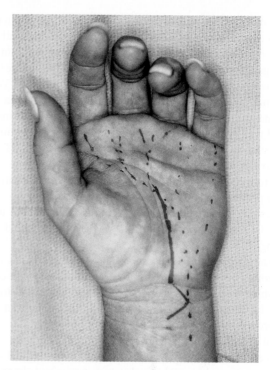

Fig. 12-2 Exposure of the carpal canal is performed through an incision represented by the solid line. Dashed lines represent the course of the ulnar artery and its branches (common digital and proper digital arteries) that must be preserved during exposure.

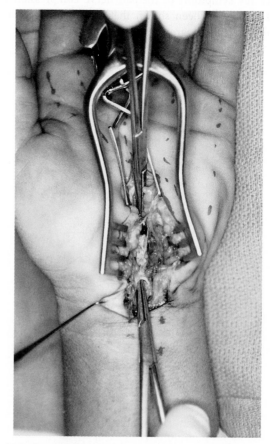

Fig. 12-3 The transverse carpal ligament has been exposed and is being tented proximally and distally by hemostats.

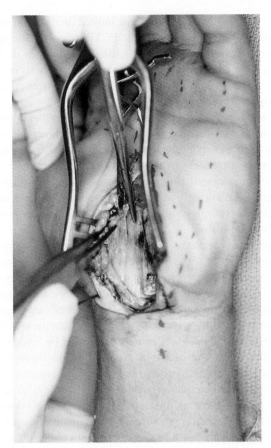

Fig. 12-4 The transverse carpal ligament has been divided, and the contents of the underlying carpal canal are exposed. The median nerve is demonstrated at the tip of the dissecting scissors.

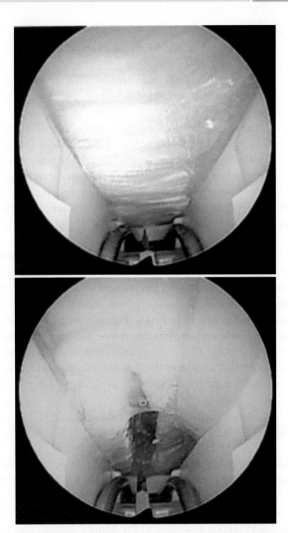

Fig. 12-5 The image above shows the transverse carpal ligament as seen from the inside of the carpal canal. The image below shows the initial cut with the integrated scalpel.

tenderness, and destabilization of the flexor tendons and the pulley effect provided by an intact TCL.

The second and less invasive procedure could be referred to as a limited open palm technique. By this method a smaller incision is made in the palm following the same course as the palm segment of the classic open technique but avoids crossing the volar flexion crease of the wrist. The distal portion of the TCL is incised under direct vision and retractors are used to complete the division proximal to the volar flexion crease. With more specialized instruments and retractors, the palmar incision can be kept quite small. The advantage of this procedure is to minimize injury to the overlying skin and cutaneous nerves, thus reducing the chance of a tender scar. Since there is less destabilization of the flexor tendons, there is less potential for prolonged weakness of grip. The disadvantage of this technique is the limited exposure and visualization of potential pathologic conditions, such as space occupying lesions within or just proximal to the carpal canal.

The third technique is endoscopic carpal tunnel release (ECTR). There are several variations of this technique including one or two portals—either one proximal to the wrist crease, one in the mid palm, or both. ECTR was introduced by Okutsu and Chow in 1989.[38,39] Chow's technique, which has become popular in the United States, employed two portals to pass the endoscope and instruments under the TCL. Agee later introduced a single proximal portal technique that employed an integrated instrument incorporating the scope and surgical knife.[40] There have since been minor modifications in technique and instrumentation for Chow's technique, but the principles remain the same.

The endoscopic techniques were developed to minimize recovery and absence from work. To this end the concept has been successful. Many studies have reported this in both the workers compensation population and the nonwork related groups.[39,40] Several studies comparing recovery rates between open carpal tunnel release and ECTR indicate that the advantages of ECTR diminish over time and there is very little difference at 3 months follow-up (Fig. 12-5).[41]

Surgery for carpal tunnel is not risk free.[42] Complications include:

- Injury to the median nerve including the motor branch
- Injury to the ulnar nerve
- Injury to digital nerves; most often the common digital nerve to the third web space
- Complex regional pain syndrome

- Infection
- Injury to superficial palmar arch and digital arteries
- Injury to the flexor tendons

Lesser complications that usually resolve with time include: hematoma, wound dehiscence, pillar pain, and weakness of grip.

The literature reports an overall higher rate of all of these complications with the endoscopic technique by a factor of two to four times. However, most of these were reports from the early and late 1990s, and although the specific techniques were rarely reported, they were probably referring to the earlier two portal techniques. There have not been any direct comparisons between the two portal and single portal techniques that compare complication rates.

Postoperatively, most surgeons will splint wrists following the open technique to allow soft tissue healing and to position the wrist in extension to prevent bowstringing of the flexor tendons, which might push the medial nerve into the area of the healing TCL. Although this was the early rationale for postoperative splinting, more recent studies have shown splinting to be less important than previously believed.[43] Wrists are often not splinted following endoscopic release, although time must still be allowed for internal healing.

PILLAR PAIN

Pillar pain is cited as a common postoperative complication and is a frequent reason to send the patient for postoperative therapy.[44] It is described as pain over either the thenar or hypothenar eminence or both. These areas correspond to the scaphoid tubercle and hook of the hamate distally, and trapezium and pisiform proximally, forming a rectangle. The three thenar muscles are anchored to the scaphoid tubercle and trapezium, and the three hypothenar muscles are anchored to the hook of the hamate and pisiform. The TCL ties the two columns together and acts as a pulley to guide the nine flexor tendons. The cause is still unclear, possibly because several different symptoms have been called pillar pain. It is unclear if the pain represents deep scar tissue, injury to sensory nerves in the TCL, loss of stability of the attached muscles, or alteration of the carpal arch. Whatever the cause, there appears to be a lowered incidence with ECTR compared with limited open releases, which further improve on the full open incision. In all cases the pain tends to resolve in 3 months.[44,45]

Failed Carpal Tunnel Surgery

Carpal tunnel surgery is highly successful in relieving the symptoms caused by compression on the median nerve at the wrist. Failures can be grouped into two categories: recurrent symptoms and residual symptoms. Both can result from incomplete or inadequate release of the TCL, progression of the underlying disease, or misdiagnosis.

Whereas the TCL is seen in its entirety in the open carpal tunnel release, it may not be when doing the ECTR. In fact, in the case of the open technique, the TCL is allowed to open

widely as much as 1 to 2 cm. The limited incision technique opens to a lesser degree and the ECTR by only a few millimeters. This latter technique is usually enough to decompress the median nerve, but there have been reports of both early and late failures that were relieved by reoperation using the open procedure.

Early return of symptoms following initial relief might be caused by tight bandages or excessive stretch on the nerve from improper splinting, hematoma, or excessive scar tissue.

Late recurrences can also result from incomplete or even full open release if the underlying condition continues to progress. Enlarging masses, trauma, edema, inflammatory conditions causing synovitis, or simply the aging process might be to blame.

Residual symptoms following carpal tunnel surgery are common, but in one of the author's experience, true recurrences and failed surgeries are very rare. Although symptoms of CTS vary depending on the individual, age, and duration of symptoms, the most common symptom of carpal tunnel is numbness in the distribution of the median nerve, which is worse at night. This is usually confirmed by evidence of significant slowing of the nerve conduction through the carpal canal. When patients with residual symptoms are properly questioned, they usually recall that they did in fact have relief of their nocturnal numbness following release of the TCL. This indicates a successful treatment of their CTS; however, they may still be dissatisfied with the result if they still have symptoms that brought them to the physician in the first place. These symptoms might include arm pain, arm numbness and tingling, shooting pains into various parts of the arm and hands, and weakness. The symptoms might be reproducible when attempting to perform specific activities, giving rise to the notion that their condition is a repetitive motion injury. In the experience of the authors of this chapter, the vast majority of these patients are no longer suffering from CTS but rather have a more proximal nerve entrapment. There are several potential points of entrapment of the median nerve at the elbow, including pronator syndrome. If cervical radiculopathy can be ruled out, the problem may be attributed to compression at the level of the brachial plexus, the so-called thoracic outlet syndrome. This diagnosis is often made by exclusion and then treated with a trial of therapy to address the thoracic outlet. Within a few weeks the patient will often notice a significant decrease in pain and an increase in strength.[46,47]

THERAPY GUIDELINES FOR REHABILITATION

Postoperative Rehabilitation

The frequency and duration of treatment is highly variable after a carpal tunnel release. In most cases minimal therapy is required, with key contributions to postoperative care being wound/scar management and proper instructions in exercises to enhance tendon gliding, obtain full active range of motion (AROM), and minimize edema. The patient may need guidance on ergonomics and other principles to facilitate full return to work or other activities.[10] All patients referred to therapy are instructed in a home exercise program appropriate to the phase of recovery and their individual needs.

In general, patients tend to do quite well after carpal tunnel release. However, because the extent of the damage to the median nerve cannot fully be known before surgery, predicting the exact outcome of carpal tunnel release is difficult. Patients with mild to moderate symptoms can expect full recovery of sensation and resolution of the numbness and tingling caused by entrapment of the nerve. Patients with more advanced disease who have significant sensibility loss and muscle weakness usually achieve significant improvement of their condition. Patients with muscle atrophy can expect a halt to progression of muscle wasting and in some cases can regain muscle mass.

The recovery of the median nerve directly relates to the success of the surgery. Ultrasonography postoperatively may be helpful in identifying the initial beneficial morphologic changes. Nerve conduction studies could take as long as 3 to 6 months to change.[48] Patients must understand that they may have some element of incisional pain after surgery, which can last as long as 3 to 6 months. They must also be informed that they will temporarily lose some strength in the hand, which usually improves after 3 to 6 months.

Postoperative Evaluation

In general, patients may be referred to therapy anywhere from 1 to 3 weeks postoperatively. The timing of the first visit will dictate which tests are appropriate to perform and which should be deferred until a later time. The initial evaluation after carpal tunnel release includes the following:

- Patient history
- Subjective pain report
- Edema measurement
- AROM measurements **(Depending on the procedure, simultaneous finger/wrist flexion may need to be deferred until 3 weeks postoperatively to avoid the risk of bowstringing.)**
- Sensibility testing
- Wound and scar assessment
- Documentation of the patient's previous and present functional status

After 3 weeks postoperatively, in addition to the above measurements, the evaluation can include:

- Grip and pinch assessment
- Finger dexterity assessment
- Neural tension testing as needed
- Manual muscle testing (MMT)

The patient's history is obtained by patient interview. Information to be noted in the history includes age, gender, hand dominance, cause of CTS, type and date of the carpal tunnel release, occupation, avocational interests, onset and description of symptoms before surgery, and notes regarding whether symptoms were unilateral or bilateral. The patient should be screened for medical or systemic problems that might contribute to the persistence of symptoms.

The patient is asked to quantify the pain on a scale from 0 (representing no pain) to 10 (indicating severe pain requiring medical attention). The patient is asked to rate the pain both at rest and with use. The quality of the patient's pain is obtained by documenting the descriptive terms the patient uses when discussing the symptoms.[49]

Edema of the hand is recorded either by volumetric circumferential or figure of eight measurements. If edema is profuse throughout the hand, then volumetric measurements can be taken provided that stitches have been removed and the patient has no open wounds. The volumetric assessment should be administered following the American Society of Hand Therapists (ASHT) guidelines. If edema is minimal or the stitches have not yet been removed, then circumferential measurements recorded in centimeters should be obtained at the distal wrist crease and the distal palmar crease (DPC). The figure of eight method for assessing hand edema has been shown to be as reliable and valid as the volumetric method, and may be easier to perform in a busy clinic than the volumetric method.[50]

AROM measurements are obtained using a goniometer for the wrist and forearm. Individual finger AROM measurements may not be necessary when motion limitations are minimal. A global measurement of finger flexibility is obtained by measuring composite finger flexion to the DPC. The distance from the middle of the pulp of a finger to the DPC is measured in centimeters for each finger. Functional thumb opposition is recorded as the ability to oppose the thumb to each fingertip, and full composite flexion/opposition as the ability to touch the thumb to the DPC of the small finger. Full motion is recorded as "zero," and lack of full motion as a negative number.

To prevent bowstringing (i.e., subluxing, or anterior displacement, of the flexor tendons through the healing TCL), simultaneous wrist/finger flexion measurements should be deferred until 3 weeks after an open incision surgery. As mentioned, bowstringing may be more of a concern with open procedures than with endoscopic procedures.[51]

"Sensibility testing is the evaluation of the ability to feel or perceive a stimulus applied to an area."[52] Sensibility assessment is completed using the Semmes-Weinstein pressure aesthesiometer kit (a five filament kit is adequate). This type of sensory test is a pressure threshold test. The patient is seated comfortably for testing with the forearm supinated and the hand supported on a towel roll. The therapist should occlude the patient's vision during the test and instruct the patient to report when a finger is stimulated and which finger feels the stimulus. The volar fingertips and thumb pulp are tested starting with the 2.83 monofilament. "Each monofilament is applied perpendicular to the skin for 1.5 seconds and lifted for 1.5 seconds."[52] The therapist should apply monofilaments 2.83 and 3.61 three times to the same spot, and apply monofilaments 4.31 through 6.65 once. The lowest-numbered monofilament felt for each digit should be recorded on the evaluation form.[52] Full hand mapping is rarely required after a carpal tunnel release.

"Two point discrimination values are most often normal in CTS, and if they are abnormal it indicates advanced disease."[53,54] The therapist should complete two-point discrimination testing only if the patient demonstrates significant deficits on the Semmes-Weinstein Monofilament Test. Two point discrimination is an innervation density test.[53] The difference between the pressure threshold test and an innervation density test is the sensitivity of the pressure threshold test to gradual loss or improvement in nerve function versus an all-or-none response on an innervation density test.

The surgical incision or scar is evaluated for its stage of healing. The therapist should document whether the scar is raised or flat, tough or soft, mobile or adherent. The color of the scar also is noted. Some authors have written that one of the principle predictors of good outcomes and successful back to work status is minimal scar tenderness.[44,55] Therapeutic interventions by physical therapists that include scar assessment and management techniques are necessary, therefore, to ensure a flat, nonadherent, nonpainful scar.

The patient's present functional status can be documented in the areas of grooming, dressing, bathing, cooking, home care, work, avocational activities, and driving. Standardized self-administered outcome measurement tools that can be employed include the DASH, the Michigan Hand Outcomes Questionnaire, and the Boston Carpal Tunnel Scales, which includes the symptoms severity scale and functional status scale. Each of these scales takes only about 5 minutes to complete. These scales have been validated for use in CTS and even reported as more responsive to clinical improvements than grip, MMT, or sensory testing by monofilaments or two-point discrimination (Fig. 12-6).[56-58]

If the patient is 3 weeks postoperation, grip strength is recorded using a dynamometer with the handle positioned at the second setting[59,60] per American Society of Surgery of the Hand (ASSH) and ASHT guidelines.

To perform a grip test, the patient should be "seated with the shoulder adducted and neutrally rotated, elbow flexed to 90°, forearm in neutral position" and unsupported.[61,62] The therapist may support the dynamometer to prevent dropping; however, the dynamometer should not be allowed to rest on the table. The therapist should document three grip measurements, alternating the right and left hands,[63] unless repetitive grasping of the dynamometer would increase the discomfort in the patient's hand. Several authors have published normal values for grip strength but because of the high standard deviation[11] and inconsistencies in the studies, "comparison of grip scores to the contralateral extremity or longitudinal comparison to earlier values for each patient is recommended by ASSH and ASHT."[60,62,64]

Three types of pinch can be recorded using a pinch meter. Finger positioning for a three-point pinch is performed with the index and middle finger on the top of the pinch meter and the thumb on the bottom. Lateral pinch positioning is performed with the pinch meter held between the radial side of the index finger and the thumb on the top of the meter. Tip pinch is thumb pulp against index finger pulp. Tip pinch has been reported as a better outcome measure of strength for postoperative carpal tunnel release than grip or lateral pinch.[65] **Early forceful pinch, however, is not recommended until 3 weeks after surgery.**

Finger dexterity can be evaluated with various instruments such as the nine hole peg test, Jebsen-Taylor hand function test, O'Connor finger dexterity test, modified Moberg pick-up test, or the Minnesota rate of manipulation test. These tests have been standardized and normative data have been established for comparison purposes.

Upper-limb tension testing of the median nerve is appropriate to determine whether the patient has restrictions in nerve gliding. Limited studies have shown a decrease in the symptoms during conservative treatment of CTS,[66,67] and neural gliding is recommended not only to minimize the potential of adhesions on the nerve, but to increase range of motion (ROM) and decrease pain.[68] Local median nerve gliding at the wrist can be addressed as well (Fig. 12-7). Readers are referred to other authors such as Butler, Coppieter, and Elvey for more detailed information on neural tensioning principles and techniques.

The hand can be assessed for any atrophy of the thenar eminence, after which MMT of the upper quarter can be performed. As mentioned previously, care is taken to avoid undue stress on the flexor tendons until at least 3 weeks after surgery. **In assessing the function of the median nerve, the "abductor pollicis brevis is the muscle of choice for clinical assessment because it is superficial, and is solely innervated by the median nerve."[69,70]**

Postoperative Splinting

The value of postoperative splinting has been debated, and physical therapists should engage the patient in a decision on the need for splint use.[43,71] Neutral wrist splinting[31,72] can be helpful for controlling tension at the wound site/scar, helping the patient to avoid simultaneous wrist/finger flexion, as well as functioning as a simple reminder for the patient to minimize use of the operative hand. However, according to one study,[43] there was less pain and scar tenderness but a greater delay in return to full activity level and less strength in patients who wore a splint postoperatively for 2 weeks compared with those who did not wear a splint.

Color	Clinical Correlation	Filament Marking
■ Green	Normal	1.65 – 2.83
■ Blue	Diminished light touch	3.22 – 3.61
■ Purple	Diminished protective	3.84 – 4.31
■ Red	Loss of protective	4.56 – 6.65
■ Red-lined	Untestable	>6.65

Fig. 12-6 Monofilament interpretation.

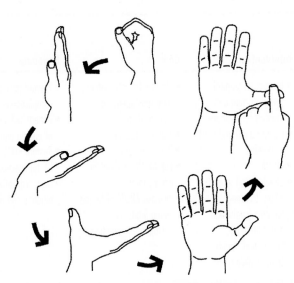

Fig. 12-7 Local median nerve glide/stretch.

AROM wrist median nerve glide

• Begin with making fist, wrist in a neutral position.
• Straighten fingers and thumb.
• Bend wrist back, move thumb away from the palm.
• Turn wrist palm up.
• Use other hand to pull thumb farther away from palm.

Perform 1 set of 1 repetitions, three times a day.

Phase I (Inflammatory Phase)

TIME: Day 1 to 3 weeks after surgery

Treatment of the patient after carpal tunnel release is based on the phases of wound healing and tissue response to stress. Treatment is directed toward patient education, edema control, scar modification, restoration of ROM, and strength and full return of hand function.

GOALS: Promote wound healing, maintain tendon excursion, and prevent median nerve from adhering to tendon, increase digit ROM to within normal limits (WNL) and maintain proximal ROM, decrease pain, decrease edema, independence with ADL, independence with home program (Table 12-1)

A light postoperative dressing is usually worn for 7 to 10 days after surgery. The patient should be instructed to elevate the hand and move fingers frequently to help decrease edema. Exercises during phase I consist of AROM to the shoulder, elbow, and digits. The patient is instructed in tendon-gliding exercises (Fig. 12-8) to prevent adhesion of the tendons through the carpal tunnel and to help decrease edema.[73] The patient is also instructed in nerve glides, which include gentle wrist flexion and extension with the UE held in a relaxed position at side of body. Many patients are not referred to formal therapy and, after instruction, can perform exercises as a home program and are instructed to use the hand as tolerated.

Phase Ia

TIME: 10 days to 3 weeks postoperative

GOALS: Promote scar remodeling, decrease hypersensitivity and pain, increase wrist ROM to WNL, begin to increase hand strength, independence in home exercise program (Table 12-2)

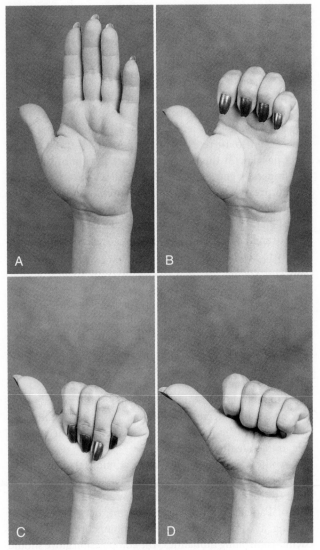

Fig. 12-8 Tendon-gliding exercises. **A,** Tendon-gliding exercises are initiated in full finger extension. The patient then completes 10 repetitions in the hook fist (**B**), straight fist (**C**), and full fist (**D**) to maximize differential tendon gliding and full excursion of the tendons through the carpal tunnel. (From Wehbe M: Tendon gliding exercises. Am J Occup Ther 41:164, 1987.)

TABLE 12-1 Carpal Tunnel Release

Rehabilitation Phase	Criteria to Progress to This Phase	Anticipated Impairments and Functional Limitations	Intervention	Goal	Rationale
Phase I Postoperative 1-10 days	• Postoperative	• Edema • Pain • Limited ROM of upper extremity • Limited functional use of upper extremity	• Instruct on surgical site protection and monitor for drainage • Elevate hand and wrist as needed • AROM • Shoulder (all ranges), elbow (all ranges), forearm (supination and pronation), fingers and thumb (tendon-gliding)	• Monitor for infection or other postoperative complications • Manage edema • Decrease pain • Full AROM of shoulder, elbow, forearm • Increase AROM of fingers within limits of postoperative dressing	• Prevent postoperative complications • Patient self-management of edema and pain • Restore ROM to prepare UE for functional use • Limit scar adhesions to tendons and nerves

AROM, Active range of motion; *ROM,* range of motion.

Within 48 hours of suture removal, scar mobilization techniques may be initiated. Begin with a light scar massage with lotion and progress to a more vigorous soft tissue mobilization as tolerated.

AROM should include composite flexion and extension of the digits, isolated blocking to the FDS and FDP, full median nerve glides, and continued tendon-gliding exercises. Seven to 10 repetitions are performed three to four times per day. At this time, **composite flexion of the wrist and fingers is generally avoided until 21 days postoperation to prevent bowstringing of the tendons through the healing carpal ligament.** Some patients may be referred for formal hand therapy for pain relief, scar desensitization, hand strengthening, and to help facilitate return to maximum activity (see Table 12-2). Modalities may be used to decrease pain and edema, to increase elasticity of tissues, and to promote tissue healing.[74] Moist heat may be used for pain control before exercise and to prepare tissues for soft tissue mobilization. The modalities of pulsed US, iontophoresis,[74] and high-voltage galvanic stimulation[74] are helpful in reducing the local swelling and pain experienced by patients after carpal tunnel release. Phonophoresis has not been shown to be any more effective than US alone for pain relief.[56]

Iontophoresis with dexamethasone sodium phosphate may be used for decreasing local edema about the incision site. However, the incision must be completely healed and able to tolerate the stimulation.

Cryotherapy, if tolerated, may be administered after exercises for 10 minutes to help in managing edema and pain. Light retrograde massage also may facilitate lymphatic return. Patients with persistent edema may benefit from wearing a compression glove in conjunction with other edema-controlling modalities. The compression glove should be worn almost continuously at first, and then worn only at night as edema decreases. As discussed, splinting is declining in favor during postoperative treatment because of the deleterious effects of immobilization on joint mobility and

muscle length. Splinting may be appropriate for patients who experience nighttime pain associated with flexed postures of the wrist and may also be used to provide rest to inflamed tissues.

The therapist should initiate scar desensitization when the surgical incision is closed. The desensitization process is initiated gently and can be performed in many ways. These methods include manual self-massage of the scar, immersion in tubs of textured particles, and rubbing the scar with different textures. When performing scar desensitization, the scar is initially rubbed lightly with soft fabrics; treatment progresses by using deeper pressure and coarser textures. Scar massage is initiated with minimal force, and the force is increased as the incision increases in tensile strength (Fig. 12-9). Scar massage can be done for 1 to 3 minutes, five times per day.

Limiting the development of scar adhesion to tendons, skin, and nerves is another important aspect of scar management after carpal tunnel release surgery. Tendon-gliding exercises are continued to move the flexor tendons differentially in the carpal tunnel. Nerve-gliding techniques are helpful in maintaining mobility of the median nerve after a carpal tunnel release.[75] The home program for median nerve gliding begins with the arm held at the side of the body, the elbow extended, and the forearm and wrist in a neutral position. The patient is instructed to extend the wrist from a neutral position in a gliding motion. The patient should be cautioned not to be overzealous with these exercises and to inform the therapist if symptoms increase.

When the incision is fully closed, a scar conformer can be fabricated from silicone elastomers or cut from silicone gel sheets (Fig. 12-10). Because the scar conformer works by applying pressure over the scar, it needs to be held firmly in place. Silicone sheeting does not need pressure wrapping, because the intervention is simply direct contact with scar tissue. Silicone gel sheeting is recommended for nightly application, for 8 to 10 hours per day. The therapist can use

TABLE 12-2 Carpal Tunnel Release

Rehabilitation Phase	Criteria to Progress to This Phase	Anticipated Impairments and Functional Limitations	Intervention	Goal	Rationale
Phase Ia Postoperative 11-21 days	• No signs of infection • Sutures removed	• Edema • Pain • Limited functional use of UE • Limited AROM of hand and wrist • Limited strength of hand and wrist • Scar sensitivity, adhesions, and thickening • Persistent paresthesia, especially at night • Limited hand function • Limited patient knowledge of neutral wrist positioning	• Hot pack • ES • Ultrasound, iontophoresis with dexamethesone sodium phosphate • Cryotherapy • Retrograde massage • Initiate pain-free isometrics—Wrist (flexion, extension) • AROM—Progress exercises as indicated and add wrist extension, radial and ulnar deviation • Finger AROM • No AROM for wrist flexion until 3 wk after surgery • Wrist splint worn as needed • Scar desensitization: gentle manual massage • Mobilization of the median nerve Instruct patient in the following: • Proper use of hand protection while performing self-care • Neutral wrist positioning • Nerve-gliding techniques • Fabricate scar conformer or have patient use silicone gel sheeting • Tendon-gliding exercises	• Decrease postoperative pain • Manage edema • Increase strength and facilitate gross grasp and wrist stabilization • Full AROM of shoulder, elbow, and forearm • AROM of wrist, radial deviation, ulnar deviation, thumb composite opposition, and finger composite flexion • Decrease sensitivity of scar • Increase mobility of scar • Decrease scar adhesion to flexor tendons, skin, and median nerve • Decrease paresthesia • Promote independent self-care • Maintain neutral wrist position during exercises • Encourage self-management of exercise program • Flatten and/or soften scar	• Modalities to manage edema and decrease pain; help in preparation for stretching and strengthening • Massage to facilitate lymphatic return • Increased wrist stabilization strength • Promote full return of UE AROM, continuation of tendon-gliding exercises to decrease scar adhesion • Wrist flexion exercises are not recommended until 21 days after surgery, depending on the type of surgical exposure, to prevent bowstringing of tendons • Strengthening and improvement of endurance of wrist and hand while maintaining neutral position • Encouragement of wrist extension with finger flexion • Neutral position to minimize pressure on median nerve • Organized sensory input normalizes sensory interpretation • Early motion organizes collagen development in scar and limits scar from restricting median nerve • Initiation of self-management • Minimizing possible development of pillar pain • Incorporation of neutral position during exercises and ADL to prevent complications • Pressure applied over a scar organizes collagen

ADL, Activities of daily living; *AROM,* active range of motion; *ES,* electrical stimulation; *UE,* upper extremity.

a self-adherent wrap such as Coban to secure the conformer or gel sheeting over the scar. The patient should be instructed not to wrap the scar conformer or sheeting too tightly with the Coban because tight wrapping will cause edema and pain in the hand. An explanation should be given to the patient regarding the purpose and importance of scar management techniques for at least 3 months. The patient should wash the scar conformer or silicone sheeting as needed to prevent skin irritation and replace the scar conformer/sheeting if it becomes worn or soiled. The patient should observe the skin closely for signs of skin maceration or heat rash. If these problems occur, then the patient should stop using the scar conformer or silicone and inform the therapist. Decreasing the amount of wear time or placing a light gauze or tissue

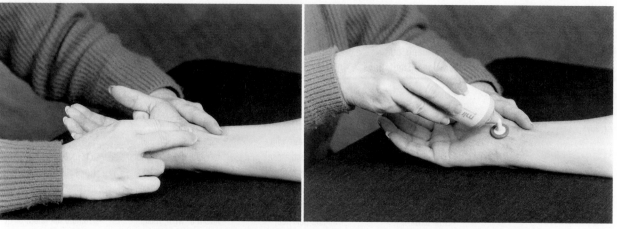

Fig. 12-9 Scar massage is initiated using manual techniques to decrease scar adhesion to the underlying tissues.

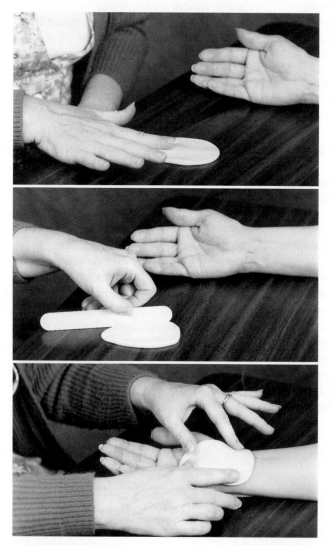

Fig. 12-10 The clinician fabricates an elastomer scar conformer by mixing the elastomer in the hands.

between the scar elastomer pad and the skin may control skin maceration and heat rash.

After 3 weeks, the therapist can also initiate isometric strengthening exercises for wrist extension and flexion. Wrist isometrics are performed in a neutral wrist position.[76] The patient applies enough resistance with the opposite hand to create a muscle contraction, which is held for 5 seconds without increasing pain. The exercises can be progressed by increasing resistance and repetitions. Instruction on ways to maintain a neutral wrist position during functional use of the hand is emphasized with paper crunch activity and isometric strengthening exercises. This education is further emphasized with ergonomic instruction in phase II.

The patient should be encouraged to use the affected hand for self-care while avoiding wrist flexion, forceful repetitive grip, and lifting more than 3 lb. Tasks that require forceful grip, such as vacuuming, handling wet laundry, putting fitted sheets on the bed, yard work, tool use, lifting, and pushing, should be avoided for 6 to 8 weeks to allow complete healing.

Phase II (Proliferation Phase)

TIME: 3 to 6 weeks after surgery
GOALS: Improve strength and endurance in hand and UE for independence in ADL, progress strength and endurance in hand to prepare for return to work, return to full-time work activities (Table 12-3)

Phase II focuses primarily on strengthening and education (see Table 12-3). It begins on day 22 after surgery and continues until day 42 (6 weeks after surgery). Phase I modalities are continued for edema and pain control. Moist heat may be continued before exercises. Scar desensitization is continued with scar massage and soft tissue mobilization. Texture desensitization techniques are continued, especially as part of the home program. Use of a gel sheeting to pad the sensitive palm may increase comfort for performing self-care and light home care. Tendon-gliding and nerve-gliding exercises and scar massage are continued to prevent or decrease scar adhesions. The pressure used for scar massage

TABLE 12-3 Carpal Tunnel Release

Rehabilitation Phase	Criteria to Progress to This Phase	Anticipated Impairments and Functional Limitations	Intervention	Goal	Rationale
Phase II Postoperative 3-6 wk	• Pain controlled • No loss of range of motion • No loss of strength • Well-healed incision	• Mild edema • Mild pain • Limited AROM of wrist, fingers, and thumb • Scar sensitivity • Scar adhesion • Scar raised or thickened • Limited UE strength • Limited ability to perform light ADL involving gripping and twisting • Limited knowledge of proper work environment organization (ergonomics) • Limited tolerance to repetitive finger and hand use	• Continuation of modalities as indicated from phase I Continuation of the following: • Scar desensitization techniques • Retrograde massage • AROM and PREs • Scar conformer or silicon at night • Progress firmness of manual scar massage • AROM — wrist flexion • Putty exercises (light resistive putty) — finger pinch, finger grip • Isotonics — upper quarter exercises Wrist — weight well, flexion and extension Forearm — pronation and supination (begin with 1-2 lb and progress as indicated.) • Patient education regarding body mechanics, joint protection, and modification of ADL using adaptive equipment (grip assistive devices) • Ergonomic evaluation as needed • Work simulated exercises, as needed	As in Tables 12-1 and 12-2 • Resolve edema in fingers • Decrease postoperative pain • Decrease sensitivity of scar and increase scar mobility • Decrease scar adhesion to flexor tendon, skin, and median nerve • AROM of wrist • Full fist to DPC with fingers • Thumb to DPC at base of small finger • Grip strength 30%-50% of uninvolved hand • Wrist strength 80%-90% • Proximal strength greater than 85% • Lift and carry 3-5 lb with involved hand • Independence with ADL using assistive devices as necessary and limiting exposure to heavy grasping activities • Organize work environment to decrease potential for reinjury and maximize efficiency • Work simulation, alternating tasks	As in Tables 12-1 and 12-2 • Decrease reliance on modalities and increase patient's ability to self-manage edema and pain • Continuation of exercises as indicated to allow progression of program as tolerated by patient response to treatment • Scar should now be able to handle increased mobilization techniques • UE stretches to elongate muscle tendon units for increased function • Healing of transverse carpal tunnel ligament is adequate to prevent bowstringing of the flexor tendons • Upper quarter strengthening as a functional unit • Initiate exercises with low repetitions to prevent development of tenosynovitis and pillar pain • Use appropriate assistive device to prevent reinjury and increase independence with ADL; avoiding heavier gripping activities; use forearms to carry versus finger grip • Promote self-management of symptoms and prevent reinjury in the work environment • Prepare for return to work

ADL, Activities of daily living; *AROM*, active range of motion; *DPC*, distal palmar crease; *PREs*, progressive resistance exercises; *UE*, upper extremity.

is increased in intensity for manual massage. Use of the scar conformer or gel sheeting is continued at night to soften and flatten the scar.

The patient can add active wrist flexion exercises after 21 days with the expectation of full wrist flexion by the end of the sixth week after surgery.

Full UE stretching exercises and neural-gliding exercises are added at this time. UE stretches include composite motions of (1) wrist flexion, forearm pronation, and elbow extension; (2) wrist extension, forearm pronation, and elbow extension; and (3) wrist extension, forearm supination, and elbow extension.[77]

Resistive gripping and pinching exercises with light resistive putty may be started 28 days after surgery. Putty exercises must be comfortably tolerated before moving to more resistive putty; however, if patients begin to complain of pillar pain, this should be discontinued for another week or two. Pillar pain is described in the literature as pain in the thenar or hypothenar areas, and should be distinguished from incisional or local scar tenderness.[44,78,79] Pillar pain occurs at the bony attachments of the TCL (the hook of the hamate, pisiform, scaphoid tubercle, and the ridge of the trapezium). Patients with pillar pain may have difficulty with gripping and palmar weight-bearing activities. Modalities may be used to decrease the inflammation and symptoms of pillar pain. Low-intensity continuous US[80] (0.5 W/cm^2, 3 MHz) has been noted to help decrease this type of pain. The therapist should instruct the patient that the *maximum* use of putty is two times a day for 5 minutes, and tell him or her to stop using the putty and notify the therapist if the pain increases significantly. Wrist isometric exercises can be continued along with the initiation of grip isometric exercises. The patient can perform grip isometric exercises by squeezing a towel roll in the hand. Light progressive resistance exercises (PREs) are added when pain is controlled. PREs are added for both wrist extension and flexion (Fig. 12-11).[76] Resistance should begin at $\frac{1}{2}$ to 1 lb and progressed to 3 lb as the patient tolerates it.

Wrist and grip strengthening are progressed to using a weight well or computerized work simulator (Fig. 12-12).

The patient starts on the weight well with no weight or on the work simulator at minimal torque and progresses as tolerated.

Proximal muscle strengthening of the forearm, elbow, shoulder, and shoulder girdle can be started on day 28 after surgery. Forearm rotation strength can be achieved using a hammer held with the elbow flexed at 90° and stabilized against the side of the body. The therapist should ask the patient to rotate the forearm from the neutral position into supination and pronation. Simply moving the hammerhead away from the hand to increase the lever arm, or toward the hand to decrease the lever arm, can change the resistance of the exercise. Bicep curls and elbow extension exercises can be performed with dumbbells beginning at 1 or 2 lb and progressing as the patient tolerates. Shoulder and shoulder girdle exercises beginning with 1 to 2 lb are important and are performed for flexion, abduction, internal and external rotation, and scapular retraction. The patient should be

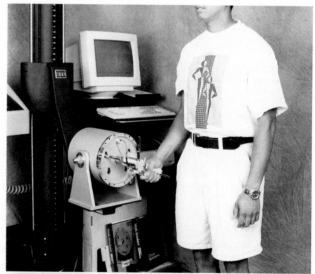

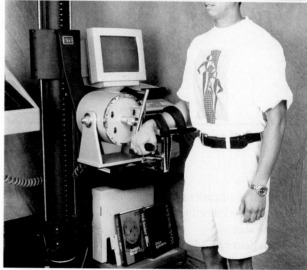

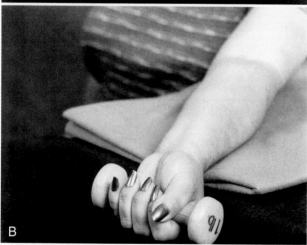

Fig. 12-11 Progressive resistance exercises are important to strengthen the wrist extensor (**A**) and flexor (**B**) musculature. The table is padded with a towel to prevent excessive pressure on the median and ulnar nerves.

Fig. 12-12 Computerized equipment is an effective way of simulating many work tasks and strengthening muscles; it requires a relatively small area in the clinic.

TABLE 12-4 Carpal Tunnel Release

Rehabilitation Phase	Criteria to Progress to This Phase	Anticipated Impairments and Functional Limitations	Intervention	Goal	Rationale
Phase III Postoperative 6 wk-1 year, until scar maturation	• Patients who perform jobs that require heavy lifting	• Limited UE and grip strength • Limited UE and grip endurance	• Continuation of exercises and stretches in phases I and II as indicated • Progress UE strengthening exercises, emphasizing endurance for return to work activities • Functional capacity evaluation • Work simulated activities	• Decrease number of exercises and stretches • Adequate strength to return to work activities full time • Self-management of symptoms	• Increase efficiency of home exercises in self-management of condition • Promote muscle balance of UE • Assess potential to return to work • Initiate appropriate program (work hardening, work conditioning, or supervised gym program)

UE, Upper extremity.

monitored closely during the advancement of the proximal strengthening program to prevent the development of other cumulative trauma disorders, such as shoulder impingement syndrome, lateral epicondylitis, de Quervain's syndrome, or trigger finger symptoms.

Treatment of the patient after carpal tunnel release surgery may also include instruction on ergonomic principles, proper posture, and body mechanics to prevent recurrence of CTS or the development of other repetitive stress injuries. Instruction should include general topics for all patients and job-specific teaching for those returning to highly repetitive or heavy-labor jobs.

Ergonomic Recommendations

Patients with jobs involving computers should be instructed in workstation setup. According to the literature, the most important factor in CTS and work is wrist position on the keyboard. Based on carpal tunnel pressure studies, in wrist extension angles greater than 15° can increase pressure in the carpal tunnel, which could result in more pressure on the median nerve. Neutral wrist extension could decrease the probability of developing other musculoskeletal disorders affecting the hand and wrist. To maintain this position, elbows should be flexed to 90° or a little less with wrists in a neutral position over the keyboard. A keyboard tray may need to be added to the desk to achieve proper positioning. Using ergonomic keyboards or negatively tilting the keyboard also may be useful for maintaining a neutral wrist position.[81] If a wrist rest is used, the patient should be instructed not to press on it during typing but to use it to rest the UEs when scanning the monitor screen.

Patients with sedentary jobs are usually discharged to a home program by the end of phase II. Heavy laborers generally progress to phase III at 6 to 8 weeks after surgery, where more emphasis is placed on increasing strength, endurance, and return to work activities.

Phase III (Remodeling and Maturation Phase)

TIME: 6 weeks after surgery, ending when the scar is mature. This phase can last for 1 year or longer.

GOALS: Adequate strength to return to full-time work activities, independent home exercise program, self-management of symptoms (Table 12-4)

The types of patients who progress to phase III are heavy laborers, construction workers, mechanics, and assembly workers. These patients should be able to progress to aerobic exercise using a bicycle, treadmill, or UE ergometer. The stretching program and scar management program from phase II is continued. Scar massage also continues, with the patient wearing the scar conformer or gel sheeting until the scar color is no longer reddened. Scar maturation can take as long as 1 year. Phase II strengthening exercises should be continued and progressed as tolerated. Large muscle group exercises using gym equipment or free weights are appropriate at this time for general body conditioning.

Work activity simulation is an important aspect of the phase III therapy protocol. These activities can include using a pipe tree or assembly boards and learning proper lifting and carrying techniques. The use of work simulation equipment can be helpful for strengthening and simulation of specific work activities (see Fig. 12-12). Full return of presurgical grip and pinch strengths often does not occur until 3 to 6 months following surgery.

Clearly, CTS affects patients physically, financially, and psychologically. Comprehensive management of the patient recovering from surgery for CTS optimizes the potential to return to ADL, work, and avocational activities.

SUGGESTED HOME MAINTENANCE FOR THE POSTSURGICAL PATIENT

The home maintenance section outlines the postoperative rehabilitation the patient is to follow. The physical therapist can use it in customizing a patient-specific program.

Suggested Home Maintenance for the Postsurgical Patient

Days 1 to 10
GOALS FOR THE PERIOD: Decrease pain, manage edema, improve AROM of UE, initiate self-management and patient education
1. Protect incision
2. Elevate the hand above the heart
3. Ice frequently
4. AROM exercises for shoulder, elbow, forearm, and thumb
5. Tendon-gliding exercises

Days 11 to 21
GOALS FOR THE PERIOD: Decrease pain, manage edema, improve AROM of UE, initiate self-management and patient education
1. Moist heat
2. Retrograde massage when incision has closed
3. Scar massage when incision has closed
4. Continue tendon-gliding exercises
5. Nerve-gliding exercises
6. Continue AROM exercises for shoulder, elbow, forearm, and thumb
7. Add AROM exercises for wrist extension, radial and ulnar deviation (avoid wrist flexion as necessary)
8. Isometric exercises for wrist extension and flexion
9. Use scar conformer or silicone gel sheeting at night
10. Use splint as needed to control symptoms
11. Ice as necessary

Days 22 to 42
GOALS FOR THE PERIOD: Decrease pain, manage edema, improve AROM of UE, initiate self-management and patient education
1. Continue all previous exercises and modalities as indicated
2. Add wrist flexion AROM
3. Add putty gripping and pinching exercises with light resistive putty
4. Add grip isometric exercises by squeezing a towel roll
5. Add PREs for wrist extension and flexion with $\frac{1}{2}$ to 1 lb
6. Add PREs for shoulder girdle and elbow with 1 to 2 lb
7. Add forearm strengthening using a hammer
8. Continue to use scar conformer at night
9. Practice ergonomic principles

Days 43 to 90
GOALS FOR THE PERIOD: Complete self-management of symptoms and home maintenance program, return to full-time work activities
1. Aerobic warm-up exercise using a bicycle or treadmill
2. Continue previous exercises as indicated, progressing intensity and duration as indicated

CLINICAL CASE REVIEW

1 Sharon had carpal tunnel release 2 months ago. She has been making good progress in therapy but continues to complain of paresthesia that was present before surgery. What could explain her continued symptoms?

It is not uncommon for patients to continue with symptoms postoperatively. The healing response of the nerve may take as much as 3 to 6 months. Besides the use of antiinflammatory modalities, wearing a night splint may help keep the wrist in a neutral position and facilitate the healing response.

2 Yvonne is a 48-year-old grocery checker who has been diagnosed with intermediate CTS; she has constant numbness and paresthesia but no thenar atrophy. She had surgery 3 weeks ago for a carpal tunnel release, and

the edema is persistent. What are some treatment techniques that may be helpful for decreasing her edema at this point?

Light retrograde massage may facilitate lymphatic return. Patients with persistent edema may benefit from wearing a compression glove in conjunction with other edema-controlling modalities. Initially the glove should be worn almost continuously. As the edema decreases, the patient only needs to wear the glove at night.

3 Yvonne tends to heal quickly after having surgery. In fact, she had difficulty regaining full knee ROM after knee surgery because adhesions quickly formed around the joint. Limiting the development of scar adhesions also is important in the patient who has had carpal tunnel

release. What are some problematic areas Yvonne may have after her carpal tunnel release? What types of treatment can be used to limit scar adhesions in this area?

Limiting the development of scar adhesion to tendons, skin, and nerves is another important aspect of scar management in the patient after carpal tunnel release surgery. Tendon-gliding exercises are continued to move the flexor tendons differentially in the carpal tunnel. Nerve-gliding techniques are helpful in maintaining mobility of the median nerve after a carpal tunnel release.

4 Lupe is returning to work (as a receptionist) 8 weeks after carpal tunnel release. Her symptoms have resolved but she is still tender over the incision. What ergonomic recommendations should be made?

In general, a worksite evaluation should be made. Close attention should be paid to the degree of wrist extension (neutral) and postural setup (i.e., head on neck, shoulder, elbow, and overall spine and pelvis position while seated) as it relates to her monitor and job duties. A padded wrist rest or padded gloves may also be useful.

REFERENCES

1. Michelson H, Posner M: Medical history of carpal tunnel syndrome. Hand Clin 18:257-268, 2002.
2. Louise DS, et al: Carpal tunnel syndrome in the work place. Hand Clin 12(2):305, 1996.
3. Tanaka S, et al: Prevalence and work-relatedness of self-reported carpal tunnel syndrome among US workers: analysis of the occupational health supplement data of 1988 National Health Interview Survey. Am J Ind Med 27:451, 1995.
4. Viera AJ: Management of carpal tunnel syndrome. Am Fam Physician 15;68(2):265-272, 2003.
5. Bickel K: Carpal tunnel syndrome. J Hand Surg Am 35A:147-152, 2010.
6. Mcdiarmid M, et al: Male and female rate differences in carpal tunnel syndrome injuries: Personal attributes or job tasks. Environ Res 83(1):23-32, 2000.
7. http://www.bls.gov/news.release/osh2.t03.htm, on July 4, 2010
8. Bureau of Labor Statistics: Survey of occupation injuries and illness in 1994, Washington, DC, 1996, US Department of Labor.
9. Kerwin G, Williams CS, Seilier JG III: The pathophysiology of carpal tunnel syndrome. Hand Clin 12(2):243, 1996.
10. Evans R: Therapist's management of carpal tunnel syndrome. In Mackin E, et al, editors: Rehabilitation of the hand and upper extremity, St. Louis, 2001, Mosby.
11. Verhagen AP, et al: Ergonomic and physiotherapeutic interventions for treating work-related complaints of the arm, neck or shoulder in adults. Cochrane Database of Systematic Reviews 2006, Issue 3. Art. No.: CD003471. DOI: 10.1002/14651858.CD003471.pub3
12. Lozano-Calderon S, Anthony S, Ring D: The quality and strength of evidence for etiology: Example of carpal tunnel syndrome. JHS 33A:525-538, 2008.
13. Boz C, et al: Individual risk factors for carpal tunnel syndrome: An evaluation of body mass index, wrist index and hand anthropometric measurements. Clin Neurol Neurosurg 106(4):294-299, 2004.
14. Cosgrove JL, et al: Carpal tunnel syndrome in railroad workers. Am J Phys Med Rehabil 81(2):101-107, 2002.
15. Gell N, et al: A longitudinal study of industrial and clerical workers: Incidence of carpal tunnel syndrome and assessment of risk factors. J Occup Rehabil 15(1):47-55, 2005.
16. Nathan PA, Istvan JA, Meadows KD: A longitudinal study of predictors of research-defined carpal tunnel syndrome in industrial workers: Findings at 17 years. J Hand Surg Br 30(6):593-598, 2005.
17. Rosecrance JC, et al: Carpal tunnel syndrome among apprentice construction workers. Am J Ind Med 42(2):107-116, 2002.
18. Werner RA, et al: Incidence of carpal tunnel syndrome among automobile assembly workers and assessment of risk factors. J Occup Environ Med 47(10):1044-1050, 2005.
19. Eversmann WW Jr: Entrapment and compression neuropathies. In Green DP, editor: Operative hand surgery, ed 3, New York, 1993, Churchill Livingstone.
20. Frymoyer J, Bland J: Carpal tunnel syndrome in patients with myxedematous arthropathy. J Bone Joint Surg 55A:78, 1973.
21. Evangelisti S, Reale V: Fibroma of tendon sheath as a cause of carpal tunnel syndrome. J Hand Surg 17A:1026, 1992.
22. Cobb T, An T, Cooney W: Effect of lumbrical incursion within the carpal tunnel on carpal tunnel pressure: A cadaveric study. JHS 20A:186-192, 1995.
23. Liu CW, et al: Relationship between carpal tunnel syndrome and wrist angle in computer workers. Kaohsiung J Med Sci 19(12):617-623, 2003.
24. Spindler H, Dellon A: Nerve conduction studies and sensibility testing in carpal tunnel syndrome. J Hand Surg 7:260, 1982.
25. Hayes E, et al: Carpal tunnel syndrome. In Mackin E, et al, editors: Rehabilitation of the hand and upper extremity, St. Louis, 2001, Mosby.
26. O'Connor D, Marshall SC, Massy-Westropp N: Non-surgical treatment (other than steroid injection) for carpal tunnel syndrome. Cochrane Database of Systematic Reviews Issue 1. Art. No.: CD003219. DOI: 10.1002/14651858.CD003219, 2003.
27. Boyer M: Corticosteroid Injection for carpal tunnel syndrome. J Hand Surg 33A:1414-1416, 2008.
28. Muller M, et al: Effectiveness of hand therapy interventions in primary management of carpal tunnel syndrome: A systematic review. J Hand Ther 17(2):210-228, 2004.
29. Werner RA, Franzblau A, Gell N: Randomized controlled trial of nocturnal splinting for active workers with symptoms of carpal tunnel syndrome. Arch Phys Med Rehabil 86(1):1-7, 2005.
30. Sailer SM: The role of splinting and rehabilitation in the treatment of carpal and cubital tunnel syndromes. Hand Clin 12(2):223, 1996.
31. Weiss ND, et al: Position of the wrist associated with the lowest carpal-tunnel pressure: Implications for splint design. J Bone Joint Surg 77A(11):1695, 1995.
32. Keir P, Bach J, Rempel D: Effects of finger posture on carpal tunnel pressure during wrist motion. JHS 23A;1004-1009, 1998.
33. Beckenbaugh RD: Carpal tunnel syndrome. In Cooney WP, Linscheid RL, Dobyns JH, editors: The wrist: Diagnosis and operative treatment, St Louis, 1998, Mosby.
34. Robbins H: Anatomical study of the median nerve in the carpal tunnel and etiologies of the carpal tunnel syndrome. J Bone Joint Surg 45A:953, 1963.
35. Zachary RB: Thenar palsy due to compression of the median nerve in the carpal tunnel. Surg Gynecol Obstet 81:213-217, 1945.
36. Cannon BW, Love JG: Tardy median nerve palsy: Median neuritis amenable to surgery. Surgery 20:210-216, 1946.
37. Goss BC, Agee JM: Dynamics of intracarpal tunnel pressure in patients with carpal tunnel syndrome, J Hand Surg 35(2):197-206, 2010, Epub 21 Dec 2009.
38. Okutsu I, et al: Endoscopic management of carpal tunnel syndrome. Arthroscopy 5:11-18, 1989.
39. Chow JC: Endoscopic release of the carpal ligament: A new technique for carpal tunnel syndrome. Arthroscopy 5:19-24, 1989.

40. Agee JM, McCarroll HR, North ER: Endoscopic carpal tunnel release using the single proximal incision technique. Hand Clin 10:647-659, 1994.

41. MacDermid JC, et al: Endoscopic versus open carpal tunnel release: A randomized trial. J Hand Surg Am 28(3):475-480, 2003.

42. Palmer AK, Toivonen DA: Complications of endoscopic and open carpal tunnel release. JHS 24(3):561-565, 1999.

43. Cook AC, et al: Early mobilization following carpal tunnel release: A prospective randomized study. J Hand Surg Br 20:228-230, 1995.

44. Ludlow KS, et al: Pillar pain as a postoperative complication of carpal tunnel release. J Hand Ther 10(4):222-282, 1997.

45. Yung PS, et al: Carpal tunnel release with a limited palmar incision: Clinical results and pillar pain at 18 months follow-up. Hand Surg 10:29-35, 2005.

46. Novak CB, Collins ED, Mackinnon SE: Outcome following conservative management of thoracic outlet syndrome. J Hand Surg 20(4):542-548, 1995.

47. Novak CB, Mackinnon SE, Patterson GA: Evaluation of patients with thoracic outlet syndrome. J Hand Surg 18(2):292-299, 1993.

48. El-Karabaty H, et al: The effect of carpal tunnel release on median nerve flattening and nerve conduction. Electromyogr Clin Neurophysiol 45(4):223-227, 2005.

49. Gretchen L, Jezek S: Pain assessment. In American Society of Hand Therapists, editors: Clinical assessment recommendations, ed 2, Chicago, 1992, The Society.

50. Leard J, et al: Reliability and concurrent validity of the figure-of-eight method of measuring hand size in patients with hand pathology. J Orthop Sports Phys Ther 34:335-340, 2004.

51. Brown R, Palmer C: Changes in digital flexor tendon mechanics after endoscopic and open carpal tunnel releases in cadaver wrists. J Hand Surg 25A:112-119, 2000.

52. Stone J: Sensibility. In American Society of Hand Therapists, editors: Clinical assessment recommendations, ed 2, Chicago, 1992, The Society.

53. Gelberman R, et al: Sensibility testing in peripheral-nerve compression syndromes: An experimental study in humans. J Bone Joint Surg 65A(5):632, 1983.

54. Macdermid J: Clinical and electrodiagnostic testing of carpal tunnel syndrome: a narrative review. Jospt 34:565-588, 2004.

55. Katz JN, et al: Predictors of return to work follwing carpal tunnel release. Am J Ind Med 31:85-91, 1997.

56. Michlovitz S: Conservative interventions for carpal tunnel syndrome. J Orthop Sports Phys Ther 34:589-600, 2004.

57. Levine D, et al: A self-administered questionnaire for the assessment of severity of symptoms and functional status in carpal tunnel syndrome. J Bone Joint Surg Am 75:1585-1592, 1993.

58. Michigan Hand Outcomes Questionnaire. Available at http://sitemaker.umich.edu/mhq/overview. Accessed September 2010.

59. American Society for Surgery of the Hand: The hand: examination and diagnosis, Aurora, Colo, 1978, The Society.

60. American Society for Surgery of the Hand: The hand: examination and diagnosis, ed 2, New York, 1983, Churchill Livingstone.

61. Fess EE, Morgan C: Clinical assessment recommendations, Indianapolis, 1981, American Society of Hand Therapists.

62. Fess EE: Grip strength. In American Society of Hand Therapists, editors: Clinical assessment recommendations, ed 2, Chicago, 1992, The Society.

63. MacDermid J, et al: Interrater reliability of pinch and grip strength measurements in patients with cumulative trauma disorders. J Hand Ther 7(1):10, 1984.

64. Mathiowetz V, et al: Grip and pinch strength: normative data for adults. Arch Phys Med Rehabil 66:69, 1985.

65. Geere J, et al: Power grip, pinch grip, manual muscle testing or thenar atrophy—which should be assessed as a motor outcome after carpal tunnel decompression? A systematic review. BMC Musculoskelet Disord 8:114, 2007.

66. Rozmaryn L, Develle S, Rothman E: Nerve and tendon gliding exercises and the conservative management of carpal tennel syndrome. JHT 11:171-179, 1998.

67. Seradge H, Bear C, Bithell D: Preventing carpal tunnel syndrome and cumulative trauma disorder: Effect of carpal tunnel decompression exercises: An Oklahoma Experience. J Okla State Med Assoc 93:150-153, 2000.

68. Walsh M: Upper limb neural tension testing and mobilization: Fact, fiction, and a practical approach. JHT 18:241-258, 2005.

69. MacDermid J: Accuracy of clinical tests used in the detection of carpal tunnel syndrome: A literature review. J Hand Ther 4(4):169, 1991.

70. Phalen GS: The carpal tunnel syndrome: Seventeen years' experience in diagnosis and treatment of six hundred and fifty-four. J Bone Joint Surg 48:211, 1966.

71. Bury T, Akelman E, Weiss A: Prospective, randomized trial of splinting after carpal tunnel release. Ann Plast Surg 35:1, 19-22, 1995.

72. Burke D: Splinting for carpal tunnel syndrome: In search of the optimal angle. Arch Phys Med Rehabil 78:1241-1244, 1994.

73. Wehbe M: Tendon gliding exercises. Am J Occup Ther 41:164, 1987.

74. Taylor Mullins PA: Use of therapeutic modalities in upper extremity rehabilitation. In Hunter JM, Mackin EJ, Callahan AD, editors: Rehabilitation of the hand: Surgery and therapy, ed 4, St Louis, 1995, Mosby.

75. Baxter-Petralia PL: Therapist's management of carpal tunnel syndrome. In Hunter JM, et al, editors: Rehabilitation of the hand: Surgery and therapy, ed 3, St Louis, 1990, Mosby.

76. Kasch M: Therapists evaluation and treatment of upper extremity cumulative trauma disorders. In Hunter JM, Mackin EJ, Callahan AD, editors: Rehabilitation of the hand: surgery and therapy, ed 4, St Louis, 1995, Mosby.

77. Pascarelli E, Quilter D: Repetitive strain injury: A computer user's guide, New York, 1994, John Wiley & Sons.

78. Brown RA, et al: Carpal tunnel release: A prospective, randomized assessment of open and endoscopic methods. J Bone Joint Surg 75A:1265, 1993.

79. Buchanan RT, et al: Method, education and therapy of carpal tunnel patients. Hand Surg Quart, Summer 1995.

80. Michlovitz S: Is there a role for ultrasound and electrical stimulation following injury to tendon and nerve? J Hand Ther 18(2):292-296, 2005.

81. Simeneau, et al: Effect of computer keyboard slope on wrist position and forearm electromyography of typists without musculoskeletal disorders. J Phys Ther 83:9, 2003.

CHAPTER 13

Transitioning the Throwing Athlete Back to the Field

Luga Podesta

"Injuries to athletes happen every day. Some can be easily treated, while others require surgery and/or lengthy rehabilitation. An arm injury to a baseball player is potentially career ending and therefore needs very special attention. Every baseball player knows the demands put on an arm in training and competition, so we also realize the need for very intense and specialized rehabilitation. During my playing career I had three serious shoulder injuries. Much time and energy was spent on the strengthening of my shoulder, but the critical time of rehabilitation was the transition from physical therapy into a throwing program. An aggressive full-body conditioning program, including plyometrics, was essential in assisting my shoulder to function correctly when throwing a baseball. This program paved the way for a smooth transition onto the field and a successful return to competition."

–Mike Scioscia, Anaheim Angels

A great deal of literature exists detailing the surgical technique and postoperative rehabilitation of the injured shoulder. However, little has been written on the difficult task of transitioning the throwing athlete from the rehabilitation setting back to throwing sports after surgery. This chapter outlines a program to return the throwing athlete back to his or her sport after surgery.

Numerous surgical procedures can be performed on a throwing athlete's shoulder for a variety of pathologic conditions (e.g., glenohumeral [GH] instability, labral tears, rotator cuff tears, impingement syndrome, acromioclavicular joint injury). Because one short appendix cannot describe each surgical procedure and the postoperative rehabilitation course recommended for it, the program described in this chapter is based on the assumption that the athlete has already been cleared to begin an advanced throwing and conditioning program.

ASSESSMENT

Regardless of the surgical procedure performed, the physical therapist (PT) must assess the athlete's overall physical condition before beginning a more aggressive conditioning and throwing program. Knowledge of the athlete's flexibility, strength, and endurance is essential for the development of a program specific for his or her needs. The athlete's throwing mechanics must be carefully evaluated throughout rehabilitation and the transition back to throwing sports.

STRENGTHENING AND CONDITIONING

In the past a great deal of emphasis was placed on developing mobility in the postoperative shoulder and developing strength in the shoulder-supporting musculature, including the rotator cuff and scapular stabilizers. Very little attention was given to the remainder of the musculature that plays a significant role in permitting the athlete to throw effectively and without injury.

Dynamic stability of the throwing shoulder requires fine, coordinated action of the GH and scapulothoracic stabilizers to facilitate synchronous function of the GH joint. After surgery, proper neuromuscular control must be reestablished to prevent asynchronous muscle-firing patterns, which can result in dysfunction.[1,2]

Neuromuscular control is defined as a purposeful act initiated at the cortical level.[3] Payton, Hirt, and Newton[3] stated that motor control is an involuntary associated movement organized subcortically that results in a well-learned skill operating without conscious guidance. The fine coordinated activity necessary for propelling a ball rapidly and accurately requires subcortical control of the muscles responsible for throwing.

Kinesthesia is the ability to discriminate joint position, relative weight of body parts, and joint movement, including speed, direction, and amplitude.[4] Proprioception is the ability to discriminate joint position.

The ability to throw requires that joint proprioceptors (muscle and joint afferents present in ligament and synovial tissues) function normally. Joint proprioceptors within the GH joint are responsible for signaling a stretch reflex when the GH capsule is taut to prevent translation at extremes of motion.[5] Many throwers recovering from surgery, especially those who have undergone procedures for instability, complain of stiffness and tightness in their shoulders. Neuromuscular controls may have been arrested by trauma and surgery, resulting in a new subcortical sense of joint tightness during throwing that was not present before the shoulder-stabilization procedure.

The upper extremity (UE) and shoulder represent the last link in the kinetic chain during the overhead-throwing motion, which begins distally as ground reactive forces are transferred caudally. Biomechanical analysis shows that tremendous forces are generated and extreme motion occurs in the shoulder with overhand throwing. Angular velocities in excess of 7000°/sec have been recorded during the transition from external rotation to internal rotation when throwing.[6,7] Shearing forces on the anterior shoulder are estimated at 400 N.[6] Approximately 500N of distraction force occurs during the deceleration phase of the throwing motion.[6] These forces are short in duration, develop quickly, occur at extremely high intensity, and must be performed repeatedly. The direction and magnitude of the forces generated when throwing a ball cause anteroposterior translational and distraction vectors that stress the GH constraints.

However, these forces are not entirely generated in the shoulder. The shoulder-supporting musculature is not capable of generating the forces and motions measured at the shoulder during throwing. Throwing a ball effectively requires the athlete to generate, summate, transfer, and regulate these forces from the legs through the throwing hand. To generate the forces measured with throwing, the shoulder relies on its position at the end of the kinetic chain. It has been reported that 51% to 55% of the kinetic energy created is generated in the lower extremities (LEs).[8,9] Use of ground reaction forces sequentially linked with the activity of the large LE and trunk muscles generate a significant proportion of the forces measured. Biomechanical data show that the shoulder itself contributes relatively little of the overall total energy necessary to the throwing motion. However, it provides a relatively high contribution to the total forces (21%), indicating that the shoulder, because of its position at the end of the kinetic chain, must effectively transfer and concentrate the developed energy. Conditioning of the shoulder and UE musculature is important in returning throwing athletes back to their sports. Moreover, the trunk and LE musculature must be adequately conditioned to provide the foundation to generate the forces required for effective and safe throwing.

When designing a program to return a throwing athlete back to sports, the physical therapist (PT) should consider two primary objectives: (1) enhancing current performance levels and (2) preventing injury. Gambetta[10] has outlined ten key principles that are basic to the development of a conditioning program for the throwing athlete (Box 13-1). The many components of the program must work together to produce optimal performance. The quality of the effort and the overall intensity should be emphasized first. The clinician should monitor each exercise and eventually scrutinize the throwing technique to ensure the optimal training effect and minimize the potential for injury.

The development of muscle balance is essential for coordinated, efficient movement to occur, especially around the shoulder where muscle imbalance can easily develop. Muscles (e.g., the rotator cuff) cannot simply be trained solely and in isolation, as in the early phases of most postoperative programs. After base strength has been developed in the postoperative shoulder, functional activities and more sport-specific exercises must be added to mimic the activities the athlete will be performing.

The development of core strength in the abdominals, trunk, and spinal-stabilizing muscles cannot be overemphasized. Without adequate core strength, the throwing athlete becomes vulnerable to improper postural alignment, which can lead to compensatory movements that place even greater stress on the shoulder, further predisposing the athlete to injury. After adequate strength has been achieved in the shoulder-supporting musculature, abdominals, spinal stabilizers, and LEs, endurance training can be added.

Only after sufficient strength and endurance have been developed and normal, synchronous muscle-firing patterns have been reestablished can a more functional and sport-specific activity such as throwing be added. The ultimate success of the training program depends on its overall design in introducing a variety of training stimuli to maximize total conditioning. An ideal conditioning program should contain a preparation period, an adaptation period, and an application period.[10] The preparation period should consist of general work, including strength and endurance training. Specialized work incorporating joint dynamics of the sport occurs during the adaptation period. Finally, the application

---

BOX 13-1 Basic Conditioning Principles

- Develop muscle synergy.
- Train for performance, not work capacity.
- Train for muscle balance.
- Train movements, not muscles.
- Develop structural (core) strength before extremity strength.
- Use body weight resistance before external resistance.
- Build strength before strength endurance.
- Develop synergists before prime movers.
- Promote joint integrity before mobility.
- Teach fundamental movement skill before specific sport skill.

period incorporates the specific joint actions and movements required to perform the sport.

ISOTONIC EXERCISES

A progressive weight- and functional-training program should start with body weight exercise. This allows the athlete to develop the proper exercise techniques and regain the synchronous muscle-firing patterns required to perform the overhand sport. This method of training also is adaptable to the more advanced plyometric exercises that follow after base strength has been gained.

Weight training is one of the most popular methods of training and can be performed with either free weights or machines. Free weight training with dumbbells is preferable, because it allows for unilateral training while permitting a full range of motion (ROM) of the extremity. Machines are better used in training the LEs. The use of rubber tubing or bands is another popular method of early strength training for the overhand-throwing athlete. These exercises can be performed as a warm-up for more strenuous weight resistance exercises or as a cool down exercise; they can accommodate all muscle actions. Rubber tubing or band exercises also allow for unilateral training of the extremity through a full ROM. They can be performed during the rehabilitation period and should continue when the thrower returns to play. Isotonic strengthening can be tailored to each athlete's needs and can be used to maintain strength in all muscle groups. Jobe's UE exercise program[11] is the most popular group of isotonic exercises performed. They can be initiated early in the rehabilitation period and continued throughout the athlete's career. However, they must be performed correctly to maximize their benefit (Table 13-1).

Core strength should first be developed using isotonic training. Only after base strength is developed should the intensity of the exercise program be increased (Table 13-2).

PLYOMETRIC EXERCISES

Plyometric training was first introduced in the late 1960s by Soviet jump coach Yuri Verkhoshanski.[12] American track coach Fred Wilt[13] first introduced plyometrics in the United States in 1975. The majority of the literature concerning plyometric exercise discusses its use in the LEs. Adapting these principles to the conditioning of throwing athletes is logical, considering the maximal explosive concentric contractions and rapid decelerative eccentric contractions that occur with each throwing cycle. Although agreement regarding the benefits of plyometric exercise in the training program is well documented, controversy exists regarding its optimal use.[14-17]

Plyometric exercise can be broken down into three phases: (1) the eccentric (or setting) phase, (2) the amortization phase, and (3) the concentric response phase. The setting phase of the exercise is the preloading period; it lasts until the stretch stimulus is initiated. The amortization phase of the exercise is the time that occurs between the eccentric contraction and the initiation of the concentric contraction. During the concentric phase the effect of the exercise (a facilitated contraction) is produced and preparation for the second repetition occurs.

Clinicians believe physiologic muscle performance is enhanced by plyometric exercise in several ways. The faster a muscle is loaded eccentrically, the greater the resultant

TABLE 13-1 Jobe's Shoulder Exercises*

Exercise	Weight (lb)	Sets/Repetitions
Shoulder flexion	3-5	3-4/10-15
Shoulder elevation	3-5	3-4/10-15
Shoulder abduction	3-5	3-4/10-15
Shoulder scaption	3-5	3-4/10-15
Military press	3-5	3-4/10-15
Horizontal abduction	3-5	3-4/10-15
Shoulder extension	3-5	3-4/10-15
External rotation I (side lying)	1-5	3-4/10-15
External rotation II (prone)	1-5	3-4/10-15
Internal rotation	1-5	3-4/10-15
Horizontal adduction	3-5	3-4/10-15
Rowing	3-5	3-4/10-1

*All exercises should be performed three times a week.
Modified from Jobe FW et al: Shoulder and arm exercises for the athlete who throws, Inglewood, Calif, 1996, Champion Press.

TABLE 13-2 Isotonic Core-Strengthening Exercises

Exercise*†	Sets/Repetitions
Chest	
Bench press (close grip)	2-3/8-10
Legs squats	2-3/8-10
Leg press	2-3/8-10
Knee extensions	2-3/8-10
Leg curls	2-3/8-10
Lunges	2-3/8-10
Calf press	2-3/8-10
Toe raises	2-3/8-10
Back	
Latissimus pull-downs	2-3/8-10
Shoulder shrugs	2-3/8-10
Seated rows	2-3/8-10
Bent-over rows	2-3/8-10
Abdominals Crunches (to be performed in sequence)	
Feet flat	3/15, rest 30 seconds
Weight on chest	3/15, rest 60 seconds
Knees bent	1/25, rest 60 seconds
Knees up with weight	1/25

*All exercises should be performed two to three times a week.
†Wide-grip bench press, behind-neck pull-down, deep squats, and behind-neck military press should not be performed.

concentric force produced. Eccentric loading of a muscle places stress on the elastic components, increasing the tension of the resultant force produced.

Neuromuscular coordination is improved through explosive plyometric training. Plyometric exercise may improve neural efficiency, thereby increasing neuromuscular performance.

Finally, the inhibitory effect of the Golgi tendon organs, which serve as a protective mechanism limiting the amount of force produced within muscle, can be desensitized by plyometric exercise, thereby raising the level of inhibition. This desensitization and the resultant raise in the inhibition level ultimately allow increased force production with greater applied loads.

Through neural adaptation, the throwing athlete can coordinate the activity of muscle groups and produce greater net force output (in the absence of morphologic change within the muscles themselves). The faster the athlete is able to switch from eccentric or yielding work to concentric overcoming work, the more powerful the resultant response. Effective plyometric training requires that the amortization phase of the exercise be quick, limiting the amount of energy wasted as heat. The rate of stretch rather than the length of stretch provides a greater stimulus for an enhanced training effect. With slower stretch cycles the stretch reflex is not activated.

Before implementing a plyometric training program, the patient must have an adequate level of base strength to maximize the training effect and prevent injury. Remedial shoulder exercises focusing on the rotator cuff and shoulder-supporting musculature are continued in order to develop and maintain joint stability and muscle strength in the arm decelerators. These exercises also should be used to warm up before the plyometric drill and cool down after it has been concluded.

Plyometric exercise is contraindicated in the immediate postoperative period, in the presence of acute inflammation or pain, in athletes with gross shoulder or elbow instability, or in both. Plyometric training also is contraindicated in athletes who do not have an adequate degree of base strength and who are not participating in a strength-training program. This form of exercise is intended to be an advanced form of strength training. Postexercise muscle soreness and delayed-onset muscle soreness are common adverse reactions that the clinician should be aware of before beginning an athlete on this type of exercise.

Tremendous amounts of stress occur during plyometric exercises; therefore they should not be performed for an extended period. A plyometric program should be used during the first and second preparation phases of training.

The plyometric training program for the UE can be divided into four groups of exercise as described by Wilk[18] (Table 13-3):

1. Warm-up exercises
2. Throwing movements
3. Trunk extension and flexion exercises
4. Medicine ball wall exercises

TABLE 13-3 Plyometric Exercises

Exercise*	Equipment	Sets/Repetitions
Warm-Ups		
Medicine ball rotation	9-lb ball	2-3/10
Medicine ball side bends	9-lb ball	2-3/10
Medicine ball wood chops	9-lb ball	2-3/10
Tubing		
IR, ER, and 90° shoulder abduction	Medium tubing	2-3/10
Diagonal patterns (D2)	Medium tubing	2-3/10
Biceps	Medium tubing	2-3/10
Push-ups		2-3/10
Throwing Movements		
Medicine ball soccer throw[†]	4-lb ball	2-4/6-8
Medicine ball chest pass[†]	4-lb ball	2-4/6-8
Medicine ball step and pass[†]	4-lb ball	2-4/6-8
Medicine ball side throw[†]	4-lb ball	2-4/6-8
Tubing Plyometrics		
IR and ER repetitions		6-8
Diagonals repetitions		6-8
Biceps repetitions		6-8
Push-ups repetitions	6- to 8-inch box	10
Trunk Extension and Flexion Movements		
Medicine ball sit-ups	4-lb ball	2-3/10
Medicine ball back extension	4-lb ball	2-3/10
Medicine Ball Exercises (Standing and Kneeling)		
Soccer throw	4-lb ball	2-4/6-8
Chest pass	4-lb ball	2-4/6-8
Side-to-side throw	4-lb ball	2-4/6-8
Backward side-to-side throws	4-lb ball	2-4/6-8
Forward two hands through legs	4-lb ball	2-4/6-8
One-handed baseball throw	2-lb ball	2-4/6-8

ER, External rotations; IR, internal rotations.
*All exercises should be performed two to three times a week.
[†]Throw with partner or pitchback device.
Modified from Wilk KE, Voight ML: Plyometrics for the shoulder complex. In Andrews JR, Wilk KE, editors: The athlete's shoulder, New York, 1994, Churchill Livingstone.

Warm-up exercises are performed to provide the shoulder, arms, trunk, and LEs an adequate physiologic warm-up before beginning more intense plyometric exercise. The facilitation of muscular performance through an active warm-up has been ascribed to increased blood flow, oxygen use, nervous system transmission, muscle and core temperature, and speed of contraction.[4,19-22] The athlete should perform two to three sets of 10 repetitions for each warm-up exercise before proceeding to the next group of exercises.

Throwing movement plyometric exercises attempt to isolate and train the muscles required to throw effectively. Movement patterns are performed similar to those found with overhead throwing. These exercises provide an advanced strengthening technique at a higher exercise level than that of more traditional isotonic dumbbell exercises. The exercises in this group are performed for two to four sets of six to eight repetitions two to three times weekly. Adequate rest times should occur between each session for optimal muscle recovery.

Plyometric exercises for trunk strengthening include medicine ball exercises for the abdominals and trunk extensor musculature. The athlete performs two to four sets of 8 to 10 repetitions two to three times weekly.

The final group of exercises, the Plyoball wall exercises, require the use of 2-lb and 4-lb medicine balls or Plyoballs and a wall or pitchback device to allow the athlete to perform this group of exercises without a partner. This group of drills starts with two-handed throws with a heavier 4-lb ball and concludes with one-handed plyometric throws using the lighter 2-lb ball. All the exercises in this phase of the program should be performed in the standing and kneeling positions to increase demands on the trunk, UE, and shoulder girdle and eliminate the use of the LEs. The same number of repetitions and sets should be performed two to three times weekly (Fig. 13-1).

Plyometric training of the LEs is essential in developing the throwing athlete's explosive strength needed for speed, lateral mobility, and acceleration. LE plyometric training also helps develop the coordination and agility necessary to compete effectively. High demands are placed on the

musculature supporting the hips, knees, and ankle joints during plyometric jump exercises. The PT must monitor exercise loads performed and allow adequate recovery time between sets. Proper technique in performing these exercises is vital to prevent injury. A variety of jump exercises can be used to train the LEs when preparing the throwing athlete to return to athletic competition (Table 13-4).

Rapid box jumps are performed to develop explosive power in the calf and quadriceps musculature. An explosive but controlled jump up onto the box, then down off the box is performed; box height can be increased as the exercise is

TABLE 13-4 LE Plyometric Exercises

Exercise*	Equipment	Sets/Repetitions
Rapid box jumps (alternating height)	Boxes of varying heights	2-3/8-10
Box jumps	12- to 24-inch boxes	3-4 sets
Depth jump and sprint[†]	24-inch box	5-8 repetitions
Depth jump and base steal[†]	24-inch box	5-8 repetitions

LE, Lower extremities.
*All exercises should be performed two to three times per week.
[†]Jump from a 24-inch box followed by an immediate 10-yard sprint.

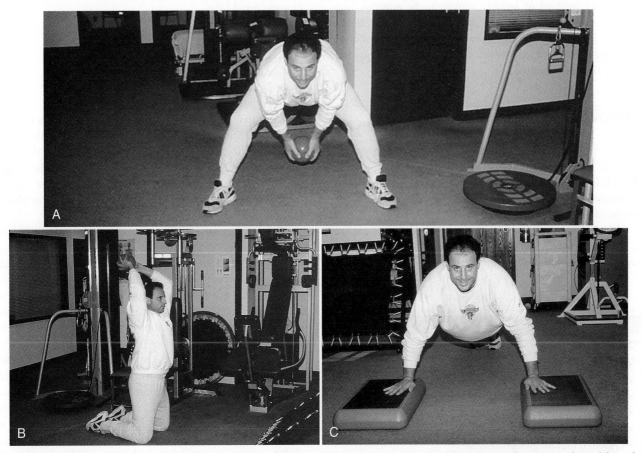

Fig. 13-1 **A,** Medicine ball wood chop warm-up exercises. **B,** Medicine ball soccer throw exercises from the knees. **C,** Plyometric push-up. (Photos by Dr. Luga Podesta, Oxnard, Calif.)

mastered. The athlete should immediately jump back on the box, spending as little time as possible on the ground.

Alternating-height box jumps train the quadriceps, hamstrings, gluteals, and calf muscles and help develop explosive power. Box jumps are performed using three to five plyometric boxes of varying heights (from 12 to 24 inches) placed in a straight line 2 feet apart from one another. Starting at the smallest box, the athlete performs controlled jumps from the box to the ground to the next tallest box, spending as little time on the ground as possible; the athlete should rest for 15 to 20 seconds between sets.

The depth jump and sprint and the depth jump with base steal focus on teaching muscles to react forcefully from a negative contraction to an explosive positive contraction. The athlete immediately explodes into a 10-yard sprint or 10-yard base steal after jumping off a 24-inch box.

AEROBIC CONDITIONING

Although the initial postoperative emphasis is on rehabilitation of the shoulder, the transition from formal therapy to return to play requires the throwing athlete to regain the preinjury aerobic condition. Therefore the aerobic conditioning component of the training program must not be neglected. Aerobic fitness can be developed using a variety of exercises (Box 13-2).

For any method of aerobic activity to be effective, the exercise should be performed continuously for 20 to 40 minutes four to five times weekly. Because this type of conditioning is long and repetitive, the athlete should enjoy the activity being performed.

THROWING

The overhead-throwing motion is not unique to throwing a baseball. Similar muscular activity is required to throw a softball, football, or javelin. However, the majority of research performed on overhead throwing has been conducted on the overhead pitch.

The clinician must appreciate the highly dynamic nature of the throwing motion to be effective in preparing and moving the rehabilitating athlete through a safe throwing program. A thorough understanding of normal and abnormal throwing mechanics and the biomechanical forces placed on the throwing arm are essential for the therapist wishing to implement a throwing program in the rehabilitation setting.

Baseball Pitching

Pitching a baseball is the most violent and dynamic of all overhead-throwing activities, producing angular velocities in excess of 7000°/sec across the shoulder. Maximal stability of the GH joint occurs at 90° of shoulder elevation.[23] Because muscle weakness can result in abnormal compression and shear forces, muscle balance is necessary to maintain stability of the humeral head in the glenoid fossa. A favorable balance between compression and shear forces occurs at 90° of shoulder elevation, placing the shoulder in the optimal position for joint stability.[1,3,23,24] All throwers therefore should maintain 90° of GH elevation relative to the horizontal surface regardless of technique or pitching style.

Dynamic control of the GH joint during throwing depends on the rotator cuff and biceps muscle strength.[1,2] An abnormal throwing pattern can result from GH instability and inadequate control of the rotator cuff and biceps tendon. Neuromuscular conditioning and control of the GH joint allows for safer throwing by facilitating the dynamic coordination of the rotator cuff and scapulothoracic stabilizers.

The throwing or pitching motion can be divided into six phases (Fig. 13-2):
1. Windup
2. Early cocking
3. Late cocking
4. Acceleration
5. Deceleration
6. Follow-through

Windup is the preparatory phase of the throwing motion. Relatively little muscle activity occurs during this phase. From a standing position, the athlete initiates the throw by shifting the weight onto the supporting back leg. The weight shift from the stride leg to the supporting leg sets the rhythm for the delivery. Windup ends when the ball leaves the gloved nondominant hand (Fig. 13-3, *A*).

The position of the stance foot is also important to help generate forces up through the ankle into the leg. Repositioning of the stance foot can significantly enhance the biomechanical forces generated at push off. It is biomechanically advantageous during push off to position the stance foot in subtalar eversion (Fig. 13-4). Greater forces can be generated in this position than if the foot is placed on the side of the pitching rubber alone.

During early cocking, the shoulder abducts to approximately 104° and externally rotates to 46°.[21] The scapular muscles are active in positioning the glenoid for optimal contact with the humeral head as the arm is abducted. The supraspinatus and deltoid muscles work synergistically to elevate the humerus. The deltoids position the arm in space, and the supraspinatus stabilizes the humeral head within the glenoid[10] (Figs. 13-3, *B-H*, and 13-5).

BOX 13-2 Aerobic Conditioning Exercises
• Running
• Bicycling
• Versa-Climber
• Stair-climbing machine
• Elliptical runner
• Cross-country ski machine
• Rowing machine
• Swimming

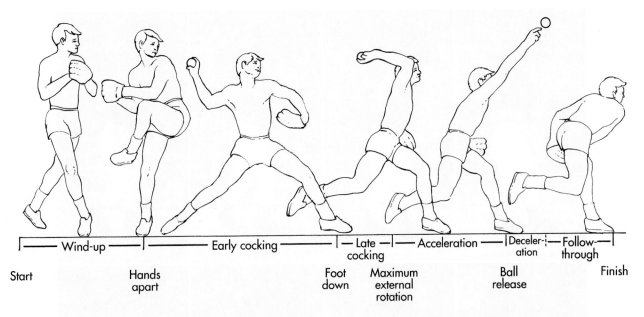

Fig. 13-2 Phases of the baseball pitch. (From Jobe FW: Operative techniques in upper extremity sports injury, St Louis, 1996, Mosby.)

The stride forward is initiated during the early cocking phase of throwing. The athlete should keep the trunk and back closed as long as possible to retain the energy stored, which later results in velocity.

As the stride leg moves toward the target, the ball breaks from the glove and the throwing arm swings upward in rhythm with the body. The positioning of the breaking hands followed by the downward then upward rotation of the throwing arm ensures optimal positioning of the arm (Fig. 13-6). Establishing this synchronous muscle-firing pattern is one of the most crucial aspects of the throw. If the throwing arm and striding leg are synchronized properly, then the arm and hand will be in the early cocked position when the stride foot contacts the ground (see Figs. 13-3, H, and 13-5, D).

The direction of the stride should either be directly toward the target or slightly closed (to the right side of a right-handed thrower) (see Figs. 13-3, H, and 13-5, E). When the stride is too closed, the hips are unable to rotate and the thrower is forced to throw across the body, losing kinetic energy from the LEs. When the stride is too open (i.e., the stride foot lands too far to the left of a right-handed thrower), the hips rotate too early, forcing the trunk to face the batter too early and dissipating stored kinetic energy. This also places tremendous stress on the anterior shoulder. After the stride leg contacts the ground, the stride is completed and cocking of the throwing arm is initiated.

During the late cocking phase of throwing the humerus maintains its level of abduction while moving into the scapular plane. The arm externally rotates from 46° to 170°.[21] In this position the humeral head is positioned to place an anterior-directed force, potentially stretching the anterior ligamentous restraints.

The trunk moves laterally toward the target, and pelvic rotation is initiated. As the trunk undergoes rotation and extension, the elbow is flexed, and the shoulder externally rotates. When the trunk faces the target, the shoulder should have achieved maximal external rotation. At the end of this phase, only the arm is cocked as the legs, pelvis, and trunk have already accelerated (see Figs. 13-3, I and J, and 13-5, F and G).

During the acceleration phase, the humerus internally rotates approximately 100° in 0.005 seconds. Tremendous torque and joint compressive forces and high angular velocities across the GH joint are present at this time.[6,21,25]

The acceleration phase begins when the humerus begins to internally rotate. Just before the beginning of internal rotation, the elbow should begin to extend (see Figs. 13-3, K, and 13-5, H and I). When ball release occurs, the trunk is flexed, the elbow reaches almost full extension, and the shoulder undergoes internal rotation (see Figs. 13-3, L, and 13-5, J). At ball release, the trunk should be tilted forward with the lead knee extending. Acceleration ends with ball release.

The deceleration phase of the throwing motion is the first third of the time from ball release to the completion of arm motion (see Figs. 13-3, M and N, and 13-5, K). During deceleration excess kinetic energy that was not transferred to the ball is dissipated. High calculated forces and torque also occur during this phase.[26,27]

Follow-through occurs during the final two thirds of the throwing motion, during which time the arm continues to decelerate and eventually stops (see Figs. 13-3, O, and 13-5, L). After ball release, the throwing arm continues to extend at the elbow and internally rotates at the shoulder. Internal angular velocities drop from their maximal level at ball release to zero. A proper follow-through is crucial in minimizing injury to the shoulder during this violent stage of throwing. Follow-through is completed when the throwing shoulder is over the opposite knee. This is achieved by

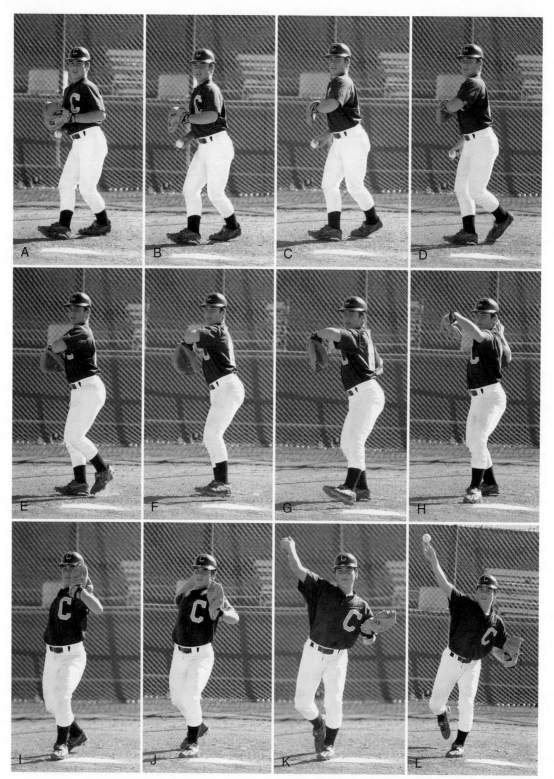

Fig. 13-3 Front view of the throwing motion. **A-E,** The crow hop step begins the throwing motion. The pelvis and chest are rotated 90° from the target. The hands separate as weight is shifted to the back leg. **F-J,** During the cocking phase of throwing, the throwing arm is elevated and externally rotated. Front view of the throwing motion. The front foot is planted in a slightly closed position as the pelvis begins to rotate. Front view of the throwing motion. **K-L,** During the acceleration phase, the elbow is above the height of the shoulder and weight is shifted to the front foot as the pelvis rotates.

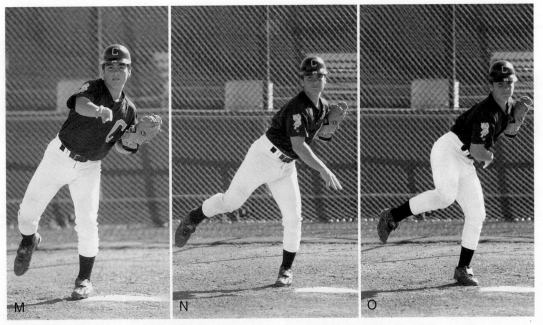

Fig. 13-3, cont'd **M-O,** The deceleration and follow-through phases. (Photos by Marsha Gorman, Camarillo, Calif.)

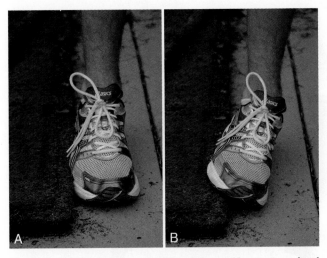

Fig. 13-4 **A,** Foot placed on side of the pitching rubber. **B,** Foot placed straddling the pitching rubber in subtalar joint eversion.

allowing the supporting leg to rotate forward, finishing the rotation of the trunk across the body.

Football

The throwing mechanics necessary to throw a football are very similar to those required to throw a baseball.[28] The most significant differences between the two are the size and weight of the ball and the positioning of the throwing hand during the acceleration and ball release phases of the throwing motion. Although the precise throwing mechanics are not well defined, studies are currently underway to determine and describe the specific mechanics. Similar forces and stresses appear to be applied to the shoulder and elbow. Dynamic control of the entire kinetic chain during the football throw is essential for the quarterback to be effective throwing to the right, left, and on the run. Neuromuscular conditioning and control of the LEs, core, and UEs allows for safer throwing by facilitating the dynamic coordination of the entire kinetic chain.

The football-throwing motion can be divided into six phases:
1. Windup
2. Early cocking
3. Late cocking
4. Acceleration
5. Deceleration
6. Follow-through

Windup is the preparatory phase of the throwing motion. From a squatting position, the quarterback steps backward from behind the center varying distances (i.e., steps) positioning the body to initiate the throw by shifting the weight onto the supporting back leg. The weight shift from the stride leg to the supporting leg sets the rhythm for the delivery. Windup ends when the ball and supporting hand separate (Fig. 13-7).

During early cocking, the shoulder abducts and externally rotates (Fig. 13-8). The stride forward is initiated during the early cocking phase of throwing. The athlete should keep the trunk and back closed as long as possible to retain the energy stored, which later results in velocity.

As the stride leg moves toward the target, the ball breaks from the hand and the throwing arm swings upward in rhythm with the body. Establishing this synchronous muscle-firing pattern from the feet to the LEs through the pelvis and trunk to the shoulder to the UE and finally the hand is one of the most crucial aspects of the throw. If the throwing arm and striding leg are synchronized properly, then the arm and hand will be in the early cocked position when the stride foot contacts the ground.

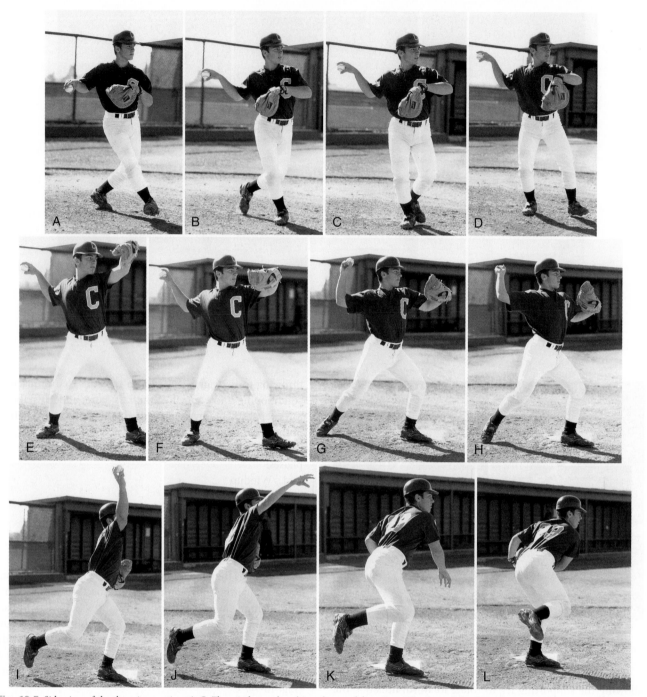

Fig. 13-5 Side view of the throwing motion. **A-C,** The windup and cocking phases of throwing. Side view of the throwing motion. **D-G,** The windup and cocking phases of throwing. **H-I,** The acceleration phases. Side view of the throwing motion. **J,** The acceleration phases. **K-L,** The deceleration and follow-through phases. (Photos by Marsha Gorman, Camarillo, Calif.)

The direction of the stride should either be directly toward the target or slightly closed (to the right side of a right-handed thrower) regardless of the direction of the throw—straight, right, or left.

During the late cocking phase of throwing (Fig. 13-9), the humerus maintains its level of abduction while moving into the scapular plane. The arm externally rotates, the trunk moves laterally toward the target, and pelvic rotation is initiated. As the trunk undergoes rotation and extension, the elbow is flexed and the shoulder externally rotates. When the

trunk faces the target, the shoulder should have achieved maximal external rotation. At the end of this phase, only the arm is cocked because the legs, pelvis, and trunk have already accelerated.

During the acceleration phase (Fig. 13-10) the humerus internally rotates, applying tremendous torque and joint compressive forces and high angular velocities across the GH.

The acceleration phase begins when the humerus begins to internally rotate. Just before the beginning of internal

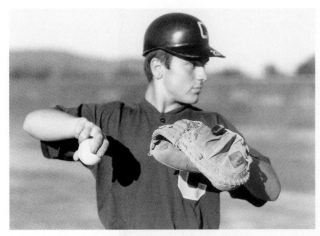

Fig. 13-6 The proper technique for gripping the ball and releasing it from the glove. The ball is gripped loosely across four seams in the fingertips of the index and middle fingers. The thumb is placed under the ball, with the index and middle fingers held together. The hands separate with a supinating motion of the forearms forcing the thumbs of both the glove and ball hand downward. (Photo by Marsha Gorman, Camarillo, Calif.)

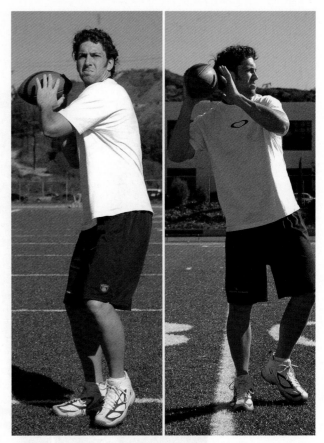

Fig. 13-8 The early cocking phase.

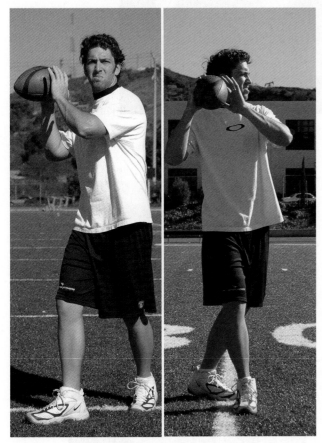

Fig. 13-7 The windup phase.

rotation, the elbow should begin to extend. When ball release occurs, the trunk is flexed, the elbow reaches almost full extension, the shoulder undergoes internal rotation, and the forearm maximally pronates (Fig. 13-11). At ball release the trunk should be tilted forward with the lead knee extending. Acceleration ends with ball release.

The deceleration phase of the throwing motion is the first third of the time from ball release to the completion of arm motion (Fig. 13-12). During deceleration, excess kinetic energy that was not transferred to the ball is dissipated.

Follow-through (Fig. 13-13) occurs during the final two thirds of the throwing motion, during which time the arm continues to decelerate and eventually stops. After ball release, the throwing arm continues to extend at the elbow and internally rotates at the shoulder. A proper follow-through is crucial in minimizing injury to the shoulder during this violent stage of throwing. Follow-through is completed when the throwing shoulder is over the opposite knee. This is achieved by allowing the supporting leg to rotate forward, finishing the rotation of the trunk across the body.

INTERVAL BASEBALL THROWING PROGRAM

The purpose of the interval throwing program is to return motion, strength, and confidence gradually to the throwing arm after injury or surgery. The interval throwing program allows the throwing patient the opportunity to reestablish timing, movement patterns, coordination, and synchronicity of muscle firing before returning to competition.[12] This is accomplished by slowly increasing the throwing distances

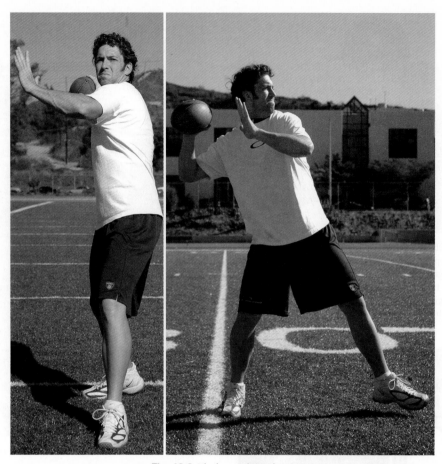

Fig. 13-9 The late cocking phase.

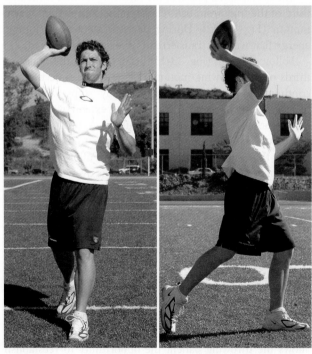

Fig. 13-10 The acceleration phase.

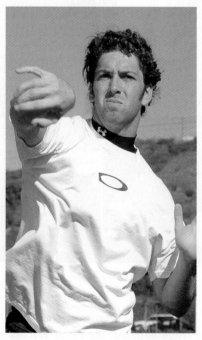

Fig. 13-11 Maximal pronation occurs toward the end of the acceleration phase.

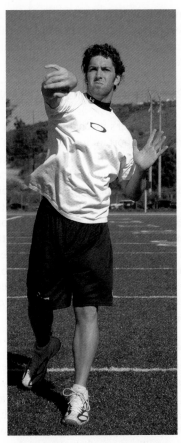

Fig. 13-12 The deceleration phase.

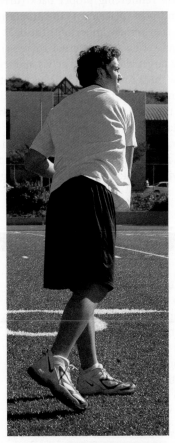

Fig. 13-13 The follow-through phase.

and eventually the velocity of the throws. The program should be individualized to each athlete. No set timetable is prescribed for the completion of the program; each patient's time spent completing the program may vary. The throwing program is designed to minimize the chance of injury by emphasizing proper prethrowing warm-up, stretching, and cool down. It should be performed in the presence of a coach, trainer, or therapist knowledgeable in throwing mechanics. Careful supervision cannot be overstressed.

The participants must resist the temptation to increase the intensity of the throwing program and understand that this may increase the incidence of reinjury, which would greatly retard the rehabilitation process.

Before initiating the interval throwing program, the athletic patient must exhibit the following criteria:

1. Full and painless ROM
2. No pain or tenderness
3. Satisfactory muscle strength and conditioning
4. Normal or clinically stable examination

Specific attention throughout the interval throwing program to the maintenance of proper throwing mechanics is crucial (Box 13-3). Participants in the rehabilitation program may find videotaping throwing sessions extremely helpful in assisting with the analysis of the athlete's throwing mechanics.

Proper warm-up before beginning to throw cannot be overemphasized. A common mistake is for the thrower to begin throwing to warm up. Instead, the thrower should increase the blood flow to muscles and joints before throwing. Running or jogging long enough to break a sweat can accomplish this.

The athletic patient must warm up to throw, not throw to warm-up.

A "crow hop" throwing technique uses a hop, skip, and throw to accentuate LE and trunk involvement in the throw. The use of the crow hop method simulates the throwing motion and emphasizes proper throwing mechanics (see Figs. 13-3, *A* to *F*, and 13-5, *A* to *D*).

BOX 13-3 Throwing Evaluation Checklist

- Foot position—Crow hop, back foot 90° to the target
- Body position—Nondominant hip and shoulder to the target
- Hand break—Ball release from glove, thumbs down
- Ball hand and glove position—Ball facing away from the target, glove side elbow points to target flexed 90°, glove down
- Arm position—Elbow above shoulder level
- Front foot plant—Step toward the target, "toes to target," slightly closed
- Trunk rotation—Hips rotate before shoulders
- Balance—Stand tall, weight back
- Finish—Stride foot posts, back leg and hip rotate through

Throwing flat-footed encourages improper throwing mechanics and places increased stress on the throwing shoulder.

The throwing athlete progresses through each step of the program, throwing every other day, or three times weekly.

The thrower progresses to the next step after the prescribed number of throws can be completed without pain or residual pain. If pain or difficulty throwing occurs, then the athlete should regress to the previous level or attempt the same level during the next session. The ultimate goal is for the athlete to throw 75 repetitions at 180 feet without pain for positional players and 150 feet for pitchers. Box 13-4 illustrates a progressive interval throwing program.[29]

When progressing through a pitcher-specific interval throwing program, it is extremely important to ensure that the person or target receiving the throws is at the same height as the thrower. When throwing on flat ground, the thrower should be throwing to a standing target. When throwing off the pitching mound, the target can get into a squatting position. Throwing on flat ground to a squatting catcher changes the point of ball release, which may lead to increased stress across the anterior shoulder and elbow. Pattern throwing (Fig. 13-14) also can be implemented to develop arm strength[10]:

1. Proper warm-up before throwing (i.e., jogging, running, bicycling)
2. Throwing from a kneeling position, facing the direction of the throw with the arm already in the abducted position for a distance of 20 feet, easy effort, for 10 repetitions, with emphasis on proper grip
3. Kneeling on one knee facing the target with the arm in the abducted position (right-handed thrower on the right knee, left-handed thrower on the left knee) from a distance of 30 feet, easy effort, 10 repetitions, with emphasis on hitting the target and maintaining proper follow-through
4. Standing with the feet in a straddle position facing the target with the shoulders turned and the ball in the glove at a distance of 40 feet, medium effort, with emphasis on follow-through

5. Standing in a regular throwing position at a distance of 40 feet, throwing medium effort for 10 repetitions, with emphasis on staying closed and pointing the front shoulder to the target

DEVELOPING THROWING MECHANICS

Once a flaw in a thrower's mechanics has been identified, it becomes extremely important for the clinician to implement a change in that patient's throwing mechanics to prevent further injury from developing. It can be very difficult to change established faulty mechanics or bad habits especially in the older thrower. Having the ability to teach proper throwing mechanics becomes extremely important. To be able to accomplish this we must provide the thrower with exercises and techniques that will sequentially reestablish the proper muscle firing patterns and muscle memory. The exercise programs are designed to reestablish proper kinematics from the feet up through the entire kinetic chain to the throwing hand.

Foot Placement (Crow Hop) Drill

To throw properly, foot placement becomes extremely important. Proper foot placement during the windup phase and early cocking phase of the throwing cycle are the foundation for development of the remainder of the sequential motion patterns. It is important to get the thrower moving toward the target. To accomplish this, we have the athlete perform a drill reinforcing proper back (drive) as well as front foot (land/post) placement. The proper positioning of the back foot is extremely important. The back foot needs to be pointed outwardly (hip external rotation) 90° perpendicular to the target allowing the pelvis and trunk to rotate. This will allow the thrower to load the back foot, sequentially transfer ground reactive forces up the kinetic chain from the foot through the pelvis into the trunk. To teach this we have the athlete start the exercise facing forward. For the right hand thrower, they would take an exaggerated step forward with his back foot turning it outward 90°. This forces the hip and then pelvis to rotate externally, positioning the throwers

---

BOX 13-4 Progressive Interval Throwing Program	
• Warm-up	**Step 2**
• Run to break sweat	a. Warm-up throwing
• Stretching	b. 45 feet (25 throws)
	c. Rest 10 minutes
45-foot Phase (half the distance to first base from home plate)	d. Warm-up throwing
	e. 45 feet (25 throws)
Step 1	f. Rest 10 minutes
a. Warm-up throwing—25 feet	g. Warm-up throwing
b. 45 feet (25 throws)	h. 45 feet (25 throws)
c. Rest 10-15 minutes	
d. Warm-up throwing	
e. 45 feet (25 throws)	

BOX 13-4 Progressive Interval Throwing Programr—cont'd

60-foot Phase (distance from home plate to pitching mound)

Step 3

a. Warm-up throwing
b. 60 feet (25 throws)
c. Rest 10-15 minutes
d. Warm-up throwing
e. 60 feet (25 throws)

Step 4

a. Warm-up throwing
b. 60 feet (25 throws)
c. Rest 10 minutes
d. Warm-up throwing
e. 60 feet (25 throws)
f. Rest 10 minutes
g. Warm-up throwing
h. 60 feet (25 throws)

90-foot Phase (distance from home plate to first base)

Step 5

a. Warm-up throwing
b. 90 feet (25 throws)
c. Rest 10-15 minutes
d. Warm-up throwing
e. 90 feet (25 throws)

Step 6

a. Warm-up throwing
b. 90 feet (25 throws)
c. Rest 10 minutes
d. Warm-up throwing
e. 90 feet (25 throws)
f. Rest 10 minutes
g. Warm-up throwing
h. 90 feet (25 throws)

120-foot Phase (distance from home plate to second base)

Step 7

a. Warm-up throwing
b. 120 feet (25 throws)
c. Rest 10-15 minutes
d. Warm-up throwing
e. 120 feet (25 throws)

Step 8

a. Warm-up throwing
b. 120 feet (25 throws)
c. Rest 10 minutes
d. Warm-up throwing
e. 120 feet (25 throws)

f. Rest 10 minutes
g. Warm-up throwing
h. 120 feet (25 throws)

150-foot Phase (distance from home plate to grass behind second base)

Step 9

a. Warm-up throwing
b. 150 feet (25 throws)
c. Rest 10-15 minutes
d. Warm-up throwing
e. 150 feet (25 throws)

Step 10

a. Warm-up throwing
b. 150 feet (25 throws)
c. Rest 10 minutes
d. Warm-up throwing
e. 150 feet (25 throws)
f. Rest 10 minutes
g. Warm-up throwing
h. 150 feet (25 throws)

180-foot Phase (distance from home plate to the outfield)

Step 11

a. Warm-up throwing
b. 180 feet (25 throws)
c. Rest 10-15 minutes
d. Warm-up throwing
e. 180 feet (25 throws)

Step 12

a. Warm-up throwing
b. 180 feet (25 throws)
c. Rest 10 minutes
d. Warm-up throwing
e. 180 feet (25 throws)
f. Rest 10 minutes
g. Warm-up throwing
h. 180 feet (25 throws)

Step 13

a. Warm-up throwing
b. 180 feet (25 throws)
c. Rest 10 minutes
d. Warm-up throwing
e. 180 feet (25 throws)
f. Rest 10 minutes
g. Warm-up throwing
h. 180 feet (25 throws)

Step 14

a. Return to position or begin throwing from the mound

Modified from Wilk KE, Arrigo CA: Interval sport programs for the shoulder. In Andrews JR, Wilk KE, editors: The athlete's shoulder, New York, 1994, Churchill Livingstone.

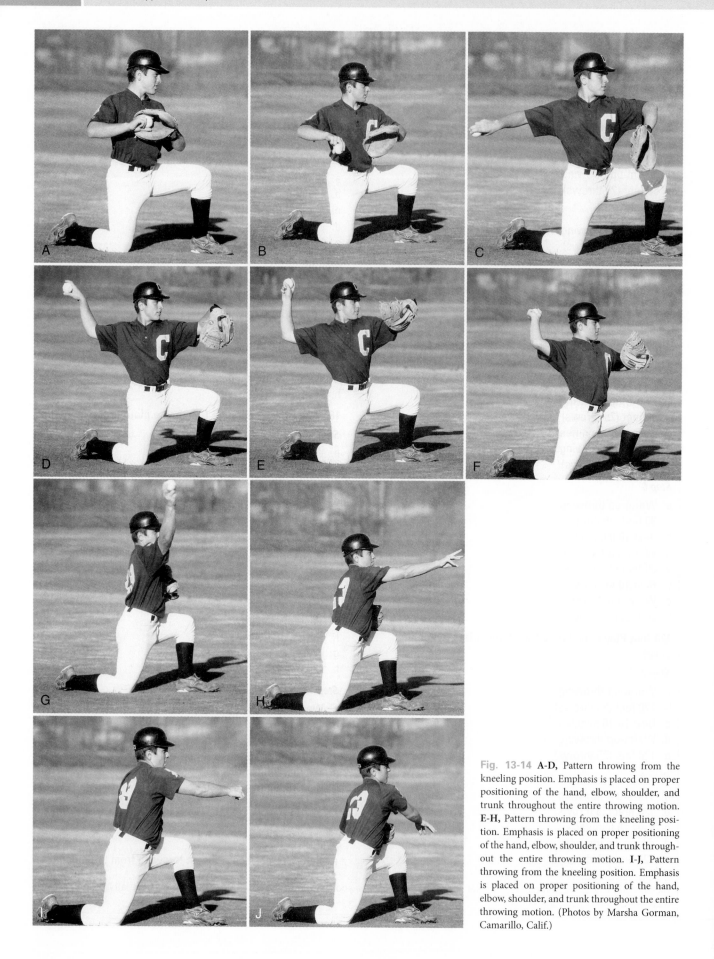

Fig. 13-14 A-D, Pattern throwing from the kneeling position. Emphasis is placed on proper positioning of the hand, elbow, shoulder, and trunk throughout the entire throwing motion. **E-H,** Pattern throwing from the kneeling position. Emphasis is placed on proper positioning of the hand, elbow, shoulder, and trunk throughout the entire throwing motion. **I-J,** Pattern throwing from the kneeling position. Emphasis is placed on proper positioning of the hand, elbow, shoulder, and trunk throughout the entire throwing motion. (Photos by Marsha Gorman, Camarillo, Calif.)

body at 90° with the nonthrowing side hip, elbow, and shoulder facing the target (Fig 13-15). The front foot or landing foot is placed in a position just inside the nonthrowing shoulder in a slightly closed position. This is repeated until the athlete is comfortable stepping to his target and rotating his back foot and trunk during the windup through the early cocking phase of the throwing cycle. This drill can then be advanced depending on the player's position, starting from a crouch with catchers and from a fielding position for position players.

Hand Position/Ball Transfer Drill

The next drill we have young throwers practice is proper hand break technique. This is accomplished by having the thrower practice transferring the baseball from the nonthrowing hand to the throwing hand pronating both wrists. This can be practiced in front of a mirror for further visual reinforcement (Fig 13-16).

Trunk Rotation/Hand Towel Drill

This next drill is designed to develop a fluid trunk rotation during the late cocking through follow-through phases of the throwing cycle. To teach proper hand placement on top of the ball, many young throwers are told during the late cocking phase of the throwing cycle to "take the ball off the shelf." This helps the athlete remember to place his hand on top of the ball but it essentially stops their trunk rotation. This drill is designed to further develop and incorporate the previous drills while maintaining the athlete's fluid trunk rotation without loosing the kinetic energy developed from the legs. The drill begins the same as the previous foot placement and hand separation drills. However, the athlete is holding a small hand towel instead of a ball while performing the drill. The drill begins with the athlete facing the target. The back foot and leg step forward and rotate as in the previous drill. The hands separate with the wrists pronating and the thumbs facing down. As the throwing arm progresses through the early cocking, late cocking, and then acceleration phases of the throwing cycle, pelvis, trunk, and shoulder motion should continue and remain fluid with stopping. The hand towel is used to provide a visual and tactile stimulus as if the athlete was waving a flag (Figs. 13-17 and 13-18). The flag should never "drop" as the thrower transitions from late cocking through the acceleration phase of throwing

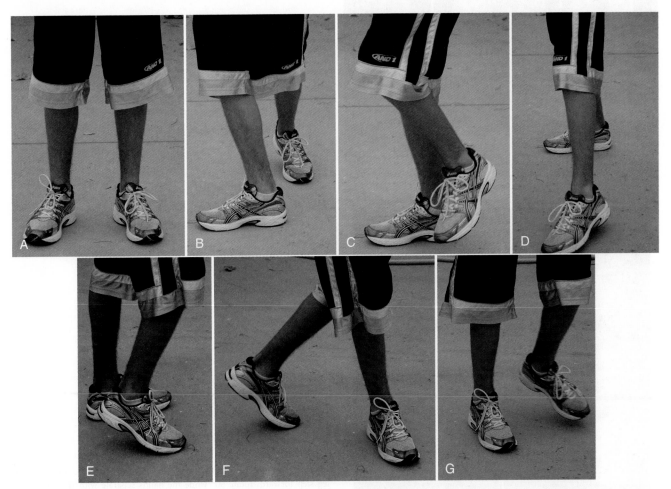

Fig. 13-15 A-D, Front view, foot placement (crow hop) drill—as the athlete moves toward the target, stepping/hopping with the back foot toward the target while rotating the foot 90°. **E-G,** Side view, foot placement (crow hop) drill—as the athlete moves toward the target, stepping/hopping with the back foot toward the target while rotating the foot 90°.

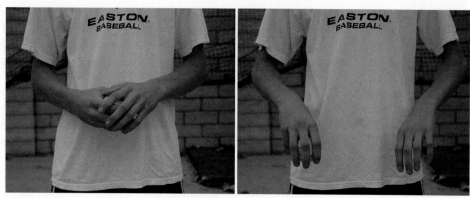

Fig. 13-16 Hand position/ball transfer drill—The athlete transfers the ball from the glove hand thumbs down, pronating the forearms.

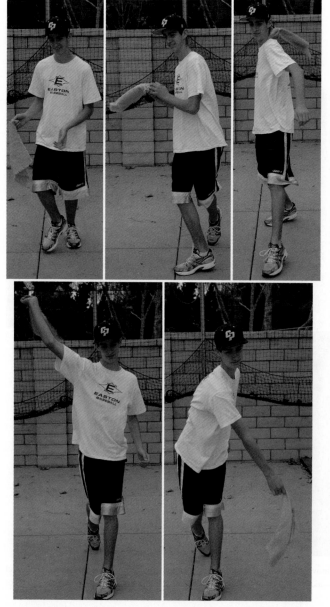

Fig. 13-17 Front view, trunk rotation-hand towel drill—The back foot and leg step forward, rotate 90° while the hands separate with the wrists and forearms pronating. The thrower progresses through the entire throwing motion with a fluid continuous movement, never allowing the towel to drop or the throwing motion to stop.

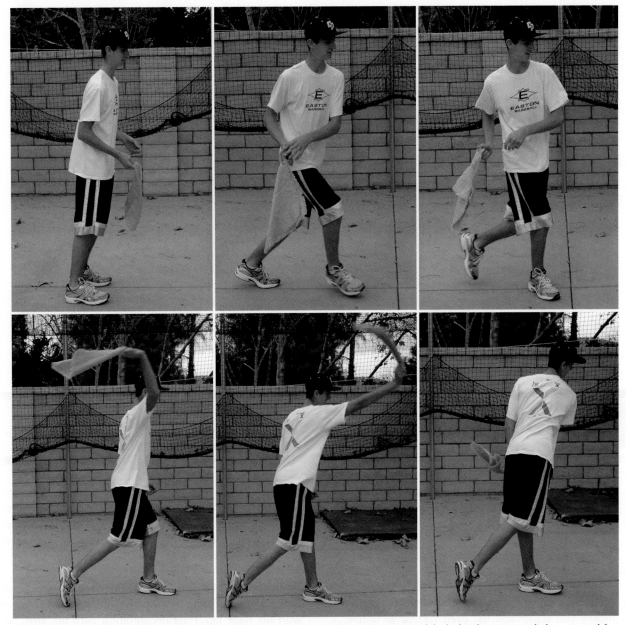

Fig. 13-18 Side view, trunk rotation-hand towel drill—The back foot and leg step forward, rotate 90° while the hands separate with the wrists and forearms pronating. The thrower progresses through the entire throwing motion with a fluid continuous movement never allowing the towel to drop or the throwing motion to stop.

(Fig 13-19). This drill should be practiced so that a fluid throwing motion is consistently performed, incorporating the feet, legs, trunk, and arms.

SUMMARY

Rehabilitation goals for the shoulder after surgery emphasize pain management, reestablishing ROM, and developing strength in the shoulder-supporting musculature. To return the throwing athlete to sports after surgery requires further intense strengthening and conditioning to regain preinjury form and performance. Progressive strengthening followed by aerobic conditioning helps prepare the thrower recovering from surgery for an eventual return to throwing. After throwing has been introduced into the rehabilitation regimen, careful attention to throwing technique is imperative to prevent reinjury. An interval throwing program is followed to establish a time frame for a safe, gradual, and progressive return to throwing.

The program described in this chapter should only serve as a guide for the progressive return of the thrower to throwing; it is not a specific postoperative protocol applicable to all Tpatient athletes. Each patient's program requires individualization and should progress at its own rate.

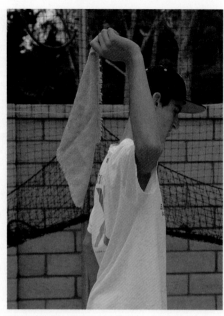

Fig. 13-19 Trunk rotation-hand towel drill—Poor technique allowing the throwing motion to stop and the towel to drop.

CLINICAL CASE REVIEW

1 When designing a program to return a throwing athlete back to sports, what two primary objectives should be considered?

(1) Enhance current performance levels and (2) prevent injury.

2 Brandon returned from postoperative rehabilitation for rotator cuff repair and has been cleared to initiate a return to throwing program. Since this is his first visit with you, what must be considered before he picks up a baseball?

A complete physical examination must be completed to assess his LE, core, and UE flexibility, strength, and coordination. An aerobic capacity test also should be performed.

3 Paul is eager to begin his baseball interval throwing program but has not been cleared by the physician yet. What factors must be met before initiating a return to throwing program (besides physician clearance)?

• Full and painless ROM
• No pain or tenderness with palpation
• Satisfactory muscle strength and conditioning
• Normal or clinically stable examination

4 Trevor is 16 years old and recovered from a UCL sprain in his throwing arm. He initiated a throwing program 1 week ago and is currently at step 3. He noted medial elbow pain in yesterday's throwing session. What should be considered?

Throwing mechanics were reviewed and subsequent video analysis found that he was not following through with his back leg, thus decelerating with his arm. As a clinician you must not take for granted that the athlete is performing the throwing motion correctly, no matter what age or level of performance. This simple correction along with backing down to step 2 for a week allowed Trevor to progress through the program successfully.

5 Kyler has completed step 10 of the interval throwing program. After yesterday's session he complained of fatigue and inability to throw the full 150 feet. What could be the problem?

Upon questioning him further it was noted that he performed his throwing exercises before performing his throwing program, thus fatiguing his throwing muscles and increasing the potential for injury (altered throwing mechanics because of fatigue). It was emphasized that if he was going to be lifting on the same day as throwing, that he should throw first and lift after.

6 During videotaping Ian's throwing motion you note that he does not fully pronate his hand during the cocking phase. What exercises can be done to improve his mechanics?

Trunk rotation/hand towel drill and hand position/ball transfer drill are two effective ways to improve mechanics during the cocking phase. This can be practiced in front of a mirror for further visual reinforcement.

REFERENCES

1. Atwater AE: Biomechanics of overarm throwing movements and of throwing injuries. Exerc Sport Sci Rev 7:43, 1979.
2. Cain PR, Mutschler TA, Fu FH: Anterior instability of the glenohumeral joint: a dynamic model. Am J Sports Med 15:144, 1987.
3. Payton OD, Hirt S, Newton RA: Scientific bases for neurophysiologic approaches to therapeutic exercise, Philadelphia, 1972, FA Davis.
4. McArdle WD, Katch FL, Katch VL: Exercise physiology: energy, nutrition, and human performance, Philadelphia, 1981, Lea & Febiger.
5. Dickoff-Hoffman SA: Neuromuscular control exercises for shoulder instability. In Andrews JR, Wilk KE, editors: The athlete's shoulder, New York, 1994, Churchill Livingstone.
6. Pappas AM, Zawaki RM, Sullivan TJ: Biomechanics of baseball pitching, a preliminary report. Am J Sports Med 13:216, 1985.
7. Perry J: Anatomy & biomechanics of the shoulder in throwing, swimming, gymnastics, and tennis. Clin Sports Med 2:247, 1973.
8. Broer MR: Efficiency of human movement, Philadelphia, 1969, WB Saunders.
9. Toyoshima S, et al: Contribution of the body parts to throwing performance. In Nelson R, Morehouse CA, editors: Biomechanics IV, Baltimore, 1974, University Park Press.
10. Gambetta V: Conditioning of the shoulder complex. In Andrews JR, Wilk KE, editors: The athlete's shoulder, New York, 1994, Churchill Livingstone.
11. Jobe FW, et al: Shoulder and arm exercises for the athlete who throws, Inglewood, Calif, 1996, Champion Press.
12. Verkhoshanski Y: Perspectives in the improvement of speed-strength preparation of jumpers. Yessis Rev Sov Phys Educ Sports 4:28, 1969.
13. Wilt F: Plyometrics what it is and how it works. Athletic J 55:76, 1995.
14. Cavagna G, Disman B, Margari R: Positive work done by a previously stretched muscle. J Appl Physiol 24:21, 1968.
15. Chu D: Plyometric exercise. Nat Strength Cond Assoc J 6:56, 1984.
16. Lundin PE: A review of plyometrics. Strength Cond J 7:65, 1985.
17. Scoles G: Depth jumping: does it really work? Athletic J 58:48, 1978.
18. Wilk KE, Voight ML: Plyometrics for the shoulder complex. In Andrews JR, Wilk KE, editors: The athlete's shoulder, New York, 1994, Churchill Livingstone.
19. Adams T: An investigation of selected plyometric training exercises on muscle leg strength and power. Track Field Q Rev 84:36, 1984.
20. Astrand P, Rodahl K: Textbook of work physiology, New York, 1970, McGraw-Hill.
21. Feltner M, Dapena J: Dynamics of the shoulder and elbow joints of the throwing arm during a baseball pitch. Int J Sports Biomech 2:235, 1986.
22. Franks BD: Physical warm up. In Morgan WP, editor: Ergogenic aids and muscular performance, Orlando, Fla, 1972, Academic Press.
23. Siewert MW, et al: Isokinetic torque changes based on lever arm placement. Phys Ther 65:715, 1985.
24. Smith RL, Brunolli J: Shoulder kinesthesia after anterior glenohumeral dislocation. Phys Ther 69:106, 1989.
25. Gainor BJ, et al: The throw: biomechanics and acute injury. Am J Sports Med 8:114, 1980.
26. Browne AO, et al: Glenohumeral elevation studied in three dimensions. J Bone Joint Surg 72B:843, 1990.
27. Ferrari D: Capsular ligaments of the shoulder anatomical and functional study to the anterior superior capsule. Am J Sports Med 18(1):20, 1990.
28. Fleisig GS, et al: Kinematic and kinetic comparison between baseball pitching and football passing. J Appl Biomech 12:207, 1993.
29. Wilk KE, Arrigo CA: Interval sport programs for the shoulder. In Andrews JR, Wilk KE, editors: The athlete's shoulder, New York, 1994, Churchill Livingstone.

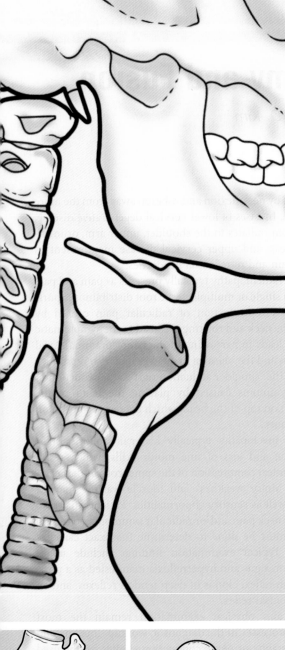

PART 3

Spine

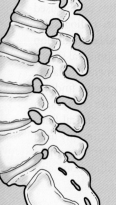

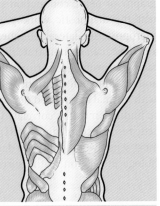

CHAPTER 14

Anterior Cervical Discectomy and Fusion

Derrick G. Sueki, Erica V. Pablo, Rick B. Delamarter, Paul D. Kim

Cervical spondylosis or degeneration presents as different clinical syndromes with the most common being degenerative disc disease, radiculopathy, and myelopathy. Cervical degenerative disc disease may present as axial neck pain, neck stiffness, or as headaches. Cervical radiculopathy classically shows symptoms of arm pain with sensory or motor deficits in the upper extremities (UEs), which is caused by disc herniation or osteophyte formation. Cervical spondylotic myelopathy (Figs. 14-1 and 14-2) may occur with gait abnormalities, hand clumsiness, or upper motor neuron signs. Studies on the natural history of degenerative disc disease demonstrate that the majority of patients suffering from axial neck pain or radiculopathy improve with conservative treatment. Cervical myelopathy, however, tends to progress with time and close clinical follow-up is warranted.

PATHOPHYSIOLOGY AND CLINICAL EVALUATION

Cervical spondylosis is a progressive degenerative cascade that occurs with aging. Annular tears and biochemical changes in the cervical disc can lead to decreased water content, shrinking or herniation of nuclear pulposus tissue, and disc collapse. This places increased stress on associated facet and uncovertebral joints, causing them to degenerate, eventually leading to axial neck pain and stiffness. In addition, this can lead to the formation of bony spurs and disc herniations that may encroach on the neuroforamina, resulting in radiculopathy.[1]

The clinical presentation of cervical spondylosis can vary and must be distinguished from referred shoulder or visceral pain. A careful history and physical examination must be done to determine the exact cause of the neck pain. Nonmechanical neck pain is less likely to be related to disc disease, and other sources including tumor and infection must be considered. Radicular symptom neck pain will often be exacerbated by neck extension and rotation to the affected side (Spurling sign). In contrast, muscular neck pain is often exacerbated by neck flexion and rotation away from the more painful side. In cases of lower cervical degenerative disease, the pain often radiates to the shoulder, upper arm, or infrascapular areas, and upper cervical disease may present as temporal pain and retroorbital headaches.[2]

Cervical radiculopathy typically presents as pain and paresthesia in a single or multiple nerve root distribution. Spurling sign is a reproduction of radicular pain caused by extending the neck and rotating the head to the symptomatic side, which leads to narrowing of the neuroforamina. Axial compression and the Valsalva maneuver may also reproduce symptoms. The "shoulder abduction sign" is the reduction of radicular symptoms caused by placing the hand of the affected arm on top of the head, which decreases tension on the nerve roots.[3]

Cervical myelopathy typically has gait abnormalities, hyperreflexia, and loss of fine motor skills, which result from mechanical compression of the spinal cord in the cervical region. Motor weakness and muscle wasting may be present, as well as sensory abnormalities. Patients may also complain of neck pain and/or radicular symptoms, so careful evaluation must be done to determine the exact cause of symptoms. Typical examination findings include upper motor neuron signs and hyperreflexia manifested as a positive Hoffman reflex, clonus of deep tendon reflexes, and an upgoing Babinski reflex.

History and physical examination remain the most important processes in the diagnostic workup. Imaging and electromyography or nerve conduction studies can be used to supplement the diagnostic workup. Plain radiographs, including anteroposterior, lateral, oblique, and lateral flexion and extension views, can demonstrate developmental stenosis, disc space narrowing, abnormal alignment, dynamic instability, and osteophyte formation. Radiographic findings may occur with normal age-related degenerative changes, so radiographic findings must be correlated with clinical findings.[4] Magnetic resonance imaging (MRI) is commonly used and is the most sensitive modality for demonstrating spinal cord morphology in relation to the surrounding bony and

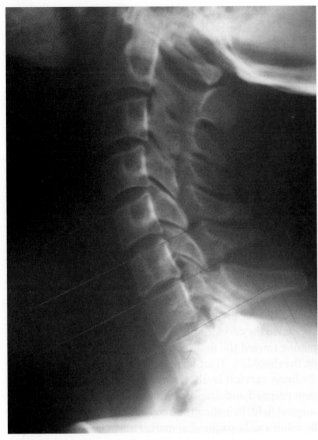

Fig. 14-1 Preoperative lateral radiograph demonstrating a small bony spur formation and disc height loss at C6-7.

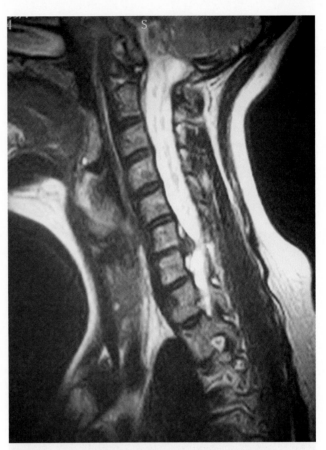

Fig. 14-2 Preoperative sagittal MRI showing C6-7 disc degeneration and a large herniation.

soft-tissue structures (Fig. 14-3). Computed tomography myelography is highly sensitive for detecting foraminal stenosis, but it is invasive and does have a risk of complications.[5] Electromyography and nerve conduction studies can help distinguish between nerve root compression and a peripheral neuropathy and are useful in patients with unclear diagnose. In cases of mechanical neck pain without radiculopathy, several studies support the use of provocative discography to confirm discogenic origin of the pain and to clarify which disc levels are appropriate to treat.[6,7]

TREATMENT AND SURGICAL INDICATIONS

The majority of patients with axial neck pain experience acceptable resolution of symptoms without surgical intervention. Cervical radiculopathy responds well to conservative treatment, but many patients progress to experience recurrent or persistent symptoms.[8] Initially, activity modification and a brief soft collar immobilization are often recommended, but prolonged inactivity may lead to deconditioning. Early pharmacologic treatment is initiated with nonsteroidal antiinflammatory drugs or acetaminophen. With severe acute pain, narcotic analgesics may be used. Paraspinal muscle spasm may be relieved with muscle relaxants but is often improved with a soft collar immobilization alone.

Some patients also may respond to oral corticosteroids.[9] All medications should be prescribed only with careful regard for the potential adverse reactions and interactions with other medications that the patient is taking. Physical therapy is an essential component of conservative treatment and includes modalities, such as traction and heat or cold therapy, as well as an isometric neck and shoulder-stabilizing exercise program. The specifics of a physical therapy program are often left up to the discretion of the particular therapist.

Surgical treatment depends on the clinical entity treated and success of nonoperative treatment. Conservative treatment is the mainstay of initial treatment for cervical radiculopathy and degenerative disc disease with acceptable results.[10] Surgical intervention for patients with cervical radiculopathy is indicated when the symptoms are persistent or recurrent or they are severe or debilitating enough to merit surgery.[11] A prolonged conservative course is recommended for treatment of axial neck pain. If surgery is being considered for axial neck pain and diagnostic evaluation has failed, a discogram is obtained to identify the exact correct level(s) responsible for discogenic pain. As with any elective surgical procedure, appropriate patient expectations and selection must be considered before any surgical intervention (Box 14-1). In general, workers' compensation patients and those involved in litigation can be expected to have

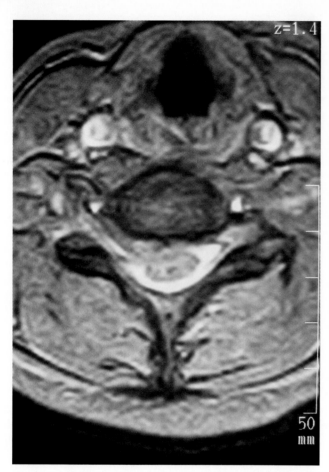

Fig. 14-3 Preoperative axial MRI showing large right-sided disc herniation at C6-7.

BOX 14-1 Indications for ACDF in Cervical Disc Disease

Strong indications:
• Progressive cervical myelopathy

Relative indications:
• Radiculopathy that has failed to respond to conservative treatment regimen of at least 6 weeks
• Recurrent radiculopathy
• Progressive neurologic deficit
• Severe, incapacitating axial neck pain that fails to respond to prolonged course of conservative treatment with consistent examination and diagnostic studies confirming cervical disc disease

---

worse outcomes even after successful fusion surgery.[12,13] Cervical myelopathy must be considered separately, however, because clinical progression usually occurs even with conservative treatment. Classically, patients with cervical myelopathy have periods of clinical stability interspersed with "stepwise degeneration" and careful follow-up must be used to monitor disease progression.[14]

SURGICAL PROCEDURE

Single-level cervical disc disease is most commonly treated with anterior cervical discectomy and fusion (ACDF). For one or more adjacent levels, some surgeons choose to perform a corpectomy of the intervening vertebral bodies instead of multilevel ACDF. After the discectomy, graft choices include an iliac crest bone graft, structural allograft, or a synthetic/metallic spacer. Currently, most surgeons use anterior cervical plating to prevent graft displacement anteriorly and to provide stability while cervical fusion occurs. In cases of severe stenosis or instability, intraoperative neuromonitoring is often used in an attempt to prevent injury and assess adequacy decompression.

Surgery begins with the induction of general endotracheal anesthesia. The patient is then placed in the supine position on a radiolucent operative table to allow imaging in both the anterior-posterior and lateral planes. A soft bump is placed beneath the scapula, and gentle traction is then applied to the cervical spine. In addition, gentle skin traction pulling toward the foot of the bed is applied with wide tape on the shoulders. Traction helps to radiographically visualize the lower cervical levels during surgery. The anterior neck is then prepped and draped, with care taken not to restrict the surgical field. Palpating the bony landmarks (or alternatively by using a radiopaque skin marker and a lateral radiograph) determines the level of the skin incision. A transverse incision is then made through the skin and subcutaneous fat, and bleeding is controlled using electrocautery. The platysma muscle is carefully cut in line with the incision to avoid cutting the large superficial veins just beneath it. Beneath the platysma muscle, the deep cervical fascia is identified and divided laterally to the anterior border of the sternocleidomastoid muscle, where it is dissected inferiorly and superiorly off of the muscle belly. A finger is then used for blunt dissection between the carotid sheath laterally and the trachea and esophagus medially down to the prevertebral fascia. Retractors are then used to retract the midline structures, allowing direct visualization of prevertebral fascia and underlying longus colli muscles and disc spaces.

Once the appropriate level is confirmed, the longus colli muscles are dissected off of the bone laterally and a self-retaining retractor is placed, exposing the disc space to the uncovertebral joints. The operating microscope, sterilely draped, is then brought into the field (Fig. 14-4). Under direct visualization using the microscope, the disc is incised with a scalpel and the anterior portion is removed using a pituitary forceps and an angled curette. A high-speed drill may be used to complete the discectomy and expose the posterior longitudinal ligament (PLL). After exposure, the PLL is elevated off of the posterior aspect of the vertebral bodies using a small 4-0 forward-angled curette; it is then excised using 1 mm and 2 mm Kerrison rongeurs. The PLL does not need to be routinely removed if no nuclear protrusion or extrusion is found, but this has to be carefully explored. The foramina can be probed with the 90° angled

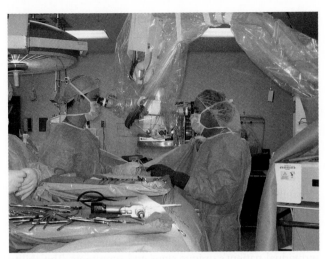

Fig. 14-4 Intraoperative photo showing primary surgeon and assistant using the microscope during discectomy.

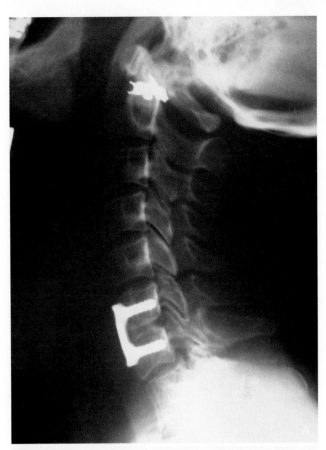

Fig. 14-5 Postoperative lateral radiograph showing solid fusion of C6 and C7 with anterior cervical plate and screws.

nerve hook to confirm adequate decompression or any remaining loose disc fragments. When the discectomy and foraminotomies are complete, the disc space is measured and an appropriately sized graft is chosen. While increased traction is applied on the halter traction device, the graft is gently impacted into position. When it is adequately positioned, all traction is removed. An appropriate-sized plate is then chosen and applied on the anterior aspect of the cervical spine. Care is taken when drilling screw holes to choose a length that will be contained in the vertebral body and be parallel with the endplate of the disc space. When the plate is in position, a lateral radiograph is obtained and graft and hardware positioning is checked (Figs. 14-5 and 14-6).

After instrumentation is complete, the wound is copiously irrigated and thoroughly checked for hemostasis. Often a drain is used even if the wound appears very dry, because a postoperative hematoma may cause significant morbidity. The platysma muscle and subcutaneous tissue are then closed with interrupted absorbable sutures. A running subcuticular layer of suture may follow this closure, followed by a sterile dressing. The patient is then placed into a rigid cervical orthosis before extubation.

Postoperatively, the head of the patient's bed is maintained in an elevated position to decrease swelling in the neck. The patient should be able to walk, void, swallow liquids, and tolerate a diet before discharge. Most patients are discharged the day after surgery. Patients commonly complain of a sore throat and pain with swallowing a few days after surgery. If these complaints seem more severe than usual, then a single dose or short course of oral corticosteroids may be given in an attempt to minimize swelling.

OUTCOMES

Postoperatively, patients with radicular symptoms will often note immediate relief of pain after surgery. Most patients report a change in the quality of their axial neck pain to one more typical of postoperative pain. Generally, patients treated for radicular symptoms achieve excellent clinical results (up to 90% satisfactory results), whereas those treated for axial neck pain achieve good results.[15,16] One concern in the postoperative period is overactivity before fusion is achieved. Solid consolidation of fusion often requires 6 to 12 weeks, so excessive motion and loading are discouraged during this period. Often patients are maintained in a rigid cervical collar for 6 to 12 weeks to restrict their activities, but patients frequently recover from surgery much sooner and desire to remove the orthosis and resume normal activities. This relative immobilization can result in significant patient deconditioning, which can be a challenge to the therapist. In the early period of return to activity and therapy, it is important to avoid injury caused by an overly strenuous exercise program or an overzealous patient.

FUTURE DIRECTIONS

ACDF is a generally well-tolerated and successful procedure; however, recent data has shown that cervical fusion may lead to less satisfying results than previously thought.[17] Concerns about adjacent segment disease has led to the development of cervical total disc replacement.[18] Recently, results of a multicenter, randomized, prospective Federal Drug Administration clinical trial of cervical disc replacement (Synthes Prodisc-C) versus ACDF has shown clinical equivalence or

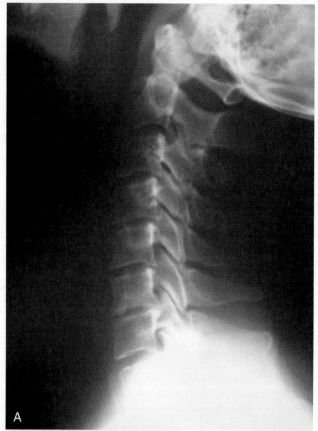

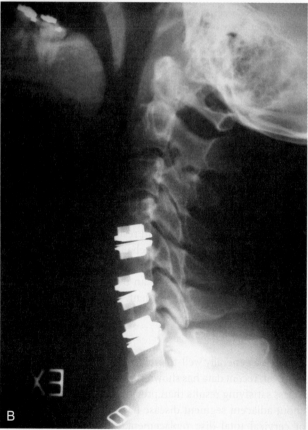

Fig. 14-6 **A,** Preoperative lateral radiograph showing multilevel cervical disc degeneration. **B,** Postoperative lateral radiograph of the same patient after three-level cervical disc replacement.

superiority of cervical disc replacement over fusion.[19] Other clinical studies have demonstrated similar consistent evidence with other cervical disc prosthese.[20,21] These treatments have the potential of offering shorter recovery times and more rapid return to activity and may help prevent the progression of adjacent-level degeneration. Our view is that cervical disc replacement is superior to fusion.

THERAPY GUIDELINES FOR REHABILITATION

Rehabilitation after a surgery is a science and an art. The science of rehabilitation relies on a solid understanding of the body's normal response to injury and trauma. The art of rehabilitation rests in the clinician's ability to interpret the individual patient's unique signs and symptoms. The ability to formulate a plan of care that maximizes an individual's healing potential relies on the ability to blend the science and the art of rehabilitation. The initial portion of this chapter is designed to provide the clinician with an understanding of the role that tissue healing plays in the development of a rehabilitation program. This will serve as a scientific foundation upon which a clinician can base his or her clinical reasoning process. This tissue-healing model will then be placed in the context of ACDF. The activities and precautions of each phase of the rehabilitation process will be rooted in current understanding of the phases of tissue healing. Specific treatment options are provided throughout the chapter, but these should only serve as a guide to treatment and should not replace sound clinical reasoning or judgment when rehabilitating after ACDF.

The decision to operate on the cervical spine may be driven by localized tissue damage and subsequent focal pain, but the majority of spinal surgeries are initiated because of damage to (or threat of damage to) the neural network of the body. Myelographic computed tomography and MRI studies have all demonstrated that 20% to 30% of people who have disc herniation and stenosis do not have radicular symptoms, and many of these people do not have neck pain.[22] It has also been shown that under anesthesia, only nerves that are inflamed will produce radicular symptoms when compressed or placed under traction. Therefore, although the intervertebral disc or stenosis can be the source of neck pain, it is generally injury to the nerve that drives the decision to undergo surgery. Protecting the nervous system from further damage and providing an environment in which the nerve can heal are primary goals of the surgery and rehabilitation thereafter.

Within the spine, injury or damage to the nerve often occurs at the spinal nerve root or the dorsal root ganglia. Anatomically, differences in the nerve root make it more susceptible to injury than at other regions of the peripheral nerve. The nerve root is not as well protected, less able to withstand deformation, and less able to repair itself than the remainder of the peripheral nerve. The other structure within the intervertebral foramen that is susceptible to damage is the dorsal root ganglia. The position of the dorsal root ganglia is not constant and can be found inside the foramen, outside the foramen, or in the spinal canal, which can increase the likelihood that it will be injured. In addition, unlike the spinal nerve root and peripheral nerve, the dorsal root ganglia do not have a blood-nerve barrier, which is necessary to prevent foreign substances from invading the nerve. These anatomic differences predispose the dorsal root ganglia to edema and mechanical compression.[22-24]

Nerves must also be able to move and glide within the tissue. For this to occur, some slack in the system must exist. The spinal cord changes length by 7 cm from flexion to extension. Studies in the arm show that a 7-mm excursion occurs in the nerves with movement. In addition to compression, increased tension of the nerve can result in nerve damage.

More specifically, tension in nerves causing a 20% to 30% increase in length will cause the nerve to break. Boyd and associates[25] demonstrated that as little as 6% strain decreases the amplitude of action potentials by 70%, and 10% to 12% strain causes complete conduction block. They have also shown that nerve stretch of as little as 8% greater than the resting length will cause a 50% decrease in blood flow to the nerve and stretch of 15% will cause 80% to 100% reduction in blood flow. Therefore, exercises that place undue stress and tension on the nerves should be avoided.[26]

Neurons are incapable of dividing and migrating; therefore regeneration occurs only through existing neurons. If the connective tissue sheathing remains intact, then a potential for nerve regrowth exists. If the sheath is disrupted, then the potential for regrowth diminishes. Initially, like any tissue, an inflammatory process is seen within the nerve. Within hours after injury, the nerves start to grow back from the distal stump at 1 to 2 mm per day. In addition to transmitting nerve impulses, the axon of the nerve functions to transmit nutrients and chemicals down its lumen. These axons are filled with axoplasm, which is necessary for nerve health and survival. Axoplasm is a viscous substance and is thixotropic, which means that it needs constant agitation or it will gel.[22-24] **Thus care must be taken to encourage movement and gliding of the nerve, but at the same time, positions that place tension on the nerve should be avoided.**

ACDF surgery affects the sternocleidomastoid, platysma, anterior scalene, middle scalene, and the longus colli muscles. It also requires the resection of the anterior longitudinal ligament, PLL, joint capsule, and synovium.[27-30] After the trauma incurred during surgery, the body is only capable of repairing small muscle lesions with regeneration of muscle tissue. Large lesions will fill in with dense connective scar tissue. Although dense connective scar tissue can function to reestablish tissue continuity, it lacks the contractile elements of normal muscle tissue and the tensile strength of normal ligament and tendon tissue. Therefore the ability to generate contractile forces or resist tensile loading through the region of repair is compromised.[31-34]

Bone grafts from the iliac crest or from bone donors are often used within the disc space, between two vertebral bodies, to aid in the mineralization and fixation of the region. The iliac crest is used as the primary source of graft material because of its cancellous bone composition. Cancellous bone has a greater potential for revascularization and osteogenesis than grafts from denser cortical bone sources. Healing after a cortical bone graft can take up to two times longer than its cancellous bone graft counterpart.[31,32] As will become apparent later in the chapter, *the healing and mineralization of bone at the site of fusion is a major factor driving progression through the rehabilitation process.*

Phase I (Inflammation)

The inflammation phase is the first phase of tissue healing. It begins with injury to the tissue, reaches its peak within the first 72 hours after injury, and is generally completed within 14 days. During these first 14 days, several events occur. Vascular structures in the immediate area constrict to prevent blood loss, and vascular tissues in the surrounding areas dilate to provide conduits through which healing materials can enter the injured site. Cells and chemical mediators are brought into the area to remove all foreign debris and dead or dying tissue and are responsible for the closure of the wound. Both of these actions are important in the prevention of infection.[31,32] During the inflammation phase in bone healing, a hematoma is formed at the site of the surgery. This begins immediately after surgery and is usually completed within 7 days. The hematoma will form around the graft and fusion site, and granulation tissue will fill any open space between the graft, the vertebral bodies, and the instrumentation.[31-34] Clinically, rehabilitation during the inflammation phase of tissue and bone healing should focus on the prevention of blood loss, reduction of inflammation, and managing the pain that accompanies tissue damage (see Table 14-1).

Phase II (Reparative)

The reparative phase is the second phase of tissue healing. This phase begins almost immediately after injury and is completed in 21 days. The primary function of this phase is the formation of the dense connective tissue needed to repair the wound and reestablish structural continuity of the affected region. The process of repairing the tissue to its original state is a time-consuming process, and little evidence supports the notion that tendons, ligaments, or large muscle injuries heal by regenerating into their original tissue. Thus the reestablishment of structural continuity and integrity of tendons, ligaments, and large muscle lesions is completed through the creation of dense connective scar tissue. Reparation with dense connective tissue patches or scar tissue is a fast process that can allow for quicker recovery of the tissue. Angioblasts and fibroblasts begin to enter the injured region within 5 days of the injury. These cells begin the process of tissue repair and the revascularization of the region. Most of the actual dense connective tissue development is completed by day 21. During bone healing at this time, a synthesis and organization of collagen is seen in the hematoma. Once the hematoma is organized, blood vessels invade the area. This allows

TABLE 14-1 Soft Tissue and Bone Healing Time Frames

Phase	Events	Time Frames
Phase I: inflammation	Vasoconstriction in immediate area Vasodilation in surrounding areas Wound closure Removal of foreign and necrotic tissue Hematoma formation in the bone	0-14 days
Phase II: reparative	Fibroblasts enter region to create dense connective tissue scars Angioblasts enter region for revascularization Soft callus formation in the bone	0-21 days
Phase IIIa: remodeling	Dense connective tissue is converted from cellular to fibrous Hard callus formation in the bone	22-60 days
Phase IIIb: remodeling	Dense connective tissue is strengthened Bone is remodeled and strengthened	61-84 days
Phase IIIc: remodeling	Dense connective tissue is strengthened Bone is remodeled and strengthened	85-360 days

osteoblasts to migrate into the region and form woven bone, which is known as a soft callus.[31-34] Clinically, the goal of rehabilitation in this phase should be to promote the development of the new dense connective reparative tissue and woven bone (see Table 14-1).

Phase III (Remodeling)

The remodeling phase is the last phase of the tissue healing process. The purpose of this phase is to strengthen the newly formed scar tissue. Two subphase make up tissue remodeling: (1) consolidation and (2) maturation. During the consolidation subphase, tissue is undergoing conversion from a cellular type to one that is fibrous in nature. The actual size of the scar stops growing by 21 days, although the scar will continue to strengthen in response to stress. This subphase lasts from 22 to 60 days. During this phase of bone remodeling, the soft callus phase begins to mineralize and form a hard callus. Variations in mineralization time exist, but generally mineralization is completed by day 64. Mineralization of the callus is used diagnostically as a marker for when it is appropriate to begin rehabilitation. The patient will not be referred for rehabilitation until radiographic evidence indicates that the callus has mineralized.[31-34] Clinically, rehabilitation should address protection and prevention of excessive motion through the fusion site.

Excessive motion at the fusion site can lead to excessive callus formation and delay of the reparative process. The goal of rehabilitation in this phase should be the strengthening of the newly formed connective tissue. Care must be taken during this phase not to exceed the mechanical limits of the newly formed tissue, because overstress of the tissue will result in tissue injury and delay healing.

The maturation subphase occurs from day 60 to 360 when the tissues are fully fibrous in nature. For this reason, a progression in the strengthening of the affected tissues may begin. For bone remodeling, the hard callus begins to adapt to the stresses placed upon it. These stressors can be internal and external and include low serum calcium levels, skeletal microdamage, and changes in mechanical stress. The bone-remodeling process generally takes 6 months from initiation to completion, but it can take up to 4 years.[31-34] Clinically, rehabilitation programs must provide appropriate levels of stress to the bone to encourage bone strengthening and remodeling without creating or exacerbating tissue injury (see Table 14-1).

Summary

Although guidelines can provide generalized time frames for healing and recovery, it is important to realize that a firm grasp of the factors listed previously will enable the clinician to individualize the rehabilitation program for each patient. No two patients are identical. Therefore no two rehabilitation programs should be identical. Solid clinical reasoning regarding the patient and the nature of the injury and surgery will ultimately drive the rehabilitation process.

Certain key components should be kept in mind during each phase of the rehabilitation process for ACDF.

Phase I:

The initial goal of rehabilitation should be the reduction of inflammation, closure of the wound, and reduction in pain.

Phase II:

The surgical site should be protected until dense connective tissue is formed and the bone shows evidence of mineralization.

Movement of the UEs below shoulder levels to promote nerve mobility and healing should be encouraged.

Phase III:

Gliding of the neural tissue through the surgical site to prevent the formation of adhesions should be promoted.

The clinician should begin placing stress on the soft tissue and bone in graded increments to promote proper soft tissue and bone growth and development.

DESCRIPTION OF REHABILITATION AND RATIONALE FOR USING INSTRUMENTATION

Phase I (Inflammatory Phase)

TIME: 1 to 2 weeks after surgery (days 0 to 14)

GOALS: Protect the surgical site, decrease pain and inflammation, maintain UE flexibility, and initiate patient education regarding neutral cervical spine mechanics (Table 14-2)

During the initial phase of rehabilitation, the primary focus of physical therapy is to protect the surgical site and make sure that the patient is educated on the mechanics of maintaining a proper neutral cervical spine (Fig. 14-7).

TABLE 14-2 Anterior Cervical Discectomy and Fusion

Rehabilitation Phase	Criteria to Progress to This Phase	Anticipated Impairments and Functional Limitations	Intervention	Goal	Rationale
Phase I Acute Inflammatory Phase Postoperative weeks 1-2 (days 0-14)	• Postoperative	• Pain • Edema • Limited neck ROM • Limited nerve mobility • Limited tolerance to upright activities • Limited cardiovascular endurance	Patient education regarding: • Proper use of cervical support • Protection of surgical site • Correct body mechanics and maintenance of neutral cervical spine • Daily walking program	• Decrease pain and edema • Protection of surgical repair (soft tissue and bone) • Restoration of UE ROM • Understand the time frame for healing structures • Understand correct body mechanics and maintenance of neutral cervical spine • Gradual increase in walking speed and duration	• Encourage self-management of pain and edema • Prevent adhesions of neural tissue • Prevent reinjury with patient education on body mechanics and maintenance of neutral cervical spine with activity • Gradually improve cardiovascular endurance

ROM, Range of motion; *UE*, upper extremity.

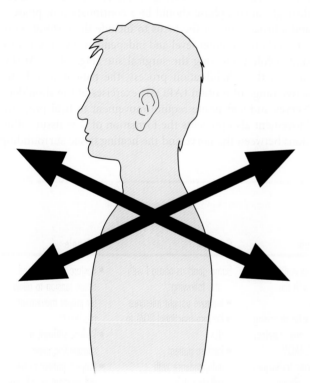

Fig. 14-7 Neutral cervical spine. Proper alignment of the cervical, thoracic, and lumbar spine in which stress to the joints, muscles, and vertebrae is minimized.

Hospitalization after ACDF in most cases will be for 1 to 2 days. During this time the patient will be given a cervical collar to wear to immobilize the neck and encourage soft tissue and bone healing. Instructions regarding the frequency of collar wear will be determined by the physician and may differ on a case-by-case basis.

Physical evaluation during this time may include wound assessment and the assessment of bed mobility and gait. **Because of the fragility of the wound and fusion sites, assessment of cervical range of motion (ROM) and UE strength are not appropriate in this phase.** The primary physical impairments that the patient is likely to experience are pain, limited cardiovascular endurance, and limited tolerance to upright activities. During this time the injured vasculature around the wound begins to close and the noninjured vessels dilate, which may lead to increased warmth and redness around the incision site. This may be accompanied by neck pain and a sore throat. Oral analgesics may be given by the physician to manage the pain and inflammation.

The inflammatory phase lasts approximately 2 weeks. During this time activities should center on resuming normal daily activities. Ambulation to and from the restroom should begin immediately, with assistance as needed, and progress until the patient is independent. The patient should be encouraged to increase the daily sitting tolerances. Pain and fatigue should guide the progression. Once discharged from the hospital, the patient will be instructed to protect the cervical region. The cervical collar issued earlier should be worn 24 hours a day unless otherwise ordered by the physician.

Before discharge from the hospital, it is important that the therapist educate the patient on proper cervical spine mechanics during activity, as well as the need to restrict large amounts of movement in the neck to prevent soft tissue and bone injury. (Refer to Box 14-2 for specific patient guidelines to follow after discharge.) Because of the many muscular attachments of the shoulder girdle to the cervical spine, the patient should be advised to refrain from

---

BOX 14-2   Discharge Instructions After ACDF Surgery

- Wear cervical collar as instructed.
- Do not pick up or carry anything heavier than a ½ gallon of milk.
- Do not sleep with arms over head.
- Do not lift anything above shoulder level.
- Sleep on a firm pillow to help support the neck.
- Avoid sitting or standing for prolonged periods of time. Change positions frequently.
- Get plenty of rest, but do not spend all of your time in bed.
- Gradually increase walking time. Do not get overtired.
- Avoid strenuous exercise or activities.
- Keep incision dry. Showering is allowed 10 days after surgery if wound is not red or draining.
- You may sleep in any position that is comfortable, except on your stomach or with arms over head.
- Do not drive until approved by your physician.

Notify your doctor if any of the following occur:

- Temperature greater than 101° F
- Redness or swelling around your incision
- Any drainage from your incision
- Separation of wound edges
- Any new bruising around the wound
- New numbness or tingling in your hands or fingers
- Increased pain in neck, shoulders, or arms
- New weakness of either arm, hands, or legs

---

heavy lifting and from activities above shoulder level. Before discharge, the need to continue a home walking program and use of the cervical collar should also be addressed.

Phase II (Reparative Phase)

TIME: 3 weeks after surgery (days 0 to 21)
GOALS: Understand neutral spine concepts, increase UE soft tissue mobility and flexibility, improve upright tolerance, improve activities of daily living (ADLs), increase cardiovascular function (Table 14-3)

In many instances, phase II of the rehabilitation process will take place independently in the patient's home. Home therapy is rarely indicated; therefore education regarding patient progression through the first month after surgery is an important aspect of hospital care. The patient will be progressed to phase III once sufficient radiographic evidence of callus formation and mineralization is seen. During the reparative phase of tissue and bone healing, the body begins to form and lay down scar tissue at the surgical site, enhancing the integrity of the musculature to withstand gradual increases in loads to the tissues. Within the bone fusion site, callus formation is nearing completion. Rehabilitation throughout this phase should be a continuation of phase I, and a broadening of the focus to include the restoration of UE ROM to shoulder level and independence with self-care skills while protecting the surgical site (Fig. 14-8). At this time in the rehabilitation process, the patient may begin active range of motion (AROM) exercises of the shoulders. Nerves and soft tissue require movement to heal properly. Movement also prevents the formation of scar tissue adhesions between the nerve and the healing tissue surrounding

TABLE 14-3 Anterior Cervical Discectomy and Fusion

Rehabilitation Phase	Criteria to Progress to This Phase	Anticipated Impairments and Functional Limitations	Intervention	Goal	Rationale
Phase II Reparative phase Postoperative week 3 (days 15-21)	• No signs of infection • Incision site is healing well	• As in phase I • Limited upper body strength • Limited upper body ROM • Limited tolerance to prolonged sitting/standing positions	Continue interventions in phase I with the following: • Initiate gentle stretching of chest (corner stretch) • Gentle UE AROM • Trunk-bracing techniques in multiple planes • Progress walking program to 15-20 minutes as tolerated	Same goals as phase I with the following: • Improve upright tolerance • Restore functional ROM to UEs • Restore patient independence with self-care skills • Improve upper body standing/sitting posture • Improve ADLs while protecting surgical site • Increase cardiovascular function • Independent with home exercise program	• Restore UE ROM and tissue tension to allow for proper movement mechanics • Reduce stiffness in surrounding joints • Prepare patient to be independent in self-care skills • Restore proper posture throughout trunk to allow patient to achieve overall neutral spine concept • Improve cardiovascular endurance

ADLs, Activities of daily living; *AROM*, active range of motion; *ROM*, range of motion; *UE*, upper extremity.

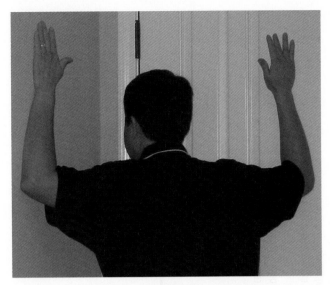

Fig. 14-8 Corner stretch. The patient stands facing a corner with the arms placed on the wall and elbows bent 90°. The patient leans the entire body forward with the knees slightly bent. Note that many patients will tend to lead with their chin into the corner, which promotes poor cervical posture. To avoid this, instruct the patient to maintain a neutral cervical spine and lead with their chest into the corner.

the surgery. Therefore movement of the arms below shoulder level should be encouraged. Exercises incorporating flexion and extension of the elbow, wrist, and fingers should also be implemented at this time. **Motion above shoulder level should still be avoided.**

Throughout all activities and exercises, the patient should be encouraged to maintain a neutral cervical spine. As neck pain and inflammation begin to subside in this phase and the patient continues to progress in activity level, trunk stabilization exercises may be introduced to allow the patient to achieve the overall neutral spine concept. Trunk stabilization exercises will allow loads to be properly distributed along the spine so as not to adversely increase loads to the cervical region during activities. Moreover, improved trunk stability and overall neutral spine will contribute to improving tolerance to upright postures.

Phase IIIa (Remodeling Phase)

TIME: 4 to 8 weeks after surgery (days 22 to 60)
GOALS: Enhance nerve healing and mobility, prevent scar tissue formation, increase UE strength and endurance, improve thoracic spine mobility (Table 14-4)

During this period of recovery, the patient (along with the soft tissues and bone of the surgical site) begins to experience numerous changes. Between the end of the fourth week and up to the sixth postoperative week, the physician will reassess the patient. Generally this reassessment will include a new radiographic study.

Protection of the surgical site and proper immobilization should continue until the physician has seen evidence of mineralization and callus formation of the bone graft.

Once the surgical site has sufficiently mineralized, the physician may permit additional rehabilitation.

Postural Rehabilitation

Rehabilitation specialists should expect to see patients in an outpatient setting at approximately 6 weeks after ACDF. Upon initial evaluation, observation of the patient's posture will give the clinician a significant amount of information concerning weakness, elongation, and strength of specific musculature, as well as the patient's ability to maintain a neutral cervical spine. According to Janda,[35] a common postural alignment seen in people with upper quarter pathology is known as upper crossed syndrome (Fig. 14-9). Regardless of the cause, this alignment will consist of an upper quarter muscle pattern in which certain muscles will be weakened and lengthened and others will be strong and shortened, resulting in an increased thoracic kyphosis, increased midcervical lordosis, and increased upper cervical extension. Protraction of the scapula will often accompany this postural deviation. More specifically, a weakening and lengthening of the rhomboids, middle and lower trapezius, deep neck flexors, supraspinatus, infraspinatus, and the deltoid musculature occurs. This is combined with a tightening and shortening of the pectoralis major and minor, levator scapulae, upper trapezius, scalenes, subscapularis, and sternocleidomastoid muscles. Thus knowledge of how each muscle has been affected after surgery is necessary to guide the rehabilitation program. Postural rehabilitation should be implemented, and interventions should focus on the stretching of shortened musculature, strengthening of the weakened muscles of the trunk and neck, and performing UE movements while maintaining a neutral cervical spine. The clinician should be constantly weighing the intervention required against the limitations imposed by healing tissue. In the case of upper cross patterns, it is appropriate for the patient to stretch the pectoralis and subclavius muscles, but stretching of the sternocleidomastoid or levator scapulae muscle should be postponed due to these muscles' proximal attachment to the cervical spine. Good evidence of fusion healing should be present before stretching of these cervical muscles commences (Fig. 14-10).

Cervical Stability

ACDF surgery requires the partial resection of the longus colli muscle.[27] From a functional recovery perspective, the longus colli has an important role in maintaining cervical stability. Although research is lacking regarding cervical stability, numerous studies have been conducted on the role of lumbar stability to control motion and stabilize spinal segments.[36] Richardson and associates[37] performed a series of studies on the ability of deep lumbar muscles to stabilize spinal segments in patients with lumbar pain. Their findings suggest that deep muscle activation is a necessary component in the reestablishment of spinal control after a low back injury. Subjects that did not reestablish segmental control continued to experience low back pain. Recently, the same group has turned its attention to the cervical spine.[38] They

TABLE 14-4 Anterior Cervical Discectomy and Fusion

Rehabilitation Phase	Criteria to Progress to This Phase	Anticipated Impairments and Functional Limitations	Intervention	Goal	Rationale
Phase IIIa Remodeling phase (consolidation) Postoperative weeks 4-8 (days 22-60)	• Patient understanding of neutral spine concepts • No increase in pain symptoms • No increase in nerve related symptoms	• Limited nerve mobility • Limited UE strength • Limited ability to perform overhead activities • Limited mobility in thoracic region • Limited cardiovascular endurance • Limited neck mobility • Poor cervical proprioception	Continue with phase II interventions as needed with the following: • PROM to shoulder above 90° • Begin gentle AROM of cervical spine as tolerated • Begin neuromobility techniques • Begin strengthening deep neck flexors • Begin progressive resistance exercise program of the UEs below 90° of shoulder elevation (biceps curls, isometric shoulder exercises) • Trunk stabilization exercises with cocontraction of scapular stabilizers • Begin gentle soft tissue mobilization of thoracic region • Begin gentle thoracic spine mobilizations to the mid or lower thoracic spine only • Thoracic AROM exercises (wall angels, scapular retractions) • Walking tolerance to 30 minutes • Cervical position sense and proprioception exercises	Same as phase II with the following: • Enhance nerve healing and mobility • Prevent scar tissue formation • Increase UE muscular strength and endurance • Increase coordination in activating trunk and scapular stabilizing muscles • Improve mobility of thoracic spine • Improve aerobic capacity • Improve cervical proprioception	• Prevent soft tissue adhesions at surgical site • Prevent neural adhesions • Increase stabilization while performing daily activities to prevent reinjury • Decrease joint stiffness to allow proper movement with decreased pain • Independence with self-care activities

AROM, Active range of motion; *PROM,* passive range of motion; *UE,* upper extremity.

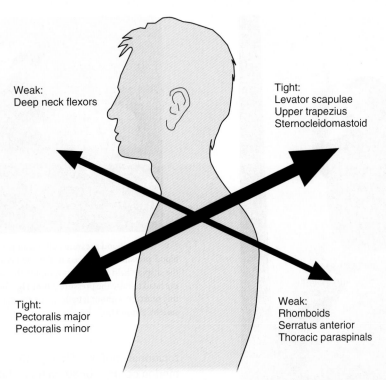

Weak:
Deep neck flexors

Tight:
Levator scapulae
Upper trapezius
Sternocleidomastoid

Tight:
Pectoralis major
Pectoralis minor

Weak:
Rhomboids
Serratus anterior
Thoracic paraspinals

Fig. 14-9 Upper crossed syndrome. An imbalance of shortened and weak musculature that are in opposition in the cervical spine region. Tightened muscles are generally the upper trapezius, sternocleidomastoid, pectoralis major and minor, and levator scapulae. Weakened muscles include rhomboids major and minor, deep neck flexors, middle and lower trapezius, and the serratus anterior. (Courtesy Tamiko Murakami.)

suggest that deep cervical muscles are necessary for normal cervical spine stability. The role may be even greater than that seen in the lumbar region because of the large role cervical spine muscles play in the maintenance and control of a region designed to provide mobility. Thus *exercises designed to recruit deep neck flexors will be imperative to provide adequate stability of a highly mobile region.* These exercises can include supine chin tucks in a neutral spine using a rolled towel or pillow if necessary, progressing to an inclined position and eventually a sitting position (Fig. 14-11). Jull[38] has proposed the use of a blood pressure cuff behind the neck as a means of monitoring the amount of cervical muscle recruitment (Fig. 14-12 and Box 14-3). A recent study by O'Leary and associates[39] showed a significant improvement in isometric craniocervical muscle performance with the use of a pressure biofeedback device. In this study, patients were initially instructed to achieve the correct cervicoflexion action without increased activity of superficial musculature. Once achieved, the use of a blood pressure cuff was used to guide the training of the craniocervical muscle contraction at different levels of pressure.[39]

A progressive resistance exercise (PRE) program for the UEs may be initiated with light weights during this phase. Biceps curls, triceps extensions, wrist and hand exercises, and isometric shoulder exercises are all appropriate at this time.

The strengthening program should still be carried out below 90° of glenohumeral elevation to ensure that the musculature of the neck is not being overstressed. Each

patient will need to begin at a different level after taking into account his or her present functional status and familiarity with the exercises. The focus should be on the use of light weights to build endurance of the musculature initially to assist with return-to-work activities and maintenance of prolonged postures.

Joint Mobilization

Decreased flexibility in thoracic spine segments and the soft tissue of the thoracic region may prevent proper body alignment, including full glenohumeral ROM. Thus treatment should include soft tissue mobilization to the mid and lower thoracic spine. **Later mobilization to the midthoracic spine can be included with the authorization of the physician.**

It is appropriate to begin AROM and passive range-of-motion activities at this time (Fig. 14-13). The clinician should keep in mind that the biomechanics of the cervical spine will be altered by cervical fusion surgery. An understanding of how it will be affected is critical in assessing a patient's progress and ultimate outcome. The cervical vertebrae are the smallest and most mobile of all spinal vertebrae. The cervical region functions to provide mobility for the head on the trunk. It also functions to protect vital structures, such as the spinal cord, as they route distally down the body. In total, the functional units of the cervical region must work together to provide 45° to 50° of flexion and 85° of extension, for a total of 130° to 135° of total sagittal plane motion. In the horizontal plane, the cervical spine must be able to provide 90° of unilateral motion and 180° of total

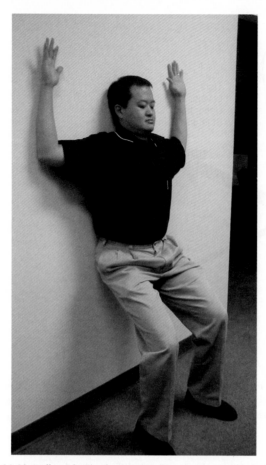

Fig. 14-10 Wall angels. The therapist has the patient stand with the head, back, and arms against the wall, knees slightly bent, chin tucked, and shoulders slightly abducted. The patient continues to elevate the arms against the wall and bring them down, making the shape of angel wings.

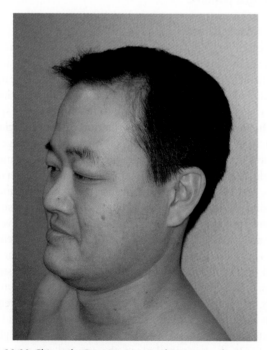

Fig. 14-11 Chin tucks. In a sitting or standing posture, the patient tucks in the chin and extends the cervical spine.

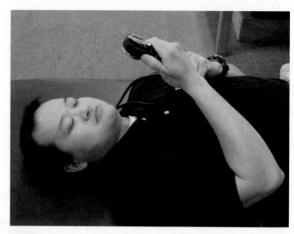

Fig. 14-12 Blood pressure cuff technique. The patient lies supine, with the blood pressure cuff placed under the neck and inflated to 20 mm Hg and the display held in front to monitor the dial. The patient nods or retracts the head to raise the pressure 2 mm Hg. Once the patient is able to maintain this pressure without fatigue, he or she may progress and increase the pressure by 2 mm Hg.

rotational motion. Finally, 40° of unilateral frontal plane motion occurs—or 80° in total (Table 14-5).[40,41] Segmentally, two adjacent spinal vertebrae and the intervertebral disc between the two comprise a functional motion segment. Each functional spinal unit provides varying degrees to the total motion seen in the cervical region. The fusing of one or several of the functional motion segments will alter the mechanics of adjacent segments. The body will eventually adjust; the result is transitional degeneration.

Therefore, initially a fusion to the C5-6 motion segment may result in a loss of 10° to 15° of unilateral rotation.[36,42] Therefore the objective goal of rehabilitation should not be to attain 90° of unilateral rotation. Instead normal unilateral rotation after fusion to C5-6 would be 65° to 70° of motion.

Mobilization techniques are a mainstay of physical therapy. In practice, they are used to increase ROM within targeted regions by moving specific joints or specific muscles. Care must be taken in choosing the appropriate time to begin implementation of soft tissue and particularly passive joint mobilization techniques because of the potential translational effect they may have on the cervical spine at the region of the fusion. Although studies are lacking in the area of mobilization of the cervical spine, several studies have addressed the effects of mobilization in the lumbar region. Researchers[43-46] studied the effects of a posterior to anterior force placed on the spinous process of L3. Their study showed a force at L3 could result in movement as far away as T8; in a follow-up study by the same group, the same posterior to anterior force resulted in an anterior rotation of the sacrum. The implications of these findings for the patient after a cervical fusion are that even mobilizations to distant segments may have a translatory effect on the fusion site. **Therefore mobilization of the spine should not be initiated until the fusion site itself has shown radiographic evidence of sufficient mineralization and callus formation. This**

BOX 14-3 Strengthening and Retraining of Deep Cervical Flexors Using Blood Pressure Cuff

Patient Position

- Patient is supine in hook-lying position.
- The head is placed in a neutral position.
- Towels may be placed beneath the patient's head to achieve neutral cervical position.
- The patient's chin may need to be tucked in and down to achieve a neutral cervical spine.

Procedure

- A pressure biofeedback unit or blood pressure cuff is placed beneath the patient's neck.
- Inflate pressure biofeedback unit or blood pressure cuff to 20 mm Hg.
- The patient holds the display in one hand and gently retracts or nods the upper cervical region until pressure rises to 22 mm Hg. This process is repeated for 24 mm Hg, 26 mm Hg, 28 mm Hg, and 30 mm Hg. Above 30 mm Hg is not relevant. The pressure that the patient can hold for several seconds without activation of the superficial neck muscles is the beginning exercise value.
- The patient is instructed to retract or nod until target pressure is achieved. This amount of force is held for 10 seconds and repeated 10 times.
- When the patient can contract for the designated duration and repetitions without fatigue or discomfort, it is appropriate to increase pressure 2 mm Hg.
- To discourage substitution with the superficial neck muscles, the patient can be instructed to place the tongue on the roof of the mouth with lips together and teeth just separated when completing the exercise.

Adapted from Jull G: Management of cervicogenic headaches. In Grant R, editor: Physical therapy of the cervical and thoracic spine, St Louis, 2002, Churchill Livingstone.

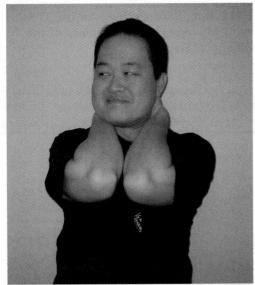

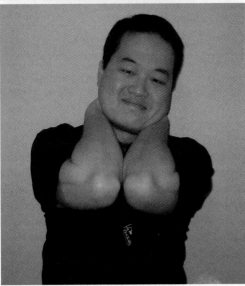

Fig. 14-13 Active cervical ROM. The patient is placed in a comfortable sitting position and asked to complete each cervical ROM movement slowly through the full ROM.

information and the authorization of mobilization to the cervical spine should come from the surgeon. Moreover, research has revealed transitional degeneration in the segments directly above and below the fusion. Once this is found, proper mobilization and joint forces may be added to begin stimulating proper formation and modeling of bone tissue.

Although it is difficult to imagine an instance when direct mobilization to the fusion site would be warranted, mobilization to adjacent structures and segments is justified to increase spinal ROM and decrease the demands placed upon the fusion site.

However, therapists should be wary of applying mobilization techniques close to the fusion site. Research has revealed transitional degeneration in the segments directly above and below the fusion.[47] Transitional degeneration is a

common long-term complication after a spinal fusion, particularly in multilevel fusions. It consists of segmental articular degeneration and spondylytic changes in the spine. It has been hypothesized that these changes are the result of the increased stress placed on these segments because of the decreased mobility of the fusion spinal segments. Goffin and colleagues[48] studied 120 patients after ACDF surgery and at a mean follow-up period of 98 months. They found that 92% of the patients demonstrated segmental degenerative changes. Eventually, when dense connective tissue and bone has been adequately strengthened and stabilized, then distant spinal segments can be mobilized when needed.

Neural Mobilization and Neural Dynamics

Neural mobility techniques should also be progressed in this phase to prevent neural adhesions to the surrounding tissue.

TABLE 14-5 Approximate ROM for the Three Planes of Movement for the Joints of the Craniocervical Region

Joint or Region	Flexion/ Extension (Degrees)	Axial Rotation— Unilateral (Degrees)	Lateral Flexion— Unilateral (Degrees)
Atlanto-occipital	Flexion: 5 Extension: 10 Total: 15	Negligible	Approximately 5
Atlantoaxial	Flexion: 5 Extension: 10 Total: 15	40 to 45	Negligible
Midcervical	Flexion: 35 Extension: 70 Total: 105	45	35
Total cervical	Flexion: 45 to 50 Extension: 85 Total: 130 to 135	90	Approximately 40

Adapted from Neumann D: Axial skeleton: osteology and arthrology. In Neumann D, editor, Kinesiology of the musculoskeletal system: Foundations for physical rehabilitation, ed 2, St Louis, 2009, Mosby.

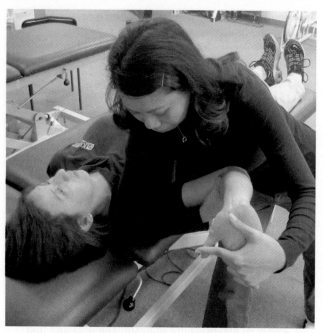

Fig. 14-14 ULNT 1 technique.

Scar tissue has the ability to restrict joints; scar tissue can adhere to nerves and affect their mobility.

Because the patient is likely to have experienced nerve-related symptoms as a contributing factor for undergoing surgery, an understanding of neurodynamics, or the relationship between the nervous system and associated connective tissues, will ensure proper interventions will be chosen that will not aggravate or overstretch the neural tissue. While the concept of neurodynamics has been around for some time, empirical data supporting its clinical use has been lacking. Neurodynamic techniques are commonly classified into two categories: techniques that glide the nerve and techniques that stretch the nerve. An example of a gliding technique in the upper quarter would be placing tension on the nerve at the wrist with wrist extension while simultaneously reducing tension at the neck by side-bending toward the same side. An example of a tensioning technique would be placing tension on the wrist with wrist extension while simultaneously side-bending the neck toward the opposite side. Research by Coppieters and associates[49] has shown that sliding techniques produce a greater amount of nerve excursion through the surrounding tissue than tensioning techniques. Furthermore, an increase in muscle activity also occurred with the addition of dorsiflexion. It has been hypothesized that muscles are recruited to protect the nerve and prevent injury when the nerve is placed in tension. Thus clinicians should ensure that soft tissue surrounding the nerve is free to achieve optimal neural movement. **Therefore treatment should address the gliding and not stretching of nerves.**

Neurodynamic testing of the upper limb enables the clinician to assess the movement capabilities of neural tissues in relation to the soft tissue structure that surrounds them. Elvy[50] developed the upper limb neurodynamic tests (ULNTs) as a method for differentiating potential sources of cervicobrachial symptoms. Upper limb neurodynamic test 1 (ULNT 1) (Fig. 14-14) was designed to assess the movement capabilities of neural tissues associated with the median nerve. Given the mechanical continuity of the nervous system, it has recently been recognized that all upper quarter neural tissues are stressed during ULNT 1; however, components of the test are specifically biased toward the median nerve trunk and C5-C7 nerve roots[51] (Table 14-6). Although originally designed to test the median nerve, clinicians are using it as a general clearing test for UE neuromobility because all three major peripheral nerves in the UE are stressed by the ULNT 1 position (Box 14-4).

Treatments using the ULNTs have generally been a point of confusion for clinicians. A positive test is indicative of restricted mobility in the nerve being tested. Therefore using the test position to stretch the nerve and release any adhesions along the course is a common treatment philosophy. Coppieters and associates[52] also found that adding positions of tension to a joint reduced the amount of nerve mobility in the adjacent joints. For example, adding wrist extension to a median nerve mobility test decreases the range of extension available at the elbow. This finding was corroborated in a study by Boyd and associates[53] in which straight leg raise ROM was reduced when dorsiflexion was added to the ankle compared with the addition of plantar flexion. Thus when using ULNT test positions to glide the nerve, therapists need to be aware that muscle tissue has the potential to elongate and stretch, whereas neural tissue is not as elastic and responds adversely to stretching as explained above (Fig. 14-15).

TABLE 14-6 Upper Limb Neurodynamic Testing (ULNT) Positions

Test	Nerve Assessed	Test Position
ULNT 1	General	Supine—leg straight and uncrossed Spine in midline position Stabilization of shoulder girdle Shoulder abduction Wrist and finger extension Forearm supination Shoulder lateral rotation Elbow extension Cervical lateral flexion away Cervical lateral flexion toward
ULNT 2a	Median	Supine—leg straight and uncrossed Spine in midline position Stabilization of shoulder girdle Shoulder girdle depression Elbow extension Whole arm lateral rotation Wrist and finger extension Shoulder abduction
ULNT 2b	Radial	Supine—leg straight and uncrossed Spine in midline position Stabilization of shoulder girdle Shoulder depression Elbow extension Whole-arm internal rotation Wrist flexion
ULNT 3	Ulnar	Supine—leg straight and uncrossed Spine in midline position Stabilization of shoulder girdle Wrist extension Forearm pronation Elbow flexion Shoulder lateral rotation Shoulder girdle depression Shoulder abduction

Adapted from Butler D: The sensitive nervous system, Adelaide, Australia, 2000, Noigroup.

Soft tissue structures along the course of the nerve can be mobilized to allow for nerve mobility. Movement of the UE can be combined with small movements of the neck to encourage gliding of the nerve rather than stretching. Finally, communication with the patient is essential, because radicular pain or paresthesia is indication that the nerve is being stretched and potentially irritated. The patient and therapist should work in ROMs that do not reproduce the patient's radicular symptoms.

Cervical Proprioception

As the healing process continues in bone and soft tissue structures, the patient may also have sensorimotor deficits, such as unsteadiness, visual disturbances, and changes in

BOX 14-4 Testing Procedure for ULNT 1

1. First, establish the patient's baseline resting symptoms. Remember to reassess baseline symptoms, resistance, and range of motion with the addition of each new component.
2. The patient is positioned in supine near edge of table.
3. Therapist position:
   a. The therapist takes a stride-stance position facing the patient's head.
   b. Next, the therapist uses a pistol grip handhold on the fingers of the limb to be tested. It is important to maintain finger extension and thumb abduction during the procedure.
   c. The therapist will then lean his or her elbow on the table for support and stabilize the patient's shoulder girdle in neutral.
   d. Alternatively, the clinician may stabilize the patient's shoulder girdle by pushing his or her fist vertically downward on the examination table with the shoulder girdle in neutral.
4. Procedure:
   a. The shoulder is abducted in the neutral coronal plane from 100° to 130°. Care must be taken to prevent any shoulder girdle elevation.
   b. Next, the therapist adds wrist extension, finger extension, and forearm supination.
   c. Add shoulder lateral rotation.
   d. Add elbow extension.
5. Sensitizing maneuvers include:
   a. Contralateral cervical lateral flexion
   b. Ipsilateral cervical lateral flexion
   c. Release of wrist extension

ULNTs, Upper limb neurodynamic tests. Adapted from Butler D: The sensitive nervous system, Adelaide, Australia, 2000, Noigroup.

postural stability and cervical joint position sense. Although the exact physiologic mechanism is not clear, these changes are believed to be the result of a traumatic injury to the nerves themselves, chemical mediators within and around the joint that inhibit the proprioceptive nerves, as well as central changes occurring at the spinal cord and cortical regions that alter the body's response to proprioceptive input. Research has shown that rehabilitation of the cervical spine thus far has traditionally focused on the strength and length of muscles in the region, as well as joint and nerve mobility, which may not be as effective in addressing proprioceptive and sensorimotor disturbances in patients with neck pain.[54] According to recent studies by Trevelean,[55,56] the abundance of mechanoreceptors in the cervical region plays an important role in providing proprioceptive input to the central nervous system. There are high densities of muscle spindles in the cervical region, especially in the suboccipital muscles, which have up to 200 muscle spindles per gram of

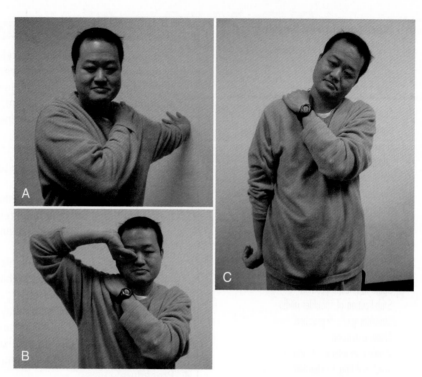

Fig. 14-15 Self-neurogliding techniques. **A,** Median. **B,** Ulnar. **C,** Radial.

muscle. This amount is significant when compared with the 16 muscle spindles per gram of muscle in the first lumbrical.[55,56] In addition, the visual and vestibular systems of the cervical spine region have been shown to influence the proprioceptive input provided by the cervical mechanoreceptors. Therefore, the visual, vestibular, and proprioception systems are integrated to provide the sensory input for proper cervical function. In terms of cervical rehabilitation, these findings suggest balance, proprioception, and visual training should be added to a patient's exercise program to address sensorimotor and proprioceptive deficits.

Symptoms of poor head and neck awareness or a "wobbling" head may be due to poor cervical position sense. To assess for disturbed joint position sense, Treleaven advocates the use of a small laser pointer mounted on a lightweight headband. The patient is seated 90 cm away from a wall and the point where the laser shines at initial setup is marked. The patient proceeds to close his or her eyes and then provides a neck motion (for example, right or left rotation). The patient is then instructed to return the head to the initial head position. A greater than 4 to 5 cm error is indicative of cervical proprioception deficits (Fig. 14-16).[57,58] This assessment technique can be used as an exercise in which the patient practices relocating the beam of light to the initial position with the eyes open, trying to improve the accuracy of the movements each time. To improve deficits in neck movement control, in which patients complain of fatigue in the neck or difficulty with AROM movements because of increased muscle contraction to protect the cervical spine, the patient may use the laser pointer to trace a pattern on the wall such as a figure eight placed 90 cm in front of the

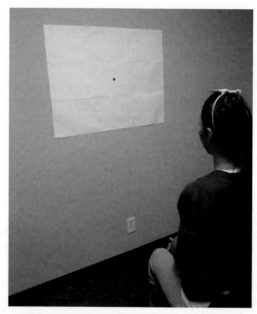

Fig. 14-16 Exercise for joint position sense retraining using a laser pointer. (Adapted from Treleaven J: Sensorimotor disturbances in neck disorders affecting postural stability, head and eye movement control. Man Ther 13:2-11, 2008.)

seated patient (Fig. 14-17). The use of joint positioning/neck movement control exercises, coupled with focused treatment on balance training, has proven to be effective in treating patients with acute and chronic neck pain.[54] Balance training to improve postural stability included exercises incorporating tandem stance and single-leg stance, with both eyes open and closed, and alterations of stance surfaces. The stance and

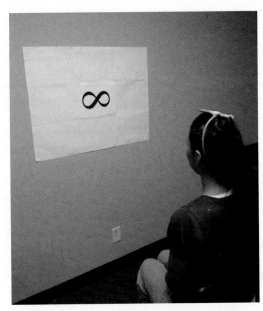

Fig. 14-17 Exercise for neck movement control using a laser pointer mounted on the head to trace a pattern on the wall. (Adapted from Treleaven J: Sensorimotor disturbances in neck disorders affecting postural stability, head and eye movement control. Part 2: Case studies. Man Ther 13:266-275, 2008.)

TABLE 14-7 Exercises and Progressions to Improve Cervical Proprioception

Task	Progression
With laser pointer on headband for feedback, relocate back to neutral head position from different head movements with eyes open	Eyes closed, check eyes open Increase speed Perform in standing
With laser pointer mounted on headband, practice tracing over a pattern placed on the wall with eyes open	Increase speed More difficult patterns Small finer movements
Balance training in standing position for 30 seconds	Eyes open and closed Change surfaces from hard to soft Different stances: comfortable, tandem, narrow, single limb
Sitting in a neutral neck position, keeping the head still and the hands on the lap, move the laser light back and forth across the wall while the patient has to follow the laser with the eyes	Eyes up and down, H pattern Increase speed Increase range of movements Perform standing Perform on uneven surfaces

surface were dependent upon the patient's capabilities. The visual training exercises consisted of asking the patient to place the head in various positions and then asking the patient to visually track objects or visual targets on the wall. Beams of light or a laser pointer provided a target that the patient could track with his or her eyes (Table 14-7). Since the patient has recently begun AROM exercises, the therapist should use sound clinical judgement as to when these exercises should be incorporated into the patient's plan of care.

In addition, balance exercises may cause increased pain or headaches, and the tasks might need to be altered to more supportive positions. Mild dizziness may occur with balance exercises to allow for vestibular habituation, but the patient's symptoms should be monitored closely. If the presence of any central nervous system signs appears without explanation or diagnosis, it may be considered a red flag and the therapist should refer the patient to a physician for further tests. Thus far, incorporating proprioceptive, balance, and visual training interventions to a cervical rehabilitation program have achieved positive outcomes.

To facilitate the return-to-work transition in this phase, cardiovascular endurance should be continued. A daily walking program should be continued and progressed as tolerated.

Phase IIIb (Remodeling Phase)

TIME: 9 to 12 weeks after surgery (days 61 to 84)
GOALS: Restoration of strength to the cervical spine, maintenance of neutral spine for prolonged periods of time with concurrent UE movement, improvement in scapulothoracic mechanics (Table 14-8)

Progression to this phase of rehabilitation should begin once the patient is able to tolerate the exercises of phase IIIa without an increase in neck or arm symptoms. Interventions from the previous phase have focused on loading the upper and lower body without directly loading the cervical spine. The purpose of this precaution is to prevent overstressing newly healed structures. This particular stage in the rehabilitation process will slowly begin to incorporate direct treatment to the cervical spine structures and therefore should not be started until the patient has adequately demonstrated tolerance to the loads placed on the neck. The patient should also be able to demonstrate proper neutral cervical spine concepts.

The thoracic spine musculature such as the rhomboids and middle and lower trapezius can be further challenged from the previous phase by adding resistance with light weights on a seated or standing rowing machine or through the use of resistance tubing (Figs. 14-18 and 14-19). Proprioceptive neurofacilitation techniques may also be used to strengthen thoracic paraspinals and scapulothoracic musculature. PREs may be increased in weight, sets, and repetitions as tolerated. Exercises above 90° shoulder elevation may be initiated to further strengthen cervical musculature. Isometric cervical spine strengthening may begin in all planes. Attention should be given to complete these exercises in the neutral cervical spine to strengthen the musculature of the cervical spine to allow for proper posture and force production of these muscles. The patient is placed in a comfortable sitting position. For flexion, the patient places both hands on the forehead and brings the forehead into the hands without moving. In extension, the patient places both hands on the back of the head and brings the head backwards into the hands without moving (Fig. 14-20). During the side bend, the patient places one hand on the side of the head and

TABLE 14-8 Anterior Cervical Discectomy and Fusion

Rehabilitation Phase	Criteria to Progress to This Phase	Anticipated Impairments and Functional Limitations	Intervention	Goal	Rationale
Phase IIIb Remodeling phase (maturation) Postoperative weeks 9-12 (days 61-84)	• Surgical site has healed • No increase in pain symptoms • Patient demonstrates neutral spine concepts	Same as phase II with the following: • Limited ability to perform activities in a prolonged sitting/standing position • Patient is not fully independent with ADLs	Continue with phase II interventions as needed with the following: • Begin isometrics of the cervical spine • Begin gentle UE strengthening above 90° of shoulder elevation • PREs: Shoulder shrugs, triceps push down, wall push-ups • Scapulothoracic and thoracic paraspinal strengthening using PNF techniques • Thoracic exercises: Scapular retractions with resistance • Progress abdominal strengthening exercises in different positions: Standing, quadruped • Initiate upper body exerciser as tolerated in neutral spine	• Restore strength to cervical spine • Improve scapulothoracic mechanics • Maintenance of neutral spine in various positions/planes with concurrent UE movement	• Independent with self-care and ADLs • Prevent reinjury with increase in dynamic activities • Knowledge of pain-relieving strategies/positions during prolonged activities

ADLs, Activities of daily living; *PNF*, proprioceptive neuromuscular facilitation; *PREs*, progressive resistance exercises; *UE*, upper extremity.

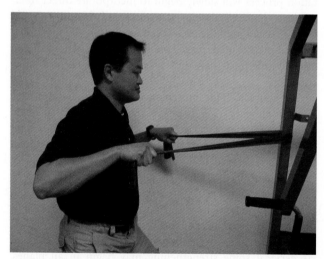

Fig. 14-18 Scapular retractions using resistance tubing. The patient sits or stands (with knees slightly bent) with resistance tubing secured in front. He or she pulls the tubing simultaneously to the sides by retracting the scapula and bending the elbows. The patient is instructed to relax the shoulders and pinch the shoulder blades together.

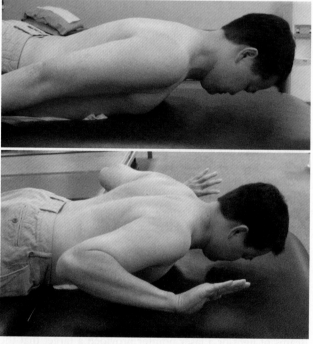

Fig. 14-19 Prone scapular retraction progression. The patient is placed in a prone position on the table with the arms at the sides. The therapist instructs the patient to lift the forehead off the table, keeping the chin tucked in a neutral cervical spine position. The patient can then perform scapular retraction exercises.

attempts to bring the ear to the shoulder without moving. In rotation, the patient places one hand to the side of the head in front of the ear and looks over the shoulder without allowing movement. Strength and trunk control can be further challenged through the addition of an unstable base of support, such as a half foam roller placed under the feet or the use of a stabilization ball. A clinician should be assisting the patient at all times during these exercises. Synchronized UE movements, such as biceps curls while balancing on an unstable support, will further challenge the trunk and neck complex simultaneously. *Placing the patient in positions such as quadruped or prone on the stabilization ball should warrant caution and be delayed if the patient has yet to demonstrate deep neck flexor strength or the ability to maintain a neutral cervical spine in an antigravity position. Proper neck alignment should be maintained during execution of all therapeutic activities.*

At this stage of rehabilitation, the patient may find it difficult to perform activities that require prolonged sitting or standing postures. It is important to assist the patient in recognizing methods or activities that have the ability to relieve some of the pain or soreness. It is also important that

he or she be assisted in the development of strategies to increase muscle endurance so that the patient may gradually build a tolerance to these positions. Strategies may include limiting the time spent in any one position, the use of cryotherapy to the neck, or active cervical ROM exercises to relieve stiffness and soreness. Cardiovascular endurance and strength should continue during this phase, and the use of an upper body exerciser may be initiated for short amounts of time.

Phase IIIc (Remodeling Phase)

TIME: 13 to 52 weeks after surgery (days 85 to 360)
GOALS: Return to presurgical strength and endurance, return to prior level of functioning, prepare for discharge from physical therapy (Table 14-9; see also Suggested Home Maintenance Box)

The remaining phase of the rehabilitation process centers on regaining presurgical strength and endurance. By the end of this phase, the patient should be able to function independently at home and in the workplace. As the patient progresses through the rehabilitation process, functional retraining of work- or sport-specific activities should be assessed. Activities that require increased loads on the cervical spine should be evaluated; pending physician approval, rehabilitation geared toward functional training can be initiated. Return to activities or sports that require contact between players or heavy lifting will require the physician's approval. At this time the physical therapist may implement a gym- or home-based exercise program to assist in maintenance of proper strength and muscle function. Discharge of the patient should occur once the patient, physical therapist, and physician have all determined that the patient has reached his or her functional goals and is able to continue the rehabilitation process safely and independently.

Clinical Pearl: Cervical Classification

In the 1980s, Sahrmann and associates began to lay the foundation for the development of a clinical reasoning method that focused on subgrouping patients of a larger entity into

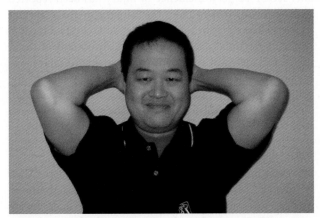

Fig. 14-20 Extension. The patient places both hands on the back of the head and brings the head backward into the hands without moving.

TABLE 14-9 Anterior Cervical Discectomy and Fusion

Rehabilitation Phase	Criteria to Progress to This Phase	Anticipated Impairments and Functional Limitations	Intervention	Goal	Rationale
Phase IIIc Remodeling phase (maturation) Postoperative weeks 13-24 (days 85-168)	• Patient able to self-manage pain • No decrease in functional ability	• Difficulty lifting heavy objects • Difficulty maintaining prolonged postures	• Progress sets and repetitions of UE-resisted exercise program as tolerated by patient • Functional retraining activities (work or sport related per physician approval)	• Return to prior level of functioning • Return to presurgical level of strength and endurance • Prepare patient for discharge	• Improve patient's ability to manage work-related schedule • Promote continuance of proper postures and home maintenance program after discharge from physical therapy

UE, Upper extremity.

smaller homogeneous groups to identify specific interventions that will address each subgroup's specific signs and symptoms.[59] Regions such as the neck and low back are large heterogeneous groups and proving efficacy of treatment with such a diversity of patients and pathology is difficult. If the characteristics of this subgroup can be identified and paired with the most effective interventions, then prognosis and the quality of patient care will improve. In recent years, the development of classification-based research has taken on renewed interest. Childs and associates proposed such a classification-based system for the treatment of the cervical region.[60] While recovery from cervical fusion surgery does not completely fit within the scope of this classification system, we can apply the principles of their findings toward the treatment of patients following cervical fusion. The study suggests five pairings of outcome goals with specific interventions. The outcome goals are mobility, centralization, conditioning and increased exercise tolerance, pain control, and reduced headaches. Of these five outcomes, pain control and conditioning and increased exercise tolerance most closely reflect the goals following a cervical spine fusion. Pain control is a primary goal in the first and second phases of cervical rehabilitation and the interventions linked to this outcome are AROM exercises within pain tolerance, ROM exercises for adjacent regions, physical modalities as needed, and activity modification. The outcome goal of increased exercise tolerance and conditioning takes place in the second and third phases of cervical rehabilitation. Strengthening/endurance exercises of the upper quarter, as well as aerobic exercises, are the interventions proposed to achieve this clinical outcome.

TROUBLESHOOTING

Red Flags

The majority of postoperative complications and red flags will occur within the first several weeks after surgery. Clinicians should be aware of these complications and should educate the patient to notify his or her physician immediately if any of the following complications should occur. Although the majority of the red flags will occur before a patient's release to outpatient rehabilitation, the outpatient clinician should be cognizant of any drastic changes that would warrant communication with the physician for further assessment and testing.

Infection

The risk of infection after cervical spine surgery is difficult to determine. Postoperative infection rates of up to 6% have been reported. Several factors affect a patient's risk for acquiring an infection, including a patient's age, duration of surgical procedure, and the patient's preoperative physical condition.[61] Obesity is also a risk factor for infection because adipose tissue is poorly vascularized. Uncontrolled diabetes also increases the risk of infection. Signs and symptoms of infections include erythema, edema, purulent wound drainage, tenderness, fever, and increased pain.

Dysphagia

The incidence of dysphagia in patients after ACDF has been reported as high as 28%.[62,63] Additional studies have noted that 51% of patients will have swallowing difficulty at 1 month after surgery, 31% at 2 months, and 15% at 6 months.[64] Therefore speech and swallowing problems after ACDF are not uncommon, although dysphagia is one of the primary symptoms accompanying plate and screw loosening. Persistent symptoms should be cause for further examination by the physician.

Esophageal Injury

Esophageal injury is rare but can occur up to 1 year after surgery.[65] The mechanism behind the injury has been attributed to laceration or pressure necrosis of the esophagus by graft displacement. Signs and symptoms of an esophageal injury include increased neck and throat pain, odynophagia, erythema, swelling, tenderness, crepitus, subcutaneous emphysema, unexplained tachycardia, sepsis, and difficulty swallowing.

Neural Injury

The recurrent laryngeal nerve is susceptible to nerve injury after ACDF surgery. Incidence of injury has been reported to be between 0.07% and 11%.[66] Injury to the recurrent laryngeal nerve may be the result of endotracheal tubing that may compress and damage the nerve. Symptoms of nerve injury include vocal cord paralysis. Spinal cord injury secondary to ACDF is 0.4%.[67] Most often the source of the spinal cord injury is posterior displacement of the bone graft. Nerve root injury is also low at 0.6%. The most affected nerve root is C5. Most incidence of injury resolved in 6 weeks.

Vascular Complications

The exact prevalence of vascular complications after ACDF is unknown. Most studies report values in the neighborhood of 0.6% or less for vertebral artery injury after ACDF surgery.[68,69] Signs and symptoms of vertebral artery injury include dizziness, dysphagia, dysarthria, diplopia, and drop attacks.

Cervical Spine Bracing

Skin breakdown and soft tissue injuries are common with the long-term use of cervical bracing. In addition, muscle atrophy, dysphagia, and gastrointestinal dysfunction have also been reported. Signs and symptoms of pressure sores or swallowing dysfunction must be monitored.[61]

Graft Failure

Graft failure after ACDF may be caused by the following: graft displacement, nonunion, instrumentation failure, host factors including osteoporosis or extreme kyphosis, and technical factors such as a short or long graft. Graft failures are highest with multilevel fusions at 60%, and graft dislodgement has been reported in 5% to 50% of multilevel surgeries without instrumentation. Nonunion rates are higher in iliac crest allografts (60%) versus autografts (17%), although they are the same rate at 5% for single level fusions.[70] Clinical symptoms for patients who are symptomatic from nonunion include increasing neck pain and worsening axial pain 6 months after surgery. Patients may have difficulty swallowing and breathing after an anterior graft displacement. Patients who experience a worsening of pain and symptoms should be referred to the physician for additional evaluation and testing procedures.

Chronic Pain

Changes in the peripheral and central nervous system occur almost immediately after an injury. Some of these changes are reversible, and other changes are nonreversible. Many of these changes have been proposed as the pathomechanisms behind the chronicity of pain. It is beyond the scope of this chapter to describe all the neural changes that occur with injury; however, from a clinician's viewpoint it is important to realize that not all patients will have full resolution of symptoms after surgery. Surgery may have addressed the structures that were originally the source of the patient's symptoms, but the adaptations that have occurred in the central and peripheral nervous system may not be reversible. Rehabilitation after ACDF has 80% to 90% satisfactory results. There remain an elusive 10% to 20% of patients who continue to experience pain despite the fact that the offending structures have been addressed through removal or

fixation. As a clinician, it is important to realize that not all pain is a reflection of actual tissue damage. Some pain is the result of tissue changes, and this will affect the ability to rehabilitate patients.[26,71-73]

SUMMARY

Rehabilitation of a patient after ACDF surgery is unique in terms of the close relationship the neck has with the shoulder region and its neural network. Unlike other regions of the body, such as the shoulder and the wrist, complete immobilization of the cervical spine is difficult, which can affect the healing potential of the fusion site. Therefore educating the patient on the need to adhere to surgical protection guidelines immediately after surgery is important. *Protection of the surgical site is the key aspect of early rehabilitation, and stressing of the fusion site should not begin before mineralization of the callus.* Moreover, the shoulder girdle and UE, unlike the hip and lower extremity (LE), rely on coordinated muscle actions to maintain function and stability. Many of these muscles have their proximal attachments at the cervical spine. **Therefore protection of the fusion must also address limiting UE activity until the surgical site is fully healed.** Finally, because radicular pain and UE paresthesia are often the symptoms driving the decision for ACDF, the prevention of neural adhesions and promotion of nerve healing should be addressed appropriately.

 ## Suggested Home Maintenance for the Postsurgical Patient

The patient can use the following home maintenance program during the rehabilitation process. The contents of the home maintenance program may change, depending on the patient's tolerance and ability to complete the exercises properly and without the onset of pain symptoms.

Weeks 1 to 3
GOALS FOR THE PERIOD: Protection of the surgical site, decrease pain and edema, understanding of proper body mechanics and posture, increase walking speed and endurance
1. Protection of the surgical incision
2. Proper use of the cervical collar per physician
3. Knowledge of correct body mechanics and cervical neutral spine during activities
4. Increase upright sitting tolerance
5. Daily walking program as tolerated

Weeks 4 to 8
GOALS FOR THE PERIOD: Increase upper extremity (UE) ROM, improve thoracic spine mobility, begin mild weight training
1. Continue use of collar per physician
2. Continue proper body mechanics and maintenance of neutral spine
3. Progress walking program
4. Active UE ROM in flexion, abduction, horizontal abduction, and adduction (maintaining ROM below 90° of shoulder elevation).
5. Wall angels
6. Scapular retractions
7. Begin biceps curls using light weights
8. Begin cervical proprioceptive training at home, including balance exercises as tolerated
9. After removal of collar, patient may begin AROM to tolerance of cervical spine in rotation, side bend, flexion, and extension (with physician approval)

Weeks 9 to 12

GOALS FOR THE PERIOD: Increase cervical strength, UE strength, independence with ADLs

1. Continue with previous exercises and progress repetitions, weight, or sets as tolerated
2. Scapular retractions with light resistance tubing
3. Wall push-ups
4. Chin tucks in sitting position
5. Tricep push-downs using light resistance tubing
6. Latissimus pull-downs using light resistance tubing
7. Home neural mobility exercises

Weeks 13 to 24

GOALS FOR THE PERIOD: Return to previous functional level and review home conditioning program

1. Continue previous exercises and progress as tolerated
2. Develop independent gym exercise program
   a. Seated or standing rows
   b. Latissimus pull-downs
   c. Tricep push-downs
   d. Bicep curls
3. Patient may perform previously mentioned exercises while sitting on stabilization ball and using resistance tubing
4. Self-resistance to cervical spine: isometrics
   a. Flexion
   b. Extension
   c. Side bend
   d. Rotation

CLINICAL CASE REVIEW

1 Angel is a 45-year-old woman who has arrived at the outpatient clinic for an initial evaluation status after ACDF. The surgery was 4 weeks ago. Her chief complaint is stiffness and soreness in her neck with difficulty sleeping at night. She also notes continued difficulty swallowing and complains of a dry mouth. She asks the therapist's opinion regarding whether she should see her doctor. What should the therapist tell her?

Angel is likely experiencing dysphagia, which is a common short-term side effect of the surgery. The therapist should ask the patient for further information on the duration and intensity of the symptoms. Mild symptoms of dysphagia may be expected, although increased symptoms related to cardiovascular signs such as difficulty breathing, shortness of breath, or symptoms of sleep apnea would warrant a physician consultation.

2 Ned is a 41-year-old man who was involved in a motor vehicle accident 2 years ago. His primary pain symptoms because of the accident included paresthesia and a burning sensation throughout his right UE. He underwent ACDF surgery 4 weeks ago and continues to have neural paresthesia in his right arm. What interventions should be administered?

Possible interventions include gentle UE AROM exercises to the elbow in flexion and extension (as well as to the wrists and fingers) below 90° of shoulder elevation to allow the nerves to glide. The therapist should encourage the patient to move the arms below shoulder level and advise the patient not to lift and only move his arms minimally above 90°.

3 Sam is a 54-year-old man who underwent ACDF 12 weeks ago. He started outpatient physical therapy services 6 weeks ago and has made significant improvements in his upper quarter ROM and strength. Recently, Sam has begun a gym exercise program as he prepares for discharge from physical therapy. However, after approximately 2 weeks at the gym, Sam reports feeling soreness in his neck and shoulders after performing the following exercises: seated scapular rows, latissimus pull-downs, biceps curls, inclined bench press, and an introductory spinning or cycling class for aerobic conditioning. Which of the previously mentioned exercises may be causing Sam's symptoms?

The introductory spinning or cycling class may be the cause of Sam's pain symptoms because of the cervical positioning this type of bike provides. This style of bike usually places the cervical spine in hyperextension and the thoracolumbar spine in flexion, causing Sam to feel soreness after maintaining this extreme position for the duration of the class. Use of a stationary upright bike may place the cervical spine in a more comfortable position and relieve Sam's symptoms. In addition, it would be prudent for the therapist to advise Sam to postpone latissimus pull-downs at this time. They can be started later in the rehabilitation process; however, at this time it is not wise to complete resisted activities above shoulder level. Finally, the therapist should assess the amount of weight the patient is using.

4 Sherry is a 50-year-old woman who had ACDF surgery 6 weeks ago and has just recently removed her cervical collar and returned to work as an accountant. She has a forward head posture, rounded and slumped shoulders, and bilateral scapular winging. She also continues to have numbness and tingling in her right UE, and her pain level reaches a 6 out of 10 (10 being the worst) by lunchtime. She is worried that the fusion has been unsuccessful. What is the therapist's response?

In this case patient education on the need for proper posture throughout the spine appears warranted. The explanation should address proper ergonomic positioning in the workplace to provide the neck and spine an optimal position for work-related activities. In addition, an explanation concerning the effects and stress her posture imposes on nerves and soft tissues will put her at ease. Tight musculature of the pectoralis major and other anterior tissues may be pinching on the brachial plexus, or the nerve roots may be affected secondary to the forward posturing. Interventions to improve her posture should be initiated to relieve undue stresses, and light strengthening of weakened muscles from upper crossed syndrome can be addressed as tolerated. The patient should also be advised to take regular breaks while at work to allow her to change positions and prevent prolonged static postures. The therapist should encourage the patient to lie down or sit in a reclined position during these breaks to allow the postural stabilizers of the neck to rest.

5 Angela underwent ACDF surgery to C5-C6 8 weeks ago. She started outpatient physical therapy last week. Her chief complaint is decreased neck mobility. She also reports that she is experiencing a nagging pain in her right anterior superior iliac crest. This is where the graft for the cervical fusion was harvested. Angela wants to know if the hip pain is normal and whether it will resolve. How should the therapist respond?

At approximately 8 weeks after surgery, bone is undergoing a transformation from a soft callus to a hard callus. Although mineralization of bone may have been completed in the cervical region based on radiographs, the affected hip rarely undergoes a series of radiographs before outpatient physical therapy is initiated. Generally, no contraindications exist to physical therapy for hip pain. The harvest site may be tender for several months after the graft removal because of the trauma of surgery and bone-remodeling process, but the pain should gradually abate. Occasionally the lateral femoral cutaneous nerve may be affected by the graft harvest. If this is the case, then the patient will experience numbness or paresthesia down the lateral aspect of the thigh. Recovery of the nerve will depend on whether the nerve was cut during the surgery or simply compressed by inflammation. If it was excised, then recovery potential is poor. If it

is simply compressed, then function of the nerve should return once the source of the compression is removed.

6 Stacey is a 52-year-old woman who underwent ACDF 8 weeks ago. She has been attending physical therapy for the last 2 weeks but continues to complain that her neck motion is limited. Although she is not currently working, she is worried that she will not be able to resume her position as a bus driver because she is unable to turn her head to look for oncoming traffic. How should the therapist address this problem?

At 8 weeks after surgery, the patient can begin active cervical ROM exercises in all planes. Stacey should be instructed in how to perform these motions beginning in neutral cervical spine position. She should also be told to monitor her symptoms and only move her head until she feels the muscles stretching. Pain should be avoided when completing cervical ROM exercises. This may be added to the patient's home exercise program, but she should be advised that if she experiences increased pain during or after the exercises, then she should stop them until she has an opportunity to talk with her physical therapist.

7 Daniel is a 40-year-old man who underwent C5-6 ACDF surgery 10 weeks ago. He has made improvements with his active cervical ROM but is still unable to side bend much or rotate his head in either direction without moving his trunk. He lacks full shoulder elevation in the sagittal and coronal plane. He also notices difficulty and discomfort while driving slightly longer distances. What form of intervention should the therapist follow?

Daniel's loss of ROM is normal after ACDF. His cervical rotation ROM will likely continue to improve given that C1-2 is a major source (accounting for up to 50%) of rotation. The therapist should keep in mind that AROM expectations for the cervical spine are less than full (65° to 70° of unilateral rotation versus 90°). The fact that he also has limits in shoulder elevation may indicate a thoracic spine mobility issue. Soft tissue mobilization techniques to the upper and midthoracic segments may relieve the tension on the shoulder and neck, allowing for increases in AROM. Improved posture should also follow, allowing a better distribution and absorption of forces while driving.

8 Joe is a 49-year-old man who has been referred to the clinic by his physician 5 months after undergoing ACDF to C4-5 and C5-6. His primary impairments include numbness and tingling in his left UE, decreased cervical ROM, and poor cardiovascular function. After 1 month of physical therapy, Joe has increased his neck ROM and aerobic capacity but still complains of numbness and weakness in his left arm. He asks if the numbness will resolve. What should the therapist tell him?

Several categories of nerve injury are based on the amount of tissue damage occurring at the nerve. A neuropraxia is a local conduction block of the nerve. It usually occurs with compression injuries in which the nerve lumen is compressed and neural and chemical transition down the nerve axon is impaired. The axon and surrounding neurium tissue remains intact. Axonotmesis refers to a condition in which a loss of axon continuity occurs. The neurium tissue remains intact, but because of the loss of axon continuity, degeneration of distal nerve occurs. This condition can be the result of traction to the nerve or severe compression. Neurotmesis is the loss of axon continuity in which the neurium tissue is damaged. Similar degeneration of distal nerve occurs, as seen in axonotmesis; however, because no neurium tissue exists, the nerve has very little chance to heal. This type of injury generally occurs with injuries in which the nerve is severed. Recovery will depend on whether the nerve axon can regrow back to its distal muscular attachment before scar tissue infiltrates the region and blocks axon growth. When the axon and neurium are damaged, little potential exists for full recovery of the nerve. Therefore the therapist should advise the patient that after 6 months, resolution of numbness and weakness is unlikely to occur. Strength can continue to increase, but this is generally the result of muscle hypertrophy and not from innervation of muscle tissue.

9 Robert is a 44-year-old man who underwent ACDF surgery 9 weeks ago. He reports that he has made significant gains in terms of overall neck pain and improvements in his original neural symptoms of burning pain in the right hand and forearm. However, since he has removed his collar over 3 weeks ago, he has complained of a "heavy" head and notes he feels "tiredness" in the back of his neck. He reports that he did not have these types of symptoms when he was wearing his collar and although he has been doing his deep neck flexor exercises, he is unsure if he is doing them correctly as he continues to have fatigue in the neck and "jerky" head movements. How should the therapist address his concerns?

The deep neck flexors have shown to be an important factor in maintaining spinal segment support. Fatigue of these muscles might cause an increase in activation of superficial neck muscles, which has the potential to overload painful cervical structures and affect cervical movement control. Furthermore, this can lead to a lack of confidence in the patient and result in increased muscle contraction to try and protect the movements of the cervical spine, which can lead to diminished active ranges of cervical motions. In this case, the therapist may want to reassess the patient's ability to perform his deep neck flexor exercises and assess the patient's cervical control by using the laser beam exercise described by Treleaven. In this case, the patient sits in a chair 90 cm away from the wall with a laser pointer mounted onto a lightweight headband. He tries to trace a pattern on the wall with the light beam. The therapist can make a subjective analysis of the accuracy and quality of movement, and if deficits exist, the therapist can use this technique as an intervention to improve joint position sense and cervical movement control.

REFERENCES

1. Connell MD, Wiesel SW: Natural history and pathogenesis of cervical disc disease. Orthop Clin North Am 23:369-380, 1992.
2. Riina J, et al: The effect of an anterior cervical operation for cervical radiculopathy or myelopathy on associated headaches. J Bone Joint Surg Am 91(8):1919-1923, 2009.
3. Davidson R, Dunn E, Metzmaker J: The shoulder abduction test in the diagnosis of radicular pain in cervical extradural compressive monoradiculopathies. Spine 6:441-446, 1981.
4. Gore DR, Sepic SB, Gardner GM: Roentgenographic findings of the cervical spine in asymptomatic people. Spine (Philadelphia 1976) 11(6):521-524, 1986.
5. Penning L, et al: CT myelographic findings in degenerative disorders of the cervical spine: Clinical significance. Am J Neuroradiol 7:119-127, 1986.
6. Garvery TA, et al: Outcome of anterior cervical discectomy and fusion as perceived by patients treated for dominant axial-mechanical cervical spine pain. Spine 27:1887-1894, 2002.
7. Roth DA: Cervical analgesic discography: A new test for the definitive diagnosis of the painful disc syndrome. JAMA 235:1713-1714, 1976.
8. Lees F, Turner J: Natural history and prognosis of cervical spondylosis. Br Med J 2:1607-1610, 1963.
9. Dillin W, Uppal G: Analysis of medications used in the treatment of cervical disc degeneration. Orthop Clin North Am 23:421-433, 1992.
10. Joghataei MT, Arab AM, Khaksar H: The effect of cervical traction combined with conventional therapy on grip strength on patients with cervical radiculopathy. Clin Rehabil 18(8):879-887, 2004.
11. Sidhu K, Herkowitz H: Surgical management of cervical disc disease: Surgical management of cervical radiculopathy. In Herkowitz H, et al, editors: The spine, Philadelphia, 1999, Saunders.
12. DeBerard MS, et al: Outcomes of posterolateral lumbar fusion in Utah patients receiving workers' compensation. Spine 27:738-747, 2001.
13. Franklin GM, et al: Outcome of lumbar fusion in Washington state workers' compensation. Spine 17:1897-1903, 1994.
14. Lees F, Turner JW. Natural history and prognosis of cervical spondylosis. Br Med J 28; 2(5373):1607-1610, 1963.
15. Gore DR, Sepic SB: Anterior cervical fusion for degenerated or protruded discs: A review of one hundred forty-six patients. Spine (Philadelphia 1976) 9(7):667-671, 1984.
16. Goldberg EJ, et al: Comparing outcomes of anterior cervical discectomy and fusion in workman's versus non-workman's compensation population. Spine J 2(6):408-414, 2002.
17. Rihn JA, et al: Adjacent segment disease after cervical spine fusion. Instr Course Lect 58:747-756, 2009.

18. Hilibrand AS, et al: Radiculopathy and myelopathy at segments adjacent to the site of a previous anterior cervical arthrodesis. J Bone Joint Surg Am 81(4):519-528, 1999.

19. Murrey D, et al: Results of the prospective, randomized, controlled multicenter Food and Drug Administration investigational device exemption study of the ProDisc-C total disc replacement versus anterior discectomy and fusion for the treatment of 1-level symptomatic cervical disc disease. Spine J 9(4):275-286, Epub 2008 Sep 6, 2009.

20. Sasso RC, et al: Artificial disc versus fusion: A prospective, randomized study with 2-year follow-up on 99 patients. Spine (Philadelphia 1976) 32(26):2933-2940; discussion 2941-2942, 2007.

21. Garrido BJ, Taha TA, Sasso RC. Clinical outcomes of Bryan cervical disc arthroplasty: A prospective, randomized, controlled, single site trial with 48-month follow-up. J Spinal Disord Tech 23(6):367-371, 2010.

22. Olmarker K, Rydevik B: Nerve root pathophysiology. In Fardon D, et al, editors: Orthopaedic knowledge update: Spine 2, Rosemont, Ill, 2002, American Academy of Orthopaedic Surgeons.

23. Posner M: Compression neuropathies. In Spivak J, et al, editors: Orthopaedics—a study guide, New York, 1999, McGraw-Hill.

24. Posner M: Nerve lacerations: Acute and chronic. In Spivak J, et al, editors: Orthopaedics—a study guide, New York, 1999, McGraw-Hill.

25. Boyd B, et al: Strain and excursion in the rat sciatic nerve during a modified straight leg raise are altered after traumatic nerve injury. J Orthop Res 23(4):764-770, 2005.

26. Butler D: The sensitive nervous system, Adelaide, Australia, 2000, Noigroup Publications.

27. Albert T: Surgical approaches to the cervical spine. In Emery S, Boden S, editors: Surgery of the cervical spine, Philadelphia, 2003, Saunders.

28. Heller J: Surgical treatment of degenerative cervical disc disease. In Fardon D, et al, editors: Orthopaedic knowledge update: Spine 2, Rosemont, Ill, 2002, American Academy of Orthopaedic Surgeons.

29. Heller J, Pedlow F, Gill S: Anatomy of the cervical spine. In Clark C, editor: The cervical spine, Philadelphia, 2005, Lippincott Williams & Wilkins.

30. Singh K, Vaccaro A: Surgical approaches to the cervical spine. In Devin V, editor: Spine secrets, Philadelphia, 2003, Hanley and Belfus.

31. Frenkel S, Grew J: Soft tissue repair. In Spivak J, et al, editors: Orthopaedics—a study guide, New York, 1999, McGraw-Hill.

32. Frenkel S, Koval K: Fracture healing and bone grafting. In Spivak J, et al, editors: Orthopaedics—a study guide, New York, 1999, McGraw-Hill.

33. Nitz A: Bone injury and repair. In Placzek J, Boyce D, editors: Orthopaedic physical therapy secrets, Philadelphia, 2001, Hanley and Belfus.

34. Nitz A: Soft tissue injury and repair. In Placzek J, Boyce D, editors: Orthopaedic physical therapy secrets, Philadelphia, 2001, Hanley and Belfus.

35. Janda V: Muscles and motor control in cervicogenic disorders. In Grant R, editor: Physical therapy of the cervical and thoracic spine, St Louis, 2002, Churchill Livingstone.

36. White A, Panjabi M: Clinical biomechanics of the spine, ed 2, Philadelphia, 1990, Lippincott.

37. Richardson C, et al: Therapeutic exercise for spinal segmental stabilization in low back pain—scientific basis and clinical approach, Edinburgh, 1999, Churchill Livingstone.

38. Jull G: Management of cervicogenic headaches. In Grant R, editor: Physical therapy of the cervical and thoracic spine, St Louis, 2002, Churchill Livingstone.

39. O'Leary S, et al: Specificity in retraining flexor muscle performance. J Orthop Sports Phys Ther 37(1): 3-9, 2007.

40. Bogduk N: Biomechanics of the cervical spine. In Grant R, editor: Physical therapy of the cervical and thoracic spine, St Louis, 2002, Churchill Livingstone.

41. Neumann D: Axial skeleton: Osteology and arthrology. In Neumann D, editor: Kinesiology of the musculoskeletal system—foundations for physical rehabilitation, ed 2, St Louis, 2009, Mosby.

42. Kapandji I: The physiology of the joints, vol 3, New York, 1995, Churchill Livingstone.

43. Lee M: Effects of frequency on response of the spine to lumbar postero-anterior forces. J Manipulative Physiol Ther 16:439-446, 1993.

44. Lee M, Gal J, Herzog W: Biomechanics of manual therapy. In Dvir Z, editor: Clinical biomechanics, St Louis, 2000, Churchill Livingstone.

45. Lee M, Kelly D, Steven G: A model of spine, ribcage and pelvic responses to a specific lumbar manipulative force in relaxed subjects. J Biomech 28:1403-1408, 1995.

46. Lee M, Lau T, Lau H: Sagittal plane rotation of the pelvis during lumbar posteroanterior loading. J Manipulative Physiol Ther 17:149-155, 1994.

47. Coe JD, Vaccaro AR: Complications of anterior cervical plating. In Clark C, editor: The cervical spine, Philadelphia, 2005, Lippincott Williams & Wilkins.

48. Goffin J, et al: Long-term results after anterior cervical fusion and osteo-synthetic stabilization for fractures and/or dislocations of the cervical spine. J Spinal Disord 8:499-508, 1995.

49. Coppieters MW, Hough AD, Dilley A: Different nerve glide exercise induce different magnitudes of median nerve longitudinal excursion: An in vivo study using dynamic ultrasound imaging. JOSPT 39(3)164-171, 2009.

50. Elvey R: Treatment of arm pain associated with abnormal brachial plexus tension. Aust J Physiother 32:225-230, 1986.

51. Butler D: Upper limb neurodynamic test: Clinical use in a "big picture" framework. In Grant R, editor: Physical therapy of the cervical and thoracic spine, St Louis, 2002, Churchill Livingstone.

52. Coppieters MW, Butler DS: Do sliders slide and tensioners tension? An analysis of neurodynamics techniques and considerations regarding their application Manual Ther 139;213-221, 2008.

53. Boyd B, Topps K: Mechanosensitivity of the lower extremity neurons system during SLR neurodynamic testing in healthy individuals. JOSPT 39(11):780-790, 2009.

54. Kristjansson E, Treleaven J: Sensorimotor function and dizziness in neck pain: implications for assessment and management. J Orthop Sports Phys Ther 39(5):364-377, 2009.

55. Treleaven J: Sensorimotor disturbances in neck disorders affecting postural stability, head and eye movement control. Man Ther 13:2-11, 2008.

56. Treleaven J: Sensorimotor disturbances in neck disorders affecting postural stability, head and eye movement control. Part 2: Case studies. Man Ther 13:266-275, 2008.

57. Revel M, et al: Cervicocephalic kinesthetic sensibility in patients with cervical pain. Arch Phys Med Rehabil 72(5):228-291, 1991.

58. Treleaven J, et al: Dizziness and unsteadiness following whiplash injury: Characteristic features and relationship with cervical joint position error. J Rehabil Med 35(1):36-43, 2003.

59. Fritz J: Clinical prediction rules in physical therapy: Coming of age. JOSPT 39(3):159-161, 2009.

60. Childs JD, et al: Proposal of a classification system for patients with neck pain. JOSPT 34 (11):686-700, 2004.

61. Wakefield A, Benzel E: Complications of cervical surgery. In Fardon D, et al, editors: Orthopaedic knowledge update: Spine 2, Rosemont, Ill, 2002, American Academy of Orthopaedic Surgeons.

62. Lowery G, McDonough R: The significance of hardware failure in anterior cervical plate fixation: Patients with 2 to 7 year follow up. Spine 23:181-186, 1998.

63. Vaccaro A: Point of view. Spine 23:186-187, 1998.

64. Winslow C, Winslow T, Wax M: Dysphonia and dysphagia following the anterior approach to the cervical spine. Arch Otolaryngol Head Neck Surg 127:51-55, 2001.

65. Hanci M, et al: Oesophageal perforation subsequent to anterior cervical spine screw/plate fixation. Paraplegia 33:606-609, 1995.

66. Bohler J, Gaudernak T: Anterior plate stabilization for fracture dislocation of the lower cervical spine. J Trauma 20:203-205, 1980.

67. Zeigman S, Ducker T, Raycroft J: Trends and complications in cervical spine surgery: 1989-1993. J Spinal Disord 10:523-526, 1997.

68. Mann D, et al: Anterior plating of unstable cervical spine fractures. Paraplegia 28:564-572, 1990.

69. Swank M, et al: Anterior cervical allograft arthrodesis and instrumentation: Multilevel interbody grafting or strut graft reconstruction. Eur Spine J 6:138-143, 1997.

70. Thongtrangan I, Balabhadra R, Kim D: Management of strut graft failure in anterior cervical spine surgery. Neurosurg Focus 15:1-8, 2003.

71. Gifford L, Butler D: The integration of pain sciences in clinical practice. J Hand Ther 10:86-95, 1997.

72. Shacklock M: Neurodynamics. Physiotherapy 81:9-16, 1995.

73. Winkelstein B, Weinstein J: Pain mechanisms: Relevant anatomy, pathogenesis, and clinical implications. In Clark C, editor: The cervical spine, Philadelphia, 2005, Lippincott Williams & Wilkins.

CHAPTER 15

Posterior Lumbar Arthroscopic Discectomy and Rehabilitation

Haideh V. Plock, Ben B. Pradhan, David Pakozdi, Rick B. Delamarter

Lumbar herniated nucleus pulposus (HNP) falls within the spectrum of degenerative spinal conditions and can occur with little or no trauma. Lumbar disc abnormalities increase with age.[1,2] The actual incidence of lumbar disc herniations is unknown because many people with herniations are asymptomatic.[1,3,4] Approximately 90% of lumbar herniations occur at the L4-L5 and L5-S1 levels.[1,5,6] More than 200,000 discectomies are performed in the United States each year, and this number is likely increasing.[7] The success of this procedure, as with all surgical procedures, depends vastly on proper patient selection and to a lesser extent on surgical technique. However, it is incumbent on the spinal surgeon to be absolutely meticulous with intraoperative technique once the decision for surgery is made. To this end, the use of a microscope is recommended for lumbar discectomy. Once the learning curve has been mastered, the microscope not only offers advantages over loupes but also forces one to think at a much higher level of clarity about what and where root encroachment pathology is present.[8] More importantly, the patient has less morbidity and an earlier hospital discharge compared with standard or limited discectomy.[5,9-14]

SURGICAL INDICATIONS AND CONSIDERATIONS

Pathophysiology

Intervertebral discs cushion and tether the vertebrae, providing both flexibility and stability. The normally gelatinous nucleus pulposus is surrounded by the ligamentous annulus broses. In the young and healthy disc, the nucleus and annulus blend. Degenerative or pathologic changes can cause separations of the two entities, as well as compromise the integrity of the annulus, such that a sufficient load can cause nuclear fragments to migrate and impinge on neural elements.[15] This pathophysiology is reflected in a clinical presentation of acute sciatica pain with a prior history of back pain. Lumbar disc herniations may occur with little or

no trauma, although patients frequently report a bending or twisting motion as the inciting event, causing the onset of symptoms. Common causes of lumbar herniations include falls, car accidents, repetitive heavy lifting, and sports injuries of all types.

Diagnosis

The radiographic diagnosis of lumbar disc herniation has been made rather simple with magnetic resonance imaging (MRI). The clinical diagnosis is frequently straightforward as well. A patient with a lumbar herniation generally has some element of low back pain with radiation into the buttocks, thigh, leg, and foot. The leg radiation almost always follows a dermatomal distribution. Patients frequently complain of numbness, tingling, or weakness in the affected dermatome. Lying down may relieve the symptoms, whereas sitting, walking, and standing may exacerbate them. Provocative maneuvers that increase abdominal pressure (coughing, sneezing, defecating) may intensify symptoms as well. Complaints of bowel and bladder dysfunction may signal a cauda equina syndrome and may necessitate emergent workup and treatment.

Physical Examination

Visual inspection may reveal lumbar muscle spasm, fasciculations, and postural changes, including listing to the side and a forward flexed position. Gait observation can reveal a listing antalgic walk. Weakness can give a dropped foot type gait (anterior tibialis), buckling of the leg (quadriceps), or Trendelenburg gait (gluteus medius). Range of motion (ROM) testing may be limited secondary to pain. Neurologic testing is extremely important and should include motor, sensory, and reflex testing. Lumbar herniations may cause varying degrees of dermatomal weakness, sensory deficits, and reflex changes. Straight-leg raises (SLRs) are a good indicator of nerve root impingement in lower lumbar herniations, and a positive femoral stretch can indicate an upper lumbar herniation.

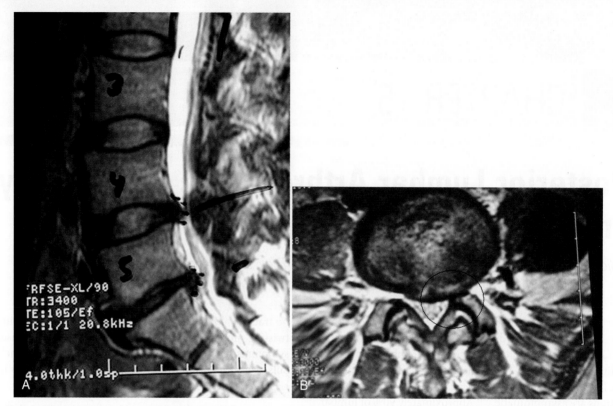

Fig. 15-1 **A,** Sagittal magnetic resonance imaging (MRI) showing herniated discs at the bottom two lumbar discs, at L4-5 and L5-S1. **B,** An axial cut of a lumbar spine MRI revealing a left-sided broad-based paracentral disc herniation effacing the thecal sac, causing left-sided lateral recess, foraminal stenosis, and neural compression.

Imaging and Other Tests

MRI is clearly the imaging study of choice to diagnose a lumbar disc herniation (Fig. 15-1). Plain radiographs should always be obtained to evaluate overall alignment, bony integrity, and stability. Patients who cannot obtain an MRI can be diagnosed using computed tomography (CT), CT myelogram, or CT discogram. These imaging tests are so sensitive that a discectomy is not indicated if a disc is not found to be herniated by one of these techniques. Other tests can include an electromyogram (EMG) or nerve conduction study.

Management

It is important to understand that most patients with symptomatic herniated lumbar discs will get better over time, regardless of the type of treatment. Weber's classic study[16] reported that sciatica from HNP would improve 60% of the time with nonsurgical methods and 92% of the time with surgery at 1 year. By 4 years out, no statistical difference was found (51% improvement in conservative group versus 66% in the surgical group), and no difference was found at 10-year follow-up. The 5-year outcomes from the Maine Lumbar Spine Study are similar to the 4-year results of the Weber study. At 1-year follow-up, 71% of surgical patients reported relief of leg symptoms compared with 43% of conservatively managed patients.[17] They reported long-term follow-up at 5 years, with 70% of patients in the operative group describing improvement versus 56% in the nonoperative group.[18] More

recently, the Spine Patient Outcomes Research Trial results have contributed to the favorable opinion of surgical outcomes as well. Treatment effects were statistically significant at 2 years and maintained at 4-year follow-up for primary outcomes in favor of surgery.[19]

In the absence of cauda equina syndrome or progressive or significant neurologic deficits, most practitioners attempt conservative care before suggesting surgical intervention.

Nonoperative Treatment

Nonoperative treatment may include:
1. Modified activity
2. Modified bed rest for 2 to 3 days (prolonged bed rest should be avoided)[20-22]
3. Analgesic, antiinflammatory medication (e.g., nonsteroidal antiinflammatory drugs, steroids, or both)
4. Physical therapy (as tolerated) or external support (e.g., corset, brace)
5. Epidural steroid injections (we recommend up to three)

Indications for Surgery

Surgical indications, as currently recommended by the North American Spine Society (NASS), include a definite diagnosis of ruptured lumbar intervertebral disc and the following[23,24]:
1. Failure of conservative treatment
2. Unbearable or recurrent episodes of radicular pain (or both)

3. Significant neurologic deficit

4. Increasing neurologic deficit (absolute indication)

5. Cauda equina syndrome (absolute indication)

Conservative treatment consists of nonoperative management and careful observation. Some may benefit from a short trial of nonoperative treatment even after 8 weeks if no prior care was given. Failed conservative treatment is the most common indication for lumbar discectomy. Those who have not improved sufficiently and are not experiencing continued improvement might then be offered treatment by surgical excision of the disc. Such patients should be advised that this is an elective operation but that delay for longer than 3 to 6 months in the face of persistent and severe symptoms may compromise the best ultimate result.[24,25] The other indications (2 to 5) are exceptions to the 4- to 8-week rule. Excruciating pain may not be relieved by nonoperative means and may require earlier surgical decompression. Recurrent sciatica should also receive consideration for surgery: the chance of recurrent sciatica after the second episode is 50% and after the third episode is almost 100%.[25] An example of a significant neurologic deficit may be a foot drop or weakness that prevents normal posture, gait, or affects the patient's profession or a particular skill. Any definite progression of neurologic deficit is an absolute indication for surgery. Cauda equina syndrome is relatively rare. It is reported in 1% to 3% of patients with confirmed disc herniations,[26,27] and it is an orthopedic or neurosurgical emergency. Features include rapid progression of neurologic signs and symptoms, bilateral leg pain, caudal sensory deficit, bladder overflow incontinence or retention, and loss of rectal sphincter tone with or without fecal incontinence.

Contraindications for Discectomy

NASS and the American Academy of Orthopaedic Surgeons have identified the following factors as absolute or relative contraindications for discectomy[24,28]:

1. Lack of clear clinical diagnosis, anatomic level of lesion, and radiographic evidence of HNP

2. Lack of trial of nonoperative treatment (with the exceptions mentioned previously)

3. Disabilities with major nonorganic components (i.e., multifocal, nonanatomic, or disproportionate signs and symptoms)

4. Systemic disease processes that can negatively influence outcome of surgery (e.g., diabetic neuropathy)

5. Medical contraindications to surgery (e.g., major comorbidities, unfavorable survival)

6. Disc herniation at a level of instability (may need additional stabilization)

SURGICAL PROCEDURES

One only has to review the natural history of lumbar disc disease to realize that spinal surgeons play a palliative role in the management of HNP.[29-33] Surgical procedures as treatment for lumbar HNP include the following:

1. Lumbar discectomy (microscopic or standard open technique)
   a. Hemilaminotomy and discectomy
   b. Laminectomy and discectomy
2. Minimally invasive percutaneous techniques
   a. Chemonucleolysis
   b. Percutaneous discectomy (suction, shaver, laser, endoscopic tools)

Use of an Operating Microscope

The attempt to improve visualization and illumination has led many spine surgeons to use loupes and a headlight. We believe the magnication and illumination built into the microscope offer many surgical advantages, the most important of which is reduced wound size and decreased tissue manipulation (Fig. 15-2). The surgeon can limit the amount of tissue dissection by working through a small exposure directly over the pathology to be removed. Microsurgical techniques can also be used to preserve the ligamentum flavum and epidural fat to minimize postoperative epidural broses and improve clinical results by preserving natural tissue planes.[8,34] With this approach, the disc herniation can be easily removed, lateral recess stenosis can be decompressed, and nerve root manipulation is kept to a minimum. The senior author has used this technique since 1986 for most lumbar disc herniations and has found the approach to be safe, with fewer dural tears and nerve root injuries and less postoperative epidural broses than with standard discectomy.[5,8,10,35]

However, the microscope is not without its disadvantages. Peripheral vision is lost, with the field of vision limited to approximately 4 to 5 cm. Because of this, the surgeon needs to know detailed anatomy of the spine. The line of vision is axed through the microscope. To look over structures (to overcome tissue overhang), the patient or microscope has to be adjusted during the surgery. This can be avoided by proper retraction or dissection of tissue away from the line of vision.

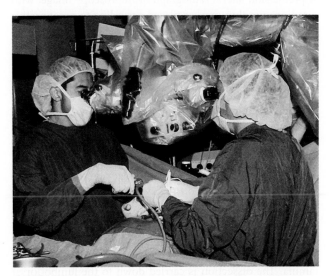

Fig. 15-2 A surgeon and an assistant surgeon using the operative microscope with a high-intensity light source and microscopic magnification. The two surgeons can work hand-in-hand with unobstructed view of the operative field.

Researchers reported increased disc space infection after microsurgery.[36,37] This was most likely caused by contamination from unsterile parts of the microscope during surgery, although no one has looked at the potential for an increased infection rate when two surgeons with loupes and headlights bump heads over the wound! Recent reports by those who have experience with the microscope do not show any increased infection rates.[5,10,14,38,]

Lumbar Microdiscectomy

Microscopic discectomy (microdiscectomy) has become the gold standard for operative treatment of lumbar disc herniations, and the latest minimally invasive percutaneous techniques have not been shown to be more effective.[8,39,40] Although no statistical differences can be shown in the ultimate long-term outcomes of microscopic versus standard open discectomies,[11,13,14,32,41-43] the microscope provides improved illumination and magni cation, and patients have less morbidity and earlier hospital discharge when compared with standard discectomies.

Operative Setup

General anesthesia is preferable because of patient comfort, as well as airway and sedation control. Another advantage is the option of hypotensive anesthesia. The procedure can also be done under epidural or local anesthesia with sedation, although this is not our preference. The patient's position is always prone with the abdomen free, thus relieving pressure on the abdominal venous system and, in turn, decreasing venous backflow through the Batson venous plexus into the spinal canal. This has the effect of decreasing bleeding from the epidural veins intraoperatively. Several frames are available for this, but we prefer a Wilson frame on a regular operating table because of the ease of setup.

Identification of Level and Side

A preincision lateral radiograph or fluoroscopy image, with a radiopaque skin marker placed according to preoperative radiographs and anatomic landmarks, will identify the appropriate incision location for the disc space to be exposed. This is best done by placing a spinal needle as straight vertically as possible, approximately 2 cm from midline contralateral to the side of surgery. The side of surgery is usually the more symptomatic side, although occasionally a midline HNP can be approached from either side.

Skin Incision and Interlaminar Space Exposure

A 2- to 3-cm incision is made midline or up to 1 cm lateral to the spinous process on the symptomatic side at a level directly over the disc space based on the localizing lateral radiograph. At L5-S1, this incision tends to be directly over the interlaminar space; but as one moves up the lumbar spine, this incision will be progressively over the cephalad lamina. The dissection is carried down to the lumbodorsal fascia, which is sharply incised. The fascial incision is placed carefully, just lateral to the spinous processes to avoid damage to the supraspinous and interspinous ligament complex. The

subperiosteal muscle dissection and elevation are confined to the interlaminar space and approximately half of the cephalad and caudad lamina. The facet capsules are carefully preserved. A Cobb elevator and Bovie cautery are used. A framed retractor is then placed. The surgeon should expose the lateral border of the pars as a landmark for preserving enough of the pars during laminotomy to prevent fracture.

At this time another localizing lateral radiograph should be obtained to confirm the proper level. A forward-angled curette can be placed underneath the cephalad lamina of the interspace. With this intraoperative radiographic verification, wrong-level surgery is impossible. The radiograph will also indicate how much of the cephalad lamina needs to be removed to expose the disc space. The microscope is then brought into position.

Spinal Canal Entry

After exposure of the interlaminar space and placement of the retractor, a high-speed burr is used to remove several millimeters of the cephalad lamina and 2 to 3 mm of the medial aspect of the inferior facet, taking care to leave at least a 6-mm bridge of bone at the level of the pars (Fig. 15-3). Once the cephalad lamina and medial aspect of the inferior facet have been removed, the ligamentum flavum is easily seen because its bony attachments are exposed. The ligamentum attaches at the very cephalad edge of the lower lamina, but approximately halfway up the upper lamina, and it attaches to the medial aspect of the superior facet. Thus the high-speed burr can be used relatively safely on top of the

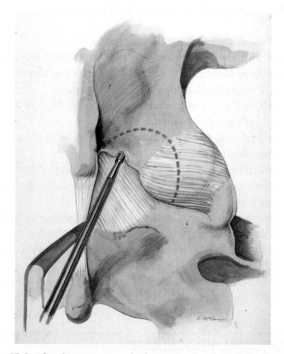

Fig. 15-3 After skin exposure and subsequent subperiosteal elevation, the retractor in position reveals the interlaminar interval, with exposure of the upper and lower laminae. Several millimeters of the cephalad lamina and 2 to 3 mm of the medial edge of the inferior facet are removed with the high-speed burr. This bone can be safely removed because the undersurface is protected by the ligamentum flavum.

bottom half of the superior lamina, as well as the medial aspect of the inferior facet.

Free Ligamentum Flavum

The ligamentum flavum is then released from the medial edge of the superior facet with a forward-angled curette. It can also be released from the undersurface of the upper and lower lamina (Fig. 15-4). It is safest to start the curette infero-laterally toward the superior aspect of the pedicle (caudal aspect of the foramen).

A ligamentum and epidural fat-sparing approach, performed by creating a flap of the ligamentum as described previously, decreases postoperative epidural broses and can improve results.[8,34] However, this can make it more difficult to get a good view of the nerve root. Certainly this is easier with a microscope than without one. The less-experienced surgeon may perform partial removal of these tissues. The ligamentum flap is also not recommended for large midline disc herniations (with or without cauda equina syndrome) and severely stenotic canals because the ligamentum itself occupies more room in the already severely compromised spinal canal and would also interfere with direct visualization for the delicate manipulation of the thecal sac.

Lateral Recess Exposure

After release of the ligamentum flavum, the medial edge of the superior facet is resected with 2- to 4-mm Kerrison rongeurs. This resection goes from the lower pedicle to the tip of the superior facet (Fig. 15-5). This medial facet resection decompresses any lateral recess stenosis at the level of the

pedicle and up into the foramen, and it allows easy access to the lateral disc space. If needed, some of the lateral ligamentum flavum, particularly into the foramen, can be removed with the Kerrison rongeurs.

Nerve Root and Ligamentum Retraction

Bipolar cautery can be used at this time to cauterize any epidural bleeding over the lateral disc space, directly cephalad to the pedicle. We recommend finding the pedicle and then using it as a guide to release the epidural nonneural tissues above the disc space. At this point a nerve root retractor can be placed on the disc space, and the ligamentum flavum, epidural fat, and nerve root are retracted toward the midline, generally exposing the herniation (Fig. 15-6). Again, the bipolar cautery can be used to cauterize any epidural veins over the disc herniation. Any free large fragments of disc can now be removed (Fig. 15-7). If needed, a forward-angled curette can be used to scrape the inferior and posterior bony margins of the foramen, using a unidirectional pulling motion. Using the bony pedicle as a starting point ensures that the end of the curette does not include any neural tissue before scraping.

Discectomy

Frequently the annular defect of the disc herniation is all that is necessary to allow cleaning out of any loose nucleus pulposus inside the disc space, although the annulotomy can be enlarged with a No. 11 blade. The herniated nuclear material is then cleaned out with straight or angled pituitary rongeurs and small back-angled curettes. Care should be taken not to

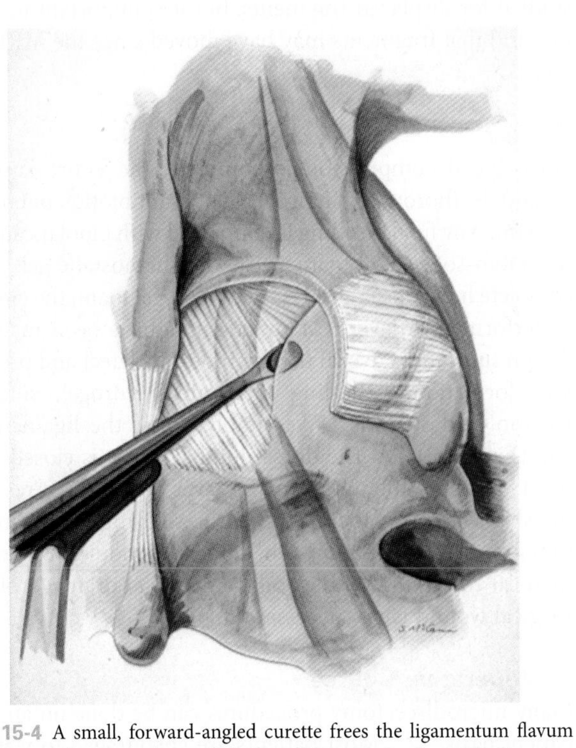

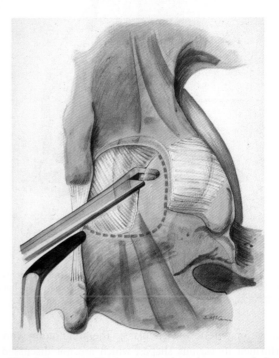

Fig. 15-4 A small, forward-angled curette frees the ligamentum flavum from its attachment to the medial edge of the superior facet. The ligamentum flavum also can be freed from the undersurface of the upper and lower laminae.

Fig. 15-5 A 3- or 4-mm Kerrison rongeur is used to remove the lateral recess (subarticular) stenosis (i.e., the medial edge of the superior facet) back to the pedicle of the lower vertebra and cephalad to the top of the superior facet. This bony resection removes the lateral recess (subarticular) stenosis and allows exposure of the lateral disc space.

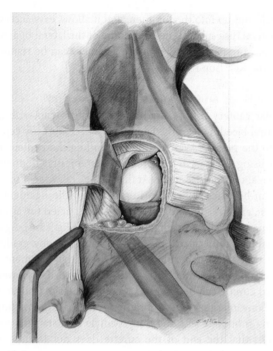

Fig. 15-6 A nerve root retractor is used to retract the ligamentum flavum, nerve root sleeve, and epidural fat toward midline over the herniated disc. Bipolar cautery can be used to cauterize the epidural plexus over the disc herniation.

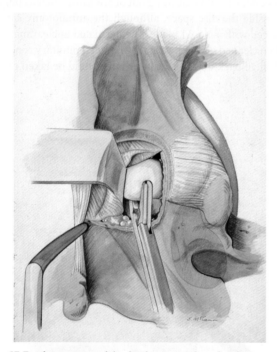

Fig. 15-7 After exposure of the disc herniation, large free fragments can be removed with a pituitary rongeur, the natural annulotomy from the disc herniation can be enlarged with a No. 11 blade, or both can be done.

damage or curette the endplates. The annulotomy can be performed in various shapes, which are not discussed in detail here.[36,44]

One unresolved issue is how much disc to remove from the disc cavity. Removal of as much disc as possible implies curettage of the interspace, including possible removal of the cartilaginous endplates. Critics of this approach point out that no matter how long the surgeon works, it is impossible to remove all disc material in this fashion. They also argue that this method increases risk of damage to anterior visceral structures and increases risk of chronic back pain induced by conditions, such as sterile discitis and instability. Although some surgeons believe that extensive intradisc débridement decreases the rate of recurrent HNP, others refute that position.[36,45-47] In the end, the only reasonable prospective controlled study is Spengler's,[48] which suggests that limited disc excision is all that is necessary. The advantages of limited disc excision are less trauma to endplates and less dissection, less nerve root manipulation, a lower prevalence of infection, reduced risk of damage to structures anterior to the disc space, and less disc space settling postoperatively (theoretically reducing the incidence of chronic back pain).

Disc Space Irrigation

After the HNP and any remaining loose material is removed, the disc space is irrigated under some pressure with a long angiocatheter; then the pituitary rongeur is again used to remove any loose fragments. The spinal canal is then palpated underneath the nerve root and across the vertebral bodies above and below for any residual fragments. In doing the limited disc excision, one must also be sure to probe under the posterior annulus (both medially and laterally) for loose fragments. This is an important step to ensure that no displaced or sequestered fragments are missed. Residual disc material will feel rough, whereas the native dural surface is quite smooth. In the end the patient must be left with a freely mobile nerve root. The preoperative MRI should be carefully studied for displaced fragments, but it is important to keep in mind that fragments may have moved since the MRI was taken.

Closure

Once the decompression is complete, the entire surgical wound is thoroughly irrigated with antibiotic-containing irrigant. Any final bleeding is controlled with bipolar cautery, thrombin-soaked gel foam, or FloSeal hemostatic gel. After complete hemostasis and removal of all gel foam, the closure is performed in layers. Many attempts have been made to design substances to seal the laminotomy defect and prevent scar formation, including fat grafts, hydrogel, silicone, Dacron, and steroids.[49] We simply prefer the ligamentum flap (Fig. 15-8).[5,8,25] The dorsal lumbar fascia is closed with No. 1-0 sutures, the subcutaneous layer with 2-0 sutures, and the skin with 3-0 subcuticular sutures. Using this ligamentum flavum–sparing approach, blood loss should be no more than 10 to 20 ml. With good hemostasis, drainage of the surgical wound is not necessary.

Postoperative Course

Many microdiscectomy procedures can be done on an outpatient basis.[12,50,51] Most patients are encouraged to walk as tolerated. Sitting is also tolerated but may be more limited. Many return to work within 5 to 10 days, especially those

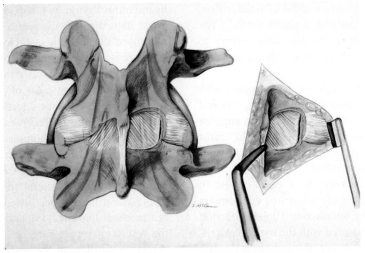

Fig. 15-8 After thorough irrigation, the nerve root retractor is released, allowing the ligamentum flavum and nerve root sleeve to return to their normal anatomic positions.

with desk type of work. All patients are required to participate in lumbar physical therapy, primary stabilization, and mobilization beginning at approximately 4 weeks after surgery. Most athletes return to their normal athletic activities within 8 weeks after surgery. However, the postoperative course is variable, and return to normal activities depends on the patient's overall medical condition, as well as neurologic and overall recovery.[16,52,53]

Unusual Disc Herniations

Herniated Nucleus Pulposus at High Lumbar Levels (L1-L2, L2-L3, L3-L4)

High lumbar HNPs are uncommon (5%). When they occur they are likely to be foraminal or extraforaminal.[25,54] Important skeletal anatomy in the higher lumbar spine for the spinal surgeon to be aware of includes the following: (1) the pars are narrower, and facet integrity is easily lost with excessive laminotomy; (2) the laminae are broader; (3) the interlaminar window is narrower; (4) the inferior border of the lamina overhangs more of the disc space; (5) at L1-L2, the conus cannot be retracted like the cauda equina at lower levels; (6) the nerve roots exit more horizontally and are less mobile; and (7) epidural veins may be more prevalent. At these levels, because of the limited size of the interlaminar space, ligamentum excision rather than sparing is recommended.

Recurrent Disc Rupture

The incidence of recurrent HNP at the same level and side of a previously operated on disc is 2% to 5%.[5,55,56] The microscope is especially valuable in this scenario because of the scar between tissue planes, including neural elements. Adequate time must be spent carefully teasing the tissues apart with a blunt instrument (e.g., bipolar, curette, Penfield) before forcefully mobilizing the nerve root. The incidence of complications is understandably higher in revision discectomies.

Cauda Equina Syndrome

The classic teaching in cauda equina syndrome is that (1) it is an orthopedic emergency, and (2) a wide decompression through a bilateral approach is necessary. We agree with the first point but not the second. Few disc herniations are too big to be addressed microsurgically. A wider hemilaminectomy may be needed. The microscope is invaluable when working in the severely stenotic canal. If the disc cannot be easily or totally excised unilaterally, then bilateral hemilaminotomies may be done.[26,27]

Herniated Nucleus Pulposus in the Adolescent Patient

The risk for recurrence of HNP after surgical excision is higher in adolescents than in adults. Because of the high proteoglycan content in adolescent discs and the prevalence of disc protrusions rather than disc extrusions, some have recommended percutaneous chemonucleolysis rather than surgical intervention in this age group.[25,57,58] Studies have been published with controversial results for surgical discectomy in this patient population.[59-61] Chemonucleolysis may have merit in the treatment of symptomatic disc protrusions, but discectomy is necessary in the setting of an extruded or sequestered disc causing significant or progressive neurologic deficit or pain. These extruded or sequestered fragments are frequently heavily collagenized.[24,62] Long-term follow-up studies of more than 12 years after discectomy in this group have reported good to excellent results in 87% to 92% of patients.[63,64]

Complications

Complications for the discectomy procedures include dural tears, neural injury, visceral injuries, postoperative infection, recurrence of herniation, inadequate decompression, and iatrogenic instability.

Dural tears occur in 1.0% to 6.7% of cases, although the incidence decreases with experience.[5,16,38,65-67] If possible, repair should be done by direct suture (5-0 to 7-0 silk, nylon, or polypropylene) with or without a dural patch.[65] The patient should be kept flat for a few days after surgery to lower the hydrostatic pressure in the lumbar thecal sac while the repair seals.

Neural injuries are rare, although the risk is greater with unusual disc herniations as described previously. Visceral injuries occur when an instrument penetrates the anterior annulus. Among these, vascular injuries are the most common.[65,68] If these are recognized, then immediate laparotomy for surgical repair is indicated.

Postoperative discitis occurs in 1% of cases or less in experienced hands, although clearly a learning curve exists in developing facility with the microscope. Higher infection rates (up to 7%) have been reported with the use of a microscope during surgery, although in experienced hands this has been shown not to be true.[65] An MRI is the best diagnostic imaging tool. An image-guided needle biopsy may be performed to assist in organism-specific antibiotic selection. Reoperation may not be necessary unless the patient develops root compression, cauda equina syndrome, or an epidural abscess.

The literature reports recurrent HNP at a previously operated site occurring anywhere from 2% to 5% after lumbar discectomy.[25,69] When reoperating for a recurrent HNP, it is important to get adequate exposure of the dural sac above and below the disc space. Then using a combination of blunt (nerve hook, Penfield, bipolar) and sharp (Kerrison) dissection, the dural sac and nerve root are exposed and mobilized above the HNP.

Iatrogenic mechanical instability is fortunately a rare occurrence after discectomy, even if a decompressive laminectomy was required for a stenotic canal or to excise a large disc.[6] Symptomatic mechanical treatment may require surgical stabilization. Suboptimal results after discectomy can be the result of several other problems that, unfortunately, do not have a straightforward medical or surgical treatment. Although very rare, these can include epidural broses, arachnoiditis, and complex regional pain syndrome.[65]

Discussion

Most modern studies using microscopic techniques for treatment of herniated lumbar discs report 90% to 95% success rates.* A multicenter, prospective trial has proved what cannot be repeated often enough: If the therapist selects patients with dominant radicular pain (compared with back pain), with neurologic changes and painful SLRs, and with a study confirming a disc rupture, then he or she can anticipate a high level of success for discectomy, with or without a microscope.[41] The rate of successful outcome drops significantly as more of these inclusion criteria are not met. Persistent back pain occurs in up to 25% of patients who undergo microdiscectomy.[66,67] This has led to the opinion that it is important to save the supraspinous and intraspinous ligament complex, remove as little lamina as possible, save the

ligamentum flavum as a flap, and do a limited discectomy. These steps theoretically reduce iatrogenic instability, epidural broses, sterile discitis, and loss of disc height. All of these steps are facilitated by the use of a microscope, but no proof exists that these steps reduce the incidence of back pain.

The most frequent cause of poor result from lumbar disc surgery is faulty patient selection because of erroneous or incomplete diagnosis. Technical errors, such as wrong-level surgery, incomplete decompression, and intraoperative complications, explain a small percentage of failures. A 1981 study assigned the following frequency of missed diagnoses as sources of failure: lateral spinal stenosis, 59%: recurrent or persistent herniation, 14%; adhesive arachnoiditis, 11%; central canal stenosis, 11%; and epidural broses, 7%. Finally, the results of repeat surgery are not as good as primary surgery, regardless of the reason or whether a microscope was used, because of scar tissue, higher incidence of complications, or larger dissections. In the past decade, a substantial increase in interest in minimally invasive procedures has occurred in all areas of medicine, particularly for spinal disorders. Several methods to remove HNP have been proposed as alternatives to standard open discectomy. Injected chymopapain can dissolve much of the central nucleus, but is not likely to act on extruded or sequestered fragments, which are often heavily collagenized.[24,57,62] Likewise, percutaneous suction discectomies and removal of nucleus (either mechanically or by laser from the center of the disc) may reduce intradisc pressure but are unlikely to influence the effects of extruded or sequestered disc material. Therefore although alternative minimally invasive techniques hold considerable promise, lumbar microdiscectomy is still the gold standard for surgical treatment of lumbar HNP with radiculopathy. However, the skills and technology to remove herniated discs by such alternatives are evolving.[24,39,40,71-73]

THERAPY GUIDELINES FOR REHABILITATION

Postoperative spine rehabilitation allows for a safer and faster return to functional activities. The early return to appropriate activities has been encouraged after surgeries of the extremities for many years. The same approach should be applied to the spine. Careful instruction and frequent reevaluation enable a therapist to progress the patient's functional activities to premorbid levels safely. The therapist should apply a functionally appropriate and suitably aggressive postoperative protocol to the patient recovering from lumbar microdiscectomy.

Lumbar disc herniations can do more than compromise the nerve root. Compensatory movement patterns, altered mechanics of the motion segment, and muscle splinting may result in misleading referred pain patterns (e.g., myofascial trigger points). Furthermore, the literature suggests that abnormal changes in paraspinal muscle activity occur after an HNP.[74,75] Triano and Schultz[76] found a high correlation between the absence of the flexion-relaxation phenomenon (i.e., the relaxation of the lumbar paraspinal muscles at

---

*References 5, 8, 9, 11-14, 29, 34, 37, 38, 42, 43, 55, 66, 69, and 70.

terminal flexion in standing) and poor results on the Oswestry Pain Disability Scale (Box 15-1).

Microdiscectomy is designed to decompress neural tissues by removing the disc material that is causing the neurologic signs and symptoms not alleviated through aggressive conservative care.[77] Surgery cannot correct poor posture and body mechanics, relieve myofascial pain syndromes, or remedy faulty motor patterns of synergistic activity accompanying muscle substitution that occur in many patients with low back pain. Additionally, Hides, Richardson, and Jull[78,79] have found that the lumbar multifidi, a primary segmental stabilizer, do not spontaneously recover after low back pain, so it is doubtful that they will spontaneously recover after the trauma of spine surgery. The loss of these crucial active segmental stabilizers may lead to recurrent lumbar pain syndromes. To avoid this and aid the patient's rehabilitation after spinal surgery, the therapist must tirelessly question and reassess, using a problem-solving approach.

The following guidelines are not intended to be a substitute for sound clinical reasoning. Rather they are intended as a guide for the successful postoperative rehabilitation of patients after lumbar microdiscectomy. The primary goals after a lumbar microdiscectomy are the reduction of pain, prevention of recurrent herniation, restoration of normal muscle activity and biomechanics, maintenance of dural mobility, improvement of function, and early return to appropriate activities. Each patient's program must be individualized to attain these goals for the following reasons:

1. Patients have slightly different pathoanatomic abnormalities and surgical procedures.
2. Patients have different levels of strength, flexibility, and conditioning after surgery.
3. Patients' goals vary.
4. Patients have varying psychosocial factors.
5. Patients possess different levels of kinesthetic-proprioceptive coordination that affect their rate of motor learning.

Each patient must therefore receive care in accordance with individual needs. To this end the guidelines should be progressed as tolerated, and the therapist should not try to keep the patient "on schedule."

 Increasing lower extremity (LE) symptoms, progressive neurologic deficit, and incapacitating pain are obvious "red flags" that require prompt reevaluation. Although the therapist must not ignore pain, an acceptable level of discomfort is reasonable if the patient is increasing functional activities and progressing in the program as anticipated. Pain should be monitored in three parameters, with the therapist carefully noting the pain pattern (e.g., left lateral thigh to knee), observing the frequency (e.g., constant, intermittent, rare), and having the patient rate the intensity (0 to 10). This allows close tracking of changes in pain with exercise and activity so that the program can be progressed or modified accordingly.

Finally, any successful spinal rehabilitation program must not ignore psychosocial factors that negatively affect the program. It has been suggested that the greatest indicator for postoperative results is preoperative psychologic testing, not MRI or clinical signs.[80-83] Additionally, patients who have active litigation or workers' compensation claims have been shown to return to activity later than patients who do not.[84] These factors must be considered in evaluating patients, progressing exercise programs, and assessing clinical results.

Phase I (Protective Phase)

TIME: 1 to 3 weeks after surgery
GOALS: Protect the surgical site to promote wound healing, maintain nerve root mobility, reduce pain and inflammation, educate patient to minimize fear and apprehension, establish consistently good body mechanics for safe and independent self-care (Table 15-1)

The first postoperative week typically consists of protective rest, progressive ambulation, and appropriately limited activities. Activity tolerance is the result of progressive activity, not rest. The patient should be encouraged to walk at a comfortable pace for short distances several times a day. Patients are usually allowed to shower 7 days after surgery, depending on wound healing.

 Driving is usually not allowed for 1 to 2 weeks, although this may be extended if the right LE is significantly compromised. Typically patients can return to office work within 1 week. Because the patient in phase I has difficulty tolerating sustained positioning, he or she may require support during driving, sitting, and lying postures. Additionally, patients may need to be directly educated in changing positions frequently. Patients may have significant incisional pain, especially with flexion movements.

 The therapist must avoid all loaded lumbar flexion in patients in phases I and II. The patient can apply cold packs to the surgical site for 15 to 20 minutes several times a day to help control pain, muscle spasm, and swelling.

The therapist may begin outpatient physical therapy as soon as the patient can comfortably come to the clinic, usually in the second or third week. Treatment begins only after the patient is evaluated to ascertain the following:

- A thorough history of the condition, including previous treatments or surgeries and time out of work
- The present pain pattern (intensity and frequency) plus activities or postures that alter these symptoms
- The status of the wound site
- Anthropometric data, and postural and body mechanics assessment

 Limited mechanical testing (Standing motion testing and end-of-range movements are not assessed until after the fifth week postoperatively.)
- Neurologic status (examination includes neural tension testing)
- *Baseline core strength testing in nonaggravating position (i.e., supine)*

 The therapist must take care during the initial evaluation to avoid any testing that may injure an already

BOX 15-1 Oswestry Low Back Pain Disability Questionnaire

This questionnaire has been designed to give your physical therapist (PT) information as to how your back pain has affected your ability to manage in everyday life. Please answer every question by marking the one box that applies. We realize you may consider that two of the statements in any one section relate to you, but please just mark the box that most closely describes your problem.

Name:

Date: Initial Interim/Discharge

1. Pain intensity
   - I can tolerate the pain I have without having to use painkillers.
   - My pain is bad, but I manage without taking painkillers.
   - Painkillers give me complete relief from my pain.
   - Painkillers give me moderate relief from my pain.
   - Painkillers give me very little relief from my pain.
   - Painkillers have no effect on my pain, and I do not use them.

2. Personal care
   - I can look after myself normally without causing extra pain.
   - I can look after myself normally, but it causes extra pain.
   - It is painful to look after myself, and I am slow and careful.
   - I need some help, but I manage most of my personal care.
   - I need help every day in most aspects of self-care.
   - I do not get dressed, wash with difficulty, and stay in bed.

3. Lifting
   - I can lift heavy objects without causing extra pain.
   - I can lift heavy objects, but it gives me extra pain.
   - Pain prevents me from lifting heavy weights off the floor, but I can manage light to medium objects if they are conveniently positioned.
   - I can lift only very light objects.
   - I cannot lift anything at all.

4. Walking
   - Pain does not prevent me from walking any distance.
   - Pain prevents me from walking more than 1 mile.
   - Pain prevents me from walking more than $\frac{1}{2}$ mile.
   - Pain prevents me from walking more than $\frac{1}{4}$ mile.
   - I can only walk using a cane or crutches.
   - I am in bed most of the time and have to crawl to the toilet.

5. Sitting
   - I can sit in any chair as long as I like.
   - I can sit only in my favorite chair as long as I like.
   - Pain prevents me from sitting more than 1 hour.
   - Pain prevents me from sitting more than $\frac{1}{2}$ hour.
   - Pain prevents me from sitting more than 10 minutes.
   - Pain prevents me from sitting at all.

6. Standing
   - I can stand as long as I want without extra pain.
   - I call stand as long as I want, but it gives me extra pain.
   - Pain prevents me from standing more than 1 hour.
   - Pain prevents me from standing more than $\frac{1}{2}$ hour.
   - Pain prevents me from standing more than 10 minutes.
   - Pain prevents me from standing at all.

7. Sleeping
   - Pain does not prevent me from sleeping well.
   - I can sleep well only by taking medication for sleep.
   - Even when I take medication, I have less than 6 hours of sleep.
   - Even when I take medication, I have less than 4 hours of sleep.
   - Even when I take medication, I have less than 2 hours of sleep.
   - Pain prevents me from sleeping at all.

8. Sex life
   - My sex life is normal and gives me no extra pain.
   - My sex life is normal but causes some extra pain.
   - My sex life is nearly normal but is very painful.
   - My sex life is severely restricted by pain.
   - My sex life is nearly absent because of pain.
   - Pain prevents any sex life at all.

9. Social life
   - My social life is normal and gives me no extra pain.
   - My social life is normal but increases the degree of pain.
   - Pain has no significant effect on my social life apart from limiting my more energetic interests, such as dancing.
   - Pain has restricted my social life, and I do not go out as often.
   - Pain has restricted my social life to my home.
   - I have no social life because of pain.

10. Traveling
    - I can travel anywhere without extra pain.
    - I can travel anywhere, but it gives me extra pain.
    - Pain is bad, but I manage journeys of more than 2 hours.
    - Pain restricts me to journeys of less than 1 hour.
    - Pain restricts me to short, necessary journeys of less than $\frac{1}{2}$ hour.
    - Pain prevents me from traveling except to the doctor or hospital.

TABLE 15-1 Microdiscectomy

Rehabilitation Phase	Criteria to Progress to This Phase	Anticipated Impairments and Functional Limitations	Intervention	Goal	Rationale

Phase I Postoperative 1-3 wk	• Postoperative	• Edema
		• Pain
		• Limited tolerance to transfers
		• Limited tolerance to strained positions
		• Limited ADLs
		• Limited nerve mobility
		• Limited LE ROM
		• Limited trunk and LE strength
		• Limited mobility of neighboring regions
		• Limited walking
		• Limited cardiovascular endurance
			• Cryotherapy
			• Electrical stimulation
			• Supportive corset or brace as indicated
			• Body mechanics training—maintenance of lumbar lordosis and avoidance of trunk flexion with the following:
			  • Sitting and driving (supported as appropriate)
			  • Sleeping (supported as necessary, avoiding fetal position)
			  • Standing and walking (limit based on symptoms)
			  • Transfers—Spine or sit-stand, in and out of car, and floor to stand
			  • Self-care
			  • Avoid lifting
			  • Bending using hip hinging and neutral spine method
			• Spine dural mobilization
			• Prone dural mobilization
			• PROM stretches—Hip (flexion [knee bent], SLR [gently], ER, standing [gastrocnemis-soleus])
			• Joint mobilization of hip and thoracic spine as indicated
			• Progressive walking program on treadmill or flat surfaces
			• Begin progressive exercise program (in unloaded positions only)
			• Pelvic rocks
			• Supine pelvic rocks (midrange lumbar flexion AROM)
			• Side-lying pelvic rocks (midrange lumbar lateral flexion)
			• Quadruped pelvic rocks (midrange lumbar AROM)
			• Prone pelvic rocks (midrange lumbar extension AROM)
			• Supine abdominal bracing (isolated transverse abdominis contraction)
			• Supine abdominal bracing with arms behind head, progressed to alternating arm raises
			• Prone abdominal bracing with alternating arm raises, progressed to unilateral arm raises
			• Partial squatting to 60°
				• Manage edema
				• Control pain
				• Decrease pain with upright postures
				• Prevent complications and reinjury
				• Good understanding and use of proper body mechanics
				• Sit up to 20 minutes
				• Resume driving after 2 wk
				• Improve sleep patterns
				• Use "log roll" technique with transfers
				• Independent with self-care
				• Improve nerve mobility
				• Prevent adhesions that limit nerve mobility
				• Restore ROM to LE
				• Improve mobility of restricted joints
				• Increase tolerance to walking level surfaces for 30 minutes
				• Establish a healthy environment for the disc
				• Good neutral control of lumbar spine while supine and prone
				• Increased LE strength
					• Promote self-management of edema and pain
					• Provide abdominal support and decompression
					• Initiate education to prepare patient for independence with ADLs, avoiding reinjury
					• Maintain lordosis and avoid flexion postures to avoid excessive longation tension on surgical site
					• Promote protective rest and resumption of limited activities
					• Transfer while avoiding unnecessary stress on surgical site
					• Avoid lifting to prevent risk of reinjury
					• Decrease stress on surgical site
					• Prevent nerve fibrosis and dural adhesions
					• Improve LE flexibility to decrease stress in the lumbar spine
					• Avoid irritating sciatic nerve
					• Maintain and improve proximal and distal mobility to reduce stress in the surgical site
					• Prepare patient to resume ADLs and promote good cardiovascular conditioning
					• Controlled lumbar movements are beneficial after microdiscectomy secondary to hydrostatic changes of the disc to promote vascularity
					• Increase strength of trunk musculature to stabilize and protect the spine from injury
					• Increase tolerance to upright postures
					• Help with maintaining good body mechanics

ADLs, Activities of daily living; *AROM*, active range of motion; *LE*, lower extremity; *PROM*, passive range of motion; *ROM*, range of motion; *SLR*, straight-leg raises.

BOX 15-2 Waddell Signs

1. Superficial tenderness to light touch in the lumbar region or widespread tenderness to deep palpation in nonanatomic distributions
2. Increased symptoms with simulated axial loading or simulated rotation tests
3. Inconsistent supine and sitting SLR tests
4. Regional weakness or sensory abnormalities that are not myotomal or dermatomal
5. Physical overreaction or disproportionate verbalization during assessment

---

compromised patient. We typically include Waddell signs[85] late in the rehabilitation process to help delineate nonorganic physical signs (Box 15-2).

The mechanical examination must be very limited in the phase I and phase II patient. It is intended to elicit symptomatic and mechanical responses that suggest mechanical problems and so dictate the treatment course. **Because weight-bearing motion testing and end-of-range movements are typically not performed until after the fifth week postoperatively, the therapist uses responses to positioning and midrange movements in prone, supine, and side-lying positions to determine mechanical problems in the initial weeks.**

Hip muscle strength testing should be postponed in the early stages of healing to prevent stressing inflamed lumbosacral tissues. Neural tension testing is an integral part of the lumbar evaluation. Therefore the therapist should have the patient perform the SLR, Cram test, femoral nerve tension test (prone knee flexion), and supine dural tension and do the appropriate measuring, recording, and comparison with the opposite limb.

Slump testing should not be performed until after the fourth or fifth week postoperatively. Core strength testing may be performed in a variety of ways; however, Lee[86] describes a nice functional approach based on grouping core musculature into slings. A good understanding of soft tissue healing rates, spinal mechanics, and the specific surgical procedure helps avoid needless soft tissue trauma. For further evaluation of the patient's physical limitations and guidance toward appropriate functional training, the therapist can use the Modified Low Back Pain Oswestry Questionnaire[87] (see Box 15-1) or the Roland-Morris Functional Disability Questionnaire.[46] These are easily administered and helpful. The therapist should document the patient's perceived disability status before treatment and at predetermined intervals to monitor functional progress and determine the appropriate direction of functional training exercises.

After evaluation the therapist thoroughly explains the existing problems and the treatment plan to the patient. Therapist and patient should work together to reach mutual agreement on realistic goals. Patient education is crucial to achieving positive results because the patient ultimately treats himself or herself several hours each day with a home exercise program and self-treatment techniques. Furthermore, avoiding reinjury is perhaps the single most important postoperative factor responsible for a rapid progression in the program and ultimately full recovery. Through patient education, a safe and relatively rapid return to activities can occur. The physical therapist (PT) should educate the patient regarding proper postures, home exercises, self-care techniques, and body mechanics for the safe performance of activities of daily living (ADLs). Proper postures and body mechanics are crucial during the postoperative healing phase. Ideally the therapist should instruct the patient before surgery, but if this does not occur, then the first postoperative task is to teach the patient correct postures and body mechanics.

Proper Postures

The PT teaches the patient to maintain normal lumbar lordosis.

Patients should avoid lumbar flexion in standing or sitting because intradisc pressures are increased and excessive shear forces occur. Intolerance to prolonged postures is typical in phase I, and frequent movement breaks are recommended. The concept of abdominal bracing should be taught early. The therapist also should investigate the ergonomics of the patient's workstation to avoid potential problems.

Sitting and Driving. The therapist should do the following:

Caution the patient to never slouch while sitting.
- Instruct the patient in the use of a lumbar roll or similar device to maintain lordosis during sitting and driving.
- Advise the patient to try to always sit on firm, straight-back chairs and **never sit on soft sofas or chairs.**
- **Caution the patient to avoid all backless seating.** If the patient eventually will need to sit in bleachers or similar backless seating, then a Nada-Chair (Nada Concepts, Inc., Minneapolis) or a similar device should be recommended that supports the lumbar spine during this type of sitting.
- Encourage frequent movement breaks. Instruct the patient to avoid sitting longer than 20 minutes at a time for the first 2 weeks. This increases in subsequent weeks, depending on tolerance to pain.
- Allow patients to return to driving for short periods after about 1 to 2 weeks. Remind the patient that safety is a priority—not a convenience.

Sleeping. The therapist should do the following:
- Teach the patient to sleep in supported supine, supported side lying, or supported prone three-quarter lying with the spine straight.

Instruct the patient to avoid sleeping in the fetal position because of the prolonged lumbar flexion.

Have the patient avoid unsupported prone three-quarter lying positions because of the rotational component.

- Caution the patient to avoid lying on soft mattresses or sofas.

Standing and Walking. The therapist should do the following:

- Advise patients to limit standing at the kitchen sink or bathroom counter to short periods and avoid bending at the waist.
- Encourage the patient to maintain lumbar lordosis during standing and walking while performing an abdominal brace.

Body Mechanics

To allow the patient to progress rapidly, the therapist should do everything possible to avoid reinjury. Minor setbacks may delay progression of the program, and a major setback may be irreparable. The therapist should pay close attention to the patient's movements. Patients may say they understand correct mechanics but display incorrect movement patterns. Frequent and critical observation allows the therapist to evaluate the patient's spinal mechanics and determine whether the patient has integrated the correct postures and mechanics. A checklist of basic functional movements (i.e., rising from lying, rising from sitting, sitting in neutral, reaching overhead, bending to knee level) is helpful to record the performance of these skills and whether the patient requires cues to complete the tasks.

Transfers. The therapist should do the following:

- Teach the patient to move correctly from supine to sitting, from standing to lying on the floor, and from sitting to standing. Rolling in bed as a unit and rising from bed must be performed correctly. In addition, give instruction on entering and exiting a car. **Remember that all twisting motions are prohibited. Instruct them to move their feet to turn instead.**

Dressing. The therapist should do the following:

- Instruct the patient in the correct way to put on pants, socks, and shoes in the supine position. Slip-on shoes are the easiest to handle in the first 2 weeks. Tying shoes can later be performed safely by putting the foot on a stool or chair.

Hygiene. The therapist should do the following:

- Explain that showering can begin after the second week. Have the patient shave her legs in the standing position, with the foot on the tub or shower seat, avoiding lumbar flexion.

Lifting. The therapist should do the following:

- Remember that correct lifting techniques should be taught early and instruct patients to try to avoid all lifting in phase I. "Swoop lifting" is usually a safe and well-tolerated technique for light lifting in phase II. The patient performs it by taking a long stride forward to the kneeling position (i.e., lunge) and then reaching to lift a light object. The exercise is then performed in reverse.

Bending. The therapist should do the following:

- **Advise the patient to avoid all bending at the waist. Lumbar flexion with loading is arguably the most hazardous movement in the first two phases.** The interdisk pressures are significantly increased, and tension on the healing posterior annulus compounds the problem. Prolonged or repetitive bending is especially injurious.[88]
- Remember that, on occasion, limited bending is necessary. Teach the patient the correct way to bend and instruct him or her to avoid lumbar flexion while bending. The patient can safely bend by simultaneously flexing at the knees and hips ("hinge at the hips"), while maintaining a neutral spine and an abdominal brace. This is easy to teach by placing a 4-foot wooden pole (1 to 2 inches in diameter) along the spine with contact at the thoracic and sacral regions. By flexing slowly at the hips and knees while maintaining a neutral spine position and viewing themselves in a mirror, patients can practice this important movement.

Occasionally, patients with low back pain possess poor kinesthetic-proprioceptive coordination. A simple technique to improve the patient's sense of lumbar movement and position involves the use of tape. First, the therapist places the patient on all fours and has him or her assume a neutral spine position. The therapist places a 12- to 18-cm long piece of tape on the paraspinals parallel to the spine (Fig. 15-9), while avoiding placing the tape directly over the incision site. The therapist then asks the patient to make small movements into flexion and extension, always returning to neutral. The additional feedback from the tape pulling or wrinkling will assist the patient in learning spinal proprioception. Various postures can then be tried, including kneeling, side lying, sitting, and standing, with small motions of the lumbar spine while in each position. The patient then progresses to functional movements (e.g., transfers, walking, bending).

Exercise

Dural mobilization (i.e., mobilization of the nervous system, neurodynamic exercise, nerve root gliding, neural tension exercises) should begin as soon as possible in the first week. The preoperative neural compromise and the postoperative inflammation in and around the epidural space contribute to neural broses and dural adhesions. They are occasionally problematic and are easily preventable. An excellent presentation of neural mobilization principles and techniques can be found in Butler.[89]

Technique. The therapist should do the following:

- Supine dural mobilization (lower lumbar neural mobilization)—Have the patient lie supine on a firm surface with both knees extended. While the patient holds the back of the thigh with both hands, he or she slowly extends the knee with the ankle dorsiflexed to the point of stretch. He or she then slowly flexes and relaxes the

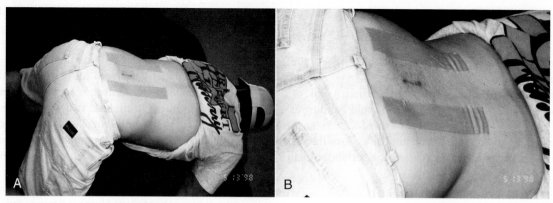

Fig. 15-9 Patient assumes a quadruped position, while the therapist places a 12- to 18-cm strip of tape on the paraspinals adjacent to the spine. The therapist should take care to avoid the incision site. **A,** Appearance of tape in squatting position. **B,** Close-up view of tape with return to standing position.

limb. Any symptoms and the maximal amount of knee extension attained should be recorded to monitor progress.

- Prone dural mobilization (upper lumbar neural mobilization)—Have the patient lie prone on a firm surface with both knees extended. Initially the patient may use a pillow under the abdomen for comfort if needed. Have the patient slowly flex the knee to the point of stretch, then slowly extend the knee and relax. *Make sure the patient maintains the abdominal brace throughout the exercise to stabilize the lumbar spine.* Alternate legs.

Dural mobilization should be done several times a day. The therapist must caution the patient that this exercise may provoke neural symptoms, and that he or she must allow the pain or tingling to resolve to baseline levels before beginning the next repetition. The patient should not overmobilize the neural tissues. **As with any exercise, self-mobilization of the nervous system at home is inappropriate until a positive response has been established from repeated movements in the clinic.** The dural mobilizations are progressed as tolerated to include other components of the affected nerve (e.g., ankle dorsiflexion, hip internal rotation [IR]). Eventually (in phase III) the patient can perform neural mobilizations while sitting ("sitting slump").

The early initiation of a progressive spinal-stabilization program is crucial to the eventual tolerance of more strenuous functional activities and sports skills. Because the lumbar spine is inherently unstable around the neutral zone, the trunk musculature must be sufficiently strong and coordinated to stabilize and protect the spine from injury.[90,91] The stabilization program progresses from unloaded spinal positions to partially loaded and eventually fully loaded functional training. The posterior pelvic tilt exercise is the least desirable exercise to obtain active lumbar stability.[90,92-94] The transversus abdominis must be isolated from the remaining abdominal musculature because it has consistently been shown to be active before the other abdominal muscles or the primary movers during limb motions, regardless of direction.[95,96] In addition, the transversus abdominis can become dysfunctional in patients with low back pain.[95,97-100] Therefore the transversus abdominis possesses a superior ability to stabilize the lumbar spine actively and locally.[38,101-103] Although

the more superficial abdominal muscles (the obliques) are important in lumbar stability, they are trained later in the program for their rotational contribution to limit lateral shear and torsional stresses and create trunk rotation. Early in phase II, the lumbar multifidi are isolated and trained because of their ability to stabilize segmentally.[102,104,105] In addition, it has been found that the lumbar multifidi atrophy in patients with low back pain and there is a decrease in muscle thickness change with activation.[100,106] Literature has also investigated the importance of the pelvic floor musculature in stabilizing the lumbar spine.[80,107,108] Evidence shows that the pelvic floor muscles cocontract with the transverse abdominus; therefore recruiting the pelvic floor muscles should be considered when instructing in bracing. Bracing has been shown to immediately increase posteroanterior spinal stiffness and stability.[109] Eventually a cocontraction of transversus abdominis, multifidus, and pelvic floor (abdominal bracing) is performed during all exercises and functional activities.[110,111] All the exercises should focus on control and technique and be progressed as tolerated to improve endurance of these primary stabilizers.

The PT should instruct the patient in the neutral spine concept and help the patient find the neutral spine position in various postures. The patient can then be taught to control the transverse abdominus with electromyographic (EMG) biofeedback, pressure biofeedback,* or rehabilitative ultrasound imaging[102,112-116] in several positions (e.g., supine, all fours, prone). Feedback available by rehabilitative ultrasound imaging has been shown to improve transverse abdominus and lumbar multifidus muscle recruitment up to 4 months posttraining.[117,118] After that, the patient can progress the postures to include sitting and standing and increase the duration of the contractions to 60 seconds.

Based on the information obtained in the history, the responses to various positions, and the limited clinical testing performed during the initial evaluation, the therapist determines which midrange lumbar movements are tolerated and are indicated for exercise. Correct and controlled lumbar movements are beneficial to the patient after microdiscectomy because hydrostatic changes of the disc promote

---

*Stabilizer, Inc., Chattanooga, Tenn.

improved vascularity.[119,120] To this end, the therapist teaches pelvic rocks in pain-free positions (e.g., all fours, prone). A pelvic rock is a repetitive and continuous pelvic tilt from an anterior to a posterior position. A bias toward lumbar extension is typical in the patient who has undergone microdiscectomy because lumbar extension reduces tangential stress posteriorly. A flexion bias is usually not recommended because the surgical entry is into the posterior disc and flexion positions tend to create stress to this area and tension on the incision. A healthy respect for soft tissue healing periods is essential.

The therapist instructs the patient in most of the following exercises in phase I, but he or she should not prescribe any exercise or position for the home program until repeated trials in the clinic have proven painless. Stabilization, flexibility, coordination, and spinal mobility exercises are included in an attempt to address all parameters. The exercise sequence is important and should be considered by the PT when adding exercises. Good technique and control of movement are essential. No exercise should increase the pain pattern or cause lingering pain. Clearly some muscular soreness may accompany the program, but this should be well tolerated and transient. The typical patient should be able to contract the transversus abdominis for 60 seconds in various positions within approximately 1 week after the initial visit.

The following exercises are taught in phase I:

1. Abdominal bracing on all fours (i.e., isolated transverse abdominis contraction, lumbar multifidus, and pelvic floor cocontraction) progressed to quadruped abdominal bracing with alternate arm raises
2. Quadruped pelvic rocks (i.e., midrange lumbar active range of motion [AROM])
3. Supine dural stretching (or prone dural stretching for upper lumbar disorders)
4. Supine abdominal bracing (isolated transverse abdominis contraction, lumbar multifidus, and pelvic floor cocontraction)
5. Supine pelvic rocks (i.e., midrange lumbar flexion AROM)
6. Supine abdominal bracing with arms behind head progressed to abdominal bracing with alternating arm raises
7. Supine gluteal, hip external rotator, and hamstring stretches to correct myofascial limitations; actively holding neutral spine during these low-load, long-hold exercises is important (Fig. 15-10)
8. Side-lying pelvic rocks (i.e., midrange lumbar lateral flexion AROM)
9. Prone pelvic rocks (i.e., midrange lumbar extension AROM)
10. Prone abdominal bracing with alternate arm raises progressed to prone abdominal bracing with bilateral arm raises
11. Gastrocnemius and soleus stretching in standing position (Fig. 15-11)
12. Partial squats to 60° of knee flexion while maintaining neutral spine with abdominal bracing

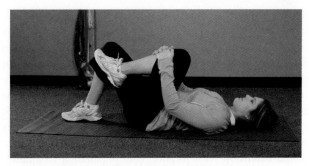

Fig. 15-10 Hip flexion is very important. When stretching the gluteals, the patient should pull the thigh toward the belly rather than toward the nose. This patient is attempting to increase the hip flexion angle rather than draw the pelvis into a posterior tilt.

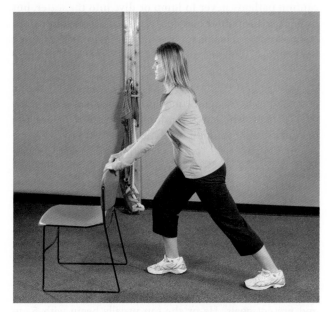

Fig. 15-11 Gastrocnemius and soleus stretching. While keeping the foot and heel of the back leg on the floor, the patient shifts the weight forward to the front leg. A stretch should be felt in the calf area. The patient should maintain the spine in neutral with an abdominal brace as the weight is shifted toward the front foot and the supporting thigh is kept directly below in the frontal plane.

Spinal Mobilization

Spinal mobilization of the lumbar spine is rarely used in phase I or II. Mobilization of the hips or thoracic spine may be needed and is best addressed on an individual basis. When progress is poor with active movements and deemed secondary to a hypomobile segment, mobilization to restore lumbar movement may be necessary in phase II. In phase III, mobilization can play an important role and is used frequently to reduce pain during specific lumbar motions, especially at end of range. A review of Maitland,[121] Mulligan,[122] and Paris[56] may assist in clinical reasoning.

Cardiovascular Conditioning

Cardiovascular conditioning is an important part of the rehabilitation program and is beneficial both for patients recovering from lumbar microdiscectomy and those with chronic low back pain.[123] In addition, endurance training of the LE musculature improves tolerance to prolonged standing and walking. When LE muscles fatigue, poor body mechanics soon follow. The patient typically performs aerobic training by progressive walking (on a treadmill or outdoors without hills), stationary cycling (on recumbent or upright bikes with the patient paying close attention to the maintenance of lordosis and avoidance of hip sway), or swimming (initially only the freestyle stroke with avoidance of "craning" during the breathing phase). Craning is suboccipital extension with rotation (occipitoatlantal to atlantoaxial) or cervical extension with rotation (C2 to C7). Swimming and aqua therapy are usually delayed until the second or third week after surgery to ensure complete wound healing and sufficient lumbar stabilization. **The PT must caution patients never to jump or dive into the water, but rather use the ladder or steps.** Aquatic therapy for postoperative lumbar rehabilitation is not covered in this chapter, but Watkins , Williams, and Watkins[124] present a good source for the interested clinician.

The therapist determines the patient's training heart rate and adheres to this guideline during all conditioning exercises. Patients who have no prior history of aerobic exercise or who are very deconditioned must progress slowly and be carefully monitored. Aerobic conditioning in phase I (with focus on correct postures and mechanics) may include walking, stationary cycling, and water exercises. Patients should avoid stair climbers and cross-country skiing machines until phase II, when adequate trunk stability is usually attained. In addition, rowing, running, and in-line skating should be avoided until phase III, when significant active lumbar stability has been achieved.

The progression of cardiovascular training is highly variable and depends on the patient's prior level of conditioning and present goals. He or she can usually begin with 5- to 10-minute bouts and progress at 5-minute intervals up to 30 or 60 minutes. The therapist must pay careful attention to patient position because correct postures deteriorate as fatigue increases. Neurologic weakness of the hip flexors or abductors, quadriceps, hamstrings, ankle dorsiflexors, and plantar flexors significantly alters gait and requires modification of the aerobic program to avoid abnormal mechanical stress.

Modalities

In general, the use of passive treatment techniques alone should be avoided; however, occasionally they may be necessary to augment the functional restoration program. The therapist should use pain control modalities only as needed to support the exercise program. Cryotherapy and interferential stimulation applied to the low back for 15 to 20 minutes after an exercise session are helpful. Some therapists may prefer electric myostimulation (EMS), microstimulation, or transcutaneous electrical nerve stimulation for muscle spasm reduction and pain control. However, EMS that is delivered too intensely in the first several weeks after surgery may unwittingly jeopardize the healing paraspinal muscle tissue and should therefore be used judiciously. The

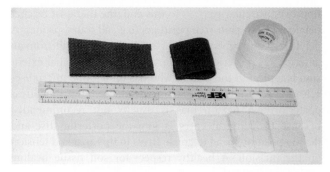

Fig. 15-12 Materials to manufacture compression patch (10- × 6-cm Neoprene pad, 2-inch elastic tape).

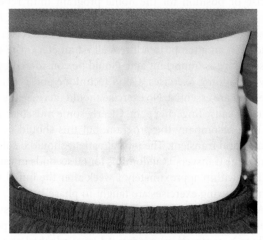

Fig. 15-13 Inspection of scar before application of compression patch.

patient's posture during modalities is always important and varies depending on positional tolerance. Supported prone lying or supported supine lying is usually quite comfortable in this phase.

Wound Care

Along with the patient's history, the inspection of the incision site during the initial evaluation helps determine whether extra measures are needed. Any signs of infection are a red flag that requires prompt medical intervention. Some patients desire "invisible" scars, whereas others are much less concerned. Because patients scar differently, the therapist should monitor their progress and offer solutions to excessive scarring or scar stretching. A compression taping technique can be used to limit hypertrophic scar formation and reduce surgical scar widening. First, the therapist folds a 10- × 6-cm Neoprene pad in half and secures it with a 2-inch wide elastic tape (Elastikon tape)* (Fig. 15-12). The pad is then affixed horizontally over the closed wound (Figs. 15-13 and 15-14) to provide both compression and approximation of the surgical scar. The patient wears the compression patch constantly for 6 to 10 weeks, removing it only to bathe. It should not be applied until the wound site is completely healed (approximately 2 weeks).

---

*Johnson & Johnson, New Brunswick, NJ

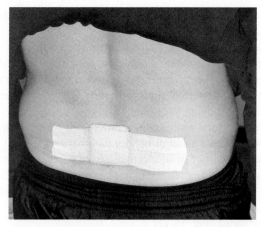

Fig. 15-14 The pad is affixed horizontally over the closed wound and held in place by 2-inch elastic tape.

Phase II (Functional Recovery Phase)

TIME: 4 to 6 weeks after surgery

GOALS: Understand neutral spine concept, improve cardiovascular condition, increase trunk strength to 80%, increase soft tissue mobility and LE flexibility and strength, maintain nerve root mobility (Table 15-2)

As surgical site pain diminishes and active spinal stability improves, the PT can increase the patient's program of functional activities and exercise. The patient in phase II should have complete wound healing, although some tenderness and paraspinal spasm may persist. Neural tension signs should be negative, but neurodynamic testing may reveal limitations. The patient should be gaining tolerance to

TABLE 15-2 Microdiscectomy

Rehabilitation Phase	Criteria to Progress to This Phase	Anticipated Impairments and Functional Limitations	Intervention	Goal	Rationale
Phase II Postoperative 4-6 wk	• No signs of infection • No increase in pain • Gradual increase in tolerance to activity • Demonstration of good knowledge of body mechanics • Performance of self-care with minimal modifications	• Pain • Limited nerve mobility • Limited trunk strength • Limited scar mobility • Limited soft tissue mobility • Limited tolerance of ADLs and sustained postures • Limited trunk stability and strength in numerous postures • Limited mobility of lumbar spine soft tissues • Poor recruitment of paraspinal muscles • Limited LE ROM • Limited cardiovascular endurance	• Continue as in phase I and progress cardiovascular activities as appropriate • Self-nerve mobilization using a belt to enhance the stretch • Isometrics with ROM—Spine abdominal bracing with alternate SLRs; progressed to cycling and dying bug when appropriate • Partial sit-ups with added rotation for obliques when appropriate • Prone (abdominal bracing with SLR extension): Begin with single leg and progress to double leg • Prone on-elbows lying, progress to partial press-ups • AROM with isometrics—All fours (abdominal bracing with single-leg raise, progress to opposite arm and leg raises); standing (abdominal bracing with squats to 60°, progress to 90° for 2-3 minutes); sitting on Swiss ball (abdominal bracing with hip flexion, arm flexion, and combinations of opposite arm and leg) • EMG training of lumbar spine multifidus muscles • PROM (stretches), then add iliopsoas and quadriceps • Soft tissue massage	• Cardiovascular exercise 20 minutes • Minimal to no neural tension signs • Trunk strength 80% • Use of neutral spine concepts in a variety of positions • Avoidance of lumbar spine extension while performing hip extension • Partial press-ups without pain • Good neutral control of lumbar spine in variety of postures • Increased strength of LEs • Improved sitting tolerance • Isolated contraction of lumbar spine paraspinal muscles • Increased LE flexibility • Increased soft tissue mobility	• Improve cardiovascular fitness • Restore neural-gliding mechanics • Prevent neural fibrosis and dural adhesions • Strengthen trunk musculature via neutral spine concepts • Perform exercises in midrange of lumbo-pelvic mobility • Stabilize and strengthen trunk while moving extremities, progressing from passive repositioning to dynamic stabilization • Restore full extension in non-weight-bearing position • Strengthen paraspinals and abdominals in a neutral position • Promote maintenance of a neutral spine in an upright posture to improve tolerance to compression positions • Increase tolerance to upright postures • Use biofeedback to improve recruitment of paraspinals • Improve flexibility of LEs to decrease stress on the spine • Improve myofascial interface and restore soft tissue mobility

ADLs, Activities of daily living; *AROM*, active range of motion; *EMG*, electromyographic; *LE*, lower extremity; *PROM*, passive range of motion; *ROM*, range of motion; *SLRs*, straight-leg raises.

functional activities and be able to perform all self-care with minor modifications. The patient's tolerance to aerobic exercise also should be improving. Correct body mechanics and postures should be maintained as functional activity increases. Patients should have confidence in their ability to stabilize the lumbar spine actively in all loaded positions. Pain-free lumbar AROM should be increasing to end-of-range strain only, although terminal flexion may still provoke pain.

The patient should continue to avoid loaded lumbar flexion. Through brief reevaluations in each treatment session, the therapist collects additional lumbar motion data. For example, if prone pelvic rocks are well tolerated, then the patient's positional tolerance to elbow lying and partial extension in lying can be assessed safely.

The therapist should avoid standing motion testing and sitting testing except for the most conditioned patients who are doing very well.

Exercise

A recent Cochrane systematic review of randomized controlled trials concluded that high-intensity exercise programs initiated 4 to 6 weeks postmicrodiscectomy lead to decreases in pain and disability faster than no treatment or low-intensity programs.[125] However, although early exercise intervention resulted in faster decreases in pain and disability, clinical outcomes at 1-year follow-up had similar results versus low-intensity or no exercise.[126,127] The therapist should instruct the patient in the correct way to contract and control the lumbar multifidus with EMG biofeedback. Special attention to the training of this important segmental stabilizer is essential.[128] Retraction of the paraspinal muscles during surgery can denervate the multifidus muscle.[129] Fortunately, lumbar microdiscectomy requires a minimal wound opening, so this complication is lessened. The patient should perform abdominal bracing (holding neutral spine with a cocontraction of the transverse abdominis, multifidus, and pelvic floor) in supine, prone, and all-fours positions, progressing to transition movements. Ultimately, the cocontraction is used to stabilize the lumbar spine during all ADLs. The therapist can progress the patient's midrange lumbar movements and spinal-stabilization program as tolerated, using Swiss ball exercises to improve balance and dynamic lumbar stabilization during sitting. **The patient should continue to avoid axial loading during end-range lumbar flexion or lateral flexion movements.** As the patient shows control and tolerance, the exercise level may be increased. Pain during exercise typically requires correction of the technique or exercise modification. In addition, muscle groups that may have been weakened by neurologic compromise (e.g., hip abductors, quadriceps, ankle plantar flexors, dorsiflexors) must be strengthened. The slow twitch fibers are most involved and are easily fatigued. The longer that neural compression and inflammation have been present, the longer the period before regeneration occurs. Careful attention to back-protected positions during strengthening exercises is crucial to avoiding reinjury.

Typical Phase II Exercises. The therapist should do the following:

1. Supine abdominal bracing with alternate SLRs, progressed to abdominal bracing with unsupported LE extension (i.e., cycling), progressed to abdominal bracing with unsupported upper extremity (UE) and LE extension (i.e., dying bug) (Fig. 15-15)
2. Supine dural mobilization, progressed to incorporate a belt or towel around the foot to enhance the effect
3. Supine partial sit-ups, progressed to partial sit-ups with rotation to facilitate oblique strengthening (Fig. 15-16)
4. Double-leg bridging, progressed to single-leg bridging and then to single-leg bridging with opposite knee extended (Fig. 15-17)
5. Prone elbow lying, progressed to partial press-ups
6. Prone abdominal bracing with single-leg raises, progressed to prone double-leg raises
7. Standing repetitive squats to 60°, progressed to 90° for 2 to 3 minutes

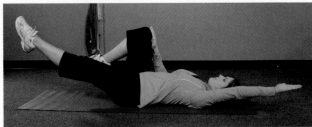
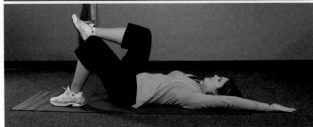

Fig. 15-15 Dying bug. This exercise teaches the patient to control extension and side-bending at the same time. The patient starts with the hands touching the knees directly over the hips and then extends the same-side arm and leg slowly and deliberately. The PT monitors the patient for side-bending or extension. The patient can modify this exercise by moving the arms and legs in smaller increments.

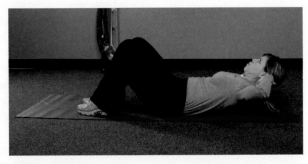

Fig. 15-16 Partial sit-ups are done in many positions. The important point is that the spine must remain in neutral, the abdominals must remain contracted throughout the exercise, and eccentric control must be emphasized. The lift is of the chest, not the head. Legs can be in extended position to bias lumbar extension.

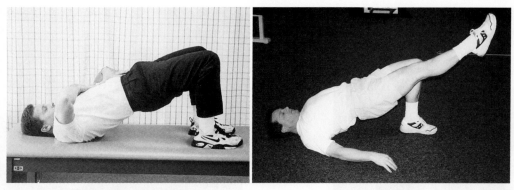

Fig. 15-17 Bridging. This exercise teaches the patient to brace the spine first, then lift the trunk as a unit. The patient is moving in and out of a hip hinge and emphasis is on coordinating the trunk and hip muscles.

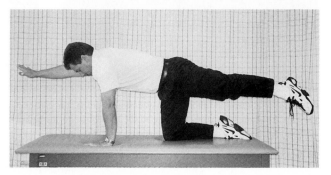

Fig. 15-18 From the quadruped position, the therapist should teach the patient to keep the hands under the shoulders and knees under the hips, extending the opposite arm and leg.

8. Abdominal bracing on all fours with single-leg raise, progressed to opposite arm and leg raises (Fig. 15-18)
9. Balance board training on both limbs, progressed in duration
10. Isolated strengthening of neurologically compromised muscles
11. Swiss ball sitting exercise progression (in neutral spine with abdominal brace)
12. Stretching of the quadriceps, gluteals, hip external rotators, iliopsoas, hamstrings, and calves as required to correct myofascial limitations (Figs. 15-19 through 15-22; see also Fig. 15-11)

Soft Tissue Mobilization

Scarring of myofascial elements with collagen cross-fibers or fibrofatty tissue limits muscle broadening during contraction and connective tissue elasticity during movement.[130] Muscle spasm and protective guarding of the gluteals and low back musculature may persist. Soft tissue mobilization of the lumbar paraspinals and buttock musculature is frequently needed to improve muscle function and reduce spasm.[131] The PT must exercise care when performing soft tissue mobilization to the paraspinals before the third or fourth week after surgery because the tissue healing is incomplete. The mechanical and reflexive effects of soft tissue mobilization are well suited for patients recovering

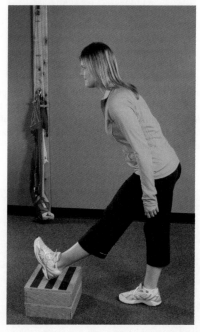

Fig. 15-19 Hamstring stretching is taught in a standing position if possible so that the patient can work on contralateral hip stability and trunk control while stretching. The patient can work the foot up and down while maintaining the stretch to increase the nerve-gliding component. A slight bend in the knee with more hip hinge will move the stretch up from the musculotendinous junction into the muscle belly.

from microdiscectomy, and certain techniques are particularly beneficial before paraspinal strengthening (e.g., sidelying paraspinal pull from midline). Careful questioning and soft tissue examination will uncover gluteal trigger points that can cause buttock or LE pain patterns.[76] These myofascial pain syndromes are not uncommon preoperatively and may linger postoperatively. With appropriate treatment they can be relieved so that the functional restoration program may progress. Scar massage to release adherent soft tissue also may be needed.

Spinal Mobilization

Spinal mobilization using nonthrust maneuvers may be beneficial for patients in phase II if they do not have protective

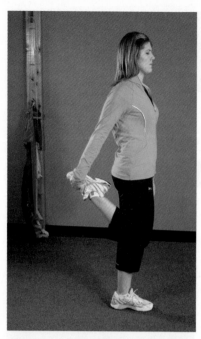

Fig. 15-20 Initially the quadriceps stretch is performed in a prone position and then is taught in standing position if possible to develop trunk control against an extension moment. If the patient does not have sufficient ROM, then he or she should modify the stretch by placing the foot on a table. Abdominal control prevents lumbar extension.

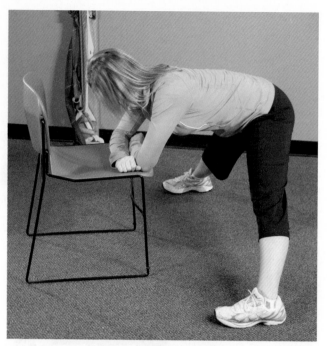

Fig. 15-22 Adductor flexibility is important for squatting. The patient can vary the trunk angle or apply pressure to the inner knee to increase the stretch.

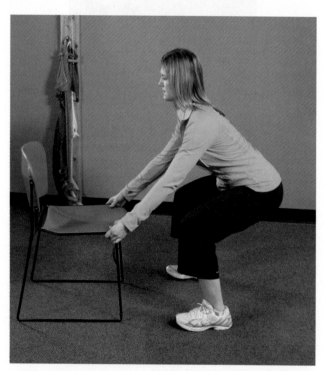

Fig. 15-21 Gracilis stretch is important for squatting to the side.

muscle spasm, bone disease of the spine, or hypermobile or irritable adjacent motion segments. Muscle energy techniques are usually well tolerated and best suited for phase II.

Thrust maneuvers (grade V or high-velocity manipulations) are not indicated.

Cardiovascular Conditioning

The PT should continue to progress the cardiovascular program in intensity and duration of aerobic training. The use of cross-country ski machines, stair climbers, and swimming for aerobic exercise is allowed if sufficient trunk stability has been achieved. **Patients should avoid rowing and in-line skating until phase III.**

Running is not recommended until after the twelfth week after surgery because of the degree of spinal stabilization required and the repetitive axial loading sustained by the disc.

Modalities

The therapist and patient should use modalities only as needed to support the exercise program. Cryotherapy and interferential stimulation to the low back after exercise may be beneficial.

Phase III (Resistive Training Phase)

TIME: 7 to 11 weeks after surgery
GOALS: Ensure patient is independent in self-care and ADLs with minimal alterations, increase tolerance to activities, progress return to previous level of function

The patient in phase III should consistently perform correct body mechanics and postures without prompting and should tolerate almost all functional activities. Prolonged positioning (e.g., unsupported sitting) may still provoke low back pain, but this should be easily relieved with change of position or simple stretching exercises. Soft tissue healing at this stage is largely complete, although some surgical site tenderness may still be present. All self-care and ADLs should be performed confidently and painlessly with minimal modifications. Patients in phase III should have good tolerance to midrange lumbar movements and sufficient spinal stabilization to perform spinal movements in loaded positions.

The resumption of lifting activities must be progressive and occur with careful instruction. Because approximately half of all workers' compensation claims for low back injury result from lifting objects, this patient group needs proportionally more instruction and functional training.

Because soft tissue healing is nearly complete by phase III, more extensive mechanical testing can be performed to ascertain tolerance to various lumbar movements, as well as the end range sensation.

Standing motion testing (without overpressure) and seated testing can be performed safely on most patients after 6 weeks. The outcome of the movement testing determines to a great extent the treatment and exercise progression. Neural tension signs should be negative unless scarring has occurred. Occasionally some neurologic signs and symptoms persist into the third phase, but with monitoring and calm encouragement the PT can reassure affected patients

that these symptoms will subside with continued neural mobilization and time.

Researchers[132] and clinicians note that flexibility, strength (stability), and coordination return at different rates after injury. During spinal rehabilitation, flexibility should precede strength, proximal strength should precede distal strength, and strength should precede coordination. This culminates in the more rapid and fluid functional movements seen in uninjured persons. The PT must be sure to consider the sequence of return of these various elements, the existing limitations uncovered during mechanical testing, and the patient's realistic goals when planning the progression of the exercise program.

Exercise

Functional training exercises (i.e., sports-specific drills, work-hardening activities) typically begin in phase III. Preset goals determine the kinetic activities that are to be the focus of rehabilitation. The therapist closely supervises the progression of these activities, paying careful attention to the quality of spinal mechanics and lumbar stabilization. Functional training is focused on trunk movements that simulate activities to which the patient will return. Sports-specific training (Figs. 15-23 through 15-26) can begin if the patient

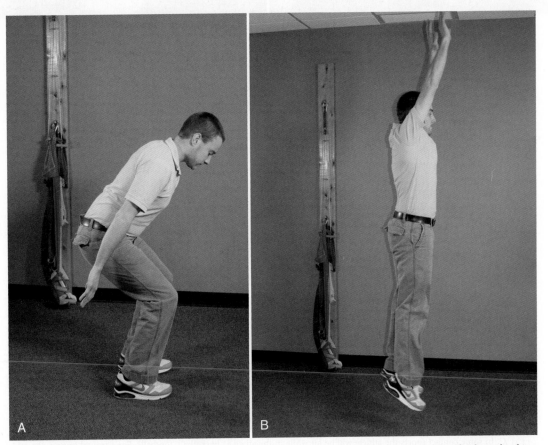

Fig. 15-23 A, Landing from a jump is invariably more difficult for jumping athletes. It is imperative that they learn to land in a hip hinge position and be trained to absorb as much shock as possible eccentrically through the hips, knees, and ankles, before it reaches the spine. Plyometric drills are helpful. **B,** While in the air with the arms overhead, the therapist should train the jumping athlete to perform a brace with the transverse abdominals to prevent extraosseous lumbar motion. When blocking a ball with the arms overhead (as in volleyball), the athlete should brace more intensely to resist the impact of the ball. Medicine ball drills are helpful.

Continued

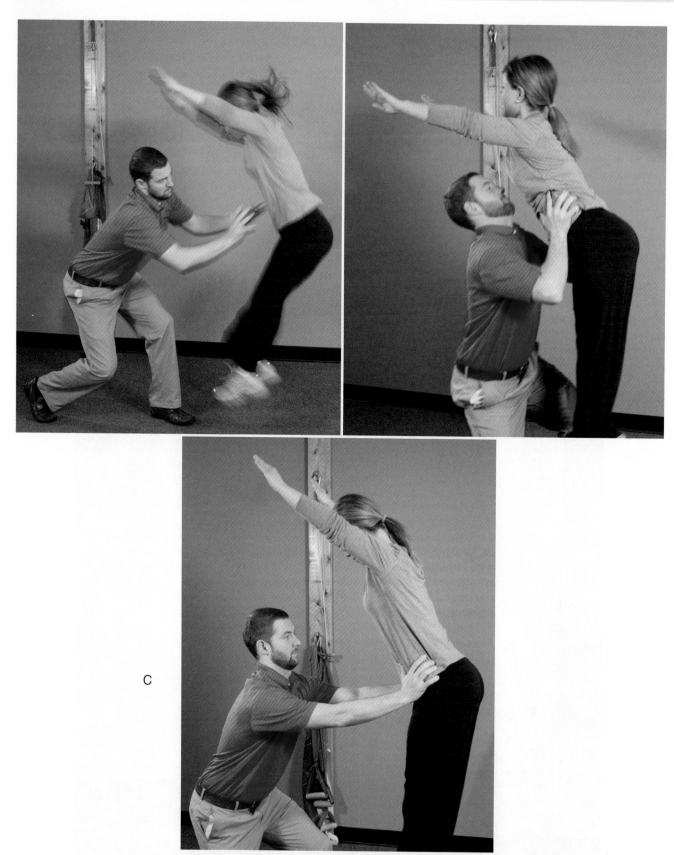

Fig. 15-23, cont'd C, In some contact sports the athlete will be hit while in the air (e.g., basketball, football). For a frontal impact, the athlete should give way at the hips; for a hit from an angle, he or she should learn to pivot away from the blow. Drills such as those shown here with progressively more difficult blows are helpful to train this specialized skill.

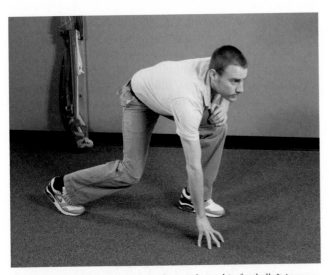

Fig. 15-24 A three-point stance is frequently used in football. It is essentially an exaggerated hip hinge. Adequate hip flexibility is essential, as well as preaction abdominal bracing.

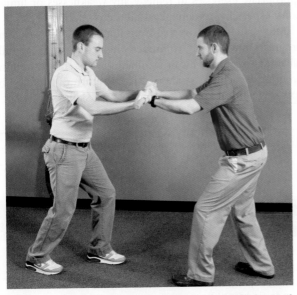

Fig. 15-25 In rugby and football, an athlete is frequently required to prevent someone from running around him or her. Stick drills such as this can teach a patient to adapt quickly to changing forces, while maintaining a neutral spine with an abdominal brace.

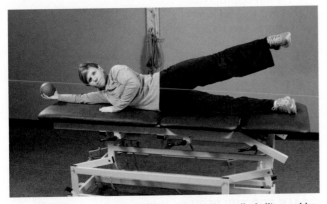

Fig. 15-26 When diving for a ball (as in baseball or volleyball), an athlete is taught to go low to the ground, stay horizontal, and land as a unit. A significant abdominal brace is required.

has achieved sufficient active lumbar stability and spinal mobility in fully loaded positions, as well as adequate myofascial flexibility and conditioning. The therapist can use proprioceptive training with balance boards and Swiss balls. Initially, athletes who take part in running and jumping activities are most safely trained with unloading devices,* during supervised treadmill running or jump training. These patients are typically well conditioned before surgery and have progressed postoperatively without setbacks.

Golfers need to be trained to hold the neutral spine dynamically during all five phases of the swing. The PT can incorporate specific strength, flexibility, and balance exercises to achieve a safe and mechanically sound golf swing.[124]

Work-hardening activities for medium to heavy work classifications typically begin at 8 weeks and include lift training from 25 to 50 lb. Workers in these fields need special attention with regard to materials handling and should have a functional capacity evaluation 10 to 12 weeks after surgery to determine appropriate return-to-work status.

The exercise program progresses in intensity and difficulty to include rotational trunk stability, overhead activities, and balance training using a balance board. Training the patient in diagonal patterns in loaded positions better simulates real-life situations. A new stabilization exercise for patients in phase III challenges the obliques and transverse abdominals with minimal stress to passive tissues.[76] McGill[133] refers to this exercise as isometric side-support on knees or on feet (depending on the degree of difficulty). Therapists should prescribe this exercise for home performance only after proving patient tolerance during clinic sessions.

The spinal mobility program attempts to restore painless and full lumbosacral ROM. The PT should prescribe appropriate exercises and incorporate mobilization to achieve full and pain-free lumbar ROM and continue the stretching exercises needed to attain normal myofascial flexibility.

Soft Tissue Mobilization

Soft tissue mobilization should continue as needed to ensure a pliable surgical scar, proper gluteal and paraspinal muscle function, and soft tissue extensibility.

Spinal Mobilization

Spinal mobilization should be used when necessary to restore motion at hypomobile segments and reduce pain associated with movement. Because the restoration of normal spinal motion is a primary goal, the therapist must identify and correct aberrant arthrokinematics. The expanded mechanical testing in phase III will reveal limitations or provoke symptoms that require attention. Maitland,[121] Mulligan,[122] and Paris[56] can be reviewed to assist in clinical reasoning.

Cardiovascular Conditioning

Cardiovascular conditioning should continue to progress in intensity and duration. The patient's aerobic fitness program is determined by the ultimate activity goals. A typical

---

*Vigor Equipment, Inc., Stevensville, Mich.

sedentary office worker obviously does not train as intensely as a professional athlete. However, the therapist should not underestimate the aerobic demands placed on a manual laborer and should encourage appropriate endurance exercises.

Aerobic conditioning (focusing on correct postures and mechanics) may include treadmill walking, stationary cycling, the use of cross-country ski machines and stair climbers, swimming, and skating (in-line or on ice). Patients who have had previous experience with rowing may resume this exercise. Attention to proper stroke form is important, and modification to maintain lordosis may be necessary.

Patients should not start a running program until after the twelfth week postoperatively because of the high compressive and repetitive axial loads at heel strike. A walk-run program should be initially implemented on a treadmill, with the therapist supervising and analyzing gait. *When the patient does resume running, it should be in the morning hours when the disc is maximally hydrated.*[124]

Modalities

Cryotherapy may still be beneficial after intensive training sessions. EMS, transcutaneous electrical nerve stimulation, microcurrent, interferential stimulation, and other modalities are seldom necessary.

Discharge Planning

When the anticipated goals and desired outcomes have been attained, the patient is discharged with a home or club exercise program (or with both). The exercise program is to be maintained indefinitely. As always, the postsurgical patient should try to return to premorbid activity levels. Because goals vary dramatically among patients, some may require substantially more training than others, such as overhead lift training, plyometric jump training, or sport-specific skill training. A reasonable level of tolerance to strenuous work activities or recreational sports should be attained before these higher activity level patients are discharged.

The comprehensive lumbar evaluation performed in phase III reveals any limitations in motion, weaknesses, neural restrictions, and painful movements that still need to be addressed. The PT can obtain additional information from computerized testing devices[132]* that provide objective data on lumbar motion speed, acceleration and deceleration, and degree of ROM. Other testing equipment, such as computerized isokinetic machines, determines objective trunk strength values at various speeds of lumbar ROM. This information can be helpful in guiding the therapist to choose appropriate exercises to remedy any weaknesses or limitations, especially in more physically active patients.

Most patients recovering from lumbar microdiscectomy progress uneventfully if properly educated and carefully rehabilitated. The PT can facilitate the systematic training program to achieve a safe and rapid return of function by applying clinical knowledge and manual skills.

---

*Lumbar Motion Monitor, Chattanooga Group, Inc., Chattanooga, Tenn.

Suggested Home Maintenance for the Postsurgical Patient

Week 1

GOALS FOR THE WEEK: Protect the surgical site to promote wound healing, maintain nerve root mobility, reduce pain and inflammation, educate patient, establish consistently good body mechanics for safe and independent self-care

1. Protect the incision site.
2. Begin gentle nerve root gliding.
3. Maintain lumbar lordosis and correct body mechanics.
4. Avoid holding positions for prolonged periods and avoid all lumbar flexion.
5. Walk daily with a gradual increase in the duration and speed.
6. Use ice as needed for discomfort.

Weeks 2-3

GOALS FOR THE PERIOD: Protect the surgical site to promote wound healing, maintain nerve root mobility, reduce pain and inflammation, educate patient to minimize fear and apprehension, establish consistently good body mechanics for safe and independent self-care

1. Progress walking program to 20 to 30 minutes.
2. Maintain nerve root mobility.
3. Begin progressive exercise program (unloaded positions only):
   a. Pelvic rocks in quadruped and prone positions
   b. Abdominal bracing in several positions
   c. Supported dying bug at end of 3 weeks or when appropriate
   d. Elbow lying to partial extension in lying
   e. Prone alternating arm raises
   f. Partial squatting (to 60°)
   g. Gentle stretching of hamstrings, calves, gluteals, hip adductors, and rotators as needed
4. Maintain proper postures and body mechanics.
5. Practice isolated contractions of transverse abdominal muscles used frequently during daily activities.
6. Begin scar compressive taping as needed.
7. Use ice as needed for discomfort.

Weeks 4-6

GOALS FOR THE PERIOD: Understand neutral spine concept, improve cardiovascular condition, increase trunk strength to 80%, increase soft tissue mobility and LE flexibility and strength

1. Maintain nerve root mobility.
2. Progress exercise program (partially loaded positions):
   a. Partial press-ups to full press-ups
   b. Prone alternating leg raises to prone double-leg raises
   c. Unsupported dying bug
   d. Double-leg bridging progressing to single-leg bridging
   e. Partial sit-ups with rotation
   f. Side-lying double-leg raises
   g. All-fours arm and leg raises
   h. Repetitive squatting (starting at 60° and progressing to 90°)
3. Strengthen neurologically compromised muscles as needed (e.g., hip abductors, ankle dorsiflexors, plantar flexors, evertors).
4. Gentle stretching of hamstrings, calves, quadriceps, gluteals, hip adductors, and rotators as needed.
5. Progress aerobic conditioning (e.g., walking, swimming, cycling) to 30 to 60 minutes.
6. Practice cocontractions of transverse abdominal muscles and multifidus frequently during daily activities.
7. Use ice as needed for discomfort.
8. Massage the scar as needed.
9. Continue compressive scar care as needed.

Weeks 7-11
GOALS FOR THE PERIOD: Ensure patient is independent in self-care and ADLs with minimal alterations, increase tolerance to activities, progress return to previous level of function

1. Progress exercise program (loaded positions):
   a. Press-ups
   b. Prone "Superman" (simultaneous arm and leg raises)
   c. Dying bug with weights
   d. Single-leg bridging with weights
   e. Partial sit-ups with rotation
   f. Side-lying double-leg raises with weights
   g. Isometric side support on elbow and knees progressed to feet
   h. All-fours arm and leg raises with weights
   i. Standing rotary-torso with resistive tubing
   j. Repetitive squatting (to 90°)
2. Begin functional training exercises (sports- and work-specific activities) at end of phase if able.
3. Continue LE myofascial stretching as needed.
4. Continue strengthening neurologically compromised muscles.
5. Develop and segue into final home or club exercise program (or into both).

CLINICAL CASE REVIEW

1 What are the goals for the first week following microdiscectomy?

(1) Protect the incision site; (2) maintain nerve root mobility; (3) reduce pain and inflammation; (4) educate the patient; (5) establish consistent body mechanics.

2 Mikayla has been progressing well over the first couple of weeks following her microdiscectomy. Today she comes in complaining of a general feeling of fatigue. She also reports that she thinks she has had a fever for about a week. What should you do?

You should inspect Mikayla's wound site for signs of infection. Look for any oozing or discharge from the wound. Note any increased redness or warmth about the incision site. Fever and malaise can be a sign of infection (or just a cold). If you suspect an infection, prompt referral back to her surgeon is indicated.

3 Myrna had microdiscectomy 2 weeks ago. She wants to go to her son's baseball game this weekend. What should her therapist tell her?

Her therapist should tell her the following:
• Caution her to avoid sitting in bleachers or on benches without any back support.
• Suggest she take some type of alternative seating device that has some back support.
• Recommend frequent changes of position (avoid sitting greater than 20 minutes at a time).
• She should avoid slouching while sitting to prevent increased intradisc pressures and shear forces that can be caused by flexing in a sitting position.

4 Rick is 41 years old. He has had progressing back pain episodes over the past 2 years. An MRI shows a herniated disc at L4-L5. Rick also has intermittent complaints of left radicular leg pain. He had microdiscectomy surgery 2 weeks ago and has come to outpatient physical therapy for evaluation and treatment. How should a spinal evaluation be altered to assess a patient who has recently had microdiscectomy surgery?

Mechanical testing should be limited (standing motion testing and end-of-range movements are not assessed until 5 weeks after surgery). Hip muscle strength testing should be postponed in the early stages of healing to prevent stressing inflamed lumbosacral tissues. Slump testing is not performed until much later. A good understanding of soft tissue healing rates, spinal mechanics, and the specific surgical procedure helps avoid needless soft tissue trauma.

5 Summer continues to have difficulty performing a proper brace. What can you do to assist her?

You can use EMG, pressure biofeedback, or rehabilitative ultrasound imaging to help Summer learn how to properly brace again.

6 Edna was a sedentary person before her surgery. You find that she is resistant to doing any exercises and appears afraid of "messing up her surgery." What should you tell Edna?

Edna should be educated on the changes in muscle function following microdiscectomy. Also, she should know that not properly rehabilitating those muscles can lead to chronic back problems in the future. Assure her that you will be tailoring her exercise program to her individual needs and will be respecting pain.

7 Verlyn is a 40-year-old woman. She had microdiscectomy surgery for the L5 disc 6 weeks ago. Back pain is minimal. LE flexibility and strength is gradually improving. Trunk strength also is progressing. She is now seeing a PT for treatment. Previous treatments have included modalities for pain control, LE flexibility exercises, trunk and general strengthening, cardiovascular conditioning, and body mechanics. Verlyn is concerned about the intermittent radicular pain in her right leg. Prolonged sitting, walking, or standing aggravates her right leg. She reports reproduction of calf pain with hamstring stretching. What treatment technique should be used to decrease calf pain frequency and intensity?

Verlyn tested positive for adverse neural tension in the right leg. After several treatments of mobilization to the nervous system, complaints of pain decreased significantly in intensity and frequency.

8 Karla has a 5-month-old daughter at home. She arrives at therapy 3 weeks after a microdiscectomy procedure. What should Karla be instructed to do immediately?

Karla should be instructed to do the following:
- She should avoid lifting and carrying her child as much as possible for the first 3 to 4 weeks after her surgery. This may require educating her family members that she will require assistance initially.
- She should be instructed in proper body mechanics and correct lifting techniques when lifting or carrying her daughter.
- She should be taught that hip hinging and swoop lifting are necessary when bending to pick up after her child.

9 Jason works in a warehouse where he must repeatedly carry heavy boxes and walk for most of the day. He had surgery 9 weeks ago and does not understand why his therapist has him riding a bicycle and walking on a treadmill as part of his lumbar microdiscectomy rehabilitation. If he has to do aerobic exercise, he would rather run. What is the therapist's rationale for these exercises?

The following explains the therapist's rationale:
- Cardiovascular conditioning is beneficial for patients recovering from microdiscectomy surgery.
- Jason's job requires prolonged walking; he will need endurance of his LEs to prevent fatigue of his legs, which can lead to poor body mechanics.
- Running should not be initiated until after the twelfth week of surgery, when the patient is able to stabilize his spine well and the repetitive axial loading is not as much of a concern.

10 Raquel is having difficulty finding a comfortable position while sleeping after her microdiscetomy. After questioning her you find that she typically sleeps on her side in the fetal position. What should you tell Raquel?

Raquel should avoid sleeping in the fetal position as this places the lumbar spine in prolonged flexion, which you want to avoid after microdiscectomy surgery.
   Recommend the following positions instead:
- Supported supine lying with a pillow under the knees
- Supported sidelying with a pillow between the knees and arms
- Supported prone three-quarter lying with the spine straight (see Fig. 16-7, A through C)

11 Summer is almost 3 months postmicrodiscectomy. She had been making excellent progress until last week when she returned to her Pilates class. Now she is complaining of low back pain, which occurs when she does a postpelvic tilt as instructed in the class. What should you tell Summer?

Posterior pelvic tilting should be avoided because it puts the lumbar spine in a flexed position. Be aware of your patients' activities and what they require so that you may adequately prepare them to return to their previous recreational or professional activities. Summer may also need to review the proper way to brace her lumbar spine by engaging her transverse abdominis, multifidi, and pelvic floor muscles.

12 Kristy is a 36-year-old mother of two who had a microdiscectomy over 3 months ago. She is currently off work from her job as a waitress where she injured her back. Objectively she appears to have made a great recovery from her surgery; however, she consistently reports high pain levels with any activity. What may be contributing to her report of pain?

Psychosocial factors need to be considered in every patient's prognosis. Patients who have workers' compensation claims have been shown to return to activity later than patients who do not.

13 Russell is ready to return to running. What is the safest way he can do this following his microdiscectomy 3 months ago?

Initially a walk-run program should be implemented on a treadmill with supervision by the PT analyzing his biomechanics. An unloading device can also be used. Advise Russell to run first thing in the morning—when he progresses to outdoor running—when his discs are maximally hydrated and can offer the most shock absorbing capability.

14 Ken had an L4 microdiscectomy 3 weeks ago. Today he has 9/10 pain and return of pain down his posterior leg. Upon examination you note that his knee jerk reflex is absent and he has weakness of his quadriceps. What should you do?

Incapacitating pain and neurologic deficit are "red flags." Joe should be referred back to his surgeon immediately for reevaluation.

15 Lynne had a microdiscectomy over 10 years ago but never had physical therapy. She is now having lower back pain and her physician has sent her to therapy. She has poor segmental motion and inability to stabilize her trunk with extremity motions. Why might this be?

Lumbar segmental stabilizers do not spontaneously recover after injury and this can lead to recurrent lumbar pain syndromes. Also, Lynne may have developed faulty motor programs and muscle substitutions, which could also contribute to her current problem.

REFERENCES

1. Boden SD, et al: Abnormal magnetic resonance scans of the lumbar spine in asymptomatic subjects: A prospective investigation. J Bone Joint Surg 72A:403-408, 1990.

2. Yasuma T, et al: Histological development of intervertebral disc herniation. J Bone Joint Surg 68A:1066-1072, 1986.

3. Buirski G, Silberstein M: The symptomatic lumbar disc in patients with low-back pain: Magnetic resonance imaging appearances in both a symptomatic and control population. Spine 18:1808-1811, 1993.

4. Jensen MC, et al: Magnetic resonance imaging of the lumbar spine in people without back pain. N Engl J Med 331:69-73, 1994.

5. Delamarter RB: Lumbar microdiscectomy: Microsurgical technique for treatment of lumbar herniated nucleus pulposus. Instr Course Lect 51:229-232, 2002.

6. Hardy RW: Lumbar discectomy: Surgical tactics and management of complications. In Frymoyer JW, editor: The adult spine: Principles and practice, ed 2, Philadelphia, 1997, Lippincott-Raven.

7. Davis H: Increasing rates of cervical and lumbar spine surgery in the United States, 1979-1990. Spine 19:1117-1124, 1994.

8. Delamarter RB, McCulloch J: Microdiscectomy and microsurgical spinal laminotomies. In Frymoyer JW, editor: The adult spine: Principles and practice, ed 2, Philadelphia, 1997, Lippincott-Raven, pp 1961-1988.

9. Caspar W, et al: The Caspar microsurgical discectomy and comparison with a conventional standard lumbar disc procedure. Neurosurgery 28:78-87, 1991.

10. McCulloch JA, Snook D, Kruse CF: Advantages of the operating microscope in lumbar spine surgery. Instr Course Lect 51:243-245, 2002.

11. Silvers HR: Lumbar disc excisions in patients under the age of 21 years. Spine 19:2387-2392, 1994.

12. Souza GM, Baker LL, Powers CM: Electromyographic activity of selected trunk muscles during dynamic spine stabilization exercises. Arch Phys Med Rehabil 82(11):1551-1557, 2001.

13. Tureyen K: One-level one-sided lumbar disc surgery with and without microscopic assistance: 1-year outcome in 114 consecutive patients. J Neurosurg 99(suppl 3):247-250, 2003.

14. Urban JPG, et al: Nutrition of the intervertebral disc. Clin Orthop Relat Res 170:296, 1982.

15. Zahrawi F: Microlumbar discectomy: Is it safe as an outpatient procedure? Spine 9:1070-1074, 1994.

16. Weber H: Lumbar disc herniation: A controlled, prospective study with 10 years of observation. Spine 8:131-140, 1983.

17. Atlas SJ, et al: The Maine Lumbar Spine Study. II. One-year outcomes of surgical and nonsurgical management of sciatica. Spine 21:1777-1786,1996.

18. Atlas SJ, et al: Surgical and nonsurgical management of sciatica secondary to a lumbar disc herniation: Five-year outcomes from the Maine Lumbar spine Study. Spine 26:1179-1187, 2001.

19. Weinstein JN, et al: Surgical versus nonoperative treatment for lumbar disc herniation: Four-year results for the Spine Patient Outcomes Research Trial (SPORT). Spine 33:2789-2800, 2008

20. Deyo RA, et al: How many days of bed rest for acute low back pain? A randomized clinical trial. N Engl J Med 315:1064, 1986.

21. Krolner B, Toft B: Vertebral bone loss: An unheeded side effect of therapeutic bed rest. Clin Sci 64:437, 1983.

22. Waddell G, et al: Non-organic physical signs in low-back pain. Spine 5:117, 1980.

23. Carragee EJ: Indications for lumbar microdiscectomy. Instr Course Lect 51:223-228, 2002.

24. Errico TJ, Fardon DF, Lowell TD: Open discectomy as treatment for herniated nucleus pulposus of the lumbar spine. Spine J 3:45S-49S, 2003.

25. McCulloch JA, Young PH: Microsurgery for lumbar disc herniation. In McCulloch JA, Young PH, editors: Essentials of spinal microsurgery, Philadelphia, 1998, Lippincott-Raven.

26. Kostuik J, et al: Cauda equina syndrome and lumbar disc herniation. J Bone Joint Surg 68:386, 1986.

27. Sihvonen T, et al: Local denervation atrophy of paraspinal muscles in postoperative failed back syndrome. Spine 18:575, 1993.

28. Hanley EN: The surgical treatment of lumbar degenerative disease. In Vaccaro AR, editor: Orthopaedic knowledge update: Spine, Rosemont, Ill, 1997, American Academy of Orthopaedic Surgeons.

29. Findlay GF, et al: A 10-year follow-up of the outcome of lumbar microdiscectomy. Spine 23(10):1168-1171, 1998.

30. Gibson JN, Grant IC, Waddell G: Surgery for lumbar disc prolapse. Cochrane Database Syst Rev (3):CD001350, 2006.

31. Hakelius A: Prognosis in sciatica: A clinical follow-up of surgical and non-surgical treatment. Acta Orthop Scand 129(suppl):1-76, 1970.

32. McCulloch JA: Focus issue on lumbar disc herniation: Macro- and microdiscectomy. Spine 21(suppl 24):45S-56S, 1996.

33. Weir BKA, Jacobs GA: Reoperation rate following lumbar discectomy: An analysis of 662 lumbar discectomies. Spine 5:366-370, 1980.

34. De Divitiis E, Cappabianca P: Lumbar discectomy with preservation of the ligamentum flavum. Surg Neurol 57(1):5-13, 2002.

35. McCulloch JA, Young PH: The microscope as a surgical aid. In McCulloch JA, Young PH, editors: Essentials of spinal microsurgery, Philadelphia, 1998, Lippincott-Raven.

36. Wilson DH, Harbaugh R: Microsurgical and standard removal of the protruded lumbar disc: A comparative study. Neurosurgery 8:422-427, 1981.

37. Wilson DH, Kenning J: Microsurgical lumbar discectomy: Preliminary report of 83 consecutive cases. Neurosurgery 4:137-140, 1979.

38. Sapsford RR, et al: Co-activation of the abdominal and pelvic floor muscles during voluntary exercises. Neurourol Urodyn 20(1):31-42, 2001.

39. Deen HG, Fenton DS, Lamer TJ: Minimally invasive procedures for disorders of the lumbar spine. Mayo Clin Proc 78(10):1249-1256, 2003.

40. Maroon JC: Current concepts in minimally invasive discectomy. Neurosurgery 51(5S):137-145, 2002.

41. Abramovitz JN, Neff SR: Lumbar disc surgery: Results of the prospective lumbar discectomy study of the Joint Section on Disorders of the Spine and Peripheral Nerves of the American Association of Neurological Surgeons and the Congress of Neurological Surgeons. Neurosurgery 29:301-308, 1991.

42. Barrios C, et al: Microsurgical versus standard removal of the herniated lumbar disc. Acta Orthop Scand 61:399-403, 1990.

43. Thomas AMC, Afshar F: The microsurgical treatment of lumbar disc protrusions. J Bone Joint Surg 69B:696-698, 1987.

44. Peterson M, Wilson J: Job satisfaction and perceptions of health. J Occup Environ Med 38(9):891, 1996.

45. Panjabi MM: The stabilizing system of the spine. I. Function, dysfunction adaptation and enhancement. J Spinal Disord 5:383, 1992.

46. Roland M, Morris R: A study of the natural history of back pain. I. The development of a reliable and sensitive measure of disability in low-back pain. Spine 8:141, 1983.

47. Williams RW: Microlumbar discectomy: A conservative surgical approach to the virgin herniated lumbar disc. Spine 3:175-182, 1978.

48. Spengler DM: Lumbar discectomy: Results with limited disc excision and selective foraminotomy. Spine 7:604-607, 1982.

49. McCulloch JA, Young PH: Wound healing and mobilization. In McCulloch JA, Young PH, editors: Essentials of spinal microsurgery, Philadelphia, 1998, Lippincott-Raven.

50. Bookwalter JW, Buxch MD, Nicely D: Ambulatory surgery is safe and effective in radicular disc disease. Spine 19:526-530, 1994.

51. Ng JKF, Richardson CA, Jull GA: Electromyographic amplitude and frequency changes in the iliocostalis lumborum and multifidus muscles during a trunk holding test. Phys Ther 77(9):954, 1997.

52. Carragee EJ, Helms E, O'Sullivan GS: Are postoperative activity restrictions necessary after posterior lumbar discectomy? A prospective study of outcomes in 50 consecutive cases. Spine 21(16):1893-1897, 1996.

53. Watkins RG, Dillin WH: Lumbar spine injury in the athlete. Clin Sports Med 9(2):419, 1990.

54. McCulloch JA, Young PH: Foraminal and extraforaminal lumbar disc herniation. In McCulloch JA, Young PH, editors: Essentials of spinal microsurgery, Philadelphia, 1998, Lippincott-Raven.

55. Loupasis GA, et al: Seven- to 20-year outcome of lumbar discectomy. Spine 24(22):2313-2317, 1999.

56. Paris SV: Mobilization of the spine. Phys Ther 49:988, 1979.

57. Gogan WJ, Fraser RD: Chymopapain: A 10-year, double blind study. Spine 17:388-394, 1992.

58. Lorenz M, McCulloch JA: Chemonucleolysis for herniated nucleus pulposus in adolescents. J Bone Joint Surg 67A:1402-1404, 1985.

59. DeLucca PF, et al: Excision of herniated nucleus pulposus in children and adolescents. J Pediatr Orthop 14:318-322, 1994.

60. Peacock EE Jr: Dynamic aspects of collagen biology. I. Synthesis and assembly. J Surg Res 7:433-446, 1967.

61. Singhal A, Bernstein M: Outpatient lumbar microdiscectomy: A prospective study in 122 patients. Can J Neurol Sci 29(3):249-252, 2002.

62. Obenchain TG: Speculum lumbar extraforaminal microdiscectomy. Spine J 1(6):415-420, 2001.

63. Parisini P, et al: Lumbar disc excision in children and adolescents. Spine 26(18):1997-2000, 2001.

64. Papegelopoulos, PJ, et al: Long-term outcome of lumbar discectomy in children and adolescents sixteen years of age or younger. J Bone Joint Surg Am 80:689-698, 1998.

65. McCulloch JA, Young PH: Complications (adverse effects) in lumbar microsurgery. In McCulloch JA, Young PH, editors: Essentials of spinal microsurgery, Philadelphia, 1998, Lippincott-Raven.

66. Shapiro S: Cauda equina syndrome secondary to lumbar disc herniation. Neurosurgery 32:743-746, 1993.

67. Travell JG, Simmon DG: Myofascial pain and dysfunction: The trigger point manual, vols 1-2, Baltimore, 1992, William & Wilkins.

68. Rogers LA: Experience with limited versus extensive disc removal in patients undergoing microsurgical operations for ruptured lumbar disc. Neurosurgery 22:82-85, 1988.

69. White T, Malone T: Effects of running on intervertebral disc height. J Orthop Sports Phys Ther 12:410, 1990.

70. Wohlfahrt D, Jull G, Richardson C: The relationship between the dynamic and static function of abdominal muscles. Aust J Physiother 39(1):9, 1993.

71. Gill K: Percutaneous lumbar discectomy. J Am Acad Orthop Surg 1(1):33-40, 1993.

72. Onik GM: Percutaneous discectomy in the treatment of herniated lumbar disks. Neuroimaging Clin N Am 10(3):597-607, 2000.

73. Onik GM, Kambin P, Chang MK: Minimally invasive disc surgery. Nucleotomy versus fragmentectomy. Spine 22(7):827-828, 1997.

74. Haig A, et al: Prospective evidence for changes in paraspinal muscle activity after herniated nucleus pulposus. Spine 17(7):926, 1993.

75. Moreland J, et al: Interrater reliability of six tests of trunk muscle function and endurance. J Orthop Sports Ther 26(4):200, 1997.

76. Triano JJ, Schultz AB: Correlation of objective measures of trunk motion and muscle function with low-back disability ratings. Spine 12(6):561, 1987.

77. McCulloch JA: Microdiscectomy: The gold standard for minimally invasive disc surgery. Spine: State Art Rev 11(2):373, 1997.

78. Hides JA, Richardson CA, Jull GA: Multifidus inhibition in acute low back pain: Recovery is not spontaneous. MPAA Conf Proc 1995;57.

79. Hides JA, Richardson CA, Jull GA: Multifidus muscle recovery is not automatic after resolution of acute, first-episode low back pain. Spine 21(23):2763-2769, 1996.

80. Scalzitti DA: Screening for psychological factors in patients with low back problems: Waddell's nonorganic signs. Phys Ther 77(3):306, 1997.

81. Schofferman J, et al: Childhood psychological trauma and chronic refractory low-back pain. Clin J Pain 9(4):260, 1993.

82. Schutz H, Watson CPN: Microsurgical discectomy: Prospective study of 200 patients. Neurol Sci 14:81-83, 1987.

83. Saberi H, Isfahani AV: Higher preoperative Oswestry Disability Index is associated with better surgical outcome in upper lumbar disc herniations. Eur Spine J 17(1):117-121, 2008.

84. Karas R, et al: The relationship between nonorganic signs and centralization of symptoms in the prediction of return to work for patients with low back pain. Phys Ther 77(4):354, 1997.

85. Waddell G: A new clinical model for the treatment of low-back pain. Spine 12(7):632, 1987.

86. Lee D: The pelvic girdle, ed 2, Edinburgh, 1999, Churchill Livingstone.

87. Hudson-Cook N, Tomes-Nicholson K, Breen A: A revised Oswestry disability questionnaire. In Roland MO, Jenner JR, editors: Back pain: new approaches to rehabilitation and education, New York, 1989, Manchester University Press.

88. Hickey DS, Hukins DWL: Relation between the structure of the annulus fibrosus and function and failure of the intervertebral disc. Spine 5(2):106, 1980.

89. Butler DS: Mobilization of the nervous system, Melbourne, 1991, Churchill Livingstone.

90. Kavcic N, Grenier S, McGill SM: Determining the stabilizing role of individual torso muscles during rehabilitation exercises. Spine 29(11):1254-1265, 2004.

91. Panjabi MM, et al: On the understanding of clinical instability. Spine 19(23):2642, 1994.

92. Richardson C, Jull G: Muscle control-pain control: What exercises would you prescribe? Man Ther 1:2, 1995.

93. Richardson C, et al: Therapeutic exercise for spinal segmental stabilization in low back pain: Scientific basis and clinical approach. St Louis, 2000, Churchill Livingstone.

94. Roberts MP: Complications of lumbar disc surgery. In Hardy RW, editor: Lumbar disc disease, New York, 1992, Raven.

95. Hodges PW, Richardson CA: Contraction of the abdominal muscles associated with movement of the lower limb. Phys Ther 77:132, 1997.

96. Yasuma T, et al: Histologic changes in aging lumbar intervertebral discs. J Bone Joint Surg 72A:220-229, 1990.

97. Ferreira PH, et al: Changes in recruitment of transversus abdominis correlate with disability in people with chronic low back pain. Br J Sports Med 44(16):1166-1172, 2010.

98. Teyhen DS, et al: Changes in lateral abdominal muscle thickness during the abdominal drawing-in maneuver in those with lumbopelvic pain. J Orthop Sports Phys Ther 39(11):791-798, 2009.

99. Teyhen DS, et al: Ultrasound characteristics of the deep abdominal muscles during the active straight leg raise test. Arch Phys Med Rehabil 90(5):761-767, 2009.

100. Kiesel KB, et al: A comparison of select trunk muscle thickness change between subjects with low back pain classified in the treatment-based classification system and asymptomatic controls. J Orthop Sports Phys Ther 37(10):596-607, 2007.

101. Hodges PW, et al: Intervertebral stiffness of the spine is increased by evoked contraction of transverse abdominis and the diaphragm: In vivo porcine studies. Spine 28(23):2594-2601, 2003.

102. Hebert JJ, et al: A systematic review of the reliability of rehabilitative ultrasound imaging for the quantitative assessment of the abdominal and lumbar trunk muscles. Spine 34(23):E848-E856, 2009.

103. McGalliard MK, et al: Changes in transverse abdominis thickness with use of the abdominal drawing-in maneuver during a functional task. PM R 2(3):187-194, 2010.

104. Barr KP, Griggs M, Cadby T: Lumbar stabilization: Core concepts and current literature. I. Am J Phys Med Rehabil 84(6):473-480, 2005.

105. McKenzie RA: The lumbar spine: Mechanical diagnosis and therapy, ed 2, Waikanae, NZ, 2003, Orthopedic Physical Therapy Products.

106. Wallwork TL, et al: The effect of chronic low back pain on size and contraction of the lumbar multifidus muscle. Man Ther 14(5):496-500, 2009.

107. Newman MH: Outpatient conventional laminotomy and disc excision. Spine 20:353-365, 1995.

108. Arab AM, et al: Assessment of pelvic floor muscle function in women with and without low back pain using transabdominal ultrasound. Man Ther 15(3):235-239, 2010.

109. Stanton T, Kawchuk G: The effect of abdominal stabilization contractions on posteroanterior spinal stiffness. Spine 33(6):694-701, 2008.

110. Hides JA, et al: Effect of stabilization training on multifidus muscle cross-sectional area among young elite cricketers with low back pain. J Orthop Sports Phys Ther 38(3):101-108, 2008.

111. Hides JA, et al: Retraining motor control of abdominal muscles among elite cricketers with low back pain. Scand J Med Sci Sports 20(6):834-842, 2009.

112. Koppenhaver SL, et al: Reliability of rehabilitative ultrasound imaging of the transverse abdominis and lumbar multifidus muscles. Arch Phys Med Rehabil 90(1):87-94, 2009.

113. Teyhen DS, et al: Changes in deep abdominal muscle thickness during common trunk-strengthening exercises using ultrasound imaging. J Orthop Sports Phys Ther 38(10):596-605, 2008.

114. Wallwork TL, Hides JA, Stanton WR: Intrarater and interrater reliability of assessment of lumbar multifidus muscle thickness using rehabilitative ultrasound imaging. J Orthop Sports Phys Ther 37(10):608-612, 2007.

115. Henry SM, Teyhen DS: Ultrasound imaging as a feedback tool in the rehabilitation of trunk muscle dysfunction for people with low back pain. J Orthop Sports Phys Ther 37(10):627-634, 2007.

116. Hides JA, et al: Ultrasound imaging assessment of abdominal muscle function during drawing-in of the abdominal wall: An intrarater reliability study. J Orthop Sports Phys Ther 37(8):480-486, 2007.

117. Herbert WJ, Heiss DG, Basso DM: Influence of feedback schedule in motor performance and learning of a lumbar multifidus muscle task using rehabilitative ultrasound imaging: A randomized clinical trial. Phys Ther 88(2):261-269, 2008.

118. Teyhen DS, et al: The use of ultrasound imaging of the abdominal drawing-in maneuver in subjects with low back pain. J Orthop Sports Phys Ther 35(6):346-355, 2005.

119. Holm S, Nachemson A: Variations in the nutrition of the canine intervertebral disc induced by motion. Spine 8(8):866, 1983.

120. Vroomen PC, et al: Lack of effectiveness of bed rest for sciatica. N Engl J Med 340(6):418-423, 1999.

121. Maitland GD, et al: Maitland's vertebral manipulation, ed 7, London, 2006, Butterworth-Heinemann.

122. Mulligan BR: Manual therapy "NAGS", "SNAGS", "MWMS", etc, ed 6, Wellington, NZ, 2010, Orthopedic Physical Therapy Products.

123. Manniche C, et al: Intensive dynamic back exercises with or without hyperextension in chronic back pain after surgery for lumbar disc protrusion. Spine 18(5):560, 1993.

124. Watkins RG IV, Williams LA, Watkins RG III: Microscopic lumbar discectomy results for 60 cases in professional and Olympic athletes. Spine 3(2):100-105, 2003.

125. Ostelo RW, et al: Rehabilitation after lumbar disc surgery: An update Cochrane review. Spine 34(17):1839-1848, 2009.

126. Danielson JM, et al: Early aggressive exercise for postoperative rehabilitation after discectomy. Spine 25(8):1015-1020, 2000.

127. Donaldson BL, et al: Comparison of usual surgical advice versus a nonaggravating six-month gym-based exercise rehabilitation program post-lumbar discectomy: Results at one-year follow-up. Spine J 6(4):357-363, 2006.

128. Williams RW: Microdiscectomy: Myth, mania, or milestone? An 18-year surgical adventure. Mt Sinai J Med 58:139-145, 1991.

129. Silvers HR: Microsurgical versus standard lumbar discectomy. Neurosurgery 22:837-841, 1988.

130. Groslin AJ, Cantu R: Myofascial manipulation: Theory and clinical management, New York, 1989, Forum Medicum.

131. Cottingham JT, Maitland J: A three-paradigm treatment model using soft tissue mobilization and guided movement-awareness techniques for a patient with chronic low back pain: A case study. J Orthop Sports Ther 26(3):155, 1997.

132. Tullberg T, Isacson J, Weidenhielm L: Does microscopic removal of lumbar disc herniation lead to better results than standard procedure? Spine 18:24-27, 1993.

133. McGill SM: Distribution of tissue loads in the low back during a variety of daily and rehabilitation tasks. J Rehabil Res Dev 34(4):448, 1997.

CHAPTER 16

Lumbar Spine Fusion

Chris Izu, Haideh V. Plock, Jessie Scott, Paul Slosar, Adam Cabalo

In the early 1900s two surgeons began performing lumbar fusions. Dr. Russell Hibbs and Dr. Fred Albee pioneered the posterior approaches for arthrodesis.[1,2] Over the subsequent decades, many surgeons improved fusion techniques, with extension of the fusion laterally to incorporate the transverse processes and the sacral ala.[3-6] The patient's autogenous iliac crest is the standard source of bone graft material.[7,8] A rapid evolution has occurred in the development and use of spinal fixation devices. Although tracing the historical evolution of these devices is beyond the scope of this chapter, they can simply be categorized as anterior or posterior fixation devices. The most common and most controversial are the pedicle screw and rod/plate systems. Anterior fixation devices include screw and rod/plate systems, as well as the recently introduced interbody cages. This chapter describes the indications for elective lumbar fusions and discusses the various methods of arthrodesis.

SURGICAL INDICATIONS AND CONSIDERATIONS

In the elective patient population, most indications for lumbar arthrodesis are based on the presence of severe, disabling back or leg pain. Posttraumatic cases of segmental instability or potential neurologic injury also may require fusions, but this chapter focuses on patients with degenerative spinal pathology.

Patients with low back pain experience symptoms resulting from tissue aggravation during the degenerative cascade.[9] Trauma or overuse causes the disc wall to begin to develop microtears; this eventually results in a loss of disc height that alters the alignment of the facet joints. This may lead to pain, with accompanying spasm and guarding. The joints begin to develop synovitis, articular cartilage degeneration, and adhesions. This alters the spinal motion mechanics at that segment, further stressing the annulus of the disc and accelerating the degenerative process of the facet. Increased wearing of the cartilage and hypermobility of the facet also occur. The superior and inferior facet surfaces begin to enlarge. As the joint becomes more disrupted, normal motion at that segment becomes impossible. The disc begins to undergo greater strain. The disc wall weakens further, begins to bulge, and can eventually herniate. The disc continues to lose fluid and height, causing narrowing of the neural foramen, or foraminal stenosis. This process is outlined in Table 16-1.

Patients with severe back pain that is refractory to conservative care may be candidates for surgical evaluation. Conservative care should include a rigorous attempt at exercise-based dynamic stabilization training, therapeutic injections, and medications. Surgical treatment should only be discussed with the patient after a firm diagnosis has been made.

Diagnostic Tests

Spinal radiographs show osteophytes and segmental disc space narrowing in patients with degenerative spondylosis. A defect in the pars interarticularis is seen in patients with spondylolysis. Anterolisthesis, or a forward slippage of one vertebra on the next, is the hallmark radiographic finding in spondylolisthesis. Flexion and extension films can help to detect hypermobility or excessive motion in degenerative lumbar conditions.

Computed tomography (CT) reliably evaluates the bone or spondylosis compression against the nerves. Computer-enhanced reformatted CT images are as effective in evaluating spinal stenosis as myelography. CT scanning is more sensitive than magnetic resonance imaging (MRI) in the evaluation of bony stenosis, whereas MRI gives useful information about the health of the discs and nerves. Combining the two imaging modalities gives a very accurate, thorough picture of the lumbar spinal pathoanatomy.

Provocative discography can be a useful diagnostic tool in the work-up of patients with painful degenerative lumbar disc disease. The lumbar discs are deep within the abdominal cavity and do not have true dermatomal pain patterns in axial discogenic cases. Overlapping sclerodermal referred pain patterns in the lumbar spine make the localization of the true pain generator difficult. Discography has evolved as

TABLE 16-1 The Degenerative Cascade

Structure	Damage at Each Stage		
	Stage 1: Dysfunction	Stage 2: Instability	Stage 3: Stability
Intervertebral disc	• Circumferential tears • Inflammatory exudates and irritation	• Radial tears • Loss of disc height • Internal disruption • Disc bulges and herniations	• Loss of proteoglycans and water, fibrotic resorbtion • Sclerosis and eventual bony ankylosis
Facet joints	• Synovitis • Minor cartilage degeneration	• Laxity of joint capsule • Moderate cartilage degeneration	• Significant bony overgrowth • Grossly degenerated cartilage
Muscles	• Spasm, guarding	• Chronic shortening and fibrosis	• Further shortening and fibrosis
Neural foramen	• Unaffected	• Narrowed through annular bulges • Disc narrowing • Bony overgrowth	• Significant stenosis • Disc narrowing

a test to examine the lumbar discs morphologically and, most importantly, provocatively. On injection into the disc, the patient must communicate to the discographer if that disc is concordantly painful. Many degenerative discs are either not painful or discordantly painful. This information can be useful for the surgeon and the patient contemplating lumbar arthrodesis. The test is not used as frequently as in the past, as authors have described conflicting results and there is emerging concern that the injection itself may cause eventual disc deterioration.[10]

Diagnosis

Among patients undergoing elective lumbar arthrodesis, painful degenerative disc disease is the most prevalent diagnosis. Confirmatory diagnostic testing often includes MRI scanning and discography for equivocal cases. Overlap occurs among patients who have had previous surgery and have a diagnosis of "failed back surgery syndrome," a nonspecific diagnosis. Before surgery is contemplated, every effort must be made to arrive at a diagnosis that specifically isolates the source of pain.

Patients often have numerous diagnoses, each of which may be valid. For example, a 45-year-old man who had a laminotomy performed 5 years ago for a herniated nucleus pulposus comes to his physician complaining of 50% low back pain and 50% right leg pain and numbness. Diagnostic imaging is significant for L4 to L5 segmental degeneration with osteophytes and narrowing of the disc space. A multiplanar CT scan reveals moderate spondylosis (bone spurs) with stenosis along the right neural foramen. Discography is concordant with pain reproduction at the L4 to L5 disc. The appropriate diagnoses include painful degenerative disc disease, lumbar spondylosis with stenosis, and postlaminectomy syndrome.

The absolute requisite for a successful lumbar surgery outcome is matching concordant patient symptoms with the appropriate surgical procedure. Patients who cannot manage their pain with conservative measures and have demonstrable, concordant pathology on diagnostic testing may benefit from lumbar arthrodesis.

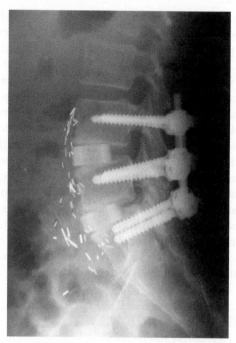

Fig. 16-1 Pedicle screw instrumentation in a circumferential lumbar fusion.

TYPES OF FUSIONS

Instrumentation Versus Noninstrumentation

The goal of a lumbar arthrodesis is the successful union of two or more vertebra. Controversy exists over the most efficient way to achieve this result. Instrumentation can be used to immobilize the moving segments while the fusion becomes solid. One of the original and most popular systems is the Harrington hook/rod construct. Although this *distraction* type of fixation immobilizes the spine in certain planes, it causes a loss of physiologic lordosis, or a "flat-back syndrome," in many patients.

Today, most spine surgeons use pedicle screw constructs to immobilize the vertebrae rigidly while preserving the normal lumbar lordosis[2] (Fig. 16-1). Typically, external orthosis bracing is not needed in these cases. As well-controlled studies emerge, data support the use of internal fixation for fusion.[11] Most studies support the use of pedicle screw fixation to obtain a more reliable bony union, although complication rates tend to be higher with these devices as well.[12,13]

Some surgeons do not routinely use pedicle screws for arthrodesis. In most of these situations (when pedicle screws are used) the patient must wear a lumbar orthosis for an extended period postoperatively. To immobilize the L5 to S1 motion segment effectively, an orthosis with a thigh-cuff extension must be applied. Patients with noninstrumented fusions may take an extensive amount of time to stabilize and become comfortable in their rehabilitation. Conversely, most patients with internal fixation become mobile and independent more rapidly, making early rehabilitation more predictable.

Posterior Fusion

Posterolateral Lumbar Fusion

Different surgeons use different techniques to perform a lumbar fusion. The traditional approach is through a midline posterior incision. If necessary the surgeon performs a laminectomy/laminotomy to address the pertinent pathology. Most surgeons perform a posterolateral fusion, which means that the transverse processes, pars interarticularis, and, if needed, the sacral alae are decorticated. The patient's own iliac crest bone graft or a bone graft substitute is then placed on the decorticated surfaces, forming a fusion bed contiguous with all the surfaces to be fused. Pedicle screws and rods or plates may be placed to immobilize the motion segments rigidly and augment the formation of a solid union.

The problems with a posterolateral fusion are both mechanical and physiologic. The fusion is attempting to form at a mechanical disadvantage because of tension. Bone heals more reliably under protected physiologic loads of compression, not tension. Also, the available area for the bone union to occur is limited to the remaining posterolateral bone surfaces. After extensive decompression of the neural elements (laminectomy), the available fusion area is reduced and often poorly vascularized. These local factors reduce the likelihood of a successful arthrodesis. Nicotine use negatively influences the formation of posterolateral lumbar fusions.

Finally, the usual source of pain in these patients is the disc itself, hence the term discogenic. In routine cases of posterolateral fusions the disc is not radically resected. Biomechanical studies have shown that people bear load through the middle and posterior thirds of the disc. Several reports describe a persistently painful disc under a solid posterior fusion.[14] As surgeons recognized the biomechanical and physiologic aspects of the discs, they began performing interbody fusions.[15]

Interbody Fusion
Posterior Lumbar Interbody Fusion. Interbody fusions evolved to address many of the drawbacks of traditional posterolateral fusions. Radical excision of the disc and anterior column support with rigid bone grafting are performed. The available area for successful bone union is greatly increased by using the interbody space.

Using a posterior lumbar approach, a surgeon performs a posterior lumbar interbody fusion (PLIF). After a wide laminectomy the posterior two thirds of the disc is resected and an interbody graft is placed into the evacuated disc space. This provides anterior interbody stability through a posterior approach. PLIF is a technically demanding procedure associated with a higher incidence of postsurgical nerve injuries.

Transforaminal Lumbar Interbody Fusion. In an effort to reduce the incidence of nerve injury performed through a PLIF, a transforaminal lumbar interbody fusion (TLIF) technique was developed. Studies have shown the results of TLIF with posterior pedicle screw instrumentation to be equivalent to that of anterior-posterior fusions with an anterior lumbar interbody fusion (ALIF). However, despite the intention of reducing nerve injury through a transforaminal approach, nerve root injury has been reported as a complication of the procedure.[16] In addition to nerve root injury, TLIFs can cause a kyphotic alignment in the lumbar spine.

After exposing the spine through either a midline or paramedian posterior approach, the facet joint and pars interarticularis above the proposed fusion level is resected. This allows access to the posterolateral aspect of the disc. Care is taken to avoid injury to both the existing and transversing nerve root. A standard discectomy and insertion of an interbody device is then performed.

Anterior Lumbar Interbody Fusion. Because the risks associated with PLIF were too great for routine use, many surgeons moved to ALIF. Using the same principles of disc excision and interbody bone grafting, many surgeons achieved excellent results. However, ALIF alone cannot withstand the forces across the grafts, so many collapse or do not fuse. Surgeons who perform ALIF have learned to protect the grafts with posterior instrumentation, leading to a predictable fusion rate and good clinical results.

From a technical standpoint, anterior lumbar surgery is most easily and safely accomplished through a retroperitoneal approach. After the anterior disc is exposed, it is relatively simple to perform a discectomy and insert the bone graft of the surgeon's choice. Posterior fusion and instrumentation can be placed through a separate posterior approach on either the same day or in a staged procedure. A circumferential fusion is accomplished in this manner (see Fig. 16-1).

Lateral Interbody Fusion. An alternative to performing an ALIF is through a lateral interbody approach. The use of a lateral approach avoids the need for exposure of the great vessels and therefore has less potential for vascular injury. However, it does not come without inherent risks, the most

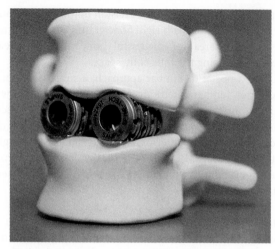

Fig. 16-2 BAK interbody cage device. (Sulzer-Spine Tech, Minneapolis).

notable of which is nerve stretch injury. The most common is an L4 nerve root injury.[17] The lateral approach cannot be used for the L5-S1 intervertebral disc as the pelvis blocks access.

With a lateral approach, the disc is accessed through the psoas muscle under neuromonitoring to avoid injury to the lumbar plexus. After gaining access to the disc, a procedure similar to an ALIF is carried out including discectomy and insertion of an interbody graft.

Interbody Cages. Ongoing technologic advances have been made in interbody cages. Essentially, these devices are hollow cylinders made of titanium, carbon, or bone (Fig. 16-2). They are filled with autogenous bone graft or a bone graft substitute and inserted between the vertebral bodies. Newer devices have implemented bone ingrowth surfaces and large footprint areas to aid in the fusion process and decrease rates of subsidence.

Research is moving rapidly to find a reliable substitute for the autogenous bone graft, most likely with the use of bone-morphogenic protein. There are other biologic alternatives available to surgeons that can be used to fill the interbody fusion cages and reduce the need for bone graft harvest.

SURGICAL PROCEDURE

The basic lumbar fusion is the posterolateral fusion. The patient is placed in a prone position on a Jackson frame, allowing the abdomen to hang free. This decompresses the lumbar epidural veins and minimizes bleeding. A skin incision is made over the operative levels, and the paraspinal muscles are stripped off the posterior elements (spinous process, lamina, and transverse processes). Deep retractors hold back the muscles to allow the surgeons to expose the bone for fusion. Using small curettes or a high-speed burr, the surgeon decorticates the dorsal aspect of the transverse processes and facet joints in preparation for the bone graft placement. Through a separate fascial incision, the surgeon

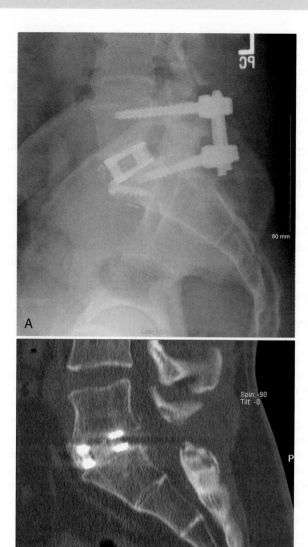

Fig. 16-3 **A,** Pedicle screw instrumentation and an anterior interbody cage in a circumferential fusion. **B,** CT scan of a titanium cage with bone formation through the center of the device.

harvests the necessary amount of cortical and cancellous bone graft from the posterior iliac crest. This bone graft material is then carefully placed in the recipient site.

If screws are used to augment the fusion, a pilot hole is made over the entry site of the pedicle with a burr (Fig. 16-3). Usually probes are placed in the pedicles and a radiograph is taken to confirm the position of the pedicle probes. After confirmation, the pedicles are tapped and appropriate length screws are placed into the pedicles. Again, an intraoperative radiograph is taken to confirm the position of the screws. The rods or plates are connected to the screws, and lordosis is preserved in the construct. The wound is usually irrigated with an antibiotic solution to minimize the chance of infection and closed over a deep suction drain. The drain is removed when the postsurgical drainage is minimal. Patients are mobilized out of bed as tolerated on the first or second day after surgery.

THERAPY GUIDELINES FOR REHABILITATION

Description of Rehabilitation and Rationale for Using Instrumentation

Opinion about the degree of rehabilitation needed after spinal surgery ranges from the optimistic view that no rehabilitation is needed to others who argue for aggressive exercise- and education-based programs. As noted earlier there has also been mounting evidence that failing to address psychosocial factors in this population may also be neglecting an integral part of the rehabilitation and recovery process. This chapter is written from the point of view that the patient who has undergone surgery needs not only a program that will protect the surgical area and create an effective healing environment, but also addresses relevant and contributing changes in motor control dealing with both the active subsystems and neural control subsystems as outlined by Panjabi[18,19] (Box 16-1). Although the surgery itself deals with improving the passive subsystem, which include such anatomic structures as the vertebral bodies, facets, and ligaments, capsule, it is our job as specialists in rehabilitation to address these other systems.[20] It is also important to realize that those individuals with more chronic pain symptoms will most likely exhibit altered pain processing, which may be addressed through including cognitive-behavioral interventions during the recovery process.

The following guidelines are not intended to substitute for sound clinical reasoning but rather serve as a foundation on which a trained physical therapist (PT) can base the rehabilitation of a patient after spinal fusion. It is assumed that the therapist will know the basics of spine and extremity evaluation in order to monitor the patient for symptoms that require prompt reevaluation, along with addressing relevant contributing factors in other body regions that have a significant impact on the lumbar spine.

Preoperative and Planning Phase

Before an individual elects to undergo lumbar spinal fusion, it is generally assumed that conservative measures have not had a significant impact on the patient's condition and that they have gone through an extensive therapy program. Hopefully the individual has been taught stabilization-based exercises and has begun to address other relevant physical and cognitive dysfunctions. Once surgery is deemed necessary by the patient and rehabilitation team, preoperative management may be very useful in determining functionally relevant outcomes along with realistic goals.[21] This is also the time to start on patient education regarding issues such as:

BOX 16-1 **Spinal Stability System Components**

1. Passive spinal column
2. Active spinal muscles
3. Neural control unit

- Postoperative precautions
- Bed mobility and transfers
- Initial postoperative exercises
- Gait training with any necessary assistive devices
- Donning and doffing any required braces
- Wound care
- General overview and prognosis of the postoperative rehabilitation process

An effective preoperative program before lumbar fusion surgery should also address any other relevant patient concerns and include other advice from the members from other disciplines included in the rehabilitation team. A tour of the facility and operating room along with meeting with individuals who have already undergone such a procedure may also help to decrease patient anxiety surrounding the surgery and hospital experience.[21] For the rehabilitation specialists, an understanding of the specific procedure performed is essential for safe rehabilitation. Before beginning a rehabilitation program, the therapist must know whether the patient has had a fusion with or without instrumentation. Patients who were operated on with instrumentation can generally be progressed more aggressively in the first phase of rehabilitation. Patients who were operated on without instrumentation require more time for the bony fusion to take place. Generally a callus should form within 6 to 8 weeks; the surgeon monitors this by radiograph and usually does not refer to outpatient therapy before a callus has formed. The therapist also must know the surgical approach and the levels fused. After a motion segment is fused, increased stress is placed on the levels above and below the fusion. This creates risk for acceleration of the degenerative cascade at the adjacent levels. Obviously the more levels that have been fused, the greater the stress placed on the remaining segments. When the fusion includes the L5-S1 motion segment, abnormal forces are then translated to the sacroiliac joints. To minimize these forces, the therapist must be sure that normal motion exists at all remaining segments, including the thoracic spine, shoulders, and lower extremities (LEs).

During a posterior fusion, the multifidi are retracted from the spine. This partially tears the dorsal divisions of the spinal nerves, resulting in partial denervation of the multifidi.[5,22] If an anterior fusion also has been performed, then a midline skin incision will be apparent and the abdominal muscular incision is lateral. The incision passes through the obliques, also partially denervating them. For this reason the therapist should teach the patient the proper way to recruit the transverse abdominis (TA), multifidi, and pelvic floor muscles and watch for any substitution patterns to promote proper spinal stabilization.

Phase I

TIME: 1 to 5 days after surgery (inpatient) and up to 6 weeks

GOALS: Patient education about daily movements, abdominal stabilization, neural mobilization, and home care principles (Table 16-2)

TABLE 16-2 Lumbar Fusion and Laminectomy

Rehabilitation Phase	Criteria to Progress to This Phase	Anticipated Impairments and Functional Limitations	Intervention	Goal	Rationale
Phase I Postoperative 1-5 days (inpatient) and up until outpatient therapy begins	• Postoperative (inpatient)	• Pain • Limited bed mobility • Limited self-care • Limited ADL • Limited tolerance to prolonged postures (sit/stand) • Limited tolerance to walking	Inpatient care • Bed mobility training, log roll technique with supine-sit-stand • ADL training with assistive devices as necessary (dressing, bathroom transfers) • Body mechanics training • Gait training, with walker if necessary • Initial training in abdominal isometric (TA and pelvic floor) • Self-neural mobilizations	Independent with the following: 1. Bed mobility 2. Don/doff clothing, and corset if indicated 3. Transfers 4. Gait, using assistive device as appropriate • Demonstrate appropriate body mechanics with self-care and basic ADL	• Promote restoration of independent function • Use log roll to avoid placing stress on the surgical site • Emphasize walking to improve tolerance to upright postures • Use proper body mechanics to avoid reinjury

ADL, Activities of daily living; *TA,* transverse abdominis.

Inpatient Phase

Most patients remain in the hospital for several days after fusion surgery. Physical therapy management during this phase consists of teaching patients the proper way to get in and out of bed, dress and perform other self-care activities, and walk (perhaps with a walker for the first 1 or 2 days). Strenuous abdominal stabilization exercises are *not* recommended at this time; however, attempts should be made to perform light TA and pelvic floor contractions to begin to practice them in different positions. The patient may use a large "sigh" or more forceful exhalation such as "blowing out a candle" to start to facilitate other abdominal muscles that assist with bracing. The therapist also can teach basic and simple neural mobilization for the nerves involving the lumbosacral plexus. Because of the sensitivity of the nervous system, more focus should be on activities such as "sliders" versus "tensioners." These are described well by Bulter.[12] Patients and their family should leave the hospital with an understanding of the home care required until they begin their outpatient physical therapy, especially in the absence of home PT during the interim. If the physician requests bracing of any kind, then the patient should understand the way to get in and out of the brace and when to wear it. **Patients will be given instructions from the physician to avoid driving, prolonged sitting, lifting, bending, and twisting.** These, along with any other specific precautions, should be understood by the patient. The PT should reinforce this information and teach patients the proper way to avoid these activities by hip hinging or pivoting. This information should be provided in written and visual form, because many patients may be medicated or overwhelmed by the recent surgery and therefore have difficulty recalling or applying what they have just been taught. Most patients are referred for physical therapy anywhere between 4 to 7 weeks after their discharge from the hospital.

Phase II

TIME: 6 to 10 weeks after surgery
GOALS: Increased activity, tissue remodeling, stabilization, and reconditioning (Table 16-3)

During phase II, patients gradually increase their activity level. While taking soft tissue healing into account, the PT can safely begin to influence the direction of tissue modeling through carefully applied stress. Patients should begin to approximate normal activities while the therapist controls the intensity of movement and exercise.

Patients progressing to the latter portion of phase II increase the intensity of the stabilization program begun in the earlier stages of the phase. They may increase repetitions and level of difficulty. Also toward the end of this phase, patients should be slowly working up to 30 minutes of exercise and physical activity at least 5 days a week as recommended by the American College of Sports Medicine.[23] They can begin a light weight-training program, avoiding exercises that inappropriately load the lumbar spine but making sure to include some exercise for the lumbar paraspinals and other muscles that attach to the thoracodorsal fascia. Patients should no longer require assistance with most daily activities.

Common restrictions are no lifting greater than 10 lb and no overhead lifting. Examples of exercises for this phase are listed in the following sections.

TABLE 16-3 Lumbar Fusion and Laminectomy

Rehabilitation Phase	Criteria to Progress to This Phase	Anticipated Impairments and Functional Limitations	Intervention	Goal	Rationale

Phase II Postoperative 6-10 wk	• Outpatient candidate
	• No signs of infection
	• Cleared by physician to begin therapy
		• Pain limited with ADL
		• Limited nerve root mobility
		• Limited trunk stability
		• Limited mobility of regions adjacent to surgical site
		• Limited endurance and tolerance to physical activity
			• Cryotherapy
			• Relative rest
			• Review of body mechanics training
			• Nerve mobilization
			• PROM/LE and UE stretches:
			  Hip flexors (gently initiate after 8 wk with physician approval)
			  Gluteals
			  Hip rotators
			  Quadriceps
			  Hamstrings
			  Calf
			  Shoulders
			• Isometrics with active range of motion:
			  Abdominal bracing with squats, transfers, and gait
			• Spinal stabilization exercises:
			  Bridging
			  Dying bug (after 8 wk, with physician approval)
			  Quadruped activities
			  Superman (after 8 wk, with physician approval)
			  Prone (much later in phase, with physician approval)
			• Walking program
			• Joint mobilization to upper and mid T/S, gentle if mobilizing lower T/S
			• Soft tissue massage after incision is closed
			• Patient education
			• Upper body ergometer
				Independent with the following:
				1. Bed mobility
				2. Don/doff clothing, and corset if indicated
				3. Transfers
				4. Gait, using assistive device as appropriate
				• Demonstrate appropriate body mechanics with self-care and basic ADL
				• Demonstrate proper motor control using transverse abdominis, pelvic floor, and multifidus
				• Demonstrate bracing and begin to incorporate this with activities
					• Self-manage pain
					• Prevent reinjury
					• Perform ADL without adding increased stress to the lumbar spine
					• Prevent neural adhesions
					• Improve mobility of LEs to decrease stress on the lumbar spine
					• Initiate trunk stabilization while performing ADL to decrease potential for reinjury
					• Perform cardiovascular conditioning and "tiny steps" to avoid excessive lumbar spine movement during gait
					• Improve mobility of thoracic spine to decrease stress on the lumbar spine
					• Improve mobility of soft tissue
					• Reduce volitional muscle guarding
					• Perform cardiovascular conditioning

ADL, Activities of daily living; LE, lower extremity; PROM, passive range of motion; T/S, thoracic spine; UE, upper extremity.

Evaluation

Before initiating treatment the therapist should perform a thorough examination to assess the patient's status and help to create an individualized program. The examination should include relevant tests and measures, such as posture, gait, range of motion (ROM), strength, balance, body mechanics, and specific functional tasks while making sure not to overload the lumbar spine. The therapist and patient can then begin to collaborate on and establish goals for treatment.

This evaluation should include ROM for the LEs and upper extremities (UEs) but not for the lumbar spine. A complete neurologic examination should be performed to establish a baseline and should include neural tension testing.

The therapist can perform strength testing for the LEs with the exception of testing hip flexor strength. He or she also can check the patient's ability to stabilize or brace the lumbar spine isometrically, which is a test of the patient's ability to recruit the core trunk muscles to control the spine. Core strength testing may be performed in a variety of ways; however, Lee[24] describes a functional approach based on grouping core musculature into "slings." The patient's spontaneous body mechanics and the way the patient responds to the challenge of daily activities should be assessed. The goals of phase II are as follows:

- Demonstrate good body mechanics for activities of daily living (ADL)
- Protect the surgical site from infection and mechanical stress
- Maintain nerve root mobility at the involved levels
- Control pain and inflammation
- Minimize patient fear and apprehension
- Begin a stabilization and reconditioning program
- Improve scar and surrounding soft tissue mobility
- Treat restrictions of thoracic, UEs, and LEs that can lead to more strain on the lumbar spine
- Education to minimize sitting time and maximize walking time

Body Mechanics Training

If body mechanics training was provided preoperatively, then it should be reviewed after surgery. If body mechanics training is new to the patient, then the therapist should go through the entire program, which is as follows:

- In and out of bed (Fig. 16-4)
- In and out of a chair (Fig. 16-5)
- Up and down from the floor (Fig. 16-6)
- Lying postures (Fig. 16-7)
- Sitting (Fig. 16-8)
- Standing
- Dressing
- Bending (Fig. 16-9)
- Reaching
- Pushing and pulling (Fig. 16-10)
- Lifting (Fig. 16-11)
- Carrying (Fig. 16-12)

Patients must perform these activities to get dressed, use the bathroom, travel to physician's appointments, and shop

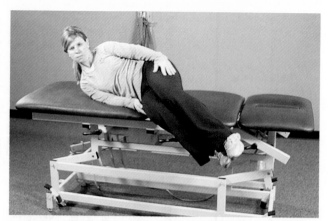

Fig. 16-4 To rise from a lying position, the patient begins with bracing to maintain a neutral spine and rolls to the edge of the bed as a unit. The patient then pivots off the elbow while throwing the legs to the ground. This momentum makes an otherwise difficult movement easier. To avoid twisting the trunk, the patient should reach toward the top foot with the top arm.

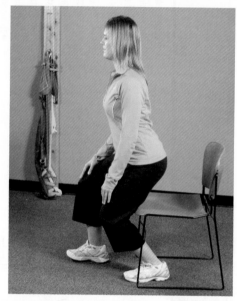

Fig. 16-5 To get out of a chair, the patient places one foot under the chair, hinges the hip, and then raises off the thigh. The hips should be the first to leave the chair and the last to land. The patient should not attempt to keep the back vertical, merely straight. To get into the chair the process is reversed. If no room is available to get the foot under the chair, such as in a couch, then the patient pivots on the hips until perpendicular to the chair. This offsets the feet and allows for easier rising.

for and prepare meals. A patient who can do these activities without stressing the surgical site will heal faster and with less discomfort. Patients can accomplish all these tasks without lumbar motion if they move their hips rather than the spine.

Instead of flexing the lumbar spine, they can "hip hinge" (see Fig. 16-9). Rather than twist in the lumbar spine, they can pivot on another body part (e.g., knees, elbows, hips). When teaching a hip hinge, the PT should point out that the hips should move back rather than down. After surgery, patients tend to guard and move cautiously. Showing them the way to use their momentum safely in many

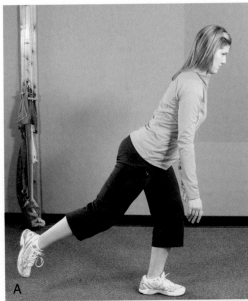

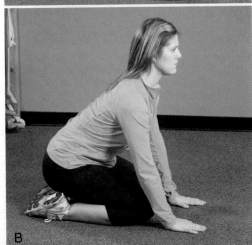

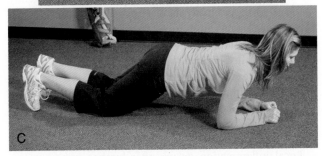

Fig. 16-6 When getting up and down from the floor, the patient moves from a single leg hip hinge (**A**) through a reverse lunge position to double kneeling (**B**). Next, the patient hinges the hips from double kneeling to about 45°. Another balance point occurs here (**C**). From this balance point, the patient rocks forward onto the elbows and rolls as a unit onto the side. To avoid uncontrolled extension, the stomach should never touch the ground. The process is reversed to rise from the ground.

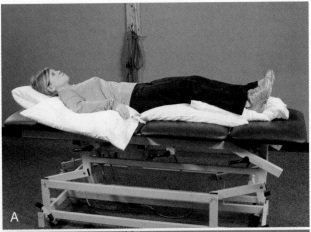

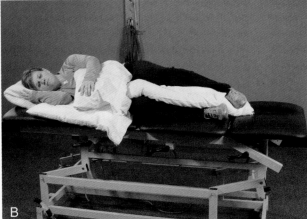

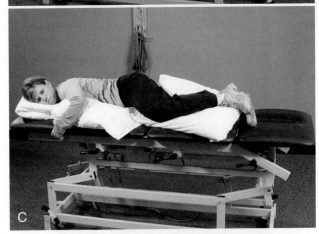

Fig. 16-7 **A,** Supported supine lying. Patients generally prefer to have the whole leg supported rather than just the knees. Any unsupported area becomes uncomfortable and causes the patient to shift and wake. The shoulders also should be supported in whatever degree of protraction exists. Any soft tissue subjected to prolonged stretch eventually becomes uncomfortable. **B,** Supported side lying. The patient needs enough pillows to support the UEs. A body pillow frequently works well. The patient should pull the support directly into the upper thigh and chest and then roll slightly onto it; he or she should not lie on the same side all night. **C,** Three-quarter prone lying is the most popular position. It is similar to supported side lying, except that the patient rolls one-quarter turn more. A wedge-shaped pillow minimizes cervical strain in this position.

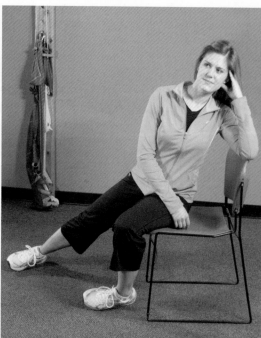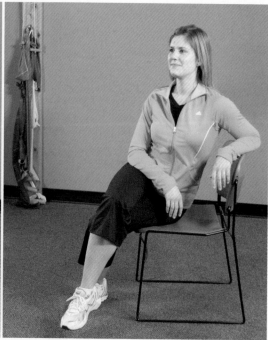

Fig. 16-8 Alternate sitting postures are important to teach, because patients will want to change sitting postures frequently. As long as a neutral spine position is maintained, the variations are limitless. These positions successfully take the weight off the left pelvis, thereby relieving pressure on the piriformis and sensitive sciatic notch.

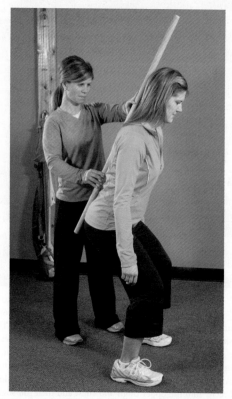

Fig. 16-9 Hip hinging is flexing the hips and knees while maintaining a neutral spine. A dowel can be helpful for patients with difficulty perceiving spinal motion. The spine should not be kept vertical but merely straight. This is one of the essential motions patients use to perform functional activities. Hip hinging also can be done on one leg (as in Fig. 16-6, A). This is especially useful when getting up and down from the ground. The position shown is a balance point that patients should learn because it requires little or no effort to maintain. Patients should attempt to move from one balance point to another.

maneuvers makes the postoperative transition easier. For example, getting out of bed requires less bracing if the legs are moved quickly to the floor, transferring the momentum to the torso (see Fig. 16-4).

Nerve Root Gliding. Patients should extend the knee while lying supine with the spine in a neutral position and the hip flexed to a 90° angle. When tension is encountered, the therapist helps the patient work the knee or ankle gently back and forth, gradually increasing the ROM (Fig. 16-13). This stretch may cause increased symptoms during the stretch, which should resolve immediately on relaxing. Education should be provided to the patient regarding expected and adverse reactions to neural gliding.

Any lingering symptom is reason to halt the stretch until the therapist can reassess the problem. Butler[12] and Shacklock[25] describe an excellent approach to evaluation and treatment of neural mobility.

Local inflammation occurs after lumbar spine surgery. Because the body forms scar tissue in response to inflammation, the nerve root can become adherent to the neural foramen or lose elasticity. It is theorized that a nerve root that is kept moving within its sheath cannot develop adhesions.[12,25] Patients with nonirritable chronic leg symptoms tend to respond well to neural mobilization. However, the patient must keep the spine stabilized while moving the leg.

Decreasing Pain and Inflammation. Patients should use medication as directed by the physician and cold packs for about 20 minutes three or four times per day to help control pain and inflammation. Patients can be taught to alternate rest periods with periods of light activity, because

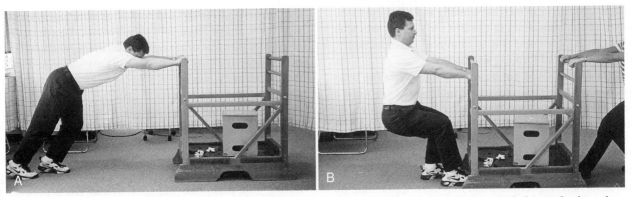

Fig. 16-10 **A,** To push an object, the patient leans into it with a hip hinge until the body weight begins to move it forward. The heavier the object, the more the patient needs to line the shoulders up behind the hands. Arms can be bent or straight. The patient should take tiny steps, because if the feet move anterior to the hips, then a lumbar flexion moment will occur. **B,** To pull an object, the patient leans back, maintaining neutral position, until the body weight begins to move the object. The heavier the object, the more the patient needs to flex at the hips and knees. The patient should take tiny steps and hold the upper body erect, because the weight tends to pull the body into flexion.

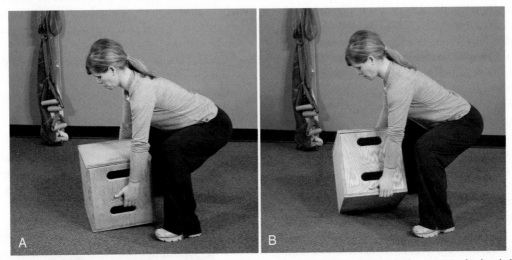

Fig. 16-11 **A,** Lifting from a hip hinge position. The spine remains straight but not vertical. This method works for conveniently placed objects. **B,** To lift a less conveniently placed object safely, the patient goes down onto one knee, then hinges the hips and tilts the object to its maximal height. The patient then locks the object to the chest, reverses the hip hinge, and places the object on the thigh. As the patient stands up, the thigh lifts the majority of the weight.

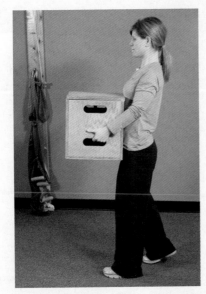

Fig. 16-12 Slight knee flexion reduces the tendency toward lumbar extension while the patient carries objects. It may feel "funny" at first, but with continued practice this flexion becomes simple.

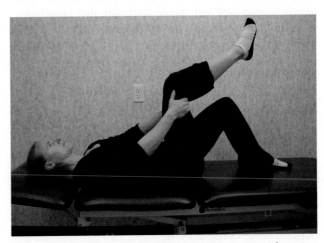

Fig. 16-13 Nerve gliding. In a hooklying or supine position, the patient can hold on to the back of the thigh or place their legs up on a bolster while slowly extending the knee until a gentle stretch is felt. In addition, ankle dorsiflexion and plantarflexion could be used to assist with nerve mobility.

sustained postures can increase swelling and pain. The therapist may apply modalities in the clinic to control pain after therapy. It is very important to minimize inflammation to decrease the risk of forming scar tissue.

Ultrasound should not be applied over a healing bony fusion. Patients with severe pain problems can try using a home transcutaneous electrical nerve stimulation (TENS) unit or interferential unit.

Minimizing Patient Fear and Apprehension. If patients know they can control their pain level, they may be less fearful of trying activities that may cause a pain flare-up or those that have been painful in the past. They will rely less on inactivity and medication to control pain. The therapist should spend some time initially discovering the patient's fears and alleviating those that are groundless. Greater progress will occur in the long run if the therapist initially allays patient fears and teaches the patient ways to control pain. More recent publications have pointed toward not only to the need for additional resources addressing pain and cognition but have also suggested that group meetings with other patients undergoing rehabilitation after lumbar fusion are an integral part of the healing process.[13,26]

Social support is suggested to help abate pain-related fear and also allow for sharing of experiences and coping strategies. Psychosocial variables have been shown to have a large influence on disability and function in individuals with chronic back pain, so ignoring these concepts could be a large detriment to the patient's functional improvement.[11] Patients are generally very fearful after lumbar spine surgery. Excessive anxiety and worry may cause increased muscular tension along with altered movement patterns and altered pain processing. Patients are typically afraid to move, thinking they will somehow disrupt the surgery. Patients can better tolerate flare-ups and variations in their symptoms if they expect them and have been instructed in self-management of these flare-ups. Patients are generally less apprehensive if the therapist is not apprehensive. Most people recover well and should start with that expectation. If the patient appears to be developing neuropathic pain, nerve root signs, symptoms from a new level, or any other complications, then the therapist should note the symptoms calmly and convey the information to the treating surgeon for advice without conveying anxiety to the patient.

Patient Education. Patients who are sensitive to load bearing through the spine should take frequent short unloading rests throughout the day. Those who cannot tolerate any one position for a length of time can learn to make a circuit of their activities, frequently changing tasks (avoiding prolonged sustained postures). Patients with specific position intolerance can benefit from learning ways to avoid that position while doing daily activities. Lumbar rolls are not recommended during this phase, because most patients cannot tolerate pressure on the incision site after surgery.

Patients should understand the expected postoperative course of events, particularly concerning postoperative pain. Increasing leg pain is not a good sign, even if low back pain

diminishes; conversely, decreasing leg symptoms is a good sign, even if low back pain is increasing. Less leg pain is consistent with less neurologic involvement, whereas the low back is expected to be sore because of the incision and altered facet mechanics.[27] Incisional pain can be expected to decrease gradually over 6 to 8 weeks. As patients begin to return to normal activities, an associated increase in muscle soreness frequently occurs. The sooner they recondition themselves, the better they will feel. Patients should be aware that their bodies will be adapting to and remodeling from the surgery for as long as 1 to 2 years. Symptoms often shift and change during that time. The therapist should teach patients to manage flare-ups using ice, rest, and resumption of previous activities within 1 or 2 days.

Stabilization, Strength, and Reconditioning. Different approaches have been suggested to improve the active stabilization system of the lumbopelvic region, and it is beyond this chapter to compare and contrast each. However, a more thorough program would include:
- Cocontraction of the TA, multifidus, and pelvic floor muscles with and without using pressure biofeedback (BFB) (Fig. 16-14)
- Abdominal breathing
- Abdominal bracing with appropriate progression (Fig. 16-15)

Abdominal bracing and supine marching are good exercises to begin strengthening the trunk. Before bracing is initiated, it is best to make sure the patient can isometrically

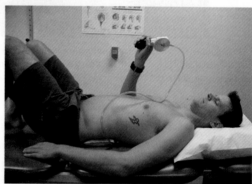
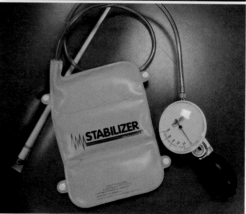

Fig. 16-14 Using pressure biofeedback can be a very helpful way to teach patients to contract their TA while minimizing a forceful contraction of the rectus abdominis.

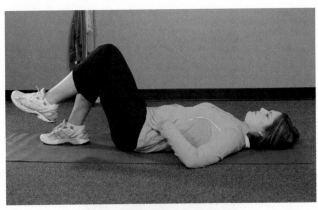

Fig. 16-15 Bracing with marching. The patient creates an abdominal brace by contracting the TA, multifidi, and pelvic floor. It is important to remember to move the abdominals without moving the spine. While maintaining the brace, the patient slowly takes the weight off one foot (removing only as much weight from the foot as possible without allowing the hips to rotate or the spine to extend). Eventually the patient should be able to lift the leg up to 90° of hip flexion with the knee bent. The patient then alternates feet.

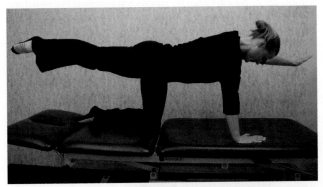

Fig. 16-16 Quadruped alternating opposite arm and leg lift. While in quadruped, the patient can draw in the deep abdominal muscles to perform an isometric contraction. Holding this contraction the patient will slowly extend the opposite arm and leg while maintaining good pelvic and lumbar spine alignment. Before this exercise the should be able to perform this activity first with just opposite arm movements and second with just leg movements.

contract the TA, multifidi, and pelvic floor muscles.[6,9,28-31] After the patient is able to do such, it is important to progress those stabilization exercises, eventually working toward functional goals that have been established. The patient should be able to contract the appropriate stabilization muscles in different postures and positions, so it is recommended that these be practiced also in sitting, standing, and quadruped. A supine progression of lower abdominal strengthening has been well outlined by Sahrmann.[32]

In quadruped (four-point kneeling) the patient should be able to more easily work on contracting TA while keeping other global muscles relaxed. Adding bracing along with arm and leg movements in this quadruped position is also a great way to activate the multifidus and lumbar spine paraspinals without placing the lumbar spine under undue axial load[32,33] (Fig. 16-16).

It has also been hypothesized that the deep stabilizers of the spine, such as the multifidus, also have a large

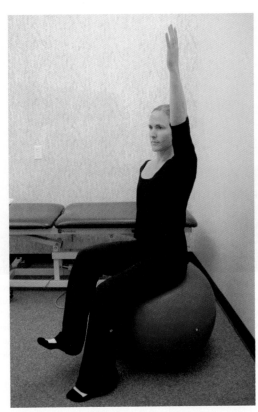

Fig. 16-17 Balance activities sitting on an exercise ball. Before starting sitting exercises on an exercise ball, the patient must demonstrate proper posture and be comfortable in this position. The therapist might want to start with postural exercises in this position while making sure to avoid excessive lumbar spine lordosis or slumped sitting. Arm or leg movements, single-leg balance activities, or resisted Thera-Band activities could provide an adequate challenge to improve balance and motor control.

proprioceptive component to the active system.[34] To add more proprioceptive feedback to the stabilizing system, it is integral to challenge the patient on both stable and unstable (but not unsafe) surfaces. General balance activities would also help with this type of challenge. Examples of these types of exercises may include:

- UE or LE activities while sitting on an exercise ball (Fig. 16-17)
- Supine/hooklying activities laying vertical on a foam roll (Fig. 16-18)
- Standing activities on a disc or rocker board (Fig. 16-19)
- Trunk or hip perturbations in sitting or standing (Fig. 16-20)

General strength and conditioning exercises should also be initiated during this phase of rehabilitation after it is cleared by the physician and the patient demonstrates appropriate stabilization. Examples of exercises would include:

- Wall squats and sit to stand
- Half lunges
- Step ups and step downs
- Walking
- Cardiovascular reconditioning (using stair climber, brisk walking, and pool exercises once the incision is closed)

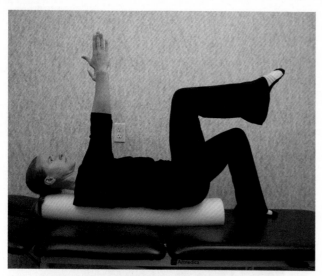

Fig. 16-18 Supine activities on foam roll. Lying on a foam roll provides opportunity to challenge the trunk muscles and improve motor control. Adding marching with bracing or arm movements can challenge the trunk and lower extremity's ability to maintain balance on the foam roll. Because of the sensitivity of the incision site or more focused pressure from the foam roll on the middle of the spine, some patients may not tolerate this position.

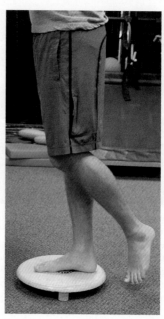

Fig. 16-19 Standing balance activities. Many varieties of standing balance activities can be done to retrain the muscles that contribute to postural and motor control of the spine. An example shown here is with a rocker board. The therapist must find an appropriate challenge for the patient by modifying variables, such as the standing surface, base or support, vision, or doing concurrent activities.

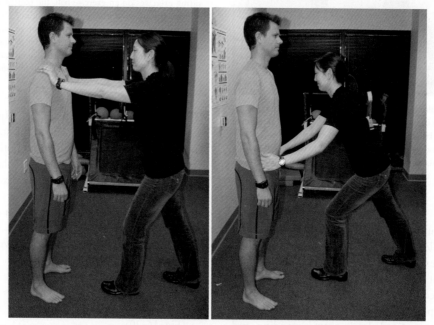

Fig. 16-20 Resisted trunk motions in standing. Here the therapist is adding perturbations to the shoulders or hips while the patient meets the resistance, maintaining good standing posture and alignment. This helps to activate stabilizing muscles. These activities should begin with very light force until the patient demonstrates the ability to tolerate more.

Care should be taken when starting more vigorous strengthening activities, because it is recommended that the patient be able to use the appropriate stabilization muscles during components of the exercise before doing the full exercise. For example, before a patient performs a wall squat, they should be able to isometrically contract the inner unit and use bracing to stabilize the spine while leaning his or her back against the wall.

Maintaining Scar and Soft Tissue Mobility. The therapist should use soft tissue techniques to maintain good scar and soft tissue mobility without disrupting the healing

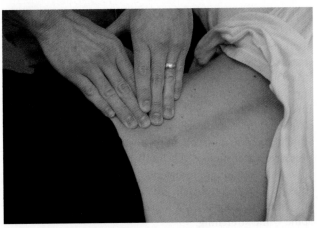

Fig. 16-21 Maintaining scar and tissue mobility. It is imperative that the healed incision and surrounding tissue/fascia have adequate movement to allow motion through the spine. The therapist may use a variety of techniques to improve mobility in different planes and at different depths of tissue.

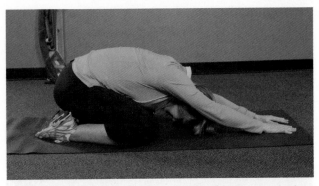

Fig. 16-23 Lumbar flexion stretch. Occasionally when the patient has been working the spinal extensor muscles hard, these muscles may get sore and tight. From an all-fours position, the patient can gradually spread the knees and sit back on the heels, allowing the spine to relax and stretch.

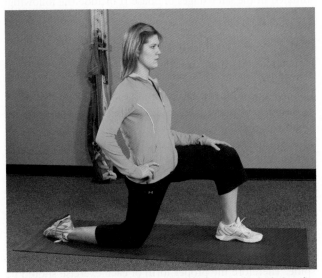

Fig. 16-22 Hip flexor stretch. The patient kneels on one leg with the other leg in front, braces the spine, and gradually begins to shift weight forward to the front foot. The patient should feel a stretch in the groin area of the kneeling leg. The spine should not be extended.

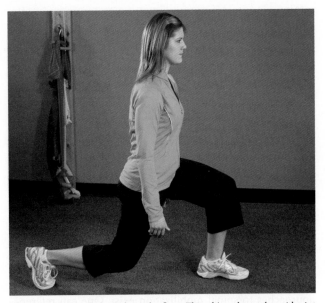

Fig. 16-24 Up and down from the floor. This photo shows the midpoint of getting up or down from the floor.

of these tissues (Fig. 16-21). Scar tissue tends to contract while healing. This can create a "tight" scar that restricts mobility.[35] In cases of prolonged incisional pain it may be beneficial to use techniques to desensitize the tissue starting with very soft and gentle surfaces progressing to more firm and vigorous materials.

Assessment and Treatment for Restrictions of Thoracic, Shoulder, and Hip Mobility. The following steps will help ease restrictions of the thoracic spine and hip:

- Manual therapy for thoracic motion restrictions
- LE and UE stretches for soft tissue restrictions
- Hamstring stretches
- Hip flexor stretches (Fig. 16-22) can be initiated in later stages with permission from the surgeon

- Quadriceps stretches (begin with prone knee flexion before progressing)
- Lumbar flexion stretch (Fig. 16-23) with surgeon approval **When initiating this stretch, the therapist must not be overly aggressive, obtaining ROM at the expense of compromising the fusion site.** Fig. 16-23 demonstrates an ideal ending position for this stretch, which may take several months to obtain.
- Up and down from the floor (Fig. 16-24)
- Hip rotator stretches (Fig. 16-25)
- Latissimus dorsi stretches (Fig. 16-26)

The loss of motion caused by the spinal fusion places additional demands for motion on the adjacent segments. *One of the most stressful motions in the lumbar spine is rotation, which causes a shearing effect across the disc. Since the thoracic spine is designed to allow more rotation, limited motion here may increase strain on the lumbar spine during twisting motions.* The PT can use manual mobilization techniques to increase thoracic spine mobility. Many different

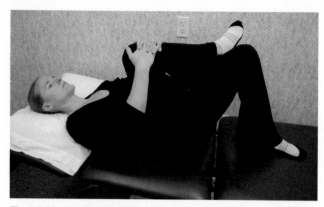

Fig. 16-25 Hip rotator stretch. While lying on the back, the patient crosses the ankle of one leg over the knee of the other leg. The patient performs the stretch by pulling the knee and ankle toward the chest. The patient should feel a stretch deep in the back of the hip.

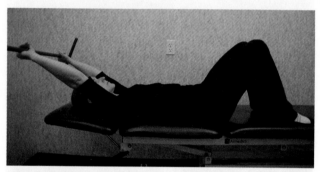

Fig. 16-26 Latissimus dorsi stretch. It is important to maintain lat mobility as short or tight lats may pull the lumbar spine into excessive lordosis with overhead arm movements. In supine, the patient should be cued to use abdominal muscles to avoid lumbar spine extension while stretching the arms overhead.

approaches to spinal mobilization exist. One can reference Maitland,[36] Mulligan,[37] and Paris[38] for some examples. PTs can teach patients to use two tennis balls taped together to form a fulcrum that can lie over a segment of the thoracic spine and localize motion to the segment above, thus maintaining good segmental mobility of the thoracic spine at home. This can be done in a standing or, later (when appropriate), in a semireclined position for the upper and midthoracic spine. A similar procedure can be done using a half or a full foam roll.

The hip joint is a large ball-and-socket joint with free motion in all planes. This joint can compensate for the lack of motion in the lumbar spine and should remain as flexible as possible. This can be achieved with stretching of the hip musculature. **Stretching throughout phase II should be very gentle and only pushed to the point the patient can brace to prevent lumbar motion.** Because these muscles attach directly to the lumbar spine or pelvis, the patient should review the principles of stretching. To stretch a muscle, one end must be fixed by something, while the other end is pulled away from the fixed end. **If patients are not stabilizing the spine while stretching the hips, then they will invariably pull on the lumbar spine, jeopardizing the**

fusion. This may also occur at the shoulder complex. If inadequate shoulder flexion/elevation exists when a patient attempts to reach overhead, they may compensate with increased lumbar spine extension. Stretches to address glenohumeral ROM or latissimus dorsi (lats) tightness should also be included if needed. All stretching should involve stabilizing one area while pulling against it with another. For example when stretching the lats the patient should perform somewhat of a posterior pelvic tilt to avoid excessive extension of the lumbar spine (see Fig. 16-26). Iliopsoas stretching is initiated in a later phase with the permission of the physician. The aggressiveness of any hip stretching is dictated by the patient's ability to control the spine while stretching.

In addition, stretches that pull on the lumbar spine or healing soft tissues should be avoided until adequate healing has occurred. Therefore permission should be obtained from the surgeon.

Examples of other exercises (performed while bracing) initiated in the later stages of phase II include the following:

- Bridging
- Heel lifts
- Superman (avoiding lumbar extension)
- Lateral pulls (light resistance with approval of surgeon) (Fig. 16-27)
- Seated upright rowing machine
- Scapular depression (avoid resisting more than 40% of body weight)
- Push-ups standing and leaning into the wall
- Stair climber
- Upper body ergometer (UBE)

A callus is forming at this stage, and patients are expected to tolerate slowly increasing their activity level and returning to normal activities. What the therapist is attempting to develop at this stage is not so much muscle power as kinesthetic sense for the muscles and their role in protecting the spine. Therefore the proper form of each exercise should be emphasized.

Phase III

TIME: 11 to 19 weeks after surgery
GOALS: Return to work, continue to advance/progress exercise program, practice specific skills program, initiate resistance training program (Table 16-4)

During this phase, patients may start to return to work, especially if they have sedentary jobs or occupations that do not require vigorous activity. They often return to work with modified duties or on a part-time schedule. At this time they should be independent with self-care duties and also with a moderately challenging home exercise program. The use of proper mechanics should be becoming a habit but will need to be continually reinforced during specific activities. Exercises that address functional movement may be a great time to reinforce those principles. More strenuous stabilization activities, such as half and full front and side planks could be added.

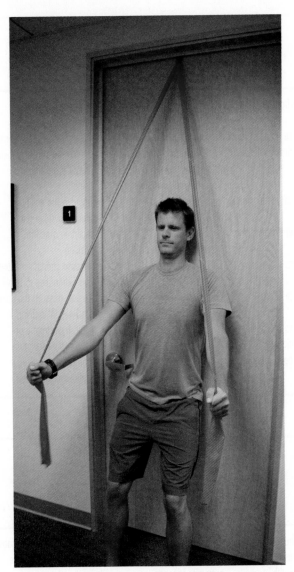

Fig. 16-27 Lat pull downs. Strengthening muscles that attach to the thoracodorsal fascia can help with improving overall trunk stability. Before using weight machines at the gym, it would be beneficial to use Thera-Bands and have the patient leaning against a supportive surface where they can use the appropriate muscles to adequately stabilize the spine.

Patients should still avoid strenuous lumbar rotation, flexion, or extension. The early development of these muscles in their role as spinal stabilizers rather than spinal movers is a crucial component of this phase. The previous trunk stabilization activities should be progressed within the patient tolerance by modifying, for example, the number of repetitions, adding Thera-Band resistance, or performing the exercise on a more challenging surface.

As long as the patient is able to perform the previous stabilization exercises, they may begin a light resistance exercise program. It is not advised to do complex weight lifting tasks, but to focus on light free weight activity and machine-based exercises that allow the patient to perform them with proper posture, technique, and bracing. Patients with a poor tolerance for any one position may do better on a circuit-training program.

Patients should be extremely careful with overhead lifting because of the axial load and compressive forces placed on the spine. Endurance and cardiovascular exercises should also be progressed at this stage and start to progress gradually. For some individuals it may be advised to do more cardiovascular or resisted exercises in an aquatic rehabilitation environment. The buoyancy of the water may help to unload the spine but allow the patient to do partial weight-bearing exercises along with core and resisted extremity activity.

At this stage the expectation is that pain continues to decrease and be at a minimal level. Those patients that continue to have an unexpected degree of pain may need to be reassessed by the PT or by the surgeon. In the absence of any physical explanation of the pain, the rehabilitation team needs to reinforce the functional improvements and minimize the importance of pain as a marker of improvement.

Phase IV

TIME: 20 weeks to 1 year after surgery
GOALS: Restore preinjury status, continue home program of conditioning and stabilization (Table 16-5)

During phase IV the body finishes remodeling and adapting to the changes induced during and after surgery. Patients should be progressing to full restoration of their preinjury level of function and be independent with conducting their previous home and gym program. They should have a good grasp of not only the exercises and physical activity required to reach their goals but also ways to modify those activities, because at this stage it might be expected that the patient may be finishing with outpatient therapy. Proper body mechanics should be consistently demonstrated during functional tasks and patients' understanding of these mechanics should allow them to maintain minimal strain on their back during novel situations. They should also have a good understanding of pain mechanisms, tactics to manage flare-ups, and time to contact the physician or therapist.

The bone continues to remodel and adapt to the fusion for as long as 1 year. *Patients with fusions frequently develop problems at the level above or below the fusion.* For these reasons, the patient should learn that spinal care is now a lifetime habit and must be maintained with regular exercise and good mechanics during all daily activities (not just those the patient perceives as stressful). It is important to consider patient motivation at this time to help design a program that will have the most realistic chance of consistent follow-through.

Patients returning to a more strenuous job or sports are now developing the extra degree of strength and skill to do so. *Later in this phase (and with clearance from the surgeon)* they may begin agility and sport-specific drills, such as running, cutting, and jumping. If a more comprehensive weight training program is called for it should be again geared to the specific activity faced by the patient. The program may require a greater focus on power, endurance, or skill, depending on the activity. Patients should work on

TABLE 16-4 Lumbar Fusion and Laminectomy

Rehabilitation Phase	Criteria to Progress to This Phase	Anticipated Impairments and Functional Limitations	Intervention	Goal	Rationale
Phase III Postoperative 11-19 wk	• No increase in pain • Improved tolerance to upright postures	• Mild pain • Limited tolerance to upright positions (sit/stand) • Limited trunk, lower extremity, and upper extremity strength	Continue intervention from phase II as indicated • Isometrics with active range of motion Abdominal bracing with the following: Bridging Dying bug Quadruped with arm and leg raise Heel lifts Superman (avoiding lumbar spine extension) Scapular depressions Push ups • Progressive resistance exercises: Lateral pull-downs Seated upright/rows triceps dips • Cardiovascular conditioning • Stair stepper upper body ergometer • Brisk walking	• Independent with most ADL • Increased trunk and extremity strength • Maintenance of neutral spine while performing strengthening exercises • Performance of 20-30 minutes of cardiovascular exercise daily	• Promote return to independent lifestyle • Develop kinesthetic sense for the muscles and their role in protecting the spine • Improve the ability to brace the spine and maintain a neutral position • Increase strength of trunk and extremities to avoid excess stress on the spine • Start weight training to begin hypertrophy of associate musculature • Promote good cardiovascular fitness

ADL, Activities of daily living.

TABLE 16-5 Lumbar Fusion and Laminectomy

Rehabilitation Phase	Criteria to Progress to This Phase	Anticipated Impairments and Functional Limitations	Intervention	Goal	Rationale
Phase IV Postoperative 20 wk-1 year	• No increase in pain • No loss in functional status • Patient has decreased reliance on formal therapy • Clearance from physician for progression to phase IV	• Limited trunk and extremity strength • Limited tolerance to sustained postures • Mild pain associated with activities • Limited with lifting and carrying	Continue exercises from previous phases as indicated • Advance exercises with regard to repetitions and weight • For appropriate patients, initiate running, cutting, and jumping progression. This would not be indicated in a majority of lumbar fusion patients. • Specific activity drills related to home, work, or sport environment • Functional capacity evaluation • Continue progression of interventions in phases II through IV • Progress home exercises • Continue patient education with regard to activity modification and performance with assistive device	• Return to work • Increase trunk and extremity strength • Increase muscular endurance • Prepare to return to more strenuous activities • Return to previous level of activity as appropriate • Discharge patient to self-management of flare-ups • Improve trunk strength to previous levels of functioning	• Patients with sedentary jobs should be able to resume their schedule • Continue reconditioning to an expected level of function while protecting the spine • Carefully apply stress to the body in tolerable doses to increase the spine's ability to withstand stress • Evaluate the ability to return to previous function • Because patients with lumbar spine fusion may continue to have problems with joints above and below the fusion site, continuation of some level of maintenance must be emphasized • Fusion patients must also maintain constant body awareness, always using proper body mechanics

maintaining control of a neutral spine during job- or sport-specific challenges during this phase, and the PT should obtain the clearance of the surgeon to begin working on these higher-level activities. The patient must demonstrate good trunk strength and control and good LE strength and flexibility before initiating agility drills. At this time it may also be necessary to perform a functional capacity evaluation and develop a work hardening program before returning the patient to full duty.

Although all therapists would like to relieve pain, some suffering is beyond the ability of current medical science to alleviate. This is a difficult concept for some patients to understand, and they may not be willing to accept it. Focus should again be on improving function and less on pain abatement. Cognitive-behavioral interventions can continue to help with pain-related fear, social adjustments, and coping strategies that may still be difficult for patients during these later stages. Therapists should make every effort to help patients accept this reality and learn to care for themselves without seeking constant medical intervention. Most people can manage chronic pain and maintain a high functional level despite the pain.

Suggested Home Maintenance for the Postsurgical Patient

Days 1 to 5 and up to starting outpatient therapy

GOALS FOR THE PERIOD: Educate patient about simple movements, teach nerve mobilization and light isometric abdominal contraction, review home care principles

1. Gentle nerve gliding
2. Initiate abdominal isometric contraction (TA, pelvic floor)
3. Walking daily as tolerated (should slowly increase in time and speed)
4. Consistent use of proper body mechanics
5. Icing as needed
6. Protection of incision
7. Ankle pumps and deep vein thrombosis (DVT) prevention

Weeks 6 to 10

GOALS FOR THE PERIOD: Initiate outpatient therapy, perform a thorough evaluation (avoid LS ROM and resisted hip flexion), patient education, neural mobilization, abdominal stabilization, begin conditioning activities and home care principles

1. Progress walking tolerance to 20 to 30 minutes
2. Isometric stabilization
   a. TA, pelvic floor, mulifidus
   b. Abdominal breathing, hollowing, bracing
   c. Bracing during light functional movements
3. Initiate light strengthening exercises
   a. Wall slides (to approximately 60° of knee flexion)
   b. Side-lying hip rotation
4. Reinforce body mechanics
5. Continue neural mobilization
6. Begin stretching hips, LEs, and shoulders while maintaining bracing
   a. Hamstrings
   b. Quadriceps
   c. Gluteals

   d. Calves (gastrocnemius and soleus)
   e. Adductors
   f. Piriformis
   g. Hip flexors (gently initiate only with physician approval)
   h. Latissimus dorsi
7. Initiate gentle balance activities

Weeks 11 to 19

GOALS FOR THE PERIOD: Increase activity, emphasize tissue modeling, stabilization, reconditioning, weight programs, and return to work

1. Progress walking tolerance to 30 to 60 minutes daily
2. Increase aggressiveness of stabilization program slowly and to patient's tolerance
   a. Supine marching
   b. Bridging
   c. Dying bug
   d. Squats (to 90° of knee flexion)
   e. Quadruped
   f. Prone over pillow or exercise ball
   g. Planks (half progressing to full) front and side
3. Continue to maintain nerve root mobility
4. Initiate resistance training using weights (generally after 12 weeks)
   a. Seated upright rowing machine
   b. Latissimus pulls
   c. Scapular depressions
   d. Dips
6. Continue cardiovascular training using the following:
   a. Stair climber
   b. Brisk walking
   c. Standing or floatation device–assisted pool exercises

Week 20 and Beyond
GOALS FOR THE PERIOD: Restore preinjury status, continue home program of conditioning and stabilization
1. Progress stabilization program to level required by patient's activity level
2. Continue to work on hip, LE, and shoulder flexibility
3. Initiate light LS flexibility exercises with proper form

4. Develop gym or home program for independent management that should include the following:
   a. Cardiovascular exercises
   b. Stabilization exercises
   c. Strengthening exercises
   d. Flexibility exercises
5. Begin sport-specific drills or work-specific activity (refer to examples in Chapter 14)

CLINICAL CASE REVIEW

1 Tom is 50 years old. He had a lumbar fusion at L4-L5 and L5-S1, 3 weeks ago. He is now in therapy. The PT gives Tom an exercise to facilitate nerve root gliding. The patient asks, "What is the significance of this exercise?" What should the therapist tell the patient?

Local inflammation occurs after lumbar spine surgery, and the body forms scar tissue in response to inflammation. It is possible for the nerve root to become restricted by surrounding scar tissue as it exits through an opening called the intervertebral foramen. Because of the inflammatory process, the nerve also can lose elasticity. By doing activities that move the nerve within its "neural container" (sheath), it may help to prevent or free-up adhesions, which can cause pain, numbness, tingling, and other symptoms.

2 The surgeon approaches the PT with some concern because the patient told the staff that the therapist was having them do "abdominal exercises" and was worried about such aggressive techniques early in the recovery period. What should the therapist tell the patient and the surgeon?

The "abdominal exercises" that the patient had been taught were not the aggressive style core exercises that might resemble gym activities. Much later in the patient's rehabilitation, they may need to perform such exercises; however, early intervention is focused on just teaching the patient how to isometrically contract the TA, which helps to stabilize the spine in a corsetlike fashion. Because these muscles do not cause the lumbar spine to flex or extend, no shearing or abnormal forces should be placed on the surgical site. In fact, being able to control (contract) these muscles should actually help to prevent those unwanted forces.

3 After being discharged from the hospital, Bill, who is 58 years old, is concerned that he is not starting outpatient therapy for another 5 to 6 weeks. He is wondering what he should do until that period. What should the therapist tell him?

After being discharged from the hospital, the physician or case manager might suggest home therapy to make sure the patient is safe and can manage the home environment without problems. In the absence of home PT, the patient should understand their precautions, which usually include avoiding bending, lifting, twisting, driving, and prolonged sitting, and know strategies to minimize strain on the lumbar spine. They should also understand all of the concepts taught in the inpatient setting, which should include bed mobility, ergonomics, body mechanics, and gait training that will help them with their ADL. During these first weeks at home, it may also be a good time to meet with others who have had the same surgery. Exercises are not recommended at this stage, but the patient should understand how to perform abdominal bracing along with a cocontraction of the TA and pelvic floor muscles.

4 Lindsey is 38 years old. She had a lumbar fusion at L4-L5 about 7 weeks ago. She tells her PT that her back pain has been increasing over the past 7 to 10 days. Lindsey has complied with all instructions and restrictions. The PT reviews her chart and exercise program. Over the past 2 weeks, Lindsey has begun doing squats and using the treadmill along with the UBE for cardiovascular exercise. She has been stretching her hamstrings, hip flexors, quadriceps, and calf muscles. She also has been doing trunk stabilization exercises in the prone, supine, and quadruped positions. Lindsey also has been strengthening her upper body with bicep curls, seated military presses, and push-ups. Which of these exercises may be aggravating her condition and why?

It is most likely that the hip flexor stretches are aggravating her condition and should not be initiated until later, when sufficient healing has occurred. The iliopsoas originates at the anterior surfaces of the T12-L5 vertebra and intervertebral discs, so a forceful contraction or stretching may cause an unwanted anterior pull on those segments. In addition, exercises such as the military press that load the lumbar spine should be avoided. Finally, all exercises should be executed correctly, with proper mechanics and abdominal bracing.

5 Jerry is 60 years old. He routinely used swimming as his form of aerobic exercise and is anxious to get back into the pool again. He just started outpatient physical therapy after his surgery 6 weeks ago and has asked the therapist about when he can begin an aquatic program and what exercises he could do. What should the therapist's response be?

The buoyancy of the water could certainly be advantageous in creating an exercise program to aid in the recovery after lumbar fusion surgery. However, there are a few concerns in regards to swimming; the incision site must be healed to prevent the increased risk of infection, and the type of exercises in the pool must not place unwanted stresses on the back. It is best practice to consult the referring physician/surgeon as to when it would be appropriate to start an aquatic program and the initial exercises should be upright and not include lap swimming. Later in the program, certain strokes like butterfly and breaststroke may still be undesirable as they require increased lumbar extension to perform efficiently.

6 During the initial outpatient treatment, what should be the main focus of the treatment?

Patient education should be emphasized to ensure protection of the surgery site and allow for a better recovery with less discomfort. Good body mechanics proper posture, and maintaining precautions are integral at this stage. In addition, the therapist must take care to avoid any testing that may irritate the condition. Lumbar spine ROM and strength testing of the hip flexors are some examples of testing that should be avoided.

7 For the second therapy visit in a row, the patient smells of smoke and although they had originally quit to have the surgery the therapist is worried that they have started smoking again. How should the therapist handle the situation?

Without accusing the patient of smoking, the therapist might confront the patient about the smell of smoke on

their clothes. It would also be a good time to remind them about the negative impact that factors such as smoking, poor nutrition, and lack of sleep have on healing, which is an integral part of the recovery from surgery. If other medical conditions such as obesity or diabetes are present, it may also be integral to assist the patient in nutritional management or direct them to other services to address these factors.

8 During outpatient therapy the therapist notices that the patient is walking with a slight antalgic gait because of pain and when asked, the patient states that the leg has been a little swollen. Why might this be a concern?

With a recent onset of pain and swelling in the patient's leg, the therapist should be concerned about the patient having thrombophlebitis or a DVT. Other signs and symptoms to look out for would be warmth and redness in the leg, especially in the calf region. In the presence of those symptoms, the patient should undergo testing as soon as possible to rule out a DVT.

9 Because psychosocial factors, such as anxiety, have an influence on pain perception, how can the therapist address this to help decrease the patient's pain levels?

Besides patient education in body mechanics and postures, the therapist needs to increase the patient's awareness of pain expectations. The patient needs to allow 6 to 8 weeks for the incision area to decrease in pain. Increased activity levels at home or in the clinic are associated with an increase in muscle soreness, which can be expected. The therapist should reassure patients that their bodies will be adapting to and remodeling for 1 to 2 years, and symptoms often change during that time. Patients also need to know how to self-manage flare-ups and that most people recover well (they should have that expectation). Meeting with other patients who share in their experiences has also been shown to be helpful during recovery from lumbar fusion. Other professionals, such as a psychologist, may help with implementing cognitive-behavioral techniques to help reduce the patient's pain.

10 Why are stabilization exercises so important for rehabilitating these patients?

While the surgery is meant to help with the passive stabilization subsystem of the lumbar spine, both the active and neural systems are addressed through stabilization exercises. In the most common lumbar spine fusion procedure, a posterolateral fusion, the paraspinal muscles including the multifidi are stripped off the posterior elements (i.e., spinous process, lamina, transverse processes). This allows for partial tears of the dorsal division of the spinal nerves, therefore having partial denervation of the multifidi. Multifidi are the primary segmental stabilizers, and they do not spontaneously recover after low back pain or back surgery. The TA is another important muscle that may be cut during a fusion surgery. Trunk stabilization exercises are important for reeducating the multifidi muscles and the other trunk-stabilizing musculature.

11 A patient asks the therapist if they should be doing back extension exercises to strengthen their lumbar spine. What should the therapist's response be?

Initially back extension exercises should be avoided as they may cause excessive shear on the lumbar spine and place unwanted stress on the surgical site. Research has shown that performing exercises in the quadruped position, such as alternate leg or arm lifts, recruits the lumbar spine extensors sufficiently to improve trunk stability. Patients that need to get back to more strenuous activities may need to do lumbar extension activities much later in the last phase of rehabilitation and should only perform them if able to stabilize appropriately.

REFERENCES

1. Abbott AD, et al: Early rehabilitation targeting cognition, behavior, and motor function after lumbar fusion: A randomized control trial. Spine 35(8):848-857, 2010.

2. Burkus K, et al: Six-year outcomes of anterior lumbar interbody arthrodesis with use of interbody fusion cages and recombinant human bone morphogenic protein-2. J Bone Joint Surg 91:1181-1189, 2009.

3. Albee FH: A report of bone transplantation and osteoplasty in the treatment of Pott's disease of the spine. N Y J Med 95:469, 1912.

4. Bourcher HH: A method of spinal fusion. J Bone Joint Surg 41B:248, 1959.

5. Hides JA, Richardson CA, Jull GA: Multifidus muscle recovery is not automatic after resolution of acute, first-episode low back pain. Spine 21(23):2763-2769, 1996.

6. Hodges PW, et al: Intervertebral stiffness of the spine is increased by evoked contraction of transverse abdominis and the diaphragm: In vivo porcine studies. Spine 28(23):2594-2601, 2003.

7. Brox JI, et al: Four-year follow-up of surgical versus non-surgical therapy for chronic low back pain. Ann Rheum Dis 69:1643-1648, 2010.

8. Brox JI, et al: Lumbar instrumented fusion compared with cognitive intervention and exercises in patients with chronic back pain after previous surgery for disc herniation: A prospective randomized control study. Pain 122:145-155, 2006.

9. Hodges PW, Richardson CA: Contraction of the abdominal muscles associated with movement of the lower limb. Phys Ther 77:132-142, 1997.

10. Carragee EJ, et al: A gold standard evaluation of the "discogenic pain" diagnosis as determined by provocative discography. Spine (Phila Pa 1976) 31(18):2115-2123, 2006.

11. Burton AK: Psychosocial predictors of outcome in acute and subchronic low back trouble. Spine 20(6):722-728, 1995.

12. Butler SD: Mobilization of the nervous system, ed 4, Melbourne, 1994, Churchill Livingstone.

13. Christensen FB, et al: Importance of the back café concept to rehabilitation after lumbar spinal fusion: A randomized clinical study with a 2-year follow-up. Spine 28(23):2561-2569, 2003.

14. Ibrahim T, et al: Surgical versus non-surgical treatment of chronic low back pain: A meta-analysis of randomized trials. Int Orthop 32(7):107-113, 2006.

15. Citation deleted in proof.

16. Karikari IO, Isaacs RE: Minimally invasive transforaminal lumbar interbody fusion: A review of techniques and outcomes. Spine (Phila Pa 1976) 35(26 Suppl):S294-S301, 2010.

17. Knight RQ, et al: Direct lateral lumbar interbody fusion for degenerative conditions: Early complication profile. J Spinal Disord Tech 22(1):34-37, 2009.

18. Panjabi MM: The stabilizing system of the spine. Part I. Function, dysfunction, adaptation, and enhancement. J Spinal Disord 5(4):383-389, 1992.

19. Panjabi MM: The stabilizing system of the spine. Part II. Neutral zone and instability hypothesis. J Spinal Disord 5(4):390-397, 1992.

20. Bardin LD: Physiotherapy management of accelerated spinal rehabilitation in an elite level athlete following L4-S1 instrumented spinal fusion. Phys Ther Sport 4:40-45, 2003.

21. Kisner C, Colby LA: Therapeutic exercise: Foundations and techniques, ed 5, Philadelphia, 2007, FA Davis.

22. Wiltse LL, et al: The paraspinalis splitting approach to the lumbar spine. J Bone Joint Surg 50A:919, 1968.

23. Thompson WR, editor: ACSM's guidelines for exercise testing and prescription, ed 8, American College of Sports Medicine, Baltimore, 2004, Lippincott Williams & Wilkins.

24. Lee D: The pelvic girdle, ed 2, Edinburgh, UK, 1999, Churchill Livingstone.

25. Shacklock M: Neurodynamics. J Physiother 81(1):9, 1995.

26. Christensen FB: Lumbar spinal fusion: Outcome in relation to surgical methods, choice of implant and postoperative rehabilitation. Acta Orthop Scand Suppl 75(313):2-43, 2004.

27. McKenzie RA: The lumbar spine, mechanical diagnosis and therapy, Upper Hutt, New Zealand, 1990, Wright and Carman.

28. Herbert JJ, et al: The relationship of transverses abdominus and lumbar multifidus activation and prognostic factors for clinical success with a stabilization exercise program: A cross-sectional study. Arch Phys Med Rehabil 91:78-85, 2010.

29. Hodges PW: Core stability exercise in chronic low back pain. Orthop Clin North Am 34(2):245-254, 2003.

30. Neumann P, Gill V: Pelvic floor and abdominal muscle interaction: EMG activity and intra-abdominal pressure. Int Urogynecol J Pelvic Floor Dysfunct 13(2):125-132, 2002.

31. Sapsford RR, et al: Co-activation of the abdominal and pelvic floor muscles during voluntary exercises. Neurourol Urodyn 20(1):31-42, 2001.

32. Sahrmann SA: Diagnosis and treatment of movement impairment syndromes, St Louis, 2002, Mosby.

33. Richardson CA, et al: Therapeutic exercise for spinal segmental stabilization in low back pain: Scientific basis and clinical approach, 1999, Churchill Livingstone.

34. Ostelo RW, et al: Rehabilitation after lumbar disc surgery. Cochrane Database of Systematic Reviews Issue 4, Article No 3007, 2010.

35. Cyriax J: Textbook of orthopedic medicine: Diagnosis of soft tissue lesions, vol 1, ed 6, Baltimore, 1975, Williams and Wilkins.

36. Maitland GD: Vertebral manipulation, ed 5, London, 1986, Butterworths.

37. Mulligan BR: Manual therapy "NAGS", "SNAGS", "MWMS," etc, ed 3, Wellington, New Zealand, 1995, Plane View Services.

38. Paris SV: Mobilization of the spine. Phys Ther 49:988, 1979.

CHAPTER 17

Lumbar Spine Disc Replacement

Derrick G. Sueki, Erin Carr, Babak Barcohana

ETIOLOGY

Low back pain is a potentially disabling condition with a lifetime prevalence of 60% to 80% in the U.S. adult population. Pain may be due to a simple muscle sprain, sciatica caused by a disc herniation, vertebral fractures, or a number of other conditions, but degeneration of the spine is often the number one cause.

Disc degeneration in the lumbar spine has a significant effect on the functional behavior of the lumbar discs. As the proteoglycan content is lost and the osmotic pressure decreases within the nucleus, there is a diminished ability to retain water within the disc. The loss of volume leads to a reduced disc height, which commonly results in intervertebral foraminal stenosis, inappropriate stress concentrations causing osteophyte formation, and central stenosis. This causes lumbar instability, axial back pain, and radicular leg pain, which can become disabling and chronic, resulting in depression, loss of work, and the inability to enjoy simple activities of daily living.

The goals of lumbar spinal surgery are to alleviate pain, restore stability, and improve neurologic injury. Lumbar disc degeneration is a continuum with a spectrum of etiologic conditions resulting in pain. Based on where in the spectrum the patient falls, various surgical techniques and approaches will be offered. This chapter focuses on artificial lumbar disc arthroplasty.

SURGICAL INDICATIONS AND CONSIDERATIONS

Patients with pain related to the lumbar spine have various complaints ranging from axial low back pain, sensation of instability, difficulty bending forward, pain with prolonged sitting or standing, inability to lift heavy items, and/or radicular leg complaints. The goal of the clinician is to identify the cause of the pain.

Various diagnostic tests are employed in the detection of the pain generator. Initially, a thorough history and physical examination are of utmost importance. The goals are to rule out other causes of pain such as infections, tumors, and visceral conditions, which may result in back pain. A careful history is taken regarding trauma, fevers, chills, weight loss, cancer history, and other associated symptoms. Questions regarding the back are also obtained, including timing of injury, aggravating factors, description of pain (sharp, dull, numbness), radicular complaints, and weakness.

Subsequently, imaging studies are obtained, including plain radiographs (Fig. 17-1), MRI studies, and CT scans. Alignment, disc heights, signs of degenerative changes, and neural compression is noted. Electrodiagnostic studies, bone densitometry, and discograms are occasionally ordered.

Once the diagnosis is established, treatment is initiated. Absent neurologic deficits and unbearable pain, nonoperative treatment is recommended. This may include physical therapy for stretching, strengthening, and modalities. Back braces may be used for short periods of time to allow the muscles to relax. Medications are prescribed, including anti-inflammatory medications, pain medications, and muscle relaxants. Acupuncture, chiropractic care, physical therapy, heat, ice, traction, epidural injections, and facet injections may be ordered as well.

When the diagnosis is certain and nonoperative measures have failed, surgery is recommended. Based on the diagnosis, various surgical procedures may be recommended. For example, for an isolated disc herniation, a lumbar microdiscectomy may be considered whereas decompression and instrumented fusion may be considered for an unstable spondylolisthesis.

There are a select group of patients for which lumbar disc arthroplasty is an option. These are patients for whom an isolated decompression or discectomy is insufficient. Additionally, these patients have symptoms arising from a single lumbar disc level with complaints of axial low back pain with disc dysfunction. Based on U.S. Food and Drug Administration (FDA) guidelines, lumbar disc replacement is approved only for one level procedures. These patients would otherwise be candidates for a lumbar fusion procedure.

Criteria for disc replacement includes degenerative disc disease with discogenic back pain isolated to one level from L3-S1 in skeletally mature patients who have failed 6 months

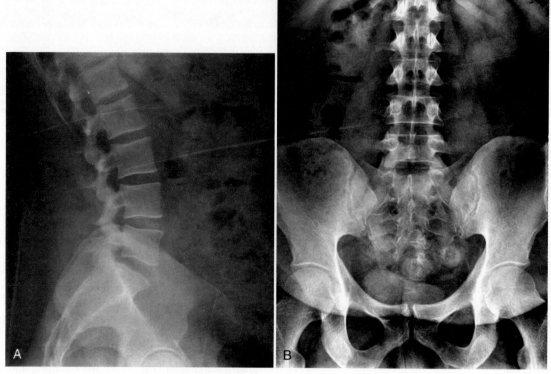

Fig. 17-1 **A,** Lateral x-ray study of the lumbar spine. **B,** AP x-ray study of the lumbar spine.

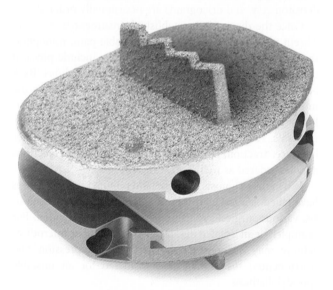

Fig. 17-2 Synthes ProDisc-L implant.

of nonoperative treatment. Contraindications include spondylolisthesis greater than grade I, significant instability or facet arthrosis, infection, bony spinal stenosis, allergy or sensitivity to implant, compromised or small vertebral bodies, isolated radicular compression syndromes, or pars defects.

As of the writing of this chapter, two lumbar artificial disc replacement devices have been granted FDA approval in the United States, including Synthes ProDisc-L (Fig. 17-2) and Charité artificial discs. These implants consist of cobalt

chromium, titanium, and ultra-high molecular weight polyethylene.

The goal and potential advantages of artificial disc replacement are to maintain motion at the operated level, thereby replicating the biomechanics of the normal disc. This serves to reduce the mechanical forces that would be transmitted to adjacent segments, which are seen with rigid fusion procedures and which may lead to early adjacent segment disease and degeneration. The device would serve to anatomic disc height while maintaining structural integrity. It would need to withstand lumbar forces with long-term stability and endurance. Given that it is not a fusion device but a motion sparing device, pseudarthrosis is not a concern. However, the implant requires integration of bone into its surfaces. There is a potential concern that fusion may still occur at the operated level.

SURGICAL PROCEDURE

The surgical approach for artificial disc procedures is similar to that performed for an anterior lumbar interbody fusion. Currently available lumbar disc replacement devices are placed from an anterior lumbar approach.

The patient is positioned on the operating room table in a supine position with all bony prominences well padded after induction of general endotracheal tube anesthesia (Fig. 17-3). Once the surgical level is identified with intraoperative C-arm fluoroscopic images, the skin is prepped and draped in the usual sterile fashion. A retroperitoneal

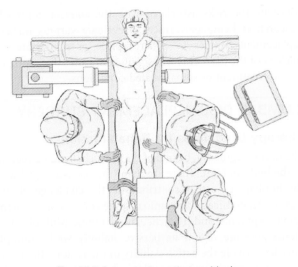

Fig. 17-3 Intraoperative patient positioning.

approach to the spine is performed. A paramedian transverse or vertical skin incision is made. The rectus sheath is incised and the rectus muscle is retracted laterally. The posterior rectus sheath is encountered and incised to reach the preperitoneal space. The abdominal muscles, including the external oblique, internal oblique, and transverses abdominis, are divided. The transversalis fascia is then divided to allow exposure of the extra retroperitoneal space. The peritoneum and its contents are carefully retracted to allow access to the retroperitoneal space. Here, various neurovascular and visceral structures are encountered, including the ureter, genitofemoral nerve and branches, psoas musculature, aorta, vena cava, sympathetic chain, and iliac vessels (Fig. 17-4).

Injury to the sympathetic nerves in males can result in retrograde ejaculation. Deep venous thrombosis may occur

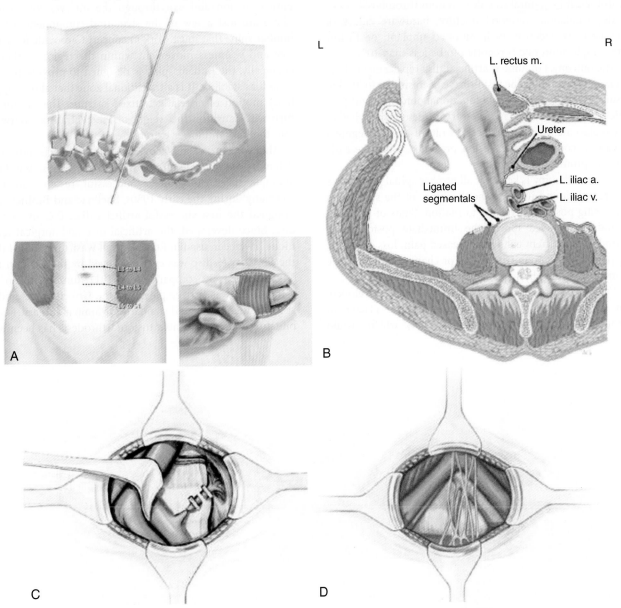

Fig. 17-4 **A,** Localization of level and approach to spine. **B,** Operative dissection to access anterior spine. **C,** Mobilization of great vessel for spinal access (L4-L5). **D,** Great vessel bifurcation (L5-S1).

in addition to injury to any of the neurovascular and visceral structures in this approach. Although many spine surgeons perform the anterior approach themselves, often general or vascular surgeons are employed to access the spine.

Once the spine is exposed and the adjacent structures are protected, a radical discectomy is performed. If necessary, neural decompression may also be performed. Next, various trials are placed to measure the size of the implant. Great care is taken to position the implant properly to maintain the appropriate center or rotation in the spine (Fig. 17-5). Multiple intraoperative images are obtained in addition to direct visualization to achieve this. The final implant is placed and is evaluated, ensuring that it is rigid with good contact (Fig. 17-6). The instruments and retractors are removed and a meticulous layered wound closure is performed.

Complications from this procedure include vascular injury, ureteral injury, wound infection, postoperative ileus, neurologic injury, dural tear, deep venous thrombosis, retrograde ejaculation, vertebral fracture, hardware failure or migration, subsidence, malpositioned implant, or fusion. The complication rate is reported to be less than 10%.

The outcomes of lumbar artificial disc replacements have been quite favorable. The results have been similar to lumbar fusion results with respect to functional outcomes and pain relief. Further research is necessary to determine whether disc replacement surgery reduces the rate of adjacent segment disease as compared with fusion procedures, but the early data are promising.

Physical therapy is key after all lumbar spinal procedures to strengthen and increase the flexibility of the spine with decreasing postoperative scar formation. Signs of infection should be watched for in the immediate postoperative period. If the patient exhibits increased pain, loss of pulses, leg pain, lower extremity swelling, or changes in neurologic examination, the physician should be contacted.

Various disc replacement products are being developed, not only for anterior approaches but also for placement through lateral or posterior approaches, which would eliminate the risks associated with the anterior approach. Research is being performed to evaluate various nucleus replacement devices to either replace or rejuvenate the nucleus of the disc. This will significantly alter the approach to and treatment of spinal related conditions.

LUMBAR DISC REPLACEMENT SURGERY

Therapy Guidelines for Rehabilitation

The lumbar spine can be one of the most challenging regions of the body to treat. There are many factors associated with the lumbar spine that contribute to the challenge of this region. Anatomically, the lumbar spine consists of 5 moving spinal segments and 10 articulating joints. Multiple ligaments give the region its passive stability while multiple muscles provide the active stability of the region. The nerve roots of the cauda equina run through the spinal canal in the lumbar region and exit through the intervertebral canal. These are just a few of the structural components of the lumbar spine that must work in concert to provide for pain-free and seamless movement within the region.[1-3] Biomechanically, the lumbar spine is designed to provide motion as well as stability. It is a transitional zone that allows upper body motion on a relatively fixed sacrum. The sacrum in turn will transition the weight of the central axis outward into the hips and lower extremities.

The concept of replacing a lumbar disc is not new. Attempts were made in the 1950s and 1960s, but both attempts failed to produce successful results.[4] In East Germany during the early 1980s, Shellnac and Buttner-Jans designed the first successful artificial disc, the SB Charité disc. Since developed, the artificial disc and surgical technique have been used in Europe, yet it wasn't until 2004 that the SB Charité disc was even approved by the FDA in the United States. By comparison, in 1911, lumbar fusion, or arthrodesis, was first employed in the United States and is still considered the gold standard for lumbar surgery. Rehabilitation following lumbar fusion/arthrodesis has been well

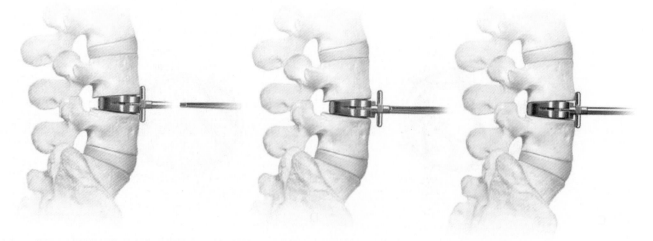

Fig. 17-5 Trial placement.

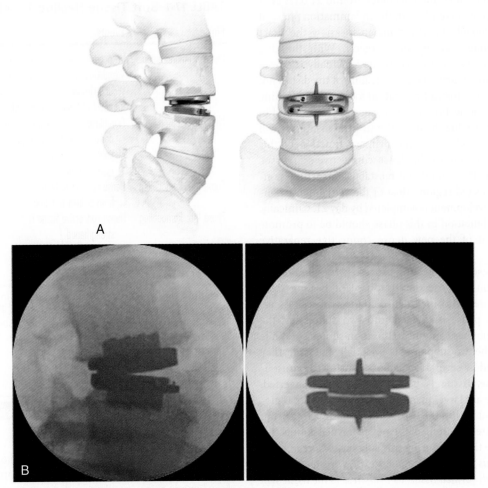

Fig. 17-6 **A,** Implant placement. **B,** Lumbar radiographs with implant in place.

established. Clinical guidelines and empirical data validating rehabilitation have also been generated for the surgery. In comparison, very few clinical guidelines have been established for lumbar disc replacement surgery and no research currently exists validating any of the suggested protocols. The guidelines that follow will be a synthesis of established tissue healing guidelines, protocols for similar spinal surgeries, and treatment geared specifically for the attributes unique to lumbar disc replacement. They are not meant to replace or supplant clinical reasoning processes. Instead they are meant as a supplement to clinical reasoning and decision-making. Each patient who has undergone total lumbar disc replacement surgery is unique. The guidelines presented should be used as a point of departure from which the clinician can customize the program to the individual's needs.

Principles of Tissue Healing[5,6]

A clinician must have a firm grasp of the tissue healing process if they are to effectively rehabilitate any patient. Variation exists in the categorization of healing; some clinicians prefer to use a system based upon symptom acuity. Acute symptoms are present for the first 3 weeks immediately following injury. The subacute phase begins at 3 weeks

and continues until 2 to 3 months after injury. Symptoms lasting longer then 2 to 3 months are considered chronic. Conversely, other systems of classification are based upon the physiologic goal of the phase. This type of physiologic based system of classification will provide the framework of this chapter.

Phase 1 is considered the inflammation phase and is so named because of the phase's physiologic goal of producing inflammation within the injured area. Inflammation is the body's initial response to any injury or surgery. Immediately after surgery, the body begins the process of repair. Inflammation occurs and intensifies in the surgical region over the course of the next several days and reaches its peak production within the first 72 hours after injury. The generation of acute inflammation is generally completed within 14 days and during these first 14 days, several events occur.[6,7] Clinically, rehabilitation during the inflammation phase of tissue healing should focus upon the prevention of blood loss, reduction of inflammation, and managing the pain that accompanies tissue damage.

The second phase of tissue healing is the reparative phase. The chief physiologic goal of this phase is to repair the injured tissue. Chronologically, this phase begins immediately after injury and concludes around 21 days after injury, running concurrently with the inflammation phase of healing. It is valuable for the clinician to know the exact surgical technique used by the surgeon. With the disc replacement surgery, the injured tissue is actually removed and replaced with an artificial disc. Healing of the disc is not an issue in this case. Instead reparation focuses on providing an environment of healing for the tissue that was incised in the process of replacing the disc. The surgical technique will influence the rehabilitation. The primary function of this phase is the formation of the dense connective scar tissue needed to repair the wound and reestablish structural continuity of the affected region. Most of the actual dense connective tissue development is completed by day 21. Clinically, the goal of rehabilitation in this phase should be to promote the development of the new dense connective reparative tissue.

The final phase of the healing process is the remodeling phase. The main purpose of this phase of healing is to strengthen the newly formed dense connective scar tissue. Classically, this phase is divided into two subphases, the consolidation subphase and the maturation subphase. While the purpose of the two subphases is essentially the same, they are characterized by several key factors. During the consolidation subphase, tissue is being formed and converted. Therefore, there are large quantities of fibroblast and angioblast cells present within the tissue. This subphase lasts from 22 to 60 days. Strengthening of the newly formed connective tissue should be the goal during this subphase. *Care must be taken during this phase so as not to exceed the mechanical limits of the newly formed tissue, as overstress to the tissue will result in tissue injury and delayed healing.* The second subphase, the maturation subphase, occurs from day 60 to 360 and is hallmarked by dense connective scar tissues that are fully fibrous in nature. For this reason, a progression in the strengthening of the affected tissues may begin more aggressively. As in the consolidation subphase, a rehabilitation programs must provide appropriate levels of stress to encourage dense connective scar tissue formation without creating or exacerbating tissue injury.

Summary Statement

Although guidelines can provide generalized timeframes for healing and recovery, it is important to realize that a firm grasp of the factors listed above will enable the clinician to individualize the rehabilitation program for each patient (also consideration is always given to the patient's signs and symptoms). No two patients are identical. Therefore, no two rehabilitation programs should be identical. Solid clinical reasoning regarding the patient and the nature of his or her injury and surgery will ultimately drive the rehabilitation process. Table 17-1 summarizes the soft tissue healing timeframe for all three phases of healing. Adequate muscle activity and protection must accompany the healing process to progress activity levels. Healing tissues may be compromised because of increased levels of strain without adequate muscle support and protection.

TABLE 17-1 Soft Tissue Healing Timeframes

Phase	Events	Timeframe
Phase I: Inflammation	Vasoconstriction in immediate area Vasodilation in surrounding areas Wound closure Removal of foreign and necrotic tissue	0-14 days
Phase II: Reparative	Fibroblasts enter region to create dense connective tissue scars Angioblasts enter the region for revascularization	0-21 days
Phase IIIa: Remodeling	Dense connective tissue is converted from cellular to fibrous	22-60 days
Phase IIIb: Remodeling	Dense connective tissue is strengthened	61-84 days
Phase IIIc: Remodeling	Dense connective tissue is strengthened	85-360 days

Data from Nitz A: Soft tissue injury and repair. In Placzek J, Boyce D, editors: Orthopaedic physical therapy secrets, Philadelphia, 2001, Hanley and Belfus; Frenkel S, Grew J: Soft tissue repair. In Spivak J, et al, editors: Orthopaedics: A study guide, New York, 1999, McGraw-Hill.

BOX 17-1 Indications for Lumbar Disc Replacement

Strong Indications

1. Progressively worsening bowel and bladder symptoms related to nerve impingement in the lumbar spine (cauda equina syndrome)
2. Saddle paresthesia (numbness and tingling in the groin in the area that would be in contact with a saddle)

Relative Indications

1. Radiculopathy that has failed to respond to conservative treatment regimen of at least 6 weeks
2. Recurrent radiculopathy
3. Progressive neurologic deficit
4. Severely limited functional ability secondary to lumbar pain or paresthesia associated with disk pathology

---

Attributes Unique to Lumbar Disc Replacement Surgery

The gold standard for surgical treatment of chronic low back pain is the lumbar fusion surgery. But like all surgeries, no surgical technique has 100% success rate and in the case of lumbar fusion surgery, 20% of patients will require additional surgery within 5 years after the initial surgical technique.[8-12] See Box 17-1 for indicators that lumbar disc replacement surgery may be required. The most common reasons for failure of the surgery are bone graft donor morbidity, the formation of pseudoarthrosis, and adjacent spinal segment degeneration. One of the major factors believed to be associated with these failure factors is the loss of normal lumbar biomechanics following spinal fusion. The lumbar disc replacement surgery has been designed to eliminate these factors. The disc replacement is designed to maintain normal spinal biomechanics at the surgical site, decompression of the lumbar facets and neural structures, and restore the normal disc height between spinal segments.[13-16] The disc replacement surgery is performed anteriorly and requires incisions through the rectus abdominis and the anterior aspect of the disc space. Following surgery, these two structures are weak and vulnerable to injury. Rehabilitation programs should address the unique aspects of this surgery and interventions designed accordingly.

Description of Rehabilitation and Rationale for Using Instrumentation

Phase I: Inflammatory Phase

TIME: Weeks 1 to 2 (Days 0 to 14)

GOALS: Protection of the surgical site, decrease pain and inflammation, initiate patient education regarding neutral lumbar spine mechanics, begin walking program (Table 17-2)

Hospital Rehabilitation. Immediately following surgery, the goals while in the hospital should focus on patient education, protection of the surgical site, reduction in pain and inflammation, and restoration of independent activities of daily living. The normal hospital stay is between 5 to 7 days, with discharge either to a home environment or a skilled nursing facility.[14,15]

While in the hospital setting, the patient will be instructed in how to protect the surgical site. This is accomplished by instructing the patient on maintaining proper neutral spine during motion. Additionally, a lumbar stabilization brace is issued to the patient for additional support and protection. Instructions regarding the duration of its use are determined by the physician and may vary on a case-by-case basis. Log rolling and abdominal bracing techniques are used to get into and out of bed, and transitioning from supine to a sitting position. Care should be taken to avoid overstressing the abdominal muscles since the rectus was surgically incised and is subsequently weak and subject to tearing or injury. Initial examination and evaluation should include assessment of the wound, hip passive range of motion (ROM) testing, bed mobility, and gait assessment.

Hospital rehabilitation should also include gentle abdominal activation/core strengthening. *The goal is not strength, but muscle recruitment.* Circulation exercises are also incorporated early in the rehabilitation process. Ankle pumping exercises and thromboembolic hose hose stockings are used to prevent pooling of blood in the lower extremities. Diaphragmatic breathing exercises can be used to mobilize the abdominal muscles and abdominal contents to stimulate the lymphatic system and encourage circulation. Since the abdominal region is the site for most of the surgery, it is not uncommon for inflammation and edema to accumulate in the abdomen.

Weight-bearing activities should also begin early in the rehabilitation process. Sit to stand and gait activities should be initiated. Initially, standing and gait training will be accomplished with the aid of a front wheel walker. By the

TABLE 17-2 Inflammatory Phase of Healing

Rehabilitation Phase	Criteria to Progress to This Phase	Anticipated Impairments and Functional Limitations	Intervention	Goal	Rationale
Phase I Inflammatory phase Postoperative wk 1-2 (days 0-14)	Postoperative	• Pain • Edema • Limited lumbar range of motion • Limited nerve mobility • Limited sitting tolerance • Limited standing tolerance • Limited walking tolerance	Patient education: • Proper use of lumbar support brace • Protection of surgical site • Correct body mechanics and maintenance of neutral lumbar spine • Splinting and guarding during coughing, sneezing, and defecating Exercise: • Daily walking program • For specific examples, refer to Table 17-8 • Avoidance of lumbar extension, rotation, and side bend	• Decrease pain and edema • Protection of surgical repair (soft tissue) • Understand the timeframe for healing structures • Understand correct body mechanics and maintenance of neutral lumbar spine • Gradual increase in walking speed and duration • Instruction on protecting lumbar spine during functional activities • Prepare patient for discharge from hospital and first month of independent home exercise and self-care	• Encourage self-management of pain and edema • Prevent adhesions of neural tissue • Prevent reinjury with patient education on body mechanics and maintenance of neutral lumbar spine with activity • Gradually improve cardiovascular endurance

end of the hospital stay, the patient should be ambulating with the aid of a single point cane. Ambulation to and from the restroom should begin immediately with assistance as needed. These activities should progress until the patient is independent. *Gentle lumbar spinal ROM can also be initiated in the hospital. Lumbar flexion exercise is the only direction of motion allowable initially.* Because the disc space and abdominal cavity was incised anteriorly, it is the weakest portion of the body. Overstressing these tissues should be avoided. **The clinician should avoid excessive and repetitive extension exercises, as well as lateral flexion and rotation. These precautions are generally in place for 6 to 8 weeks. Prone lying should also be avoided during this time period because of weakness and sensitivity of the anterior tissues.**

Before discharge from the hospital, it is important that the clinician educates the patient on proper lumbar spine mechanics during activity and the need to avoid excessive trunk extension, side bend, or rotation. Refer to Box 17-2 for specific patient guidelines to follow after discharge. *The patient should be advised to refrain from heavy lifting, bearing down during defecation, and abdominal splinting during*

BOX 17-2 Hospital Discharge Instructions Following Lumbar Disc Replacement Surgery

- Wear lumbar brace continuously unless instructed otherwise.
- Do not pick up or carry anything heavier than 5 lb.
- Limit twisting or bending backward. You may bend forward as tolerated with physician approval.
- Keep your low back braced and stabilized as instructed when completing daily activities
- Avoid sitting or standing for prolonged periods of time. Change positions frequently.
- Get plenty of rest, but do not spend all of your time in bed.
- Gradually increase walking time. Do not get overtired.
- Avoid strenuous exercise or activities.
- Keep incision dry. Showering is allowed 10 days following surgery if wound is not red or draining.
- You may sleep in any position that is comfortable, except sleeping on your stomach or with arms overhead.
- Do not drive until approved by your physician.
- Continue home exercise program.
  Notify your doctor if any of the following occur:
- Temperature greater than 101° F
- Redness or swelling around your incision
- Any drainage from your incision
- Separation of wound edges
- Any new bruising around wound
- New numbness or tingling in your hands or fingers
- Increased pain in low back or legs
- New weakness in the legs
- Changes in bowel or bladder function

---

coughing or sneezing. Before discharge, the need for a continued home exercise program should also be addressed. Patients can be discharged once they are able to walk unassisted or with minimal assistance depending on their post-surgical care and rehabilitation plans. They also must be free of complications, have normalized their bowel and bladder function, and show a good understanding of their surgical precautions and activity limitations.

Initial Posthospital Rehabilitation. The second postoperative week will occur at home or a skilled nursing facility. Activities during this later stage of the inflammation phase are a continuation of the care received while in the hospital. During this time, activities should center on resuming protected normal daily activities. The patient should be encouraged to increase their daily sitting, standing, and walking tolerances. Pain and fatigue should guide the progression. The lumbar stabilization belt should be worn 24 hours a day unless otherwise ordered by the physician. Patient exercises may progress. The patient can begin gentle neutral spine lumbar stabilization exercises. Once again care must be taken to avoid overstressing the abdominal muscles. The goal is muscle recruitment, not strengthening. The patient may begin gentle lower extremity strengthening exercises, but care must be taken to stabilize the lumbar region. The clinician should keep in mind throughout this phase that the primary goal of this phase of rehabilitation is protection of the surgery, pain abatement, and restoration of protected daily activities.

Phase II: Reparative Phase
TIME: Week 3 (Days 0 to 21)
GOALS: Understand neutral spine concepts, increase lower extremity mobility, improve upright tolerance, improve protected activities of daily living, increase cardiovascular function (Table 17-3)

In many instances, phase II of the rehabilitation process will take place independently in the patient's home. Home therapy is rarely indicated. Therefore, education regarding patient progression through the first month following surgery is an important aspect of hospital care. The clinician's advice and instructions will be followed for the next 3 to 4 weeks. During the reparative phase of tissue healing, the body begins to form and lay down scar tissue at the surgical site, thus enhancing the integrity of the musculatures, ligaments, and capsule to withstand gradual increases in loads to the tissues. Therefore, as time progresses, increasing load can be placed upon the surgically repaired tissue. Rehabilitation should be a continuation of phase I and progress restoring lower extremity ranges of motion and independence with self-care skills. Movement improves circulation and prevents the formation of scar tissue adhesions between the nerve and the healing tissue surrounding the surgery. Following lumbar disc replacement surgery, scar tissue formation is inevitable in and around the surgical site. In certain instances, scar tissue can adhere to surrounding tissues,

TABLE 17-3 Reparative Phase of Healing

Rehabilitation Phase	Criteria to Progress to This Phase	Anticipated Impairments and Functional Limitations	Intervention	Goal	Rationale
Phase II Reparative phase Postoperative wk 3 (days 15-21)	• No signs of infection • Incision site is healing well	As in phase I • Limited upper body and lower body strength • Limited walking tolerance • Limited tolerance to prolonged sitting/standing positions	Continue interventions in phase I Exercise: • Initiate gentle ROM of the hip • Begin core/lumbar stabilization exercises in supine (see Fig. 17-7) • Progress walking program to 15-20 minutes as tolerated • For specific examples, refer to Table 17-8 • Increase lumbar flexion ROM as tolerated	Same goals as phase I with the following: • Improve upright tolerance • Restore functional ROM to lower extremities • Restore patient independence with self-care skills • Improve activities of daily living while protecting surgical site • Increase cardiovascular function • Independent with home exercise program	• Restore lower extremity ROM and tissue tension to allow for proper movement mechanics • Prepare patient to be independent in self-care skills • Restore proper posture throughout trunk to allow patient to achieve overall neutral spine • Improve cardiovascular endurance

ROM, Range of motion.

impacting mobility of any structure to which it attaches. Therefore, movement of the lower extremity and lumbar region should be encouraged to promote circulation and prevent adhesion formation. Throughout all activities and exercises, the patient should be encouraged to maintain a neutral lumbar spine. Activities should not increase symptoms. Protection of the surgical site and proper immobilization should continue until the physician has seen evidence that the prosthetic is well situated. At this time, the physician will approve additional lumbar motion and activities.

Phase IIIa: Remodeling Phase
TIME: Weeks 4 to 8 (Days 22 to 60)
GOALS: Enhance nerve healing and mobility, prevent scar tissue formation, increase lower extremity strength and endurance, improve thoracic spine and sacral mobility, begin normalization of functional daily activities, restoration of lumbar ROM (Table 17-4)

Between the end of the fourth week and up to the sixth postoperative week, the patient's physician will reassess the patient. Generally, this reassessment will include a new radiographic study. Most physicians will release the patient to begin outpatient rehabilitation following this reassessment. This decision will be dependent upon several factors, including patient symptoms and function. At 4 to 6 weeks following surgery, it is anticipated that the patient will continue to have mild (possibly moderate) low back pain and achiness. This will most likely be present in the morning and at the end of the day. Functionally, the patient should be walking limited community distances with a single point cane for balance. Neurologic symptoms that are the result of spinal compression or inflammation should be improving

and stabilizing. Objectively, the physician will order a spinal radiograph to assess the position of the prosthetic. If all of these factors are acceptable, the physician will allow the patient to begin outpatient rehabilitation.

The first postoperative outpatient examination should include evaluation of the patient's scar, assessment of posture and gait, balance testing, and active range of motion assessment. ROM can be tested in all directions of motion, but end range extension, rotation, and side bending must be avoided for 6 weeks. Additionally, the clinician should conduct a neurologic examination if nerve involvement is suspected. The clinician should also assess the patient's lumbar soft tissue, looking for muscle guarding and atrophy. Quick screening of the patient's lower extremity should also be completed. Once the patient has been screened and deemed appropriate for phase III rehabilitation, the clinician can begin to design his or her treatment plan.

Postural Rehabilitation. Upon initial evaluation, observation of the patient's posture will give the physical therapist a significant amount of information concerning weakness, elongation, and strength of specific musculature as well as the patient's ability to maintain a neutral lumbar spine. According to Janda, a common postural alignment seen in people with lower quarter pathology is known as the lower cross syndrome.[17] Regardless of the cause, this alignment will consist of a lower quarter muscle pattern in which certain muscles will be weakened and lengthened and others will be strong and shortened, resulting in an increased lumbar lordosis and increased hip flexion. *More specifically, there is a weakening and lengthening of the gluteal and abdominal muscles. This is combined with a tightening and shortening of the hip flexors and lumbar extensors.* Although a very common posture following spinal surgery, this position is

TABLE 17-4 Remodeling Phase of Healing 1

Rehabilitation Phase	Criteria to Progress to This Phase	Anticipated Impairments and Functional Limitations	Intervention	Goal	Rationale
Phase IIIa Remodeling phase (consolidation) Postoperative wk 4-8 (days 22-60)	• Patient understanding of neutral spine concepts • No increase in pain symptoms • No increase in nerve-related symptoms • Follow-up visit with physician and approval to progress rehabilitation	• Limited nerve mobility • Limited upper extremity strength • Limited ability to perform overhead activities • Limited mobility in thoracic region • Limited cardiovascular endurance • Continued pain or discomfort with sustained postures (i.e., standing and sitting)	Continue with phase II interventions as needed with the following: Exercise: • Progress lumbar stabilization activities • At 6 wk, begin gentle AROM/PROM of lumbar spine as tolerated (see Fig. 17-8) • Begin progressive resistive exercise program of the upper and lower spine while maintaining lumbar stability • Increase walking tolerance to 30 minutes Neuromobility: • Begin neuromobility techniques (see Box 17-5 and Table 17-6) Mobilization: • Begin soft tissue mobilization • Begin joint mobilization to the thoracic spine and sacroiliac joint at 4 wk • Begin joint mobilization to the lumbar spine at 8 wk • For specific examples, refer to Table 17-8 • Initiate gentle LE flexibility for hamstrings and quadriceps near end of phase in protected postures • Initiate soleus and gastrocnemius stretches	Same as phase II with the following: • Enhance nerve healing and mobility • Prevent scar tissue formation • Increase upper and lower extremity muscular strength and endurance • Increase lumbar range of motion • Improve mobility of thoracic spine and sacrum • Correct abnormal lumbar movement patterns • Improve functional ability • Improve aerobic capacity	• Prevent soft tissue adhesions at surgical site • Prevent neural adhesions • Increase stabilization while performing daily activities to prevent re-injury • Decrease joint stiffness to allow proper movement with decreased pain • Correct abnormal lumbar movement patterns • Independence with self-care activities

AROM, Active range of motion; *LE,* lower extremity; *PROM,* passive range of motion.

not advisable for the patient because it places the lumbar spine in an extended or lordotic position. During gait, the clinician may notice that the patient walks with a shortened stride length because with long strides the spine is further extended during the terminal stance phase of gait if tight hip flexors are present. **Physiologically, lumbar extension should be avoided because of the increased stress it places upon the prosthetic and the weakened anterior musculature.**

Postural rehabilitation should be implemented and interventions should focus upon the stretching of shortened hip flexor and lumbar extensor muscles and strengthening of the weakened gluteal and abdominal muscles of the lumbar region. **Posturally, the patient should be instructed to avoid anterior pelvic tilt that will lead to increased lumbar lordosis.**

Therapeutic Exercise. While no research or clinical practice guidelines have been developed specifically for lumbar disc replacement surgery, systematic reviews and clinical practice guidelines have been developed for the rehabilitation after lumbar disc surgery and can be extended to rehabilitation after lumbar disc replacement surgery. While most studies are mixed in terms of intervention efficacy, the one intervention that is uniformly beneficial is therapeutic exercise.

Lumbar Stabilization. Core stabilization, lumbar stabilization, transverse abdominis training, and multifidus training are all rehabilitation programs developed to activate local muscle groups, stabilize the lumbar region, and normalize the recruitment of lumbar musculature. Normal muscle activity involves a coordinated recruitment of both local and global muscle groups. Local muscles work to stabilize the region while global muscles function as movers of the body. In the lumbar spine, the local muscles, such as the multifidus and transverse abdominis, engage to stabilize spinal segments. The global muscles, such as the quadratus lumborum and hip flexors, function as primary movers of the lumbar region. When injury occurs, local muscle groups are inhibited, requiring global muscles to activate and stabilize the region. Theoretically, localized inflammation inhibits neuromuscular control systems. Richardson and associates performed a series of studies on the ability of deep lumbar muscles to stabilize spinal segments in patients with lumbar pain.[18] Their findings suggest that deep muscle activation is a necessary component in the reestablishment of spinal control following a low back injury. Subjects that did not reestablish segmental control continued to experience low back pain. Therefore, whether the clinician chooses to use core stabilization, lumbar stabilization, transverse abdominis training, or multifidus training, the program should have a component of deep local muscle activation. Once the local muscle can be recruited, rehabilitation should progress to coordinating local and global muscle activation. Exercises focused upon the recruitment of local muscle groups are appropriate for this phase of healing.[19-21] See Fig. 17-7 for

examples of therapeutic exercises appropriate for this phase of healing.

Stretching. Following most surgeries, tissue mobility in and around the surgical area will be tight and restricted. In the presence of tissue injury or damage, muscles play a primary role of protection. Muscle tightness is commonly found in the hip flexors, quadratus lumborum, and the erector spinae of disc replacement patients. Stretching and ROM exercises should target these muscles, because normalization of muscle length is a key component of the restoration of muscle function and of normal lumbar mechanics. Normalization of lumbar motion should occur by 8 weeks following disc replacement surgery. Although individual variations will occur, by 6 weeks, the patient should have exercises that actively and passively promote normal spinal motion in all directions, including rotation, side bend, and extension. Care should be taken when initiating each of these motions, and patients should be advised to stretch slowly and within pain tolerances. All stretches should be pain free. See Fig. 17-8 for examples of therapeutic exercises appropriate for this phase of healing. Typical ROM exercises for this phase of rehabilitation include single knee to chest, seated flexion, prone press ups, prayer stretch, supine piriformis stretch, hip flexor stretch, supine and seated trunk rotations, and lateral side bend exercises. See Boxes 17-3 and 17-4 for normal sequencing of motion during lumbar flexion and for normal ranges of motion in the lumbar spine during lumbar flexion.

Soft Tissue Mobilization. As a lone intervention, massage and soft tissue mobilization have been shown largely to be ineffective at reducing a patient's symptoms or improving a patient's functional capacities. When used in

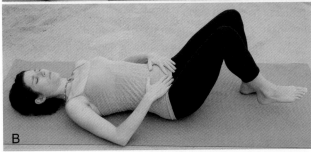

Fig. 17-7 Therapeutic exercises. **A,** Transversus abdominis strengthening. In hooklying, isometrically contract the transversus abdominis by drawing in your belly button. Make sure to maintain a neutral spine and not posteriorly tilt the pelvis causing lumbar flexion. Normal breathing should also be maintained. **B,** Transversus abdominis and hip dissociation. Contract the transversus abdominis in hooklying with a neutral spine. Lift one leg off the ground 1 to 2 inches. Alternate legs. Transversus abdominis contraction should be maintained throughout concentric and eccentric movement of both legs.

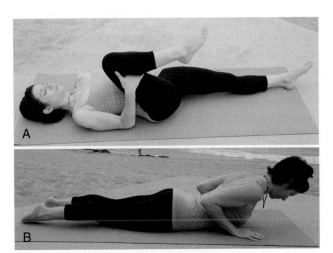

Fig. 17-8 Therapeutic exercises. **A,** Single knee to chest. Begin in hooklying position. Hug one knee to chest allowing pelvis to posteriorly tilt. Opposite knee can stay flexed in early phase of healing and can be progressed to knee extension. **B,** Prone press-ups. Begin in prone position with hands placed under shoulders. While maintaining chin tuck, push-up, promoting lumbar spine extension. This exercise can be progressed with elbow extension, therefore increasing lumbar spine extension.

BOX 17-3 Normal Sequencing of Motion for Lumbar Forward Bend

1. When the patient initiates the forward bend, the first event that occurs is a posterior sway of the pelvis. This occurs as the body attempts to maintain its center of gravity within its base of support.
2. As the body continues to bend forward, the hips begin to flex and the lumbar spine begins to reverse its lordotic curve.
3. The lumbar curve fully reverses and the hips continue to flex forward to complete the forward bending motion.
   NOTE: The lumbar spine should not complete more than 50% of its motion before hip flexion motion is initiated.

Data from Delilitto A, Woolsey NB, Sahrmann S: Comparison of two noninvasive methods for measuring lumbar spine excursion which occurs in forward bending. Phys Ther 67:743, 1987; Sahrmann S: Diagnosis and treatment of movement impairment syndromes, St Louis, 2002, Mosby.

BOX 17-4 Lumbar Spine Motion With Forward Bend

The lumbar spine is typically positioned between 20° and 30° of lumbar extension with a normal standing posture. With a full lumbar forward bend, the patient should reverse the lumbar lordosis. The final position of lumbar flexion is between 20° and 30° of lumbar flexion.

Data from Loebl WY: Measurement of spinal posture and range of spinal movement. Ann Phys Med 9(3):103-110, 1967.

TABLE 17-5 Approximate Range of Motion for the Three Planes of Movement for the Joints of the Lumbar Region

Joint or Region	Flexion/ Extension (Degrees)	Axial Rotation— Unilateral (Degrees)	Lateral Flexion— Unilateral (Degrees)
L1-L2	12	2	6
L2-L3	14	2	6
L3-L4	15	2	8
L4-L5	16	2	6
L5-S1	17	1	3
Total Lumbar	74	9	29

Adapted from White AA III, Panjabi MM: The basic kinematics of the human spine: A review of past and current knowledge. Spine 2:12, 1978; White AA, Panjabi MM: Clinical biomechanics of the spine, Philadelphia, 1990, Lippincott.

---

conjunction with other intervention, soft tissue mobilization can be an effective adjunct to allow the body to recover mobility and function. Muscles will contract to protect any area of the body vulnerable to injury. Chronically, this protective contraction can result in postural changes and these postural changes can result in abnormal forces being placed upon normal tissue. Over time these alterations in posture and loads can result in tissue breakdown and pathology. Retraining and maintaining muscles and soft tissue tension is an important aspect of normalizing lumbar motion. Soft tissue mobilization to the hip flexors, quadratus lumborum, and the erector spinae can be used effectively as an adjunct to normalizing lumbar motion and mechanics.

Joint Mobilization. Normalization of the biomechanics of the lumbar spine should be a large consideration in any rehabilitation program that is developed for disc replacement surgery. Mobilization techniques have taken on increased prominence in rehabilitation programs. In practice, they are used to increase ranges of motion within

targeted regions by moving specific joints or specific muscles. Care must be taken in choosing the appropriate time to begin implementation of joint mobilization techniques because of the potential translational effect they may have on the lumbar spine and more specifically at the replacement site. Research has studied the effects of a posterior to anterior force placed on the spinous process of L3. Studies by Lee et al showed a force at L3 could result in movement as far away as T8, and in follow-up studies by the same group, the same posterior to anterior force resulted in an anterior rotation of the sacrum.[22-25] The implications of these findings for the patient following a lumbar disc replacement surgery is that even mobilizations to distant segments may have a translatory impact upon the surgical site. Initially, the clinician must use caution when directly mobilizing the lumbar spine. **The anterior aspect of the joint and the prosthetic are particularly vulnerable to injury. Posterior to anterior mobilization of the lumbar spine is not advisable for the first 8 weeks following surgery.** After that time, the lumbar spine can be mobilized in this direction. Posterior to anterior mobilization should focus on segments adjacent to the prosthetic. Mobilization of adjacent segments can be used to normalize motion in these segments and decrease the demands placed upon the replacement site. **There is no need to mobilize the segment with the prosthetic in a posterior to anterior manner since the prosthetic is a fixed unit and posterior to anterior motion of the prosthetic does not occur.** The more appropriate mobilizations for the prosthetic segment are techniques focused on improving segmental flexion, extension, and rotation, for these are the motions provided by the new prosthetic. Mobilization in flexion can begin before mobilization into other ranges of motion. As with any mobilization, the clinician should use patient symptoms and status as a guide for how much mobilization to use. See Table 17-5 for normal ranges of motion for lumbar spinal segments.

Lumbar pain and pathology can lead to or be the result of movement dysfunction and compensations in other regions of the body. While mobilization of the lumbar spine may not be advised immediately because of postsurgical tissue weakness, mobilization of regions adjacent to the lumbar spine is appropriate. Initially, the clinician can begin to mobilize the thoracic spine or sacrum. Decreased flexibility in thoracic spine segments and the soft tissue of the thoracic region may prevent proper body alignment, including normal lumbar lordosis. Thus treatment should include soft tissue mobilization to the thoracic spine musculature and passive joint mobilization techniques to the thoracic spine.[26,27] Mechanics and proper functioning of the sacrum can also directly impact the functioning of the lumbar spine. The sacrum is required to provide a stable base from which the rest of the spine can move. The sacrum and sacroiliac joint are an important link between the lower extremities and the spine. If they are not functioning correctly, the forces are transmitted to the lumbar spine. Mobilization of the thoracic and sacral regions can help to alleviate the pressure placed upon the disc. Both mobilizations are an appropriate early intervention for this phase of rehabilitation.

Neural Mobilization. At this phase of rehabilitation, neural mobilization should show progress. The clinician should assess the mobility of neural structures. The common base test for neural mobility is the straight leg raise test. This test can be used as a starting point from which the clinician can test specific peripheral nerves of the lower extremity. Fibular, tibial, sural, and femoral all have specific test positions that place the nerve into a position of tension.[28] See Figs. 17-9 through 17-11 for examples of neural mobility testing and testing sequences. If the nerve does not glide through its surrounding tissue, the nerve is stretched. In response to the tensile load, symptoms such as numbness, tightness, and tingling are produced. These symptoms lessen when tension is removed from the nerve. A positive test is

indicative of restricted mobility in the nerve being tested. Using the test position to stretch the nerve and release any adhesions along its course is a common treatment philosophy. See Box 17-5 and Table 17-6 for lower limb nerve test positions and methods. Unlike muscles, neural tissue is not as elastic and responds adversely to stretching.[29] Neural mobility techniques are commonly classified into two categories: techniques that glide the nerve and techniques that stretch the nerve. Sliding techniques produce a greater amount of nerve excursion through the surrounding tissue than tensioning techniques. Joint motions can influence the mobility of the nerve.[30,31] Muscle activity in the test leg also increases when the ankle is placed in a tensile position.[32,33] It has been hypothesized that increased muscle activity could indicate the muscles plays a protective role with regard to nerve mobility testing. When the nerve is placed in tension,

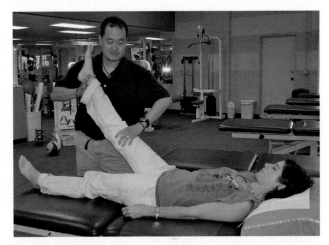

Fig. 17-9 Straight leg raise base test. This test is designed to assess the mobility of the sciatic nerve. The knee is kept in extension and the foot ankle in a neutral position. The leg is lifted up until tightness or the patient's symptoms are reported. Pillow is optional, but should be consistent between testing sessions.

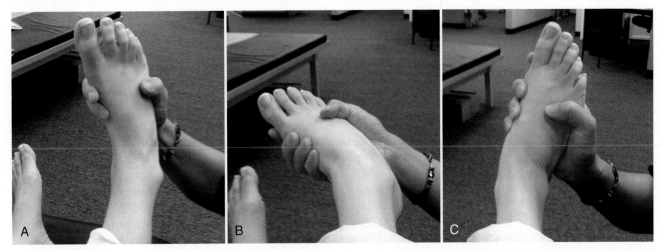

Fig. 17-10 Straight leg raise test foot positions for biasing peripheral nerves. **A,** Position for the sural nerve (dorsiflexion and inversion). **B,** Position for the peroneal nerve (plantar flexion and inversion). **C,** Position for the tibial nerve (dorsiflexion and eversion).

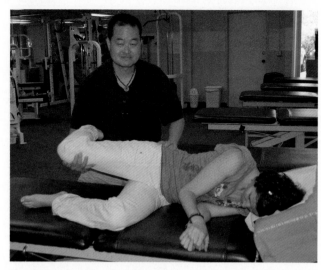

Fig. 17-11 Side-lying femoral nerve test. This test is also known as the side-lying slump test. The patient is positioned in side lying. The cervical and thoracic regions are flexed forward. The clinician takes the upward lower extremity from a position of hip flexion toward hip extension. The leg is extended until the patient reports the onset of tightness or symptoms are reproduced.

muscles are recruited to protect the nerve and prevent injury to the structure. Nerves are sensitive structures and can be easily damaged.

Treatment, therefore, should address the gliding and not stretching of nerves. Before gliding the nerve, soft tissue structures along the course of the nerve can be mobilized to allow for nerve mobility. Movement of the lower extremity can be combined with small movements of the neck to encourage gliding of the nerve rather than stretching. Finally, communication with the patient is essential since radicular pain or paresthesia are indications that the nerve is being stretched and potentially irritated. **The patient and therapist should work in ranges of motion that do not reproduce the patient's radicular symptoms. Neural mobilization techniques, as well as all techniques mentioned in this book, should only be used by therapists specifically trained in the technique.**

Summary Comments. At this stage of rehabilitation, the patient may find it difficult to perform activities that require prolonged sitting or standing postures. These limitations are normal. It is important to assist the patient in recognizing methods or activities that have the ability to relieve some of the pain or soreness. It is also important that they be assisted in the development of strategies to increase muscle endurance so that they may gradually build a tolerance to these positions. Strategies may include limiting the time spent in any one position, the use of cryotherapy to the back, or active lumbar ROM exercises to relieve stiffness and soreness. Improving protected functional abilities and normalizing nerve mobility are appropriate for this phase of healing. Cardiovascular endurance and strength should continue during this phase.

Phase IIIb: Remodeling Phase
TIME: Weeks 9 to 12 (Days 61 to 84)
GOALS: Restore strength and ROM in the lumbar spine, maintenance of neutral spine with concurrent upper and lower extremity movements, improve and normalize function movements, improve the coordinated recruitment of local and global muscle, address musculoskeletal issues that may have contributed to the patient's low back pain (Table 17-7)

The primary goal of this phase of rehabilitation is restoration of function. Progression to this phase of rehabilitation should begin once the patient is able to tolerate the exercises of phase IIIa without an increase in low back or lower extremity symptoms. Interventions from the previous phase have focused on loading the body in a manner that protected the lumbar spine. The purpose of this precaution was to prevent overstressing newly healed structures. By week 9 after surgery, most scar tissue should have been formed. Edema and inflammation should be minimal and patient function should be returning to normal. From a tissue perspective, the newly laid dense connective tissue requires appropriate loading to promote strength in the tissue. Basic strengthening and protection should be continued but progressed to include movement outside the basic framework of the core. The goal is protected restoration of function and functional motion.

Functional Retraining. Functional retraining is not a new concept in rehabilitation. It challenges strength, balance, and coordination in functional positions. It involves systems of core training and lumbar stabilization in a weight-bearing, functional environment. At this phase of rehabilitation, it is appropriate to begin to train the body to work in outside of its center of mass (Fig. 17-12). Earlier in the chapter, it was discussed how local muscles are inhibited and global muscles recruited in response to injury. Initial exercises involved recruitment of local muscles such as the transverse abdominis and the multifidus muscles. As the patient continues his or her progress and rehabilitation, it becomes appropriate to start to challenge the patient outside of midline and in upright functional positions. Patients need to operate outside of a neutral spine and perform normal function where strength, flexibility, motor control, and proprioception are all required. Activities such as front lunges and side lunges can be progressed to include upper extremity motions and upper body rotation or side bends. Near the end of this phase, patients can be evaluated for advanced strengthening (i.e., planks, pointer dog, and supine bicycle). Squats and sit to stand can incorporate trunk rotation. Single-leg balance can be combined with single-leg squats and forward or side reaching. By changing position of the upper body and lumbar spine, and adding active functional based activities, the body can begin to recruit the local muscles while at the same time selectively targeting weakened groups of muscles. Various positions of the hip and trunk can force the selective

---

BOX 17-5 Straight Leg Raise and Side-Lying Femoral Nerve Testing Procedure

Testing Procedure for Straight Leg Raise Testing

1. First, establish the patient's baseline resting symptoms. Remember to reassess baseline symptoms/resistance/range of motion with the addition of each new component.
2. Patient is positioned in supine near edge of table.

Therapist position

1. The clinician is positioned adjacent to the patient's thigh.
2. Next, the clinician will grasp the patient's foot with one hand while the other hand is placed on the patient's knee and will be used to keep the knee straightened.
3. Alternatively, the clinician may grasp the patient's ankle with one hand while the other hand is placed on the ball of the patient's foot and will be used to control the patient's foot position.

Procedure

1. The clinician positions the foot and ankle to test specific nerves.
2. The patient's leg is raised into flexion while the knee is kept in an extended position.
3. The clinician raises the leg until the patient reports the initial onset of tightness in the leg.
4. The clinician next releases the foot and ankle position to see if the symptoms in the leg change. If neural structures are involved, the symptoms should lessen.
5. The clinician can vary the sensitizing positions to further implicate the nerve as the source of the motion restriction.

Sensitizing positions

- Contralateral cervical lateral flexion should increase patient symptoms.
- Ipsilateral cervical lateral flexion should decrease patient symptoms.

- Hip abduction should decrease patient symptoms.
- Hip adduction should increase patient symptoms.

Testing Procedure for Femoral Nerve Testing

1. First, establish the patient's baseline resting symptoms. Remember to reassess baseline symptoms/resistance/range of motion with the addition of each new component.
2. Patient is positioned in side lying with a pillow placed beneath the head to maintain a midline position.

Therapist position

1. The clinician is positioned adjacent to the patient's gluteal region.
2. Next, the clinician will support the patient's knee and lower extremity with the hand and forearm of one arm. The other hand is placed on the patient's hip to stabilize the pelvis.

Procedure

1. The clinician pre-positions the patient's thoracic and cervical spine into flexion.
2. The clinician takes the hip from a flexed position to an extended position until the patient reports the initial onset of tightness in the leg.
3. The clinician next extends the patient's head while maintaining the hip position. If neural structures are involved, the symptoms should lessen.
4. The clinician can vary the sensitizing positions to further implicate the nerve as the source of the motion restriction.

Sensitizing positions

- Cervical flexion should increase patient symptoms.
- Cervical extension should decrease patient symptoms.
- Hip abduction should decrease patient symptoms.
- Hip adduction should increase patient symptoms.

Adapted from Butler D: The sensitive nervous system, Adelaide Australia, 2000, Noigroup Publications.

---

recruitment of one muscle group while inhibiting others. See Fig. 17-13 for examples of therapeutic exercises appropriate for this phase of healing. *Progression to this phase of rehabilitation should not be permitted until the patient shows good motor recruitment and control of the basic set of exercises and the patient's symptoms are minimal.*

Lumbar Proprioception. Proprioceptive training has played a large role in the rehabilitation of individuals following injury. In the lower extremities, it has been established for quite some time that injury impacts joint proprioception. The mechanism of this impairment can vary and in some cases the exact physiologic mechanism behind the

proprioceptive changes is not clear. Regardless of the exact physiologic mechanisms, research has shown that rehabilitation can improve joint proprioception. In response to these findings, rehabilitation experts have included proprioceptive training in rehabilitation programs to address and change the proprioceptive system.[34]

While a mainstay in many extremity rehabilitation programs, proprioceptive training has not factored into most spinal programs. Recently, research has surfaced that suggests that proprioception should play a larger role in spinal rehabilitation programs.[35-39] In response to these findings, as a patient's functional and physical capabilities progress, it is appropriate and necessary to begin to progress exercises in

TABLE 17-6 Lower Limb Nerve Testing Positions

Test	Nerve Assessed	Test Position	Test Motion
Straight leg raise	General	Supine: Leg straight and uncrossed Spine in midline position Arms resting at the patient's side No pillow under head	Knee in extension Foot in neutral position Hip flexed until initial onset of symptoms Check sensitizers: ankle DF/PF, cervical flexion, hip abduction/adduction
Straight leg raise with peroneal bias	Peroneal	Supine: Leg straight and uncrossed Spine in midline position Arms resting at the patient's side No pillow under head Shoulder abduction	Knee in extension Foot in DF and inversion Hip flexed until initial onset of symptoms Check sensitizers: inversion/eversion, ankle DF/PF, cervical flexion, hip abduction/adduction
Straight leg raise with tibial bias	Tibial	Supine: Leg straight and uncrossed Spine in midline position Arms resting at the patient's side	Knee in extension Foot in DF and eversion Hip flexed until initial onset of symptoms Check sensitizers: ankle inversion/eversion, ankle DF/PF, cervical flexion, hip abduction/adduction
Straight leg raise with sural bias	Sural	Supine: Leg straight and uncrossed Spine in midline position Arms resting at the patient's side No pillow under head	Knee in extension Foot in PF and inversion Hip flexed until initial onset of symptoms Check sensitizers: ankle inversion/eversion, ankle DF/PF, cervical flexion, hip abduction/adduction
Femoral nerve	Femoral	Side lying: Bilateral hips and knees flexed Thoracic and cervical spine in flexed position Pillow under head to maintain neck in midline	Knee in flexion Foot/ankle in neutral Hip extended until initial onset of symptoms Check sensitizers: cervical flexion/extension, hip abduction/adduction

DF, Dorsiflexion; *PF*, plantar flexion.
Adapted from Butler D: The sensitive nervous system, Adelaide Australia, 2000, Noigroup Publications.

TABLE 17-7 Remodeling Phase of Healing 2

Rehabilitation Phase	Criteria to Progress to This Phase	Anticipated Impairments and Functional Limitations	Intervention	Goal	Rationale
Phase IIIb Remodeling phase (maturation) Postoperative wk 9-12 (days 61-84)	• Surgical site has healed • No increase in pain symptoms • Patient demonstrates neutral spine concepts • Correct abnormal lumbar movement patterns • Patient able to complete most normal daily activities while maintaining lumbar stability and without an increase in symptoms	Same as phase II with the following: • Limited ability to perform activities in a prolonged sitting/standing position • Patient is not fully independent with ADL • Walking tolerance still limited by lumbar fatigue	Continue with phase II interventions Exercise: • Progressive resistive exercises with lumbar stabilization at the end of the phase, if appropriate (see Fig. 17-13, *D*) • Begin functional retraining (see Fig. 17-12) Balance training: • Begin balance and proprioceptive training Mobilization: • Progress thoracic, lumbar, and sacral joint and soft tissue mobilization	• Restore strength to upper and lower extremities • Normalize lumbar range of motion • Improve lumbar mechanics • Maintenance of neutral spine in various positions/planes with concurrent upper and lower extremity movement • Begin to increase motion and function outside of the base of support • Improve proprioception in the lumbar spine	• Independent with self-care and ADL • Prevent reinjury with increase in dynamic activities • Knowledge of pain-relieving strategies/positions during prolonged activities

ADL, Activities of daily living.

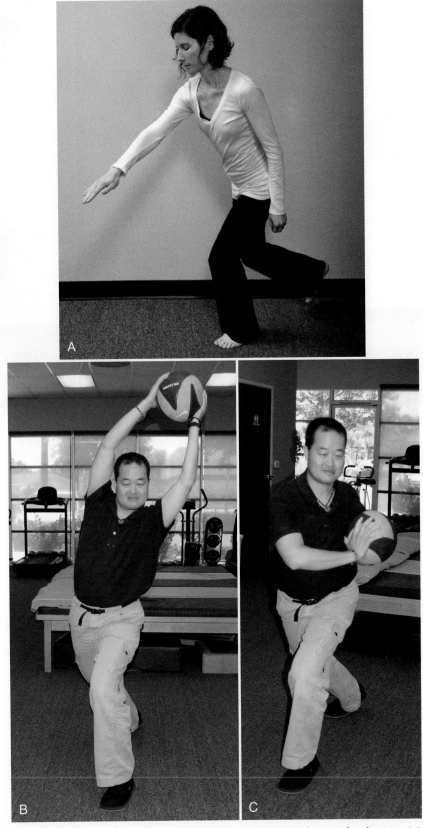

Fig. 17-12 Functional retraining. **A,** Single-leg reach. Begin exercise with single-leg balance. Flex knee, as if performing minisquat. While knee is flexing, simultaneously extend opposite arm and leg. Rotate trunk toward the side of the standing limb. **B,** Forward lunge with ipsilateral side bend. Exercise can be varied and the upper body can be positioned in contralateral side bend, extension, or flexion. Each position will selectively recruit different muscle groups. **C,** Forward lunge with ipsilateral rotation. Exercise can also be completed with contralateral rotation. Weighted medicine ball is used in this picture, but exercise can be completed with a variety of objects and weights to simulate work and sports-related environments.

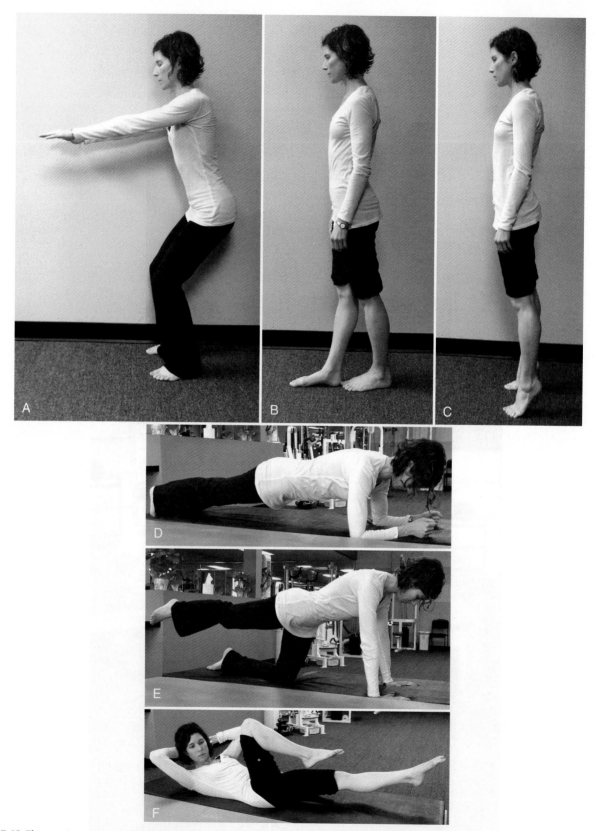

Fig. 17-13 Therapeutic exercises. **A,** Minisquats. Feet are placed a hip width apart. While maintaining abdominal contraction, squat with 30° to 45° of knee flexion as if sitting in a chair. **B,** Tandem balance. Place one foot in front of the other while maintaining trunk control. Hold position 30 to 45 seconds in each direction. **C,** Heel raises. Standing with knees and ankles, hip width apart, lift up onto balls of feet. Weight should be placed over the first digit on each foot. **D,** Planks. Begin in the prone position with elbows in-line with shoulders. Contract transversus abdominis and push up onto forearms as well as toes. Isometrically contract abdominals, maintain neutral spine and chin tuck. **E,** Pointer dog. Begin in quadruped position (hips and knees in 90° of flexion), neutral spine, chin tucked. While maintaining trunk control and transversus abdominis contraction, extend one lower extremity with opposite upper extremity. Lower each limb and repeat with opposite limbs. **F,** Bicycles. Begin in hooklying position. Place hands behind head. Bring both legs into 90° of hip and knee flexion. Contract transversus abdominis, bring right armpit to left knee promoting slight trunk rotation. Extending opposite lower extremity simultaneously. Do not lift scapulas off mat.

manners that challenge proprioception and balance. See Figures 17-12 and 17-13, *F*, for examples of therapeutic exercises appropriate for this phase of healing.

Summary Comments. As the patient progresses, it is important for him or her to begin to normalize lumbar motion with functional activities. Functional activities that change balance and proprioception while at the same time challenging strength and endurance are the most appropriate types for this phase of healing. Patients do not function in a small, limited amount of lumbar motion. They must bend, twist, and rotate through large ranges of motion and their backs must be capable of functioning during these larger ranges of motion. See Table 17-8 for a list of therapeutic exercises for the various phases of rehabilitation.

Phase IIIc: Remodeling Phase

TIME: Weeks 13 to 52 (Days 85 to 360)
GOALS: Return to work or sport, return to prior level of functioning, preparation for discharge from physical therapy (Table 17-9). Some of these goals may be reached at 6 months and some may be reached at 1 year.

From a prognostic standpoint, it takes a full year for a patient to totally recover from lumbar surgery. That is not to say that it will take a full year for the patient to restore function and return to normal daily activities. It is simply that the remodeling phase takes a full year and that changes in tissue can take up to year to reach their ultimate strength. The remodeling phase of the rehabilitation process focuses on return to work, sport, or normal daily activities. By the end of this phase, the patient should be able to function independently at home and in the workplace. As the patient progresses through the rehabilitation process, functional retraining of work or sport-specific activities should be assessed. Activities that require increased loads on the lumbar spine should be evaluated and, pending physician approval, rehabilitation geared towards functional training can be initiated. *Return to activities or sports that require contact between players or heavy lifting will require a physician's approval.* At this time, the clinician may implement a gym- or home-based exercise program to assist in maintenance of proper strength and muscle function. Discharge of the patient should occur once the patient, rehabilitation personnel, and physician have all determined that the patient has reached his or her functional goals and is able continue the rehabilitation process safely and independently.

Troubleshooting

Red Flags

There is a 30% to 40% chance complications will occur during and/or after lumbar spine surgery because of exposure and mobilization of anterior structures.[40] Those requiring multilevel versus single level exposure are at a higher risk

---

TABLE 17-8 Therapeutic Exercise List

Phase	Appropriate Therapeutic Exercises
Phase I: Inflammation	Neutral spine abdominal bracing with bed mobility
	Lumbar stabilization/transverse abdominis muscle activation (see Fig. 17-7)
	Single knee to chest hip ROM exercise
	Ankle pumps
	Abdominal breathing
	Gait training
	Transfer training
	Bed mobility training
	Hooklying isometric abdominal contractions
Phase II: Reparative	Lumbar stabilization/transverse abdominis exercises in supine
	Progress walking program
	Increase sitting and walking tolerances
Phase IIIa: Remodeling	Progress supine stabilization and walking programs
	Add standing core and lumbar stabilization exercises:
	• Squats (see Fig. 17-13, *A*)
	• Heel raises (see Fig. 17-13, *C*)
	• Sit to stand
	• Standing bicep curls
	Add movement assessment and correction of abnormalities:
	• Seated knee flexion and extension
	• Quadruped rocking
	• Supine
	Add lumbar ROM exercises:
	• Prone extension (see Fig. 17-8, *B*)
	• Supine trunk rotation
	• Seated trunk rotation
	• Seated flexion
	Add straight leg neural gliding techniques in supine (see Table 17-6)
	Add recumbent bicycle and treadmill as tolerated
Phase IIIb: Remodeling	Continue and progress phase IIIa exercises:
	• Planks (see Fig. 17-13, *D*)
	• Side planks
	• Standing rows
	Add functional training:
	• Single-leg squats
	• Single-leg squat reaches (see Fig. 17-12, *A*)
	• Forward lunges with trunk side bend (see Fig. 17-12, *B*)
	• Side lunges with trunk side bend
	• Lunges with shoulder flexion
	Add balance and proprioception training:
	• Single-leg stance
	• Standing on air discs or BOSU balls
	• Single-leg squats with eyes closed
	Progress walking and recumbent bicycle
Phase IIIc: Remodeling	Continue with phase IIIb exercises
	Add sports- and work-related training
	Add running on treadmill, elliptical trainer
	Add work simulated activities

ROM, Range of motion.

TABLE 17-9 Remodeling Phase of Healing 3

Rehabilitation Phase	Criteria to Progress to This Phase	Anticipated Impairments and Functional Limitations	Intervention	Goal	Rationale
Phase IIIc Remodeling phase (maturation) Postoperative wk 13-24 (days 85-168)	• Patient able to self-manage pain • No decrease in functional ability	• Difficulty lifting heavy objects • Difficulty maintaining prolonged postures • Unable to complete work- or sports-related activities	Exercise: • Progress sets and repetitions of upper and lower extremity resisted exercise program as tolerated by patient • Functional retraining activities (work or sport related per physician approval) • Preparing to run with treadmill, minitrampoline	• Return to prior level of functioning • Return to presurgical level of strength and endurance • Prepare patient for discharge	• Improve patient's ability to manage work-related schedule • Promote continuance of proper postures and home maintenance program after discharge from physical therapy

for such complications, as are the elderly, obese, and those with cardiovascular disease.[40,41] It is important the clinician is aware of these potential complications to educate the patient on the importance of reporting any signs or symptoms to his or her physician immediately.

Infection

Infection has been reported in approximately 1% to 2.4% of patients undergoing lumbar spine surgery.[42] Incisional hernias, sterile discharge, and other superficial wounds at the incision site can occur.[43] Periincisional abdominal bulges can also occur because of intercostal denervation.[40] Deeper infection can also occur, leading to more serious complications including bone destruction and resorption as well as osteomyelitis in vertebrae adjacent to the surgical site.[42] Signs and symptoms of infection include fever, hypotension, tachycardia, tachypnea, increased pain, edema, wound drainage, tenderness, and general malaise.[44]

Vascular Complications

Injury to vascular structures is the most common complication when using an anterior approach for lumbar spine surgery.[40,41,45] Potential damage to the arterial and venous systems occurs in 2.8% of cases because of mobilization of the aorta, inferior vena cava, and iliac arteries.[46-48] Thrombosis is the most likely postoperative arterial complication, yet can be prevented with use of anticoagulants, compressive hoses, and calf pumps.[40] When exposure of the L4-L5 lumbar spine segments is required, mobilization of renal, iliac, and iliolumbar veins is necessary, placing an increased risk for complications. With this in mind, intraoperative bleeding can occur when venous structures are damaged. Individuals who are diabetic, obese, elderly, or have cardiovascular disease are not only at a higher risk for experiencing such complications, but they are also at risk for postoperative ischemia.[40] Signs and symptoms of arterial or venous damage may include calf pain, lower extremity edema, diminished pedal pulses, temperature changes, discoloration, and heaviness in the lower extremities.

Neural Complications

There are a variety of nerves that can be injured during lumbar spine surgery. The lumbar sympathetic chain runs along the spine, controlling genitourinary organs. If damaged, one may be left with a warm lower extremity, often mistaken for vascular damage, and a variation of incontinence.[40] The iliohypogastric, ilioinguinal, and genitofemoral somatic nerves are also at risk for damage resulting in decreased sensation to the groin and external genitalia.[40] After surgery, increased radicular pain may occur because of epidural fibrosis causing nerve root traction during surgery.[49,50] This has been shown to resolve by the third month postoperatively.[50]

Genitourinary Complications

Genitourinary complications can occur from damage from the mobilization of the hypogastric sympathetic plexus. Injury to urinary tract organs, decreased genital sensation, retrograde ejaculation, and impotence in males can result.[40,51] Damage to ureters occurs in 0.3% to 8.0% of cases and can be injured whether spine surgery requires an anterior or posterior approach.[40] Retrograde ejaculation occurs in up to 28% of males undergoing lumbar spine surgery with an anterior approach.[40,51] When this occurs during lumbar spine surgery it is often irreversible. Elderly men, diabetics, and those with vascular disease are at a higher risk for such complications.[40]

Spontaneous Fusion and Heterotropic Ossification

Unlike spinal fusion surgery, the goal of total disc replacement (TDR) surgery is to preserve movement and restore disc height and segmental lumbar lordosis. Spontaneous interbody fusion of segments above and below the surgical site has occurred in greater than 60% of patients after a 17-year follow-up.[48,50] Approximately 1.4% to 15.2% of patients have also experienced heterotropic ossification with the use of ProDisc and SB Charité prostheses.[48]

Implant Materials

The polyethylene metal used in TDR is the same type of metal used in total knee and hip replacements. Although there haven't been any reported cases of wear debris, creep, or osteolysis occurring in disc replacement surgery, there is a potential for permanent deformation and wear of the metal similar to total knee and hip replacements.[45,48] This may take as little as 1 year or as long as 10 years to occur, both leading to a necessary anterior and posterior spinal fusion of the involved segments.[45,48,50] Possible dislocation or loosening of the polyethylene metal can also occur over time, resulting in chronic pain and requiring spinal fusion because of biomechanical failure.[52]

Biomechanics

The purpose of having a TDR rather than spinal fusion is to preserve the normal movement of the lumbar spine.[48] During surgery, malpositioning of the disc implant, whether anterior or posterior, can occur.[48] This can ultimately cause decreased ROM and/or an increase in load to posterior structures. Malpositioning also affects the sagittal balance of the lumbar spine, resulting in decreased lumbar lordosis and possible degeneration of adjacent segments.[48]

Chronic Pain

Changes in the peripheral and central nervous system occur almost immediately following an injury. Some of these changes are reversible and other changes are nonreversible. It is beyond the scope of this chapter to describe all the neural changes that occur with injury, but from a clinician's viewpoint it is important to realize that not all patients will have full resolution of symptoms following surgery. Surgery may have addressed the structures that were originally the source of the patient's symptoms, but the adaptations that have occurred in the central and peripheral nervous system may not be reversible. It is important to realize that not all pain is a reflection of actual tissue damage. As a result, not all patients will have full resolution of symptoms.[28,53,54] See Box 17-6 for factors that contribute to chronic pain.

SUMMARY

Rehabilitation of a patient following a TDR is unique, considering its goal is to maintain lumbar ROM and overall mobility. Although it is pertinent to begin mobility exercises early on in the rehabilitation process, it is just as important

---

BOX 17-6 Factors Contributing to Chronic Pain

Peripheral Changes
- Changes in tissue sensitivity at the site of injury and along the peripheral nerve

Spinal Cord Changes
- Inhibition and processing changes at the spinal cord level

Alteration In Midbrain Function
- Changes in midbrain process leading to changes in:
  - Immune function
  - Autonomic function
  - Motor control
  - Endocrine function

Alteration In Cortical Processing
- Changes in ways pain is interpreted and processed
- Changes in memories, emotions, and stress in the interpretation and the processing of pain

Data from Butler D: The sensitive nervous system, Adelaide, Australia, 2000, Noigroup Publications; Gifford L, Butler D: The integration of pain sciences in clinical practice. J Hand Ther 10:86-95, 1997.

---

to allow the surgical site to heal. Therefore, patient education regarding surgical protection guidelines immediately following surgery is a must. Aside from healing the surgical site, specific rehabilitation protocols and guidelines created for TDR surgery are similarly based on protocols for other lumbar spine surgeries (i.e., microdiscectomies and fusions). Balancing abdominal stability and lumbar mobility in conjunction with lower extremity strength and cardiovascular exercise is most important. Considering the variety of individuals requiring a lumbar disc replacement surgery, it is necessary to create and progress a program specific to each patient's needs. Finally, since radicular pain and lower extremity paresthesia are often the symptoms driving the decision for lumbar disc replacement surgery, prevention of neural adhesions and promotion of nerve healing should be addressed appropriately.

Suggested Home Maintenance for the Postsurgical Patient

The patient can use the following home program during the rehabilitation process. The contents of the home maintenance program may vary depending on the patient's prior level of function, single versus multilevel TDR and tolerance and ability to complete the exercises properly without the onset of pain symptoms or aberrant motions.

Inflammation and Reparative Phases I and II (Weeks 1 to 3)

Goals For This Period: Protection of the surgical site, decrease pain and edema, understand proper body mechanics and posture, increase walking tolerance, speed, and endurance. Extension exercises past neutral should be avoided during this phase of the healing process.[55]

---

1. Protection of the surgical site
2. Manage swelling/edema in lower extremities
   a. Ankle pumps
   b. Compression stockings
   c. Leg elevation
3. Bracing as needed during seated and standing activities to encourage healing
4. Knowledge and understanding the need for regaining normal lumbar spine ROM
5. Gentle flexion exercises encouraged,[56] performed after 2 weeks in supine
   a. Hook lying isometric abdominal contractions emphasizing transverse abdominis and multifidus recruitment[55]
   b. Bed mobility
6. Lower extremity strengthening for quadriceps and gluteal muscles
   a. Sit to stands
   b. Minisquats
   c. Heel raises
   d. Daily walking program
7. Neuromuscular reeducation
   a. Tandem balance
   b. Single-leg balance

Remodeling Phase IIIa (Weeks 4 to 8)

Goals For This Period: Increase lumbar spine ROM in all directions and begin to return to normal activities of daily living

1. Increase lumbar flexion mobility
   a. Progress abdominal strengthening with hip dissociation, (i.e., hip flexion, hip internal/external rotation in hook lying)
   b. Single knee to chest stretch
   c. Quadruped rocking
2. Begin upper extremity and lower extremity strengthening exercises with proper abdominal bracing
   a. Rows
   b. Bicep curls
   c. Hamstring curls
   d. Step-ups
   e. Squats

3. Begin lumbar extension, side bend, and rotation ROM exercises between week 6 and 8 as long as incision site has healed; begin progressing to end of range movements after 6 weeks[55]
   a. Prone press ups
4. Nerve gliding
   a. Nerve gliding for those experiencing radicular symptoms (i.e., sciatica) into lower extremities postsurgery.[55] Perform with caution, careful not to stretch the nerve.
5. Cardiovascular
   a. Progress walking program
   b. Recumbent bike
6. Return to performing basic activities of daily living including reaching, stooping, and squatting Avoid heavy lifting and high impact activities such as jumping and running.

Remodeling Phases IIIb (Weeks 9 to 12)

Goals For This Period: Progress lower extremity strength, aerobic capacity, and functional activities.

1. Progress abdominal, erector spinae and gluteal strength
   a. Planks (initiate near end of phase)
   b. Pointer Dog
   c. Abdominal bicycles (must have enough muscle control to perform correctly)
   d. Latissimus dorsi pull downs
   e. Bosu ball squats
   f. Lunges
   g. Single-Leg reach

Remodeling Phase IIIc (Weeks 13 to 24)

Goal For This Period: Independence with progressive home exercise program, return to sport.

1. Continue previous exercises and progress reps and weights as tolerated
2. Begin sport-specific drills
3. Increase walking speed and distance
4. Preparations for running and more aggressive exercises may begin at week 12
5. Lifting mechanics with weight; twisting and bending may begin after 12 weeks if ready

CLINICAL CASE REVIEW

1 Your patient is a 34-year-old male who underwent a L4-L5 lumbar disc replacement surgery 1 day ago. The physician states that the surgery was a complete success and that the patient is ready to begin in-hospital rehabilitation. You have been asked to evaluate and begin the rehabilitation process. What will your evaluation and initial treatment involve?

Initial evaluation in the hospital will involve taking the patient's vital signs and assessing the patient's wounds. Given that both of these objective measures are satisfactory, the clinician should have several goals on day 1. First is to educate the patient on neutral spine bracing and mechanics. The patient should be educated on how to move in bed and progress from lying to sitting with the lumbar region braced. The patient should be fitted with a lumbar support brace and shown how to use the brace. The brace is worn 24 hours a day unless otherwise ordered by the physician. Sit to stand mobility should be assessed using the front wheel walker for support. The patient should be able to walk from the hospital bed to the bathroom with minimal assistance. A front wheel walker will be used for support. The patient should be encouraged to sit, walk, and stand for limited times initially. No position should be held for greater than 15 minutes. The patient should be advised not to transfer, stand, or walk without assistance for the first day.

2 Your patient is a 53-year-old male who underwent an L4-L5 TDR 4 weeks ago. He has type II diabetes and is 100 lb overweight. During his initial evaluation for outpatient physical therapy, he reports that he ran out of his blood thinners 1 week ago and has been experiencing right lower extremity leg pain and swelling for the past 5 days. Symptoms seem to be progressively worsening. The patient has not yet spoken with his physician.

Red Flag: This patient is at risk for a deep vein thrombosis. He is diabetic and overweight, both predisposing him to vascular complications during and after surgery. Symptoms including lower extremity pain, severe edema, discoloration, temperature changes, diminished pedal pulses, and heaviness are all signs of deep vein thrombosis. This patient should be advised to see his physician or go to the nearest hospital as soon as possible to prevent further complications, including a pulmonary embolus.

3 Your patient is a 42-year-old female who underwent a lumbar disc replacement surgery 5 days ago. She is progressing well and without complications and is preparing for discharge from the hospital tomorrow. She will be returning to her home where her husband and family will help care for her. What must be done with the patient before her discharge tomorrow?

The patient will mostly likely not have home rehabilitation care. The instructions given in the hospital at time of discharge should be followed until the patient is released to physical therapy in approximately a month. Therefore, several instructions need to be purveyed to the patient. The patient should be given the hospital discharge instructions (See Box 17-2). The patient should be instructed to maintain the lumbar stabilization program and joint protection precautions. A progressively increasing walking program should be encouraged. Lumbar flexion should be promoted and lumbar extension, rotation, and side bend avoided. A lumbar brace should be worn 24 hours a day unless otherwise ordered by the physician. Lumbar core stabilization should be used with all daily activities.

4 Your patient is once again the 42-year-old female who underwent a lumbar disc replacement surgery. She is now in an outpatient orthopedic clinic 5 weeks following her surgery. She saw her doctor yesterday and has been cleared to begin outpatient orthopedic rehabilitation. What will your evaluation and initial treatment involve?

The patient will guide your initial evaluation. Most patients will have a little low back pain and stiffness, but the symptoms are getting better. The initial evaluation will involve assessing posture and motion. ROM can be tested in all directions of motion, but end-range extension, rotation, and side bend should be avoided until 6 weeks. Lower extremity ROM and lower extremity strength should also be tested. Care must be taken not to overtax the patient's injured regions. A neurologic examination should be completed to determine the amount of nerve damage sustained during surgery. The patient should avoid lying on her stomach for the first 6 weeks following surgery. Interventions will include reviewing the patient's current exercises and the progression of exercises as needed. Walking tolerance should be encouraged. Lumbar and core stability exercises should be included and progressed at week 6. Soft tissue mobilization in side lying may begin at this time. The patient should be warned to avoid trunk extension, rotation, and side bend. The patient may begin to wean off of the lumbar brace at 6 weeks pending physician approval. The weaning process should involve coming out of the brace for 1 hour on day 1, 2 hours on day 2, 3 hours on day 3, etc.

5 Your patient is a 29-year-old female who is 5 weeks postsurgical L4-L5 lumbar disc replacement. She is in your clinic for her first outpatient rehabilitation session. You are assessing her posture and ROM. She stands with increased hip flexion and increased lumbar lordosis. When asked to forward flex, her motion is guarded and she is unable to fully flex because of low back tightness and pain. What are the implications of these finding in your clinical decision-making process?

Pain and guarding are normal symptoms at 5 weeks postoperation. Lumbar lordosis should be avoided in patients following disc replacement. The patient should be taught abdominal bracing and lumbar protection strategies. Neutral lumbar spine positioning should be incorporated to avoid lumbar lordosis. With lumbar flexion, the patient should be able to bend forward and the lumbar spine should flatten or reverse its lordotic curve. The patient has a normal response for her phase of healing. The clinician should begin manual therapy and exercises to restore normal lumbar motion.

6 Your patient is a 65-year-old male who underwent a TDR surgery with dynamic stabilization 5 weeks ago.

He complains of shooting pain and numbness down his left lower extremity. He has difficulty when transitioning from supine to sit and sit to stand, and can only walk 100 feet before having to sit and rest because of pain. He asks why this is happening after surgery and wonders how long it will take for these symptoms to resolve.

Radicular symptoms into the lower extremity following disc replacement surgery are not an uncommon complaint. Multiple factors can be the cause of the symptoms. In certain instances, the radicular symptoms can be the result of nerve root traction during surgery secondary to epidural fibrosis. Such symptoms usually resolve by the twelfth week, postoperatively. It is important that the clinician educates the patient on such symptoms, so he also knows what to expect and to follow up with his physician in case symptoms worsen.

7 Your patient is a 37-year-old male who is 6 weeks postsurgical L3-L4 lumbar disc replacement. He is progressing well but continues to experience limitation in ROM. Low back pain is improving, but stiffness in the lumbar region continues to persist. You decide to incorporate joint mobilization into your treatment plan. What joints and techniques should you use in your treatments?

At 6 weeks after surgery, prone techniques are appropriate for the patient. The clinician can begin mobilization of the thoracic region at 4 weeks and mobilization of the lumbar spine at 6 weeks. The patient's symptoms will be your guide to mobilization intensity and duration. Posterior to anterior mobilization can be used at the thoracic and lumbar spine, but is not appropriate at the L3-L4 spinal segment. Sacral mobilization can also be incorporated. Rotational and flexion/extension mobilization techniques are most appropriate for the L3-L4 spinal segment.

8 Your patient is a 55-year-old female who had L2-L3 lumbar disc replacement surgery 2 months ago. She is progressing well with her initial exercises and would like to begin further exercise progression. What and how can she progress her exercises?

Lumbar exercises can be progressed in the following manner:
- Increase the number of repetitions for each exercise
- Increase the amount of resistance the patient is using for each exercise
- Progress core stabilizing exercises from supine to more functional positions such as standing
- Decrease base of support while completing exercises and begin to challenge balance
- Begin to work outside of the patient's base of support and begin functional-based exercises

9 Your patient is a 35-year-old male who had lumbar disc replacement surgery 3 months ago. He is progressing well and would like to begin running. What is your advice for the patient and should he be allowed to begin running?

Generally, running can begin in some patients at 3 months following surgery, but most people will begin at a running regime at 5 to 6 months following surgery. Before that time, the patient can begin prerunning activities. Prerunning would include several weeks of walk/running on the treadmill, use of an elliptical trainer, and running on a minitrampoline before beginning running on the street. In the beginning, the patient should only begin running for 10 to 15 minutes and then increase the running time 5 minutes a day as tolerated. Ultimately the decision to begin running will need to be approved by the surgeon, but will be based upon the patient's symptoms and whether he can complete daily activities with good lumbar control and stability.

10 Your patient is a 34-year-old male who has been making steady progress in physical therapy. He is 9 weeks postlumbar disc replacement surgery at L4-L5 and wants to know when he can return to surfing and snowboarding.

Surfing and snowboarding are considered extreme sports. It is recommended to postpone participation in such activities for at least 6 months post-TDR and in most cases it is closer to 9 months. This time frame is variable and depends upon the nature of the sport and the patient's functional and symptom progression. At 12 weeks, he is able to begin light running, lifting, twisting, and bending activities. Sport-specific activities can begin when the patient can run pain free. The patient will require clearance from his physician before returning to sports. This patient needs to be educated on the proper exercise progression to prepare for such recreational activities and requires clearance from his physician to participate in such activities.

11 Your patient is a 38-year-old male who had lumbar disc replacement surgery 6 months ago. He is now running for short distances and has not noticed any increase in symptoms. His chief limitation is running greater than 30 minutes. The physician has approved him to return to work and discontinued outpatient orthopedic rehabilitation. What is his program and what is your advice to him in terms of his ultimate prognosis?

If the patient is running and has been approved to return to work. He is now appropriate for discharge. He will continue to heal and strengthen for up to 1 year following the surgery. So, he should continue to progress his exercises at home and in a gym setting. He can begin to return to playing sports at 6 months, but this will be dependent upon the nature of the sport and the patient's symptoms. Higher impact sports that require contact or repetitive jumping may require additional time. These athletes may require 9 to 12 months of time before return to the sport. The patient should be given a home- and gym-based program to continue for the next 6 months. The patient should also be advised to respect his pain and symptoms, and to progress his home program in a pain-free manner.

REFERENCES

1. Kapandji I: The physiology of the joints, vol 3, New York, 1995, Churchill Livingstone.
2. Marco R, An H: Anatomy of the spine. In Fardon D, et al, editor: Orthopaedic knowledge update: Spine 2, Rosemont, Ill, 2002, American Academy of Orthopaedic Surgeons.
3. Neumann D: Axial skeleton: Osteology and arthrology. In Neumann D, editor: Kinesiology of the musculoskeletal system—foundations for physical rehabilitation, St Louis, 2009, Mosby.
4. Frelinghuysen P, et al: Lumbar total disk replacement. Part I: Rationale, biomechanics, and implant types. Orthop Clin North Am 36(3):293-299, 2005.
5. Nitz A: Soft tissue injury and repair. In Placzek J, Boyce D, editors: Orthopaedic physical therapy secrets, Philadelphia, 2001, Hanley and Belfus.
6. Frenkel S, Grew J: Soft tissue repair. In Spivak J, et al, editor: Orthopaedics—a study guide, New York, 1999, McGraw-Hill.
7. Frenkel, S, Koval, K: Fracture healing and bone grafting. In Spivak J, et al, editors: Orthopaedics—a study guide, New York, 1999, McGraw-Hill.
8. Eck JC, Humphreys SC, Hodges SD: Adjacent-segment degeneration after lumbar fusion: A review of clinical, biomechanical, and radiologic studies. Am J Orthop 28(6):336-340, 1999.
9. Deyo RA, Nachemson A, Mirza SK: Spinal fusion surgery—The case for restraint. N J Med 350:722-726, 2004.
10. DeBerard MS, et al: Outcomes of posterolateral lumbar fusion in Utah patients receiving workers' compensation. Spine 27:738-747, 2001.
11. Delamarter RB, Bae HW, Pradhan BB: Clinical results of ProDisc-II lumbar total disk replacement: Report from the United States clinical trial. Orthop Clin North Am 36(3):301-313, 2005.
12. Franklin GM, et al: Outcome of lumbar fusion in Washington State workers' compensation. Spine 17:1897-1903, 1994.
13. Delamarter RB, et al: Artificial total lumbar disk replacement: Introduction and early results from the United States clinical trial. Spine 28:S167-S175, 2003.
14. Young MS: Total disk replacement. InTouch 3:9, 2006.
15. Gilber P, et al: Spinal disk replacement. InTouch 3:10-11, 2006.
16. Guyer RD, et al: Prospective randomized study of the Charité artificial disc: Data from two investigational centers. Spine J 4:252S-259S, 2004.
17. Janda V: Muscles and motor control in low back pain: Assessment and management. In Twomey LT, editor: Physical therapy of the low back, New York, 1987, Churchill Livingstone.
18. Richardson C, et al: Therapeutic exercise for spinal segmental stabilization in low back pain—scientific basis and clinical approach, Edinburgh, 1999, Churchill Livingstone.
19. Hebert JJ, et al: Postoperative rehabilitation following lumbar discectomy with quantification of trunk muscle morphology and function: A case report and review of the literature. JOSPT 40(7):402-412, 2010.
20. Ostelo RWJG, et al: Rehabilitation after lumbar disk surgery (Review). The Cochrane Collaboration, 2008, John Wiley & Sons.
21. Philadelphia Panel Members Clinical Specialty Experts: Philadelphia Panel evidence-based clinical practice guidelines on selected rehabilitation interventions for low back pain. Phys Ther 81(10):1641-1674, 2001.
22. Lee M: Effects of frequency on response of the spine to lumbar posteroanterior forces. J Manipulative Physiol Ther 16:439-446, 1993.
23. Lee M, Lau T, Lau H: Sagittal plane rotation of the pelvis during lumbar posteroanterior loading. J Manipulative Physiol Ther 17:149-155, 1994.
24. Lee M, Kelly D, Steven G: A model of spine, ribcage and pelvic responses to a specific lumbar manipulative force in relaxed subjects. J Biomech 28:1403-1408, 1995.
25. Lee M, Gal J, Herzog W: Biomechanics of manual therapy. In Dvir Z, editor: Clinical biomechanics, St Louis, 2000, Churchill Livingstone.
26. Cleland J, et al: Immediate effects of thoracic manipulation in patients with neck pain: A randomized clinical trial. Man Ther 10:127-135, 2005.
27. Mintken P, Cleland J: Thoracic clinical decision making. In Sueki D, Brechter J, editors: Orthopedic rehabilitation clinical advisor, St Louis, 2010, Mosby.
28. Butler D: The sensitive nervous system, Adelaide, Australia, 2000, Noigroup Publications.
29. Butler D: Upper limb neurodynamic test: clinical use in a "big picture" framework. In Grant R, editor: Physical therapy of the cervical and thoracic spine, St Louis, 2002, Churchill Livingstone.
30. Coppieters MW, Butler DS: Do sliders slide and tensioners tension? An analysis of neurodynamics techniques and considerations regarding their application. Man Ther 139:213-221, 2008.
31. Coppieters MW, Hough AD, Dilley A: Different nerve glide exercises induce different magnitudes of median nerve longitudinal excursion: An in vivo study using dynamic ultrasound imaging. JOSPT 39(3)164-171, 2009.
32. Boyd B, Topps K: Mechanosensitivity of the lower extremity neurons system during SLR neurodynamic testing in healthy individuals. JOSPT 39(11):780-790: 2009.
33. Boyd B, et al: Strain and excursion in the rat sciatic nerve during a modified straight leg raise are altered after traumatic nerve injury. J Orthop Res 23:764-770, 2005.
34. Treleaven J, Jull G, LowChoy N: The relationship of cervical joint position error to balance and eye movement disturbances in persistent whiplash. Manual Ther 11(2):99-106, 2006.
35. Treleaven J: Sensorimotor disturbances in neck disorders affecting postural stability, head and eye movement control. Manual Ther 13:2-11, 2008.
36. Treleaven J: Sensorimotor disturbances in neck disorders affecting postural stability, head and eye movement control. Part 2: Case studies. Manual Ther 13:266-275, 2008.
37. Treleaven J, et al: Dizziness and unsteadiness following whiplash injury: Characteristic features and relationship with cervical joint position error. J Rehabil Med 35(1):36-43, 2003.
38. Revel M, et al: Cervicocephalic kinesthetic sensibility in patients with cervical pain. Arch Phys Med Rehabil 72:228-291, 1991.
39. Revel M, et al: Changes in cervicocephalic kinesthesia after a proprioceptive rehabilitation program in patients with neck pain: A randomized controlled study. Arch Phys Med Rehabil 75:895-899, 1994.
40. Ikard RW: Methods and complications of anterior exposure of the thoracic and lumbar spine. Arch Surg 141:1025-1034, 2006.
41. Zindrick MR, et al: An evidence-based medicine approach in determining factors that may affect outcome in lumbar total disc replacement. Spine 33(11):1262-1269, 2008.
42. Hayeri MR, Tehranzadeh J: Diagnostic imaging of spinal fusion and complications. Appl Radiol 38(7/8):14-25, 2009.
43. Mirovsky Y, et al: Lumbar disk replacement with ProDisc prosthesis. Orthopedics 31(2):1-5, 2008.

44. Hoppes CW, Mills JT: Total disk arthroplasty. In Joint arthroplasty: Advances in surgical management and rehabilitation. Orthopedic Section. Independent study courses. APTA 1-32, 2010.

45. Punt IM, et al: Complications and reoperations of the SB Charité lumbar disk prosthesis: experience in 75 patients. Eur Spine J 17:36-43, 2008.

46. Boden SD, et al: An AOA critical issue: Disk replacements: This time will we really cure low-back and neck pain? J Bone Joint Surg 86(2)411-423, 2004.

47. Gamradt SC, Wang JC: Lumbar disk arthoplasty. Spine J 5:95-103, 2005.

48. Mayer HM: Total lumbar disk replacement. J Bone Joint Surg 87(8):1029-1038, 2005.

49. Freeman BJC, Davenport J: Total disk replacement in the lumbar spine: A systematic review of the literature. Eur Spine J 15(3):S439-S447, 2006.

50. Tropiano P, et al: Lumbar total disk replacement: Seven to eleven-year follow-up. J Bone Joint Surg 87(3):490-497, 2005.

51. Hagg O, Fritzell P, Nordwall A: Sexual function in men and women after anterior surgery for chronic low back pain. Eur Spine J 15:677-682, 2006.

52. Robinson Y, Sanden B: Spine imaging after lumbar disk replacement: Pitfalls and current recommendations. Patient Safety Surg 3:15-21, 2009.

53. Kim PK, Branch CL: The lumbar degenerative disc: Confusion, mechanics, management. Clin Neurosurg 53:18-25, 2006.

54. Gifford L, Butler D: The integration of pain sciences in clinical practice. J Hand Ther 10:86-95, 1997.

55. Keller J: Rehabilitation following total disk replacement surgery. In Butler Janz, editor: The artificial disc. Berlin, 2003, Springer Verlag.

56. Rodts MF: Total disk replacement arthroplasty. Orthop Nurs 23(3):216-220, 2004.

ADDITIONAL READING

Bajnoczy S: Artificial disk replacement—Evolutionary treatment for degenerative disk disease. AORN J 82(2):192-196, 2005.

Bradford DS, Zdeblick TA: Master techniques in orthopaedic surgery: The spine, Philadelphia, 2004, Lippincott Williams and Wilkins.

Bridwell KH, DeWald RL, editors: The textbook of spinal surgery, ed 2, Philadelphia, 1997, Lippincott-Raven.

Hoppenfeld S, Thomas H: Physical examination of the spine and extremities, Norwalk, Conn, 1976, Appleton-Century-Crofts.

Lee CK: Accelerated degeneration of the segment adjacent to lumbar fusion. Spine 13:375-377, 1988.

Lee D: The pelvic girdle, ed 3, 2004, Churchill Livingstone.

Sahrmann S: Diagnosis and treatment of movement impairment syndromes, St. Louis, 2002, Mosby.

Spivak JM, Connolly PJ: Orthopaedic knowledge update: Spine 3. Rosemont, Ill, 2006, American Academy of Orthopedic Surgeons /North American Spine Society.

Szpalski M, Gunzburg R, Mayer M: Spine arthroplasty: A historical review. Eur Spine J 11(suppl 2):S65-S84, 2002.

Vaccaro A: Spinal Arthroplasty with DVD, Philadelphia, 2007, Saunders.

Yue JJ, et al: Motion preservation surgery of the spine: Advanced techniques and controversies, Philadelphia, 2008, Saunders.

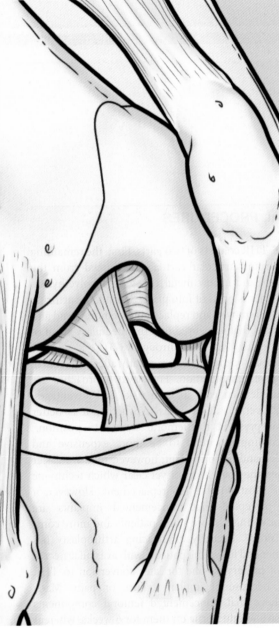

PART 4

LOWER EXTREMITY

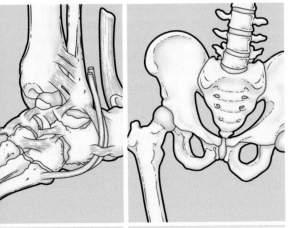

CHAPTER 18

Total Hip Arthroplasty

Patricia A. Gray, Edward Pratt

Each year in the United States approximately 250,000 people undergo a total hip replacement (THR) procedure[1] hoping to eliminate persistent pain and to improve their ability to function in daily life. The majority of these people have failed to find relief from their symptoms with conservative medical intervention.

SURGICAL INDICATIONS AND CONSIDERATIONS

THR is used to correct intractable damage resulting from osteoarthritis, rheumatoid arthritis, avascular necrosis, and the abnormal muscle tone caused by cerebral palsy.[2] Nonelective THR procedures are performed for fractures in which open reduction internal fixation is deemed inappropriate.

Contraindications for THR surgery include inadequate bone mass, inadequate periarticular support, serious medical risk factors, signs of infection, and lack of patient motivation to observe precautions and follow through with rehabilitation. Surgery also is contraindicated if it is unlikely to increase the patient's functional level.[2]

The prostheses used currently have a projected life span of less than 20 years. Therefore candidates for THR are usually more than 60 years old. Younger patients elect this surgery when their functional status is severely compromised and their pain becomes intolerable. In the case of a fracture, younger patients are treated with an open reduction internal fixation whenever practical. Given the projected life span of current prostheses, younger THR candidates may require a revision surgery later in life.

THR predictably improves function and reduces pain in virtually all patients with disabling disease. Patient satisfaction (with a rating of very good or excellent) regarding pain relief and improvement of function has been measured as high as 98% at 2 years after THR. The long-term survivability rate has been reported as high as 87.3% to 96.5% at 15 years.[2-4]

SURGICAL PROCEDURES

In its essence, THR consists of two parts. First, the remaining arthritic bone and articular cartilage is reamed from the acetabular cup, and a new metal cup with a polyethylene plastic inner liner is press fit into place. Second, the arthritic femoral head is removed and replaced by a femoral head and stem component that is secured into the medullary canal of the proximal femur (Figs. 18-1 through 18-3).

Several aspects of the procedure greatly affect the course of postoperative rehabilitation. First, two approaches are commonly used, each with its own risks and advantages. Second, controversy still exists as to whether it is better to cement or press fit the femoral stem into position.[5] Noncemented implants tend to be more expensive and technically demanding to implant; however, they are easier to revise when they fail. It is not yet clear which technique produces the most durable hip replacement. However, it is generally accepted that noncemented implants are best suited for younger, more active patients and more complicated revisions.[6] Recently, resurfacing arthroplasty has been recommended for young patients with avascular necrosis, because it preserves bone for later conversion to THR if necessary because of implant failure or pain. Many surgeons believe that noncemented femoral components should not have weight borne on them for 6 weeks, whereas cemented femoral components can support weight immediately after surgery. This has been contested recently, and many surgeons now allow patients with noncemented hips to bear weight from the outset.[7] Both approaches have in common the creation of instability around the hip during the early postoperative period. The release of muscle, bone, and joint capsule during accessing of the joint renders the hip vulnerable to dislocation at its extreme ranges of motion. Patient education of "hip precautions" becomes extremely important during early convalescence and is alluded to later in this chapter. Controversy remains as to which approach provides the lowest postoperative

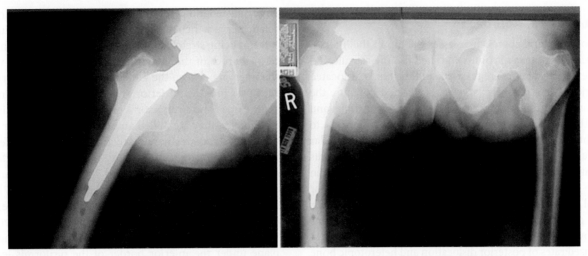

Fig. 18-1 Hybrid cemented total hip arthroplasty. (From Biomet Integral Design, Warsaw, Ind.)

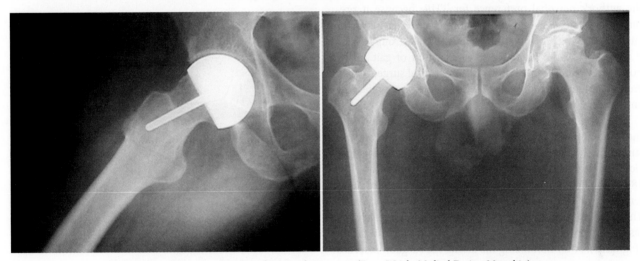

Fig. 18-2 Resurfacing arthroplasty for avascular necrosis. (From Wright Medical Design, Memphis.)

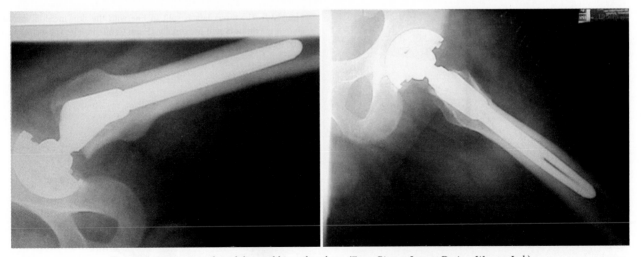

Fig. 18-3 Noncemented modular total hip arthroplasty. (From Biomet Impact Design, Warsaw, Ind.)

dislocation rate, the shortest operative time, and the least blood loss.[8] Because of problems with trochanteric nonunion and long-term abductor weakness, the original transtrochanteric approach (in which the greater trochanter or the gluteus medius is completely released) is used most often today in revision surgery. Its main advantage lies in an excellent view of the proximal femoral shaft. The two exposures discussed in the following paragraphs are the posterolateral approach (Gibson) and the anterolateral approach (Watson-Jones).

Posterolateral Approach

The posterolateral approach accesses the hip in the interval between the gluteus maximus and medius. The capsule and short external rotators are released, and the hip is dislocated posteriorly. In extremely large or contracted patients, the surgeon must occasionally release the gluteus maximus and even the adductor magnus at their femoral insertions to translate the proximal femur anteriorly, gaining acetabular exposure. This exposure places traction on the gluteus maximus, medius, and tensor fascia lata. Care must be taken not to place traction on the sciatic nerve or the superior gluteal nerve and artery, which may cause nerve palsy. Repair of the posterior capsule and short external rotators remains controversial, although several recent reports suggest decreased rates of posterior dislocation and heterotopic bone formation when this is done. The posterolateral approach is the author's personal preference for THR, because it preserves the gluteus medius and minimus, as well as the vastus lateralis, making rehabilitation of these muscle groups easier. It also provides for a quicker normalization of gait in the postoperative period, although this is personal surgeon preference and may be disputed by surgeons who prefer the anterolateral approach.

The patient is placed in the lateral decubitus position with the affected hip up; the entire limb is washed, prepared, and surgically draped. The incision is begun 4 to 5 inches superior and medial to the top of the greater trochanter (Fig. 18-4). The line of incision runs down to the greater trochanter, then 3 or 4 inches along the course of the posterior femur. The skin and subcutaneous tissues are incised, and the deep fascia is exposed and divided in line with the skin incision (Fig. 18-5). After mobilizing the fascia, the surgeon inserts a large self-retaining retractor to hold the fascia apart. The sciatic nerve is then either exposed or palpated to ensure that it is not being stretched or traumatized (Fig. 18-6). The posterior border of the gluteus medius is identified, as well as the interval between the gluteus minimus and piriformis as they pass into the posterior greater trochanter. This interval is developed and a retractor is placed around the medius and minimus as they are pulled anteriorly. The remainder of the posterior structures is released from the posterior femoral neck and intertrochanteric line, including the piriformis, obturator internus, superior and inferior gemelli, and the superior half of the quadratus femoris (Fig. 18-7). The surgeon releases the posterior hip capsule with the short external rotators, allowing them to retract together (Fig. 18-8). This decreased dissection around the crucial nervous plane under the inferior border of the piriformis leaves a stronger posterior cuff of tissue to repair at the end of the

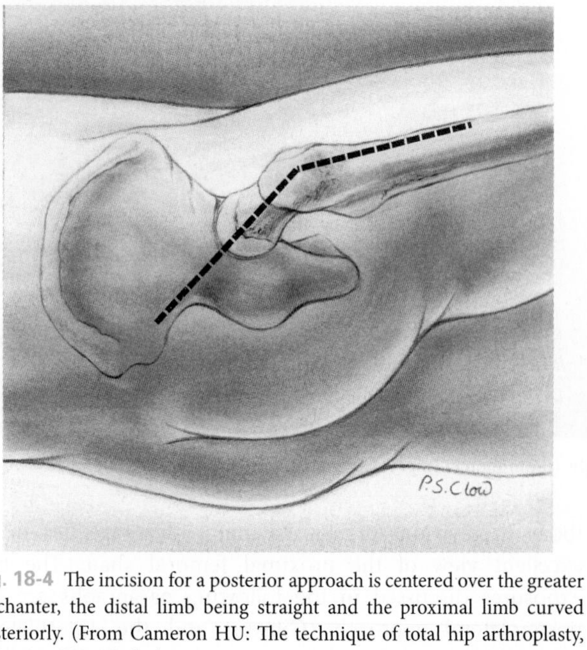

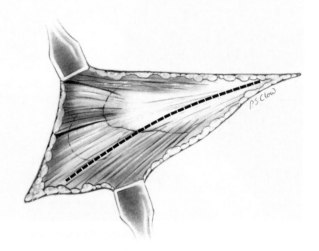

Fig. 18-5 The fascia lata is split in line with the skin incision, and the gluteus maximus is split proximally. (From Cameron HU: The technique of total hip arthroplasty, St Louis, 1992, Mosby.)

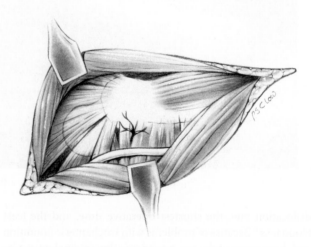

Fig. 18-6 The short external rotators are exposed by blunt dissection. The sciatic nerve lies superficial to the external rotators. (From Cameron HU: The technique of total hip arthroplasty, St Louis, 1992, Mosby.)

Fig. 18-4 The incision for a posterior approach is centered over the greater trochanter, the distal limb being straight and the proximal limb curved posteriorly. (From Cameron HU: The technique of total hip arthroplasty, St Louis, 1992, Mosby.)

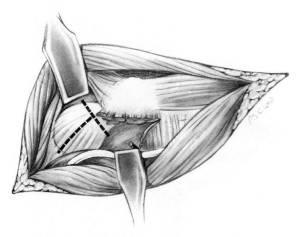

Fig. 18-7 The short external rotators are divided. When the upper part of the quadratus is released, brisk bleeding usually ensues from the medial circumflex femoral artery. (From Cameron HU: The technique of total hip arthroplasty, St Louis, 1992, Mosby.)

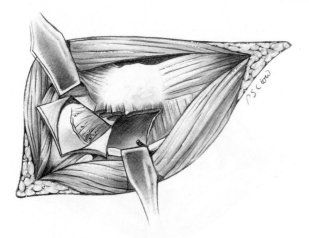

Fig. 18-8 Retraction now exposes the hip joint capsule. (From Cameron HU: The technique of total hip arthroplasty, St Louis, 1992, Mosby.)

procedure. The limb is next measured for its length between the ilium and greater trochanter, and the hip is posteriorly dislocated. A reciprocating saw is used to cut through the femoral neck, and the arthritic femoral head is delivered from the field. The hip annulus is débrided sharply, and a minimal anterior capsulotomy is performed to help mobilize the proximal femur. As mentioned previously, the surgeon must sometimes go back and release the gluteus maximus, adductor longus, and occasionally even the adductor magnus from the proximal femur so that it can be translated anteriorly. A cobra retractor is placed under the femur and over the front edge of the acetabulum, allowing the femur to be levered anteriorly out of the way of the acetabulum. The acetabulum is then reamed and the acetabular component inserted.

The clinician begins femoral preparation by placing a large retractor under the femur and levering it out of the wound. The surgeon then reams the femoral shaft, increasing the reamer size by 2 mm each pass until good bony contact is made. The intertrochanteric area is then broached or rasped in the same manner until good proximal fill of the femur is obtained. A provisional head is applied, and the joint is placed back together and ranged to check for stability and length. At this stage a stable hip should allow 80° to 90° of flexion, 60° to 80° of internal rotation (IR), and 20° to 30° of external rotation (ER) while being held in neutral abduction. After this the surgeon press fits or cements the implant in place and begins closure. Many surgeons prefer repair of the capsule and short external rotators as a single cuff of tissue held by large No. 2 nonabsorbable sutures through drill holes in the bone. The gluteus maximus and hip adductors are repaired if they were released, and the deep fascia is repaired again with nonabsorbable suture. After closure of subcutaneous tissue and skin, the patient is placed in a triangular-shaped pillow that holds the hip in approximately 30° of abduction. The pillow straps should not be tightened to the point that they compress the common peroneal nerve.

Rehabilitation begins as soon as the patient is coherent. Ankle pumps, quadriceps sets, and leg lifts help reestablish the distal venous circulation, minimizing the risk of thromboembolic disease and helping with postoperative edema. Standing, sitting, and walking can be started on the first day after surgery if hip precautions are followed carefully.

Anterolateral Approach

The anterolateral approach, made popular by Smith-Peterson,[3] provides better visibility without the risk of posterior dislocation associated with the posterolateral approach. It avoids the need for postoperative abduction pillows and can allow the patient greater freedom of movement during the initial postoperative period, because hip precautions become less crucial. Because of the reported decreased incidence of posterior dislocation, the anterolateral approach is sometimes preferred in patients who have suffered strokes or those who have cerebral palsy and therefore have a significant muscle imbalance or spasticity that induces flexion and IR of the hip. This approach has been associated with a greater incidence of heterotopic bone formation, greater blood loss, and longer operative times. However, individual surgical expertise seems to have a greater influence on these variables than the exposure chosen.[9,10]

The anterolateral approach uses the interval between the gluteus medius and tensor fascia lata. The superior gluteal nerve near the ilium innervates both of these muscles. Injury to this nerve can result in a partial or complete abductor paralysis that can vary from a temporary neurapraxia to complete and permanent paralysis. In addition, the femoral nerve can be injured through overretraction of soft tissues in the front of the hip, leaving significant quadriceps weakness. This approach preserves the short external rotators of the hip and prevents direct exposure of the sciatic nerve. The tissues violated include the gluteus medius and minimus, the tensor fascia lata, the vastus lateralis, the referred head of the rectus femoris, the anterior hip capsule, and the iliopsoas tendon.

The patient is placed in the lateral decubitus position with the affected hip up (Fig. 18-9, A); a lateral incision is made

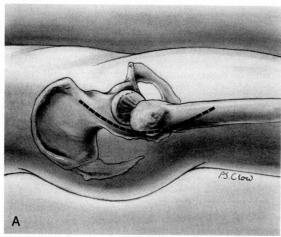

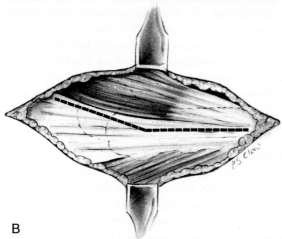

Fig. 18-9 A, The skin incision is roughly C-shaped and centered over the back of the greater trochanter. **B,** The fascia lata is divided over the summit of the greater trochanter. (From Cameron HU: The technique of total hip arthroplasty, St Louis, 1992, Mosby.)

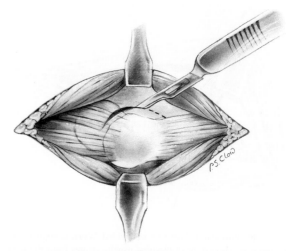

Fig. 18-10 The anterior fibers of the gluteus medius are released from the greater trochanter. The muscle incision is not extended proximally. (From Cameron HU: The technique of total hip arthroplasty, St Louis, 1992, Mosby.)

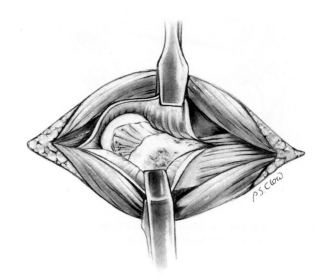

Fig. 18-11 An anterior capsulectomy is carried out with a blunt Homan retractor above and below the femoral neck and a medium Homan retractor placed on the pelvic brim. (From Cameron HU: The technique of total hip arthroplasty, St Louis, 1992, Mosby.)

with a slight anterior curvature in its proximal aspect. After dividing the subcutaneous tissue, the surgeon incises the lateral fascia and finds and develops the interval between the gluteus medius and the tensor fascia lata (Figs. 18-9, *B,* and 18-10). The surgeon must be careful not to extend the incision too far proximally, because the investing nerve of both muscles (the superior gluteal nerve) can be injured, resulting in paralysis of the tensor. The vastus lateralis origin is often dissected off its vastus ridge origin to access the anterior hip capsule fully. The capsule is then bluntly released from the front of the femoral neck to gain access to the hip joint itself (Fig. 18-11). The last deep layer of exposure requires the release of the anterior aspect of the gluteus medius off the greater trochanter and the reflection of the rectus femoris off the anterior acetabulum (Fig. 18-12). The gluteus release can be done either through the tendon or through trochanteric osteotomy (although trochanteric osteotomy has fallen out of favor to some extent because of the incidence of non-union). After the gluteus release, the hip can be dislocated anteriorly and joint replacement begun much as in the posterolateral approach.

ER and flexion must be avoided postoperatively to prevent dislocation. Hip range of motion (ROM) precautions remain important, especially during the first 6 weeks. Normalization of gait via abductor and quadriceps strengthening remains the focus during early rehabilitation. Pool exercise appears to be extremely helpful in this regard.

Generally a walker or crutches is required for 3 weeks after THR. A cane is used for an additional 3 weeks before unassisted walking is allowed. This varies depending on the age and preoperative condition of the patient. Driving and a return to sedentary activities may be allowed at 3 weeks, and some of the hip precautions can be relaxed at 6 weeks. Improvement in strength and ROM can be expected for as long as 6 months with a motivated patient.

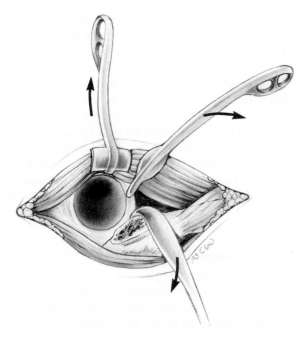

Fig. 18-12 The acetabulum is exposed with a medium Homan retractor on the pelvic brim, a long sharp Homan retractor inferiorly, and a bent Homan retractor posteriorly levering down on the stump of the femoral neck. (From Cameron HU: The technique of total hip arthroplasty, St Louis, 1992, Mosby.)

THERAPY GUIDELINES FOR REHABILITATION

The following text can be used as guidelines for rehabilitation after a THR. Flexibility on the part of the therapist is essential because individual surgeons may impose their own protocols.

The therapist's role is crucial at the postsurgical stage. Santavista's study[11] revealed that the majority of THR patients report that they received most of their information regarding their surgical recovery phase from physical therapists. These patients will depend on their therapists for encouragement and advice. A therapist should set the patient's expectations toward independence and wellness early on. Each client should anticipate his or her own unique recovery progression and avoid comparisons with other patients.

Phase I (Preoperative Training Session)

TIME: a few days before surgery

GOALS: To teach THR precautions so that patients will transfer and move safely after surgery and avoid dislocation of the prosthetic joint, to teach a basic exercise program for the postoperative phases of recovery

Many institutions have initiated preoperative THR training sessions to increase their patients' confidence and reduce the length of their hospital stays. These sessions may take place in the physical therapy department or in the patient's home through a home care agency's physical therapist. Educational videos are now available as an adjunct teaching tool.

The preoperative session generally includes an assessment of the patient's strength (including upper-extremity [UE] potential), ROM, neurologic status, vital signs, endurance, functional level, and safety awareness. Any existing edema, contractures, and leg length discrepancies should be noted at this time, as well as knowledge of the patient's scar healing ability.[12] If the assessment takes place in the patient's home, check the stairways, hallways, sidewalks and elevators (or lack of) and recommend the necessary safety adaptations (e.g., moving furniture and electrical cords). Evaluate the need for durable medical equipment such as a shower chair, walker, or bedside commode.

Instruction in THR precautions should begin during the preoperative session and be repeated throughout the rehabilitation process as necessary. **The precautions after a posterolateral approach to THR prohibit flexion of the hip past 90°, adduction past the body's midline, and IR of the hip. After an anterolateral THR, the patient should observe these precautions and avoid hip ER (especially with flexion).** A review of proper body mechanics for safe functional mobility at home, along with appropriate postoperative sleeping and sitting positions should accompany the precautions training. Often a patient is able to recite these precautions but will still move in a dangerous fashion. Ask the patient to demonstrate an understanding of these precautions with safe transitional movements and transfer techniques.

Teach the proper use of assistive devices such as walkers and crutches according to the patient's projected weight-bearing status. **A non–weight-bearing (NWB) order may be given if the prosthesis is noncemented. Maintain adherence to both weight-bearing and ROM precautions throughout the entire rehabilitation process**.

Postoperative exercises can be taught at this time. These exercises may include the following:
- Ankle pumps (Fig. 18-13)
- Quadriceps sets
- Gluteal sets
- Active hip and knee flexion (heel slides) while maintaining hip ROM within the physician's recommended guidelines for the surgical technique performed
- Isometric hip abduction
- Active hip abduction

The patient should not perform hip abduction if a trochanteric osteotomy was performed. A dislocation of the THR prosthesis is possible if inappropriate stresses are placed on the new joint.

Traditional THR exercise programs have become controversial in recent years. The contact pressure on the hip joint during specific activities has been measured and compared with pressure on the hip during gait. Although some practitioners dispute the methodology used, the results of these studies have caused many to question the prescription of some of the standard THR exercises. Consult the surgeon regarding exercise programs that include straight-leg raising.

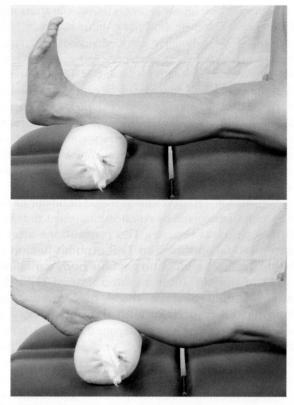

Strickland found that active hip flexion and isometric hip extension produced the greatest stresses on the joint. Based on these findings, Lewis and the consensus group recommend performing gluteal sets at submaximal levels of contraction to avoid the possibility of dislocation.

Givens-Heiss and colleagues[13] found that a maximal isometric hip abduction contraction generated greater peak pressure than both the straight leg raise (SLR) and unsupported gait. The Krebs study[14] also found that maximal contraction during exercise generated greater pressure at the hip than did gait. Lewis and Knortz[15] recommend that isometric hip abduction be done at submaximal levels based on the results of these studies and suggests slow, supine hip abduction as an alternative.

Phase IIa (Hospital Phase)

TIME: 1 to 2 days after surgery
GOALS: To prevent complications, to increase muscle contraction and improve control of the involved leg, to help patient to sit up for 30 minutes, to reinforce understanding of the THR precautions

Day of Surgery

Postoperative physical therapy (Table 18-1) may begin on the day of surgery when the patient regains consciousness. The patient will be resting in the supine position and wearing

Fig. 18-13 Ankle pumps. The patient lies supine with both knees straight and pumps the feet up and down as far as possible.

TABLE 18-1 Total Hip Replacement

Rehabilitation Phase	Criteria to Progress to This Phase	Anticipated Impairments and Functional Limitations	Intervention	Goal	Rationale
Phase IIa Postoperative 1-2 days	• Postoperative (inpatient) • No signs of infection • Medically stable	• Pain • Immobilized postoperatively in bed with abduction pillow • Limited respiratory exchange	• Adjust abduction pillow ankle straps • Order foot cradle • Provide patient education regarding total hip precautions • Isometrics—Quadriceps sets, gluteal sets • AROM—Ankle pumps • Encourage use of cough and incentive spirometer On postoperative day 2, begin the following: • Bed mobility training • Transfer training • Gait training (weight bearing per physician's orders) as appropriate	Avoid the following: • Peripheral nerve damage • Heel ulcers • Dislocations of prosthesis • Pooling of fluid in legs • Fluid buildup in lungs • Improve volitional control of involved leg • Initiate mobility training • Sit up in chair 30 minutes • Maintain precautions while performing mobility activities	• Decrease strap pressure on legs • Decrease prolonged, unchecked pressure against heels • Prevent excessive stresses on hip • Promote distal venous circulation • Initiate muscle contractions • Prevent respiratory complications • Reinforce precautions to avoid complications • Prepare patient to perform transfers independently • Use assistive device during ambulation for safety and protection of hip

AROM, Active range of motion.

thromboembolic disease (TED) hose with the legs abducted and strapped to a triangular foam cushion. To avoid damage to the peripheral nerves, the therapist is expected to check the tightness of the cushions around the patient's legs.

Pulmonary hygiene exercises typically begin immediately after awakening. The patient's lower-extremity (LE) exercise program also may be initiated at this point with ankle pumps, quadriceps sets, and gluteal sets. The heel booties which are used to prevent bedsores can be removed for these exercises.

Since the client may be groggy and unable to remember the THR precautions at this point, a review is in order. Some may benefit from a sign placed by the bed that lists the ROM precautions. A knee immobilizer placed on the affected leg can reduce the possibility of making dangerous movements.

Repositioning of the patient every 2 hours (with the abductor pillow in place) is critical at this stage to avoid pressure ulcers. Foot cradles are often attached to the foot of the bed to avoid IR of the operated hip and to prevent the heel sores that may develop as a result of pressure from the blankets. Many hospitals' protocols will assign these functions to the nursing staff and then begin physical therapy intervention on the first day after surgery. All personnel rendering care to the patient should monitor changes in the limb's vascular and neurologic status closely.

Postoperative Day 1

Acute care physical therapy sessions vary in frequency from one to three times per day and from 5 to 7 days per week, depending on the medical center's protocol.[16] The therapist will proceed after being informed of the surgical approach used, any special precautions, and the patient's weight-bearing status. Assessment and treatment are conducted at the patient's bedside while the patient is situated as described previously.

The THR precautions should be repeated at this time. These precautions remain in place until the scheduled follow-up visit with the orthopedist 3 to 6 weeks later. The surgeon may then relax the precautions or decide to continue them for another 6 weeks.

The physical therapist can initiate ankle pumps (see Fig. 18-13), quadriceps sets, and gluteal sets if the patient did not begin them on the day of surgery. Bilateral UE exercises can also begin at this time. **Ankle circles are not indicated, because the patient may inadvertently internally rotate the affected extremity while performing the exercise. As stated previously, submaximal contraction of the muscles is recommended.** Ideally these exercises should be repeated 10 times every hour.[17] Be aware that some patients may not meet this expectation.

Transfer training begins by assisting the patient to move safely from a supine to a sitting position and then from sitting to a standing position while observing precautions. Frequently patients are struggling with pain and anxiety and need encouragement. The physical therapist should allot a considerable amount of time for this task and emphasize the use of the UEs when shifting weight. **Avoid pivoting on the operative leg.** Surgeons usually allow a patient to transfer to an appropriate bedside chair and sit up as tolerated, **rarely more than 30 to 60 minutes.** The therapist then supervises the return to bed.

If a patient is not complaining of excessive pain, fatigue, or dizziness, then gait training may begin on the first postoperative day. More frequently, gait training begins on day 2.

Postoperative Day 2

Treatment on postoperative day 2 includes a review of the previous day's activities. The client must maintain hip ROM within the physician's recommended guidelines. The physical therapist expands the exercise program to include heel slides and isometric or active assistive hip abduction. Short arc quadriceps sets may require active assistance at this time. Again, *submaximal force is recommended for isometric hip abduction.* Assistance from the therapist may be necessary for some exercises. The use of verbal cues such as "point the moving knee or big toe toward the ceiling" to avoid rotation of the leg may also be helpful.

Gait training usually begins during this session. The patient's assistive device is adjusted to the client's height before instruction and practice begin. Older patients are typically issued a front-wheeled walker. Younger patients may be issued crutches and instructed in the three-point crutch pattern. Patients who have undergone bilateral THR are instructed in the four-point crutch pattern.

The weight-bearing status after a noncemented THR is up to the surgeon's discretion. A NWB order on the operative extremity may be in effect for several weeks. Most patients with cemented prostheses are instructed to bear weight as tolerated at this stage.

Complex surgeries may require more caution. When the postoperative order calls for only touch down weight bearing (TDWB), taping a "cracker" to the sole of the patient's operative forefoot with instruction not to break the cracker can be helpful in teaching this concept. Stepping onto a bathroom scale with the affected extremity helps the partial–weight-bearing (PWB) patient to determine the appropriate amount of pressure (usually 50% of body weight or less) to be put on that leg. Those who are still experiencing difficulty can practice weight shifting at the parallel bars before using a walker.

Patients who have undergone THR frequently walk with the affected leg in abduction. Encourage normalization of their gait pattern early in the recovery phase. Most facilities set a short-term goal for discharge at walking on a level surface for 100 feet with an appropriate assistive device.

Phase IIb

TIME: 3 to 7 days after surgery
GOALS: To promote transfer and gait independence (using assistive devices as indicated), to reinforce THR precautions, to discharge to home

Postoperative Day 3 (Until Discharge)

Patients are often moved from the acute care section to a rehabilitation center or skilled nursing facility on day 3 (Table 18-2). Some patients (usually those who are younger and more fit) may be discharged to home care at this time.

Treatment at the rehabilitation center is conducted in the physical therapy gym. Stair training generally begins on day 3. A step-to gait pattern with minimal weight bearing on the affected leg is taught for ambulation on even surfaces; on steps or stairs, the patient leads up the stairs with the unaffected leg and down the stairs with the affected leg. Patients should become comfortable climbing the number of stairs demanded by the home situation. When the patient is not competent with stair climbing, arrangements are sometimes made for the patient to live on the ground floor.

Refinement of these skills continues daily at the rehabilitation center until the time of discharge. By the discharge date, family members or other caregivers must be trained to assist the patient safely whenever necessary.

Common discharge criteria for THR are as follows:
- The patient is able to demonstrate and state the THR precautions.
- The patient is able to demonstrate independence with transfers.
- The patient is able to demonstrate independence with the exercise program.
- The patient is able to demonstrate independence with gait on level surfaces to 100 feet.

- The patient is able to demonstrate independence on stairs.

Written instructions with illustrations pertaining to these criteria are included in a discharge packet for home use. Patients are typically discharged between 5 to 10 days after surgery. Zavadak and colleagues[18] found that independence in functional activities required the following number of physical therapy sessions:
- Supine to sit: 8.1
- Sit to stand: 5.5
- Ambulate to 100 feet: 8.1
- Independent on stairs: 9.5

However, the therapist's expectations should not be unduly influenced by statistics. Munin and colleagues[19] found that fewer than 40% of patients who undergo THR are independent in performing all the basic tasks at the time of discharge from the rehabilitation center. Approximately 80% of patients were at the supervision level of performance. Advanced age, solitary living conditions, and an increased number of comorbid conditions were the factors that predicted the duration of a patient's treatment stay.[19]

Phase III (Return to Home)

TIME: 1 to 6 weeks after surgery

GOALS: To evaluate the safety of the home, to assure patient independence with transfers and ambulation, to plan the client's return to work or previous community activities as appropriate

TABLE 18-2 Total Hip Replacement

Rehabilitation Phase	Criteria to Progress to This Phase	Anticipated Impairments and Functional Limitations	Intervention	Goal	Rationale
Phase IIb Postoperative 3-7 days	• Good tolerance to phase IIa • No signs of infection • No significant increase in pain • Medically stable • Gradual improvement in tolerance to inpatient program	• Limited bed mobility • Limited transfers • Limited gait • Limited understanding of postoperative precautions	• Continue interventions from phase IIa with progression of activity as tolerated • AROM—Heel slides, hip abduction (if able; otherwise do active assisted hip abduction), terminal knee extension, UE exercises • Bed mobility training • Transfer training; initiate car transfers when appropriate • Gait training; initiate stair training when indicated ("up with good, down with bad") • Evaluation of equipment needs at home • Caregiver training	• Maintain postoperative precautions • Improve involved LE AROM within boundaries of precautions • Improve arm strength • Become independent with transfers • Become independent with gait using appropriate assistive device • Promote carryover of precautions at home	• Prevent prosthesis dislocation • Restore volitional control of involved LE • Prepare arms to assist during transfer and gait • Emphasize restoration of independence with self-care activities (bed mobility, transfers) • Promote independence with activities of daily living • Ambulate safely and decrease stress on the involved LE • Ensure patient and caregiver safety (reinforce precautions) and prevent falls

AROM, Active range of motion; *LE*, lower extremity; *UE*, upper extremity.

Home Care Phase

Physical therapy home assessment usually occurs within 24 hours after hospital discharge. The elements to be assessed are those listed in the preoperative section, with the addition of the status of the surgical incision. The number of visits authorized by the patient's insurance company may limit the goals set by the therapist. Medicare coverage at this stage is restricted to patients who are homebound or severely limited in their ability to go out. Most patients are no longer homebound after 3 to 4 weeks.

Because managed care insurance has placed constraints on the number of nursing visits allowed, physical therapists are now being trained to remove staples, traditionally a nursing function. Staple removal normally occurs 12 to 14 days after surgery.

After hospital discharge, expect to advise the patient regarding appropriate sitting and sleeping positions, furniture adjustments, and other home safety issues such as slippery rugs or strung-out electrical cords. A home care agency admission assessment includes a review of patient medications. Check to see if the patient and/or caregiver have the appropriate medications in the home and are taking them as prescribed.

A postural assessment should be done and contractures noted should be addressed through a cautious stretching program. Careful straight leg hamstring stretches done with the therapist's assistance may be added to the supine exercise series (not to exceed 90° of hip flexion). The Achilles tendon stretch can be done at a kitchen countertop, walker, or at the wall. Closed kinetic chain exercises (with involved leg firmly planted on the ground or on exercise equipment), such as heel raises and minisquats, can also be done at the countertop. Open chain exercises done while standing at this location include hip flexion, hip abduction, and hip extension. Sidestepping is a functional abduction exercise that stimulates both sets of glutes and engages eccentric hip rotators in stance phase.

Frequently patients will substitute hip flexion for true abduction. They have difficulty firing the glut medius and glut minimus because of chronically flexed posture. Good hip extension and good concentric and eccentric control of the hip rotators are needed for a normal gait pattern.[20] Lunges, done standing in a doorway with elevated arms on either side of the door frame, can effectively stretch the plantar flexors, hip flexors, arms, and trunk while strengthening the opposite LE quads.[20] Stronger, more mobile patients may be able to assume a prone position to stretch shortened hip flexors.

Progress the client to wall slides done with the patient's back resting against a wall and feet placed about 12 inches in front of the wall. Balance training and a core/trunk strengthening program to reinforce good postural habits may begin now or in the outpatient clinic depending on the patient's level of progress. Exercise equipment already in the patient's home may be added to the existing program if it can be used safely.

Shoes often adapt in shape to the stresses imposed by an abnormal gait pattern and may encourage a return to the old pattern if worn after THR surgery. Replace the patient's old misshapen shoes if possible.

Progression from the use of a front-wheeled walker or crutches to a single-point cane usually occurs at 3 to 4 weeks after surgery. Occasionally, a four-point cane is used as an interim device. Use of the cane is usually discontinued 3 to 4 weeks later. The patient should walk safely on level and sloped surfaces, jagged sidewalks, curbs, and stairs before discharge.

Enough strength may have been recovered to allow step-over-step stair climbing during the home phase. At first, the patient can practice stepping up onto books or other household items that provide a stable, shallow rise. A modified lunge with the affected extremity placed on the upper step is another helpful prestair climbing exercise.

Driving is allowed 3 to 6 weeks after surgery at the orthopedist's discretion. Permission may be given sooner, depending on the patient's lifestyle requirements and rate of progress. Instruct the patient in getting on and off a bus or in and out of a car safely. A clean plastic trash bag placed over the seat of a car provides a surface that allows the patient to glide-pivot around on the seat to assume the rider's position more easily.

Outpatient Clinic

Physical therapy intervention often ends with the home care phase. Patients with physically demanding lifestyles may require additional strength and endurance training. Some patients are referred to the clinic because of lingering gait problems, others because they didn't meet homebound requirements at the time of hospital discharge. The outpatient therapist should check with the surgeon for the status of precautions and activity level before designing an aggressive exercise program.

The patient reassessment at this point includes posture, balance, strength (both concentric and eccentric at the hips), gait pattern, and core control. A stretching and exercise regime begun in the home or hospital can be expanded upon in the clinic. Continue to improve posture with trunk and hip flexor stretching. Normalize the gait pattern with weight shifting and hip strengthening exercises. Core strengthening to support good posture should be present in the program. Pool exercise is recommended after THR. Equipment such as a treadmill, exercise bike, and elliptical cross-trainer can be incorporated into a home program so that the patient may continue at his or her own gym later on.

As in home care, the goals at this stage depend on the number of visits authorized by the patient's insurance company. Quick independence with a home exercise program should be encouraged.

After Rehabilitation Intervention

The surgeon will determine the patient's return-to-work date. Job modification may be needed and some may not be allowed to return to their previous jobs. Heavy manual labor is not permitted after THR surgery and vocational counseling may be necessary.[21]

High-impact sports such as running, waterskiing, football, basketball, handball, karate, soccer, and racquetball traditionally have been contraindicated after THR.[22] The results of the 2007 Survey[23] also list snowboarding and high-impact aerobics as "not allowed." Activities "allowed with experience" are downhill skiing, cross-country skiing, weightlifting, ice-skating/rollerblading, and Pilates.[23] The sports "allowed" by the 2007 Survey[20] respondents are swimming, scuba, golf, walking, speed walking, hiking, stationary cycling, bowling, road cycling, low-impact aerobics, rowing, dancing (ballroom, jazz, square), weight machines, stair climber, treadmill, and elliptical.[23] Doubles tennis is considered less stressful than singles tennis.[14] The survey results were undecided regarding singles tennis and the martial arts.

Patient compliance with home exercise programs is often questionable after the first few weeks and especially after discharge from therapy services. No agreement seems to exist among surgeons as to how long exercise programs should be continued. The surgeon may release the patient from the home exercise program at his or her discretion.

Sheh and colleagues[24] state that flexion showed the slowest rate of recovery in diseased hips. Persistence of weakness was noted in all patients for at least 2 years after hip surgery despite the return of normal stride and phasic activity of muscles. Gluteus maximus or minimus weakness can result in aching near the hip during endurance activities. Sheh states that muscular weakness reduces the protection of the implant fixation surfaces during endurance activities. This may contribute to higher loosening rates reported in active patients.[24] Therefore, therapists should encourage long-term continuation of exercise programs when this does not contradict the surgeon's orders.

TROUBLESHOOTING

The THR procedure has been refined so that patient progress is now fairly certain and predictable. However, most complications call for a referral back to the surgeon. Examples include the following:

- Thigh pain with walking that clears quickly with sitting down, possibly indicating intermittent claudication
- A positive Trendelenburg sign that does not resolve with treatment, possibly caused by damage to gluteal innervation
- Severe rubor and swelling at the surgical site with accompanying fever, possibly indicating a wound infection
- Unexplained swelling of the limb that does not dissipate with elevation, possibly indicating TED hose
- General systemic effects, possibly indicating an allergy to the implant materials (rare), postoperative anemia, pulmonary embolus, or other medical complications
- Persistent, severe pain (even referred medial knee pain, unexplained limb shortening or extreme rotation, or pain with rotation of the limb), possibly resulting from dislocation of the prosthesis, heterotopic ossification, or a fracture of the adjacent bone or reflex sympathetic dystrophy

Many times the therapist is the first to see a developing complication; therefore, good communication with the surgeon is extremely important. Leg length discrepancy is an example. The patient can continue gait training with a temporary shoe insert or with shoes of different heel heights. The surgeon may later prescribe a permanent orthotic. Persistent edema may be treated with medication. Patients should be advised to elevate their legs, rest more often, wear TED hose, pump their ankles, and apply ice to swollen areas. Pain flare-ups in unaffected areas of the body are usually managed with medication. Possible side effects of the medication include nausea, constipation, and hypertension. The therapist can assist in pain reduction with modalities, exercises, and positioning. Significant abnormalities should always be reported to the surgeon.

CONCLUSION

A rapid, substantial improvement in quality of life can be expected after THR surgery. Better physical function, sleep, emotional behavior, social interaction, and recreation are usually experienced in the first few months. At 2 years after surgery, patients who had undergone THR have reported greater satisfaction with their results than they had predicted in their best preoperative hypothetical scenarios.[25]

Suggested Home Maintenance for the Postsurgical Patient

Days 1 to 2 (in Hospital)
GOALS FOR THE PERIOD: Protect healing tissues, prevent postoperative complications, improve volitional control of involved lower extremity (LE)
Isometric Exercises
1. Gluteal sets
2. Quadriceps sets
Active Range of Motion (AROM) Exercises
3. Ankle pumps

Days 3 to 7 (in Hospital)
GOALS FOR THE PERIOD: Improve lower-extremity (LE) and upper-extremity (UE) strength
AROM Exercises
1. Heel slides
2. Hip abduction
3. Terminal knee extension
Resistive Exercises
4. Resisted shoulder IR and ER with Theraband

5. Shoulder depressions and triceps dips while seated

Weeks 1 to 6 (after Discharge to Home Setting or as Appropriate in Interim Setting)
GOALS FOR THE PERIOD: Improve strength and balance of LEs, promote return to activities and hobbies as indicated

1. Closed-chain exercises (progression to gym equipment and inclined sled): step-ups, minisquats, heel raises, SLRs, and hip abduction
2. Pool therapy
3. Treadmill (as part of gym program)
4. Heel cord stretches

CLINICAL CASE REVIEW

1 Anita had a minimally invasive THR. How will the rehabilitation process change because her procedure was less invasive?

Pain and swelling will be less because the trauma to soft tissue is less. The procedure is performed using a smaller opening. This may allow the patient to progress with bed mobility and transfers more quickly and with greater ease and comfort. The surgeon will determine weight-bearing status and rehabilitation progression. However, the hip precautions remain and the rehabilitation is usually similar (because the procedure is similar but performed with a smaller opening and in a smaller area). New materials such as metal-on-metal implants or ceramic implants are starting to be used. It is hoped that these prosthetic hips will have a longer life span.

2 Sabrina had a noncemented THR surgery 3 days ago. She is TDWB with a walker but continues to place a moderate amount of weight on her affected LE. Because she has difficulty maintaining TDWB during gait, what can be done to help her?

A cracker can be taped to the sole of the patient's forefoot. If the patient still has difficulty maintaining TDWB, then she should try using a thick-soled shoe only on the affected leg. If the patient is PWB, say 50%, then a scale can be used to give feedback regarding how it feels to bear 50% of the weight on the LE.

3 Before having severe hip pain, Tracy was biking 20 to 30 miles a day, 4 days a week. She also competed in bicycle races and worked out in the gym with light weights three times a week. Should Tracy participate in a long-term exercise program after having a THR if it does not contradict the surgeon's orders? Why?

Sheh and associates[26] state that muscular weakness reduces the protection of the implant fixation surfaces during endurance activities. This may contribute to higher loosening rates reported in active patients. Therefore Tracy and other active patients should continue on a long-term exercise program to maintain good muscular strength around the hip.

4 Karen is a 75-year-old female who had a THR 3 weeks ago. She is receiving physical therapy at home and has had two treatments. Today is her third treatment. Her main complaint is the swelling in her foot. Her last treatments emphasized mobility training. She lives with her daughter. She demonstrates stand by assist for most transfers; however, she requires minimal assistance for her affected LE when getting in and out of bed. What should be addressed during today's treatment?

The patient was sitting upon arrival of the therapist. Physical therapy performed transfer training back to bed. When the patient was supine, the therapist massaged her foot and lower leg, milking the fluid up toward the heart. The therapist followed up with AROM for SLR with eccentric lowering of the LE using minimal assistance for guidance. In addition, active assistive hip abduction and adduction (before reaching midline and within the area of hip precautions) were done. Heel cord stretching was also addressed. A discussion regarding using a TED hose and maintaining LE elevation while sitting and in bed followed. In addition, the therapist encouraged the patient to do ankle pumps every hour throughout the day.

5 Why is it not enough to quiz the patient about THR precautions?

Frequently, patients are able to recite the precautions correctly but they do not demonstrate their understanding of them through safe movement. They may still turn their bodies in a way that creates "relative" IR at the hip or flex their hips to greater than 90° while sitting down or standing up. Sitting surfaces often need to be raised up to be used safely. Many patients with NWB orders will put their foot on the ground while turning. Explain the difference between NWB and TDWB to the client as many times as necessary to change this behavior.

6 Following her THR operation, Mary is concerned that her surgical cement may not adhere at the joint and asks if this will cause a dislocation of her prosthesis.

The THR surgery disrupts the integrity of the hip's joint capsule. Movement beyond the limitations of the THR precautions places too much strain on the compromised joint capsule. This is the most frequent cause of postsurgical dislocation. Surgical cement is dry and at its full strength within 10 minutes of its application and is not a factor in dislocation although many patients worry about it. Knowledge of this can motivate the patient to adhere to his or her precautions and to the strengthening program.

7 Why should the surgeon be consulted about the prescription of SLR exercises?

Enloe's consensus group[16] eliminated the SLR from their "ideal" THR rehabilitation plan, because Strickland and colleagues[27] found that it created greater stresses than the amount incurred at the hip during normal unsupported gait. Lewis and Knortz[15] found that SLRs should be initiated when the patient has regained partial or full weight bearing in the operative leg. Gilbert believes that SLRs are unnecessary and may cause dislocation; he warns therapists against using them.[28]

8 Upon the physical therapist's arrival at the patient's home, the patient's operative limb is found to be ruborous, warm, severely swollen, and very painful in spite of elevation and the use of ice. What needs to be done?

Be sure that the patient was discharged with the appropriate number of enoxaparin syringes and has followed through with these injections as prescribed. The patient may have a clot in his leg. Check the status of the surgical scar. There is the possibility of an infection. Make sure that the patient has taken any antibiotics prescribed

since other causes of infection may be due to dental work or other medical procedures unrelated to the THR. Refer the patient back to the surgeon for further evaluation.

9 Robert is having difficulty with transferring into and out of his car safely. What adjustments can help him?

A clean plastic trash bag placed over the passenger's seat provides a slippery surface, which allows the patient to glide-pivot around on the passenger's seat and assume the rider's position more easily. If the height of the seat is adjustable, then raise the seat to the highest possible position. The back of the seat may need to be tilted backward to maintain the precaution of less than 90° flexion at the hip.

10 John was running 3 to 5 miles a day before hip pain necessitated a THR surgery. Should he resume running at the end of his rehab phase?

Running is not recommended following a THR surgery. Alternatives for John could include speed walking, the treadmill, stair climber, and the elliptical cross-trainer. John should be set up with a stretching program that will allow him to pursue his activities showing good posture. This could help to avoid the uneven wear and tear on joints that can encourage further deterioration.

11 What advice can be given when the patient asks about sexual activity following a THR?

Sexual activity after an uncomplicated THR may resume in approximately 1 to 2 months with the surgeon's approval. Studies have shown that most patients feel uncomfortable asking for this type of information. Women tend to prefer the supine position or side lying on the nonoperated side. Men prefer the supine position. The patient is advised to take the more passive role and the prone position may be resumed in 2 to 3 months after surgery.[9]

REFERENCES

1. Buckley R, MD: Total joint replacement: What you really need to know, John Muir MC Orthopedic Update presentation 2008.
2. Hicks JE, Gerber LH: Rehabilitation of the patient with arthritis and connective tissue disease. In DeLisa JA, editor: Rehabilitation medicine: Principles and practices, Philadelphia, 1988, Lippincott.
3. Smith-Peterson MN: A new supra acetabular subperiosteal approach to the hip. Am J Orthop Surg 15:592, 1917.
4. Stern FH, et al: Sexual function after total hip arthroplasty. Clin Orthop 269:228, 1991.
5. Mulroy RD Jr, Harris WH: The effect of improved cementing techniques on component loosening in total hip replacement: An 11-year radiographic review. J Bone Joint Surg 72B:757, 1990.
6. American Academy of Orthopaedic Surgeons: Orthopedic knowledge update 3, Rosemont, Ill, 1987, the Academy.
7. Whitesides L: Personal communication (Total Hip Conference). St Louis, 1993.
8. American Academy of Orthopaedic Surgeons: Orthopedic knowledge update 4: home study syllabus, Rosemont, Ill, 1992, the Academy.
9. Roberts JM, et al: A comparison of the posterolateral and anterolateral approaches to total hip arthroplasty. Clin Orthop 187:205, 1984.

10. Vicar AJ, Coleman CR: A comparison of the anterolateral, transtrochanteric, and posterior surgical approaches in primary total hip arthroplasty. Clin Orthop 188:152, 1994.

11. Santavista N, et al: Teaching of patients undergoing total hip replacement surgery. Int J Nurs Stud 31(2):135, 1994.

12. Petty W: Total joint replacement, Philadelphia, 1991, Saunders.

13. Givens-Heiss DL, et al: In vivo acetabular contact pressures during rehabilitation. II. Postacute phase. Phys Ther 72(10):700, 1992.

14. Krebs D, et al: Exercise and gait effects on in vivo hip contact pressures. Phys Ther 71(4):301, 1991.

15. Lewis C, Knortz K: Total hip replacements. Phys Ther Forum May 20, 1994.

16. Enloe LJ, et al: Total hip and knee replacement programs: A report using consensus. J Orthop Sports Phys Ther 23(1):3, 1996.

17. Jan MH, et al: Effects of a home program on strength, walking speed, and function after total hip replacement. Arch Phys Med Rehabil 85(12):1943-1951, 2004.

18. Zavadak KH, et al: Variability in attainment of functional milestones during the acute care admission after total hip replacement. J Rheumatol 22:482, 1995.

19. Munin MC, et al: Predicting discharge outcome after elective hip and knee arthroplasty. Am J Phys Med Rehabil 74:294, 1995.

20. O'Halloran J: Are you boomer ready—Joint replacement rehabilitation, Birlingame, Calif, 2010, Cross Country Education.

21. McGrorey BJ, Stewart MJ, Sim FH: Participation in sports after hip and knee arthroplasty: a review of the literature and survey of surgical preferences. Mayo Clin Proc 70B:202, 1995.

22. Engh CA, Glassman AH, Suthers KE: The case for porous-coated hip implants: the femoral side. Clin Orthop 261:63, 1990.

23. Klein G, et al: Return to athletic activity after total hip arthroplasty: Consensus guidelines based on a survey of the Hip Society and American Association of Hip and Knee Surgeons. J Arthroplasty 22(2) 171-175, 2007.

24. Sheh C, et al: Muscle recovery and the hip joint after total hip replacement. Clin Orthop 302:115, 1994.

25. Kavanagh BF, et al: Charnley total hip arthroplasty with cement: Fifteen year results. J Bone Joint Surg 71A:1496, 1989.

26. Munin M, et al: Rehabilitation. In Callaghan J, Rosenberg A, Rubash H, editors: The adult hip, Philadelphia, 1998, Lippincott-Raven.

27. Strickland EM, et al: In vivo acetabular contact pressures during rehabilitation. I. Acute phase. Phys Ther 72(10):691, 1992.

28. Gilbert R: Personal communication. June 10, 1998.

CHAPTER 19

New Approaches in Total Hip Replacement: The Anterior Approach for Miniinvasive Total Hip Arthroplasty

Lisa Maxey, Joel M. Matta

SURGICAL TECHNIQUE

After administration of general or regional anesthesia, both feet are placed in the boots. The patient is placed in the supine position on the PROfx or HANA table, a perineal post is placed, and the boots are attached to the table (Fig. 19-1). The hip that will not be operated on is placed in neutral or mild internal rotation (to maximize offset), neutral extension, and slight abduction and will serve as a radiographic reference for the operated side. Avoiding external rotation (ER) of the hip to be operated on will make the external landmarks of the hip more reliable and enhance the landmark of the natural bulge of the tensor fascia lata muscle.

The typical team consists of the surgeon, an assistant, an anesthesiologist, a scrub nurse, a circulating nurse table operator, and a radiograph technician. Although the incision is normally small (8 to 10 cm), the author prefers to drape a relatively wide area. The normal incision starts 2 to 3 cm posterior and 1 to 2 cm distal to the anterosuperior iliac spine. This straight incision extends in a distal and slightly posterior direction to a point 1 to 3 cm anterior to the greater trochanter. On thinner people the bulge of the tensor fascia lata muscle marks the center of the line of the incision. After incision of the skin and subcutaneous tissue, the tensor can be seen through the translucent fascia lata. The author places a vinyl circumferential skin retractor (Protractor) undermining slightly the fat layer off the underlying fascia. The fascial lata should be incised in line with the skin incision over the tensor where the fascia lata is translucent and anterior to the denser tissue of the iliotibial tract. The fascial incision should be continued slightly distal and proximal beyond the ends of the skin incision (Fig. 19-2).

The surgeon should lift the fascia lata off the medial portion of the tensor and follow the interval medial to the tensor in a posterior and proximal direction. Dissection by feel is most efficient at this point, and the lateral hip capsule can be easily palpated just distal to the anteroinferior iliac spine. A cobra retractor should be placed along the lateral hip capsule to retract the tensor and gluteus minimus laterally, and the sartorius and rectus femoris muscles should be retracted medially with a Hibbs retractor. The reflected head of the rectus that follows the lateral acetabular rim will be visible. A small periosteal elevator placed just distal to the reflected head and directed medial and distal elevates the iliopsoas and rectus femoris muscles from the anterior capsule. The elevator opens the path for a second cobra retractor placed on the medial hip capsule. Using this technique, a view of 180° of the circumference of the hip capsule is obtained within a few minutes (Fig. 19-3).

The medial and lateral retraction of the cobras brings the lateral femoral circumflex vessels into view as they cross the distal portion of the wound. These vessels are clamped, cauterized, and transected. Further distal splitting of the aponeurosis that overlies the anterior capsule and vastus lateralis muscle (and at times excision of a fat pad) enhances exposure of the capsule and the origin of the vastus lateralis. The anterior capsule may be either excised or opened as flaps and repaired as part of the closure. (The author prefers to retain the capsule in most cases.) The surgeon should open the capsule with an incision that parallels the anterolateral femoral neck. The proximal portion of this incision crosses the anterior rim of the acetabulum and the reflected capsular origin of the rectus femoris. The distal portion exposes the lateral shoulder of the femoral neck at its junction with the anterior greater trochanter. The junction of the capsule and the origin of the vastus lateralis muscle identify the intertrochanteric line. The distal anterior capsule should be detached from the femur at the anterior intertrochanteric line and suture tags placed on the anterior and lateral capsule at the

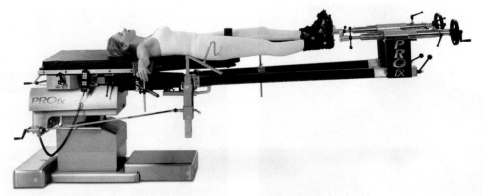

Fig. 19-1 Patient positioned supine on PROfx table.

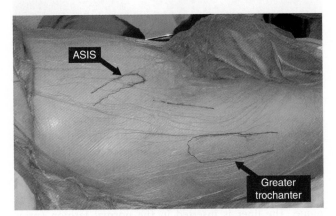

Fig. 19-2 Eight-centimeter incision.

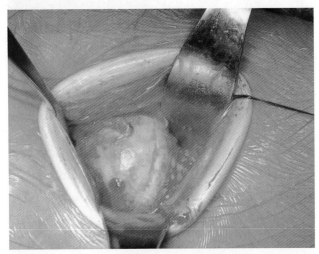

Fig. 19-4 Ninety-degree external rotation allows femoral head dislocation for further exposure.

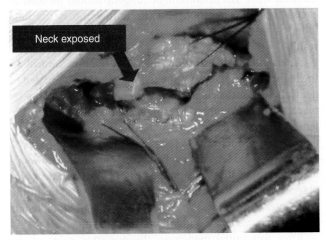

Fig. 19-3 Incision of anterolateral capsule.

distal portion of the incision that separates them. The cobra retractors should be placed intracapsular medial and lateral to the neck. Exposure of the base of the neck is facilitated by a Hibbs retractor that retracts the vastus and distal tensor.

A narrow Hohmann retractor is now placed on the anterolateral acetabular rim. With this exposure, the antero-lateral labrum (and often associated osteophytes) is excised. Distal traction on the extremity will create a small gap between the femoral head and the roof of the acetabulum. A femoral head skid is placed into this gap and then placed in

a more medial position. The traction is partially released. The patient's hip should be externally rotated about 20°, and a femoral head corkscrew should be inserted into the head in a vertical direction. As the extremity and hip are externally rotated and leverage is applied to the skid and corkscrew, the hip should be dislocated anteriorly and the femur externally rotated 90° (Fig. 19-4).

After dislocation, the surgeon should place the tip of a narrow Hohmann retractor distal to the lesser trochanter and beneath the vastus lateralis origin. The capsule should be detached from the medial neck and the lesser trochanter, and the medial posterior neck exposed. The patient's hip is then internally rotated and reduced, the cobra retractors are replaced around the medial and lateral neck, and the vastus origin and distal tensor are retracted with a Hibbs. The surgeon cuts the femoral neck with a reciprocating saw at the desired level and angle as indicated by the preoperative plan (Fig. 19-5). The neck cut is completed with an osteotome that divides the lateral neck from the medial greater trochanter and is directed posterior and slightly medial to avoid the posterior greater trochanter. The head is extracted with the corkscrew. Light traction will distract the neck osteotomy and facilitate this extraction.

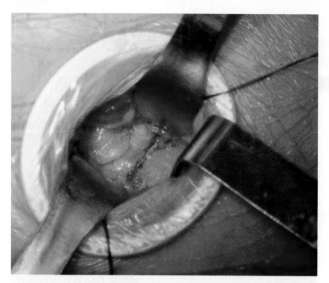

Fig. 19-5 Lateral neck cut finalized with osteotome. Head removed.

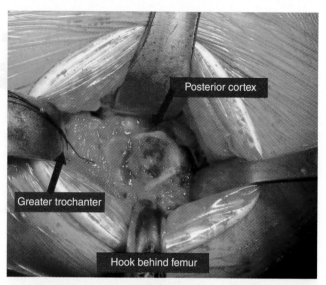

Fig. 19-7 Hip hyperextended and adduction with external rotation allows delivery of proximal femur for femoral broaching.

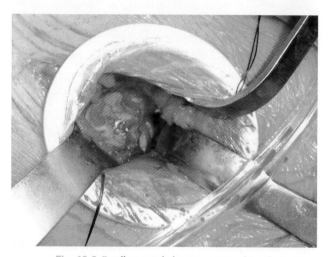

Fig. 19-6 Excellent acetabular exposure is achieved.

Throughout the procedure the surgeon will find that the tensor fascia lata muscle is potentially vulnerable to injury. If an initial injury to the muscle fibers is avoided, then the muscle seems to hold up well through the procedure. On the other hand, an early laceration to the surface of the tensor seems to hurt its capability of resisting further damage.

The acetabulum is now visualized and prepared. ER of the femur of about 45° usually facilitates acetabular exposure (Fig. 19-6). Light traction also limits femoral interference. The author prefers to use a bent Hohmann retractor above the distal anterior rim of the acetabulum to retract the anterior muscles. The surgeon should take care to place the tip of this retractor on bone and not into the anterior soft tissues. The author places a cobra retractor with the tip on the mid posterior rim. The labrum is then excised circumferentially. A transverse release of a prominent band of inferior capsule will facilitate later placement of the acetabular liner. The author usually begins reaming under direct vision and later checks with the image intensifier to confirm depth of reaming

and adequate circumference. The indicators of torque and acetabular appearance are also used. The author then inserts the acetabular prosthesis. Most experienced surgeons can easily recognize a properly positioned cup on a radiograph (40° to 45° abduction and 15° to 25° anteversion), and good position can be achieved consistently with the image technique. The liner is inserted in the normal fashion (prior excision of labrum and the inferior capsule release will facilitate this). An osteotome or rongeur should be used to excise projecting osteophytes. The radiograph is the final judge as to whether computer guidance led to the correct result.

After acetabular insertion, the gross traction control on the leg spar is released and the femur is internally rotated to neutral. The vastus ridge is palpated, and the femoral hook placed just distal to this and around the posterior femur. The femur is then externally rotated 90° and the hip hyperextended and adducted.

For proximal femoral exposure, the author uses a long-handled cobra with the tip on the posterior femoral neck and places the tip of a trochanteric retractor over the tip of the trochanter. The femoral hook now raises the proximal femur until the tissues come under moderate tension.

After this initial maneuver, the posterior ridge of the greater trochanter may lie posterior to the posterior rim of the acetabulum. The femur needs to be mobile enough so that lateral and anterior displacement brings the posterior edge of the trochanter lateral and anterior to the posterior rim of the acetabulum. The lateral capsular flap and its tag suture will be clearly visible distal to the trochanteric retractor and attaching to the remnant of the lateral neck. Detachment of this flap from the base of the neck in an anterior to posterior direction facilitates visualization of the medial greater trochanter and enhances femoral mobility (Fig. 19-7). The surgeon should use a rongeur to excise the remnant of the lateral neck.

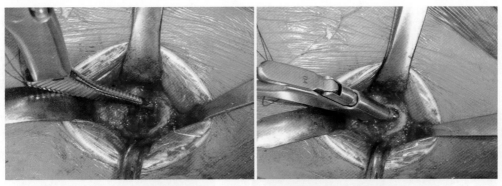

Fig. 19-8 Broach insertion easily accomplished through anterior incision.

It should be remembered that the obturator internus and piriformis tendons insert on the anterior superior greater trochanter. After release of the lateral capsule, the surgeon should place the tip of the trochanteric retractor closer to the upper border of the trochanter to retract the gluteus minimus muscle and piriformis, and obturator internus tendons. Depending on the requirements for femoral mobility, the surgeon may choose to release one or more of the short external rotator tendons and the obturator internus tendon, particularly when it cannot be flipped over the posterior tip of the trochanter. However, the author prefers to preserve all tendon attachments and strives in particular to preserve the attachment of the obturator externus tendon, because its medial pull on the proximal femur is an important active restraint against dislocation.

In general, prostheses with less prominence in the proximal lateral area will be easier to insert, will allow preservation of the rotator attachments, and will present a lower risk of trochanteric fracture. However, the instrumentation required most determines the applicability of a stem to the anterior approach. The tip of the first broach enters the neck near the posterior medial cortex (Fig. 19-8). When the broaching is complete, a trial reduction is made, with the neck length estimated from the preoperative template.

During trial phase I, the surgeon should check for hip stability in extension and ER with the traction released. The surgeon should also check for impingement with osteophytes and excise appropriately. The author of this chapter feels that it is best to rely on the radiograph for length and offset decisions rather than soft tissue tension and intraoperative stability.

After the decision is made for the femoral prosthesis, the femoral hook is replaced behind the proximal femur, traction is applied to distract the head, and the hip is dislocated with ER. The femur is then placed into the preparation position (i.e., 90° ER, hyperextension, adduction, proximal elevation). The femoral prosthesis is then inserted in the normal fashion. The appropriate-length permanent head can be placed at this time (Figs. 19-9 and 19-10). With the hip flexed to neutral, the acetabulum is visualized before reduction to ensure that it is clear of bone or cement fragments. Another transparency printed with the image intensifier confirms leg

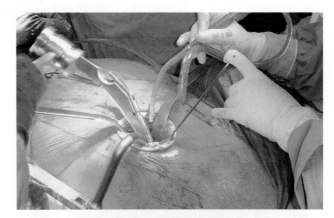

Fig. 19-9 Broaching easily accomplished through anterior incision.

length and offset and serves as the immediate postoperative radiograph. Before discharge, radiographs are obtained in the radiology department (Fig. 19-11).

A check is made for bleeding and the wound is irrigated. The closure is simple. The anterior and lateral capsular tag sutures are tied together, and further capsular closure is performed if desired. The fascia lata is closed with a running suture, followed by subcutaneous tissue and skin.

After surgery the patient does not follow antidislocation precautions. The patient is encouraged to weight bear immediately, use the hip, and discard external support as symptoms permit.

From November 1996 to April 2005, the author of this chapter performed 657 primary anterior total hip arthroplasties (THAs), including 67 bilateral THAs. This series of 657 anterior approaches is unselected and consecutive. The surgeries were performed on a Judet or Tasserit table until 2003. Beginning in 2003 the PROfx table became available and is now preferred. The average patient age is 66 and ranges from 29 to 91. The average operative time is 1.2 hours. Average blood loss is 345 mL. The median hospital time is 4 days, and the mode is 3 days. Two early anterior dislocations and one posterior dislocation occurred that were reduced closed and did not recur or require revision. The median time to doing some ambulation without external support is 8 days. The median time for doing all ambulation without external support is 15 days. It is the author's impression that pain is

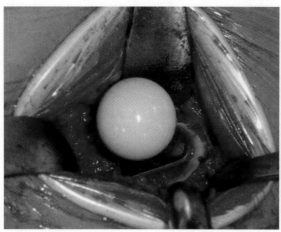
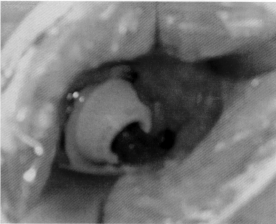

Fig. 19-10 Delta ceramic head placed and reduced.

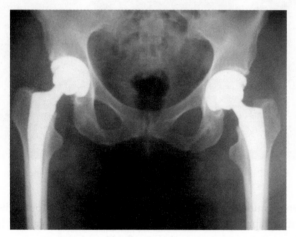

Fig. 19-11 Intraoperative imaging ensures length and cup position.

reduced and the recovery rate greatly enhanced. (See the THA slide show at www.hipandpelvis.com for more detailed statistics.[1])

REHABILITATION AFTER ANTERIOR TOTAL HIP ARTHROPLASTY

With this procedure tendon attachments, such as the obturator externus, rotator attachments, and gluteus medius, have been preserved. In fact, all the muscle attachments are preserved. The obturator externus has a medial pull on the proximal femur and is an important active contractor against hip dislocation. With the preservation of these muscle attachments and other soft tissues, total hip precautions are not required. Pain is reduced and the recovery rate is enhanced. Weight bearing is immediately encouraged, and assistive devices are discarded when possible.

The rehabilitation process is similar to most total hip replacement regimens. However, the patient will progress through the process more quickly and with a lower risk of hip dislocation.

In the hospital bed, mobility, transfer training, and gait training are done during the initial treatments. The patient is instructed in ankle pumps. Isometrics such as hip abduction, hip adduction, quadriceps sets, and gluteus sets can also be started immediately. In addition, heel slides are encouraged with assistance, then without any assistance. The patient then progresses to active range of motion for hip abduction, adduction, and straight leg raises. Patients can be taught pelvic tilts and knee to chest (using the unaffected lower extremity) for low back discomfort. Heel cord stretches can be done carefully with the leg slightly back and a wedge under the forefoot. Closed-chain exercises like minisquats, step-ups, and heel raises are begun when the patient can safely perform them.

GENERAL COMMENTS REGARDING HIP REPLACEMENT

The first very successful hip prosthesis was designed and implanted in the 1960s by John Charnley of England. Charnley's design used a one-piece metal stem with a 22-mm diameter head that was cemented into the proximal femur. The acetabular component was made entirely of polyethylene and cemented into the acetabulum. Follow-up studies of the Charnley prosthesis and other similar cemented designs have shown sufficient longevity that the majority of prostheses in surviving patients are still functioning 20 years after implantation. Despite the great success of these hip prostheses, it is recognized that the failure rate increases over time. The mode of failure is typically loosening of the secure bond between the prosthesis and the bone and bone loss associated with this process.

Because of the recognized limits to longevity of these early designs, continued work to improve the design has been conducted, and thereby longevity of hip prostheses has been achieved. Currently the U.S. Food and Drug Administration (the federal agency regulating hip prostheses) has over 750 approved designs for hip prostheses on file. The majority of new designs, however, have proven to be not as good as Charnley's hip. In addition, some new designs have been shown to equal the longevity of the Charnley hip but have not proven superior to it.

What is the significance of this history for today's hip replacement patient? Just because a hip prosthesis is the latest design does not mean it is better; in fact, it could be worse. Time gives us the answers. We need to continue to look for prostheses with improved longevity; however, a quantum improvement may not be just around the corner, and the current expected longevity may be with us for some time to come.

What has changed? The acetabulum is now almost always implanted without cement. The results of the uncemented acetabulum appear equal to cement, and clinicians hope that the longevity will prove better over time. Some designs of uncemented femoral stems have also shown good longevity comparable with the best-proven cemented stems. It is widely felt that the bearing surfaces have been improved, which means that this surface wears at a slower rate. Although metal against extremely high-density polyethylene is the best-proven bearing, evidence also supports the use of metal-on-metal and ceramic bearings.

Today, development of hip replacement surgery is not limited to efforts to improve the prostheses. Improvements also include surgical approaches that limit the surgical trauma to the soft tissue, thereby accelerating recovery and limiting the possibility of dislocation. The author applauds this trend because it is the basis of the anterior approach for hip replacement described herein.

Possible complications of hip replacement surgery include infection, injury to nerves and blood vessels, fracture of the femur or acetabulum, hip dislocation, and need for revision surgery. Patients should remember that recovery means not only recovery from the surgical procedure but also time to recover from the condition they were in before surgery.

REFERENCE

1. Matta JM, Klenck RE, Hipandpelvis.com: Available at: http://www.hipandpelvis.com/.

FURTHER READING

Matta JM, Ferguson TA: The anterior approach for hip replacement. Orthopedics 28(9):927, 2005.

Matta JM, Shahrdar C, Ferguson T: Single-incision anterior approach for total hip arthroplasty on an orthopaedic table. Clin Orthop Rel Res 441:115, 2005.

Yerasimides JG, Matta JM: Primary total hip arthroplasty with a minimally invasive anterior approach. Semin Arthroplasty 16(3):186, 2005.

CHAPTER 20

Hip Arthroscopy

Jonathan E. Fow

ETIOLOGY

Arthroscopy of the hip has been performed for many years, but has become more mainstream over the last few years. Initially, it was used as a minimally invasive method of removing loose bodies. As we have learned more about variations in hip morphology, both congenital and acquired, the useful applications of hip arthroscopy have grown. Overall, hip arthroscopy can improve pain and function in 68% to 96% of surgical patients[1] (Fig. 20-1).

ANATOMY

Femoral acetabular impingement (FAI) is a cause of hip pain and debility. An anomalous, aspherical femoral head or anterosuperior "bump" on the femoral head and neck are features of controlled action motion (CAM) impingement (Fig. 20-2). An anterosuperior acetabular lip or retroverted acetabulum causes pincer impingement (Fig. 20-3). There is often a mixed morphology involving attributes of both CAM and pincer impingement. Femoral osteoplasty to reshape the femoral head and neck can treat CAM impingement, whereas acetabular osteoplasty can reshape the acetabular rim to improve pincer impingement.[2] Both osteoplasty procedures result in improved range of motion (ROM) and function. Hip arthroscopy can address labral tears by both débridement and repair. Surgeons may perform microfracture or abrasion chondroplasty on the acetabulum also to débride cartilage lesions, and extraarticular pathology, such as gluteus medius tears, chronic iliotibial (IT) band snapping syndrome, and snapping psoas syndrome, can also be addressed endoscopically.

The complex mechanical interrelationships of the lumbar spine, hip, and lower extremity can functionally cause FAI despite near normal architecture. There can be functional impingement caused by hyperlordosis or the type of stress or activity imposed on the joint. In addition, often there exists multiple sources of pain such as degenerated discs, sacroiliac disorders, hip bursitis and IT band syndrome, hip flexor strains, and hernias. Diagnosis of FAI, loose bodies, and other causes of intraarticular or extraarticular hip pain must be confirmed while other possible sources of pain are ruled out. At the very least, patients should be aware of the risk that hip pain can be, and often is, multifactorial. Arthroscopy of the hip may only be able to address a percentage of the pain they experience.

INDICATIONS/CONSIDERATIONS

Patients who are seen in the office with hip pain are initially examined, their history reviewed, and radiographs taken. History of the patient's hip pain may include chronic psoas strains, lumbar spine, and sacroiliac joint dysfunction. Transitioning to a higher or different level of activity (e.g., high school to college track) may precipitate hip pathology, as well as previous involvement and previous injuries in sports. FAI can also become symptomatic with changes in equipment, which affect body position such as shoes and bicycles.

Hip pathology is often described by a patient as groin or gluteal pain. Because hip pain can also radiate to the thigh and knee, patients may have had inappropriate knee arthroscopy.

PHYSICAL EXAMINATION: Examining the lumbar spine, hip, and knee and observing posture and gait are very important in evaluating a patient with hip pain. Consider pursuing evaluation in functional positions, especially during sporting activities (e.g., running, pushing, jumping, skating, lunging). Observe the relationship of the pelvis to the lower extremities, then examine the extremities. Examine the patient walking, standing, supine, lateral, and prone.

Standing:

Gait: Observe stride length, foot progression angle, pelvis rotation, stance phase, foot drop, clicking, popping, antalgic gait, Trendelenburg gait, pelvic wink (external rotation >40), short leg limp (IT band pathology, true/false leg length discrepancy).

Patient recreation of click: Psoas or IT band.

Alignment: Note shoulder height, scoliosis, pelvic tilt; grossly measure anterosuperior iliac spine (ASIS) to medial malleolus; note spinal alignment posterior and lateral (flat

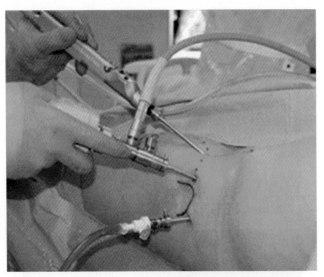

Fig. 20-1 Arthroscopy of the hip uses small incisions to address an increasing range of pathology via small incisions.

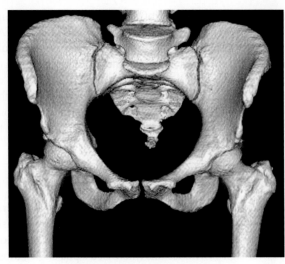

Fig. 20-3 Computed tomographic 3-D reconstruction of the pelvis helps gain appreciation for acetabular pathology, such as pincer lesions, retroversion, and os acetabuli.

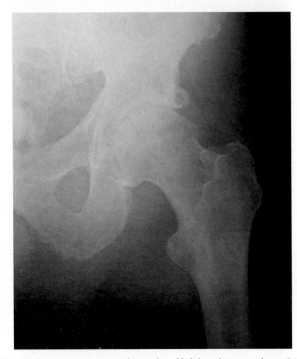

Fig. 20-2 Anteroposterior radiographs of left hip showing a large CAM lesion.

lumbar spine) hyperlordotic; and consider that which would functionally affect pelvic and acetabular orientation (e.g., weak abdominal musculature, gluteus, lumbar spine, tight hamstrings). Observe single-leg stance for pelvic balance.

Sitting:

Leg length, rotation, neurologic (motor: abduction: superior gluteal nerve L4 to S1; adduction: obturator nerve L2 to 4; knee extension: L2 to 4; knee flexion: L4 to S3 sciatic nerve; great toe extension: L5; extensor hallucis longus, plantar flexion: L4 to S1; sensory: dermatomal sensation).

Supine:

ROM: External rotation, internal rotation in hip neutral and 90° of hip flexion, popliteal angle, supine abduction, frog leg abduction (knee height), adduction.

Palpate: Inguinal region, pubis, ASIS, anteroinferior iliac spine (AIIS), Stinchfield test (straight leg raise versus resistance causing pain indicates iliopsoas and/or intraarticular pathology), inferior to AIIS (labrum, anterior capsule, rectus reflected). Note: Nondisplaced or stress fracture will also hurt with straight leg raise, heel strike, and log roll.

Provocative: FADIR (flexion, adduction, internal rotation) indicates FAI and labral pathology, FABER (flexion, abduction, external rotation) or Patrick test for groin, iliopsoas, lateral FAI, lateral-FAI flexion to extension in abduction (abduction), posterior labrum, and sacroiliac pathology); Thomas test: click may indicate labral tear and tightness represents iliopsoas contracture; McCarthy: full ROM from extension to flexion with external/internal rotation; Scour test: full flex and palpate superior acetabular rim for irregularity.

Lateral:

Palpate ischial tuberosity, greater trochanter, tensor fascia lata, IT band, piriformis, gluteus, sacrum, coccyx, sciatic nerve.

Ober (knee flexion and extension), test strength gluteus medius, gluteus minimus, Ely test in lateral tight quadriceps mechanism.

Prone:

Palpate sacroiliac joint, ischial tuberosity, spine, musculature. Ely test: rectus/quadriceps contracture.

OTHERS

ROM is examined with the hip in flexion and extension. The hip is fully passively ranged and observed for pain with FADIR and FABER. Popliteal angle is evaluated to check for hamstring tightness. A loss of the arc of motion of the hip, especially internal rotation, is suspicious for significant FAI or arthritis. A low lumbar spine examination can help rule out or reveal concurrent lumbar spine pathology. Strength of abductors, adductors, hip flexors, and extensors, as well as knee and ankle muscles, can be very revealing about the functional contributions of deficits and imbalance that contribute to hip pain. Even a foot drop can contribute to overuse of hip flexors and subsequent hip pain.

IMAGING

Radiographs include AP pelvis, cross-table, and frog lateral hip views. Simple radiographs can demonstrate dysplasia (decreased center-edge angle), acetabular retroversion (crossover sign), CAM lesions (increased alpha angle), loose bodies, and radiographic signs of arthritis (joint space narrowing, osteophyte formation, subchondral sclerosis, and cysts) (Fig. 20-4). Newer studies suggest that joint space narrowing with less than 3 mm of space remaining, inferior osteophytes, and a center-edge angle of less than 20° (measure of dysplasia/shallow acetabulum) are reasons to *not* perform a hip arthroscopy but rather prepare the patient for a hip replacement when symptoms warrant the procedure despite conservative treatment.[3] Other considerations are lumbar spine and sacroiliac pathology.

If examination and radiographs support the diagnosis of a hip problem, an MRI can be performed to observe for labral pathology, chondral injury, and loose bodies (Fig. 20-5). An arthrogram at the time of the MRI improves the accuracy of the examination, and allows injection of a local anesthetic and cortisone type of medication into the joint and observation for pain relief. If pain relief occurs, then intraarticular causes of hip pain are suggested. More specifically, response to the injection implies chondral damage.[4] Depending on the cause, a computed tomographic scan with 3-D reconstructions may help better analyze the pincer impingement lesion and how much "rim trimming" may need to be performed to correct that pathology (Fig. 20-3).

Hip arthroscopy is an excellent, minimally invasive method of addressing femoral acetabular pathology previously only addressed with open hip disarticulation.

SURGICAL PROCEDURE

Hip arthroscopy can be performed from two surgical positions: supine and lateral. Arthroscopic portals are identical in both positions, and the choice is really based on surgeon training and preference.

Supine hip arthroscopy can be performed with easier operating room setup. However, the posterior lateral portal is difficult to establish, and the entire procedure can be more difficult in an obese to large patient (Fig. 20-1).

Lateral hip arthroscopy requires a more complex room setup with a specialized table attachment to apply traction and position the leg. It does provide excellent access to the hip joint anterior and posterior, even in large patients.

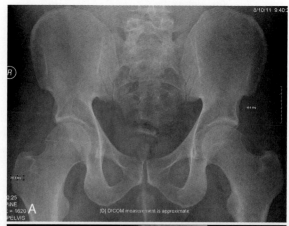
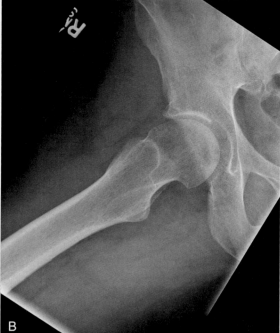

Fig. 20-4 Anteroposterior radiographs of pelvis (**A**) and frog lateral (**B**) are useful for observing crossover sign, CAM lesions, alpha angle, center-edge angle, inferior osteophytes, joint space narrowing, and other bony pathology.

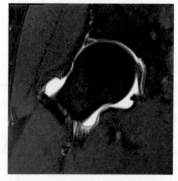

Fig. 20-5 MRI arthrograms of the hip help identify labral tears, as seen here on the superior acetabulum, as well as loose bodies, CAM lesions, bone cysts, some cartilage lesions, and ligamentum teres pathology.

Once the patient is positioned, the anterolateral portal is established first. Various arthroscopic portals penetrate the tensor fascia lata, gluteus medius, and sartorius and rectus femoris. After careful placement with fluoroscopic guidance, the anterior portal is established next, with care taken to avoid injury to the lateral femoral cutaneous nerve. The capsule is opened between the portals and then split in a "T" or "H" shape to gain access to the femoral CAM lesion. Most surgeons start in the central compartment to look for loose bodies, cartilage injuries, ligamentous injuries, and notch osteophytes (Fig. 20-6). Cartilage injuries are often adjacent to labral injuries. In the peripheral compartment, the labrum, acetabular rim, and anterosuperior femoral neck are evaluated. Labral tears can be débrided or repaired with suture anchors. At the same time, a "rim-trimming" or acetabular osteoplasty can be performed where the pincer impingement is removed and the acetabular retroversion is improved. Care is taken via preoperative planning not to remove so much acetabulum as to destabilize the hip by respecting the CEA. The femoral CAM lesion can also be removed via a femoral osteoplasty (Figs. 20-7 and 20-8). Multiple portals can be used to access the central and peripheral compartments. A posterolateral portal, accessory anterolateral portal, and the mid anterolateral portal can be used to assist with the femoral osteoplasty, rim trimming, or anchor placement.

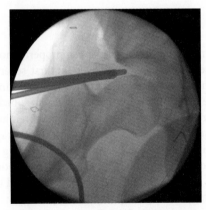

Fig. 20-6 Initial arthroscopy often starts with the hip distracted to observe the central compartment where a cartilage injury is often identified.

The anterior portals may put branches of the lateral femoral cutaneous nerve at risk; thus the portals are carefully closed with absorbable and/or nonabsorbable suture. A bulky dressing and an abduction pillow are placed. The surgery can be performed outpatient in a surgery center or a hospital. The surgical time can be quite prolonged, and an overnight stay may be considered.

The protocol for postoperative management varies based on whether microfracture or labral repairs are performed. Indomethacin is given for 2 weeks to help prevent postoperative heterotopic ossification (HO).[5] Extra effort is taken to lavage the joint and soft tissues after the femoral osteoplasty, but HO is still possible and one reason for reoperation. After surgery, the patient can be sent home with arrangements for a continuous passive motion machine, crutches or walker, and a hip cryo-sleeve.

OUTCOMES

Depending on the condition of the acetabular cartilage and possibly the labrum, patients can do quite well. Long-term outcomes can be very satisfying, delaying or preventing the need for hip replacement. A more severe or involved acetabular cartilage damage predicts a poorer outcome and earlier need for arthroplasty.

Surgical challenges are related to the acetabular cartilage damage, severity of the CAM impingement, and labral takedown and rim-trimming for pincer impingement. Recent studies suggest superior outcomes in labral repair (Harris Hip Score 89.7% vs. 66.7% good to excellent results). Although it may make sense to recreate the labral "gasket," a large definitive study needs to be published.[6] The labrum contributes to hip stability. Hip stability is not reduced until 2 cm has been removed.[7]

Although hip arthroscopy is safer and has a faster rehabilitation rate than an open procedure, complications can still occur. Various studies quote an up to 18% complication rate.[8] They include neuropraxia of the sciatic, femoral, or lateral femoral cutaneous nerve; HO (1.6%); portal wound bleeding; and instrument breakage. Other case reports describe complications that include femoral neck fracture,[9]

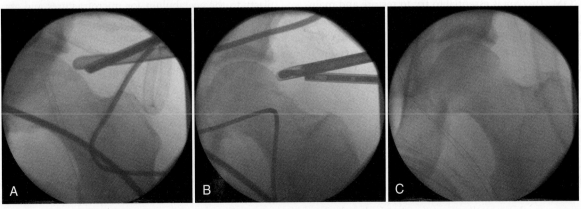

Fig. 20-7 In the peripheral compartment, distraction can be discontinued as CAM lesions are identified (**A**) and removed with the assistance of fluoroscopy (**B** and **C**).

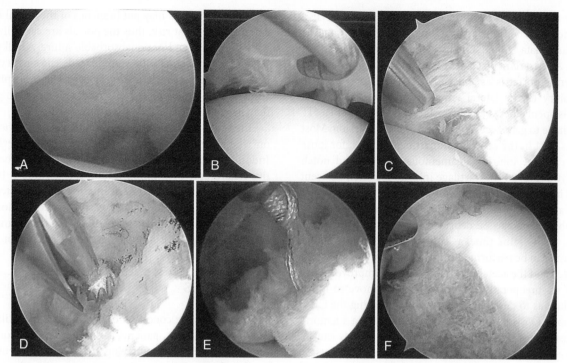

Fig. 20-8 Arthroscopy shows the central compartment labrum and the inverted horseshoe of articular cartilage around the fovea (**A**). Labral tears are identified (**B**) and débrided with capsular, anteroinferior iliac spine pathology. The acetabulum is débrided then burred (**D**) to remove diseased tissue and to allow the labral repair (**E**) to heal into healthy bone. The burr can also be used to remove pincer lesions and os acetabuli in a similar process. CAM lesions are removed (**F**) under fluoroscopic guidance.

dislocation,[10] trochanteric bursitis, abdominal compartment syndrome,[11] intrathoracic extravasation of fluid,[12] avascular necrosis,[13] and penetration of the acetabulum by anchors.[14] A common reason for reoperation is underresection of the CAM lesion. Postoperative radiographs can show the improvement in CAM lesions and elimination of the crossover sign. The need for a conversion to a total hip arthroscopy is as high as 26%.

Neuropraxias can be related to portal placement or distraction. Symptoms are usually short-lived and resolve completely. HO can occur, and indomethacin is given after surgery to help prevent its formation. Patients can develop painful stiffness several weeks after surgery despite early good ROM. Therapy is essential to try to restore and maintain ROM at this point. If HO forms and is symptomatic, it can be resected. The patient is given indomethacin and radiation to help prevent recurrence at the time of the resection of HO. After labral repair, care must be taken to avoid impingement, which may stress the repair before healing (≥6 weeks). Furthermore, after microfracture in the hip, it is recommended to limit weight bearing, and many surgeons advocate the use of a postoperative continuous passive motion for reasons similar to its use after microfracture in the knee.

POSSIBLE COMPLICATIONS

In addition to the complications previously listed, there are a few other potential rehabilitation concerns. Pain control

is important so that the therapist can properly mobilize the hip; this seems to be a focus over the first several weeks. Maintaining weight-bearing status is also important for protecting the healing labrum and microfracture bed. Sudden stiffness or mechanical signs may forebode reinjury of the labrum, worsening cartilage injury (or frank rapid-onset osteoarthritis), avascular necrosis, or developing HO and would necessitate communication with the surgeon.

Various types of procedures can be performed to correct hip pathology through hip arthroscopy surgery. Cartilage and lesions can be débrided. For example, labral tears can be débrided or repaired. Osteoplasty procedures can be done to improve ROM and function, including chondroplasty to the acetabulum for microfractures and abrasions. Also, extraarticular pathology, such as gluteus medius tears, chronic IT band snapping syndrome, and snapping psoas syndrome, can also be addressed. The rehabilitation progression will vary depending on the hip pathology and procedure.

SUMMARY

This chapter equips the rehabilitation professional with an understanding of the various procedures performed using hip arthroscopy. Also, a description of a hip arthroscopy is provided so that the reader can appreciate the different tissues that are compromised, altered, or repaired during this surgery.

REFERENCES

1. Clohisy JC, St John LC, Schutz AL: Surgical treatment of femoroacetabular impingement: A systematic review of the literature. Clin Orthop Relat Res 468(2):555-564, 2010.

2. Colvin AC, Koehler SM, Bird J: Can the change in center-edge angle during pincer trimming be reliably predicted? Clin Orthop Relat Res 469(4):1071-1074, 2011.

3. Larson CM, Giveans MR, Taylor M: Does arthroscopic FAI correction improve function with radiographic arthritis? Clin Orthop Relat Res 469(6):1667-1676, 2011. Epub 2010 Dec 22.

4. Kivlan BR, Martin RL, Sekiya JK: Response to diagnostic injection in patients with femoroacetabular impingement, labral tears, chondral lesions, and extra-articular pathology. Arthroscopy 27(5):619-627, 2011.

5. Randelli F, et al: Heterotopic ossifications after arthroscopic management of femoroacetabular impingement: The role of NSAID prophylaxis. J Orthop Traumatol 11(4):245-250. Epub 2010 Nov 30, 2010.

6. Larson CM, Giveans MR: Arthroscopic debridement versus refixation of the acetabular labrum associated with femoroacetabular impingement. Arthroscopy 25(4):369-376. Epub 2009 Mar 5, 2009.

7. Smith MV, et al: Effect of acetabular labrum tears on hip stability and labral strain in a joint compression model. Am J Sports Med 39(Suppl):103S-110S, 2011.

8. Botser IB, et al: Open surgical dislocation versus arthroscopy for femoroacetabular impingement: A comparison of clinical outcomes. Arthroscopy 27(2):270-278, 2011.

9. Ayeni OR, et al: Femoral neck fracture after arthroscopic management of femoroacetabular impingement: A case report. J Bone Joint Surg Am 4;93(9):e47, 2011.

10. Matsuda DK: Acute iatrogenic dislocation following hip impingement arthroscopic surgery. Arthroscopy 25(4):400-404. Epub 2009 Feb 1, 2009.

11. Fowler J, Owens BD: Abdominal compartment syndrome after hip arthroscopy. Arthroscopy 26(1):128-130, 2010.

12. Verma M, Sekiya JK: Intrathoracic fluid extravasation after hip arthroscopy. Arthroscopy 26(9 Suppl):S90-S94. Epub 2010 Aug 5, 2010.

13. Scher DL, Belmont PJ Jr, Owens BD: Case report: Osteonecrosis of the femoral head after hip arthroscopy. Clin Orthop Relat Res 468(11):3121-3125. Epub 2010 Feb 10, 2010.

14. Hernandez JD, McGrath BE: Safe angle for suture anchor insertion during acetabular labral repair. Arthroscopy 24(12):1390-1394. Epub 2008 Oct 10, 2008.

CHAPTER 21

Open Reduction and Internal Fixation of the Hip

Patricia A. Gray, Mayra Saborio Amiran, Edward Pratt

Hip fractures are the bony injuries that require surgical intervention in the United States most frequently. The annual expense for the treatment of these patients has been estimated as high as $7.3 billion. Because the incidence of osteoporosis in our steadily aging population is increasing, the number of hip fractures is expected to increase from 275,000 per year in the late 1980s to more than 500,000 by the year 2040.[1]

SURGICAL INDICATIONS AND CONSIDERATIONS

Numerous classification systems have been devised to describe hip fractures. However, in the context of surgical exposure, soft tissue injury, and rehabilitation potential, they can be simplified into five main categories:

1. Nondisplaced or minimally displaced femoral neck fractures
2. Displaced femoral neck fractures
3. Stable intertrochanteric fractures
4. Unstable intertrochanteric fractures
5. Subtrochanteric fractures

All categories of these fractures can demonstrate good outcomes with surgical intervention and early mobilization.[2] This is true regardless of age, gender, or comorbidities. The rare exception is an incomplete or impacted femoral neck fracture in a nonambulatory or extremely ill individual. The expected postoperative stability of the hip is directly proportional to the severity of the injury, the quality or density of the bone to be repaired, and the technical expertise of the surgeon.

The patient's overall preinjury physical and mental condition is also a predictor of postoperative success. Patients with major cardiopulmonary afflictions, obesity, poor upper body strength, osteoporosis, or dementia in its various forms have increased risk for complications in the treatment of hip fractures. Overall mortality rates of 20% after 1 year, 50% at 3 years, 60% at 6 years, and 77% after 10 years have been

reported.[3] This is not surprising, because most hip fractures occur in the older adult population.

The traditional goal of rehabilitation has been to restore patients to the level of function that they had before the injury. In many cases this may not be realistic. Only 20% to 35% of patients regain their preinjury level of independence. Some 15% to 40% require institutionalized care for more than 1 year after surgery. Many—50% to 83%—require devices to assist with ambulation.[4]

Rehabilitation goals must be individualized, with the therapist taking into account all comorbidities, fracture severity, and motivational level of the patient.

Displaced or minimally displaced femoral neck fractures represent the least severe injuries in the spectrum of hip fractures. They are stable and can bear the full weight of the patient immediately after surgery. Moreover, they require no limitations on range of motion (ROM) or exertion in the immediate postoperative period. The preferred surgical procedure is a fluoroscopically aided placement of cannulated 6.5-mm screws through a limited or percutaneous lateral approach. This approach violates the skin, subcutaneous fat, deep fascia of the fascia lata, and fascia and muscle fibers of the vastus lateralis. Typically blood distends the joint capsule, creating some limitation in hip ROM and pain. No major nerves or vessels are at risk in this approach.

The patient is brought to the operating room, and anesthesia is induced. The patient is positioned supine on a fracture table capable of distracting and manipulating the affected limb. After satisfactory position of the fracture fragments is verified with an image intensifier, surgery is begun.

A 2-cm incision is made along the lateral femur in line with the fractured femoral neck. A guide pin is then placed percutaneously through the lateral musculature at or about the level of the lesser trochanter. The pin is introduced up the femoral neck and across the fracture into the subchondral bone of the femoral head. After two to four guide pins have been placed, the outer cortex is drilled with a cannulated drill and cannulated screws are introduced over the

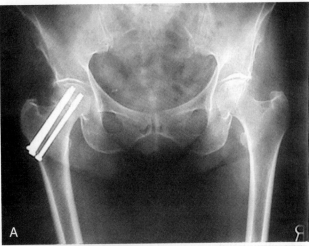

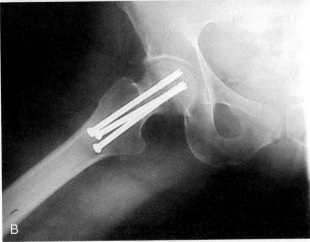

Fig. 21-1 **A,** Anteroposterior radiograph of the pelvis showing proper placement of three cannulated screws across a minimally displaced subcapital femoral neck fracture. **B,** Lateral view of the case illustrated in **A.**

guide pins (Fig. 21-1). The soft tissues are repaired, and a dressing is applied. Femoral neck fractures that occur more toward the base of the femoral neck require fixation that is able to resist the bending movement between the femoral neck and shaft. These are treated much like intertrochanteric fractures, and the operative procedure is described in that section.

Displaced Femoral Neck Fractures

Femoral neck fractures in which the femoral head has been separated widely from the neck do not heal if reduced and fixed by screws or pins. In these fractures the vascular supply to the femoral head (specifically the medial and lateral femoral circumflex arteries) are often severed. In younger patients it is still desirable to attempt fixation despite the high rate of nonunion and osteonecrosis. When open reduction is attempted, the anterolateral exposure of Watson-Jones is preferred because it preserves the blood supply to the femoral head, which enters through the posteroinferior femoral neck.[5] This approach is discussed in the section on total hip replacement (THR). Older adult patients are often best treated by bipolar, endoprosthetic, or THR procedures using a posterolateral approach.

The posterolateral approach involves violation of the skin; subcutaneous tissue; fascia lata; gluteus maximus; and short external rotators of the hip, including the piriformis, obturator internus, gemelli, and quadratus femoris. The capsule is incised posteriorly and often released anteriorly. Traction is applied on the gluteus maximus, gluteus medius, and gluteus minimus throughout the procedure. Nerves and vessels at risk include the sciatic nerve, the superior gluteal nerve, the inferior gluteal nerve, and their accompanying vessels. Although the psoas is left alone, it is often inflamed and can scar down and across the anterior hip capsule if adequate postoperative mobilization is not encouraged. Generally incisions are healed by 2 weeks, deep soft tissue healing is well advanced by 6 weeks, and full bony healing is expected at 12 weeks.

The patient is anesthetized and placed in the lateral decubitus position with the injured hip up (see Fig. 15-4); the torso is stabilized, and the hip and affected leg are draped to move freely. The initial incision is centered over the greater trochanter and taken distally 3 inches along the femoral shaft, then proximally and medially 4 inches along the course of the fibers of the gluteus maximus. The deep fascia is incised over the greater trochanter and carried distally along the same line as the skin incision, exposing the origin of the vastus lateralis without violating it. The surgeon digitally palpates the interval between the gluteus maximus and tensor fascia lata proximally, then extends the deep incision in this interval. A large, self-retaining retractor is then positioned to hold the deep fascia apart. The greater trochanteric bursa is incised to expose the short external rotators. The interval between the piriformis, gluteus medius, and gluteus minimus is identified, and the glutei are retracted anteriorly. Carefully the short external rotators are taken off the posterior femoral neck along the posterior hip capsule as a single cuff of tissue for later repair. Alternatively the capsule can be released separately with a T incision. Generally the surgeon must release the piriformis, gemelli, obturator internus, and half of the quadratus to expose the femoral neck to the level of the lesser trochanter. The hip is then flexed and internally rotated to bring the fracture into view. A saw is used to cut the femoral neck smoothly at the proper level, and the femoral head is retrieved from the acetabulum. The acetabulum is examined, and bone fragments are removed along with the ligamentum teres. After exposure is completed, the prosthesis is installed. It is often inserted in 15° to 20° more anteversion than was present with the biologic hip to minimize the risk of dislocation. This occasionally limits external rotation (ER) after surgery but usually not enough to create a functional impairment.

Closure is somewhat more controversial. The author prefers to repair the capsule and short external rotators with a large No. 2 nonabsorbable suture extending through drill holes in the greater trochanter and intertrochanteric line. This limits the formation of heterotopic bone, decreases the incidence of postoperative dislocation, and improves proprioception during rehabilitation. The deep fascia is then repaired, followed by the subcutaneous tissue and skin.

The initial postoperative rehabilitation is predicated on early mobilization to prevent morbidities associated with recumbency, such as deep venous thrombosis, atelectasis, pneumonia, decubiti, and loss of muscle strength and joint mobility. Full weight bearing is encouraged. After arthrotomy each patient must be educated and drilled regarding potentially dangerous hip positions that can lead to dislocation. The risk inherent in the posterolateral approach is greatest with hip flexion greater than 90° and internal rotation (IR), adduction, or both across the midline.

Patients with prosthetic hips should be instructed to follow their hip precautions religiously for the first 6 weeks after surgery, at which time the soft tissue has regained most of its tensile strength. Even then they are at greater risk of dislocation than they were before surgery.

Intertrochanteric Hip Fractures

Intertrochanteric hip fractures tend to be the most technically challenging. The intertrochanteric region joins the femoral shaft and neck at an angle of about 130°. **The angular movement created by weight bearing is greatest here, and often weight bearing in the initial postoperative period is not feasible.** Morbidity tends to be higher after these fractures, owing to significant comminution of bone and the resultant inadequate stabilization provided by the internal fixation.

These patients often must remain at touch down weight bearing (TDWB) or non–weight bearing until fracture healing is demonstrated. The most important prognosticator in this subset of patients is the evaluation of fracture stability (i.e., the tendency of the fracture to collapse or angulate under physiologic loads after surgery). Fractures with an intact posteromedial cortex and those at the base of the femoral neck are stable. These fractures tolerate limited weight bearing in the initial postoperative period without shifting. Surgeons best treat patients with these fractures by placing a sliding compression hip screw device in an anatomically aligned fracture.

The best surgical approach for the unstable fracture is controversial. Suggested approaches include hip screw devices with or without medial displacement, third-generation intermedullary reconstruction nail fixation, and calcar replacement endoprostheses. The surgical exposure for placement of a calcar replacement prosthesis is as described under the use of endoprostheses for displaced femoral neck fractures. The exposure and morbidity involved in the placement of an intermedullary nail are discussed in the section on subtrochanteric fractures. The exposure for placement of a dynamic compression hip screw is the same regardless of whether a stable or unstable fracture is being addressed. Typically a long lateral approach is used. This approach violates the skin, subcutaneous tissue, fascia lata, vastus lateralis fascia, and muscle belly. Generally in unstable fractures the lesser trochanter and inserting psoas tendon are

left free, limiting hip flexion strength in the initial postoperative period.

Controversy exists as to whether it is better to align unstable fractures anatomically with a highly angled 145° to 150° compression plate and allow them to collapse into stability under physiologic loads or to perform a "medical displacement" osteotomy to obtain good posteromedial cortical abutment and stability during surgery (Fig. 21-2).

Both methods can lead to stability or instability; therefore each case must be discussed with the surgeon to ascertain the degree of stability obtained and the permitted amount of weight bearing. In addition, both methods shorten the distance between the insertion of the hip abductors in the greater trochanter and the center of rotation of the hip, creating a mechanical disadvantage for the abductors. This can lead to Trendelenburg gait, which must be overcome during the postoperative rehabilitation period.

The patient is placed supine on a fracture table with the afflicted limb in the traction boot. Care is taken to place the correct rotation on the distal limb to prevent malalignment. Reduction is carried out under an image intensifier until satisfactory reduction is achieved. Occasionally a satisfactory preoperative reduction is not possible because of posterior sag of the bony fragments, and further reduction must be done manually. After the limb has been prepared and draped, a lateral incision is made from the level of the greater trochanter distally approximately 7 inches, depending on the length of plate to be used. The incision is developed in the same line through skin, subcutaneous fat, and fascia lata. At this point the fascia of the vastus lateralis is followed posteriorly to its origin in the linea aspera. By incising it here the surgeon limits the amount of muscle denervated by the exposure and protects the main muscle mass from damage. The surgeon accesses the lateral cortex of the femoral shaft and places a retractor to maintain anterior retraction of the vastus lateralis, exposing the lateral femoral shaft. After exposure is completed, placement of the fixation device is begun (Fig. 21-3). Closure involves interrupted repair of the fascia of the vastus lateralis, fascia lata, subcutaneous tissue, and skin. The dynamic-compression screw device was not designed to hold the head and neck segment firmly (Fig. 21-4). Rather it allows the ambient muscle forces across the hip joint to pull the fracture fragments together until encountering good bony resistance. In many comminuted osteoporotic fractures, the ability of the screw device to contract is exceeded before good cortical abutment is obtained between the fracture fragments.

In such cases weight bearing must be curtailed until bony healing ensues, or the screw will "cut out" and all stabilization will be lost. Again, the skin is healed by 2 weeks, the deep fascia and soft tissues are healed by 6 weeks, and good bony healing is expected by 12 weeks. In older adult osteoporotic patients with severely comminuted fractures, bony healing can sometimes be delayed for as long as 4 to 6 months. In patients with obviously unstable fractures, weight bearing should be delayed until good bony healing is demonstrated on radiographs. The resultant collapse can

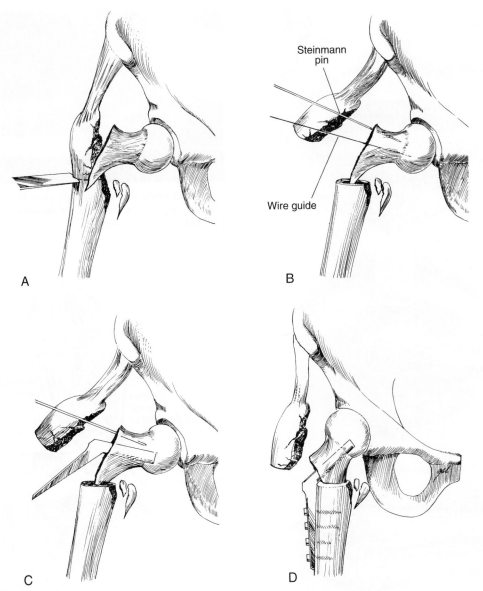

A

B
Steinmann
pin

Wire guide

C

D

Fig. 21-2 Dimon-Hughston method of internal fixation of unstable trochanteric fractures. **A,** Transverse osteotomy of the lateral shaft. **B,** Insertion of a guide pin with a Steinmann pin for control of fragment. **C,** Insertion of nail in the proximal fragment. **D,** Fixation of the side plate to the shaft. (From Hughston JC: Intertrochanteric fractures of the hip. Orthop Clin North Am 5[3]:585-600, 1974.)

often leave a limb significantly shorter. Leg length should be checked after healing and a lift provided if appropriate.

Subtrochanteric Hip Fractures

The use of advanced intermedullary nailing techniques has revolutionized the treatment of subtrochanteric fractures. Traditionally, these fractures have been difficult to fix because of the extreme angular force centered in this region, as well as the muscular deforming forces and minimal bony inter-face between the two fragments available for healing (Fig. 21-5).

Moreover, the bone in this region is more cortical in character, with a poorer blood supply and less osteogenic activity than in the intertrochanteric region. The use of a sliding compression screw device has yielded a higher

implant failure and nonunion rate than in other regions. The femur can be stabilized with a static locked intermedullary nail without exposing the fracture or disturbing its periosteal blood supply. The two preferred methods of fixation for patients with these fractures are a routine lateral approach for the placement of an extended compression screw device and the placement of a static locked intermedullary nail. The exposure for the lateral compression plate is discussed in the section on intertrochanteric fractures and deviates only in that the exposure must be taken more distally, causing more damage to the fascia lata and the vastus lateralis.

Although this design stabilizes the fracture, weight bearing usually must be delayed, soft tissue exposure is extensive, and healing is often delayed because of destruction of periosteal blood supply around the fracture.

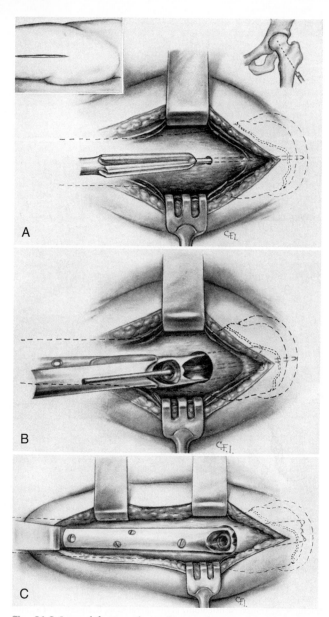

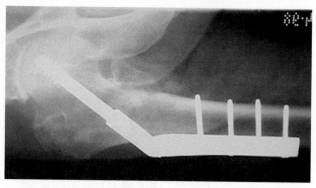

Fig. 21-4 Unstable intertrochanteric fracture of the hip treated with a four-hole compression screw device. The lesser trochanter is often left floating, which can lead to weakness.

Fig. 21-3 Internal fixation of a trochanteric fracture. **A,** A guide pin is inserted, and its position and that of the fracture are checked by roentgenograms. A cannulated Henderson reamer, placed over the guide pin, is used to make a hole through the lateral cortex. *Left insert,* skin incision; *right insert,* proper position of guide pin in anteroposterior view. **B,** A Jewett nail is inserted over the guide pin. **C,** The plate part of the Jewett nail has been fixed to the femoral shaft with screws.

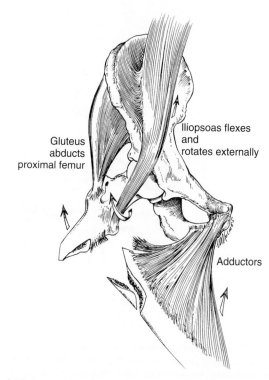

Fig. 21-5 Diagram of pathologic anatomy of subtrochanteric fracture. The proximal fragment is flexed, abducted, and externally rotated, whereas the femoral shaft is shortened and adducted. (From Froimson AI: Treatment of comminuted subtrochanteric fractures of the femur. Surg Gynecol Obstet 131[3]:465-472, 1970.)

The more limited exposure for a static locked or reconstruction nail runs more proximally through the abductors, with a second stab incision for the interlocking screws at the level of the greater or lesser trochanter and a third stab incision laterally along the supracondylar femur. The newer reconstruction nails run the more proximal interlocking screws from the lateral femoral cortex (at the level of the lesser trochanter), and across and through the prefabricated holes in the nail in the intermedullary canal. The nails then run up the femoral neck, ending in the hard bone of the subarticular femoral head. The distal interlocking screws

pass lateral to medial through the lateral cortex of the femur the nail, and finally the medial femoral cortex. This design effectively neutralizes deforming forces across the subtrochanteric femur, allowing full weight bearing from the outset (Fig. 21-6).

The patient is placed supine on a fracture table with both legs inserted into traction boots. Traction is applied over a perineal post. The legs are positioned with the involved leg adducted across the midline and slightly flexed at the hip. The uninvolved leg is abducted and extended at the hip, lying adjacent to the operative leg (Fig. 21-7). An incision is started

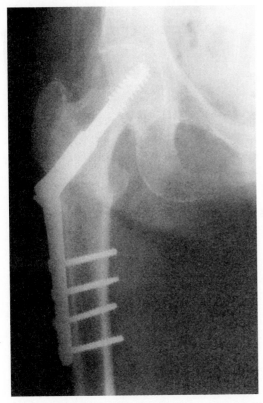

Fig. 21-6 A subtrochanteric fracture of the femur fixed with Richards compression screw-plate device. (From Crenshaw AH: Campbell's operative orthopaedics, vol 3, ed 7, St Louis, 1987, Mosby.)

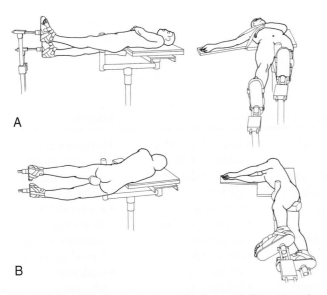

A

B

Fig. 21-7 Russell-Taylor interlocking nail technique. **A,** Patient in supine position. **B,** Patient in lateral decubitus position. (From Crenshaw AH: Campbell's operative orthopaedics, vol 3, ed 7, St Louis, 1987, Mosby.)

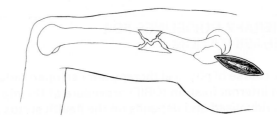

Fig. 21-8 Skin incision at the greater trochanter. (From Crenshaw AH: Campbell's operative orthopaedics, vol 3, ed 7, St Louis, 1987, Mosby.)

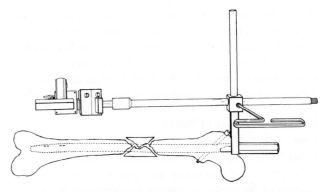

Fig. 21-9 Distal-locking block assembly is attached to the handle of the proximal drill guide. (From Crenshaw AH: Campbell's operative orthopaedics, vol 3, ed 7, St Louis, 1987, Mosby.)

1 inch proximal to the greater trochanter (Fig. 21-8). It is developed proximally and slightly medially 3 inches. The surgeon then extends the incision through the skin and subcutaneous tissue to the fascia of the gluteus medius, which is divided for about 2 inches in line with the skin incision and the fibers of the gluteus medius. Using a small guide pin and fluoroscopy, the surgeon makes a small entry point at the base of the superior posterior femoral area, the piriformis fossa. The guide pin is passed down the femoral shaft approximately 6 inches, and a cannulated reamer is placed over the guide pin to enlarge the entry hole and begin the reaming process. A larger ball-tip guide that is run down across the fracture and down the intermedullary canal to the intercondylar notch replaces the initial guide pin. After this the canal is reamed with flexible reamers in progressively larger sizes until obtaining a good cortical fit. After overreaming a millimeter or two, the surgeon carefully inserts the nail across the fracture under fluoroscopic guidance and then inserts the interlocking screws. The screws at the proximal end of the nail are aimed with the use of a special jig that attaches to the proximal end of the nail (Fig. 21-9). They are inserted percutaneously through the deep fascia and vastus lateralis. The distal screws are usually placed freehand, again percutaneously, using the image to visualize the holes in the nail passing through the iliotibial band and vastus lateralis. Closure consists of repairing the deep fascia, subcutaneous tissue, and skin.

Rehabilitation efforts during the initial postoperative period should consist of regaining control of the proximal hip musculature. Good functional quadriceps contraction and the ability to lift and maneuver the hip against gravity are prerequisites to adequate ambulation. Because of the strength of the fixation, patients can begin full weight bearing immediately after intermedullary reconstruction nailing. Healing normally requires 3 months (Fig. 21-10); nail removal should not be considered before 18 to 24 months.

THERAPY GUIDELINES FOR REHABILITATION

The course of physical therapy after an open reduction internal fixation (ORIF) procedure at the hip is individualized and depends on the health status of the patient before the fracture, the type of ORIF procedure used, and the precautions ordered by the surgeon. This chapter provides some general guidelines for the rehabilitation process. The physical therapist (PT) must manage the patient's progress, keeping in mind the patient's ability to heal and the constraints of the patient's insurance carrier. The rehabilitation process can be described in three phases: (1) hospital, (2) home care, and (3) outpatient. In many cases, depending on lifestyle demands, the patient may only go through one or two of these phases.

Phase I (Hospital Phase)

TIME: 1 to 7 days after surgery
GOALS: To help the patient become independent with transfers and gait using appropriate assistive devices, to ready the patient for discharge from acute care (Table 21-1)

Treatments performed on the day of surgery, such as incentive spirometry exercises, management of air

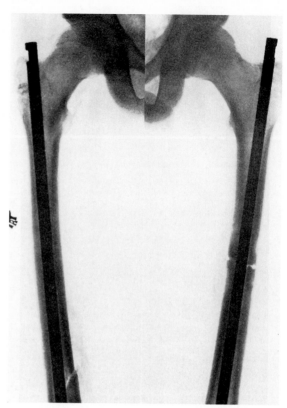

Fig. 21-10 Appearance 2 months after closed reduction of dislocations and medullary nailing of fractures. (From Crenshaw AH: Campbell's operative orthopaedics, vol 3, ed 7, St Louis, 1987, Mosby.)

TABLE 21-1 Hip Open Reduction Internal Fixation

Rehabilitation Phase	Criteria to Progress to This Phase	Anticipated Impairments and Functional Limitations	Intervention	Goal	Rationale
Phase I Postoperative 1-7 days	• Postoperative (inpatient)	• Pain • Limited bed mobility • Limited transfers • Limited gait • Limited strength of involved LE	• Inpatient on pain medication • Bed mobility training • Transfer training • Gait training • Isometrics—Quadriceps sets, gluteal sets • A/AROM—Hip (flexion, extension, abduction, adduction) • AROM—Heel slides, ankle pumps • Patient education emphasizing safety with all mobility training	• Independent or stand-by assistance with bed mobility transfers and gait 200 feet using front-wheel walker • Independent with home exercise program • Caregiver trained to assist with basic skills • Discharge to home	• Emphasize restoration of independence with self-care activities (bed mobility, transfers) • Ambulate safely to return to home environment with some degree of independence • Provide exercises to help patient regain muscular control of involved LE • Provide assistance to patient to perform hip range of motion • Ensure patient and caregiver safety and prevent falls

A/AROM, Active assistive range of motion; *AROM*, active range of motion; *LE*, lower extremity.

compression equipment, and donning thromboembolic disease (TED) hose, are generally assigned to the nursing staff. When a good recovery from surgical trauma is demonstrated, hospital-phase physical therapy usually begins on the first day after surgery.

Physical therapy treatment on postoperative day 1 consists of an evaluation, bed mobility, transfer training, gait training, and a beginning exercise program. The patient's initial goal is to transfer out of bed safely and walk to the bathroom independently using a front-wheel walker (FWW). Some confusion or an emotional reaction to the event that precipitated the surgery may be encountered on the first postoperative day, and the patient may be groggy or in a great deal of pain. Because ORIF is normally an emergency surgery, the patient does not have the advantage of a preoperative training session. However, bed mobility and transfer training may be easier here than with a patient who has undergone THR, because usually no ROM precautions are in place.

Patients who received sacral anesthesia may show a faster initial rate of progress than those who were administered general anesthesia. The patient's pain medications should be timed to reach peak effectiveness during therapy sessions.

The PT should be informed of the patient's weight-bearing status, the type of fracture and surgery performed, and any special ROM restrictions. On the first postoperative day, the patient will attempt to walk to a chair and then sit up for approximately 1 hour before returning to bed. This may be repeated two to three times on the first day. The patient will be encouraged to sit up longer each day.

The patient's skin should be checked daily for pressure sores, especially at the heels. Be sure the patient is placed properly in bed to preclude the tendency to lie in a frog-legged position with the hips in extreme ER and flexion.

Ankle pumps are the first exercises to be assigned. They help to prevent blood clots and to decrease edema in the legs. The patient should perform at least 10 to 20 repetitions every 30 minutes. Quadriceps sets with and without adductor squeezes (Fig. 21-11), gluteal sets, hamstring sets, and hip abduction sets should be performed three times per day with 10 repetitions of each exercise to begin restoration of proximal hip strength. This program may be expanded to include active assistive and then active hip abduction, adduction, and hip-knee flexion. Encourage the client as much as necessary to complete the program.

Ankle proprioceptive neuromuscular facilitation patterns done in both diagonal planes can help prepare the patient for weight bearing. Lower extremity (LE) stretching may be done to avoid contractures and to prepare the patient for a normal gait pattern. The patient can strengthen the upper extremities (UEs) using a Theraband or the hospital bed's triangle as a pull-up bar. Pelvic tilts and single knee-to-chest stretches of the uninvolved extremity can help decrease lumbar soreness and stiffness.

The patient's weight-bearing status, assigned by the surgeon, will vary depending on the type of procedure performed. An FWW is recommended for patients with

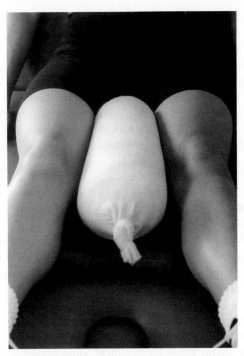

Fig. 21-11 Quadriceps set with the adductor squeezed. The patient sits with legs stretched out in front. With a pillow between the knees and thighs, the patient squeezes the knees together and tightens the top of the thighs at the same time, holding for a count of 10 seconds.

weight-bearing restrictions. However, patients who are assigned non–weight bearing status may feel more secure using a pick-up walker. A platform walker may be appropriate if UE injuries are present. Agile patients are issued axillary crutches immediately regardless of weight-bearing status.

Patients having difficulty with TDWB, defined as less than 10 lb of pressure through the affected leg,[6] or with partial weight bearing (PWB), approximately 40% of normal weight bearing on the involved extremity, will benefit from weight shift training on the parallel bars. A very thick-soled shoe worn on the uninvolved leg helps to lift the patient (to facilitate TDWB with the involved leg). With PWB status, stepping onto a bathroom scale helps the patient to determine the appropriate amount of pressure to place on the involved extremity.

Electrical galvanic stimulation is sometimes used to manage edema and electrical stimulation (ES) in the muscle reeducation mode can help facilitate quadriceps (especially the vastus medialis oblique) contraction. **However, electrical modalities tend to be very uncomfortable for most patients, especially those with metal implants.** These treatments may be more appropriate at the outpatient stage. The surgeon, as always, should be consulted before the application of these modalities.

Transfer to the skilled nursing facility from acute care is expected on the third day after surgery. Patients are discharged from the hospital when they are medically stable and demonstrate independence with bed mobility, transfers, and ambulation (using an appropriate assistive device). Home caregivers should be trained to assist with these tasks safely before the patient leaves the hospital.

Discharge goals are usually attained within 1 or 2 weeks after surgery. Patients may be kept in an extended-care wing longer if no home caregiver is available and assistance is still required for basic mobility. A written exercise program for home use is presented at the time of discharge. The visiting PT in the home will reinforce the skills learned in the hospital.

Phase II (Home Phase)

TIME: 2 to 4 weeks after surgery
GOALS: To improve hip active range of motion (AROM) to 90°, to educate patient regarding a home maintenance program, to help the patient become independent with transfers and to ambulate at home with appropriate assistive devices, to encourage limited community ambulation (Table 21-2)

Home care physical therapy is normally authorized for patients who are homebound or would incur undue hardship by leaving home for treatment. Homebound status is a requirement for reimbursement through Medicare and most other insurance plans. PTs usually schedule visits two to three times per week until the patient is no longer homebound or until goals have been met. This is usually achieved within 2 to 4 weeks of the patient's returning home from the hospital.

Typically the goal of the home care therapist is to ensure the patient's safety at home and to enable a return to previous community activities with the use of an appropriate walking device. These goals may depend on the patient's overall health status, motivation level, or previous level of function. In such a case, the patient is discharged when the PT determines that no more progress can be made.

During the initial home care visit, the PT evaluates the patient's ROM, strength, bed mobility, transfer ability, gait pattern, stair-climbing ability, ability to perform the home exercise program, endurance, pain level, leg length, overall safety awareness, and skin status. The ability of caregivers to assist the patient will also be assessed.

A home care admission assessment will include a review of the patient's medications. If enoxaparin injections are prescribed to avoid blood clots, be sure that the patient has the appropriate number of syringes and follows through with the injection series.

Equipment needs can include a bedside commode, a raised toilet seat (if the patient has not attained 90° of hip flexion), a shower chair, grab bars installed in the bathroom, railings installed by stairways, and appropriate assistive devices for the progression of gait. Furniture and electrical cords may need to be moved to ensure a clear pathway.

The patient's understanding of any weight-bearing restrictions and ROM precautions prescribed should be recited and demonstrated. Caregivers should be present during this review.

TABLE 21-2   Hip Open Reduction Internal Fixation

Rehabilitation Phase	Criteria to Progress to This Phase	Anticipated Impairments and Functional Limitations	Intervention	Goal	Rationale
Phase II Postoperative 2-4 wk	• No signs of infection • No increase in pain • Usually home health status but may be transitioned to outpatient when appropriate	• Limited hip ROM • Limited LE strength • Limited with transfers in and out of car • Limited gait	• Continuation of exercises as in phase I • PROM—Stretches as indicated (calf, hamstring, quadriceps, single knee to chest) • AROM—Standing (hip flexion, extension, abduction, adduction); minisquats, lunges, heel raises, wall slides; sitting (long arc quadriceps, pelvic tilt) • Elastic tubing exercises for UEs • Gait/stair training • Standing balance training (balance boards) with assistance as needed • Car transfers	• Increase AROM to hip flexion 90°, abduction 20°, knee flexion 90° • Independent with home exercises • Increase strength in hip to 60%, knee to 70% • Initiate UE strengthening program • Gait—Independent with cane at home; SBA with cane in community (1000 feet) • Improve balance • Perform independent transfers	• Develop flexibility to improve sitting posture and tolerance • Improve strength to ensure safety with ambulation and transfers, decreasing dependence on uninvolved LE • Restore presurgical UE strength • Promote independence with community ambulation • Improve balance to prevent falls • Encourage return to previous activities of daily living and community activities

AROM, Active range of motion; *LE,* lower extremity; *PROM,* passive range of motion; *ROM,* range of motion; *UE,* upper extremity; *SBA,* stand by assist.

PTs are now being trained to remove staples because of constraints imposed on nursing visits by insurance carriers. Staples are usually removed at about the fourteenth postoperative day. Proper sanitary technique protocols must be followed. Consult the physician if any irregularity is noted in scar healing.

Advance the patient from isometric to active ROM exercises during the home phase. Patients who require an active assist should soon be performing their exercises independently. Bilateral tiptoes (plantarflexion) (Fig. 21-12) and heel cord stretches (Fig. 21-13) while standing can be performed while using a walker or countertop for support. Closed kinetic chain exercises (with the involved leg firmly planted on the ground or on exercise equipment), such as heel raises and minisquats, can also be done at the countertop. Open chain exercises done while standing at this location include hip flexion, hip abduction, and hip extension. Other closed-chain exercises such as modified lunges and wall slides (Fig. 21-14) are added as appropriate.

Hip flexion, extension, and abduction performed while standing are beneficial for the involved leg. They may be alternated bilaterally, depending on the patient's weight-bearing restrictions. With a status of weight bearing as tolerated (WBAT), the patient may attempt balancing exercises on the involved leg.

The PT should address chronic deficits in flexibility, strength, and balance that may have precipitated the patient's injury. The postsurgical program should focus on restoring proximal hip strength.

The integrity of the abductors is especially compromised by ORIF surgeries and often the hip abductors were weak before the injury that precipitated the surgery. It may be necessary to stretch chronically flexed hip and trunk muscles before the abductors can be in a position to fire effectively.

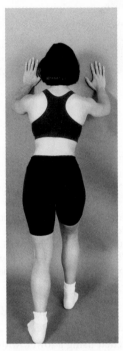

Fig. 21-13 Heel cord stretch. The patient stands with the involved leg and foot back, with the toes turned in slightly. He or she then places the hands against a wall and leans forward until a stretch is felt. The patient keeps the heel down, holds for 20 seconds, and slowly releases.

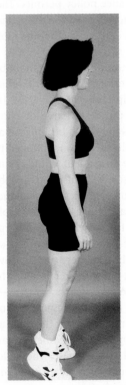

Fig. 21-12 Bilateral tiptoes. The patient stands on the floor with the knees straight and then lifts onto the toes, holds for 5 seconds, and slowly releases downward.

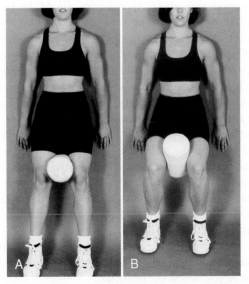

Fig. 21-14 Wall slides using an adductor pillow. A, The patient stands with the back against a wall, feet shoulder-width apart, with a pillow between the thighs. B, He or she then bends the knees to a 45° angle, tightens the thighs, and squeezes the pillow. The patient holds for 10 seconds, then extends the knees and slides up the wall.

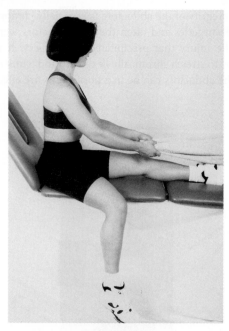

Fig. 21-15 Sitting hamstring stretch. The patient sits with the involved leg straight and the other leg bent off the edge of a table or bed. He or she then hooks a towel around the foot, keeps the back straight, and leans forward until a stretch is felt. The patient holds this position for 20 seconds and slowly releases. Older patients with less flexibility may simply lean back on their hands, initially.

Hamstring and calf stretches may be done in the supine or the sitting position using a towel (Fig. 21-15). The quadriceps can be stretched using a towel, with the patient lying prone with knees bent. Pelvic tilt, knee-to-chest, hip rotator stretches, and trunk rotation exercises benefit the low back and the hip.

The patient progresses from using an FWW or two crutches to a cane during this phase. The ability to ambulate safely without an assistive device is sometimes attainable within the time period authorized. Special care should be taken to correct uneven stride length (leading with the involved extremity and stepping-to with the uninvolved extremity), knee flexion in the late stance phase, forward flexion at the waist, and overstriding with crutches.[6] Trendelenburg signs in gait following an ORIF are common because of disruption of the abductors. Be sure to cue and facilitate the engagement of the abductors in both exercises and gait.

Gait training includes stair climbing. Initially the patient should walk up the stairs leading with the strong leg and descend the stairs leading with the operative leg in a step-to pattern.

Training to step up and down safely from curbs, to walk on uneven surfaces, and to transfer in and out of cars also is provided in the home phase.

A balance retraining program may benefit patients who have vestibular or neurologic involvement. Vision problems should be referred to the physician.

Home health physical therapy is usually finished within 2 to 4 weeks. The patient should have 90° of hip flexion and 20° of hip abduction at this point. The quadriceps and hip abductor strength should be fair to fair plus (3/5 to 3+/5 with a manual muscle test), and the patient should be able to perform all exercises actively.

The majority of ORIF patients are older people with fairly sedentary lifestyles. They may refuse further rehabilitation past the home care phase. Walking programs should be strongly encouraged with these patients. Swimming and bicycle riding are recommended, when realistic, for long-term exercise programs; tai chi has been shown to decrease the risk of falls in older adults.[7] Active patients with more rigorous lifestyle requirements should go on to outpatient therapy for further strengthening.

With osteoporosis so prevalent in this population, the patient may be advised to consult the primary care physician regarding the propriety of a calcium replacement program or hormone replacement therapy.

Phase III (Outpatient Phase)

TIME: 5 to 8 weeks after surgery
GOALS: To encourage patient self-management of exercises, to help the patient become independent in community ambulation, to increase the strength of the LEs (Table 21-3)

Outpatient physical therapy is intended to increase the involved extremity's flexibility toward full ROM and increase its strength to at least the good minus level (4-/5 manual muscle test). Gait pattern irregularities are to be normalized. Cardiovascular capacity also may be improved. These treatments should be conducted two to three times per week if the patient's insurance policy permits. The duration of outpatient rehabilitation depends on the patient's ability to make objective progress and on whether the intervention or treatment requires the skill of a PT.

All exercises should be done actively by this time. Exercises previously performed in gravity-eliminated positions, such as supine hip abduction (Fig. 21-16) and adduction (Fig. 21-17), are progressed to side-lying gravity-resisted positions. Ankle weights can be added if appropriate.

The closed-chain exercises mentioned previously also are performed in the outpatient clinic. Minisquats and wall slides can emphasize a vastus medialis oblique contraction with the addition of an isometric hip adductor squeeze using a pillow or small ball. Lunges with the involved leg on a small step can progress to stair climbing on larger, more normal-sized steps. If the patient is still doing stairs in a step-to pattern, progress him or her to a step-over-step pattern if possible. Standing balance exercises on the affected leg are appropriate with WBAT status.

Cardiovascular exercise is important during this phase to increase circulation throughout the body and endurance for ambulation. An upper body ergometer or a stationary bicycle can be introduced at this phase. The patient's tolerance for these activities could be built up to a combined 15 to 30 minutes, if possible.

The modalities mentioned in the hospital phase may be performed here with the approval of the surgeon. Balance

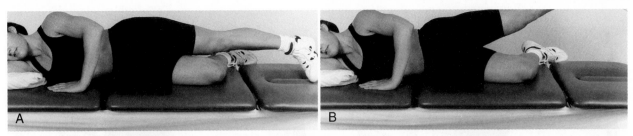

Fig. 21-16 Active hip abduction. **A,** The patient lies on the uninvolved side with the bottom knee bent. **B,** Keeping the top leg straight, he or she lifts upward, holds for 5 seconds, then slowly returns to the starting position.

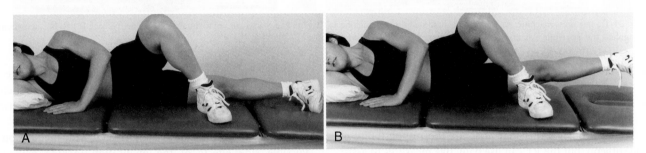

Fig. 21-17 Active hip adduction. **A,** The patient lies on the involved side with the bottom leg straight. **B,** He or she then bends the top knee and places the foot in front of the bottom leg. The patient lifts the bottom leg up approximately 6 to 8 inches and holds for 5 to 10 seconds before slowly returning the leg to the starting position.

TABLE 21-3 Hip Open Reduction Internal Fixation

Rehabilitation Phase	Criteria to Progress to This Phase	Anticipated Impairments and Functional Limitations	Intervention	Goal	Rationale
Phase III Postoperative 5-8 wk	• Independence with transfers in and out of car • No loss of hip ROM	• Limited AROM and strength of involved LE • Limited tolerance to community ambulation • Limited tolerance to cardiovascular exercises • Limited with resuming more advanced activities	• Progression of exercises in phases I and II, adding resistance where appropriate • Modalities as necessary: heat, ice, electrical stimulation • Trunk stabilization exercises • Upper body ergometer • Stationary bicycle • Treadmill • Gait training for uneven surfaces and stairs	• Control pain • Regain full AROM of involved LE • Increase LE strength to 75% • Become independent with community ambulation	• Progress strength and ROM of involved LE • Use modalities to control any residual activity or prepare tissue for stretching • Promote safety with ambulation on all types of surfaces • Regain cardiovascular conditioning • Resume all activities of daily living and community activities

AROM, Active range of motion; *LE,* lower extremity; *ROM,* range of motion.

retraining programs may be expanded to include various balance boards. Spine stabilization exercises can include those done in the prone and quadruped positions. Core strengthening should be included, as well as Pilates exercises when realistic.

Inclusion of the leg press (Fig. 21-18) and other weight-training equipment may be appropriate in the clinic phase. At the PT's discretion, a treadmill also may be used to contribute to balance and gait retraining. The therapist should consider activities that the patient can carry on in life when the rehabilitation phase is over.

TROUBLESHOOTING

Complications may arise in the course of rehabilitation. Examples that should be referred to the surgeon include the following:

- Thigh pain with walking that clears with sitting (may represent intermittent claudication)
- A positive Trendelenburg sign that does not resolve with treatment (may result from damage to the gluteal innervation)

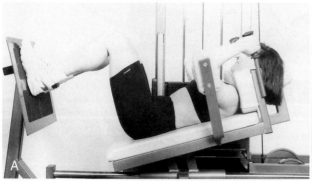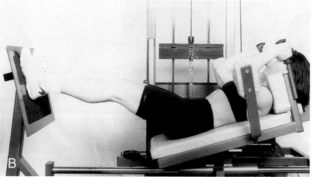

Fig. 21-18 Leg press machine. **A,** The patient should adjust the machine so that the knees are bent approximately 90° while the back is flat. **B,** The patient straightens the legs while exhaling without locking the knees, then slowly releases.

- Severe rubor and swelling at the surgical site with accompanying fever (may indicate a septic infection)
- Persistent, severe pain (may result from an expansion of the fracture or loosening of the fixation devices)

Other problems that may arise are the responsibility of the surgeon, but the PT can use palliative measures to assist the patient. Leg length discrepancy is an example. The patient can continue gait training with a temporary shoe insert or with shoes of different heel heights. The surgeon may later prescribe a permanent orthotic. Persistent edema is treated with medication. Patients should be advised to elevate their legs, rest more often, wear TED hose, pump their ankles, use kinesio tape, and apply ice to swollen areas.

Pain exacerbations are usually treated with medication. Possible side effects of the medication include nausea, constipation, and hypertension. The therapist can assist in pain reduction with modalities, exercise, ice, and positioning.

Suggested Home Maintenance for the Postsurgical Patient

Days 1 to 7 (in Hospital)
GOALS FOR THE PERIOD: Increase volitional control of involved LE, improve and maintain ROM
Isometric Exercises
1. Quadriceps sets
2. Gluteal sets
AROM Exercises
3. Heel slides
4. Ankle pumps

Weeks 2 to 4
GOALS FOR THE PERIOD: Increase LE strength and functional ROM, initiate upper-extremity strengthening program
1. Stretching as indicated by evaluation

AROM Exercises
2. Standing hip flexion, extension, abduction, and adduction
3. Minisquats
4. Lunges
5. Wall slides
6. Pelvic tilt
7. Long-arc quadriceps
8. Upper body exercises as indicated

Weeks 5 to 8
GOALS FOR THE PERIOD: Promote return to previous level of function (as cleared by physician)
1. Continue exercises from weeks 2 to 4
2. Progress to gym activities as indicated and prepare for discharge to community or home gym (treadmill, stationary bicycle)

CLINICAL CASE REVIEW

1 Why do ORIF patients differ emotionally from other postsurgical orthopedic patients?

They cannot prepare for their surgery because it is an emergency surgery. Some have sustained their injury in an accident where other loved ones have been injured. Their situation needs to be appreciated and respected. The mortality rate following a hip fracture is high and elderly patients are aware of this. They may be worried that they will not recover or may not be able to return to their homes. Expect to give these patients a lot of encouragement.

2 How can the treadmill be useful at the outpatient phase?

At slow speeds, the hip abductors, core trunk muscles, and glutes are forced to engage during the stance phase on the unstable surface of a treadmill. Placement of a mirror in front of the treadmill can help the patient to observe and correct gait pattern irregularities. The treadmill may be a beneficial activity following discharge from the outpatient clinic.

3 Upon the PT's arrival at the patient's home, the patient's operative limb is found to be ruborous, warm, severely swollen, and very painful despite elevation and the use of ice. What needs to be done?

Be sure that the patient was discharged with the appropriate number of enoxaparin syringes and has followed through with these injections as prescribed. The patient may have a clot in his leg. Check the status of the surgical scar. There is the possibility of an infection. Make sure that the patient has taken any antibiotics prescribed since other causes of infection may be due to dental work or other medical procedures unrelated to the THR. Refer the patient back to the surgeon for further evaluation.

4 Why do so many patients have difficulty performing hip abduction exercises?

Frequently patients will substitute hip flexion for true abduction. They have difficulty firing the glute medius and glute minimus because of their chronically flexed posture. Good hip extension is needed for true abduction to occur and good concentric and eccentric control of the hip rotators are needed for a normal gait pattern. Lunges, done standing in a doorway with elevated arms on either side of the door frame, can effectively stretch the plantar flexors, hip flexors, arms, and trunk while strengthening the opposite LE quads. Stronger, more mobile patients may be able to assume a prone position to stretch chronically shortened hip and trunk flexors. Sidestepping is a functional abduction exercise that challenges balance and stimulates both sets of glutes and engages eccentric hip rotators in stance phase. Backstepping can challenge even more aspects of balance and posture.

5 Mary, 73 years old, had an R hip ORIF and has a chronically flexed trunk and hips. What should the therapist consider in designing a rehab program for Mary?

A postural assessment should be done and the contractures noted should be addressed through a cautious stretching program. Careful straight leg hamstring stretches done with the therapist's assistance may be added to the supine exercise series. The Achilles tendon stretch can be done at a kitchen countertop, walker, or at the wall. The patient can stand in a doorway and perform a lunge while her UEs are placed on either side of the doorframe to stretch a chronically tight trunk, shoulder, and hip flexors.

6 What should a PT consider when performing a home safety evaluation for a patient who has sustained a fracture from a fall?

Are steps, floorboards, and tiles secure?
Are rugs, especially carpet on stairs, secure?
Which scatter rugs should be removed?
Are railings and banisters secure?
Which electrical cords should be taped down or removed?
Are stairways, hallways, and entryways clear of obstacles?
Are pets and small children under control when near the patient?
Are grab bars available in the bathroom?
Are there nonskid mats in the shower/tub?
Is durable medical equipment adjusted to proper height? Should home furniture be raised?
Is lighting adequate? Are night lights available?
Is the patient wearing nonslippery shoes or slippers?
Are emergency numbers posted near the telephone?
Is an occupational therapy evaluation needed for home adjustment?
Should the patient have an emergency call system installed?
Are caregivers well trained to assist?
Are the eyeglasses that the patient is wearing clean? Many patients who think that they have lost most of their vision are trying to see through filthy eyeglasses.

7 During gait training Julie has difficulty maintaining TDWB on the affected LE. She tends to place approximately 20% of her weight onto her affected leg. She attempts to respond to verbal cues but is unsuccessful. A scale was placed under the affected leg so that Julie could see and feel how much weight she was transferring onto her leg. Although she improved after using the scale, she still could not maintain a safe level of TDWB through the affected leg. What is another way to assist her in maintaining TDWB status?

A very thick-soled shoe worn on the uninvolved foot helps lift the patient and facilitates TDWB status. Also a saltine cracker packet taped to the bottom of the operative foot can give the necessary feedback during stance phase. When the patient progresses to PWB, use the bathroom scale again to help the patient determine how much weight to put on the operative LE.

8 Ruth is 70 years old. She sustained a hip fracture at home when she tripped and fell. She had an ORIF on her left hip 3 months ago. Before her fall, she could walk without

an assistive device. Presently she walks at home without an assistive device but needs a cane to ambulate around the community. She rarely goes out because she is so fearful of falling. She has maintained a strengthening home exercise program. Ruth feels that her leg remains weak despite all her exercising. Her LE flexibility is generally restricted throughout. The left leg is more restricted than the right. Ruth's balance and coordination also are impaired. Movements other than forward gait appear labored and slow. Left hip strength is generally 4-/5. Should strengthening, stretching, ROM, balance training, or coordination training be emphasized initially during treatment?

The therapist ascertained the conditions that were hampering progress with strength, balance, and ease of movement during gait. LE flexibility exercises with the guidance and careful assistance of the therapist were emphasized during the first four visits. Balance, coordination, gait, and strength issues also were addressed. As the flexibility of the LEs increased, advances with strength could be obtained more easily. In addition, the patient was able to move her LEs more freely during lateral or backward movements. Therefore balance and coordination also progressed. Ruth's confidence grew, and in a few weeks she was safely walking and maneuvering around the community without an assistive device.

9 Robert is having difficulty with transferring into and out of his car safely. What adjustments can help him?

A clean plastic trash bag placed over the passenger's seat provides a slippery surface, which allows the patient to glide-pivot around on the passenger's seat and assume the rider's position more easily. If the height of the seat is adjustable, then raise the seat to the highest possible position. The back of the passenger seat may need to be tilted backward if a precaution of less than 90° flexion at the hip is in place.

10 What activities are recommended following discharge from outpatient physical therapy?

By the end of the outpatient phase, the patient should have a well-rounded program that can be continued at home or at a fitness center. Bicycling, recreational walking, tai chi, and swimming are excellent long-term options for the active patient recovering from hip ORIF surgery. Wii Fit or Wii Sport, now being featured at nursing homes and senior center exercise programs, are recommended for home use to improve balance, strength, and endurance.

11 How can a patient build enough hip strength to allow normal stair climbing?

The patient with WBAT status can practice step-ups onto a book or a step with a very narrow rise using the operative leg (Fig. 21-19). An initial isometric contraction can precede the step-up onto progressively taller rises until the patient is able to walk up and down stairs in a normal step-over-step pattern while holding a railing.

12 How can problems because of abductor weakness manifest in the hip ORIF patient?

Surgical disruption of the abductor tendons can cause traction neurapraxia on the superior gluteal nerve. A shortened abductor lever arm can cause a Trendelenburg sign to appear with gait. With abductor weakness, secondary joint pain can develop at the spine, knees, and opposite hip because of the added stresses of the shifting of the center of gravity while ambulating.

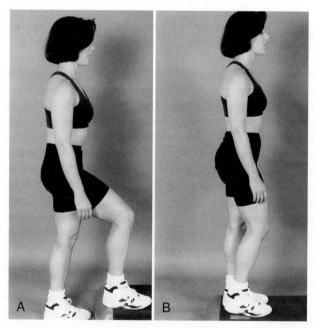

Fig. 21-19 Step-ups. **A,** The patient slowly steps onto a step with the involved extremity while tightening the muscles of the thigh. **B,** The patient must control the knee while stepping up.

REFERENCES

1. American Academy of Orthopaedic Surgeons: Orthopedic knowledge update 3: home study syllabus, Rosemont, Ill, 1990, the Academy.

2. American Academy of Orthopaedic Surgeons: Orthopedic knowledge update 4: home study syllabus, Rosemont, Ill, 1992, the Academy.

3. Elmerson S, Zetterberg C, Andersson G: Ten-year survival after fractures of the proximal end of the femur. Gerontology 34:186-191, 1988.

4. Jette AM, et al: Functional recovery after hip fractures. Arch Phys Med Rehabil 68:735-740, 1987.

5. White BL, Fisher WD, Laurin CA: Rate of mortality of elderly patients after fracture of the hip in the 1980s. J Bone Joint Surg Am 69(9)1335-1340, 1987.

6. Fagerson TL: The hip handbook, Newton, Mass, 1998, Butterworth-Heinemann.

7. Clark GS, Siebens HC: Geriatric rehabilitation. In DeLisa JA, editor: Rehabilitation medicine: Principles and practice, ed 3, Philadelphia, 1988, Lippincott.

CHAPTER 22

Anterior Cruciate Ligament Reconstruction

Jim Magnusson, Richard Joreitz, Luga Podesta

nterior cruciate ligament (ACL) injuries can occur at any stage of life from 5 to 85 years old.[1-3] However, most often they occur in the relatively young active (athletic) population. The age group more commonly associated with ACL ruptures is between 14 and 29 years old.[3-8] The extent of the injury and desired level of activity usually dictate when surgical intervention is required. This chapter describes the current surgical considerations, techniques, and rehabilitative guidelines with supportive rationale. The individual clinician must determine the speed and intensity appropriate for each patient.

SURGICAL INDICATIONS AND CONSIDERATIONS

Cause and Epidemiologic Factors

ACL injury has been well documented and classically involves a noncontact mechanism involving rapid deceleration in anticipation of a change of direction (i.e., pivoting motion) or landing motion.[9-13] Boden and colleagues[14] reported that 72% of ACL tears occurred as a result of noncontact. Most injuries are sustained at foot strike, with the knee close to full extension and with the ground reaction forces lateral to the knee joint causing a "valgus collapse[9,15]"; sagittal plane motion seems to have less influence on the ACL during injury.[9,16,17] The incidence of individuals sustaining a ruptured ACL has been reported at 1 in 3000.[12]

Patients describe feeling and sometimes hearing a "pop[18]" and are 1000 times more likely to be participating in a sporting event.[4] Swelling is immediate, which implicates a ligamentous injury because of its associated vascularity. Patients exhibiting instability of the knee that affects pivot shift demonstrate a positive Lachman test; positive magnetic resonance imaging (MRI) for ACL rupture should be thoroughly evaluated for surgical considerations. Functionally, these patients have difficulty performing pivoting and deceleration related to activities of daily living (ADLs) or sports. Although individuals who have sustained isolated rupture of the ACL may continue to be functional, their level of function is compromised and may require future surgical intervention

because of secondary restraint pathology.[19-21] The surgeon should thoroughly evaluate the patient's desired level of activity to ensure a successful outcome. Multiple studies have made reference to the sequelae of degenerative arthritis and potential for meniscal tears in the ACL-deficient knee.[21-25]

Both anatomic and physiologic risk factors have been researched. Some of the anatomic risk factors that may predispose an individual to ACL injury include the following: hypermobility (laxity of joints), hormonal influences on hypermobility, a narrow intercondylar notch, ligament width, tibial rotation, pronated feet, and increased width of the pelvis in the female athlete.[26] Although some causes exist to suggest certain anatomic features, conclusive evidence has not been established between ligament failure and the anatomic risk factors. Physiologic risk factors include poor core strength, lower extremity (LE) deficits in muscular strength and coordination, and foot wear–ground interface. It may be a combination of the previously listed factors that leads to ACL injury, but women are two to eight times more likely to sustain injury than males.[13,27-29] Hormonal influences that affect ligament laxity have been explored, with evidence leaning toward this as a nonfactor. However, menstrual hormones may indirectly contribute to injury by influencing neuromuscular performance and muscle function.[29,30] Although there may be some influence on laxity, more compelling arguments point to strength and coordination differences. Many researchers have further studied the relationship of neuromuscular performance as a potential risk factor. They have identified significant differences in neuromuscular control after the onset of maturation. This deficit was observed in females landing after a jump. The neuromuscular deficit allowed migration of the knee into a valgus collapse position, placing the ACL at risk.[9,30-32] Hewett, Myer, and Ford[30] also noted that after maturation (i.e., neuromuscular spurt) males regained their control; however, females did not make similar adaptations. The "drop jump" screening test is a useful examination to help prevent and further understand the mechanisms of an ACL injury.[33] Leetun and associates[34] looked at lumbopelvic (core) stability as a risk factor for LE injury in female athletes. They concluded that athletes who did not sustain an injury demonstrated better hip abduction and external rotation strength, and that hip external rotation strength was the only useful predictor of injury status.

Overall, the therapist must be aware of the potential risk factors that were present leading up to the ACL injury. In this way, the rehabilitation program can safely return the patient to the sport and prevent future injury.

Treatment Options

The timing of when to perform reconstruction (acute versus chronic) has been a source of debate. It has been accepted that a higher risk for complications exists if surgery is performed (1) before obtaining a homeostatic environment, (2) if range of motion (ROM) is limited (especially extension), and (3) when quadriceps and hamstring contraction is inadequate (i.e., unable to perform a straight leg raise [SLR]).[23,35] It is also apparent that with postponing reconstruction in an active population, the risk is higher for meniscal and chondral surface damage.[22,36-38]

A topic of debate is how soon after injury should reconstructive surgery be performed. When using a bone-patella tendon-bone (BPTB) autograft, evidence exists that surgery should not occur before 3 weeks after injury to decrease the risk of arthrofibrosis.[23,39-41]

Other authors propose that loss of motion is not dependent upon time when performing surgery after an injury.[42-45]

Bottoni and associates also showed through a randomized controlled trial that early ACL reconstructions with a hamstring autograft can be performed and will not increase the likelihood of arthrofibrosis because long rehabilitation emphasizes extension and early ROM.[45] Sterett and associates did not find an association between incidence of motion loss and timing of surgery but used the minimal criteria of active ROM of 0° to 120°, active quadriceps control, and the ability to perform an SLR without a lag as determinants of successful outcome. In a systematic review, Smith and associates did not find a consensus for the optimal time after injury to perform reconstructive surgery to return to activity faster with limited complications.[46,47]

Typically, surgeons will require the patient to achieve full extension, be able to do an SLR without a lag, and have minimal to no swelling present before operating.

Researchers have speculated about an age when reconstruction is not recommended; however, to date no literature has noted any detrimental outcomes based on the age of the patient. In fact, studies have shown no significant difference in outcomes in comparing individuals at the age breaks of 35 and 40 years.[7,48-50] Reconstruction of the skeletally immature (SI) patient remains controversial, but the current literature appears to be leaning toward performing reconstruction. Younger populations are sustaining ACL tears; although it has been generally advisable to await physeal closure before reconstruction, some surgeons are having successful outcomes.[51,52] Appropriateness for reconstruction should be evaluated based on chronologic age, Tanner stage, radiologic

findings in the knee, and developmental-psychologic factors.[53,54] Drilling across the physis has not been advocated because of the risks of arresting bone growth. However, Shelbourne and colleagues[51] presented information on a small group of SI patients (Tanner stage 3 or 4 with clearly open growth plates) who underwent intraarticular patella tendon graft. Surgery emphasized the importance of not overtensioning the graft and meticulous placement of the bone plugs proximal to the physes. The patients had no growth disturbances on follow-up; when confronted with the potential of new meniscal tears, recurrent instability, effusion, and pain, ACL reconstruction in the SI patient appears to be a viable option.[26,55]

The anticipated functional limitations (modification of activities involving pivoting and deceleration) must be explored and explained to the patient who chooses not to have an ACL-deficient knee reconstructed. Ciccotti and associates[56] reported on nonoperative management of patients from 40 to 60 years. They found that 83% of the patients had a satisfactory result with guided rehabilitation. However, they also mentioned that surgery might be an option for individuals wishing to continue sporting and pivoting activities.

Surgical techniques to replace the deficient ACL continue to evolve. Advances in arthroscopic surgery provide surgeons with the ability to perform these reconstructive procedures using a one-incision endoscopic technique. Research continues in the search for the optimal graft, fixation technique, and surgical reconstructive procedure. In 1920, Hey-Groves[57] and Campbell[58] (in 1939) first described the use of the patella tendon as an ACL graft. Because of these original surgical descriptions, numerous procedures to repair or reconstruct the ACL have been advocated. Attempts at primary repair of the ACL with and without augmentation[59-61] were of limited success.[37] Extraarticular ACL reconstruction also was suggested as a technique to reconstruct the ACL-deficient knee.[62,63] However, long-term results were disappointing.[64,65] Intraarticular ACL reconstruction using various tissues, including the patellar tendon, iliotibial band, and combinations of hamstring tendons (semitendinosus, semitendinosus-gracilis), has been extensively described in the literature.[20,66-69]

The biologic grafts most widely used today are the central third patellar tendon (i.e., BPTB complex) or multistrand hamstring tendon grafts. Although the hamstring graft has some advantages,[70,71] both procedures are equally successful (surgeon preference dictates choice if problems such as patella dysfunction are not present).[72-75]

In general the endoscopic patellar tendon autograft reconstruction remains the most popular.[10,76-78]

Graft Selection

The selection of the appropriate graft to replace the ACL is crucial to the ultimate success of the reconstruction. Primary concerns in the selection of an autogenous graft to replace the incompetent ACL include the biomechanical properties of the graft (e.g., initial graft strength and stiffness relative to the normal ACL), ease of graft harvest and fixation, potential for donor-site morbidity, and individual patient concerns. Other factors that ultimately influence graft performance include biologic changes in graft materials over time and their ability to withstand the effects of repetitive loading and stress.[79] Noyes and colleagues[80] studied the biomechanical properties of a number of autograft tissues and showed that an isolated 14-mm-wide BPTB graft has 168% the strength of an intact ACL. A graft 10 mm wide is about 120% as strong. The study also determined that a single-strand semitendinosus graft displayed only 70% of the normal ACL strength. The data show that BPTB grafts have comparable tensile strength but increased stiffness in relation to the normal ACL, whereas single-strand semitendinosus grafts have decreased tensile strength but comparable stiffness. Other researchers have shown that multiple strands of semitendinosus or semitendinosus-gracilis composite grafts are stronger relative to the normal ACL.

The graft of choice varies among surgeons. They currently include BPTB autografts and allografts; single-, double-, and quadruple-stranded semitendinosus autografts; and composite grafts using semitendinosus-gracilis autografts. The enthusiasm surrounding the use of allograft replacement of the ACL has recently declined because of the small but tangible risk of infectious disease transmission. The risk of human immunodeficiency virus transmission has been estimated to be 1 in 1.6 million using currently available bone- and tissue-banking techniques.[81] Sterilization by means of fresh freezing of allograft tissue may have an advantage over gamma radiation and ethylene oxide. Fielder and associates[82] have determined that 3 mrads or more of gamma radiation are required to sterilize HIV. Furthermore, sterilization procedures have been associated with alterations in graft properties and shown to cause a significant average decrease in stiffness (12%) and maximal load (26%),[83] and a marked inflammatory response with ethylene oxide use. Further studies must be conducted regarding poststerilization ACL allograft performance. Although the use of allografts as ACL replacements can diminish operative time and prevent graft harvest site morbidity, they are not recommended for routine use in primary ACL deficiency. Currently, either BPTB or multistrand semitendinosus autografts are the most widely used ACL substitutes to reconstruct the ACL-deficient knee.

Graft Fixation

Adequate fixation of the biologic ACL graft is crucial during the early postoperative period after ACL reconstruction. Fixation devices must transfer forces from the fixation device to the graft and provide stability under repetitive loads and sudden traumatic loads. Various techniques are now available for fixation, including interference screws, staples, sutures through buttons, sutures tied over screw posts, and ligament and plate washers. Kurosaka, Yoshiyas, and Andrish[84] determined the interference screw to be the strongest method of fixation of BPTB grafts. Interference screw strength depends on compression of the bone plug,[79] bone quality,[79,84] length of screw thread-bone contact,[85] and direction of ligament forces.[79] Robertson, Daniel, and Biden[86] studied soft tissue fixation to bone and determined the screw with washer and the barbed staple to be the strongest methods of fixation.

Graft Maturation

Graft maturation has an influence on the patient whose goals include a return to sports, most of which require pivoting and cutting. The healing properties of autografts have been discussed in the literature.[14,87-90] Although a majority of the studies we have reviewed describe the maturity of the graft at 100% 12 to 16 months postoperatively, return to sports participation in some protocols occurs at 6 months (if functional tests and isokinetics meet criteria).[91,92]

The graft maturation process begins at implantation and progresses over the next 1 to 2 years. Autografts are strongest at the time of implantation. The implanted graft undergoes a process of functional adaptation (ligamentization), with gradual biologic transformation. The tendon graft undergoes four distinct stages of maturation[14,87,89]:

1. Necrosis
2. Revascularization
3. Cellular proliferation
4. Collagen formation, remodeling, and maturation

Within the first 3 weeks after implantation, necrosis occurs in the patella tendon intrinsic graft cells. The graft consists of a collagen network that to this point has relied on a blood supply. As this blood supply is interrupted, the graft undergoes a necrotizing process. Necrosis commences immediately and generally lasts 2 weeks.[88-90] Native patella tendon (graft) cells diminish, and replacement cells can be present as early as the first week. Cellular repopulation occurs before revascularization. These cells are thought to arise from both extrinsic sources (i.e., synovial cells, mesenchymal stem cells, bone marrow, blood, ACL stump) and intrinsic sources (i.e., surviving graft cells). Early full ROM is desirable because as new collagen is formed, its formation and strength are dictated by the stresses placed on it.

As the new cells find their way to this frame and add stability to this weak structure, rehabilitation must be careful not to disrupt or stretch them. Necrosis of the graft allows the metamorphosis of the graft from tendon to ligamentous process. Necrosis of the graft is highlighted by the formation of granulation tissue and inflammation. The bone blood supply and synovial fluid nourish the graft by synovial diffusion.[93] Revascularization occurs within the first 6 to 8 weeks after implantation. By this time the graft is revascularized via the fat pads, synovium, and endosteum,[88-90] and the inflammatory response should be under control. Further inflammatory problems signify a delayed healing process and potential graft problems; the physician and therapist should be alert for them.[94,95]

Amiel and colleagues[93] in 1986 described ligamentization of the rabbit patella tendon ACL graft. However, the graft never obtained all the cellular features of normal ACL tissue. Although the graft takes on many of the physical properties of the normal ACL, the cellular microgeometry of the remodeling graft does not closely resemble that of a normal

ACL. The revascularization process progresses from peripheral to central.

Bone plugs incorporate into their respective bone tunnels over a 12-week period but are felt to near completion by approximately the sixth postoperative week. The comparative strength of the healed tendon-to-bone attachment versus the healed bone-plug attachment is unknown. Tendon-bone healing begins as a fibrovascular interface develops between the bone and tendon. Bony ingrowth occurs into these interfaces, which extends into the outer tendon tissue. A gradual reestablishment of collagen fiber continuity between bone and tendon occurs, and the attachment strength increases as collagen fiber continuity increases. These ACL autografts approximate 30% to 50% of the normal ACL strength 1 to 2 years postoperatively.[89]

Cellular proliferation and collagen formation take place as a continuing process throughout the maturation process. The function of collagen in the ligament is to withstand tension, and certain types of catalysts are present during the healing process. Transforming growth hormone factor b1 has been isolated during the healing of the medial collateral ligament in rats. Administration of this growth hormone during the first 2 weeks after injury was found to increase strength, stiffness, and braking energy of the ligament.[90] Other catalysts of collagen formation (platelet-derived growth factor 1 [basic fibroblast growth factor]) have had equally good results in improving the tensile strength of healing ligaments. Since our last edition, more human studies are being presented with varying degrees of success.[96] With the relatively recent expansion of platelet rich plasma injections to assist in soft tissue repair, more research is coming out on its use in anterior cruciate ligament reconstruction (ACLR). Recent studies have looked at the use of platelet rich growth factor in assisting the reconstruction.[97] Future studies should be performed to validate this intervention.

During the rehabilitation program, pain and edema should dictate the speed at which the patient may progress. In clinics in which it is available, an assessment using the KT-1000 (Medmetric, San Diego) is helpful as well.[4,23,98-102]

SURGICAL PROCEDURE

Endoscopic Bone-Patella Tendon-Bone Complex Anterior Cruciate Ligament Reconstruction

The procedure begins with a complete examination of the knee under anesthesia followed by a thorough diagnostic arthroscopic evaluation. The menisci, joint surfaces, and ligamentous structures are evaluated and additional injuries assessed arthroscopically. The leg is then exsanguinated, and a tourniquet is inflated with 350 mm of pressure. A medial parapatellar incision is made from the inferior pole of the patella to the tibial tuberosity. The skin is dissected down to the peritenon, and skin flaps are made superiorly, inferiorly, medially, and laterally. The peritenon is incised and the patella tendon is exposed. The width of the patellar tendon is noted (Fig. 22-1), and a 10-mm graft is measured from the

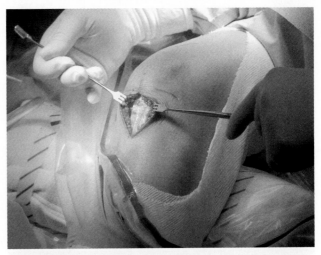

Fig. 22-1 Exposure of the patella tendon in preparation for harvesting.

midpatellar tendon. Two small incisions 10 mm apart are made in the patellar tendon and then extended superiorly and inferiorly with a hemostat. The patellar and tibial bone plugs are measured to provide graft lengths of 20 to 25 mm of patella and 25 to 30 mm of tibial bone. To facilitate bone graft harvest, the corners of the bone plugs are predrilled with a 2-mm drill to decrease stress risers. The perimeters of the bone plugs are then sawed out with a reciprocating saw to a depth of 10 to 11 mm, depending on the size of the patella and tibial tubercle. The graft (Fig. 22-2, *A* and *B*) is then taken to the back table, where it is prepared and fashioned to allow passage through the appropriate guides. The surgeon completes the graft by placing one No. 5 Tycron suture in the femoral and three No. 5 Tycron sutures into the tibial bone plugs to facilitate graft passage through the knee. The graft is preserved in a saline-moistened gauze sponge for later use.

The remnant of the ACL is resected, along with any hypertrophic tissue. Arthroscopically, the intercondylar notch is then prepared with the aid of a burr to prevent graft impingement. A site is chosen for placement of the tibial tunnel. Through the midline incision, a small area medial to the tibial tubercle is prepared with subperiosteal elevation. Using a tibial guide and under direct visualization, the surgeon drills a guide pin into the knee from the outside in, exiting within the knee at a site chosen anteromedial to the ACL insertion. The tibial tunnel is reamed to the size of the harvested graft. A curette placed over the guide pin during reaming helps protect the articular cartilage and posterior cruciate ligament from damage. The tibial tunnel must be larger than the femoral tunnel to allow passage of the graft into the knee. The tibial tunnel edges are smoothed with a rasp to prevent graft abrasion after implantation. A fenestrated plug is then placed into the tibial tunnel to prevent fluid extravasation yet allow passage of instruments.

The femoral isometric point is determined on the medial aspect of the lateral femoral condyle, usually 3 to 5 mm anterior to the posterior cortex near the superior intercondylar notch margin (over-the-top position); it is marked with

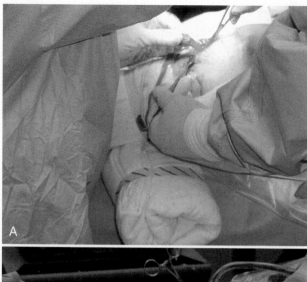

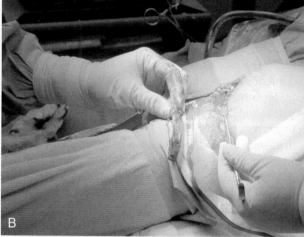

Fig. 22-2 Removal of the bone-tendon-bone graft from the patella. **A,** Graft removed from the distal patella. **B,** Graft completely removed.

a curette or burr. With the knee flexed past 90°, a fenestrated guide pin is inserted into the knee through the tibial tunnel and drilled through the femoral isometric point and out through the skin with the aid of an over-the-top guide. The femoral tunnel is then reamed to the size of the femoral bone plug to a depth of 30 mm.

The sutures from the femoral bone plug are inserted into the femoral pin and pulled out through the skin. The graft is delivered into the knee, through the tibial tunnel, and into the femoral tunnel under direct visualization. A cannulated interference screw is then inserted into the knee over a nidal guide pin and screwed into the femoral tunnel, compressing the femoral bone plug within the tunnel. Graft isometry is evaluated. The tibial bone plug within the tibial tunnel is secured with interference screw fixation. ROM and stability testing are then performed. The graft is evaluated arthroscopically to assess graft excursion and placement within the intercondylar notch.

The tourniquet is released, hemostasis is obtained, and the knee is irrigated. Loose closure of the patellar tendon is performed with the peritenon approximated to close the anterior defect. The subcutaneous tissue is approximated,

and a continuous subcuticular skin closure is performed. The wounds are dressed sterilely. A light compressive wrap and continuous ice water cryotherapy system are applied, and the patient is taken to the recovery room with the knee in a knee immobilizer in full extension.

PHYSICAL THERAPY GUIDELINES FOR REHABILITATION

Rehabilitation following ACL reconstruction has dramatically changed over the past 20 years. While the gold standard of graft choice still remains a BPTB autograft, previous rehabilitation protocols were tailored for this surgery.[89,91,94,102-119]

Physical therapy therefore must adapt its rehab protocols and tailor them to the individual patient based on graft choice and concomitant injuries and/or surgery. Regardless of the surgical procedure, the rehab protocol must be based on biologic healing. This section will discuss preoperative management following injury, including decision making for conservative management, and postoperative management from the acute inflammatory phase to return to activity.

Preoperative Management (Table 22-1)
Goals:
* Decrease swelling and inflammation
* Increase ROM
* Increase quadriceps strength
* Evaluate the entire LE

Regardless of when surgery is scheduled, the patient almost always is evaluated and receives treatment to increase ROM, especially extension, increase quadriceps/hamstrings strength, and achieve a normal gait pattern. The evaluation commonly begins with an assessment of gait when the patient enters the premises. The patient will often exhibit a flexed-knee gait or a quadriceps avoidance pattern.[120] The patient will commonly have a rehabilitation brace locked in extension and will use two crutches. While the brace is thought to limit ROM and varus-valgus forces to the knee,[121] the evidence is inconclusive that braces improve extension, and decrease pain and graft strain following ACL reconstruction.[122] Clinically speaking, the brace is used preoperatively and postoperatively to limit external forces that may cause further damage to the knee. For example a patient before having ACL reconstruction may fall and tear their meniscus or have some osteochondral damage. Active and passive knee ROM, patella mobility, presence of edema, hamstring and gastrocnemius flexibility, quadriceps strength, and weight-bearing capacity should be assessed. During the preoperative phase, the patient's whole kinetic chain should be evaluated. Strength, flexibility, and mobility of the foot, ankle, hip, and core should be assessed. Particular attention should be given to the mechanism of injury to start planning prevention strategies for postoperative rehabilitation. Assessing the entire kinetic chain before the surgery is easier and more comfortable for the patient than after surgery because of the amount of pain and how inflamed the knee will be. Exercises and modalities should be used to decrease

TABLE 22-1 Preoperative Anterior Cruciate Ligament Reconstruction

Rehabilitation Phase	Criteria to Progress to This Phase	Intervention	Goal	Rationale
Phase 1a Preoperative 1-4 wk	• Preoperative	• Cryotherapy 20-30 min • Elevation with ankle pumps (10 repetitions per minute) 20-30 min • Gait training (emphasizing normal gait pattern weight shift) • PROM stretches—supine knee extension, prone hangs, supine wall slides, seated knee flexion • Isometric exercise—quadriceps/hamstring sets (cocontraction) • A/AROM—seated knee flexion • AROM-PREs—heel raises, hip abduction/adduction, external rotation • Joint and soft tissue mobilization	By the end of 4 wk: • Self-manage pain • Decrease edema • ROM 0° extension to 130° flexion • Independent straight leg raise • Full weight bearing (brace as appropriate) • Good isometric quadriceps contraction • Maintain hip and ankle strength	• Pain control • Edema management • Gait training for safety and ease with transition postoperation • ROM stretches to prevent complications going into surgery • Muscle pump to assist lymph drainage • Graduated exercise to improve neuromuscular coordination • Emphasize self-management of ROM program • Prepare for transfers (supine-sit) • ROM and muscle contraction to assist with edema management and improve ROM • Decrease pain through soft tissue and joint mobilization techniques

A/AROM, Active assistive range of motion; *AROM,* active range of motion; *PREs,* progressive resistance exercises; *PROM,* passive range of motion; *ROM,* range of motion.

inflammation and swelling, restore patellofemoral mobility and increase quadriceps strength as well as global LE strength and flexibility.

Phase 1: 0 to 4 Weeks (Table 22-2)

Goals:
- Protect the healing graft
- Decrease swelling and inflammation
- Attain full extension
- Increase quadriceps strength

Rehabilitation following ACL reconstruction can be broken down into phases. Phase 1 begins immediately after surgery and lasts 4 weeks. In this phase, emphasis is placed on decreasing pain and inflammation, protecting the healing graft, and restoring strength and ROM. While inflammation after surgery is normal, the swelling and subsequent pain must be reduced as soon as possible. Swelling can increase pain and quadriceps muscle inhibition.[123,124]

Hopkins and associates showed that transcutaneous electric neuromuscular stimulation can be used to control pain and edema.[125] Jarit and associates showed that home interferential current therapy can help to reduce pain and swelling, and increase ROM following knee surgery.[126] However, the time parameters for transcutaneous electric neuromuscular stimulation[125] was 30 min/day and interferential current therapy treatment[126] was 3 sessions per day for 28 minutes per session, which may not be feasible for both the patient and treating physical therapist. Cryotherapy, whether in the form of continuous flow cold therapy, crushed ice, or commercial cold gel packs, is effective at reducing secondary hypoxia, pain, and edema.[125,127] When available, continuous flow cold therapy should be used over crushed ice.[128,129] Elevation with muscle pumping (ankle pumps, quad sets) can help the lymph system remove tissue debris and inflammatory byproducts (free-floating proteins too large to filter through the capillaries).[127] Cryotherapy with compression and elevation should occur after each treatment session, as well as up to 5 times daily for 20 minutes when pain, inflammation, and swelling are present. Girth measurements should be taken at the midpatella, as well as proximally and distally, to monitor progress of swelling reduction.

Patients will typically have two crutches and a postoperative brace locked in extension for the first week following surgery. After 1 week, the brace can be unlocked for exercise and gait. If the patient demonstrates a normal pain-free gait pattern, they may wean from two to one crutch, and then discharge them entirely. The brace will typically be discharged once the patient has approximately 100° of flexion, is able to do an SLR without a lag, and has a normal pain-free gait cycle. This process usually occurs 4 to 6 weeks after surgery. Table 22-3 shows commonly used guidelines for using and discharging the brace and crutches.

As previously stated, there should be an emphasis on early ROM following surgery. Full passive knee extension should be achieved within the first week to decrease abnormal joint arthrokinematics and prevent arthrofibrosis.[130,131] Bracing in extension[22,132] or hyperextension[133] can be used as a means to prevent flexion contractures. Patellar mobilizations, especially superiorly and inferiorly, should be applied to regain full mobility. Patellar immobility could result in ROM complications and difficulty recruiting quadriceps contraction.[4,92,100,134-145]

TABLE 22-2 Phase 1 Anterior Cruciate Ligament Reconstruction

Rehabilitation Phase	Criteria to Progress to This Phase	Intervention	Goal	Rationale
Phase 1 Postoperative 1-4 wk	• Postoperative	• Brace should be worn for all exercises in **bold** type • Edema and pain management program • PROM—supine knee extension, prone heel hangs, supine wall slides • Isometrics—quadriceps/hamstring sets, coconcoction, towel squeeze • AROM—heel slides **SLR (brace locked at 0°)**; hip (flexion, extension, abduction, adduction); standing hamstring curls • PREs—**supine leg press (0°-45° as indicated)**, heel raises, bicycle, and when appropriate (full weight bearing pain free), step-up exercises (initiate on a 2-inch step) • Gait training using crutches: weight bearing as tolerated, normalize gait (use small obstacle [foam cup] to emphasize hip and knee flexion in conjunction with ankle dorsiflexion) • Weight shifting—joint mobilization as indicated • Patella glides tibia-femoral (posterior) glides	Achieve the following by the end of wk 4: • ROM 0°-125° • Transfers (supine-sit) without assisting involved leg (SLR independent) • Good quality thigh and calf muscle contraction • Full weight bearing • Walk without crutches or cane (household and limited community distances) • Self-manage edema/pain	• Provide support and proprioceptive feedback • Prevent complications • Control pain • Manage edema • Provide PROM to improve joint mobility and decrease pain • Initiate home exercise program • Teach isometrics to improve muscle recruitment in preparation for functional activities • Provide AROM to improve neuromuscular coordination, strength, transfers, and gait • Promote self management of pain • Educate on positions/movements that will stress the graft • Provide gait training to progress independent ambulation without assistive device • Increase strength and tolerance to weight bearing • Joint mobilization to restore ROM and improve arthrokinematics

AROM, Active range of motion; *PREs,* progressive resistance exercises; *PROM,* passive range of motion; *ROM,* range of motion; *SLR,* straight leg raise.

TABLE 22-3 Guidelines for Using and Discharging Brace and Crutches

Brace	Locked in full extension for the first week
	Unlocked for exercises in physical therapy
	Discharged when the patient has full extension, no lag with an SLR, and at least 100° of flexion
Crutches	Bilateral crutches following surgery for first 4 wk
	After 4 wk, wean to one crutch and then discharge as long as the patient has a normal gait pattern without pain

SLR, Straight leg raise.

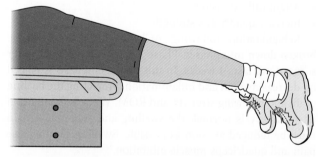

Fig. 22-3 Prone heel hangs. Patient is in the prone position with the involved leg hanging over the edge of the table or bed. Care is taken to avoid pressure on the patella.

Exercises to achieve full extension include, but are not limited to, hamstring and gastrocnemius stretching, quad sets with the heel propped under a wedge, superior patella mobilizations, a prone or supine (Figs. 22-3 and 22-4) hang, and overpressure of up to 10 lb. Remember that the ACL prevents anterior tibial translation and posterior femoral translation. With joint mobilizations, take caution with overpressure to avoid pushing the joint in the direction that the healing ACL graft limits (Fig. 22-5). The heel should also be propped up when icing and/or resting at home. You must educate the patient to avoid putting a pillow under the knee when resting at home so that the patient does not develop a flexion contracture. Tables 22-4 and 22-5 show examples of commonly used exercises to increase ROM.

Within the first 2 weeks following isolated ACL reconstruction, the patient should achieve 100° to 120° of flexion. If a concomitant meniscal repair is performed, the patient will be limited to 90° flexion for the first 4 to 6 weeks following surgery. Common causes of decreased flexion include

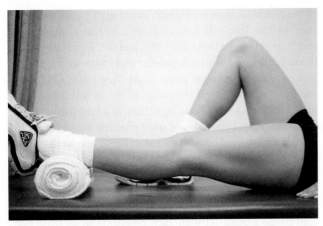

Fig. 22-4 Passive knee extension. Patient is supine or sitting with involved leg straight, into full extension. A towel is placed under the heel, allowing the knee to hang. Care is taken to avoid rotating the hip.

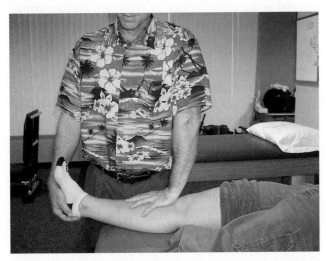

Fig. 22-5 Mobilization for extension range of motion. A posterior glide of the tibia on the femur can be accomplished, avoiding stress to the graft and donor site. Care must be taken to avoid unprotected hyperextension of the knee.

TABLE 22-4 Knee Extension Exercises

Active exercises	Quad sets
	SLRs
	Terminal knee extensions (closed chain)
Passive exercises	Hamstring and gastrocnemius stretches
	Prone hang
	Supine or long-sitting with heel propped
Manual therapy	Superior patella mobilizations
	Overpressure <10 lb

SLR, Straight leg raise.

arthrofibrosis, patella immobility (particularly with the inferior glide), posterior capsular hypomobility, decreased quadriceps flexibility, and excessive swelling. Exercises to increase knee flexion include active and active-assisted heel slides, posterior tibial and inferior patella mobilizations (in non–bone-tendon-bone autograft graft patients), and pedaling on

TABLE 22-5 Knee Flexion Exercises

Active exercises	Active heel slides
	Standing heel slide curls
	Bicycle
Passive exercises	Passive heel slides
	Use of continuous passive motion machine
Manual therapy	Inferior patellar mobilizations on non–bone-tendon-bone graft patients
	Posterior tibial mobilizations

a stationary bicycle. It is difficult to stretch the quadriceps when there is decreased knee flexion. However, the physical therapist can stretch the patient in the side-lying position with the knee flexed as much as tolerated and stretching into more hip extension. Despite conflicting evidence of long-term benefits,[146-148] the use of a continuous passive motion device may also be used at home for 4 hours per day until the patient reaches 120° flexion.

Increasing quadriceps strength is another goal of phase 1. A hallmark in the early rehabilitation process is the ability to perform an SLR without a lag. To achieve full active extension, the patient must also have full passive extension and adequate superior patella mobility. As mentioned previously, there should be minimal pain and swelling to decrease quadriceps inhibition.[55,123,124,127]

Early initiation of quadriceps strengthening has been shown to increase ROM and quadriceps muscle torque safely.[149]

Debate exists on the most appropriate type of strengthening. Closed kinetic chain (CKC) exercises are more functional and were previously thought to be safest for the healing graft.[92,150-155]

CKC exercises can begin with isometrics (Fig. 22-6) and progress to include minisquats and the leg press in the range of 0° to 45° to minimize patellofemoral joint stress (Fig. 22-7).[47,156] However, it has been shown that controlled open kinetic chain (OKC) quadriceps strengthening is both safe and advantageous following ACL surgery.[157-161] These authors[157-161] reported that active OKC knee extension without resistance did not strain the ACL from 90° to 40° of flexion. Mikkelsen and associates[159,162] showed that it was safe to add OKC knee extension exercises from the sixth week postsurgery in the range of 90° to 40°, and progressing to 90° to 10° by the twelfth week. Steinkamp and associates[156] showed that OKC knee extension can be performed with minimal patellofemoral joint stress from the range of 90° to 45°. Heijne[163] began OKC knee extension exercises at 4 weeks and 12 weeks for both hamstring tendon and patellar tendon grafts. Quadriceps muscle torque was not significantly different for any group. But the early addition of OKC exercises for patients receiving hamstring tendon autografts resulted in significant increased laxity over time. They therefore concluded that further studies are needed to determine the optimal time to add OKC quadriceps strengthening following ACL reconstruction with a hamstring graft. Because

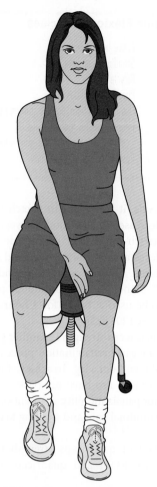

Fig. 22-6 Spider killers. Patient is seated with the involved knee (in this case the left) flexed to a comfortable position (70° to 90°). The patient is instructed to palpate over the vastus medialis oblique while applying pressure down through the heel (ankle dorsiflexed), eliciting a quadriceps and hamstring cocontraction.

of the potential increased strain to the graft with OKC exercises in low levels of flexion (<30°), isometric quadriceps exercises should be done at 0°, 90°, and 60°. Emphasis should be on achieving a superior patellar glide with each quad set, and an inferior patellar glide when they relax. OKC knee extension should be in the range of 90° to 40° in the early weeks following ACL reconstruction. If a hamstring graft is used, the patient should wait until after the fourth week. If a lag is present, an SLR will cause strain to the healing graft because the quadriceps is active with the knee in low levels of flexion. Therefore, the patient should wear their postoperative brace with it locked in extension for the exercise until the lag is gone. When performing SLRs, the patient should actively do a quad set with each repetition to increase neuromuscular control.

Even in the acute phase, the entire kinetic chain can be strengthened. OKC hamstring curls and/or CKC hamstring sets and bridges may be used to strengthen the hamstrings. Caution should be given, if a hamstring autograft was used, when strengthening the hamstrings. If, for example, the patient receives a concomitant meniscal repair, weight-bearing and/or hamstring strengthening exercises may be delayed for 4 to 6 weeks. Four-way SLRs hip external rotation and abduction can be used to strengthen the hip. Weight-bearing heel and toe raises or use of a resistance band or cuff weight can be used to strengthen the ankle. Weight shifting side-to-side and front-to-back should be employed as the precursor to gait training.

Neuromuscular electrical stimulation (NMES) should be used to increase quadriceps strength and improve gait[164] following ACL reconstruction. Their protocol used a 2500-Hz alternating current, with intensities that induced at least 50% of maximum voluntary isometric torque measured by a dynamometer positioned at 60° to 85° of flexion. The contraction time was for 10 seconds followed by a 50-second rest, for a duration of 10 to 15 contractions. Their results demonstrated a greater increase in quadriceps strength than voluntary exercise alone.[164-166]

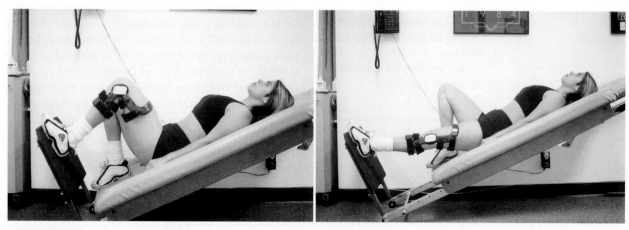

Fig. 22-7 Inclined sled. The use of an inclined sled can be initiated early to recruit volitional muscle contraction in a limited weight-bearing (resistance) environment.

Fitzgerald and associates[167] modified the protocol described by Snyder-Mackler and associates in which the patient receives the NMES with the knee in full extension. The NMES and exercise group demonstrated moderately greater quadriceps strength at 12 weeks and moderately higher levels of self-reported knee function at both 12 and 16 weeks postsurgery compared with the exercise only group. If a dynamometer is available, the physical therapist should apply the parameter described by Snyder-Mackler and associates.[164,166] However, Fitzgerald and associates demonstrated positive gains with his modified protocol.[167]

Some patients are given portable NMES units to use at home in addition to exercises, depending on whether they are unable to receive formal physical therapy twice per week or are having difficulty achieving adequate volitional quadriceps strength. The Empi 300PV (Empi, St. Paul, Minn.) has been shown to produce comparable levels of average peak torque for quadriceps strengthening.[44]

Because of the limited number of physical therapy visits paid for by insurance, the patient may only be treated once per week for the first 4 to 6 weeks. It is therefore imperative

that the patient be educated on the importance of doing his or her home exercise program. It is the job of the treating physical therapist to provide the patient with a detailed yet easily understood list of exercises to perform, teach the patient the proper form for each exercise, and maximize time spent in each physical therapy appointment.

Phase 2: 4 to 16 Weeks (Table 22-6)
Goals
- Increase LE strength
- Increase neuromuscular control
- Normalize gait
- Prepare for running

Phase 2 begins when the patient has full passive ROM and normalized pain-free independent gait and lasts until the patient begins to run (if and when appropriate).

In phase 2, the primary focus of rehabilitation is to increase strength and neuromuscular control in preparation for dynamic tasks and be independent with ADLs.

Strength training should follow the principle of progressive overload, which means to gain strength, the muscles

---

TABLE 22-6 Phase 2 Anterior Cruciate Ligament Reconstruction

Rehabilitation Phase	Criteria to Progress to This Phase	Intervention	Goal	Rationale
Phase 2 Postoperative 4-16 wk	• Postoperative	• Braces should be worn (if indicated) for all exercises in **bold** type • Continue phase 1 exercises (patient may have functional brace by 6 wk, depending on physician) • Exercise intensity progressed from AROM to PREs • PREs—**step up/down, progress to 6-inch step** • **Isokinetics—limited range (90°-30°)** • **Walking program inclusive of boxes and figure eights** • **Balance exercises** • Patient education • Continue joint mobilization • Brace should be worn if any quadriceps insufficiency is present • Phase I and II exercises as indicated • PREs using closed and open chain (isokinetic) (open chain 90°-30°) • Trampoline jogging progressing to single-leg balance/hopping, initially bilateral, progressing to unilateral in later phase • Initiate running when cleared by physician (usually by third month) • Sport- and activity-specific drills as appropriate	Achieve the following by the end of wk 8: • Range of motion 0°-135° • 100% single-leg squat 90°-0° • Gait with functional brace 1 mile • Transfer sit-stand (equal weight bearing) • Self-manage pain • Stand for 1 hour Achieve the following by the end of wk 16: • Come within 10% of full range flexion • Isokinetic test within 25% of uninvolved knee • Run 1 mile without pain (patient dependent) • Initiate sport- or activity-specific training, modifying appropriately	• Wear brace for additional proprioceptive input to the knee and to increase stability • Increase muscle strength to progress functional activities • Use limited range on open-chain exercises to protect graft • Prepare for return to sport or activity • Increase patient self-reliance for exercise and self-management • Improve joint mechanics and normalize arthrokinematics • Increase stability of the knee while limiting stress on the graft • Prepare for functional activities such as jumping and hopping • Prepare to return to sports

AROM, Active range of motion; *PREs*, progressive resistance exercises.

must be gradually loaded beyond the point to which they are normally loaded.[168] However the clinician must keep in mind that the reconstructed joint (mechanics), patellofemoral control, and joint surfaces may be the limiting factors for progressing exercise intensity.

Ideally, a one repetition maximum (RM) can be found for each exercise, and exercise prescription can be based on that. Initially, strength training in the early phases after surgery will start with 1 to 3 sets of 8 to 12 repetitions with 70% to 80% of 1 RM. Once this initial goal is met, muscle endurance should be progressed, consisting of 3 to 5 sets of 15 to 25 repetitions with 50% to 70% of 1 RM.

To build muscular power, exercise prescription should change to 1 to 3 sets of 3 to 6 repetitions (with >80% of 1 RM) but also performed at a fast velocity (usually performed during phase 3).[169] Exercises should be both concentric and eccentric, and isolate specific muscles as well as combine the entire kinetic chain. However, it is still important to remember to protect the healing graft by keeping exercises in the protected ranges. Approximately 6 to 8 weeks after surgery, the mechanical strength of the healing graft is at its weakest.[170] However, during that time, bony plugs from BPTB grafts heal within the tibial and femoral tunnels.[171] It is not until 8 to 12 weeks after surgery that the soft tissue to bone healing within the tunnels occurs with hamstring grafts.[172]

Recently, Gerber and associates[173] demonstrated increased quadriceps and gluteus maximus strength after a 12-week eccentrically focused resistance training program at 1 year following ACL reconstruction compared with standard rehabilitation. Lately, neuromuscular training protocols are being integrated into the rehabilitation process. Neuromuscular training is such that enhances unconscious motor responses by stimulating both afferent signals and central mechanisms responsible for dynamic joint control. The goal is to induce compensatory changes in muscle activation patterns.[174]

Previous studies show positive results following ACL injury.[93,175-177] These programs consist of balance exercises, dynamic joint stability exercises, plyometric exercises, agility drills, and sport-specific exercises. Risberg and associates[178] showed that a 6-month neuromuscular training program versus a traditional strength training program resulted in significantly improved Cincinnati Knee Scores and visual analog scales for pain and function. Risberg and associates[179] also showed that at a 2-year follow-up, there were no significant differences between a neuromuscular exercise training protocol and a traditional strength training protocol for the Cincinnati knee score but there was significantly improved knee function and reduced pain. It is the opinion of the authors of this chapter that rehabilitation programs after ACL reconstruction should include traditional strength training, both concentrically and eccentrically focused, as well as neuromuscular training.

Balance exercises can begin as soon as the patient is comfortable with weight bearing. They can begin with forward and lateral weight-shifts and transition to tandem standing. Single-leg stance exercises can be performed in a variety of ways: on the floor, on unstable surfaces such as foam, a trampoline, a tilt-board, and rocker-board, and with the eyes open or closed.[180,181]

Dynamic single-leg stance exercises can include doing another task while balancing, such as throwing and catching a ball or reaching in multiple directions like a "star.[182]"

Isolated quadriceps strengthening should progress from simple quad sets and SLRs to knee extensions in the protected ranges. Quadriceps strengthening that incorporates the entire kinetic chain should include double- and single-leg squats, forward and lateral step-ups, wall squats and lunges in multiple planes (Figs. 22-8 through 22-12). Global hip strengthening should progress from SLRs on the table to use of a machine, or sidestepping and diagonal stepping with a resistance band. Hamstring strengthening should progress from prone or standing curls with cuff weights to use of a machine, Romanian deadlifts, and curls with a Physioball while doing a bridge. Core strengthening should include double- and single-leg bridges, prone and side planks, and the chop and lift[183] in a lunge position. By the ninth week postoperation, patients should have close to full ROM, be able to perform a unilateral squat with 100% body weight (0° to 90°), walk up to 1 mile, tolerate standing for at least 1 hour, and demonstrate independence in self-management of exercises. The hallmark of this phase is progression from being a functionally independent person with ADLs to initiating exercises/activities in preparation of returning to the previous level of physical activity (Return to running, hiking, and sport-specific activities which will be progressed in phase 3).

We suggest a simple progression for the return to running based on activity or sport need and allowing a rest day between runs (as shown in Box 22-1). For a more complete return to a running program refer to Chapter 34.

Phase 3: 16 Weeks to 6 Months (Table 22-7)
Goals:
- Continue to increase muscle strength, power, and endurance
- Initiate/progress return to running program

Phase 3 begins when the patient is cleared to run, but there is no consensus about when to start following ACL reconstruction. During phase 3, the patient should progress all exercises to increase LE flexibility and muscular strength, power, and endurance. Commonly, the surgeon will wait between 3 to 6 months following surgery to clear the patient for running based on graft healing and concomitant surgeries.[142,170,172,184]

Few studies are available that give criteria to begin running following ACL reconstruction. Myer and associates,[185] however, used the criteria of: (1) minimum Internation Knee Documentation Committee subjective knee form score of 70, (2) either no postsurgical history of giving way or a negative pivot shift, and (3) a minimum baseline strength knee extension peak torque/body mass of at least 40% (male) and 30% (female) at 300°/sec, and 60% (male) and 50% (female) at 180°/sec. A major obstacle to using their guideline can be if the treating physical therapist does not have access to a dynamometer. The authors of this chapter recommend that

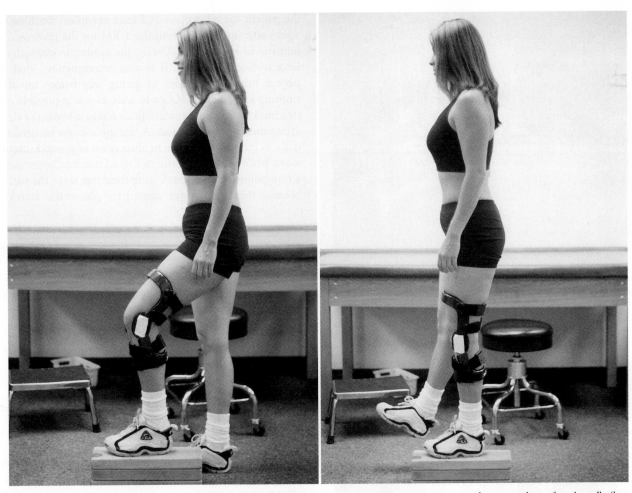

Fig. 22-8 Step up and down. Patients progress from 2-inch to 6-inch high steps. Care is taken to prevent increased stress on the graft and patella (knee is kept in line with the foot and not allowed to migrate anterior to the toes during the exercise).

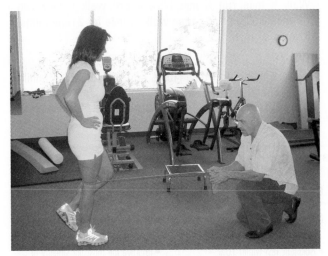

Fig. 22-9 Single-limb balance into terminal extension. This exercise can be initiated with both feet on the floor and resistance band around the distal femur pulling into flexion. The patient should maintain terminal knee extension while avoiding any pain. This exercise can be progressed to allow the patient to perform terminal knee extension movements maintaining balance.

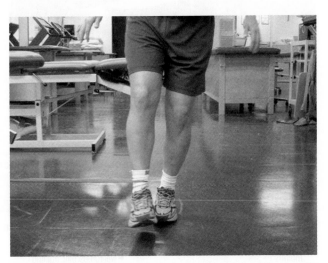

Fig. 22-10 Single-limb balance using elastic band. Standing on the involved leg (in good alignment), the patient performs hip movements (i.e., flexion, extension, abduction, adduction) with the uninvolved leg. Resisted hip adduction is pictured here.

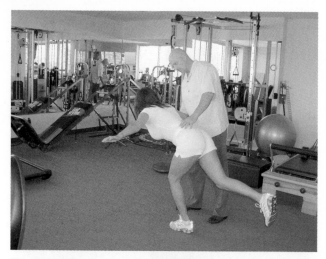

Fig. 22-11 The skater—single-limb balance on the involved leg with partial knee flexion. Slowly (maintaining a neutral spine with slight extension bias) have the patient flex at the hip, maintaining alignment of the knee in both the coronal and sagittal planes. Progress the degree of difficulty by increasing hip flexion so that the torso is parallel to the floor.

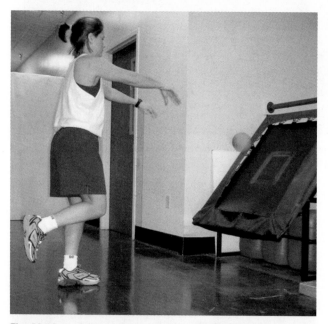

Fig. 22-12 Single-limb balance using medicine ball. Toss and catch activity, maintaining good alignment and slight knee flexion.

the patient use a leg press and knee extension machine (12 weeks after surgery) to find the 1 RM for the involved and uninvolved leg and use 70% for the minimum strength criteria to begin running. It is also recommended that the patient have no episodes of giving way before initiating running and have the ability to walk as fast as possible on a treadmill for 15 minutes without an increase in pain or signs/symptoms of inflammation. A trampoline can be used initially to increase tolerance to absorption of ground reaction forces before running. Patients should simulate bouncing on a trampoline but without letting their feet leave the surface because they are not yet cleared for plyometric activities,

---

BOX 22-1 Running Program

Week 1

Walk $\frac{1}{4}$ mile; then run $\frac{1}{4}$ mile (50% effort) for four repetitions, three times a week.

Week 2

Walk $\frac{1}{4}$ mile; then run $\frac{1}{2}$ mile (50% effort) for two repetitions, three times a week.

Week 3

Walk $\frac{1}{4}$ mile, run 1 mile (50% effort); then walk $\frac{1}{4}$ mile for one repetition, three times a week.

Week 4

Walk $\frac{1}{4}$ mile, run $\frac{1}{4}$ mile (50% effort), walk $\frac{1}{4}$ mile, run $\frac{1}{2}$ mile (75% effort); then walk $\frac{1}{4}$ mile for two repetitions, three times a week.

Week 5

Walk $\frac{1}{4}$ mile, run 1 mile (75% effort); then walk $\frac{1}{4}$ mile for two repetitions, three times a week.

Week 6

Walk $\frac{1}{4}$ mile, run $\frac{1}{4}$ mile (75% effort), walk $\frac{1}{4}$ mile, run $\frac{1}{2}$ mile (100% effort); then walk $\frac{1}{4}$ mile for 2 repetitions, 3 times a week.

Week 7

Walk $\frac{1}{4}$ mile, run 1 mile (100% effort); then walk $\frac{1}{4}$ mile for 2 repetitions, three times a week.

TABLE 22-7 Phase 3 Anterior Cruciate Ligament Reconstruction

Rehabilitation Phase	Criteria to Progress to this Phase	Intervention	Goal	Rationale
Phase 3 16 wk-6 months	• Same as in phase 2	• Continuation of exercises from phases 1-2 as indicated • Neuromuscular training • Plyometrics — hopping and jumping activities • Sport-specific activities	Achieve the following before return to sport or activity: • Isokinetic test within 10% • Functional tests within criteria to return to sport • Return to sport by 8-12 months	• Improve LE neuromuscular response to sports-related activity • Improve the muscular stability of the knee • Return to sport/activity safely and confidently

LE, Lower extremity.

much less activities on an unstable surface. Running should begin at a comfortable pace for short durations (1 to 2 minutes), followed by walking for 30 seconds to 1 minute. The running duration should increase as tolerated. The physical therapist should look for any evidence of pain, such as audible differences from foot to foot or different stride lengths. The patient should not progress in time or speed of running if there are any complaints of pain, instability, or signs/symptoms of inflammation.

Phase 4: 6 to 9 Months

Goals:

- Normalize running pattern
- Begin agility exercises
- Begin plyometric exercises
- Prepare for return to sport

The last phase of rehabilitation focuses on the actual return to the activity or sport. The correct timing of when to release an athlete back to sport participation has been controversial. Although criteria for return to sport may be fulfilled before the desired time frame, the clinician must discuss and weigh short-term and long-term risks and rewards with the athlete should he or she desire to participate. A recent study found that only 63% of National Football League players who underwent ACLR returned to play. The 63% who returned to play took an average 10.8 months to do so.[78]

Phase 4 is the final phase of rehabilitation, focusing on preparation for return to sport. In this phase, rehabilitation will focus on sport-specific exercises such as agility, plyometrics, and sprinting. The rehabilitation protocol should be individualized to meet the demands of not only the patient's sport, but also their position. A receiver in football has different physical demands than a lineman; just as a shortstop has different demands versus a centerfielder in softball. It is difficult to decide when to initiate each of these exercises because there is little evidence available. While there are some guidelines available,[138,186,187] they may not apply to your patient based on machines needed, graft type, and/or concomitant surgery. The further direction of initiating functional exercises is the opinion of the treating clinician. Once the patient can tolerate running 1 to 2 miles, they can begin low level agility drills such as forward/backward shuttle runs, lateral shuffling, and carioca. Speed should start at 50% of the patient's self-perceived effort and increase as tolerated. The physical therapist should look for any compensation when the patient decelerates and pushes off the involved LE. Plyometric training should begin next in all planes of motion. Jumping (two feet) should begin forward, at short distances. Emphasis must be placed on avoiding a valgus collapse when loading before the jump, as well as landing. When the patient demonstrates adequate dynamic control of forward jumps, they should progress in distance jumped, jumping in the frontal and transverse planes, jumping onto boxes, and consecutive jumping. Hopping (one foot) should follow the same progression after the patient demonstrates dynamic control with jumping. The last functional exercises that should be added are high-level agility drills such as cutting,

pivoting, and cut-and-spinning. Again, the physical therapist should look for any compensation when decelerating.

Returning to sport should be a collaborative decision made between the surgeon and the physical therapist. It is the responsibility of the physical therapist to prepare the patient for all tasks they could encounter in their particular sport. The patient must demonstrate each exercise at 100% effort with no episodes of giving way, increased pain, or signs/symptoms of inflammation. The patient should return to practice (if applicable) and perform at 100% effort without episodes of giving way, increased pain, or signs/symptoms of inflammation before participating in games. Although the time frame varies with the demands of the activity, Malone and Garrett[94] note that it is possible to return to the sport at 6 months if the patient has successfully completed "controlled physiologic rehabilitation." Thus initiating the training at the 4-month point allows 2 months of functional training and progression. Isokinetic testing is another piece of the puzzle used to determine whether the patient is ready to return to sport.[188] Shelbourne and associates[136] described criteria for return as follows:

- Full ROM
- Strength at 65%
- Completion of prescribed running and agility drills

The factors that most rehabilitation programs use to evaluate readiness for return to sport are KT-1000 stability, isokinetic equivalence, and functional tests.[4,91,92,135,189-191] **The** **most useful of these, without denying the importance of others, is functional testing. By using a complement of functional and isokinetic tests, the therapist and physician can determine when return to sport is appropriate.** An average timeframe for functional exercises is running at 4.3 months, jumping at 6.5 months, return to light sports at 5.0 months, return to moderate sports at 5.8 months, and return to strenuous sports at 8.1 months.[142]

Currently, there is not a specific, validated return to sport criteria following ACL reconstruction. There are, however, a variety of tests that have been described in the literature. Neeter and associates[184] showed a high ability to determine deficits in leg power 6 months after both ACL injury and ACL reconstruction using a test battery of OKC knee extension, OKC knee flexion, and CKC single-leg press. Reid and associates[160] found the use of the single hop for distance, a 6-m timed hop, a triple hop, and crossover hops for distance to be reliable and valid following ACL reconstruction with intraclass correlation coefficients for limb symmetry index values ranging from 0.82 to 0.96. The tuck jump may be used to identify LE valgus and side-to-side differences.[192]

Intrarater within-session reliability was 0.84 (range, 0.72 to 0.97) when scoring the tuck jumps.[186] Ground reaction forces can be assessed via hopping on force plates. A decrease in quad strength could result in decreased knee flexion angles when landing, which would increase the force at landing.[193] Maximum vertical ground reaction force shows high within-session reliability on both the dominant (r = 0.823) and nondominant (r = 0.877) sides.[194]

It is recommended that athletes have a side-to-side discrepancy of less than 10%.[194]

Differences in drop landing[195] and drop vertical jump[196] should be addressed to within 10%. Because unsuccessful ACL reconstruction can range from 3% to 52%,[197] ACL injury prevention techniques should be incorporated throughout the rehabilitation process.

In an effort to avoid excessive genu valgum, the hip abductors should be strengthened. The responsibility of the hip abductors is to prevent and control the excessive Trendelenburg position and subsequent dynamic valgus position at the knee. Studies have found this to be predictive of ACL injuries.[15,198]

It has been shown that athletes are more injury prone if side-to-side strength and flexibility differences are present.[199] In conclusion, rehabilitation following ACL reconstruction must prepare the patient to return to his or her prior level of function. This long process begins immediately following injury with accurate diagnosis and determination if the patient will be a potential "coper."[180,200] Following surgery, protecting the healing graft, immediately decreasing swelling, increasing ROM, and strengthening in protected ranges is warranted. Global kinetic chain strengthening and neuromuscular training, as well as injury prevention tactics, should be incorporated to best prepare the patient to safely return to the prior level of function.

TROUBLESHOOTING

Carson and associates[201] reviewed 90 failed ACL reconstruction surgeries. Based on their findings, a majority of the failures were the result of surgical technical errors. The most common complications from ACL reconstruction are joint stiffness, flexion contractures, patellar irritability (as high as 34%), and quadriceps weakness.[95,202-204] Less frequently, complications include reflex sympathetic dystrophy (less than 1%), neurovascular injury (less than 1%), deep venous thrombosis, infection and possible fluid extravasation, and compartment syndromes (especially with endoscopic techniques).

The incidence of stiffness is reduced after ACL reconstruction by using proper surgical technique combined with an aggressive rehabilitation program. Improper graft placement with the tibial tunnel too far anterior or inadequate notchplasty can cause graft impingement, blocking terminal knee extension. Intraoperative inspection of the graft throughout a full ROM should always be conducted to ensure that the graft is not impinging within the intercondylar notch.[205]

Arthrofibrosis

One of the most devastating complications after ACL reconstruction is the development of arthrofibrosis. The knee synovium and fat pad become inflamed, leading to a thickened joint capsule. This in turn begins to obliterate the medial and lateral gutters and suprapatellar pouch. The patellar tendon can shorten, produce patella baja, and

eventually cause articular damage. Paulos and colleagues[206] have defined three stages in the arthrofibrotic knee:

1. In the early stage, stage 1 (2 to 6 weeks), decreased extension is noted, in addition to quadriceps lag, diminished patellar mobility, joint swelling, and failure to progress in rehabilitation.
2. The active stage, stage 2 (6 to 30 weeks), is defined by a marked decrease in ROM, decreased patellar mobility, quadriceps atrophy, skin changes, and osteopenia. These patients walk with a significant limp.
3. The residual stage, stage 3 (beyond 8 months), is defined by a marked decrease in ROM, patellar rigidity, quadriceps atrophy, patella baja, osteopenia, and possibly arthrosis.

The physical therapist should manage arthrofibrosis early to attempt restoration of full mobility.

A knee with a significant flexion contracture can cause greater impairment than an ACL-deficient knee. Antiinflammatory agents, aggressive physical therapy, and patellar mobilization are the initial treatments for all stages of arthrofibrosis. Arthroscopic débridement, open débridement, and dynamic splinting are usually required in the later stages.[207]

Another potential complication in obtaining and maintaining full-extension ROM is the presence of a cyclops lesion.[208,209] This lesion is usually the result of the proliferation of fibrous tissue surrounding the graft and has been shown to be a cause of failure to regain or to lose full extension in the early postoperative period. Some patients who have achieved full extension will develop a gradual loss of full extension and joint line pain with terminal extension. MRI can verify the presence of this nodule that ultimately must be surgically removed. The patient responds quite well once the lesion is débrided. The therapist must be alert for the patient with delayed onset of ROM loss, especially in extension. They should undergo careful evaluation, including radiographs and MRI. If a cyclops lesion is confirmed, then arthroscopic resection should be performed.[208]

Anterior Knee Pain

Patellofemoral (PF) pain commonly occurs after ACL reconstruction, although it occurs more frequently after BPTB autograft reconstructions than with hamstring autograft reconstructions. Bach and colleagues[42] reported an 18% incidence of mild PF symptoms in a 2- to 4-year follow-up study, whereas Kartus and associates[202] reported a 33.6% incidence. Emphasis should be placed on quadriceps strengthening in protected ranges of 0° to 45° for CKC and 90° to 45° for OKC, and avoidance of pain.

Patellar fractures have been reported in the literature as a late complication of BPTB graft harvest. These are believed to be stress fractures that develop because of the decreased vascularity of the patella. Patellar fracture also can occur intraoperatively during graft harvest and has been reported after surgery. Brownstein and Bronner[210] reported the incidence of patellar fractures at 0.5% and noted that it usually occurs as a result of a fall. They put the patella at highest risk for fracture during rehabilitation at 10 to 14 weeks postoperation. Pain over the tibial tubercle is less frequently encountered but may occur in those with prominent tibial tubercles. If the patient has limited joint motion before surgery, especially in extension, then a continuous passive motion device should be used immediately after surgery.[189]

During the first postoperative phase, ROM complications, if present, usually occur in extension. If mobilization and home exercises are not effective, then the patient should try adding weight to the ankle during the prone hanging exercises. Duration and intensity are determined individually, but the authors of this chapter generally start with 3 to 5 lb for a 5-minute increment and have the patient follow through at home three to five times a day. In addition, the patient can add weights to the knee while performing supine knee extension (towel propped under the heel) and progress in a similar manner.

Treatment for Complications and Troubleshooting

Phases 1 and 2

Strength complications are addressed using NMES over the affected muscles in conjunction with exercise. The physical therapist also can initiate biofeedback on the vasti to assist with balanced muscle contraction. Anterior knee pain related to PF dysfunction can be treated with modalities (i.e., cryotherapy and ultrasound), soft tissue mobilization, patella taping (after the incision has healed), emphasis on proper LE alignment during the offending activity, and hip strengthening; assessment of foot biomechanics (the need for orthotics) can also be useful in addressing PF issues.

Persistent swelling may indicate hemarthrosis, synovitis, reinjury, or infection.[201] If by 4 to 6 weeks the patient has not gained full extension, then the cause may be patellar entrapment. Use of patellar mobilization to a greater extent and with more vigor and serial casting may be considered. Arthroscopy is usually considered if full extension is not obtained by the eighth week.[63] If reflex sympathetic dystrophy occurs, then it is usually seen by the fifth week after surgery.

Motion limitations are of primary concern and require aggressive management, as mentioned earlier. Some patients may need to be manipulated or evaluated for surgery during phase 2. As the patient progresses with strengthening exercises, the physical therapist should pay careful attention to any residual pain or edema. The PF mechanism must be continually evaluated as the resistance of the exercises is progressed.

Phase 2

Complications 9 weeks or more after surgery are usually the result of edema or pain after activity. This can result from the addition of new stressors (e.g., exercises) on the knee joint and soft tissue. If not already initiated, then pool exercises may be a helpful adjunct in continuing to develop strength, maintain ROM, and improve mechanics of the LE in a less than full weight-bearing posture. Exercises in the form of deep-water running and activity-specific drills are a good adjunct to land-based rehabilitation.

SUMMARY

In conclusion, rehabilitation following ACL reconstruction must prepare the patient to return to his or her prior level of function. This long process begins immediately following injury with accurate diagnosis and determination if the patient will be a potential "coper."[9,211] Following surgery, protecting the healing graft, immediately decreasing swelling, increasing ROM, and strengthening in protected ranges is warranted. Global kinetic chain strengthening and neuromuscular training, as well as injury prevention tactics, should be incorporated to best prepare the patient to safely return to the prior level of function.

Suggested Home Maintenance for the Postsurgical Patient

Home exercises are progressed through the four phases of rehabilitation based on the patient's tolerance to activity. Any increase in edema, pain, or laxity should be addressed early, and exercises should be modified to eliminate complications.

Weeks 1 to 4

GOALS FOR THE PERIOD: Manage pain and edema, improve quadriceps/hamstring contractions, improve ROM

Pain and Edema
1. Cryotherapy with elevation 20 to 30 minutes with ankle pumps (10 repetitions every minute)
2. Use of home electrical stimulation unit

Strength
1. Isometrics: quadriceps and hamstring sets isolation and cocontraction, 10 to 30 repetitions (can also be done with elevation)

ROM Exercises
1. Supine knee extension
2. Prone heel hangs
3. Heel slides
4. Supine wall slides (supine with involved foot against the wall, gravity assisted into flexion)

Active Range of Motion Exercises (Brace Locked)
1. Hip: flexion, extension, abduction, adduction, abduction with external rotation
2. Standing hamstring curls

Gait Training

1. Gait training using crutches: weight bearing as tolerated, weaning as appropriate
2. Use small obstacles to work on swing phase of gait clearing involved leg (hip flexion, knee flexion, and ankle dorsiflexion)
3. Once full weight bearing obtained, work on single-limb balance activities
   (Perform exercises three times a day with repetitions and sets determined by strength— usually two sets of as many as 30 repetitions.)

Weeks 5 to 8

GOALS FOR THE PERIOD: Progress ROM, increase functional strength of hip, knee, and ankle

ROM Exercises

1. Continue passive range of motion (PROM) exercises on an as-needed basis (ROM as needed, progress to prescribed duration with weight on top of knee if full extension is not reached at this time).
2. Add seated passive flexion.

Strength

1. Add step up and down with appropriate-height object (local phone book versus county phone book) and single-limb balance activities.
2. Follow a walking program (as much as 45 minutes of continuous walking on level surfaces daily).
3. Progress back into therapy or community gym environment for cardiovascular exercises: bike, elliptical, treadmill (forward and reverse). Progress upper extremity exercise program to weight-bearing position gym activities (progressed to include cardiovascular and proprioceptive and neuromuscular training techniques).

Gait Training

1. Work on single-limb balance and walking figure-eight and box patterns.
2. Try walking box and figure-eight patterns.

Weeks 9 to 16

GOALS FOR THE PERIOD: Progress functional activities, prepare to return to sport or activity

ROM Exercises

1. Should be close to full ROM by this time. Maintenance program should be initiated.

Strength

1. Periodize gym program; initiate running program when appropriate (usually about 3 months).
2. Progress neuromuscular (balance and coordination) training emphasizing proper LE alignment with activities.
3. Progress balance and coordination activities and continue education on injury prevention with return to specific sport or activity.
4. Add one-legged hopping and jumping activities once cleared for running (usually about week 12).
5. Begin foundational exercises for return to sport emphasizing LE control and neuromuscular training principles.

Week 17 and Beyond

GOALS FOR THE PERIOD: Progress back to sport or activity

ROM Exercises

1. Maintenance

Strength

1. Gym-based workouts continuing to emphasize proprioceptive and neuromuscular training techniques
2. Perform exercises specific to sport
3. Reassess and progress the periodization program for the athlete to adequately prepare for return to sport

CLINICAL CASE REVIEW

1 Michelle is 3 weeks post-ACLR and wants to know when she can discontinue her postoperation knee brace.

The brace should be discharged when the patient has full extension, no lag with an SLR, and at least 100° of flexion. This typically occurs 2 to 3 weeks after surgery. Most rehabilitation protocols require crutch use with weight bearing as tolerated for 4 weeks following surgery. After

4 weeks, the patient may be weaned from two crutches to one, and then ultimately discharged. A requirement for discharging crutches is that the patient must have a normal pain-free gait pattern. In both situations, consultation and approval from the surgeon should take place.

2 When strengthening the quadriceps, what range is safe for exercises? Why is this important?

For OKC exercises, the quadriceps should be strengthened in the range of 90° to 45° to guard against straining the healing ACL graft and to protect against patellofemoral pain. OKC exercises should begin 4 weeks after surgery. Before that, the patient can perform isometric quadriceps exercises at 90° and 60°. When performing CKC exercises, the patient should stay in the range of 0° to 45° to guard against straining the healing ACL graft and to protect against patellofemoral pain. CKC exercises may be incorporated into the treatment regime when the patient can be full weight bearing without pain.

3 Charlie is 10 weeks post-ACLR and demonstrates good ROM and strength. He is eager to begin running again. In terms of graft healing, when is it generally safe to begin running following ACL reconstruction?

The mechanical strength of the healing graft is at its weakest from 4 to 8 weeks. Bone-to-bone healing, as with the use of a BPTB autograft, occurs approximately at 10 weeks. Soft tissue to bone healing, as with the use of a hamstring or quadriceps autograft, occurs approximately at 12 weeks. Therefore, running should never be initiated before 3 months postsurgery because of the lack of healing. Additionally, the patient must demonstrate adequate strength and neuromuscular control of the LE with particular emphasis on the quadriceps. This typically occurs at 4 to 6 months postsurgery. A collaborative decision with the surgeon as to when the patient should begin running is necessary.

4 George is 4 months post-ACLR and wants to return to playing soccer. How do you best prepare the patient to return to sport following ACL reconstruction?

Given that there are no complications along the way, sport-specific exercises can be introduced into the program (**at low intensity**) beginning at 3 to 4 months. The best way to prepare the patient is to gradually expose the patient to everything he or she will encounter. Therefore, the patient must be able to tolerate running, going up/down steps, and figure eights, again starting at a low intensity level (walk figure eights before jog, jog before run, etc.). Plyometrics are introduced (usually around 5 months) as the patient begins to show that he or she are able to tolerate and have eccentric as well as concentric control of the LE before agility, plyometric, and cutting exercises are progressed. The patient should eventually perform all of the exercises in all three planes of motion. For example, jumping should be forward/backward, to each side, and clockwise/counterclockwise. Also, the patient should be able to perform any and all exercises at 100% effort in physical therapy before returning to practice. To return to competition, the patient must be able to participate in full practice and perform at 100% effort without any complaints of pain, giving way episodes, or signs/symptoms of inflammation.

5 Tracy is 50 years old and had ACLR 1 week ago. She arrives at her first outpatient visit with moderate edema about the knee and ankle. She states that she has been compliant with weight bearing and uses her crutches and brace as instructed. What further questions can help the therapist provide a successful edema management program?

The most effective way to manage swelling (at home) is with elevation, compression, and ice. Upon further questioning she has not been elevating her leg (above heart level) regularly or performing ROM or isometric exercises. A program was initiated consisting of elevation an ice (20 minutes, four times a day) with ankle pumps (10 repetitions every minute).

6 Randy is 45 years old and tore his ACL while horseback riding. He had ACLR 3 weeks ago. Knee flexion ROM is progressing nicely. Knee extension is limited, with a PROM of −10°. Inflammation is decreasing. He has pain while performing quadriceps sets and SLRs. What treatment techniques can be used to gain knee extension?

Tibiofemoral anterior-posterior mobilization movements into resistance at end range (using grades III and IV) can be performed with the knee in extension. Care must be taken not to elicit any increased tension on the graft. Full extension will decrease stress on the patellofemoral and tibiofemoral articulations.

7 Steve is a 45-year-old fireman. He had an ACLR 9 weeks ago on his left knee. Because of mishaps and personal reasons, physical therapy was not initiated until 5 weeks ago. Presently (9 weeks after surgery) PROM for knee flexion is 110°. The end range is beginning to feel leathery. Soft tissue restrictions appear to be present in the quadriceps. Swelling and complaints of pain are usually minimal. Strength is gradually progressing. What treatment techniques could be used to promote increased knee flexion?

Tibiofemoral posterior glides can also be performed with the knee in flexion (into resistance, grade IV), followed by PROM into flexion with overpressure. Patellofemoral glides can be performed. While PF glides superiorly will assist in gaining extension, PF glides inferiorly will assist with knee flexion and should be mobilized accordingly. In the prone (better for rectus femoris [RF]/Psoas) and supine positions, gentle contraction and relaxation stretches can be performed with the quadriceps. Also, soft tissue mobilization to the distal quadriceps and lateral retinaculum can be performed to address PF restrictions.

8 Nancy is making excellent progress in therapy. However, at 10 weeks after surgery the therapist notices a palpable "clunk" with her AROM, and extension has become quite painful. What could be the origin of her problem?

Limitations with extension usually are the result of posterior capsule or notch problems. The presence of crepitation or a palpable clunk in addition to pain with extension could signify an ACL "nodule." Nancy was referred back to her surgeon and an MRI confirmed the presence of a cyclops lesion (nodule). Surgery was scheduled to remove the fibroproliferative tissue.

REFERENCES

1. Miller MD, Sullivan RT: Anterior cruciate ligament reconstruction in an 84-year-old man. Arthroscopy 17(1):70-72, 2001.
2. Shea KG, et al: Anterior cruciate ligament injury in pediatric and adolescent soccer players: An analysis of insurance data. J Pediatr Orthop 24(6):623-628, 2004.
3. http://emedicine.medscape.com/article/307161-overview.
4. Dietrichson J, Souryal TO: Physical therapy after arthroscopic surgery: "Preoperative and post operative rehabilitation after anterior cruciate ligament tears." Orthop Phys Ther Clin N Am 3(4):539-554, 1994.
5. Drez D, Faust DC, Evans IP: Cryotherapy and nerve palsy. Am J Sports Med 9:256, 1981.
6. McLean DA: The use of cold and superficial heat in the treatment of soft tissue injuries. Br J Sports Med 23:53, 1989.
7. Novak PJ, Bach BR Jr, Hager CA: Clinical and functional outcome of anterior cruciate ligament reconstruction in the recreational athlete over the age of 35. Am J Knee Surg 9(3):111, 1996.
8. Sandberg R, Balkfors B: Reconstruction of the anterior cruciate ligament: A 5-year follow-up of 89 patients. Acta Orthop Scand 59(3):288, 1988.
9. Boden BP, et al: Mechanisms of anterior cruciate ligament injury. Orthopedics 23(6):573-578, 2000.
10. Bradley JP, et al: Anterior cruciate ligament injuries in the National Football League: Epidemiology and current treatment trends among team physicians. Arthroscopy 18(5):502-509, 2002.
11. Cerulli G, et al: In vivo anterior cruciate ligament strain behaviour during a rapid deceleration movement: Case report. Knee Surg Sports Traumatol Arthrosc 11(5):307-311, 2003.
12. Frank CB, Jackson DW: The science of reconstruction of the anterior cruciate ligament. J Bone Joint Surg Br 79A(10):1556, 1997.
13. Boden BP, et al: Noncontact anterior cruciate ligament injuries: Mechanisms and risk factors. J Am Acad Orthop Surg 18(9):520-527, 2010.
14. Arnoczky SP: Blood supply to the anterior cruciate ligament and supporting structures. Orthop Clin North Am 16(1):15-28, 1985.
15. Hewett TE, et al: Biomechanical measures of neuromuscular control and valgus loading of the knee predict anterior cruciate ligament injury risk in female athletes: A prospective study. Am J Sports Med 33(4):492-501, 2005.
16. Imwalle LE, et al: Relationship between hip and knee kinematics in athletic women during cutting maneuvers: A possible link to noncontact anterior cruciate ligament injury and prevention. J Strength Cond Res 23(8):2223-2230, 2009.
17. Harrison AD, et al: Sex differences in force attenuation: A clinical assessment of single-leg hop performance on a portable force plate. Br J Sports Med 45(3):198-202, 2011.
18. Gould JA, Davies GJ: Orthopedic and sports physical therapy, vol 2, St Louis, 1985, Mosby.
19. Bellabarba C, Bush-Joseph CA, Bach BR Jr: Patterns of meniscal injury in the anterior cruciate-deficient knee: A review of the literature. Am J Orthop 26(1):18-23, 1997.
20. Insall JJ, et al: Bone block iliotibial-band transfer for ACL insufficiency. J Bone Joint Surg Br 63:560, 1981.
21. Maffulli N, Binfield PM, King JB: Articular cartilage lesions in the symptomatic anterior cruciate ligament-deficient knee. Arthroscopy 19(7):685-690, 2003.
22. Foster A, Butcher C, Turner PG: Changes in arthroscopic findings in the anterior cruciate ligament deficient knee prior to reconstructive surgery. Knee 12(1):33-35, 2005.
23. Shelbourne KD, Patel DV: Timing of surgery in anterior cruciate ligament-injured knees. Knee Surg Sports Traumatol Arthrosc 3(3):148-156, 1995.
24. Oiestad BE, et al: The association between radiographic knee osteoarthritis and knee symptoms, function and quality of life 10-15 years after anterior cruciate ligament reconstruction. Br J Sports Med, 45(7):583-588, 2011.
25. Sutherland AG, et al: The long-term functional and radiological outcome after open reconstruction of the anterior cruciate ligament. J Bone Joint Surg Br 92(8):1096-1099, 2010.
26. McCarroll JR, Shelbourne KD, Patel DV: Anterior cruciate ligament injuries in young athletes: Recommendations for treatment and rehabilitation. Sports Med 20(2):117-127, 1995.
27. Arendt E, Dick R: Knee injury patterns among men and women in collegiate basketball and soccer: NCAA data and review of literature. Am J Sports Med 23(6):694-701, 1995.
28. Huston LJ, Greenfield ML, Wojtys EM: Anterior cruciate ligament injuries in the female athlete: Potential risk factors. Clin Orthop Relat Res (372):50-63, 2000.
29. Rozzi SL, et al: Knee joint laxity and neuromuscular characteristics of male and female soccer and basketball players. Am J Sports Med 27(3):312-319, 1999.
30. Hewett TE, Myer GD, Ford KR: Decrease in neuromuscular control about the knee with maturation in female athletes. J Bone Joint Surg Am 86-A(8):1601-1608, 2004.
31. Hewett TE, Myer GD, Ford KR: Reducing knee and anterior cruciate ligament injuries among female athletes: A systematic review of neuromuscular training interventions. J Knee Surg 18(1):82-88, 2005.
32. Hewett TE, et al: A review of electromyographic activation levels, timing differences, and increased anterior cruciate ligament injury incidence in female athletes. Br J Sports Med 39(6):347-350, 2005.
33. Noyes FR, et al: The drop-jump screening test: Difference in lower limb control by gender and effect of neuromuscular training in female athletes. Am J Sports Med 33(2):197-207, 2005.
34. Leetun DT, et al: Core stability measures as risk factors for lower extremity injury in athletes. Med Sci Sports Exerc 36(6):926-934, 2004.
35. Millett PJ, et al: Early ACL reconstruction in combined ACL-MCL injuries. J Knee Surg 17(2):94-98, 2004.
36. Andriacchi TP, Dyrby CO: Interactions between kinematics and loading during walking for the normal and ACL deficient knee. J Biomech 38(2):293-298, 2005.
37. Jones HP, et al: Meniscal and chondral loss in the anterior cruciate ligament injured knee. Sports Med 33(14):1075-1089, 2003.
38. Sherman MF, et al: The long-term follow up of primary anterior cruciate ligament repair: Defining a rationale for augmentation. Am J Sports Med 19:243, 1991.
39. Harner CD, et al: Loss of motion after anterior cruciate ligament reconstruction. Am J Sports Med 20:499-506, 1992.

40. Shelbourne KD, Johnson GE: Outpatient surgical management of arthrofibrosis after anterior cruciate ligament surgery. Am J Sports Med 22:192-197, 1994.

41. Wasilewski SA, Covall DJ, Cohen S: Effect of surgical timing on recovery and associated injuries after anterior cruciate ligament reconstruction. Am J Sports Med 21:338-342, 1993.

42. Bach BR Jr, et al: Arthroscopy-assisted anterior cruciate ligament reconstruction using patellar tendon substitution: Two-to-four-year follow-up results. Am J Sports Med 22(6):758, 1994.

43. Hunter RE, et al: The impact of surgical timing on postoperative motion and stability following anterior cruciate ligament reconstruction. Arthroscopy 12:667-674, 1996.

44. Majors RA, Woodfin B. Achieving full range of motion after anterior cruciate ligament reconstruction. Am J Sports Med 24:350-355, 1996.

45. Marcacci M, et al: Early versus late reconstruction for anterior cruciate ligament rupture: Results after five years of followup. Am J Sports Med 23:690-693, 1995.

46. Bottoni CR, et al: Postoperative range of motion following anterior cruciate ligament reconstruction using autograft hamstrings: A prospective, randomized clinical trial of early versus delayed reconstructions. Am J Sports Med 36(4):656-662, 2008.

47. Sterett WI, et al: Decreased range of motion following acute versus chronic anterior cruciate ligament reconstruction. Orthopedics 26:151-154, 2003.

48. Barber FA, et al: Is an anterior cruciate ligament reconstruction outcome age dependent? Arthroscopy 12(6):720, 1996.

49. Kuechle DK, et al: Allograft anterior cruciate ligament reconstruction in patients over 40 years of age. Arthroscopy 18(8):845-853, 2002.

50. Grood ES, et al: Biomechanics of the knee-extension exercise: Effect of cutting the anterior cruciate ligament. J Bone Joint Surg Am 66:725, 1984.

51. Shelbourne KD, Patel DV, McCarroll JR: Management of anterior cruciate ligament injuries in skeletally immature adolescents. Knee Surg Sports Traumatol Arthrosc 4(2):68-74, 1996.

52. Finlayson CJ, Nasreddine A, Kocher MS: Current concepts of diagnosis and management of ACL injuries in skeletally immature athletes. Phys Sportsmed 38(2):90-101, 2010.

53. Brewer BW, et al: Age-related differences in predictors of adherence to rehabilitation after anterior cruciate ligament reconstruction. J Athl Train 38(2):158-162, 2003.

54. Paletta GA Jr: Special considerations: Anterior cruciate ligament reconstruction in the skeletally immature. Orthop Clin North Am 34(1):65-77, 2003.

55. Millett PJ, Willis AA, Warren RF: Associated injuries in pediatric and adolescent anterior cruciate ligament tears: Does a delay in treatment increase the risk of meniscal tear? Arthroscopy 18(9):955-959, 2002.

56. Ciccotti MG, et al: Non-operative treatment of ruptures of the anterior cruciate ligament in middle-aged patients: Results after long term follow-up. J Bone Joint Surg Br 76A(9):1315, 1994.

57. Hey-Groves EW: The crucial ligaments of the knee joint: Their function, rupture, and operative treatment of the same. Br J Surg 7:505, 1920.

58. Campbell WC: Reconstruction of the ligaments of the knee. Am J Surg 43:473, 1939.

59. Cabaud ME, Rodkey WG, Feagin JA: Experimental studies of acute anterior cruciate ligament injury and repair. Am J Sports Med 7:18, 1979.

60. Marshall JL, Warren RJ, Wickiewicz TL: The anterior cruciate ligament: A technique of repair and reconstruction. Clin Orthop 143:97, 1979.

61. Marshall JL, Warren RJ, Wickiewicz TL: Primary surgical treatment of anterior cruciate ligament lesions. Am J Sports Med 10:103, 1982.

62. Ellison AE: Distal iliotibial-band transfer for anterolateral rotatory instability of the knee. J Bone Joint Surg Br 61:330, 1979.

63. MacIntosh DL, Tregonning RJA: A follow-up and evaluation of the over-the-top repair of acute tears of the anterior cruciate ligament. J Bone Joint Surg 59B:511, 1977.

64. Garcia R Jr, et al: Lateral extra-articular knee reconstruction: Long-Term patient outcome and satisfaction. J South Orthop Assoc 9(1): 19-23, 2000.

65. Teitge RA, Indelicato PA, Kerlan RK: Iliotibial band transfer for anterolateral rotatory instability of the knee: Summary of 54 cases. Am J Sports Med 8:223, 1980.

66. Alm A, Lijedahlso SO, Stromberg B: Clinical and experimental experience in reconstruction of the anterior cruciate ligament. Orthop Clin North Am 7:181, 1976.

67. Cho KO: Reconstruction of the ACL by semitendinosus. J Bone Joint Surg 68B:739, 1986.

68. Jones KG: Reconstruction of the anterior cruciate ligament using the central one-third of the patella ligaments: A follow-up report. J Bone Joint Surg Br 63A:1302, 1970.

69. Nicholas JA, Minkoff J: Iliotibial band transfer through the intercondylar notch for combined anterior instability. Am J Sports Med 6:341, 1978.

70. Giron F, et al: Anterior cruciate ligament reconstruction with double-looped semitendinosus and gracilis tendon graft directly fixed to cortical bone: 5-year results. Knee Surg Sports Traumatol Arthrosc 13(2):81-91, 2005.

71. Ibrahim SA, et al: Clinical evaluation of arthroscopically assisted anterior cruciate ligament reconstruction: Patellar tendon versus gracilis and semitendinosus autograft. Arthroscopy 21(4):412-417, 2005.

72. Dopirak RM, Adamany DC, Steensen RN: A comparison of autogenous patellar tendon and hamstring tendon grafts for anterior cruciate ligament reconstruction. Orthopedics 27(8):837-842, 2004.

73. Herrington L, et al: Anterior cruciate ligament reconstruction, hamstring versus bone-patella tendon-bone grafts: A systematic literature review of outcome from surgery. Knee 12(1):41-50, 2005.

74. Svensson M, et al: A prospective comparison of bone-patellar tendon-bone and hamstring grafts for anterior cruciate ligament reconstruction in female patients. Knee Surg Sports Traumatol Arthrosc 14(3):278-286, 2006. Epub 2005 Nov 16.

75. Laxdal G, et al: A prospective comparison of bone-patellar tendon-bone and hamstring tendon grafts for anterior cruciate ligament reconstruction in male patients. Knee Surg Sports Traumatol Arthrosc 15(2):115-125, 2007. Epub 2006 Sep 9.

76. Gladstone JN, Andrews JR: Endoscopic anterior cruciate ligament reconstruction with patella tendon autograft. Orthop Clin North Am 33(4):701-715, 2002.

77. Hospodar SJ, Miller MD. Controversies in ACL reconstruction: Bone-patellar tendon-bone anterior cruciate ligament reconstruction remains the gold standard. Sports Med Arthrosc 17(4):242-246, 2009.

78. Shah VM, et al: Return to play after anterior cruciate ligament reconstruction in National Football League athletes. Am J Sports Med 38(11):2233-2239, 2010.

79. Daniel DM: Principles of knee ligament surgery. In Daniel DM, Akeson WH, O'Connor J, editors: Knee ligaments: Structure, function and repair, New York, 1990, Raven.

80. Noyes FR, et al: Biomechanical analysis of human ligament grafts used in knee ligament repairs and reconstructions. J Bone Joint Surg 66A:344, 1984.

81. Bock B, Malinin T, Brown M: Bone transplantation and human immunodeficiency virus: An estimate of the risk of acquired immunodeficiency syndrome (AIDS). Clin Orthop 240:129, 1989.

82. Fielder B, et al: Effect of gamma irradiation on the human immunodeficiency virus. J Bone Joint Surg Br 76A:1032, 1994.

83. Rasmussen T, et al: The effects of 4 mrad of gamma irradiation on the internal mechanical properties of bone-patella tendon-bone grafts. Arthroscopy 10:188, 1994.

84. Kurosaka M, Yoshiyas S, Andrish JT: Biomechanical comparison of different surgical techniques of graft fixation in anterior cruciate ligament reconstruction. Am J Sports Med 15:225, 1987.

85. Bolga LA, Keskula DR: Reliability of lower extremity functional performance tests. J Orthop Sports Phys Ther 26(3):138, 1997.

86. Robertson DB, Daniel DM, Biden E: Soft tissue fixation to bone. Am J Sports Med 14:398, 1983.

87. Arnoczky SP, Tarvin GB, Marshall JL: Anterior cruciate ligament replacement using patellar tendon. J Bone Joint Surg Am 643:217, 1982.

88. Corsetti JR, Jackson DW: Failure of anterior cruciate ligament reconstruction: The biologic basis. Clin Orthop Relat Res 323:42, 1996.

89. Fu FH, Woo SLY, Irrgang JJ: Current concepts for rehabilitation following anterior cruciate ligament reconstruction. J Orthop Sports Phys Ther 15(6):270, 1992.

90. Liu SH, et al: Collagen in tendon, ligament, and bone healing: A current review. Clin Orthop Relat Res 318:265, 1995.

91. DeCarlo MS, et al: Traditional versus accelerated rehabilitation following ACL reconstruction: A one-year follow-up. J Orthop Sports Phys Ther 15(6):309, 1992.

92. Shelbourne KD, Nitz P: Accelerated rehabilitation after anterior cruciate ligament reconstruction. J Orthop Sports Phys Ther 15(6):256, 1992.

93. Amiel D, et al: The phenomenon of "ligamentization": anterior cruciate ligament reconstruction with autogenous patellar tendon. J Orthop Res 4:162, 1986.

94. Malone TR, Garrett WE Jr: Commentary and historical perspective of anterior cruciate ligament rehabilitation. J Orthop Sports Phys Ther 15(6):265, 1992.

95. Tomaro JE: Prevention and treatment of patellar entrapment following intra-articular ACL reconstruction, athletic training. J Athl Train 26:11, 1991.

96. Vogrin M, et al: Effects of a platelet gel on early graft revascularization after anterior cruciate ligament reconstruction: A prospective, randomized, double-blind, clinical trial. Eur Surg Res 45(2):77-85, 2010.

97. Sánchez M, et al: Ligamentization of tendon grafts treated with an endogenous preparation rich in growth factors: Gross morphology and histology. Arthroscopy 26(4):470-480, 2010.

98. Aglietti P, et al: Patellofemoral problems after intraarticular anterior cruciate ligament reconstruction. Clin Orthop Relat Res 288:195, 1993.

99. DeLorme TL, Watkins A: Progressive resistance exercise, New York, 1951, Appleton-Century.

100. Shelbourne KD, Patel DV: Treatment of limited motion after anterior cruciate ligament reconstruction. Knee Surg Sports Traumatol Arthrosc 7(2):85-92, 1999.

101. Spencer JD, Hayes KC, Alexander IJ: Knee joint effusion and quadriceps reflex inhibition in man. Arch Phys Med Rehabil 65:171, 1984.

102. Tegner Y: Strength training in the rehabilitation of cruciate ligament tears. Sports Med 9(2):129, 1990.

103. DeMaio M, Noyes FR, Mangine RE: Principles for aggressive rehabilitation after reconstruction of the anterior cruciate ligament. Sports Med Rehabil Orthop 15(3):385, 1992.

104. Dietrichson J, Souryal TO: Physical therapy after arthroscopic surgery, "preoperative and post operative rehabilitation after anterior cruciate ligament tears," Orthop Phys Ther Clin N Am 3(4):539-554, 1994.

105. Hardin JA, et al: The effects of "decelerated" rehabilitation following anterior cruciate ligament reconstruction on a hyperelastic female adolescent: A case study. J Orthop Sports Phys Ther 26(1):29, 1997.

106. Johnson RJ, et al: Five to ten year follow-up evaluation after reconstruction of the anterior cruciate ligament. Clin Orthop 83:122, 1984.

107. Mangine RE, Noyes FR: Rehabilitation of the allograft reconstruction. J Orthop Sports Phys Ther 15(6):294, 1992.

108. Mangine RE, Noyes FR, DeMaio M: Minimal protection program: Advanced weight bearing and range of motion after ACL reconstruction—weeks 1-5. Orthopedics 15(4):504, 1992.

109. Noyes FR, Barber-Westin SD: Revision anterior cruciate ligament surgery: Experience from Cincinnati. Clin Orthop Relat Res 325:116, 1996.

110. Paulos L, et al: Knee rehabilitation after anterior cruciate ligament reconstruction and repair. Am J Sports Med 9(3):140, 1981.

111. Rubenstein RA, et al: Effect on knee stability if full hyperextension is restored immediately after autogenous bone-patellar tendon-bone anterior cruciate ligament reconstruction. Am J Sports Med 23(3):365, 1995.

112. Seto JL, et al: Rehabilitation of the knee after anterior cruciate ligament reconstruction. J Orthop Sports Phys Ther 11(1):8, 1989.

113. Shelbourne KD, et al: Correlation of remaining patellar tendon width with quadriceps strength after autogenous bone-patellar tendon-bone anterior cruciate ligament reconstruction. Am J Sports Med 22(6):774, 1994.

114. Shelbourne KD, et al: Ligament stability two to six years after anterior cruciate ligament reconstruction with autogenous patellar tendon graft and participation in accelerated rehabilitation program. Am J Sports Med 23(5):575, 1995.

115. Shelbourne KD, Klootwyk TE, DeCarlo MS: Update on accelerated rehabilitation after anterior cruciate ligament reconstruction. J Orthop Sports Phys Ther 15(6):303, 1992.

116. Shelbourne KD, Nitz P: Accelerated rehabilitation after anterior cruciate ligament reconstruction. J Orthop Sports Phys Ther 15(6):256, 1992.

117. Silverskiold JP, et al: Rehabilitation of the anterior cruciate ligament in the athlete. Sports Med 6:308, 1988.

118. Wilk KE, Andrews JR: Current concepts in the treatment of anterior cruciate ligament disruption. J Orthop Sports Phys Ther 15(6):279, 1992.

119. Wilk KE, Reinold MM, Hooks TR: Recent advances in the rehabilitation of isolated and combined anterior cruciate ligament injuries. Orthop Clin North Am 34(1):107-137, 2003.

120. Torry MR, et al: Mechanisms of compensating for anterior cruciate ligament deficiency during gait. Med Sci Sports Exerc 36(8):1403-1412, 2004.

121. France EP, Paulos LE: Knee bracing. J Am Acad Orthop Surg 2:281-287, 1994.

122. Wright RW, Fetzer GB: Bracing after ACL reconstruction: A systematic review. Clin Orthop Rel Res 455:162-168, 2007.

123. Hart JM, et al: Quadriceps activation following knee injuries: a systematic review. J Athl Train 45(1):87-97, 2010.

124. Hopkins JT, et al: Effect of knee joint effusion on quadriceps and soleus motoneuron pool excitability. Med Sci Sports Exerc 33(1):123-126, 2001.

125. Hopkins J, et al: Cryotherapy and transcutaneous electric neuromuscular stimulation decrease arthrogenic muscle inhibition of the vastus medialis after knee joint effusion. J Athl Train 37(1):25-31, 2002.

126. Jarit GJ, et al: The effects of home interferential therapy on postoperative pain, edema, and range of motion of the knee. Clin J Sport Med 13(1):16-20, 2003.

127. Knight KL: Cryotherapy in sport injury management, Champaign, Ill, 1995, Human Kinetics.

128. Barber FA: A comparison of crushed ice and continuous flow cold therapy. Am J Knee Surg 13(2):97-101, 2000.

129. Schröder D, Pässler HH: Combination of cold and compression after knee surgery: A prospective randomized study. Knee Surg Sports Traumatol Arthrosc 2(3):158-165, 1994.

130. Cosgarea AJ, Sebastianelli WJ, DeHaven KE: Prevention of arthrofibrosis after anterior cruciate ligament reconstruction using the central third patellar tendon autograft. Am J Sports Med 23(1):87, 1995.

131. Noyes FR, et al: Prevention of permanent arthrofibrosis after anterior cruciate ligament reconstruction alone or combined with associated procedures: A prospective study in 443 knees. Knee Surg Sports Traumatol Arthrosc 8:196-206, 2000.

132. Melegati G, et al: The role of the rehabilitation brace in restoring knee extension after anterior cruciate ligament reconstruction: A prospective controlled study. Knee Surg Sports Traumatol Arthrosc 11:322-326, 2003.

133. Mikkelsen C, et al: Can a post-operative brace in slight hyperextension prevent extension deficit after anterior cruciate ligament reconstruction? A prospective randomized study. Knee Surg Sports Traumatol Arthrosc 11:318-321, 2003.

134. Mangine RE, Noyes FR, DeMaio M: Minimal protection program: Advanced weight bearing and range of motion after ACL reconstruction—weeks 1-5. Orthopedics 15(4):504, 1992.

135. Noyes FR, Barber-Westin SD: Revision anterior cruciate ligament surgery: Experience from Cincinnati. Clin Orthop Relat Res 325:116, 1996.

136. Shelbourne KD, et al: Ligament stability two to six years after anterior cruciate ligament reconstruction with autogenous patellar tendon graft and participation in accelerated rehabilitation program. Am J Sports Med 23(5):575, 1995.

137. Wilk KE, Andrews JR: Current concepts in the treatment of anterior cruciate ligament disruption. J Orthop Sports Phys Ther 15(6):279, 1992.

138. Wilk KE, Reinold MM, Hooks TR: Recent advances in the rehabilitation of isolated and combined anterior cruciate ligament injuries. Orthop Clin North Am 34(1):107-137, 2003.

139. Allum R: Aspects of current management, complications of arthroscopic reconstruction of the anterior cruciate ligament. J Bone Joint Surg Br 85-B:12-16, 2003.

140. Beynnon B, et al: Treatment of anterior cruciate ligament injuries. Part I. Am J Sports Med 33:1579-1602, 2005.

141. Beynnon B, et al: Treatment of anterior cruciate ligament injuries. Part II. Am J Sports Med 33:1751-1767, 2005.

142. Cascio B, Cult L, Cosgarea A: Return to play after anterior cruciate ligament reconstruction. Clin Sports Med 23:395-408, 2004.

143. Gale T, Richmond J: Bone patellar tendon bone anterior cruciate ligament reconstruction. Tech Knee Surg 5:72-79, 2006.

144. McCarty L, Bach B: Rehabilitation after patellar tendon autograft anterior cruciate ligament reconstruction. Tech Orthop 20:439-451, 2005.

145. Potter N: Complications and treatment during rehabilitation after anterior cruciate ligament reconstruction. Oper Tech Sports Med 14:50-58, 2006.

146. Richmond JC, Gladstone J, MacGillivray J: Continuous passive motion after arthroscopically assisted anterior cruciate ligament reconstruction: Comparison of short versus long-term use. Arthroscopy 7(1):39, 1991.

147. Gaspar L, Farkas C, Szepeski K: Therapeutic value of continuous passive motion after anterior cruciate ligament replacement. Acta Chir Hung 36(1-4):104-105, 1997.

148. Rosen MA, Jackson DW, Atwell EA: The efficacy of continuous passive motion in the rehabilitation of anterior cruciate ligament reconstruction. Am J Sports Med 20(2):122-127, 1992.

149. Shaw T, Williams MT, Chipchase LS: Do early quadriceps exercises affect the outcome of ACL reconstruction? A randomized controlled trial. Aust J Physiother 51(1):9-17, 2005.

150. Beutler AI, et al: Electromyographic analysis of single-leg, closed chain exercises: Implications for rehabilitation after anterior cruciate ligament reconstruction. J Athl Train 37(1):13-18, 2002.

151. Bynum EB, Barrack RL, Alexander AH: Open versus closed chain kinetic exercises after anterior cruciate ligament reconstruction: A prospective randomized study. Am J Sports Med 23(4):401-406, 1995.

152. Jansson KA, et al: A prospective randomized study of patellar versus hamstring tendon autografts for anterior cruciate ligament reconstruction. Am J Sports Med 31(1):12-18, 2003.

153. Palmitier RA, et al: Kinetic chain exercise in knee rehabilitation. Sports Med 11(6):402-413, 1991.

154. Panni AS, et al: Clinical and radiographic results of ACL reconstruction: A 5- to 7-year follow-up study of outside-in versus inside-out reconstruction techniques. Knee Surg Sports Tramatol Arthrosc 9(2):77-85, 2001.

155. Pinczewski LA, et al: A five-year comparison of patellar tendon versus four-strand hamstring tendon autograft for arthroscopic reconstruction of the anterior cruciate ligament. Am J Sports Med 30(4):523-536, 2002.

156. Steinkamp LA, et al: Biomechanical considerations in patellofemoral joint rehabilitation. Am J Sports Med 21:438-444, 1993.

157. Fitzgerald GK: Open versus closed kinetic chain exercises: Issues in rehabilitation after anterior cruciate ligament reconstructive surgery. Phys Ther 77(12):1747, 1997.

158. Beynnon BD, Johnson RJ: Anterior cruciate ligament injury rehabilitation in athletes: Biomechanical considerations. Sports Med 22(1): 54-64, 1996.

159. Mikkelsen C, Werner S, Eriksson E: Closed kinetic chain alone compared to combined open and closed kinetic chain exercises for quadriceps strengthening after anterior cruciate ligament reconstruction with respect to return to sports: A prospective matched follow-up study. Knee Surg Sports Traumatol Arthrosc 8(6):337-342, 2000.

160. Morrissey MC, et al: Effects of open versus closed kinetic chain training on knee laxity in the early period after anterior cruciate ligament reconstruction. Knee Surg Sports Traumatol Arthrosc 8(6):343-348, 2000.

161. Beynnon et al: Beynnon BD, Fleming BC. Anterior cruciate ligament strain in-vivo: A review of previous work. J Biomech 31:519-525, 1998.

162. Fu FH, Schulte KR: Anterior cruciate ligament surgery 1996: State of the art? Clin Orthop Relat Res 325:19, 1996.

163. Heijne A, Werner S: Early versus late start of open kinetic chain quadriceps exercises after ACL reconstruction with patellar tendon or hamstring grafts: A prospective randomized outcome study. Knee Surg Sports Traumatol Arthrosc 15:402-414, 2007.

164. Snyder-Mackler L, et al: Strength of the quadriceps femoris muscle and functional recovery after reconstruction of the anterior cruciate ligament: A prospective randomized clinical trial of electrical stimulation. J Bone Joint Surg Am 77:1166-1173, 1995.

165. Delitto A, et al: Electrical stimulation versus voluntary exercise in strengthening thigh musculature after anterior cruciate ligament surgery. Phys Ther 68:660-663, 2000.

166. Snyder-Mackler L, et al: Use of electrical stimulation to enhance recovery of quadriceps femoris muscle force production in patients following anterior cruciate ligament reconstruction. Phys Ther 74:901-907, 1994.

167. Fitzgerald GK, Piva SR, Irrgang JJ: A modified neuromuscular electrical stimulation protocol for quadriceps strength training following anterior cruciate ligament reconstruction. J Orthop Sports Phys Ther 33(9):492-501, 2003.

168. Ratamess NA, et al: American College of Sports Medicine position stand: Progression models in resistance training for healthy adults. Med Sci Sports Exerc 41(3):687-708, 2009.

169. Kraemer WL, et al: Progression models in resistance training for healthy adults. Med Sci Sports Exerc 34:364-380, 2002.

170. Parker MC: Biomechanical and histological concepts in the rehabilitation of patient with anterior cruciate ligament reconstruction. JOSPT 20(1):44-50, 1994.

171. West RV, Harner CD: Graft selection in anterior cruciate ligament reconstruction. J Am Acad Orthop Surg 13:197-207, 2005.

172. Rodeo SA, et al: Tendon-healing in a bone tunnel: A biomechanical and histological study in the dog. J Bone Joint Surg Am 75:1795-1803, 1993.

173. Gerber JP, et al: Effects of early progressive eccentric exercise on muscle size and function after anterior cruciate ligament reconstruction: A 1-year follow-up study of a randomized clinical trial. Phys Ther 89:51-59, 2009.

174. Risberg MA, et al: Design and implementation of a neuromuscular training program following anterior cruciate ligament reconstruction. JOSPT 31(11):620-631, 2001.

175. Beard DJ, Dodd CA, Simpson AH: Proprioception enhancement for anterior cruciate ligament deficiency: A prospective randomized trial of two physiotherapy regimes. J Bone Joint Surg Br 76:654-659, 1994.

176. Fitzgerald GK, Axe MJ, Snyder-Mackler L: The efficacy of perturbation training in nonoperative anterior cruciate ligament rehabilitation programs for physically active individuals. Phys Ther 80:128-140 2000.

177. Ihara H, Nakayama A: Dynamic joint control training for knee ligament injuries. Am J Sports Med 14:309-315, 1986.

178. Risberg MA, et al: Neuromuscular training versus strength training during first 6 months after anterior cruciate ligament reconstruction: A randomized clinical trial. Phys Ther 87(6):737-750, 2007.

179. Risberg MA, Holm I: The long-term effect of 2 postoperative rehabilitation programs after anterior cruciate ligament reconstruction: A randomized controlled clinical trial with 2 years of follow-up. Am J Sports Med 37(10):1958-1966, 2009.

180. Fitzgerald GK, Axe MJ, Snyder-Mackler, L: Proposed practice guidelines for nonoperative anterior cruciate ligament rehabilitation of physically active individuals. JOSPT 30(4):194-203, 2000.

181. Knott M, Voss DE: Techniques for facilitation. In Knott M, Voss DE, editors. Proprioceptive neuromuscular facilitation: Patterns and techniques, ed 2, Hagerstown, Md, 1968, Harper & Row.

182. Gray GW: Lower extremity functional profile. Adrian, Mich, 1995, Winn Marketing.

183. Voight ML, Hoogenboom BJ, Cook G: The chop and lift reconsidered: Integrating neuromuscular principles into orthopedic and sports rehabilitation. NAJSPT 3(3):151-159, 2008.

184. West RV, Harner CD: Graft selection in anterior cruciate ligament reconstruction. J Am Acad Orthop Surg 13:197-207, 2005.

185. Neeter C, et al: Development of a strength test battery for evaluating leg muscle power after anterior cruciate ligament injury and reconstruction. Knee Surg Sports Traumatol Arthrosc 14:571-580, 2006.

186. Myer GD, et al: Rehabilitation after anterior cruciate ligament reconstruction: Criteria-based progression through the return-to-sport phase. JOSPT 36(6):385-402, 2006.

187. van Grinsven S, et al: Evidence-based rehabilitation following anterior cruciate ligament reconstruction. Knee Surg Sports Traumatol Arthrosc 18(8):1128-1144, 2010.

188. Grace TG, et al: Isokinetic muscle imbalance and knee-joint injuries. J Bone Joint Surg Am 66:734, 1984.

189. DeMaio M, Noyes FR, Mangine RE: Principles for aggressive rehabilitation after reconstruction of the anterior cruciate ligament: Sports medicine rehabilitation series. Orthopedics 15(3):385, 1992.

190. Juris PM, et al: A dynamic test of lower extremity function following anterior cruciate ligament reconstruction and rehabilitation. J Orthop Sports Phys Ther 26(4):184, 1997.

191. Mangine RE, Noyes FR: Rehabilitation of the allograft reconstruction. J Orthop Sports Phys Ther 15(6):294, 1992.

192. Myer GD, Ford KR, Hewett TE: Rationale and clinical techniques for anterior cruciate ligament injury prevention among female athletes. J Athl Train 39:352-364, 2004.

193. Lephart SM, et al: Gender differences in strength and lower extremity kinematics during landing. Clin Orthop Relat Res (401):162-169, 2002.

194. Brent JL, et al: Reliability of single leg landings on a portable force platform. Med Sci Sports Exerc 37:400, 2005.

195. Decker MJ, et al: Landing adaptations after ACL reconstruction. Med Sci Sports Exerc 34:1408-1413, 2002.

196. Paterno, MV, et al: Biomechanical limb asymmetries in female athletes 2 years following ACL reconstruction. J Orthop Sports Phys Ther 35:A75, 2005.

197. Cheatham SA, Johnson DL: Anatomic revision: ACL reconstruction. Sports Med Arthrosc 18(1):33-39, 2010.

198. Padua DA, et al: Predictors of knee valgus angle during a jump-landing task. Med Sci Sports Exerc 37:S398, 2005.

199. Knapik JJ, et al: Preseason strength and flexibility imbalances associated with athletic injuries in female collegiate athletes. Am J Sports Med 19:76-81, 1991.

200. Fitzgerald GK, Axe MJ, Snyder-Mackler L: A decision-making scheme for returning patients to high-level activity with nonoperative treatment after anterior cruciate ligament rupture. Knee Surg Sports Traumatol Arthrosc 8:76-82, 2000.

201. Carson EW, et al: Revision anterior cruciate ligament reconstruction: Etiology of failures and clinical results. J Knee Surg 17(3):127-132, 2004.

202. Kartus J, et al: Complications following arthroscopic anterior cruciate ligament reconstruction: A 2-5-year follow-up of 604 patients with special emphasis on anterior knee pain. Knee Surg Sports Traumatol Arthrosc 7(1):2-8, 1999.

203. McHugh MP, et al: Preoperative indicators of motion loss and weakness following anterior cruciate ligament reconstruction. J Orthop Sports Phys Ther 27(6):407-411, 1998.

204. Wilk KE, Andrews JR, Clancy WG: Quadriceps muscular strength after removal of the central third patellar tendon for contralateral anterior cruciate ligament reconstruction surgery: A case study. J Orthop Sports Phys Ther 18(6):692, 1993.

205. Howell SM, Taylor MA: Failure of reconstruction of the anterior cruciate ligament due to impingement by the intercondylar roof. J Bone Joint Surg 75A:1044, 1993.

206. Paulos LE, et al: Infrapatellar contracture syndrome: An unrecognized cause of knee stiffness with patella entrapment and patella infera. Am J Sports Med 15:331, 1987.

207. Biggs A, Shelbourne, KD: Use of knee extension device during rehabilitation of a patient with type 3 arthrofibrosis after ACL reconstruction. N Am J Sports Phys Ther 1(3):124-131, 2006.

208. Nuccion SL, Hame SL: A symptomatic cyclops lesion 4 years after anterior cruciate ligament reconstruction. Arthroscopy 17(2):E8, 2001.

209. Tonin M, et al: Progressive loss of knee extension after injury: Cyclops syndrome due to a lesion of the anterior cruciate ligament. Am J Sports Med 29(5):545-549, 2001.

210. Brownstein B, Bronner S: Patella fractures associated with accelerated ACL rehabilitation in patients with autogenous patella tendon reconstructions. J Orthop Sports Phys Ther 26(3):168, 1997.

211. Boland AL: Rehabilitation of the injured athlete. In Strauss RH, editor: Sports medicine and physiology, Philadelphia, 1979, Saunders.

CHAPTER 23

Arthroscopic Lateral Retinaculum Release

Daniel A. Farwell, Andrew A. Brooks

SURGICAL INDICATIONS AND CONSIDERATIONS

While surgical treatment (lateral patellar retinacular release) for maltracking of the patella has shown promising results,[1] it is becoming less popular as an isolated procedure.[2] The surgery appears less successful in patients that have severe chondromalacia, patella instability, or evidence of trochlear dysplasia.[3-5] Latterman and associates[6] state that "isolated lateral retinacular release has little or no role in the treatment of acute or recurrent patella instability. This procedure should be reserved for the few patients with a clearly identified lateral patella compression syndrome in presence of a tight lateral retinaculum and clearly discernable lateral retinacular pain." Currently it appears that lateral patellar retinacular release is usually performed as an adjunct to other knee surgeries where patellofemoral misalignment is an issue.[6] This chapter will deal with patellofemoral rehabilitation that should be considered an adjunct to any knee surgery where patella pain is an issue.

Adaptation resulting from chronic compression in the patellofemoral joint can lead to significant arthrosis in a wide variety of patients, both young and old. Pain, attributed to increased patellofemoral compression, occurs in different aspects of the joint, but the most common site is along the lateral aspect. This patellofemoral pain can originate from mechanical malalignment, the static or dynamic soft tissue stabilizers, or increased load placed across the joint as a result of various activities.[7] Symptoms may include diffuse aches and pains that are exacerbated by stair climbing or prolonged sitting (i.e., flexion of the knees). Crepitus and mild effusion are often associated with patellofemoral arthralgia. Although complaints of "giving way" or collapse are more often linked with ligamentous instability, these symptoms also can be associated with patellofemoral pain. Patients may even complain of joint pain and "locking" when they are experiencing poor patella stabilization during flexion of the knee.

In examining the way lateral retinacular release procedures may affect the arthrokinematics of the patellofemoral joint, the focus should be on the relationship between patella tilt compression and associated tightness in the lateral retinaculum. The function of the patella is to increase the lever of the quadriceps muscle, thus increasing its mechanical advantage. For functional and efficient knee motion, the patella must be aligned so that it can travel in the trochlear groove of the femur. The ability of the patella to track properly depends on the bony configuration of the trochlear groove and the balance of forces of the connective tissue surrounding the joint.

Weakness and stiffness from the hip are factors that appear to influence poor patella alignment (gluteus medius weakness and iliotibial band [ITB] tension). Tensor fascia latae and gluteus maximus fibers combine to form a very thick, fibrous structure that attaches distally into the lateral tibial tubercle (Gerdy tubercle).[8] The ITB slips into the lateral border of the patella, which interdigitates with the superficial and deep fibers of the lateral retinaculum. This design often leads to excessive compression over the lateral condyle and lateral border of the patella during dynamic activity.

Tilt compression is a clinical radiographic condition of the patellofemoral joint that can lead to retinacular strain (i.e., peripatellar effect) and excessive lateral pressure syndrome (i.e., articular effect).[9] A case can definitely be made for a cause-and-effect relationship between tilt compression and retinacular strain. Chronic patella tilting and associated retinacular shortening cannot only produce significant lateral facet overload but also a resultant deficiency in medial contact pressure. This tilt compression syndrome may have simple soft tissue pain related to the shortening of the lateral retinacular tissue. If left untreated, then histologic studies of painful retinacular biopsies may reveal degenerative fibroneuromas within the lateral retinaculum of patients with chronic patellofemoral malalignment.[10] Excessive lateral pressure syndrome results from chronic lateral patella tilt, adaptive lateral retinacular shortening, and resultant chronic imbalance of facet loads. It is prevalent in active, middle-aged adults. In younger patient populations, excessive lateral pressure during growth and development can alter the shape and formation of both the patella and trochlea.[10]

Nonoperative treatment of patella tilt should focus on mobilization of tight quadriceps muscles and the lateral retinaculum. Patellofemoral taping, bracing, and antiinflammatory medications also are quite helpful. Gait deviation and excessive foot pronation should be corrected to eliminate possible secondary influences on patellofemoral malalignment.[7] The use of resistant weight training or isokinetic exercise (in conjunction with patella taping) can be beneficial in building quadriceps muscle strength.[11]

Patellofemoral Taping

McConnell patellofemoral taping has become a useful technique in the conservative (nonsurgical) rehabilitation of patellofemoral pain; it can also benefit patients after surgical lateral release as well. Controversy exists as to the mechanism behind the pain relief from taping. Whether via cutaneous stimulation, enhancement of patellofemoral ligaments, or improved vastus medialis oblique (VMO) timing, clinically we know that patellofemoral pain can be reduced or eliminated via its appropriate application.[12,13]

Patellar taping has been shown to increase vasti muscle activity[14,15] and may enhance knee joint proprioception after surgery.[16] The McConnell patellofemoral program emphasizes closed-chain exercises to correct patella glide (Fig. 23-1), tilt (Fig. 23-2), and rotation, (Fig. 23-3) and allows for pain-free rehabilitation. The patient is evaluated dynamically during a functional activity such as walking, stepping down, or squatting. According to Maitland,[17] "The aim of examining movements is to find one or more comparable signs in an appropriate joint or joints." These comparable signs, or reassessment signs, are reevaluated after each patella correction to determine the effectiveness of the treatment. After an assessment of patella orientation, a specifically designed tape is used to correct for each patella orientation. The patellofemoral joint is principally a soft tissue joint, which suggests that it can be adjusted through appropriate mechanical means (i.e., physical therapy). Two primary components (glide and tilt) may be present either statically or dynamically. Patella orientation varies among patients and even from left to right extremities.

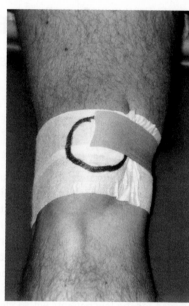

Fig. 23-2 Patella tilt. Place the tape on the medial superior half of the patella. Pull the tape medially to lift the lateral border. Lift the soft tissue over the medial femoral condyle toward the patella to ensure a more secure fixation.

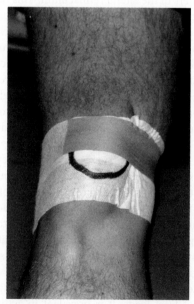

Fig. 23-1 Patella glide. Place a piece of tape on the superior half of the lateral border of the patella and pull the tape medially. Lift the soft tissue over the medial femoral condyle toward the patella to ensure a more secure fixation and less tape slippage.

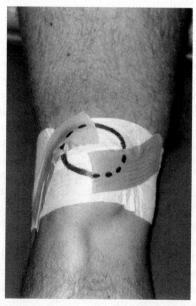

Fig. 23-3 Patella rotation. Place a piece of tape on the inferior-medial quarter of the patella and perform an upward rotation movement of the patella. Place another piece of tape on the superior-lateral half of the patella and perform a downward rotation movement of the patella.

Glide Component

The amount of glide correction depends on the tightness of the structures and the relative amount of activity in the entire quadriceps musculature. The corrective procedure involves securing the edge of the tape over the lateral border of the patella and pulling or gliding the patella more medially. Although this technique is useful for most patellofemoral pain, it is not often used in the postoperative care of patients recovering from lateral retinacular release (see Fig. 23-1).

Tilt Component

Tilt correction is quite often used to stretch the deep retinacular fibers along the lateral borders of the knee. Increased tension in the lateral retinaculum along with a tight ITB (which inserts into the lateral retinaculum) can produce a lateral "dipping," or tilt, of the lateral border of the patella (see Fig. 23-2).

When focusing on patients recovering from lateral retinacular release, the physical therapist (PT) should remember that the very tissues these taping techniques address have been surgically released. Although patella orientations have definitely been altered in patients after surgical release, muscle recruitment patterns and joint loading characteristics that may have contributed to the symptoms are still present.

McConnell taping procedures produce improved joint loading and allow the patient to return to a more active, pain-free lifestyle when used in conjunction with closed-chain functional exercises.[18,19]

Although conservative management remains the cornerstone of treatment for patients with anterior knee pain, some patients will not respond and continue to have pain and functional disability. If conservative (nonsurgical) treatment is unsuccessful in providing the patient with appropriate pain relief and function, then surgical intervention should be considered.[20]

In addition to subjective complaints and functional limitations, other indications for surgery include dislocation, subluxation, and failure of previous surgery with or without medial patella position.

Operative procedures that modify patella mechanics are most successful in treating patients with patella articular cartilage lesions. Lateral release procedures should ultimately produce a mechanical benefit to the patient, such as relieving documented tilt.[21]

SURGICAL PROCEDURE

Review of the literature suggests strict indications for lateral release[9]:

1. Chronic anterior knee pain despite a trial of a nonoperative program for at least 3 months
2. Minimal or no chondrosis (Outerbridge grade 2 or less)
3. A normal Q angle
4. A tight or tender lateral retinaculum with clinically and radiographically documented lateral patella tilt

Results may be disappointing for lateral release in the presence of the following conditions:

1. Patellofemoral pain syndrome (anterior knee pain)
2. Advanced patellofemoral arthritis
3. A Q angle greater than 20°

Patients with instability may require medial retinacular imbrication or a distal realignment in addition to an isolated lateral release.

The Southern California Orthopedic Institute (SCOI) technique of arthroscopic lateral release is performed in the supine position without the use of a leg holder; the tourniquet is inflated only when necessary. The procedure is performed with the arthroscope in the anteromedial portal. Routine arthroscopic fluid is used. An 18-gauge spinal needle is inserted at the superior pole of the patella and is used as a marker for the proximal extent of the release. The needle must be withdrawn as the electrosurgical electrode approaches it. With experience, the surgeon can omit the needle marker. The electrosurgical lateral release electrode is inserted through the inferior anterolateral portal using a plastic cannula to protect the skin. The procedure is performed with the generator setting at approximately 10 to 12 W of power. With the patient's knee extended, the surgeon performs the release approximately 1 cm from the patella edge, progressing from distal to proximal using the cutting mode. The deep and superficial retinaculum, as well as the lateral patellotibial ligament, are released under direct visualization until subcutaneous fat is exposed. The extent of the proximal release is only to the deforming tight structures and should never extend beyond the superior pole of the patella.

An incomplete release is often secondary to inadequate release of the patellotibial ligament. Again, the tourniquet is not inflated during the procedure, and vessels are coagulated as they are encountered. An adequate release is confirmed by the ability to evert the patella 60°. After the release, the knee is passively moved through a range of motion (ROM) and correction of lateral overhang during knee flexion is confirmed. The arthroscope should be switched back to the accessory superolateral portal for this assessment. Usual postoperative dressings are applied after the arthroscopic procedure (sterile dressings and an absorbent pad held in place by an elastic toe-to-groin support stocking previously measured for the patient).

Postoperative rehabilitation includes muscle strengthening and ROM exercises the day of surgery, including quadriceps sets and straight leg raising. The patient continues to do these exercises at home the night of surgery and is given weight bearing as tolerated status with crutches immediately. Crutches are discontinued when adequate quadriceps muscle control has been obtained and patients can walk safely. The vast majority of patients use their crutches for less than 7 days, although some may need them for 2 to 3 weeks depending on quadriceps control.

The SCOI experience with arthroscopic lateral retinaculum release (ALRR) has been reported previously.[22] The researchers monitored 39 patients with a history of recurrent patella subluxation or dislocation in 45 knees for an average of 28 months and noted good to excellent results in 76% of patients. Similar experiences with ALRR have been reported in the literature, with favorable results in 60% to 85% of cases.[23] Arthroscopic treatment compares favorably with open realignment and has a lower complication rate. No postoperative hemarthrosis occurred in the SCOI series; hemarthrosis is the main complication reported in the literature, occurring in 2% to 42% of cases. Small's review[24] of 194 cases of ALRR, performed by 21 arthroscopic surgeons, found hemarthrosis associated with 89% of the 4.6% total complications. Careful coagulation of vessels without an inflated tourniquet can reduce hemarthrosis. If strict criteria are met and proper surgical techniques are used, then a consistent result can be obtained with these patients.

The complexity of the patellofemoral articulation and its associated disorders are evident by the significant body of literature on the subject and the abundant surgical procedures involving the joint. A thorough clinical evaluation, including history and physical and radiographic examination, helps to clarify the diagnosis of patellofemoral disorder. Use of the arthroscope for the electrosurgical lateral release is an effective component in the armament of knee surgeons for patients with persistently symptomatic patellofemoral disorders who meet the surgical indications described.

THERAPY GUIDELINES FOR REHABILITATION

Phase I (Acute Phase)

TIME: 1 to 2 weeks after surgery
GOALS: Decrease pain, manage edema, increase weight-bearing activities, facilitate quality quadriceps contraction (Table 23-1)

After knee surgery the goal of rehabilitation is to prevent loss of muscle strength, endurance, flexibility, and proprioception. These issues often are difficult to address immediately after lateral release. The procedure is often associated with significant hemarthrosis resulting from sacrifice of the lateral geniculate artery.[25] Therefore the acute phase of treatment should focus on managing edema and decreasing pain. The use of vasopneumatic compression, electrical stimulation, ice, and intermittent elevation of the limb can assist in decreasing the patient's swelling.

Other strategies to both decrease joint effusion and begin restoring joint mobility include grade II (mobilizations performed shy of resistance in an effort to decrease pain)[26] patella mobilizations, active calf pumping exercises, and the application of McConnell taping[27] specific to acute lateral release rehabilitation (Fig. 23-4). This procedure places a very mild tilt on the patella, providing a small amount of length to the repair site or lateral retinacular tissue. The tape maintains the new alignment, preventing adhesions that may bind down the released retinaculum during tissue healing. Other taping procedures such as unloading the lateral soft tissue may assist in decreasing pain and discomfort during exercise (Fig. 23-5). This procedure is beneficial in decreasing joint effusion and adds joint stability. It is often used in combination with a patella tilt correction.

Phase II (Subacute Phase)

TIME: 3 to 4 weeks after surgery
GOALS: Continue to manage edema and pain, improve sit-to-stand transfer activities, improve strength and stability of the patellofemoral joint, progress functional training to return activity to previous levels (Table 23-2)

TABLE 23-1 Lateral Retinaculum Release

Rehabilitation Phase	Criteria to Progress to This Phase	Anticipated Impairments and Functional Limitations	Intervention	Goal	Rationale
Phase I Postoperative 1-2 wk	• Postoperative	• Postoperative pain • Postoperative edema • Gait deviations • Limited tolerance to weight-bearing activities • Limited range of motion • Limited strength	• Ice • Vasopneumatic compression • Grade II patella mobilization • Neuromuscular stimulation • Patellar taping • Knee AROM—ankle pumps • Knee PROM—hamstring and iliotibial band stretches • Isometrics—quadriceps/hamstring sets, quadriceps sets at 20°-30° • Home exercises (refer to Suggested Home Maintenance Box)	• Decrease pain • Manage edema • Decrease gait deviations • Increase tolerance to weight-bearing activities • ROM 0°-135° • Quality contraction of the quadriceps	• Decrease edema and pain • Increase neuromuscular coordination with muscle contraction • Restore joint mechanics • Improve joint mobility and stability • Prevent adhesions • Initiate volitional muscle control and increase strength • Increase patient self-management

AROM, Active range of motion; *PROM,* passive range of motion.

As the patient's swelling and pain subside (1 to 2 weeks), the patient moves into a subacute phase. During this phase a more direct and aggressive type of treatment is implemented for the knee. Heat modalities (i.e., moist heat, ultrasound) are used to assist in the absorption and removal of waste products within the joint. Their influence on the cardiovascular system produces increased capillary permeability and vasodilation. The vasodilation brings increased oxygen and nutrients to the knee, which assist in the healing and repairing of the surgically altered tissue.[28] Increased blood flow produces increased capillary hydrostatic pressure. Therefore heat modalities can be very beneficial at this stage of rehabilitation, but only if the patient's effusion is

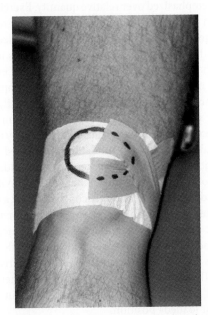

Fig. 23-4 Stabilization taping. After surgery the lateral tissue is often hypersensitive to any type of stretching or pulling. The application of a taping correction for both internal rotation and external rotation results in a low-level patella stabilization that the patient finds much easier to tolerate. Taping enables the patient to perform normal knee flexion-extension activity without pain or with less pain. It also decreases effusion.

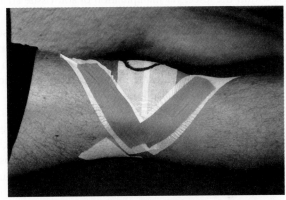

Fig. 23-5 Unloading of lateral soft tissue structures. Taping allows for a decrease in the tension produced over the surgical repair site by inhibiting the effective pull from the ITB and vastus lateralis. Unloading the lateral retinaculum may significantly reduce the patient's symptoms. Tape from the posterior aspect of the lateral joint line down to the tibial tubercle and from the posterior lateral joint line to the distal midthigh (approximately 2 to 3 inches above the patella). The tissue inside the tape should be pulled toward the joint line as you pull and secure the tape. The tape should look like a wide V lateral to the knee and should not inhibit active motion.

TABLE 23-2 Lateral Retinaculum Release

Rehabilitation Phase	Criteria to Progress to This Phase	Anticipated Impairments and Functional Limitations	Intervention	Goal	Rationale
Phase II Postoperative 3-4 wk	• Incision healed • Edema controlled • Full weight bearing, although full ROM and strength may be deficient	• Pain with squatting and sit-to-stand • Gait deviations • Limited stability of patellofemoral joint • Limited tolerance (if any) to prolonged walking, standing, running, or jumping	Continuation of interventions from phase I, progressed as indicated: • Moist heat and ultrasound (if edema is under control) • Soft tissue mobilization when pain is significantly diminished on palpation • Neuromuscular stimulation • Closed-chain exercises, lunges, standing wall slides, and step-downs (see Figs. 23-6 to 23-8) • Biofeedback in conjunction with exercises • Patellofemoral taping (refer to Patellofemoral Tape-Weaning Protocol) • Home exercises	• Achieve full ROM • Decrease pain • Increase mobility • Increase strength • Sit-to-stand without pain • Decrease gait deviations • Increase stability of patellofemoral joint • Tape only for skill-specific activity	• Decrease swelling and pain • Increase neuromuscular coordination with muscle contraction • Restore joint mechanics • Functional strengthening using closed-chain exercises • Biofeedback with exercise to improve tonic activity of vastus medialis oblique • Improve joint mobility and stability • Increase patient self-management

ROM, Range of motion.

under control. If the patient's effusion is displacing the patella from the trochlear groove or the patient cannot perform active isometric quadriceps contractions, then the joint effusion is significant.

Heat applications may be contraindicated until edema is no longer a concern. Soft tissue mobilization can be beneficial at this stage to increase circulation, decrease swelling, mobilize healing tissue, and decrease hypersensitivity in the knee joint.[10] Deep massage can assist in the reabsorption of fluid within the knee, yet manipulation of soft tissue structures over the lateral aspect of the knee should be avoided to prevent aggravation of the trauma from surgery. **Soft tissue mobilization should not be initiated in the area of lateral structures before the tissues have begun to heal (1 to 2 weeks) and pain is significantly diminished on palpation of the entire patellofemoral joint.**

Electrical stimulation (ES) is used to assist in activation of the quadriceps muscle. Specific benefits include decreasing joint edema, increasing local blood flow to the muscle, promoting increased muscle tone, and controlling postoperative pain.[29,30] Electricity also can be used to retard quadriceps atrophy, which results from immobilization or inhibition of the muscle.[31] When used in combination with active isometric and isotonic exercises, ES retrains transposed muscles and promotes muscle awareness in regaining volitional muscle control postoperatively.[28]

Experiments conducted by scientists in the USSR in the 1970s examined the possibility of producing greater intensity of muscle contraction with electrical current. Some studies have found the use of ES during immobilization produces a significant increase in muscle strength.[24,27] By using ES early in the rehabilitative process, PTs can prevent the loss of oxidative capacity, thus shortening postoperative rehabilitation and conditioning time and allowing a more rapid return to functional activities.[32] Although ES can be of great benefit, it should not be used as a replacement for postoperative rehabilitation and strengthening exercise programs.[33]

In summary, the use of modalities is beneficial in aiding healing by decreasing acute reactions and altering blood flow, which may provide low-level analgesic effects.[29,34] Understanding the action of these modalities and the way they influence healing is important in predicting their usefulness and appropriateness in the rehabilitation of patients after lateral retinacular release.

Strengthening

Strengthening of the entire lower kinetic chain is the goal in most patients suffering from anterior knee pain. This goal is no different for patients after lateral retinacular release. Although special attention is paid to the quadriceps muscle, particularly the VMO, it is the balanced contraction in the vasti group as a whole that is the ultimate goal. Richardson[20] examined the activity level of the quadriceps, specifically the VMO, to better understand the activation patterns of the quadriceps during dynamic motion. The quadriceps were monitored with surface electromyography through a full arc of motion in both patients suffering from patellofemoral pain and normal patients. The VMO produced a tonic

(constant) pattern of activation throughout a full (0° to 135°) arc of motion in pain-free patients; a phasic (intermittent) activity pattern was observed in patients with patellofemoral pain. A consistent activation of the entire quadriceps is the goal in quadriceps strengthening. Quality of motion should be emphasized over relative quantity. Exercise beyond 20° flexion (20° to 135°) increases the surface area of contact and gives better stability within the trochlear groove. Although the development of muscle strength is important, it is not the only goal of rehabilitation. Muscle endurance, flexibility, and the development of correct proprioceptive loading through the entire lower extremity (LE) must be addressed as well. These goals can be accomplished in patients recovering from surgical lateral release by protecting the surgical repair through modalities that speed the tissue repair process and protective taping that adds stability and promotes early functional rehabilitation. Wittingham, Palmer, and Macmillan[35] recently concluded that a combination of patellar taping and exercise was superior to the use of exercise alone. Early quadriceps activation includes isometric quadriceps sets in varying degrees of flexion produced by a proximal load-bearing shift with increased knee flexion.[36] This allows for early muscle strengthening even while joint effusion may still be causing pain in a closed-chain (joint loaded) position.

When effusion and pain have been eliminated for 7 to 14 days, a gradual increase in activity may begin, with cryotherapy being used after activity. During LE rehabilitation, after the patient can stand or load the joint, the emphasis should be on closed-chain activity because of its relevance to function. The goal is to advance the patient toward functional activities and then slowly introduce a patient-specific exercise program. Specific closed-chain exercises allow for the selection and stimulation of the appropriate muscles at the proper time.[37] These factors, combined with gradual muscle inhibition of the antagonist, produce smooth, coordinated loading of the entire LE.

Although McConnell patellofemoral taping is the modality of choice used by the authors of this chapter to bolster stability at the onset of exercise, a variety of braces may be beneficial in supporting the patellofemoral joint after surgery. Almost any elastic, compressive support around the patellofemoral joint produces an improved ability to exercise. The concept of proprioceptive feedback, together with comfort and affordability, makes postoperative McConnell patellofemoral taping or nonspecific bracing of the knee desirable in patients who do not respond to exercise alone.

Phase III (Advanced Phase)

TIME: 5 to 6 weeks after surgery
GOALS: Patient self-manages edema and pain, performs gait without deviations, and has unlimited ambulation (Table 23-3)

By phase III patients should have their pain under control using little if any external support (brace or tape). They may continue to benefit from stretching, patella mobilization, and taping in addition to ice after exercise. However, this phase

TABLE 23-3 Lateral Retinaculum Release

Rehabilitation Phase	Criteria to Progress to This Phase	Anticipated Impairments and Functional Limitations	Intervention	Goal	Rationale
Phase III Postoperative 4-6 wk	• Pain-free during functional activity (sit-to-stand, squat 0°-90°) • Limited tolerance to walking, running, and standing	• Limited endurance with prolonged functional activities • Mild instability of patellofemoral joint during skill-specific exercises • Continued reliance on patellofemoral taping	• Closed-chain and stretching exercises as listed in Tables 23-1 and 23-2 • Patella taping • Patella mobilization • Lunges with weights, increased repetitions and speed with exercises • PREs on leg press • Functional specific activity isokinetic training • Knee flexion and extension 270°-300°/sec, 10 repetitions at each speed is one set (2-10 sets) • Home exercises	• No gait deviations • Good patella stability without taping • Unlimited community ambulation • Leg press body weight • Pain-free with specific activity • Increase strength and velocity of muscle contraction • Patient can self-manage symptoms	• Functional strengthening • Decrease pain with functional activities • Improve joint mechanics • Improve joint mobility and stability • Improve endurance of vastus medialis oblique • Increase strength • Specificity of training and progression to community-based gym program (if appropriate) • Use isokinetic principles of strength training • Discharge patient

PREs, Progressive resistance exercises.

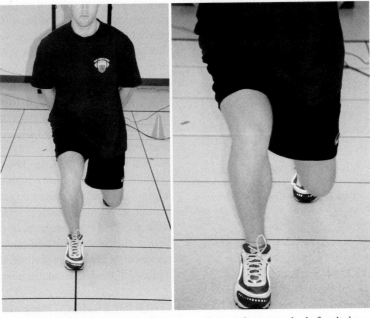

Fig. 23-6 Closed-chain lunge. Instruct the patient to take a "normal" step forward. Have the patient slowly flex the knee to 30° flexion, hold for 3 seconds, and return to 0° extension while maintaining proper postural alignment (i.e., anterosuperior iliac spine over midpatella and second toe). The patient should be able to activate the quadriceps tonically (constantly) during the entire motion.

is designed to take the patient back to the preinjury level of function. Exercises are progressed through specificity of training principles. By breaking down the activity into its core components, the PT can assess patellofemoral and LE function for any deviations or barriers to performance.

Again, any exercise that increases knee pain and/or swelling needs to be modified or discontinued. After further progress has been gained, the therapist can reassess the patient and attempt the exercise again.

Closed kinetic chain progression consists of the following:

1. Lunges with 5 lb weights in a long-stride position (Fig. 23-6)—Patients must activate the quadriceps and hold the contraction from 0° to 30° eccentrically and back to 0° concentrically without stopping, while moving slowly and maintaining proper alignment.
2. Wall slides at various degrees of flexion with 1-minute holds to promote fatigue (Fig. 23-7)—The patient

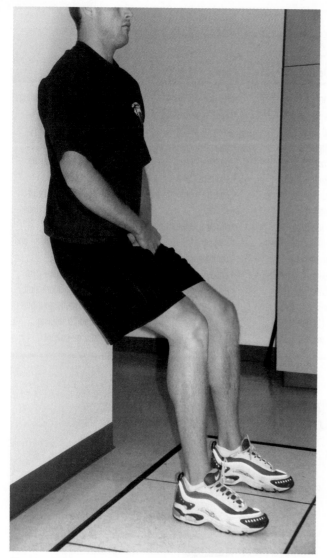

Fig. 23-7 Closed-chain wall slide. This exercise allows the patient to maintain better alignment simply by locking in pelvic tilt. The patient can then move through a particular ROM or the PT can have the patient perform isometric contractions at various ranges of weakness.

should progress from 0° to 45°; if a certain angle in the arc of motion appears weaker, then the patient can perform isometric holds at the angle of weakness.

3. Functional single-limb squats from 0° to 30°—Deep flexion squats can be performed by two different methods. In the first, both LEs are aligned directly below the hips, and bilateral knee flexion is initiated. The patient should maintain proper patella alignment directly over the midfoot. The second method is a shortened stride position with the involved LE forward. The patient initiates the squat until the knee is flexed 90° and then rises back to full extension.

4. Functional double-limb squats with elastic tubing

5. Sit-to-stand at increased speed and repetition—The patient initiates sit-to-stand activity (and stand-to-sit activity) without upper extremity assistance. This exercise can be adjusted from easier to more difficult by lowering the height of the chair.

6. Step-down exercises with an increase in height of step and speed of movement—Proper alignment is crucial, along with slow, controlled movement. The patient must activate the quadriceps before motion is initiated and hold the contraction until heel contact with the opposite leg (Fig. 23-8).

7. Resistive leg press using progressive resistance exercise protocols for weight[38,39]

8. Standing (four-wall) elastic tubing exercises for hip flexion, extension, abduction, and adduction (the involved knee acts as the stabilizing leg)—The LE that anchors the body is the "working" leg. The patient should activate the quadriceps and hold throughout the entire active motion of the opposite leg. This may be performed in terminal extension or 10° to 20° of knee flexion of the involved (stabilizing) leg.

Activity-specific exercises (Fig. 23-9) may include the following: stationary cycle, stair-climbing machine, slide board, and treadmill. The authors of this chapter recommend a 6-week progression to presurgery activity level. Isokinetic exercise is introduced in this phase at a training velocity spectrum protocol between 270° and 300°/sec.[40] The patient performs 10 repetitions at each speed in a ladder progression (50 repetitions equal one set). Patient tolerance for exercise determines the number of sets performed (2 to 10 sets). After patients can perform the exercises with good control of the patellofemoral joint, they are weaned from formal physical therapy and encouraged to continue their home exercise program as appropriate.

Once you have arrived at the decision to move the patient into a home program, it is important to understand how variable the long-term results can be following this procedure. Recent studies describe favorable results (73% to 86%) after 1 year.[41] This same study indicates that the results are far less favorable (29% to 30%) if the follow-up period is extended to 4 or 5 years. Questions exist concerning the appropriateness of an isolated lateral release procedure alleviating the biomechanical symptoms it is designed to address.[42] This evidence underscores the importance in identifying muscle strength and muscle length imbalances in the entire lower limb. Any abnormal LE alignment needs to be addressed in advance of discharge to a self-guided program.

TROUBLESHOOTING

Postural Alignment

A lateral retinacular release procedure produces immediate effects on the patella orientation of the knee, yet the entire lower kinetic chain may still have alignment issues that need to be addressed. When assessing a patient's functional status, the PT should consider equalizing leg lengths, balancing foot posture, restoring normal gait, and regaining appropriate muscle flexibility and strength, which will lead to a restoration of normal posture and balance.[10] By observing static alignment issues, PTs can gather valuable information regarding the way the patient will function dynamically. The interaction of poor alignment measures and quadriceps

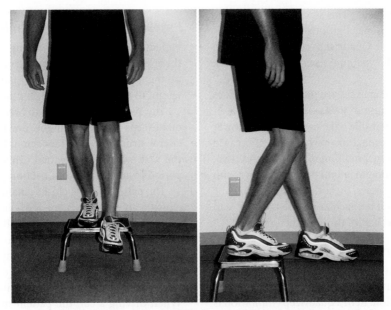

Fig. 23-8 Closed-chain step-down. Patients need to begin on a low-level step (3 to 4 inches) and work up to a standard step (8 inches). Patients must focus on improved alignment. Because the patient is now performing single-limb support activity, he or she should focus on gluteal muscle activation to better stabilize the femur during dynamic activity.

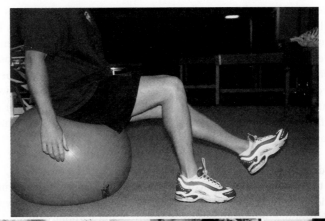

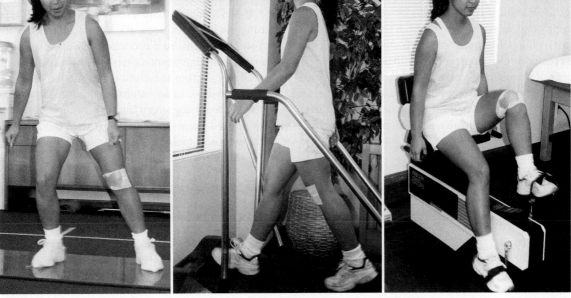

Fig. 23-9 Skill-specific training. After the patient is without pain and has developed a quality contraction that is consistent throughout full knee ROM, a sport- or activity-specific exercise program is needed to aid in the development of an improved loading pattern and promote coordinated balance in patellofemoral mechanics.

contraction has been examined.[43] This study compared static and dynamic patellofemoral malalignment measures in subjects with anterior knee pain. Quadriceps contraction altered the malalignment in both type and severity in more than 50% of cases.

The literature suggests that excessive pronation at the foot is a primary problem because of its association with patellofemoral pain, which inhibits the balance of the entire lower kinetic chain.[7] Increased pronation may lead to increased valgus, compensatory external rotation of the foot and tibia, and a resultant predisposition to lateral patella tracking with dynamic activity.[44] In such cases, orthotic correction may be indicated even after a lateral retinacular release procedure to restore proper loading mechanics through the knee.

Quadriceps Inhibition

Many clinicians tend to use the term quadriceps inhibition as though it were synonymous with quadriceps weakness, which is not an accurate description. Reflex quadriceps inhibition is defined as the inability to perform a quadriceps contraction voluntarily because of direct neurologic suppression.[30,45]

Does true quadriceps inhibition exist? Numerous research articles on the subject describe several mechanisms that could produce a neurogenic influence on voluntary control of the quadriceps.[46,47] The effect of pain on the overall activation of the quadriceps has been examined as a possible cause.[48,49] Effusion also can impair activation of the quadriceps muscle.[50,51] Mechanical receptors within the patellofemoral joint may influence quadriceps function through proprioceptive input.[52,53] Other factors may include training methods, joint position, aging, and even the possible effects of medication.

 Any problem resulting in decreased activation of the quadriceps is detrimental to the rehabilitation process. With full activation of the quadriceps femoris muscle, proper strengthening exercises should produce excellent results. However, if voluntary control is absent or compromised, then atrophy and weakness may result. If this situation persists, then volitional exercise protocols may be ineffective and thus temporarily inappropriate for these patients.

Because of the nature of a lateral retinacular release procedure, pain and especially effusion are quite common after surgery. Therefore any treatment techniques that address pain and swelling will ultimately assist in improved recruitment of the quadriceps femoris muscle.

Patellofemoral Tape-Weaning Protocol

Patients using McConnell taping need to learn how to tape themselves. The tape loosens according to the aggressiveness of the patient's activity. The patient should therefore be taught to tighten the tape when necessary.

The patient only needs to wear tape while training the quadriceps to maintain the newly acquired length in the lateral structures. The tape should be removed at night and the skin should be cleaned. This gives the skin a resting period from the pull and friction produced by the tape.

The patient begins closed-chain exercises when pain and effusion are under control. Early home exercises stress "little bits often," meaning multiple VMO sets or quadriceps contractions are performed throughout the day and are linked with a patient's lifestyle. For example, the PT may instruct a patient to perform a quadriceps contraction every time he or she sits down in a chair, palpating the VMO for feedback. When driving a car, the patient may perform a quadriceps set at every stoplight, taking care to leave the foot firmly on the brake. As the patient begins to recruit a quality quadriceps contraction successfully, goal setting enters into the program and the patient is asked to attempt repetitions of closed-chain exercises (i.e., lunges, wall slides, squats, step-downs). The more the patient practices, the faster the skill to activate a quality quadriceps muscle contraction is learned.

The patient is ready to be weaned off the taping protocol and continue the program with specific sports-related activity and training when he or she can do the following:

1. Sustain a quarter squat for 1 minute against the wall without pain.
2. Sustain a half squat for 1 minute against the wall without pain.
3. Perform 10 step-downs (off an 8-inch step) for at least 5 seconds per step with good control and alignment and without pain.

If functional activity produces pain and the patient is using patella taping, the PT should first assess the taping procedure to ensure it is correct. The clinician may need to make small adjustments in tension and direction. At the time of discharge from the clinical facility, the patient needs to remember how to self-mobilize the patella (Fig. 23-10), as well as proper alignment and the postural issues associated with closed-chain exercises; the patient should be reminded that exercise should be painless.

Suggested Home Maintenance for the Postsurgical Patient

Weeks 1 to 2
GOALS FOR THE PERIOD: Decrease pain, manage edema, increase weight-bearing activities, and facilitate quality quadriceps contraction
1. Elevate and ice at home two to three times per day (preferably after exercises).
2. Perform ankle pumping and hamstring stretches while elevated on ice (20 to 30 minutes).
3. Perform gentle patella self-mobilizations (Fig. 23-10).
4. Perform active heel slides: 1 set of 10 repetitions performed three to four times per day.

5. Perform quadriceps sets: 2 sets of 10 repetitions performed three to four times per day.

The PT should always remember that even though general protocols such as this one may prescribe a number of sets and repetitions, if the patient fatigues and cannot continue to recruit a quality quadriceps contraction, then the exercise is over. Patients are only to count repetitions with quality quadriceps contractions. Quadriceps sets are performed in the sitting or long-sitting position with the knee positioned at 20° to 30° flexion. The heel stays on the floor. Quadriceps sets also may be performed standing if the patient finds it is easier to activate the quadriceps in this position. The key to early strengthening is to find which position gives the patient the most success in recruiting a quality quadriceps contraction.

Weeks 3 to 4
GOALS FOR THE PERIOD: Continue to manage edema and pain, improve sit-to-stand transfer activities, improve strength and stability of the patellofemoral joint, progress functional training to return activity to previous levels

1. Perform the same exercises as in weeks 1 to 2, but increase the number of repetitions. Generally the patient should perform two sets of 10 to 20 repetitions per day (more or less depending on fatigue).
2. Perform closed-chain exercises (see Figs. 22-6 to 22-9) at home depending on quadriceps and LE control.
3. Perform self-taping as deemed appropriate by the therapist. Taping should be tailored to the activity.
4. Continue using ice after exercises.

Weeks 5 to 6
GOALS FOR THE PERIOD: Patient self-manages edema and pain, performs gait without deviations, and has unlimited ambulation

1. Depending on remaining deficits, exercises from weeks 1 to 4 are continued. The need for taping should be minimal; however, if continued taping is required, then patients should be instructed in self-taping techniques.
2. Patient should gradually return to functional activities, with both patient and therapist monitoring for pain and joint effusion.

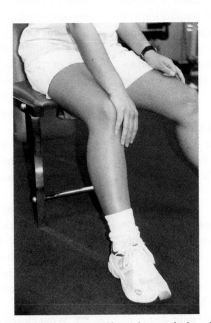

Fig. 23-10 Self-mobilization. The patient should be able to perform active self-stretching to the lateral retinacular tissues. The patient is instructed to place the heel of the hand over the medial half of the patella and push the medial border of the patella down into the trochlear groove. If the exercise is done properly, then the lateral border tilts anteriorly, stretching the lateral retinacular tissue. The knee should be placed in at least 30° of flexion to ensure stability in the trochlear groove and guard against lateral gliding of the patella. The patient progresses into deeper ranges of flexion as pain and lateral tissue tension subside. Each stretch should be held for 5 seconds for two to three repetitions, three to four times a day.

CLINICAL CASE REVIEW

1 George has been having chronic anterior (patellofemoral) knee pain with recurrent subluxation. He is seeing you for his shoulder rehabilitation and wants to know if surgery (ALRR) is an option for him. What should you consider in your response?

Isolated lateral retinacular release has little or no role in the treatment of acute or recurrent patella instability. This procedure should be reserved for the few patients with a clearly identified lateral patella compression syndrome in the presence of a tight lateral retinaculum and clearly discernable lateral retinacular pain.

2 Kathy is a 17-year-old soccer player that underwent ALRR because of chronic anterior knee pain. She comes for her 2-week postoperative evaluation. What should be the main focus of her postoperative rehabilitation?

Given the chronicity of her symptoms, the therapist should evaluate LE mechanics during gait and with dynamic activities when appropriate. The clinician should focus initially on hip strength and ankle mechanics (pronation dysfunction). Hip weakness can cause a valgus position of the knee, creating increased patellofemoral stress. The hip external rotators and abductors (especially the gluteus medius) are a major component in positioning the knee in proper alignment. Ankle mechanics should also be fully explored and orthotics initiated if appropriate.

3 Rebecca is 24 years old. She had ALRR performed on her right knee 18 days ago. Treatment has focused on decreasing joint effusion, pain, and discomfort. Over the past 2 days her pain has increased, with redness around the knee. What should be done?

Because of the increase in temperature and redness (signs of potential infection), the clinician should notify the physician immediately.

4 Sarah is a 17-year-old basketball player who had ALRR 3 weeks ago. She is complaining about her knee "giving out" during walking. She notes minimal pain, but continues to note pronounced swelling around the knee, especially laterally.

In exploring her situation further, it was noted that she was not able to perform an adequate quadriceps contraction. Quadriceps inhibition is a result of the continued edema. A more aggressive edema management program (i.e., elevation, compression, ES three times a day) was initiated along with therapy treatment consisting of ES in conjunction with quadriceps isometrics. A single-point cane was used in the interim until she could demonstrate adequate quadriceps control with walking.

5 Diane is 33 years old. She has a history of anterior knee pain for 2 years. Before having ALRR, she used orthotics because she overpronated during gait. She had surgery 6 weeks ago. Complaints of pain are minimal to nonexistent if she avoids all aggravating factors. However, she generally has some soreness from activities of daily living around the home and from taking care of two young children. Diane is performing all the exercises mentioned in phase I and most exercises in phase II without pain. However, she has pain during functional double-leg squats with knee flexion exceeding 60° and knee pain with step-downs from a 4-inch step. What may help Diane progress with her exercise program?

Diane was evaluated for patellofemoral symptoms and treated with the McConnell method of taping. She was able to progress with the closed-chain exercises when the appropriate McConnell taping procedure was used. She was able to perform double-limb squats to 80° of knee flexion without pain. She also could perform two sets of 10 repetitions of step-downs on the 4-inch step without pain. Pain with the single-limb squat persisted but lessened. Therefore, single-limb squats were not performed until they could be done without pain.

6 Travis is 3 weeks postoperation and is having trouble with maintaining a good quadriceps contraction. What exercises can be performed to address this issue?

Early quadriceps activation should include isometric quadriceps sets in varying degrees of flexion produced by a proximal load-bearing shift with increased knee flexion. This allows for early muscle strengthening even while joint effusion may still be causing pain in a closed-chain (joint loaded) position.

7 What closed-chain exercises are appropriate to perform once ROM is obtained and pain is under control?

- Lunges in a long-stride position (see Fig. 23-6)
- Wall slides at various degrees of flexion with 1-minute holds to promote fatigue (see Fig. 23-7)
- Functional single-limb squats from 0° to 30° directly over the midfoot
- Functional double-limb squats with elastic tubing

- Sit-to-stand at increased speed and repetition
- Step-down exercises with an increase in height of step and speed of movement (see Fig. 23-8)
- Resistive leg press using progressive resistance exercise
- Standing (four-wall) elastic tubing exercises for hip flexion, extension, abduction, and adduction

8 Brian is making good progress in his rehabilitation program with the adjunct of patella taping (medial glide). He asks how long can he leave the tape on and will he have to tape his knee forever?

The patient only needs to wear tape while training the quadriceps to maintain the newly acquired length in the lateral structures. The tape should be removed at night and the skin should be cleaned. This gives the skin a resting period from the pull and friction produced by the tape. Patients using McConnell taping will need to learn how to tape themselves. The tape will loosen according to the aggressiveness of the patient's activity. The patient should therefore be taught to tighten the tape when necessary.

The patient is ready to be weaned off the taping protocol and continue the program with specific sports-related activity and training when he or she can do the following:

- Sustain a quarter squat for 1 minute against the wall without pain
- Sustain a half squat for 1 minute against the wall without pain
- Perform 10 step-downs (off an 8-inch step) for at least 5 seconds per step with good control and alignment and without pain

REFERENCES

1. Gerbino PG, et al: Long-term functional outcome after lateral patellar retinacular release in adolescents: An observational cohort study with minimum 5-year follow-up. J Pediatr Orthop 28(1):118-123, 2008.
2. Ricchetti ET, et al: Comparison of lateral release versus lateral release with medial soft-tissue realignment for the treatment of recurrent patellar instability: A systematic review. Arthroscopy 23(5):463-468, 2007.
3. Panni AS, et al: Long-term results of lateral retinacular release. Arthroscopy 21(5):526-531, 2005.
4. Schöttle PB, et al: Arthroscopic medial retinacular repair after patellar dislocation with and without underlying trochlear dysplasia: A preliminary report. Arthroscopy 22(11):1192-1198, 2006.
5. Fabbriciani C, Panni AS, Delcogliano A: Role of arthroscopic lateral release in the treatment of patellofemoral disorders. Arthroscopy 8(4):531-536, 1992.
6. Lattermann C, Toth J, Bach BR Jr: The role of lateral retinacular release in the treatment of patellar instability. Sports Med Arthrosc 15(2):57-60, 2007.
7. Steine HA, et al: A comparison of closed kinetic chain and isokinetic joint isolation exercise in patients with patello-femoral dysfunction. J Orthop Sports Phys Ther 24(3):136, 1996.
8. Krivickes LS: Anatomical factors associated with overuse sports injuries. Sports Med 24(2):132, 1997.
9. Fu F, Maday M: Arthroscopic lateral release and the patellar compression syndrome. Orthop Clin North Am 23:601, 1992.
10. Fulkerson JP: Disorders of the patellofemoral joint, ed 3, Baltimore, 1997, Williams and Wilkins.
11. Vuorinen OP, et al: Chondromalacia patellae: Results of operative treatment. Arch Orthop Trauma Surg 104(3):175, 1985.
12. Christou EA: Patellar taping increases vastus medialis oblique activity in the presence of patellofemoral pain. J Electromyogr Kinesiol 14(4):495-504, 2004.
13. Lesher JD, et al: Development of a clinical prediction rule for classifying patients with patellofemoral pain syndrome who respond to patellar taping. J Orthop Sports Phys Ther 36(11):854-866, 2006.
14. Christou EA: Patellar taping increases vastus medialis oblique activity in the presence of patellofemoral pain. J Electromyogr Kinesiol 14(4):495-504, 2004.
15. Macgregor K, et al: Cutaneous stimulation from patella tape causes a differential increase in vasti muscle activity in people with patellofemoral pain J Orthop Res 23(2):351-358, 2005.
16. Callaghan MJ, et al: The effects of patellar taping on knee joint proprioception. J Athl Train 37(1):19-24, 2002.
17. Maitland GD: Peripheral manipulation, ed 5, Newton, Mass, 1986, Butterworth-Heinemann.
18. Spencer JDC, Hayes KC, Alexander IJ: Knee joint effusion and quadriceps reflex inhibition in man. Arch Phys Med Rehabil 65:171, 1984.
19. Aminaka N, Gribble PA: Patellar taping, patellofemoral pain syndrome, lower extremity kinematics, and dynamic postural control. J Athl Train 43(1):21-28, 2008.
20. Richardson C: The role of the knee musculature in high speed oscillative movements of the knee. In Proceedings of the MTAA 4th Biennial Conference, Brisbane, Australia, 1985.
21. Tiberio D: The effect of excessive subtalar joint pronation on patellofemoral mechanics: A theoretical model. J Orthop Sports Phys Ther 9:160, 1987.
22. Shelton GL: Conservative management of patellofemoral dysfunction. Prim Care 19(2):331, 1992.
23. Aglietti P, et al: Arthroscopic lateral release for patellar pain or instability. Arthroscopy 5:176, 1989.
24. Small NC: An analysis of complications in lateral retinacular release procedures. Arthroscopy 5:282, 1989.
25. Armato DP, Czamecki D: Geniculate artery pseudoaneurysm: A rare complication of arthroscopic surgery. AJR Am J Roentgenol 155(3):659, 1990.
26. Lutz GE, et al: Rehabilitative techniques for athletes after reconstruction of the anterior cruciate ligament. Mayo Clin Proc 65(10):1322, 1990.
27. McConnell DF: Patellofemoral Program course notes, 1997.
28. Kues JM, Mayhew TP: Concentric and eccentric force-velocity relationships during electrically induced submaximal contractions. Physiother Res Int 1(3):195, 1996.
29. Lehmann JF, et al: Effect of therapeutic temperatures on tendon extensibility. Arch Phys Med Rehabil 51:481, 1970.
30. Meunier S, Pierrot-Deseilligny E, Simonetta-Moreau M: Pattern of heteronymous recurrent inhibition in the human lower limb. Exp Brain Res 102(1):149, 1994.
31. Gould N, et al: Transcutaneous muscle stimulation to retard disuse atrophy after open meniscectomy. Clin Orthop Relat Res 178:190, 1983.
32. Currier DP, Petrilli CR, Threlkeld AJ: Effect of graded electrical stimulation on blood flow to healthy muscle, Phys Ther 66(6):937, 1986.
33. Currier DP, Lehmon J, Lightfoot P: Electrical stimulation in exercise of the quadriceps femoris muscle. Phys Ther 59(12):1508, 1979.
34. Morrissey MC: Reflex inhibition of thigh muscles in knee injury: Cases and treatment. Sports Med 7:263, 1989.

35. Whittingham M, Palmer S, Macmillan F: Effects of taping on pain and function in patellofemoral pain syndrome: A randomized controlled trial. J Orthop Sports Phys Ther 34(9):504-510, 2004.

36. Sherman OH, et al: Patellar instability: treatment by arthroscopic electrosurgical lateral release. Arthroscopy 3:152, 1987.

37. Lui HI, Corrier DP, Threlkeld AJ: Circulatory response of digital arteries associated with electrical stimulation of calf muscles in healthy subjects. Phys Ther 67(3):340, 1987.

38. DeLorme TL: Restoration of muscle power by heavy resistance exercise. J Bone Joint Surg 27:645, 1945.

39. Wild JJ, Franklin TD, Woods GW: Patellar pain and quadriceps rehabilitation: An EMG study. Am J Sports Med 10:12, 1982.

40. Davies GJ: A compendium of isokinetics in clinical usage and rehabilitation techniques. ed 2, 1984, S&S Publishers.

41. Panni AS, et al: Long-term results of lateral retinacular release. Arthroscopy 21(5):526-531, 2005.

42. Fithian DC, et al: Lateral retinacular release: a survey of the International Patellofemoral Study Group. Arthroscopy 20(5):463-468, 2004.

43. Guzzanti V, et al: Patellofemoral malalignment in adolescents: computerized tomographic assessment with or without quadriceps contraction. Am J Sports Med 22(1):55, 1994.

44. Heckman TP: Conservative vs. postsurgical patellar rehabilitation. In Mangine R, editor: Physical therapy of the knee, New York, 1988, Churchill Livingstone.

45. Hensyl WR: Steadman's pocket medical dictionary. Baltimore, 1987, Williams and Wilkins.

46. Chaix Y, et al: Further evidence for non-monosynaptic group I excitation of motoneurons in the human lower limb. Exp Brain Res 115(1):35, 1997.

47. McMiken DF, Todd-Smith M, Thompson C: Strengthening of human quadriceps muscles by cutaneous electrical stimulation. Scand J Rehabil Med 15(1):25, 1983.

48. Arvidsson I, et al: Reduction of pain inhibition on voluntary muscle activation by epidural analgesia. Orthopedics 9:1415, 1986.

49. Werner S, Knutsson E, Ericksson E: Effect of taping the patella and concentric and eccentric torque and EMG of knee extensor and flexor muscles in patients with patello-femoral pain syndrome. Knee Surg Sports Traumatol Arthrosc 1(3-4):169, 1993.

50. DeAndrade JR, Grant C, Dixon ASJ: Joint distension and reflex muscle inhibition in the knee. J Bone Joint Surg Am 47A:313, 1965.

51. Soo CL, Currier DP, Threlkeld AJ: Augmenting voluntary torque of healthy muscle by optimization of electrical stimulation. Phys Ther 68(3):333, 1988.

52. Hurley MV, et al: Rehabilitation of the quadriceps inhibited due to isolated rupture of the anterior cruciate ligament. J Orthop Rheumatol 5:145, 1992.

53. Johansson J: Role of knee ligaments in proprioception and regulation of muscle stiffness. Electromyography 1:158, 1991.

CHAPTER 24

Meniscectomy and Meniscal Repair

Morgan L. Fones, George F. Rick. Hatch III, Timothy Hartshorn

Although meniscal repair was introduced more than 100 years ago, only within the past 10 to 20 years has the meniscus successfully outlived its characterization as a "functionless remain of leg muscle.[1]" Only a few years ago it was standard practice to excise the meniscus with impunity because of the perception that it played little role in the function of the knee. Fairbanks[2] called attention to the frequency of degenerative changes after removal of the meniscus and stimulated a new era of research into the anatomy and function of this poorly understood structure. Researchers eagerly investigated the role of the meniscus in load transmission and joint nutrition, and soon the pendulum of orthopedic popular opinion swung in the direction of determining new ways to preserve the injured meniscus.

With the advent of arthroscopic surgery, partial meniscectomy rapidly supplanted total meniscectomy, and research continued to determine the healing capacity of the torn meniscus. From these efforts, meniscal repair has evolved as a successful technique. Ultimately, recognition of the intact meniscus as a crucial factor in normal knee function has led to widespread acceptance of preservation of torn menisci through partial meniscectomy or repair.

SURGICAL INDICATIONS AND CONSIDERATIONS

When assessing the suitability of a meniscal tear for repair, the surgeon must consider several factors: patient age; chronicity of the injury; type, location, and length of the tears (the blood supply of the meniscus exists primarily at the peripheral 10% to 25%); and associated ligamentous injuries.[3] The perfect candidate for a meniscal repair is a young individual with an acute longitudinal peripheral tear of the meniscus that is 1 to 2 cm long, to be repaired in conjunction with an anterior cruciate ligament (ACL) reconstruction. Success rates for meniscal repairs in conjunction with ACL reconstruction has been as high as 90% compared with 75% for isolated meniscus repairs.[4] It appears that the medial meniscus is more suitable for repair than the lateral meniscus. Shelbourne and Dersam[5] performed a repair of

partially excised lateral meniscus tears. The surgery was performed in conjunction with ACL reconstruction and the repair was performed using an inside-outside technique. They noted that although no significant statistical difference existed between the two groups (International Knee Documentation Committee grade), the partial meniscectomy group had more pain.[5] Shelbourne and Heinrich[6] also noted that certain types of lateral meniscus tears could be successfully treated with abrasion and trephination or just left in situ. Noyes and Barber-Westin[4,7] studied two different age groups and their response to meniscus repair. They used an inside-outside technique with a majority of the patients undergoing concomitant ACL reconstruction. In looking at the outcomes, 87% of the older (over 40 years old) group, and 75% of the younger (under 20 years old) group were asymptomatic for medial compartment symptoms. They also noted significant improvement in outcomes when the repair was done in conjunction with an ACL reconstruction. Age may not be as significant a factor as the type of tear (degenerative or nondegenerative).[8] The current trend appears to lean toward the preservation of the meniscus whenever possible based on the patient's current and future activity levels. More research is being performed looking at the long-term results and categorizing further the indications for meniscus repair.[9] Outside of these parameters, little consensus exists regarding the relative indications for meniscal repair.

The arthroscopic surgeon should be prepared to perform meniscal repair at the time of any knee arthroscopy. The identification of reparable menisci is usually not possible preoperatively, but often magnetic resonance imaging (MRI) can help demonstrate the location of tears.

Four techniques for repair currently exist:
1. Open meniscal repair
2. Arthroscopic inside-out repair
3. Arthroscopic outside-in repair
4. All-inside arthroscopic repair

Each of these techniques has advantages and disadvantages; application of individual techniques is largely a matter of individual preference.

SURGICAL PROCEDURE

Open Meniscal Repair

Open meniscal repair (Fig. 24-1) is the oldest technique for meniscal repair and has been popularized by Dr. Ken DeHaven.[10] It has a good record of success, even at 1-year follow-up.[11] Open meniscal repairs are best suited for extremely peripheral tears. DeHaven still advocates routine arthroscopic evaluation before considering open repair. The arthroscope is removed from the joint and the knee is prepared. After exposing the capsule through a longitudinal incision, the surgeon prepares the meniscal rim and capsular attachment, and places vertically oriented sutures at 3- to 4-mm intervals. The incision is closed in a layered fashion. Long-term follow-up has shown success rates of 70% to 79%.[12-14]

Inside-Out Meniscal Repair

The inside-out meniscal repair technique was popularized by Henning[15] in the early 1980s and is the most popular technique for meniscus repair. The surgeon uses long, thin cannulas to allow placement of vertical or horizontal sutures. After identifying the tear arthroscopically, he or she prepares the tear by using a meniscal rasp to create a better biologic environment for healing. A small posterior incision is carried down to the capsule, and sutures are placed arthroscopically using specially designed long Keith needles to pass the suture. The assistant protects the popliteal structures with a retractor while grasping the suture needles. After placing all sutures, the surgeon ties them over the capsule. Success rates have been noted to be 75% to 88%.[14,16]

Outside-In Meniscal Repair

The outside-in meniscal repair technique allows suture placement using an 18-gauge spinal needle placed across the tear from outside the joint to inside. Absorbable polydioxanone suture[17] is passed through the needle into the joint; it is secured with a mulberry knot tied to the end of the sutures. These sutures are tied to adjacent sutures at the end of the procedure over the joint capsule; separate small incisions are made for each pair of sutures. Morgan and colleagues[18] noted an 84% success rate and found the primary reason for failure was an associated ACL deficiency.

All-Inside Meniscal Repair

All-inside meniscal repair allows the meniscus to be repaired without any additional incisions outside the knee. This is truly an all-arthroscopic technique. It is popular because it avoids additional incisions and therefore diminishes neurovascular risk and decreases operative time.[14] Success rates have been noted as high as 90%.[14,19]

All-inside meniscal repair can be accomplished with either suture or biodegradable "darts."[20] The suture technique is accomplished using a specially designed cannulated suture hook to pass suture through both sides of the tear. The sutures are then tied arthroscopically using a knot pusher.

The biodegradable darts are passed across the tear using specially designed cannulas. After preparing the torn meniscal surface, the surgeon reduces the tear and holds it in place with a cannula. A thin cutting instrument is used to make a pathway across the meniscal tear, and the biodegradable dart is passed through the same cannula, fixing the tear. The darts generally completely resorb by 8 to 12 weeks.

THERAPY GUIDELINES FOR REHABILITATION

Limited research is available regarding physical therapy protocols after meniscus repair and long-term outcomes. Clinic protocols vary with the degree of weight bearing, duration of immobilization, control of range of motion (ROM), and time frame for a return to sports or work. Recent studies have shown the success rates after accelerated rehabilitation programs to be similar to those in conservative rehabilitation programs. These studies found no statistically significant difference in success and repair failure rates between groups using conservative or accelerated programs. The hallmarks of accelerated programs are early full weight-bearing tolerance, unrestricted ROM, and return to pivoting sports.[21-23] Recent studies have shown that dynamic loading can help meniscal repair healing in inflammatory environments.[24]

Several crucial factors must be considered before initiating a rehabilitation program. These factors influence the speed and aggressiveness of the rehabilitation program. The size of the tear, repair stabilization technique, suture material, number of sutures, and location of the meniscal repair influence initial postoperative weight-bearing tolerance,

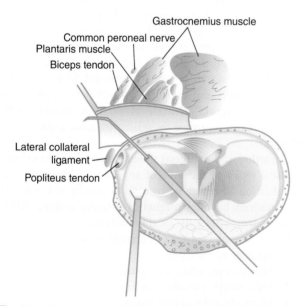

Fig. 24-1 Meniscus repair. (From Noyes FR, Barber-Westin SD: Meniscus tears: diagnosis, repair techniques, clinical outcomes. In Noyes FR, Barber-Westin SD, editors: Noyes' knee disorders: surgery, rehabilitation, clinical outcomes, Philadelphia, 2009, Saunders.)

ROM, and exercise restrictions. Other factors to consider before initiating a rehabilitation program include degenerative pathology in the weight-bearing articulations or patellofemoral joint, previous patella dysfunction, concomitant injuries, possible joint laxity (i.e., ACL deficiency or reconstruction, medial collateral ligament injury), and severe kinetic chain movement dysfunctions proximally or distally that alter knee alignment and forces. These injuries do not necessarily indicate a potentially unsatisfactory result, but accommodations may be required in the protocol to accommodate the effects of these pathologies. Barber and Click[21] evaluated the results of 65 meniscal repairs in patients who underwent an accelerated rehabilitation program. Successful meniscal healing occurred in 92% of patients with a concomitant ACL reconstruction, compared with 67% of patients with ACL-deficient knees and 67% of patients with meniscal pathology alone.

An understanding of the clinical implications of knee and meniscus biomechanics helps guide the therapist through the rehabilitation process. Communication among all rehabilitation team members—the physician, therapist, patient, family, and coach—is crucial to a successful rehabilitation outcome. Most importantly, the meniscal repair rehabilitation protocol must be individually tailored to the patient's needs.

The rehabilitation process can be broken down into three phases: initial, intermediate, and advanced. These phases may overlap and should be based on objective and functional findings rather than time.

The early phase of the rehabilitation program should emphasize decreasing postoperative inflammatory reaction, restoring controlled ROM, and encouraging early weight bearing as tolerated. Exercise intensity is increased in the later phases of rehabilitation. Closed kinetic chain exercises are progressed through a variety of positions, from simple linear movements to complex multidirectional, multiplanar motions. The final phase of treatment is directed toward return to normal activity (sport or work).

The length of rehabilitation varies among patients. Treatments may be equally distributed among each of the phases of rehabilitation if the number of patient visits must be managed. Fewer treatments are required in the initial phases of rehabilitation if swelling and pain are adequately controlled and ROM is progressing without complications.

Preoperative Care

Ideally the patient should be seen at a preoperative visit, which includes a brief clinical evaluation to record baseline physical data and identify potential latent biomechanical deficits. The evaluation format encompasses a subjective history as outlined in Maitland,[25] and objective data are gathered primarily to record baseline measurements. The lower extremity (LE) is evaluated as a functional unit. Strength and ROM are recorded for the hip, knee, ankle, and foot. Foot mechanics also are evaluated for any biomechanical faults that may lead to excessive tibial motions in the frontal or transverse planes. For example, pes planus has the

potential to drive tibial internal rotation, creating a mechanism for excessive transverse friction at the knee joint. In addition, hip abduction and external rotation strength need to be examined to avoid excessive femoral adduction and internal rotation distally. Reassessment continues postoperatively with each progression of weight bearing. Girth measurements also are taken about the knee. The remainder of the preoperative visit should include instruction in proper use of crutches, education regarding ROM (heel slides with a 30-second hold for 10 repetitions), instruction in antiembolic exercises (ankle pumps with a 30-second hold for 10 repetitions), and prescription of LE strengthening exercises in the form of isometrics (quadriceps sets, hamstring sets, and cocontraction of quadriceps and hamstrings; all three exercises should be held for 10 seconds for 10 to 20 repetitions) and active range of motion (AROM) of the hip (working the adductors, abductors, and external rotators for 10 to 20 repetitions). Cryotherapy and elevation (for 15 to 30 minutes) and compression wrapping should be reviewed for postoperative pain and swelling management. Depending on individual clinic and physician preference, the patient may be instructed in the use of electrical stimulation (ES). The patient should be instructed in activities of daily living, such as bathing and dressing, as appropriate. Home exercises are to be performed three times a day until return for the initial postoperative physical therapy evaluation.

Phase I (Initial Phase)

TIME: 1 to 4 weeks after surgery
GOALS: Manage pain and swelling, increase ROM and strength, increase weight-bearing activities and prevent excessive loads/stresses through the joint surfaces (Table 24-1)

The patient is typically seen for physical therapy 4 to 7 days after surgery. He or she may complain of mild to moderate pain, swelling, impaired balance, and decreased weight-bearing tolerance. The patient may or may not be using pain medication.

Generally, patients undergoing partial or total meniscectomy may be weight bearing as tolerated immediately or soon after surgery whereas those undergoing repair are usually non–weight bearing (NWB) or partial weight bearing (PWB) with crutches for a period of 2 to 6 weeks. Noyes recommends 4 weeks of PWB for complex and avascular tears, with up to 6 weeks of toe touch weight bearing when the patient has a radial tear.[26] Tibiofemoral loads induce a circumferential stress (so-called "hoop stress") in the meniscus, which would distract the radial tear margins.[27] Based on physician preference, the patient may have a postoperative hinged knee brace, which will either be statically locked at a particular setting for 7 to 10 days or set between certain parameters to allow for immediate postoperative ROM. Meniscal repairs in the "red-red zone" and larger peripheral repairs may be braced up to 90° for up to 14 days. "White zone" repairs may be braced at 20° to 70°. Extension

TABLE 24-1 Meniscus Repair

Rehabilitation Phase	Criteria to Progress to This Phase	Anticipated Impairments and Functional Limitations	Intervention	Goal	Rationale
Phase I Postoperative 1-4 wk	Postoperative	• Mild to moderate pain • Peripheral repairs: Partial weight bearing by 2 wk, weight bearing to tolerance at 3-4 wk • Complex tears: Partial weight bearing by 6 wk, weight bearing to tolerance at 7-8 wk • Decreased strength • Minimal to moderate effusion • Decreased ROM	• Cryotherapy, heat and ice contrast, ES • PROM—Hamstring stretches, gastrocnemius-soleus stretches • Wall slides or passive heel slides (see Fig. 24-2) • Isometrics—Cocontraction quadriceps and hamstring (depending on the repair site), quadriceps sets, hip adductor sets, hamstring sets, resistive exercises • Four-quad program, weight added distally as tolerated • Elastic tubing exercises • Gait training • Low-resistance, moderate-speed stationary cycling • Aquatic therapy; closed kinetic chain activities (initiate near end of phase for peripheral tears only) • Leg press machine • Partial squats • Heel raises • Standing terminal knee extension with tubing	• Manage pain and swelling • Knee ROM 0°-120° • Increased muscle strength and endurance • Normalization of gait within healing and weight-bearing limitations	• Decrease pain and minimize swelling • Prevent ROM complications • Assist in restoration of joint mechanics • Facilitate return of neuromuscular control • Minimize disuse atrophy • Strengthen knee musculature while protecting the repair site • Increase muscle endurance • Use the properties of water during exercise performance • Functional strengthening

ES, Electrical stimulation; *PROM*, passive range of motion; *ROM*, range of motion.

is increased to 0°, and flexion is increased to 90° after 7 to 10 days as healing allows.

On the first postoperative visit a comprehensive evaluation is performed, with the physical therapist collecting the new objective data and reviewing and updating the previous subjective data.[25] Subjective data that need to be reviewed postoperatively include medication usage, sleep pattern, pain levels at rest and during activity, and aggravating and easing factors. In addition, the therapist should review the postoperative report dictated by the operating surgeon that describes the extent and nature of the repair, as well as any unique patient-specific postoperative instructions. Goals and rehabilitation expectations are established and reviewed with the patient during the initial visit.

The new and updated objective and clinical data should include visual examination, gait assessment, ROM measurement, strength assessment, palpation, and girth measurement (as described in the section on the preoperative initial visit). Visual observation should focus on areas of atrophy, in particular the quadriceps and gastrocnemius; healing status of incision sites; and swelling about the knee joint and

distal LE. Depending on the patient's weight-bearing status or tolerance, gait assessment is either brief or detailed. Gait assessment should focus on proper mechanics and weight-bearing tolerance. If the patient is NWB or PWB, the assessment is brief and focuses primarily on safety, correct mechanics (with crutches), and includes a discussion regarding weight-bearing restrictions. If the patient does not have weight-bearing limitations and has good gait tolerance, then a more detailed assessment of gait can be made. The patient's ability to ambulate with normal mechanics throughout each phase of gait is very important and should be assessed. Remedial corrective actions are required to decrease potentially harmful loading onto healing structures. Typically patients require cueing to avoid hip external rotation during the stance phase, because this puts abnormal stresses through the knee, ankle, and foot. Crutches should be used throughout the initial phase of treatment until adequate strength, ROM, and normal gait mechanics are achieved. Static and dynamic foot function (as related to normal gait mechanics) continues to be assessed during this phase of rehabilitation. Dysfunctions must be addressed to decrease abnormal tensile or compressive force affecting healing of the meniscus repair.

Flexibility of the hip musculature, hamstring, and gastrocnemius-soleus complex should be assessed. The patellofemoral joint should be assessed, especially if the patient reports previous or present patella symptoms. Patella tracking and glides are part of this assessment. Joint mobilization or patellofemoral taping may be helpful in mitigating these symptoms.[28] All major muscle groups in the LE should be assessed bilaterally for strength capacity. In addition, visible observation and palpation of the quadriceps during an isometric quad set or straight leg raise (SLR) can give the clinician insight into the patient's ability to be safe and secure in an upright position. The remaining LE musculature should be assessed, with the therapist identifying any potential weakness that may alter normal closed kinetic biomechanics and therefore increase tensile or compressive forces across the meniscus repair site.

No standard method has been established for assessing girth about the knee joint. Consistency among the team members providing patient care is important when reassessing the patient's condition. Atrophy as measured by girth measurements is not diagnostic of weakness or atrophy in a specific muscle group. Circumference measurement assesses girth of all muscle and joint structures underlying the measurement area. Typical measurement sites for a bilateral comparison include the midpatella, 5 and 10 cm above the knee joint and 5 and 10 cm below the knee joint.

Treatment is initiated after the clinical evaluation is completed (see Table 24-1). Initial phase treatment goals are to decrease pain and manage swelling, restore ROM, increase muscle strength and endurance, and normalize gait within healing and weight-bearing limitations.

Pain and Edema Management

Minimal to moderate effusion will likely be evident at the evaluation. Modalities such as cryotherapy, heat and ice contrast, and ES can be used to decrease pain and swelling.[29-31] Instructions in home use of cryotherapy, compression wrapping, and elevation as discussed in the section on preoperative management is initiated for postoperative pain and swelling. The importance of home cryotherapy cannot be overemphasized. The study of Lessard and colleagues[30] on the use of cryotherapy after meniscectomy found statistically significant differences between groups with and without postoperative cryotherapy. Patients reported decreased pain ratings per the McGill pain questionnaire, decreased medication consumption, improved exercise compliance, and improved weight-bearing status.

Range of Knee Motion and Flexibility

Restoration of ROM is vital to a return to the patient's prior level of function. Typically on initial evaluation, the patient exhibits a loss of extension of 5° to 10°; flexion ROM is typically 70° to 90°. The patient usually exhibits a guarded end feel with motion improving with repetition. The time parameter to achieve full ROM is longer with meniscal repair than it is in partial arthroscopic meniscectomies. Although early restoration of ROM is important to normalize joint function, the healing process of the meniscus repair dictates caution, especially with full circumferential peripheral repairs.

Any exercises used to increase ROM should not be forced because of the risk of stressing healing repair sites. Wall slides, sitting passive knee flexion, or passive heel slides (Fig. 24-2) may be used to increase knee flexion. ROM exercises are to be performed within pain tolerance, held at least 30 seconds, and repeated as tolerated (generally 5 to 10 times). As part of the home exercise program, ROM activity can be repeated three to five times per day.

Appropriate remedial flexibility exercises can be implemented as tolerated in this phase, with the patient avoiding forced knee flexion and rotation about the knee joint. Patients should perform slow static stretches, avoiding ballistic movements, to maintain control of the lower limb and minimize the chance of affecting the healing meniscus repair.[32,33] Hamstring and gastrocnemius-soleus flexibility exercises are typically indicated at this time. Stretches should be held at least 30 seconds and repeated 5 times, three times a day. Stretches should be sustained and passive in nature, allowing the patient or therapist to control knee joint motions, avoiding potential complications from ballistic type of stretching.[34] The hamstring group can be stretched passively using

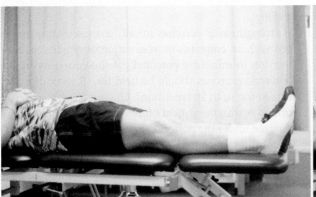
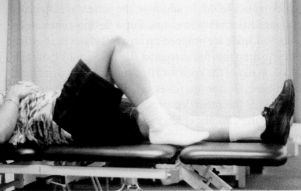

Fig. 24-2 Heel slides. While lying supine the patient slides the involved heel toward the buttock, maintaining the knee in a straight plane and avoiding any hip or tibial rotation.

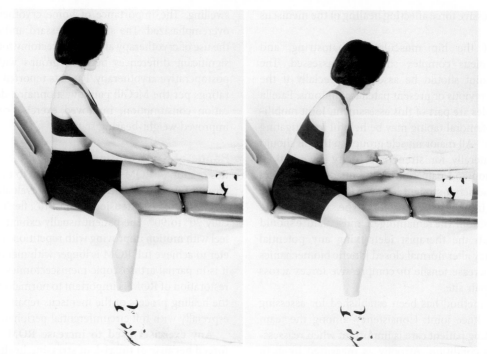

Fig. 24-3 Hamstring stretching. In a long-sit position, the patient leans forward from the hip, avoiding lumbar flexion.

supine position. A towel can be used to assist with the raising of the leg (Fig. 24-3). The gastrocnemius-soleus can be stretched using a towel or strap in the early phases of rehabilitation. Progression to stretching of the hip musculature and quadriceps can be performed as the patient's increase in knee ROM dictates. The knee needs to be kept in a relative neutral position to avoid any rotational or compressive forces on the repaired meniscus site. Standing gastrocnemius-soleus stretching can be initiated as weight-bearing tolerance increases.

It is important to keep the foot in a neutral position to avoid any tibial rotation caused by supination or pronation, which may increase knee joint compression and tensile forces across the repaired meniscal site.

Patients who develop limitations in either flexion or extension of the surgical knee require manual patella mobilizations (Fig. 24-4) and home exercises for aggressive long static stretches. Patella mobilizations should be done in the superior, inferior, medial, and lateral directions and are vital to achieving full ROM. In addition, the patient is instructed in prolonged flexibility stretches. For a flexion contracture, the foot and ankle are propped up on a rolled towel, allowing the knee to drop into full extension. Then a 5- to 10-lb weight is placed on top of the knee for 10 minutes. This is done daily 6 to 8 times. Flexion exercises can be done in the seated position with the other leg providing overpressure. Other ways are to use a rolling chair, a supine wall slide, or a quadriceps stretch.

Strengthening

Initial strengthening is performed as tolerated in open-chain positions. Closed kinetic strengthening can be initiated, depending on the weight-bearing status and tolerance of

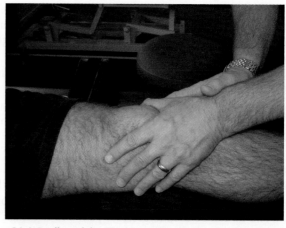

Fig. 24-4 Patella mobilizations. Aggressive Maitland grade IV mobilizations are typically needed if there are ROM concerns early on.

the patient. *All strengthening exercises should be closely monitored for potential adverse reactions and increased pain or swelling.*

Strengthening exercises for all LE musculature are initiated with an emphasis on restoration of quadriceps muscle function to minimize potential patellofemoral dysfunction. Isometric exercises should be held for 10 seconds and performed for 10 to 20 repetitions. Quadriceps sets can be performed within the patient's tolerance. A small towel may be required under the posterior aspect of the knee if the patient lacks full extension or if muscle setting in full extension is painful to the knee joint area. The patient is instructed to extend at the hip while tightening the quadriceps muscle, straightening the knee as tolerated. This exercise also may help restore knee extension. The towel should be removed as knee extension increases or becomes less painful. Adductor isometric contractions can be performed isolated or in conjunction with quadriceps sets.[35]

Hamstring isometrics can be performed; they should initially be performed at a submaximal level, with vigor increased based on patient tolerance and response.

Caution should be exhibited when performing hamstring exercises early in rehabilitation, especially with larger peripheral rim or posterior horn meniscus repairs. Active knee flexion pulls the medial and lateral meniscus posterior. Because the lateral meniscus is more loosely attached, it can migrate posteriorly as much as 1 cm as a result of pull from the popliteus muscle. The medial meniscus may move a few millimeters via the posterior attachment to the joint capsule and influence from the nearby semimembranosus attachment.[3] Cocontraction isometrics of the quadriceps and hamstrings may be used in the first 2 to 4 weeks in patients with the aforementioned repairs to allow adequate meniscal healing.[36]

Short arc quadriceps exercises can be added if the patient tolerates end-range extension movement. Resistance should be added carefully, with the therapist remaining mindful of the role of the quadriceps in pulling the meniscus anteriorly by way of the meniscopatellar ligament, as well as the anterior posterior compressive force exerted by the femoral condyle during knee extension.[28] Another effective open chain exercise for the quadriceps is active assisted knee extension in sitting from 90° to 30°. An open-chain (SLR) "4 quad" program (i.e., four quadrants: hip flexion, abduction, adduction, and extension) can be initiated with the knee fully extended if the patient has adequate LE and quadriceps control. The "4 quad" program is a series of SLR exercises held for 10 seconds and 10 to 20 repetitions:

1. Supine SLR
2. Side-lying hip abduction
3. Side-lying hip adduction
4. Prone hip extension

Progression of this program is based on patient signs and symptoms. Resistance can be added distally as tolerated. The DeLorme strength progression protocol[37] can be used, with gradual increases in resistance based on patient signs and symptoms.

Weight-bearing status and patient tolerance may limit the ability to strengthen the distal musculature. Strengthening of the ankle can be aided by exercises using elastic tubing; the patient should perform three sets of 10 to 20 repetitions. Ankle movements of dorsiflexion, plantar flexion, inversion and eversion, and hip proprioceptive neuromuscular facilitation (PNF) patterns (with the knee extended) can be performed to the patient's tolerance. As with other healing collagen structures, controlled tensile and compressive loading may assist in scar conformation, revascularization, and improvement in the tensile properties of the meniscal repair through the maturation process.[38] Gradual progression and reassessment of activity is crucial.

When initiating any of the closed kinetic chain exercises, the patient must keep the knee and LE in a neutral position. In normal gait the compressive forces on the knee joint may be two to three times normal body weight. The meniscus assumes 40% to 60% of the weight-bearing load. Variations in knee joint angulation or rotation can increase the force across the meniscus 25% to 50%.[1] Variations in foot mechanics that cause rotation or angulation of the knee into varus or valgus can have potentially significant effects on meniscal compressive and tensile forces that may affect the repair site. As a result, some physicians recommend initiating closed-chain exercises only for peripheral tears during this phase while waiting until phase II (5 to 11 weeks) for complex tears[39] (Table 24-2).

Partial weight-bearing, closed kinetic chain activities using leg press or inclined squat machines, partial squats, and heel raises can be initiated later in the initial phase. Standing terminal knee extension with tubing can be added to increase quadriceps strength and control with full weight bearing.

Aquatic therapy is an additional treatment option during the third and fourth week of the initial phase, especially if the patient has limited weight bearing and cannot tolerate traditional therapy because of pain.[40]

Balance and Proprioceptive Training

When patients achieve PWB, balance and proprioceptive training can begin. Crutches are used to assist during these exercises. Initially, the patients begin with tolerable weight shifts in the sagittal and frontal planes. Tandem balancing can also be initiated during the partial weight-bearing phase. Gait training with small obstacles like water cups can help develop adequate stance phase stability, symmetry between the surgical and contralateral limbs, and improved proprioception. Some patients may be able to progress to a single-leg balance exercise, where the knee is held at 20° to 30° of flexion. Different surfaces can be added as needed.

Conditioning

A conditioning program can be initiated 2 to 4 weeks postoperatively with an upper body ergometer. Low-resistance, moderate-speed stationary cycling can be initiated when knee flexion ROM is around 110°. Toe clips may be optional if hamstring activity is to be minimized because of the location of the repair. Progression is determined by the patient's tolerance to stationary cycling. The goal of initial phase cycling is to increase muscle endurance.

Complications in the initial phase of treatment include persistent pain and swelling, arthrofibrosis, adhesions at the porthole sites, patella tendonitis, and patellofemoral pain. Activity modification, use of modalities, heat and cold contrast, cryotherapy, and ES may be helpful in decreasing pain and swelling. Adhesion of the porthole sites within the distal fat pads may cause painful limitation of knee flexion and active knee extension. Ultrasound or phonophoresis, along with soft tissue mobilization of incision sites, may be helpful in mitigating distal patella symptoms. Assessment of patellofemoral mechanics (active and passive) is an ongoing process. Patellofemoral taping should be used to control pain and dysfunction.[41]

TABLE 24-2 Meniscus Repair

	Postoperative Weeks					Postoperative Months			
	1-2	3-4	5-6	7-8	9-12	4	5	6	7-12
Brace: long-leg postoperative	C, T	C, T	C, T						
Range of Motion Minimum Goals									
0°-90°	X								
0°-120°		X							
0°-135°			X						
Weight Bearing									
Toe touch to ½ body weight	P								
¾ to full body weight		P							
Toe touch to ¼ body weight	C, T								
½-¾ body weight		C, T	C						
Full body weight				T	C				
Patellar mobilization	X	X	X						
Stretching									
Hamstring, gastrocnemius, soleus, iliotibial band, quadriceps	X	X	X	X	X	X	X	X	X
Strengthening									
Quadriceps isometrics, straight leg raises, active knee extension	X	X	X	X	X	X	X	X	X
Weight bearing: gait retraining, toe raises, wall sits, minisquats		P	C	X	X	X	X	X	
Knee flexion hamstring curls (90°)			P	C	X	X	X	X	X
Knee extension quads (90°-30°)			X	X	X	X	X	X	X
Hip abduction-adduction, multihip			X	X	X	X	X	X	X
Leg press (70°-10°)			P	P	X	X	X	X	X
Balance/Proprioceptive Training									
Weight-shifting, minitrampoline, BAPS, KAT, plyometrics		P	X	X	X	X	X	X	X
Conditioning									
UBE	X	X	X						
Bike (stationary)			X	X	X	X	X	X	X
Aquatic program				X	X	X	X	X	X
Swimming (kicking)					P, C	X	X	X	X
Walking					X	X	X	X	X
Stair-climbing machine					P, C	P, C	P, C	P, C	X
Ski machine					P, C	P	P	C	X
Running: straight*						P	P	C	X
Cutting: lateral carioca, figure 8s*							P	P	X
Full sports*							P	P	X

BAPS, Biomechanical Ankle Platform System (Camp, Jackson, Mich); *C*, complex meniscus repairs extending into central one-third region; *KAT*, Kinesthetic Awareness Trainer (Breg, Inc., Vista, Calif); *P*, peripheral meniscus repairs; *T*, transplants; *UBE*, upper body ergometer, *X*, all meniscus repairs and transplants.

*Return to running, cutting, and full sports based on multiple criteria. Patients with noteworthy articular cartilage damage are advised to return to light recreational activities only.

ROM gradually increases during the initial phase of treatment, approaching full ROM by the end of this phase. Passive and dynamic splints may be helpful in gaining ROM if the joint does not respond to conservative treatment. **Initiation of vigorous stretching or knee joint mobilization should be discussed with the patient and physician.** The therapist should be aware of knee joint symptoms, pain, and swelling as attempts to increase ROM (especially knee flexion) continue.

In addition, the therapist should be cognizant of and recognize meniscus lesion signs and symptoms. These include persistent joint effusion, joint line pain, and locking or giving way of the knee (as opposed to buckling or weakness from decreased LE or quadriceps strength).

If activity modification and use of modalities does not improve the patient's symptoms and objective findings, or if the patient exhibits classic signs of a meniscus tear, then referral to the physician is indicated.

Phase II (Intermediate Phase)

TIME: 5 to 11 weeks after surgery
GOALS: Gain full ROM and 90% to 100% strength, progress functional activities, progress to gym program (Table 24-3)

Objective findings rather than time ranges give an indication of progression into the intermediate phase of rehabilitation. In general this phase occurs around 4 to 6 weeks, in part based on improved patient signs and symptoms but also because enough time has elapsed to allow sufficient healing of the meniscal repair. This phase lasts until the patient is ready to enter a return-to-sport program (usually by week 12). Pain and swelling should be minimal and easily controlled before initiation of this phase. ROM should be full. However, the patient may have a slight restriction of knee flexion, with discomfort at the end ROM. Unless the patient is being treated conservatively secondary to repair of a complex or avascular tear, they should be able to tolerate full weight bearing without pain or swelling. The patient should exhibit normal gait mechanics. Good control of the LE musculature should be evident before activity is progressed. The goals of the intermediate phase are to normalize strength, ROM, gait, and endurance, as well as progress the patient into functional activities. Muscle flexibility exercises are continued as needed during this phase. Quadriceps and iliopsoas stretching to improve knee flexion and hip extension can be initiated. Strength exercises are continued and advanced as tolerated. Hamstring strengthening (with isotonic exercise) can be advanced during this phase. Progression is based on DeLorme's principles.[37] Resistance can be applied to the hamstring group gradually, based on patient tolerance.

Closed-chain activity can be advanced during this phase of rehabilitation. Progression of activity should be from simple linear movements to complex multidirectional movements. Patients are instructed to perform three sets of 10 to 30 repetitions as indicated. *The patient must demonstrate adequate control of LE mechanics and not have adverse*

TABLE 24-3 Meniscus Repair

Rehabilitation Phase	Criteria to Progress to This Phase	Anticipated Impairments and Functional Limitations	Intervention	Goal	Rationale
Phase II Postoperative 5-11 wk	• Minimal pain and swelling 4 to 6 wk to allow sufficient healing • Full weight bearing for peripheral tears; complex tears begin at 7-8 wk • Normal gait mechanics • Good control of the LE musculature	• Decreased strength • Minimal effusion • Decreased ROM (flexion)	• Continue exercises as outlined in phase I Resistive exercise: • Isotonics—Hamstrings • Isokinetics—A submaximal multispectrum isokinetic program • Closed-chain exercises (now can begin for complex tears as well), heel raises, lateral step-up, forward step up/down, wall squats, knee flexion at 45°-60°, minisquats, partial lunges, progression in knee flexion ROM • Balance/proprioceptive training: Weight shifting, minitrampoline, BAPS, BBS, balance board • Elastic tubing activity, T kicks (see Fig. 24-5) • At 9 wk can begin stationary cycling, aquatic program, swimming, stair-stepping machine, ski machine (wait until 5-6 months for complex tears), or treadmill	• Full ROM • 90%-100% LE strength • Normal gait and standing tolerance • Progression to functional activities • Prepare patient for discharge	• Restore knee and LE function • Increase muscle strength • Use specificity of training principles to return the patient to previous level of functional activity • Enhance response of joint proprioceptors and neuromuscular coordination • Emphasize stability/strengthening of involved leg • Improve cardiovascular fitness

BAPS, Biomechanical Ankle Platform System (Camp, Jackson, Mich); *BBS,* Biodex Balance System (Shirley, NY); *LE,* lower extremity; *ROM,* range of motion.

reactions (pain and swelling) from the simple linear movements before progressing to complex multidirectional movements. Variables of time, repetitions, ROM, and resistance are used in functionally progressing the rehabilitation program. Full weight-bearing heel raises, lateral step-ups, wall squats, minisquats with tubing, and partial lunges can be performed. ROM should be limited initially, with most activity being from 0° to 90°.

Constant reassessment should occur, and patient tolerance to the particular activity must be demonstrated before any exercise progression. Balance and coordination exercises can be added to the rehabilitation program during the intermediate phase. Initial training is done bilaterally and progressed as tolerated to unilateral activities. Balance boards, trampolines, and elastic cords can be used. Single-limb balance and control can be performed with exercise tubing "T kicks" (Fig. 24-5). The uninvolved extremity has a cord attached distally; the involved extremity remains stationary with the knee in about 10° of flexion. The patient moves the uninvolved extremity into flexion, extension, abduction, adduction, and diagonal planes. Initially the patient performs 10 to 15 repetitions for two sets in each plane of movement. The patient may require support for balance. The exercise can be progressed by altering the tubing resistance, increasing the repetition or time (up to 30 seconds in each plane), and altering the speed of movement (Fig. 24-6).

Cycling can be continued, with the patient modifying the workload parameters of speed, resistance, and duration based on response to the activity. Additional cardiovascular activity (e.g., stair-stepping machine, cross-country ski machine, treadmill) can be added based on patient response and tolerance.

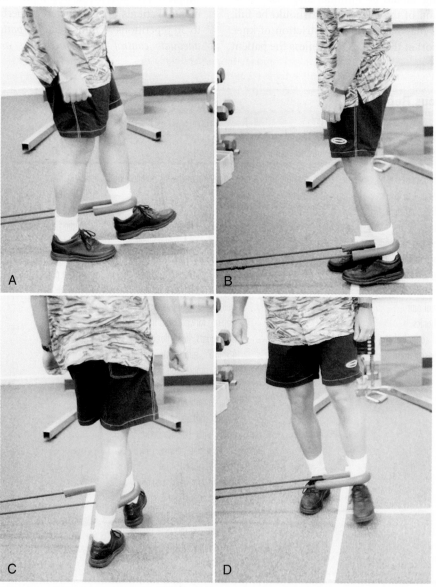

Fig. 24-5 T kicks. This exercise is performed in a standing position, with elastic tubing around the ankle of the uninvolved LE (foot off ground). The uninvolved LE moves into flexion (**A**), extension (**B**), adduction (**C**), and abduction (**D**). The emphasis is on maintaining proper LE alignment and avoiding tibial rotation.

A gradual walking-to-running program can be established toward the end of this phase based on weight-bearing tolerance and adequate closed-chain control and LE strength. (Refer to Chapter 34 for a detailed progressive running program.) Assessment of foot function with appropriate modifications may be helpful in minimizing abnormal joint and meniscus stress before initiating a running program. The running program can start with jogging in place on a trampoline and be progressed to treadmill running. Continued progression is based on patient tolerance and absence of pain and swelling.

Isokinetics strength and endurance training can be initiated during this phase. Tolerance to resisted quadriceps and hamstring strengthening must be demonstrated before an isokinetic program is initiated. A submaximal multispectrum program with a lower velocity speed of 180°/sec (three sets of 15 to 20 seconds) and higher velocity speed of 300°/sec (three sets up to 30 seconds) can be initiated. Progression is based on patient tolerance and adequate response to training.

Phase III (Advanced Phase)

TIME: 12 to 18 weeks after surgery
GOALS: Return to sport or preinjury activities, establish an ongoing training program (Table 24-4)

Progression to the advanced phase of rehabilitation is based on tolerance to intermediate phase treatment. Typically this phase is initiated around 12 to 18 weeks. ROM should be complete without pain.

Caution should be exhibited with full squat or lunge activity. These activities should be avoided early in the advanced phase and gradually introduced with progressive loading toward the end of the phase. Normal strength in all major muscle groups should be exhibited. The patient should exhibit good closed-chain control in linear and multidirectional activity. The goals of this phase are to establish a training program and return to sports or preinjury activity levels.

Progression of strength and endurance training continues. New loads and demands are placed on the LE through running, agility, and plyometric training. Depending on previous activity level and functional requirements, agility, sprinting, and track running can be initiated. An indicator of patient progress in these activities is the ability to jog on a treadmill 10 to 15 minutes at a pace of 7 to 8 mph without adverse signs and symptoms. As with other knee disorders, adequate isokinetic strength (70% of the uninvolved extremity) can be used as an indication for progression to a running, agility, and plyometric program. A deficit of 10% or less is a reliable indicator of return to sport or activity participation.[23] An initial plyometric program may include squat jumps in water. It serves as an effective alternative to dry land jumps by keeping adequate intensity while limiting the loads placed through the joint.[42] However, other functional tests need to be assessed to ensure safe return. Refer to Chapter 34 for a more complete return to running program.

SUGGESTED HOME MAINTENANCE FOR THE POSTSURGICAL PATIENT

An exercise program has been outlined at the various phases. The physical therapist can use it in customizing a patient-specific program.

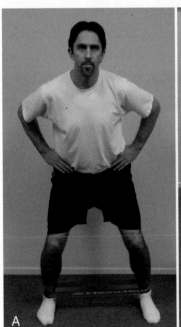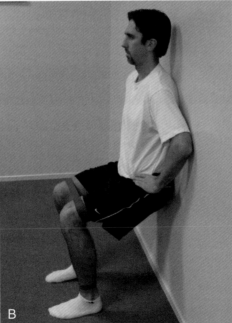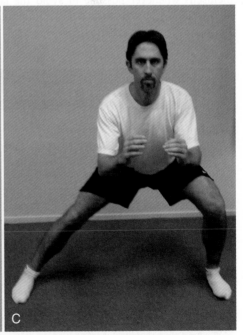

Fig. 24-6 **A,** Side steps with resistance loop. Starting position is an athletic stance. Slowly side step 50 to 100 feet, avoiding trunk compensations and dragging of nonlead leg. **B,** Wall squat with resistance loop. Squats are done to varying degrees of knee flexion depending on what is indicated at that time. Mirror is recommended so patient can see faulty movement patterns. **C,** Frontal plane lunges. Step length and knee flexion are to patient comfort and therapist discretion. Patient can avoid hip external rotation with step or emphasize it depending on the forces wanted in the knee.

TABLE 24-4 **Meniscus Repair**

Rehabilitation Phase	Criteria to Progress to This Phase	Anticipated Impairments and Functional Limitations	Intervention	Goal	Rationale
Phase III Postoperative 12 wk-12 months	• Tolerance to intermediate phase treatment • Full ROM • Normal manual muscle test • Good closed-chain control in linear and multidirectional activity • Treadmill 10-15 minutes at a pace of 7-8 mph without adverse signs and symptoms • Isokinetic strength 70% of the uninvolved extremity	• Isokinetic strength and endurance deficit • Decreased ability to perform full squat or lunge • Fair balance and control with higher level activity	• Progression and continuation of exercises as listed in phases I and II, depending on previous activity level and functional requirements • For peripheral tears, running straight at 4 months, cutting at 5 months, full sports at 5-6 months. • For complex tears, running straight at 6 months, cutting at 7-12 months, full sports at 7-12 months • Isokinetics—Strength and endurance training	• Establish an ongoing training program • Return to preinjury activity or sport • Appropriate performance functional and isokinetic tests as indicated for return to sport or activity	• Continued progression of endurance and strength training • Safe return to functional activity

ROM, Range of motion.

CONCLUSION

Meniscal repair is an effective technique for preserving certain types of tears. Long-term results are still unknown, but the current literature supports preservation of the meniscus whenever possible to avoid the late sequelae of meniscectomy: progressive degeneration of the articular cartilage, flattening of the articular surfaces, and subchondral bone sclerosis. Numerous techniques are available to achieve this goal and selection is primarily a matter of surgeon preference. *A rehabilitation program must be individually tailored based on tear specifics (size, location, repair technique), scientific evidence, clinical signs and symptoms, and patient needs.*

 Suggested Home Maintenance for the Postsurgical Patient

Weeks 1 to 2
GOALS FOR THE PERIOD: Manage pain and swelling, increase ROM and strength, increase weight-bearing activities
1. Heel slides—10 repetitions to be held 30 seconds; pressure within patient's tolerance
2. Ankle pumps—20 to 30 repetitions
3. Isometric muscle contractions—quadriceps, hamstring (if appropriate), adductor, and gluteal isometric contractions (10 to 20 repetitions to be held 10 seconds)
4. Cryotherapy with elevation to be performed as needed throughout the day for 10 to 15 minutes
5. Additional compression garment or wrapping may be helpful

Weeks 3 to 4
GOALS FOR THE PERIOD: Manage pain and swelling, increase ROM and strength, increase weight-bearing activities
1. Supine wall slides or passive heel slides, 10 repetitions to be held 30 seconds; pressure within patient's tolerance
2. Cocontraction isometrics of the quadriceps and hamstrings, 10 to 20 repetitions to be held 10 seconds (depending on the repair site)
3. Isometric quadriceps, adductor, and hamstring contractions, 10 to 20 repetitions to be held 10 seconds
4. Flexibility exercises for the hamstring and gastrocnemius-soleus; stretches should be held at least 30 seconds and repeated 5 to 10 times

5. Four-quad program, two to three sets of 10 repetitions, weight added distally as tolerated
6. Elastic tubing exercises (dorsiflexion, plantar flexion, inversion and eversion, and hip PNF patterns), two to three sets of 10 repetitions
7. Low-resistance, moderate-speed stationary cycling
8. Home aquatic therapy (performing AROM exercises of the hip, knee, and ankle in chest-high water)
9. Continued cryotherapy with elevation to be performed as needed throughout the day for 10 to 15 minutes

Weeks 5 to 11

GOALS FOR THE PERIOD: Gain full ROM and 90% to 100% strength, progress functional activities, progress to gym program
1. Continued open-chain exercise program, four-quads, short arc quadriceps, and PNF patterns with tubing
2. Hamstring, gastrocnemius-soleus, quadriceps, and iliopsoas stretching, 5 to 10 repetitions to be held at least 30 seconds
3. Heel raises, two to three sets of 10 repetitions; lateral step-ups and forward step up and down (using 2-inch height progressions), two to three

sets of 10 repetitions; wall squats, knee flexion at 45° advanced to 60°, two sets of 10 repetitions to be held 10 seconds; minisquats, partial lunges, and progression in knee flexion ROM (add tubing or weight to progress resistance as tolerated), two to three sets of 10 repetitions to be held 5 to 10 seconds
4. Balance activities (bilateral progressed as tolerated to unilateral)—balance board, trampoline (side-to-side and forward-to-back steps), two sets of 1 minute each
5. Exercise cords activity, T kicks, two to three sets of 10 repetitions
6. Stationary cycling, modifying the workload parameters of speed, resistance, and duration based on the response to the activity
7. Stair-stepping machine, cross-country ski machine, or treadmill, with workload progression based on patient response and tolerance

Weeks 12 to 18

GOALS FOR THE PERIOD: Return to sport or preinjury activities, establish an ongoing training program
1. Progression of strength and endurance training
2. Functional or sport-specific drills
3. Agility, sprinting, and track running

CLINICAL CASE REVIEW

1 Jonathan is a 52-year-old man who underwent an inside-out repair of a medial meniscus posterior-horn tear. On his first postoperative visit, he complains of numbness on the inside of his calf extending down the medial side of his leg. What do you tell the patient?

The patient underwent an inside-out repair of a medial meniscus tear, so the surgeon likely made a posteromedial incision through which he or she gained access to tie the sutures. The saphenous neurovascular structures lie an average of 22.6 mm away from this incision[43] and is at risk during this approach (the peroneal nerve is at risk during the posterolateral incision). The patient's nerve injury is likely a neuropraxia (stretching of the nerve but still in continuity) and should return, but the therapist should direct these types of questions to the operating surgeon.

2 Martha is a 47-year-old woman who had a partial lateral meniscectomy for a complex tear approximately 3 weeks ago. This is her second visit, and she is complaining of pain, moderate knee swelling, and limited

knee AROM (30° to 70°). What is most concerning at this point and why?

The patient has a 30° extension lag, and this is very concerning. The inability to fully extend affects gait biomechanics and can lead to the development of permanent flexion contractures if not addressed early. The patient may benefit from more aggressive stretching exercises, as well as a dynamic extension brace. Knee swelling and pain can persist a few weeks after surgery and should be evaluated, but this patient should have obtained full extension within the first week or two after surgery. Also, the patient underwent a partial meniscectomy and not a meniscal repair, so it would be extremely unlikely that the patient has sustained a new meniscal tear this early after surgery.

3 Marek is a 49-year-old golfer who had a lateral posterior horn meniscal repair 3 weeks ago. You find his hamstring musculature remains weak. What would be an appropriate strengthening exercise. At what point will you apply a prone hamstring curl and why?

Bridging with a gym ball requires hip extension while maintaining knee ROM from 0° to 30°. Therefore, both gluteal and hamstring musculature are active in the hip extension role, without any active knee flexion. Active knee flexion pulls the medial and lateral meniscus posterior. The lateral meniscus migrates 1 cm posterior, because the popliteus muscle pulls it during knee flexion. This activity places increased stress on the repaired and healing tissues.

4 Silvia is 40 years old. Before tearing her meniscus, she had two episodes of anterior knee pain over the past 3 years. Silvia had a medial meniscal repair 5 weeks ago. She has been progressing nicely with exercises, and the exercises have been advanced. After treatment she reports pain in the anterior inferior patella region with most of the exercises. Silvia is concerned because she almost slipped and fell after her last physical therapy visit. She denies any episode of her knee locking or becoming stuck. What might be the source of her pain?

Silvia's history, along with the pain distribution pattern, indicates a patellofemoral joint problem that may have become irritated. Meniscal pain often produces complaints of pain near the joint line. Of course, a detailed assessment should be made and the physician notified. In this case the patellofemoral joint was the source of the anterior inferior knee pain. Therefore the patient should be treated for both the patellofemoral symptoms and the meniscal repair. Necessary restrictions should be maintained for each condition. After the patellofemoral symptoms have been significantly reduced or eliminated, the exercise program for the meniscal repair can again be the focus, with consideration of the patellofemoral joint.

5 Darby is a 19-year-old female soccer player who had medial meniscal repair and ACL reconstruction of her right knee. She is 6 weeks postoperation but has noted progressive episodes of clicking in her knee with sit-to-stand transitions. Her swelling has increased, and she has had increased difficulty with walking and standing. What course of action should be taken?

She was reinstructed in an edema management program (i.e., elevation, compression, ice). Her therapeutic exercises and home exercise program were reevaluated for any provocative weight-bearing activities. The physician was called and an MRI was ordered (which revealed that the repair had torn). Complex tears have a higher incidence of failures than simple tears.

6 Angie had a complicated radial repair of her right medial meniscus 7 weeks ago. You want to initiate weight-bearing frontal plane exercises without stressing the repair site. Prescribe three exercises with rationale.

Side steps with resistance band to her right only, so no valgus force is placed through her medial collateral ligament and medial meniscus. Frontal plane lunges with glut dominant movement pattern, placing the knee at no more than 90° flexion. Wall squats with a resistance band around the distal thigh. This requires an isometric hip abduction contraction, strengthening the patient in the frontal plane.

7 John is a 44-year-old recreational tennis player who underwent repair of his medial meniscus 8 weeks ago. He has progressed rapidly through his exercise program without any significant obstacles. He notes a sudden onset of swelling in his knee, which he relates to performing yard work (i.e., raking leaves, squatting down). Although his knee is swollen, no crepitation or locking is seen. His mild pain symptoms appear localized to the medial joint line. What changes should be made in his program?

It appears that he aggravated his repair site with squatting and pivoting activities. This activity should be avoided until he can clinically demonstrate tolerance to this stress. Use of minisquats or an inclined sled allows for the careful control of how much compression is delivered to the knee. Pivoting should be avoided for 6 months. John was cautioned about the risk of retearing his meniscus and his swelling was managed with relative rest, ES, ice, and elevation.

8 Tammy is an active 45-year-old female who had a medial meniscal repair for a radial tear of the posterior horn 2 months ago. She has active knee ROM of 0° to 120° and is currently beginning closed-chain exercises to increase quadriceps and hamstring strength. She asks you if she can return to her Pilates class, which requires deep flexion squats without weight. What should the therapist tell her?

There are many reasons why Tammy should not return to Pilates at this time. First, she has not yet completed the closed-chain portion of her strengthening regimen, which includes toe raises, wall sits, and minisquats. After sufficient strength has been obtained, she must then progress to open-chain knee extension and flexion exercises and ultimately to balance/proprioceptive training before any type of strenuous activity can be initiated. Second, she underwent repair of a radial tear, and this type of tear should be treated more conservatively as it is more difficult to heal than longitudinal or peripheral tears. Third, the load-sharing percentage of the meniscus increases from 50% in full extension to 90% in 90° of flexion, with most of the force transmitted to the posterior horns of the menisci. This patient should refrain from forceful deep knee flexion activities for a period of 4 to 6 months.

9 Tim is 3 months out of medial meniscal repair. He is progressing well except for the medial pain he feels as he approaches 90° of knee flexion while doing wall squats. Your movement analysis reveals excessive femoral adduction and internal rotation during the wall squat. What is your strategy to correct this?

Tim's faulty movement pattern is most likely stressing his repair. The femoral adduction and internal rotation is a result of weak gluteal musculature, both hip abductors and external rotators. Therefore exercises based on recruitment of these muscles is optimal for correcting the alignment. These exercises would progress to weight-bearing exercises with resistance. For example, squats with resistance tubing wrapped around the distal thigh promotes recruitment of hip abductors, and cues the patient to maintain proper form while squatting.

REFERENCES

1. Norkin CC, Levangie PK: Joint structure and function: A comprehensive analysis. Philadelphia, 1992, FA Davis.

2. Fairbanks TJ: Knee joint changes after meniscectomy. J Bone Joint Surg 30B:664, 1948.

3. Arnoczky SP, Warren RF: Microvasculature of the human meniscus. Am J Sports Med 10:90, 1982.

4. Noyes FR, Barber-Westin SD: Arthroscopic repair of meniscal tears extending into the avascular zone in patients younger than twenty years of age. Am J Sports Med 30(4):589-600, 2002.

5. Shelbourne KD, Dersam MD: Comparison of partial meniscectomy versus meniscus repair for bucket-handle lateral meniscus tears in anterior cruciate ligament reconstructed knees. Arthroscopy 20(6):581-585, 2004.

6. Shelbourne KD, Heinrich J: The long-term evaluation of lateral meniscus tears left in situ at the time of anterior cruciate ligament reconstruction. Arthroscopy 20(4):346-351, 2004.

7. Noyes FR, Barber-Westin SD: Arthroscopic repair of meniscus tears extending into the avascular zone with or without anterior cruciate ligament reconstruction in patients 40 years of age and older. Arthroscopy 16(8):822-829, 2000.

8. Shelbourne KD, Carr DR: Meniscal repair compared with meniscectomy for bucket-handle medial meniscal tears in anterior cruciate ligament-reconstructed knees. Am J Sports Med 31(5):718-723, 2003.

9. McCarty EC, Marx RG, DeHaven KE: Meniscus repair: Considerations in treatment and update of clinical results. Clin Orthop Relat Res Sept:(402):122-134, 2002.

10. DeHaven KE: Peripheral meniscal repair: An alternative to meniscectomy. J Bone Joint Surg Br 63:463, 1981.

11. DeHaven KE, Stone RC: Meniscal repair. In Sahiaree H, editor: O'Connor's textbook of arthroscopic surgery. Philadelphia, 1983, Lippincott.

12. DeHaven KE, Lohrer WA, Lovelock JE: Long-term results of open meniscal repair. Am J Sports Med 23(5):524-530, 1995.

13. Rockborn P, Gillquist J: Results of open meniscus repair: Long-term follow-up study with a matched uninjured control group. J Bone Joint Surg Br 82(4):494-498, 2000.

14. Rockborn P, Messner K: Long-term results of meniscus repair and meniscectomy: A 13-year functional and radiographic follow-up study. Knee Surg Sports Traumatol Arthrosc 8(1):2-10, 2000.

15. Henning CE: Arthroscopic repair of meniscus tears. Orthopedics 6:1130, 1983.

16. Spindler KP, et al: Prospective comparison of arthroscopic medial meniscal repair technique: Inside-out suture versus entirely arthroscopic arrows. Am J Sports Med 31(6):929-934, 2003.

17. Johnson LL: Diagnostic and surgical arthroscopy. The knee and other joints, ed 2, St Louis, 1981, Mosby.

18. Morgan CD, et al: Arthroscopic meniscal repair evaluated by second-look arthroscopy. Am J Sports Med 19(6):632-637, 1991.

19. Gill SS, Diduch DR: Outcomes after meniscal repair using the meniscus arrow in knees undergoing concurrent anterior cruciate ligament reconstruction. Arthroscopy 18(6):569-577, 2002.

20. Morgan CD: The all "inside" meniscus repair: Technical note. Arthroscopy 7:120, 1991.

21. Barber FA, Click SD: Meniscus repair rehabilitation with concurrent anterior cruciate reconstruction. Arthroscopy 13:433, 1997.

22. Rubman MH, Noyes FR, Barber-Westin SD: Technical considerations in the management of complex meniscus tears. Clin Sports Med 15:511, 1996.

23. Shelbourne KD, et al: Rehabilitation after meniscal repair. Clin Sports Med 15:595, 1996.

24. McNulty AL, et al: Dynamic loading enhances integrative meniscal repair in the presence of interleukin-1. Osteoarthritis Cartilage 18(6):830-838, 2010.

25. Maitland GD: Peripheral manipulation, ed 3, London, 1991, Butterworth-Heinemann.

26. Noyes FR, Barber-Westin SD: Repair of complex and avascular meniscal tears and meniscal transplantation. J Bone Joint Surg Am 92:1012-1029, 2010.

27. Starke C, et al: Meniscal repair. Arthroscopy 25(9):1033-1044, 2009 Sep.

28. McConnell J: The management of chondromalacia patellae: A long term solution. Aust J Physiother 32(4):215, 1986.

29. Cohn BT, Draeger RI, Jackson DW: The effects of cold therapy on postoperative management of pain In patients undergoing anterior cruciate ligament reconstruction. Am J Sports Med 17(3):344, 1989.

30. Lessard LA, et al: The efficacy of cryotherapy following arthroscopic knee surgery. J Orthop Sports Phys Ther 26(1):14, 1997.

31. Whitelaw GP, et al: The use of the Cryo/Cuff versus ice and elastic wrap in the postoperative care of knee arthroscopy patients. Am J Knee Surg 8(1):28, 1995.

32. DeVries HA: Evaluation of static stretching: Procedures for improvement of flexibility. Res Q Exerc Sport 33:222-229, 1962.

33. Kottke FJ, Pavley DJ, Ptakda DA: The rationale for prolonged stretching for corrections of shortening of connective tissue. Arch Phys Med Rehabil 47:345, 1966.

34. Zachazewski JE: Flexibility for sports. In Saunders B, editor: Sports physical therapy, Norwalk, CT, 1990, Appleton & Lange.

35. Bose K, Kanagasuntheram R, Osman MBH: Vastus medialis oblique: An anatomic and physiologic study. Orthopedics 3:880, 1980.

36. Mangine R, Heckman T: The knee. In Saunders B, editor: Sports physical therapy, Norwalk, CT, 1990, Appleton & Lange.

37. DeLorme TL, Watkins A: Progressive resistance exercise. New York, 1951, Appleton-Century.

38. Kvist M, Jarvinen M: Clinical, histological and biomechanical features in repair of muscle and tendon injuries. Int J Sports Med 3:12, 1982.

39. Heckmann TP, Barber-Westin SD, Noyes FR: Meniscal repair and transplantation: Indications, techniques, rehabilitation, and clinical outcome. J Orthop Sports Phys Ther 36(10):795-814, 2006.

40. Tovin BJ, et al: Comparison of the effects of exercise in water and on land on the rehabilitation of patients with intra-articular anterior cruciate ligament reconstruction. Phys Ther 74(8):710, 1994.

41. McConnell J, Fulkerson J: The knee: Patellofemoral and soft tissue injuries. In Zachazewski JE, Magee DJ, Quillen WS, editors: Athletic injuries and rehabilitation, Philadelphia, 1996, Saunders.

42. Colado JC, et al: Two-leg squat jumps in water: an effective alternative to dry land jumps. Int J Sports Med 31(2):118-122, 2010.

43. Pace JL, Wahl CJ: Arthroscopy of the posterior knee compartments: Neurovascular anatomic relationships during arthroscopic transverse capsulotomy. Arthroscopy 26(5):637-642, 2010. Epub 2010 Mar 12.

CHAPTER 25

Autologous Chondrocyte Implantation

Karen Hambly, Kai Mithoefer, Holly J. Silvers, Bert R. Mandelbaum

Since its first description by Brittberg in 1994,[1] chondrocyte implantation (also known as chondrocyte transplantation) has been performed in more than 15,000 patients worldwide and many studies have clinically validated this technique as a reliable method for biologic restoration of injuries of articular cartilage surfaces.[2-12] Based on the recent evolution and better understanding of the treatment of articular cartilage defects and cell-based implantation techniques, this challenging surgical technique has undergone several technical modifications. These recent developments can help to reduce patient morbidity and technique-specific complications as chondrocyte implantation techniques continue to evolve using modern tissue engineering technologies.

PREOPERATIVE CONSIDERATIONS

History and Clinical Symptoms

Obtaining a thorough history in patients with chondral defects presents a critical first step in the treatment process and selection of patients that are appropriate candidates for chondrocyte implantation. Articular cartilage defects may present acutely after joint trauma such as knee ligament tears, or more chronically as part of a degenerative process. Pain is often present with weight bearing and impact activities. Joint effusion is frequently reported, particularly after demanding impact activities. Cartilage defects of the femoral condyles may produce point tenderness over the femoral condyle rather than the joint line. Catching and locking sensation can occur from cartilage flaps or larger cartilage defects but are nonspecific and may also result from other knee pathology such as meniscal tears. Defects of the patella or trochlea usually lead to pain when ambulating stairs, driving a car, or getting out of a chair or squatting position. Symptoms of patellar instability may be reported. Patients considered for chondrocyte implantation techniques may have undergone prior cartilage repair procedures and a detailed evaluation of the prior surgical procedures should be performed. The time since the initial injury and the type of previous surgeries should be recorded since these factors have been shown to affect the outcome after chondrocyte implantation.

Physical examination includes the evaluation of the patient's gait pattern and lower extremity alignment. Hip, knee, and ankle range of motion (ROM) should be assessed and any joint effusion noted. Since articular cartilage lesions are frequently found in patients with acute hemathrosis, acute or chronic ligamentous instability, patellar dislocation or maltracking, or lower extremity malalignment, these factors should be routinely evaluated. Depending on the defect's location and size, mechanical symptoms may or may not be present and may overlap with meniscal tests. The patient's body mass index should be assessed because it has been shown to correlate with functional outcome after articular cartilage repair.

Diagnostic Imaging

Plain radiographs including weight-bearing anterior/posterior and lateral views, Rosenberg and tunnel views, long-leg films, and Merchant views can help to identify osteochondral lesions, joint space narrowing, patellar maltracking, or lower extremity malalignment. Cartilage sensitive magnetic resonance imaging (MRI) presents a sensitive, specific, and accurate tool for noninvasive diagnosis of articular cartilage injury.[13,14] Cartilage sensitive MRI provides useful information about meniscal and ligamentous status, subchondral bone, lesion size, location, and depth. Because of the pathologic changes in the surrounding cartilage, the final size of the defect intraoperatively usually is larger than defect size measured on a preoperative MRI. Besides its use for preoperative diagnosis, cartilage sensitive MRI can be very helpful for postoperative evaluation of cartilage repair. Routine postoperative MRI is recommended to evaluate the cartilage repair tissue and detect potential complications such as graft hypertrophy. If available, newer technologies such as T2 mapping, delayed gadolinium enhanced MRI of cartilage, or T1 rho relaxation mapping can be used to obtain additional detail about cartilage morphology before and after surgery.[14]

Indications and Contraindications

Chondrocyte implantation is indicated for symptomatic, high-grade chondral and osteochondral defects of the knee in active patients that are physiologically too young for arthroplasty. This technique can be successfully used as a first-line treatment for lesions more than 2 cm² of femoral condylar, trochlear, and patellar lesions or used as a revision technique for failed prior cartilage repair procedures.[2,10-12] The technique can be successfully used for isolated, multiple, and kissing cartilage defects. Prerequisites for successful autologous chondrocyte implantation (ACI) include adequate ROM, appropriate axial alignment or patellar tracking, ligamentous stability, and the ability to comply with the postoperative rehabilitation. Adjuvant procedures may be indicated to correct coexisting knee pathology and can be performed simultaneously with chondrocyte implantation without negative effects of these complex procedures on the postoperative functional outcome and activity level.

Absolute contraindications for ACI include generalized osteoarthritis, inflammatory arthropathies, or joint sepsis. Patients unable to comply with the postoperative rehabilitation and weight-bearing protocol should also not be treated with this technique. A body mass index greater than 30 kg/m² has been associated with limited improvement after knee articular cartilage repair and presents a relative contraindication. Patients with severe meniscal deficiency should be considered for meniscal allograft transplantation at the time of chondrocyte implantation.

Preoperative Patient Counseling

Based on the history, physical examination, and radiologic information, the indication for ACI or adjuvant procedures is discussed with the patient. In-depth preoperative patient counseling is critically important to determine the patient's demands, to assess his or her ability to comply with the postoperative rehabilitation plan, and to create realistic expectations and goals for postoperative knee function and activity level.

SURGICAL TECHNIQUE

Stage 1: Chondrocyte Harvest

Step 1: Diagnostic Joint Arthroscopy

ACI of the knee presents a two-stage procedure. The first stage involves a complete arthroscopic evaluation. Besides identification of the index cartilage defect, the entire articular cartilage surface is inspected to rule out any additional cartilage pathology. During the first-stage arthroscopy, the cartilage defect is identified and existing cartilage flaps are débrided back to a stable and healthy peripheral margin. Following thorough débridement, the size of the articular cartilage lesion is measured and its containment documented. The knee is taken through a full ROM and the arc of motion, during which the lesion articulates with the opposing joint surface, is carefully recorded (Fig. 25-1). The opposing joint surface should always be carefully inspected for the presence

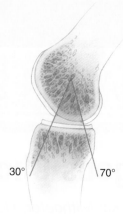

Fig. 25-1 The exact location and range of articulation of the defect is noted carefully to facilitate postoperative rehabilitation in the nonloading "safe zone"

of a kissing lesion or signs of low-grade cartilage injury. Partial meniscectomy and meniscal repair can be performed because it minimally affects the course after the initial arthroscopy and decreases operative time during the second-stage procedure. However, surgical treatment of meniscal deficiency or ligamentous pathology should be performed simultaneously with ACI to avoid repetitive operative joint trauma and prolonged rehabilitation.

Step 2: Chondrocyte Harvesting

Following initial arthroscopic evaluation, 200 to 300 mg of normal articular cartilage is obtained from a lesser weight-bearing area of the injured knee, generally the medial or lateral superior ridge of the femoral condyle or intercondylar notch. The intercondylar notch is preferred for patellofemoral lesions. Using cartilage that has been débrided from the cartilage defect as graft is not recommended because chondrocyte quality from this area has been shown to be inferior. The grafted cartilage tissue is sent for standardized commercial isolation and culturing of chondrocytes. Implantation of cultured chondrocytes is performed after 2 to 4 weeks when a sufficient number of cells have been obtained for the size of the defect (range, 4 to 12 million cells). Chondrocyte viability is routinely tested and should be more than 95% before implantation.

Stage 2: Chondrocyte Implantation

Step 1: Adjuvant Procedures

Ligamentous instability, meniscal injury and deficiency, or malalignment have been shown to contribute to the development of articular cartilage lesions, and surgically addressing these concomitant pathologies is critical for an effective and durable articular cartilage repair.[10-12] Concomitant ligament reconstruction, meniscal allograft, or osteotomy should be performed before ACI. Isolated or combined adjuvant procedures do not negatively affect postoperative activity levels after ACI.[8] Concomitant rather than staged adjuvant procedures avoid prolonged rehabilitation, promote postoperative activity, and provide a significant cost benefit.

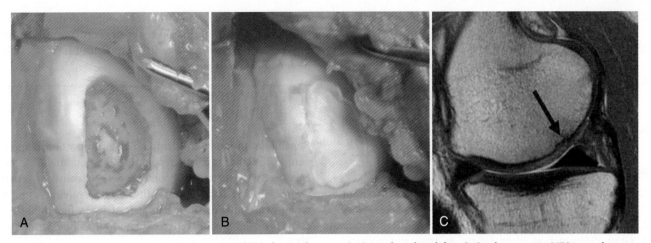

Fig. 25-2 A, Articular cartilage defect of the femoral condyle before implantation. **B,** Covered cartilage defect. **C,** Cartilage sensitive MRI image demonstrating complete fill of the cartilage defect after 36 months.

Step 2: Autologous Chondrocyte Implantation

Following parapatellar arthrotomy, the cartilage defect is débrided back to a healthy cartilage margin and the calcified cartilage and intralesional osteophytes are carefully removed without violating the subchondral bone (Fig. 25-2, *A*). If bleeding is encountered, hemostasis of the defect bed can be achieved by application of thrombin or fibrin glue. A template of the defect is created to then harvest an appropriately sized periosteal flap from the proximal medial border of the tibia. When using periosteum, the tissue patch should be slightly larger than the defect because of a tendency of the periosteum to contract. Any adherent fatty or connective tissue needs to be carefully removed to minimize the potential for graft hypertrophy. The periosteal flap is then sutured flush to the articular cartilage defect using interrupted 6-0 Vicryl* with the cambium layer facing into the defect. As an alternative to the periosteum, a type I/III collagen membrane can be used to cover the defect (Fig. 25-2, *B* and *C*). This allows for smaller incisions, reduces patient morbidity, and minimizes the potential for graft hypertrophy. The rim of the periosteal flap or collagen membrane is sealed watertight with fibrin glue except for one corner, where the implanted chondrocytes are injected into the defect. Following cell injection, the remaining corner of the periosteal flap is secured with sutures and sealed with fibrin glue. Drains are not normally used to prevent injury to the periosteal cover or fibrin seal of the defect from direct abrasion by the drain during postoperative joint mobilization. A compression dressing is placed over the involved joint and cryotherapy is used routinely. Bracing is not indicated for isolated chondrocyte transplantations but may be used if simultaneous adjuvant procedures require postoperative protection.

Deep Chondral or Osteochondral Defects

In patients with lesions deeper than 1 cm, autologous bone grafting should be performed in combination with ACI. Implantation of chondrocytes in these cases is performed using the "sandwich technique." The osseous defect is filled with a cancellous bone graft from the iliac crest or proximal tibia to the level of the subchondral plate. One periosteal flap or collagen membrane—sized for the defect—is then anchored using fibrin glue applied between the patch and the bone graft. A second sized periosteal flap or membrane is then placed facing into the defect and sutured to the surrounding cartilage. The rim is again sealed with fibrin glue and the cultured chondrocytes are then implanted between the two periosteal flaps or collagen membranes (sandwich technique).

POSTOPERATIVE MANAGEMENT

Complications

Complications after chondrocyte implantation include stiffness and adhesions in up to 10% of patients. Graft hypertrophy is seen in 25% to 63% of postoperative magnetic resonance images but described as clinically symptomatic in only 13% to 15%.[1-12] Symptomatic hypertrophy can be effectively treated by arthroscopic chondroplasty. Hypertrophy may lead to partial detachment or graft delamination. Substituting the periosteum with collagen membranes or second generation matrix-associated chondrocyte implantation (MACI) effectively reduce the risk for periosteal hypertrophy.[15] Graft failure has been described in 6% to 7% of cases. Grafts usually fail between 12 to 24 months after surgery and frequently show central degeneration. Treatment with revision chondrocyte implantation has been shown to be effective in many cases.[12] All patients with graft failure should be carefully evaluated for the presence of subtle instability, axial malalignment, or patellar maltracking, which has been shown to lead to lower success rates after ACI.

SURGICAL PEARLS AND PITFALLS

Pearls

1. Assess for and address concomitant joint pathology (alignment, instability, and meniscal pathology).

*Ethicon Inc., New Brunswick, N.J.

2. Avoid staging adjuvant procedures to reduce prolonged rehabilitation and facilitate return to activity.

3. Record location and articulation of defect to facilitate postoperative rehabilitation in "safe zone".

4. Substitution of periosteum with collagen membrane or MACI can reduce invasiveness and risk for graft hypertrophy.

5. Sandwich technique useful for deep chondral/osteochondral defects.

Pitfalls

1. Failure to recognize and treat concomitant joint pathology

2. Limited success rate for tibial defects and kissing lesions

3. Graft delamination from failure to treat symptomatic graft hypertrophy

Surgical Summary

ACI has been successfully used for hyaline-like restoration of full-thickness articular cartilage lesions in the knee with long-term durability of functional improvements of up to 11 years.[10,11] Good to excellent results were found in 92% of isolated femoral condyle lesions, 89% of osteochondritis dissecans, 75% of femoral condyle lesions with concomitant anterior cruciate ligament reconstruction, 67% of patients with multiple lesions, and in 65% of patella lesions.[1-12] Return to sport is possible in 33% to 96%, with best return rates in competitive and adolescent athletes. Patients with single lesions, younger age, and short preoperative intervals have the best results.[8,9] Correcting axial malalignment, patellar maltracking, and ligamentous laxity is critical for the functional improvement. Limitations of this technique include its invasiveness, long postoperative rehabilitation, and periosteal hypertrophy, which may lead to acute graft delamination. This cartilage repair technique provides significant functional improvement with high return rates to demanding sports and excellent durability even under high athletic demands both in the primary and revision setting.

Scaffold-associated second-generation autologous cartilage implantation techniques use three-dimensional biodegradable scaffolds to temporarily support the chondrocytes until they are replaced by matrix components synthesized from the implanted cells. MACI has been used with promising results in Europe and Australia but is not routinely available for use in the United States.[15,16] The use of the biomatrix seeded with chondrocytes reduces surgical invasiveness and has the theoretic advantages of less chondrocyte leakage, more homogeneous chondrocyte distribution, and less graft hypertrophy. Arthroscopic MACI has been described with improvement of knee function up to 90%.[16] Future developments are aimed at improving cellular matrix production by using more productive "characterized" chondrocytes and more sophisticated bioactive scaffolds that include growth factors and stimulate a more natural spatial distribution of chondrocytes within the repair cartilage.[17,18] Other promising future approaches include identification and selective expansion of specific chondrocyte subpopulations capable of producing more hyaline-like repair cartilage tissue or implantation of neocartilage tissue produced in specifically designed bioreactors.[19,20]

THERAPY GUIDELINES FOR REHABILITATION

Rehabilitation has been identified as an important component in articular cartilage repair with the potential to influence both the patient outcome and the quality of repair tissue.[21] In the last 10 years, the fastest evolving surgical repair of articular cartilage has been ACI. The first published review of ACI postoperative care and rehabilitation was in 2006.[22]

The goal of any ACI rehabilitation program is to provide a mechanical environment for the local adaptation and remodeling of the repaired tissue that will enable the patient to safely return to the optimal level of function. The challenge is to construct an individualized rehabilitation program that matches mechanical loading to the status of the repair tissue at any postoperative time point. Successful ACI rehabilitation is reliant on a collaborative environment, with thorough communication between the surgeon, therapist, and patient. A graded rehabilitation program incorporating preoperative counseling, progressive weight bearing,[30] and controlled exercise[31] is generally recommended following ACI. An understanding of applied clinical biomechanics and appreciation of the forces and loads that will be exerted on the repair tissue are essential in the design of an ACI rehabilitation program. This chapter focuses on the principles behind effective ACI rehabilitation and the rationale behind the components of the rehabilitation.

There are a number of elements that are essential in the designing of an individualized ACI rehabilitation program, including the following:

1. Recognition of factors that led to the acute or chronic degeneration of the articular cartilage surface

2. Recognition of factors that affect functional outcome after ACI

3. Respect for the biologic timeframes for healing

4. Application of exercise programming knowledge

5. Establishment of criteria for modification or progression of exercise

6. Acknowledgement and incorporation of the expectations and goals of the patient

The three main components required within an ACI **rehabilitation program are progressive weight bearing; restoration of ROM; and enhancement of muscle control, proprioception, and strength.**[22-25] The ACI-specific evidence base to directly support the frequency, intensity, type, and timing of exercise modalities during rehabilitation is limited. Studies have advocated avoidance of certain ranges of knee movement, for example, active knee flexion between 40° and 70° in the early stages after patellofemoral ACI.[22] However, virtually all exercise activities, including common activities such as walking, cycling, and rowing, involve a knee flexion/extension pattern within this range.[31] The incorporation of exercises into the ACI rehabilitation program may be better considered in terms of minimizing joint stress as opposed to the complete avoidance of specific ranges of movement. This can be achieved through the selection, introduction, and progression of exercise activities that are appropriate for the graft status, size, and location. Exercises should complement and not replace functional movement retraining.

The guidelines that follow are designed to help guide therapists through the rehabilitation process. It should be noted that these guidelines are for first-generation ACI using either periosteal flap or collagen membrane and that there is currently considerable variation in rehabilitation practice between clinical centers. The therapist should evaluate each patient on an individual basis and select appropriate rehabilitation content and criteria for progressions for the individual, working around any restrictions imposed by the surgeon.

Initial Evaluation

Several factors have been associated with superior functional outcome following cartilage repair surgery.[26] These include:

- Younger age of patient
- Shorter preoperative duration of symptoms
- Fewer number of previous surgeries
- Smaller size of defect (cm$_2$)
- Medial femoral condyle repairs do better than patellofemoral repairs
- Isolated defects do better than multiple and/or kissing defects.
- The correction of mechanical malalignment before surgery
- Professional/competitive athletes do better than recreational athletes.
- Participants of low impact sports do better than participants of high-impact sports.

A preoperative evaluation should be made for each patient. Overt muscle imbalances should be noted and addressed in a home exercise program before surgery. The patient's occupational demands and their access to rehabilitation facilities and modalities is extremely useful information when designing an individualized rehabilitation program.

PREOPERATIVE MANAGEMENT

A preoperative session is beneficial for both patient and therapist. To maximize the benefits of ACI surgery, it is essential for patients to understand and consequently comply with their ACI rehabilitation program. Preoperative assessment should include ROM, muscle strength, proprioception, function, gait, and an assessment of problematic activities of daily living (ADL). A preoperative therapy session provides an ideal opportunity to explain the rehabilitation program; teach ambulation with crutch(es); and demonstrate early home exercises to the patient.

POSTOPERATIVE REHABILITATION

The repair site is at its most vulnerable during the first few months after ACI. Although chronologic time frames have been established for the rehabilitation phases, it is more important that the patient achieves the qualitative goals of each phase. An important rehabilitation principle is program individualization. Patients may progress through rehabilitation at different paces because of multiple factors, including lesion size, lesion location, preoperative duration of symptoms, preoperative baseline physical condition, age, and patient motivation. When a patient achieves all the functional goals of a particular rehabilitation phase, they may advance to the next phase of the rehabilitation.

Phase I: Recovery and Protection

TIME: 0 to 6 weeks
GOALS: Protection of the repair tissue, restoration of joint homeostasis, and improving ROM (Table 25-1)

The evidence basis for optimal timing of return to full weight bearing (FWB) following ACI is limited. Historically, as with most new surgical interventions, rehabilitation has been conservative and has included lengthy periods of non–weight bearing and partial weight bearing (PWB). Newly emerging research indicates that it is possible to accelerate weight-bearing loads in certain patient populations with good clinical and functional outcome after 2 years without jeopardizing the graft.[27,28] Research indicates that moderate dynamic compression and shear loading are beneficial to extracellular matrix biosynthesis; chondrocyte proliferation; and repair tissue maturation, whereas static compression and immobilization are associated with adverse effects.[29,32] **High shear stress may lead to mechanical failure of ACI grafts in the early postoperative rehabilitation phase and it is therefore necessary to implement a graded increase in loading.** Weight-bearing status should be predicated based on the location of repair, secondary to the biomechanical differences between ACI to a tibiofemoral joint surface and a patellofemoral joint surface.

For femoral condyle defects:
- Toe-touch weight bearing for 1 to 2 weeks at minimal body weight (<10%) and as tolerated
- Begin heel-toe touch down weight bearing (approximately 10 to 15 kg) at week 2
- Progress to PWB (approximately 30% of body weight) at week 4
- Aim for FWB by weeks 8 to 10

For trochlea and patella defects:
- Immediate heel-toe touch down weight bearing in full extension with approximately 25% body weight as tolerated
- Progress to 50% body weight in full extension at week 2
- Progress to 75% body weight in full extension at week 4
- Aim for FWB by weeks 6 to 8

TABLE 25-1 **Autologous Chondrocyte Implantation**

Rehabilitation Phase	Criteria for Progress to This Phase	Anticipated Impairments and Functional Limitations	Intervention	Goal	Rationale
Phase I Postoperative 0-6 wk	• Postoperative and cleared by the surgeon to initiate therapy • There may be specific precautions	• Edema • Pain • Limited ROM • Limited strength • Limited weight bearing • Altered gait	• Weight-bearing control with crutches • CPM • AROM exercises (ankle, knee, and hip) • Education and coaching • Quadriceps setting exercises • Cryotherapy, elevation, and compression • Patellar mobilization • Biofeedback and electric muscle stimulation • Aquatic therapy once incision has healed • Balance for control of PWB	• Avoid excessive stress on ACI • Restore full PROM knee extension • Gradually increase pain-free knee flexion • Ensure safe transfers for home and transportation • Regain quadriceps control • Gradual increase in weight bearing • Improve PF mobility	• Protection of repair tissue from excessive load and shear forces • Allow cell adherence • Prevent adhesions • Improve ROM • Gradual increase in ROM and weight bearing for protection of repair tissue • Restore proprioception • Increase reliance on patient self-management

ACI, Autologous chondrocyte implantation; *AROM*, active range of motion; *CPM*, continuous passive motion; *PF*, patellofemoral; *PROM*, passive range of motion; *PWB*, partial weight bearing; *ROM*, range of motion.
Exercises: Lateral hip (abduction) side-lying, hip extension work (glut activation) without knee flexion, isometric glut squeezes.

It is important to note that patients are not completely reliable in PWB and tend to overestimate weight in the early rehabilitative stages even after instruction.[33] The accuracy of weight bearing can be practically assessed, taught, and reinforced with patients using two pairs of identical scales (Fig. 25-3).[22] This is also a useful technique for controlling weight shift exercises and for the correction of body posture, and any residual unloading of the involved limb later in the rehabilitation process.

Continuous passive motion (CPM) is reported to increase the quality of chondral repair tissue[34-36] and stimulate the metabolism of proteoglycan 4.[37] Consequently, CPM is a standard inclusion in ACI rehabilitation in many centers.[25] However, for patients with small, isolated defects of the femoral condyle, results may not be negatively affected by the replacement of CPM with graded weight bearing and active ROM (AROM); however, the evidence base is limited.[38,39] The recommendation for the use of CPM is currently based on basic science, usual practice, case series, and disease-orientated evidence.[25] Once again, there is a need to differentiate the rehabilitation based on the defect location:

For femoral condyle defects:
- Initiate CPM day 1 for a total of 6 to 8 hours per day at 0° to 60°
- Progress CPM by 5° to 10° per day as tolerated
- Continue CPM for a total of 6 to 8 hours per day for 6 weeks
- Knee flexion ROM goal is 90° by week 2; 105° by week 3; 115° by week 4; and 125° by week 5.

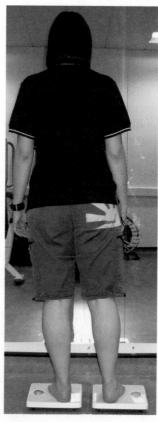

Fig. 25-3 PWB can be practically assessed, taught, and reinforced using standard bathroom scales.

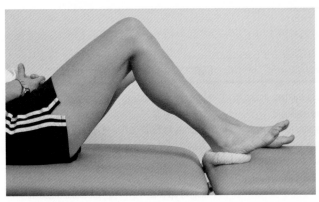

Fig. 25-4 Heel slides using a crepe bandage "donut" under involved limb to assist sliding.

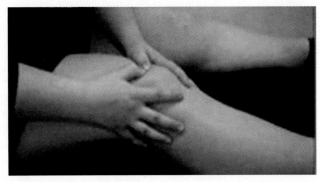

Fig. 25-5 Patellar mobilizations can be taught to the patient for self-management on a daily basis.

For trochlea and patella defects:

- Initiate CPM day 1 for a total of 6 to 8 hours per day at 0° to 40°
- Progress CPM by 5° to 10° per day as tolerated
- Continue CPM for a total of 6 to 8 hours per day for 6 weeks
- Knee flexion ROM goal is 90° by week 3; 105° by week 4; and 120° by week 6.
- No active open kinetic chain (OKC) knee extension exercises during this phase.

CPM is not consistently used across cartilage repair centers and is often not available to patients. Where CPM is not available, it can be substituted by 500 active assisted heel slides performed three times per day with the same ROM progressions and goals as indicated for CPM (Fig. 25-4). **ROM exercises should progress through a controlled increase in ROM through passive, active-assisted, and then active movements.** Repetitive dynamic movement through the available ROM provides mechanical stimulation to chondrocytes, as well as increasing synovial fluid flow over the graft.[40,41]

In addition to weight bearing, CPM, and ROM guidance, most rehabilitation guidelines will provide further information regarding exercise and therapeutic modalities. In the early postoperative time period, the application of cryotherapy, compression, and elevation are important to lower tissue temperature, slow metabolism, decrease secondary hypoxic injury, and reduce edema formation.[42] Gentle patellar mobilizations in all directions 4 to 6 times per day are important to prevent adhesions and arthrofibrosis (Fig. 25-5).[43-46] Knee surgery results in proprioceptive deficits[47] that should be addressed at the earliest postoperative opportunity. Proprioception can be initiated in phase I of rehabilitation as long as weight-bearing restrictions are applied. This may require adaptation of exercises to PWB. Gait training focuses on crutch walking to minimize soft tissue constrictions (especially tightness in hamstrings, gastrocnemius, and soleus muscles) and increasing the acceptance of load on the involved leg through controlled weight shifting. Aquatic therapy to enhance gait training and improve lower extremity strength/ROM can commence once the surgical incision has healed and the patient is able to safely transfer in and out

of the pool. The water depth should reflect the weight-bearing status of the individual. Stationary cycling can be introduced with minimal resistance once knee flexion ROM is at least 100°.[22] There is currently no evidence-based consensus to support or refute the use of postoperative bracing for ACI. Some centers will use bracing for patellofemoral ACI repairs for the first 4 to 6 weeks, especially if the defects are large or kissing or if there is a quadriceps lag. Neuromuscular electrical stimulation can be introduced and is a valuable adjunct to the program, especially where voluntary control of the quadriceps mechanism is limited.

Phase II: Transition

TIME: 6 to 12 weeks

GOALS: Inauguration of the repair tissue, restoration of full ROM, and initiation and progression of muscle strengthening (Table 25-2)

During the transition phase, many of the interventions from phase I are continued and incorporated into a maintenance program. AROM exercises can be progressed to light resistance in "safe ranges" while simultaneously maintaining no resistance over the repaired area. Safe ranges will be dictated by the articulation surfaces, contact area, and size and location of the graft. For example, as the posterior aspect of the medial femoral condyle contacts the tibia between 90° and 120°,[48] light resistance in the range from 0° to 80° may be appropriate. Several research articles provide detailed information on the clinical biomechanics of the tibiofemoral and patellofemoral joints.[11,49-52] Once FWB has been restored, forward lunges and forward and lateral step-ups can be introduced and treadmill walking can be initiated within safe ranges as dictated by the repair location and size.

Quadriceps setting exercises can be progressed from isometric multiangle exercises. Gluteal muscle retraining is an important component of ACI rehabilitation, especially where patients have altered lower extremity kinematics.[53] Gluteus medius and minimus play an important role in the neuromuscular and valgus control of the knee[54] and consequently normal posture and gait patterns, so exercises should be targeted at these muscles (Fig. 25-6, *A* and *B*).[55,56] Proprioception and balance exercises can be progressed in line with

TABLE 25-2 Autologous Chondrocyte Implantation

Rehabilitation Phase	Criteria for Progress to This Phase	Anticipated Impairments and Functional Limitations	Intervention	Goal	Rationale
Phase II Postoperative 6-12 wk	• Minimal pain and swelling • Able to perform daily joint circulation exercises within homeostasis • Surgical incisions healed • Full passive knee extension • Voluntary quadriceps activity and able to perform quadriceps setting exercise with no lag • Active, pain-free knee flexion of 120°	• Edema • Pain • Reduced ROM • Limited strength • PWB • Altered gait	• WB control with crutches moving to FWB in control conditions • Stretching program for the hip, ankle, and knee (as appropriate) • AROM exercises (no resistance over repaired zone and light resistance in safe ranges) • Education and coaching • Quadriceps setting exercises progressing to isometric multiangle exercises • Balance for control of weight bearing for ADL • Patellar mobilization • Biofeedback and electric muscle stimulation • Quadriceps isometric multiangle exercises • Aquatic therapy • Gluteal muscle retraining—hip extension, external rotation, abduction	• Increase to full active, pain-free ROM • Progress to FWB • Regain full quadriceps control • Increase ADL • Regain optimal coordination for walking and stairs • Increase proprioception • Improve PF mobility • Increase neuromuscular control and muscle activation • Increase quad strength and overall joint stability • Increase strength, endurance, and stamina while diminishing WB	• Quadriceps control and coordination • Aquatic therapy for gait coordination and joint circulation exercises • Restore proprioception • Gradual increase in weight bearing and ROM for protection of repair tissue • Gradual increase in functional activities • Improve coordination in multidirectional tasks • Increase reliance on patient self-management • Improve gait while limited with WB • Improve single-limb stance

ADL, Activities of daily living; *AROM,* active range of motion; *FWB,* full weight bearing; *PF,* patellofemoral; *PWB,* partial weight bearing; *ROM,* range of motion; *WB,* weight bearing.
Exercises: Gluteal strength: standing hip extension (with appropriate knee angle), standing abduction—use mild resistance (i.e., Thera-Band) to address gluteus medius and gluteus maximus deficiencies.

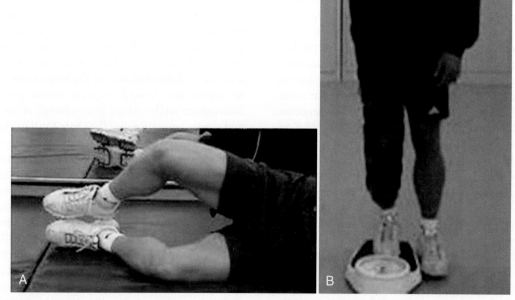

Fig. 25-6 Gluteal muscle exercises can be adapted for the repair location. **A,** For tibiofemoral joint repairs, a side-lying "clam" exercise can be used. **B,** For patellofemoral joint repairs, a hip hike exercise can be used during standing, with the involved knee in full extension.

increased weight-bearing status. The therapist must monitor any progressions in exercises and check that symptoms are not increased.

Phase III: Remodeling

TIME: 12 to 26 weeks
GOALS: Improvement of muscle strength and endurance and reintroduction of functional activities (Table 25-3)

Phase III continues with the maintenance program of exercises within phase II with appropriate progressions in resistance, repetitions, sets, and frequency, with close monitoring of patient response. Proprioception and balance training can be progressed to involve multidirectional functional tasks. Feed-forward muscular control exercises, such as lunges and unilateral step up/downs (Fig. 25-7) in a controlled therapy environment will not only assist in strengthening and restoring dynamic control but will also help to enhance the patient's confidence in the involved knee. Gait analysis allows the therapist to assess the patient dynamically, identifying asymmetries in pressure transfer, compensatory mechanisms, and movement-related problems during the gait cycle (Fig. 25-8). Cardiovascular and muscular

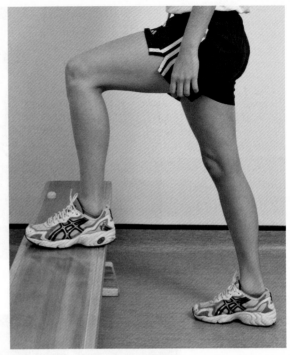

Fig. 25-7 Single-leg steps are a good way to evaluate neuromuscular control and body posture.

TABLE 25-3 Autologous Chondrocyte Implantation

Rehabilitation Phase	Criteria for Progress to This Phase	Anticipated Impairments and Functional Limitations	Intervention	Goal	Rationale
Phase III Postoperative 12-26 wk	• Minimal pain and swelling • Full ROM • Full voluntary quadriceps activity • Acceptable muscle strength—hamstrings within 20% of contralateral leg and quadriceps within 30% of contralateral leg • Balance testing within 30% of contralateral leg • Able to walk 1-2 miles (level ground) or bike for 30 minutes (stationary cycle low resistance)	• Reduced strength • Altered gait • Reduced endurance • Reduced balance • Reduced confidence in knee • Possible kinesiophobia	• AROM exercises (no resistance over repaired zone and light resistance in safe ranges) • FWB control in exercise conditions • Preparatory (feed-forward) neuromuscular control exercises • Gait reeducation • Gluteal muscle retraining • Single-limb stance exercises as appropriate • Patellar mobilization • Aquatic therapy, further progression of gait training, and single-limb stance activities in the water	• Increase muscle strength • Restore gait • Increase ADL • Progress OKC strengthening with minimal resistance over angles where defect articulates • Progress walking—distance, cadence, and incline • Continue maintenance program • Decrease gait deviations in stance phase	• Improve control in exercise conditions • Increase reliance on patient self-management • Improve coordination in multidirectional tasks • Increase functional activities • Aquatic exercises help reduce stress with weight-bearing activities

ADL, Activities of daily living; *AROM,* active range of motion; *FWB,* full weight bearing; *OKC,* open kinetic chain; *ROM,* range of motion.
Exercises: Increase progressive resistive therapeutic exercise for quadriceps (knee extension with appropriate knee angles), knee flexion, hip extension/flexion/abduction/adduction in standing with resistance at ankle joint, supine core/trunk stability work (i.e., Pilates), physioball (supine and prone), and proprioceptive work on unstable surface (wobble boards, Bosu, Airex mat).

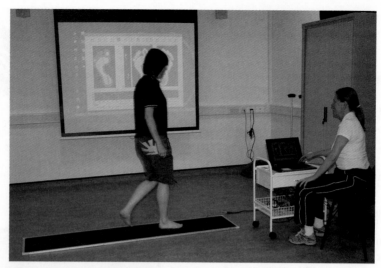

Fig. 25-8 Clinical gait analysis is very useful for revealing abnormal patterns of functional movement and residual asymmetries.

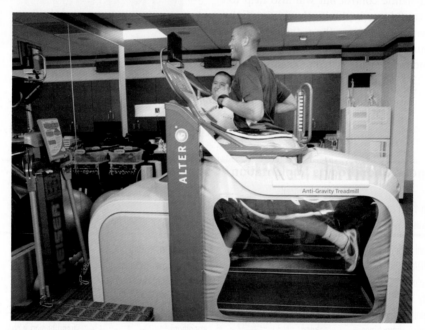

Fig. 25-9 Positive air pressure treadmills can provide an opportunity for an earlier return to jogging and running in a PWB environment.

endurance can be increased with the introduction of low impact exercise activities, such as swimming, rowing, or elliptical training, and through the progression of the walking program with increases in distance, cadence, and incline.

Phase IV: Maturation

TIME: 26 weeks onward
GOALS: Returning the patient to full unrestricted
activity (Table 25-4)

During the maturation phase, return to work times will depend on the demands of the occupation. Sedentary work can be resumed earlier than manual labor. A phased return to work allows for a more controlled return, with initial recovery time for the body to adapt. Return to driving times

will depend on which leg is involved and whether the vehicle is manual or automatic transmission.

Return to sport times will depend on the type of sport that the individual wants to return to and the ability of the individual to accept the demands of that sport without short- or long-term adverse effects. Low impact exercise activities such as swimming, cycling, and rowing can be started at 4 to 6 months. Higher impact exercise activities, such as jogging, running, and aerobics, may be performed from 8 months. Jogging can be introduced earlier for athletes by using a positive air pressure treadmill at reduced body weight (Fig. 25-9). High impact sports such as basketball, ice hockey, badminton, tennis, football, and soccer are allowed at 12 to 18 months. Return to sport rates after ACI from published clinical studies average 67%, but there is a considerable range

TABLE 25-4 Autologous Chondrocyte Implantation

Rehabilitation Phase	Criteria for Progress to This Phase	Anticipated Impairments and Functional Limitations	Intervention	Goal	Rationale
Phase IV Postoperative 26-52+ wk	• Full nonpainful ROM • Strength within 80%-90% of contralateral leg • Balance within 75%-80% of contralateral leg • No pain, inflammation, or swelling • Able to perform daily joint exercises for at least 60 minutes within homeostasis	• Limited endurance • Reduced confidence in knee • Asymmetry in lower limb strength and flexibility • Possible kinesiophobia	• Impact loading program individually designed for patient's needs • Balance exercises in challenging, coordinative tasks • Aquatic therapy swimming (kick emphasis) for general endurance • Functional and sport-specific agility training • Functional strength training (progressing to full resistance over repaired zone for both OKC and CKC) • Presports conditioning (if appropriate) • Education and coaching	• Progress maintenance program • Progress resistance as tolerated • Emphasis on entire lower limb strength and flexibility • Return to sports activities if appropriate • Improve confidence in knee • Increase intensity, load, and volume of exercise • Aim for unrestricted function • Restore symmetry including lower limb strength and flexibility • Prevent further damage/injury	• Preparing patient for return to full unrestricted functional activities • Prevent further injury • Gradually restore loading to repair tissue • Prepare patient for return to sports activities if appropriate

CKC, Closed kinetic chain; *OKC,* open kinetic chain; *ROM,* range of motion.
Exercises: Address any pathokinematics during joint loading (i.e., dynamic valgus). Improve single-leg balance with combined balance/strength activities. Increase intensity, duration, and resistance of therapeutic exercise for core/trunk, hip, knee, and ankle joints. Increase time duration for supine plank work. Aerobically (cardiovascular), incorporate interval work for incline and speed to return to prior level of fitness.

(33% to 96%).[26] Average time to return to sport is reported to be 18 months (range, 12 to 36 months), varying on the individual factors and the nature of the sport.[26] It is important to note that not all individuals will return to sport after ACI and this will be key to managing patient expectations.

REHABILITATION PEARLS AND PITFALLS

Pearls

1. Agree on realistic expectations and goals with the patient.
2. Obtain details on the surgery, size, location, and articulation of the defect.
3. Address the faulty pathokinematics that may have led to the defect in the first place.
4. Focus on what the patient can do rather than the restrictions.
5. Closely monitor clinical signs of pain or swelling; modify or regress rehabilitation as appropriate.
6. Accelerated postoperative weight-bearing protocol can help to promote postoperative function and the patient's overall satisfaction with the procedure.
7. Provide emotional support for the patient through the rehabilitation process.

8. Recognize that not all patients will return to sports activities.

Pitfalls

1. Failure to recognize and adjust rehabilitation to individual patient presentation
2. Biologic timescales for cartilage repair not fully understood
3. Functional rehabilitation principles not consistently applied
4. Rehabilitation not differentiated based on location and size of defect

SUGGESTED HOME MAINTENANCE FOR THE POSTSURGICAL PATIENT

The rehabilitation following ACI is a lengthy process that requires considerable input from the patient. The home maintenance suggested for the postsurgical ACI patient is integral within the general rehabilitation guidelines as presented earlier. The therapist needs to provide guidance on the progression and the exercise parameters (intensity, frequency, repetitions, duration) based on the individual patient's age, needs, and rehabilitative status. Where particular facilities and modalities are not available to a patient, the therapist should recommend suitable alternatives that allow the patient to achieve the rehabilitation goal. Individualization of the rehabilitation program is critical to patient compliance.

TROUBLESHOOTING

Mechanical complications are fairly common after ACI.[57] Graft failure and delamination accounted for almost half of the adverse events reported to the United States Food and Drug Administration up until 2003.[57] Tissue hypertrophy was shown to be one of the more common adverse events,[57] but this is predominantly associated with periosteal ACI. The introduction of second generation ACI has resulted in lower levels of hypertrophy.[15] One of the complications of ACI surgery that potentially has the most impact on the patient is the development of arthrofibrosis.[43-46] ACI rehabilitation is lengthy and noncompliance to the rehabilitation program can be an issue with some patients. Education and counseling regarding the rehabilitation program and why restrictions are imposed can be useful.

The rehabilitation guidelines provided in this chapter should provide a framework for ACI rehabilitation but should not be viewed as strict protocols. Monitoring of patient status and progression throughout the rehabilitation

process is critical and referral back to the surgeon should be considered where appropriate. Signs that the rehabilitation program should be reviewed include the following:

- Increased levels of pain, especially pain after cessation of activity
- Swelling or joint effusion
- Sustained plateau or reduction in ROM, weight bearing, or strength
- Increased difficulty in performing functional activities

If concomitant surgical procedures such as ACL reconstruction or meniscus repair are performed, the rehabilitation program should be revised on an individual basis to incorporate the requirements of the concomitant procedure in concert with the ACI requirements.

SUMMARY

This chapter has focused on the principles behind effective ACI rehabilitation and the factors in developing an individualized rehabilitation program. A general rehabilitation guideline has been provided for first generation ACI. The emergence of newer, cell-based articular cartilage repair technologies and variations of ACI surgery are likely to require modification to the existing rehabilitation guidelines.

REFERENCES

1. Mandelbaum BT, et al: Articular cartilage lesions of the knee. Am J Sports Med 26:853-861, 2000.
2. Brittberg M, et al: Treatment of deep cartilage defects in the knee with autologous chondrocyte transplantation. N Engl J Med 331:889-895, 1994.
3. Bentley G, et al: A prospective, randomised comparison of autologous chondrocyte implantation versus mosaicplasty for osteochondral defects in the knee. J Bone Joint Surg Br 85:223-230, 2003.
4. Fu F, et al: Autologous chondrocyte implantation versus debridement for treatment of full-thickness chondral defects of the knee: an observational cohort study with 3-year follow-up. Am J Sports Med 33:1658-1666, 2005.
5. Horas U, Pelinkovic D, Aigner T: Autologous chondrocyte implantation and osteochondral cylinder transplantation in cartilage repair of the knee joint: A prospective comparative trial. J Bone Joint Surg Am 85:185-192, 2003.
6. Knutsen G, et al: A randomized trial comparing autologous chondrocyte implantation with microfracture. Findings at five years. J Bone Joint Surg Am 89:2105-2112, 2007.
7. Mandelbaum B, et al: Treatment outcomes of autologous chondrocyte transplantation for full thickness articular cartilage defects of the trochlea. Am J Sports Med 35:915-921, 2007.
8. Mithöfer K, et al: Articular cartilage repair in soccer players with autologous chondrocyte transplantation: Functional outcome and return to competition. Am J Sports Med 33(11):1639-1646, 2005.
9. Mithöfer K, et al: Functional outcome of articular cartilage repair in adolescent athletes. Am J Sports Med 33:1147-1153, 2005.
10. Peterson L, et al: Two- to 9-year outcome after autologous chondrocyte transplantation of the knee. Clin Orthop Relat Res 374:212-234, 2000.
11. Peterson L, et al: Autologous chondrocyte transplantation: Biomechanics and long-term durability. Am J Sports Med 30:2-12, 2002.
12. Zaslav K, et al: A prospective study of autologous chondrocyte transplantation in patients with failed prior treatment for articular cartilage defect of the knee: Results of the study of the treatment of articular repair (STAR) clinical trial. Am J Sports Med 37:42-55, 2009.
13. Brown WE, et al: Magnetic resonance imaging appearance of cartilage repair in the knee. Clin Orthop 422:214-223, 2004.
14. Potter HG, Chong LR: Magnetic resonance imaging assessment of chondral lesions and repair. J Bone Joint Surg 91, Suppl 1:126-131, 2009.
15. Bartlett W, et al: Autologous chondrocyte implantation versus matrix-induced autologous chondrocyte implantation for osteochondral defects of the knee: A prospective, randomized study. J Bone Joint Surg Br 87:640-645, 2005.
16. Kon E, et al: Arthroscopic second-generation autologous chondrocyte implantation compared with microfracture for chondral lesions of the knee: Prospective nonrandomized study at 5 years. Am J Sports Med 37:33-41, 2009.
17. Saris DBF, et al: Comparison of characterized chondrocyte implantation versus microfracture in the treatment of symptomatic cartilage defects of the knee: Results after three years. Proceedings of the 8th World Congress of the International Cartilage Repair Society P175, Zurich, 2009.
18. Saris DBF, et al: Characterized chondrocyte implantation results in better structural repair when treating symptomatic cartilage defects of the knee in a randomized controlled trial versus microfracture. Am J Sports Med 36(2):235-246, 2008.
19. Mithoefer K, et al: Emerging options for treatment of articular cartilage injury in the athlete. Clin Sports Med 28:25-40, 2009.
20. Crawford D, et al: An autologous cartilage tissue implant NeoCart for treatment of grade III chondral injury to the distal femur: prospective clinical safety trial at 2 years. Am J Sports Med 37:1334-1343, 2009.
21. Minas T, Peterson L: Advanced techniques in autologous chondrocyte transplantation. Clin Sports Med 18(1):13-14 v-vi, 1999.

22. Hambly K, et al: Autologous chondrocyte implantation postoperative care and rehabilitation: Science and practice. Am J Sports Med 34(6):1020-1038, 2006.

23. Reinold MM, et al: Current concepts in the rehabilitation following articular cartilage repair procedures in the knee. J Orthop Sports Phys Ther 36(10):774-794, 2006.

24. Riegger-Krugh CL, et al: Autologous chondrocyte implantation: Current surgery and rehabilitation. Med Sci Sports Exerc 40(2):206-214, 2008.

25. Howard JS, et al: Continuous passive motion, early weight bearing, and active motion following knee articular cartilage repair: Evidence for clinical practice. Cartilage 1(4):276-286, 2010.

26. Mithoefer K, et al: Return to sports participation after articular cartilage repair in the knee: Scientific evidence. Am J Sports Med 37(1):167S-176S, 2009. http://ajs.sagepub.com/citmgr?gca=amjsports;37/1_suppl/167S.

27. Wondrasch B, et al: Effect of accelerated weightbearing after matrix-associated autologous chondrocyte implantation on a femoral condyle on radiographic and clinical outcome after 2 years: A prospective, randomized controlled pilot study. Am J Sports Med 37(Suppl 1):88S-96S, 2009.

28. Ebert JR: Post-operative load bearing rehabilitation following autologous chondrocyte implantation, Perth, Australia, 2008, School of Sport Science, Exercise and Health and School of Surgery and Pathology, University of Western Australia.

29. Arokoski J, Jurvelin J, Vaatainen U: Normal and pathological adaptations of articular cartilage to joint loading. Scand J Med Sci Sports 10(4):186-198, 2000.

30. Hinterwimmer S, et al: Cartilage atrophy in the knees of patients after seven weeks of partial load bearing. Arthritis Rheum 50(8):2516-2520, 2004.

31. Eckstein F, Hudelmaier M, Putz R: The effects of exercise on human articular cartilage. J Anat 208(4):491-512, 2006.

32. Klein L, et al: Prevention of ligament and meniscus atrophy by active joint motion in a non-weight-bearing model. J Orthop Res 7(1):80-85, 1989.

33. Ebert JR, et al: Accuracy of partial weight bearing after autologous chondrocyte implantation. Arch Phys Med Rehabil 89(8):1528-1534, 2008.

34. Salter RB, et al: The biological effect of continuous passive motion on the healing of full-thickness defects in articular cartilage: An experimental investigation in the rabbit. J Bone Joint Surg Am 62(8):1232-1251, 1980.

35. Alfredson H, Lorentzon R: Superior results with continuous passive motion compared to active motion after periosteal transplantation: A retrospective study of human patella cartilage defect treatment. Knee Surg Sports Traumatol Arthrosc 7(4):232-238, 1999.

36. Salter RB: The biologic concept of continuous passive motion of synovial joints: The first 18 years of basic research and its clinical application. Clin Orthop Relat Res 242:12-25, 1989.

37. Nugent-Derfus GE, et al: Continuous passive motion applied to whole joints stimulates chondrocyte biosynthesis of PRG4. Osteoarthritis Cartilage 15(5):566-574, 2007.

38. Marder RA, Hopkins G, Jr, Timmerman LA: Arthroscopic microfracture of chondral defects of the knee: a comparison of two postoperative treatments. Arthroscopy 21(2):152-158, 2005.

39. Allen M, et al: Rehabilitation following autologous chondrocyte implantation surgery: Case report using an accelerated weight-bearing protocol. Physiother Can 59:286-298, 2007.

40. Ikenoue T, et al: Mechanoregulation of human articular chondrocyte aggrecan and type II collagen expression by intermittent hydrostatic pressure in vitro. J Orthop Res 21(1):110-116, 2003.

41. Wong M, Carter DR: Articular cartilage functional histomorphology and mechanobiology: a research perspective. Bone 33(1):1-13, 2003.

42. Macauley DC: Ice therapy: how good is the evidence? Int J Sports Med 22(5):379-384, 2001.

43. Creighton RA, Bach BRJ: Arthrofibrosis: Evaluation, prevention, and treatment. Tech Knee Surg 4(3):163-172, 2005.

44. Seyler TM, et al: Functional problems and arthrofibrosis following total knee arthroplasty. J Bone Joint Surg Am 89(suppl_3):59-69, 2007.

45. Noyes FR, et al: Prevention of permanent arthrofibrosis after anterior cruciate ligament reconstruction alone or combined with associated procedures: a prospective study in 443 knees. Knee Surg Sports Traumatol Arthrosc 8(4):196-206, 2000.

46. Noyes FR, Mangine RE, Barber SD: The early treatment of motion complications after reconstruction of the anterior cruciate ligament. Clin Orthop Relat Res 277:217-228, 1992.

47. Hewett TE, Paterno MV, Myer GD: Strategies for enhancing proprioception and neuromuscular control of the knee. Clin Orthop 402:76-94, 2002.

48. Irrgang JJ, Pezzullo, D: Rehabilitation following surgical procedures to address articular cartilage lesions in the knee. J Orthop Sports Phys Ther 28(4):232-240, 1998.

49. Martelli S, Pinskerova V: The shapes of the tibial and femoral articular surfaces in relation to tibiofemoral movement. J Bone Joint Surg Br 84(4):607-613, 2002.

50. McGinty G, Irrgang JJ, Pezzullo D: Biomechanical considerations for rehabilitation of the knee. Clin Biomech (Bristol, Avon) 15(3):160-166, 2000.

51. Grelsamer RP, Klein JR: The biomechanics of the patellofemoral joint. J Orthop Sports Phys Ther 28(5):286-298, 1998.

52. Eckstein F, et al: In vivo cartilage deformation after different types of activity and its dependence on physical training status. Ann Rheum Dis 64(2):291-295, 2005.

53. Powers CM: The influence of altered lower-extremity kinematics on patellofemoral joint dysfunction: a theoretical perspective. J Orthop Sports Phys Ther 33(11):639-646, 2003.

54. Shields RK, et al: Neuromuscular control of the knee during a resisted single-limb squat exercise. Am J Sports Med 33(10):1520-1526, 2005.

55. Ayotte NW, et al: Electromyographical analysis of selected lower extremity muscles during 5 unilateral weight-bearing exercises. J Orthop Sports Phys Ther 37(2):48-55, 2007.

56. Bolgla LA, Uhl TL: Electomyographic analysis of hip rehabilitation exercises in a group of healthy subjects. J Orthop Sports Phys Ther 35:487-494, 2005.

57. Wood JJ, et al: Autologous cultured chondrocytes: Adverse events reported to the United States Food and Drug Administration. J Bone Joint Surg Am 88(3):503-507, 2006.

CHAPTER 26

Patella Open Reduction and Internal Fixation

Daniel A. Farwell, Craig Zeman

Patella fractures can occur in a wide variety of individuals. Both genders have similar fracture rates. Age-related incidence of patella fractures tends to be shifted to a mature population. Patella fractures are usually caused by direct trauma or a blow to the patella,[1-4] or can be a postoperative complication from ACL or total knee replacement surgery.[5-8] Depending on the force of the injury, the fracture can be nondisplaced or highly comminuted with significant injury to the extensor mechanism complex. Active extension of the knee is usually preserved with a nondisplaced fracture. However, in a displaced fracture the extensor mechanism is disrupted to the extent that active extension is not possible. Displaced fractures require open reduction internal fixation (ORIF) to maximize active extension of the knee and decrease the incidence of posttraumatic arthritis.

SURGICAL INDICATIONS AND CONSIDERATIONS

Physicians use two main criteria to determine whether surgery is indicated:
1. Fracture displacement of more than 3 or 4 mm
2. Loss of ability to extend the knee actively

Different surgical treatments are based on the type or severity of the fracture. Tension band wiring is still the most accepted treatment for displaced patella fractures.[9-11] Weber and colleagues[12] noted that if stability and early range of motion (ROM) is to be performed, there must be a stable repair of the fracture site to avoid displacement of the repair. They noted increased stability by repairing cadaveric patella fractures with a technique in which the wire is anchored directly in bone. They also noted that the retinaculum should be repaired because it added to stability. Bostman and colleagues[13] examined several different approaches and techniques to repair patella fractures and discovered the tension band wiring procedure to be far superior to other methods,

but using screws with tension band technique appears the strongest.[14-16] With the production of Kevlar sutures, the use of sutures to fix patella fractures has been reported.[17-19]

Smith and associates[20] performed a retrospective review of postoperative complications after ORIF of patella fractures. They followed 51 patients treated with the tension band fixation technique until complete healing had occurred at a minimum of 4 months. The authors' objective was to focus on acute, short-term complications after ORIF of patella fracture. Although the study did not specifically assess clinical parameters, such as pain or strength, it did point out two important factors to consider during rehabilitation. Approximately 22% of the patella fractures treated with modified tension band wiring and early ROM displaced significantly during the early postoperative period.

Failure of fixation was related to unprotected ambulation and noncompliance. Patient noncompliance in restricting early ROM and weight bearing can cause failure of even technically correct tension band wire fixation.[3,13,21-23]

Joint congruity must be restored to decrease the development of arthritis, and the extensor mechanism must be restored to regain full extension. Most patients with displaced fractures are candidates for ORIF. If the patient was ambulatory before the injury and can medically tolerate surgery, then surgery should be performed regardless of age. Situations in which nonambulatory patients with patella fractures lack lower-extremity (LE) function and sensation (neurologic impairment) can be managed conservatively.

Patients with simple two-part fractures have a better chance of a successful outcome than those with highly comminuted fractures. The variability of outcomes relates to the degree of fixation and the ability of the fracture site or sites to consolidate. In some cases of irreducible comminution, the fragments may have to be removed, resulting in a partial or total patellectomy.[4,21,24-32] Patellectomy procedures have a lower success rate than stable internal fixation procedures.[33-36]

SURGICAL PROCEDURE

Most methods of ORIF incorporate tension band wiring techniques.[12,21,22,37,38] Makino and associates described an arthroscopically assisted technique.[39] The tension band wire is placed around the proximal and distal pole of the patella through the quadriceps and patella tendons. This wire compresses the fracture site. The surgeon maintains rotational control with one or two screws placed across the fracture site from the proximal to the distal pole. The tension band wire is passed under the k-wires or screws to add compressive and rotational stability to the fixation. Another method is to use cannulated screws through which the tension band wire may be passed. Suture can be used instead of wire in certain cases.[17-19]

The integrity of the skin over the patella must be evaluated before surgery because of its potential to produce postoperative complications. The therapist should assess this area continually for infection and poor healing because vascular supply may have been disrupted during the trauma that caused the patella fracture.

Surgery is performed under either general or regional anesthesia. The patient is positioned supine, and a tourniquet is applied to the thigh. It is important that the knee can fully flex and extend so that the surgeon can determine the stable postoperative ROM. The leg is then prepped and draped in sterile fashion. If the skin allows, then a longitudinal midline incision is made over the patella. This incision (Fig. 26-1) is carried down to the peritenon, and full-thickness flaps are developed both medially and laterally to expose the entire patella and extensor mechanism. The peritenon is then incised to expose the fracture and the tendons. The fracture hematoma is débrided from the fracture site, and the raw cancellous bone is delineated to aid in fracture reduction. Two k-wires are then run from the fracture site of the proximal fragment and out the proximal pole of the patella (Fig. 26-2, A to C). The proximal and distal fragments of the patella are brought together to reduce the fracture. The fracture is then held together with bone-holding forceps while the knee is in extension (Fig. 26-2, D). The k-wires are passed back through the middle of the patella and out the distal pole. The bone-holding forceps are then removed (Fig. 26-2, E). Next the tension band wire is placed around the patella and k-wires. It should be positioned as close to the bone and k-wires as possible to minimize complications after ROM is initiated postoperatively (Fig. 26-2, F).

To place the tension wire as close to the bone and k-wire as possible, the surgeon usually passes a hollow needle under the k-wire and over the bone to guide the tension band wire. The tension band wire is then passed through the needle and brought around the patella. The two ends of the tension band wire are then twisted together with pliers to add tension to the system. The surgeon must be careful not to add too much tension to the wire because this may cause the wire to break early in the rehabilitation process (Fig. 26-2, G and H).

The surgeon then repairs the extensor mechanism. The medial and lateral retinacula are commonly torn in line with the fracture. These tears are simply repaired using nonabsorbable sutures. After this last repair, the surgeon checks the ROM to ensure that the patient can easily obtain full extension and at least 90° of flexion. The surgical site is then closed in the following order: first the peritenon, then the subcutaneous tissue, and finally the skin. The wound is dressed with a bulky dressing and placed in an immobilizer. A postoperative water-cooling system or ice pack may be used to assist with pain control immediately.

A partial patellectomy may be performed in patients with comminuted displaced fractures who have at least 50% of the patella remaining.[33] The inferior pole of the patella usually suffers the most trauma, resulting in its removal (Fig. 26-3, A). To do a partial patellectomy, the surgeon débrides the bone fragments from the tendon end and then weaves two large 5-0 nonabsorbable sutures into the tendon (5-0 Fiber-Wire is now available that has the strength of 18-gauge wire and the flexibility of suture). The surgeon then drills two holes longitudinally into the remaining piece of the patella. The sutures in the tendon are brought through the holes in the patella and tied over the bone bridge formed by the two holes (Fig. 26-3, B and C).

Most patients require a second operation to remove the hardware placed in the patella.[40] The wires and sutures can become prominent and bother the patient during rehabilitation, slowing progress in gaining ROM.

The fixation of simple fractures is usually the most stable immediately after surgery. If the tension band wire is not placed right next to the screw, then the wire can cut through the tendon until it butts up against the screw, decreasing the compressive effect of the wire and possibly allowing the fracture to displace. Stable fixation of a simple fracture is usually strong enough to allow early passive range of motion (PROM). The amount of ROM is dictated by the surgical procedure and pain tolerance. Time frames to initiate physical therapy vary depending on the degree of comminution. The repair is most vulnerable between 4 to 6 weeks when the bone and tendon have not completely healed and the pins and wires have loosened. After 8 weeks, the repair should be stable enough to allow aggressive therapy with the goal of regaining full ROM.[41]

The exception to this time frame is the patient who has a comminuted fracture with unstable fixation. This type of situation may require 12 weeks before the initiation of therapy. Most patients return to preinjury activities (sports) by 6 months after surgery.

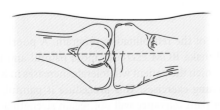

Fig. 26-1 The incision line from which repair of the fracture is initiated.

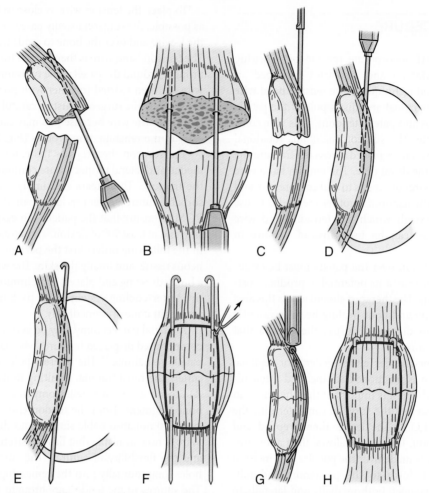

Fig. 26-2 The open reduction internal fixation procedure for transverse fracture of the patella. **A** to **C,** The patella is prepared for the k-wires by drilling congruent holes through both pieces of the fracture. **D** and **E,** Bone forceps are used to approximate the fracture while wires are placed through the drill holes. **F** to **H,** The surgeon finishes the process of tension band wiring, creating stable postoperative fixation.

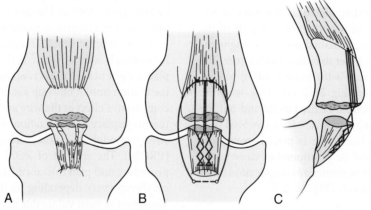

Fig. 26-3 The process of partial patellectomy. **A,** Comminuted fracture involving the inferior pole of the patella. Front view (**B**) and side view (**C**) after débridement of inferior fragments; sutures are woven into the tendon.

Outcomes

A successful outcome is a knee with full active extension, full ROM, and without significant pain. The things that can prevent a successful outcome are unstable fixation, incongruous reduction, poor patient compliance, and delays in early PROM exercises. Unstable fixation will decrease the

aggression of the rehabilitation program. A poorly reduced joint will make ROM exercises more painful and limit the speed at which the patient will tolerate increases in ROM and strengthening exercises. This procedure is painful. Patients with poor pain tolerance will not regain strength and ROM as easily as patients who are motivated and who can handle an aggressive rehabilitation program. Some early postoperative ROM exercises need to be started to get the best results. If ROM exercises are delayed in the first few weeks for any reason, then it will be more difficult to get back full ROM and strength.

Maximal function after patellar fracture is usually not achieved until 1 year after sugery.[42] Stiffness and anterior knee pain especially with stair climbing or prolonged sitting with the knee flexed are common.[*] Total patellectomy patients can have an extension lag. Around 70% to 80% of patients with ORIF will end up with a good to excellent result and 20% to 30% with a fair to poor result.[3] A loss of 20% to 49% of extensor mechanism strength can be expected.[36,43,44] About 70% of patients followed long-term will have some complaint about the knee. Long-term results after total patellectomy range from 22% to 85% (good to excellent) and 14% to 64% (fair to poor).[†]

The therapist should call the surgeon with any signs of wound infection. Wound infections after ORIF in patella fractures need to be dealt with quickly because the hardware is superficial and can easily become infected, which can lead to a deep infection requiring long-term antibiotics.

If in the course of therapy the patient develops an extension lag greater than he or she had earlier in rehabilitation, the surgeon should be called because a loss of fixation has possibly occurred. To help confirm this, the fracture site can be palpated for a gap.

THERAPY GUIDELINES FOR REHABILITATION

The treatment of patients who have undergone ORIF for patella fractures requires a cooperative approach from the orthopedist and the physical therapist (PT). This concept is most evident when considering the challenge in treating patients after surgery. The goal of treatment is to provide a structurally stable patellofemoral joint and allow for full functional recovery of the involved LE. Factors that influence the choice of treatment include the following:

1. The overall health of the patient and the way it may influence wound and fracture healing
2. The location and configuration of the fracture
3. Immobilization after surgery (osteopenia of the entire LE, muscle atrophy, and possible contracture of the knee joint) versus ORIF (which allows for early ROM and patella mobilization)
4. Patient compliance with the prescribed treatment plan (home program)

Although rehabilitation after a patella fracture treated with ORIF is crucial, a wide range of protocols may be used depending on the factors listed previously, the physician's chosen fixation technique, and the patient's goals (which differ among athletes, sedentary adults, and children). The information the PT collects from both the physician and the patient aids in determining the design and time parameters of the rehabilitation program.

The remainder of this chapter deals only with the simple transverse fracture. However, the clinician is reminded to respect the previously discussed four factors influencing treatment when planning rehabilitation for all patella fractures.

Phase I (Acute Phase)

TIME: 1 to 4 weeks after surgery
GOALS: Control pain, manage edema, gain 0° to 90° of PROM, improve quadriceps and hamstring contraction (Table 26-1)

The acute phase of rehabilitation (the first 4 weeks) after ORIF of the patella is the time when reinjury is most likely. Attention to detail and communication with the treating physician are crucial during this period.

Controversy exists over when to initiate ROM. Hung and colleagues[10] initiate knee motion 1 week after surgery, whereas Lotke and Ecker[47] often immobilize patients for as long as 3 weeks before beginning any type of motion. Bostman and associates[9,13] not only immobilize their patients an average of 38 days but also state that they see no correlation between the initial time of immobilization and the final outcome. Biomechanical studies that have demonstrated the appropriateness of tension band wiring and early ROM have generally used a simple transverse fracture pattern as the model.[48] Complications such as poor bone quality and comminuted patella fractures may prevent the desired fixation and thus preclude any early joint ROM.

The PT performs an evaluation on the first postoperative visit, respecting the surgical procedure and any restrictions noted by the surgeon. Observation of the surgical site is documented and continually assessed to prevent wound complications.

If the surgical site shows any signs of infection, then the PT should notify the surgeon immediately. Crutches are used postoperatively, and weight bearing is as tolerated with the immobilizer in place. Patients may eventually progress to independent ambulation (with the immobilizer still in place) after they tolerate full weight bearing (FWB) and are cleared by the physician (usually between 3 to 6 weeks). Smith and associates[20] reported four complete failures after ORIF with tension band wiring. No inadequacies were detected during the initial procedures, and all four failures resulted from falls while walking unprotected in the early postoperative period.

ROM measurements of the knee are taken passively, with the PT again observing any restrictions. Quality of muscle contraction in the extensor mechanism is noted, and active knee flexion is assessed. Girth measurements may be taken to assess atrophy of the thigh and calf; however, this has little overall benefit compared with functional assessment.

Early ROM is the goal in any operative treatment of patella fractures, yet the definition of early ROM varies,

---

[*]References 24, 29, 34, 36, 43, 44.
[†]References 3, 29, 34, 36, 43, 44-46.

TABLE 26-1 Patella Open and Reduction Internal Fixation

Rehabilitation Phase	Criteria to Progress to This Phase	Anticipated Impairments and Functional Limitations	Intervention	Goal	Rationale
Phase I Postoperative 1-4 wk	• Postoperative and cleared by physician to initiate therapy • There may be specific precautions, depending on stability of fixation (communicate with physician)	• Edema • Pain • Limited ROM • Limited strength • Limited transfers • Limited gait	• Cryotherapy • ES for muscle stimulation • PROM—knee extension, knee flexion, supine wall slides • Isometrics—quadriceps/hamstring sets, quadriceps sets at 20°-30° • AROM—standing hamstring curls, supine heel slides • Gait training using crutches and weight bearing as tolerated in immobilizer • Weight shifting • Gentle joint mobilization to the patella (resistance free)	• Control pain • Manage edema • Improve muscle contraction • PROM—knee extension 0°, flexion 90° • Initiate volitional muscle contraction • Improve tolerance to flexion ROM • Avoid excessive stress on the extensor mechanism during ambulation • Decrease pain	• Initiate self-management of pain • Use ES to improve muscle contraction • Restore joint ROM as indicated by physician • Prepare for independence with transfers (SLR independent) • Begin to prepare extensor mechanism to accept load • Restore independence with ambulation • Improve stability of involved LE • Control pain through resistance-free mobilization to the patella

AROM, Active range of motion; *ES,* electrical stimulation; *LE,* lower extremity; *PROM,* passive range of motion; *ROM,* range of motion; *SLR,* straight-leg raising.

depending on who performs the procedure.[9,10,13,47] Although the acute phase of rehabilitation tends to focus on knee joint range, gait deviations can produce problems later in rehabilitation if they are not addressed early. Patients often are treated in some type of immobilizer. A hinged brace can be used to allow for motion while stabilizing the fracture.

Initial treatments focus on restoring ROM (0° to 90°), improving quadriceps activation and hamstring muscle control, progressing gait (weight-bearing tolerance), managing edema, and controlling pain. A program of elevation and ice (20 to 30 minutes three times a day) is used as necessary to manage edema and control pain.

Electrical stimulation (ES) for pain control is avoided because of the proximity of the screw and wires. However, ES can be used to assist in quadriceps contraction when appropriate. Gentle mobilization (grades 1 and 2 shy of resistance) of the patella also is used to control pain.

Initial exercises of the knee involve PROM, limited active range of motion (AROM), and isometrics. Passive stretches are performed to restore flexion and extension. The vigor of the stretch should be in concert with the guidelines established by the surgeon. In general, patients are expected to reach 90° of flexion and full extension by 4 weeks. Supine wall slides can be easily performed in the clinic or at home. (See the section on Suggested Home Maintenance for the Postsurgical Patient.) Regaining full extension is usually not a problem; however, limitations of extension can be treated quite successfully.

Active exercises primarily focus on using the hamstrings to flex the knee. Heel slides and standing hamstring curls

are initiated to aid in increasing muscle control and progressing ROM.

Isometric exercises involve quadriceps and hamstring cocontraction and isolated quadriceps contractions at 20° to 30° flexion. Quality is observed and ES is helpful in recruitment.

Gait training focuses on increasing the acceptance of weight on the involved leg. Weight shifting can be given as part of the home program. After the incision is healed and the surgeon allows it, aqua therapy can be initiated with an emphasis on proper weight shifting and gait mechanics.

Phase II (Subacute Phase)

TIME: 5 to 8 weeks after surgery

GOALS: Self-manage pain, increase strength, increase ROM to 90%, initiate quadriceps AROM (6 to 8 weeks), have minimal gait deviations on level surfaces (Table 26-2)

The subacute or midphase of rehabilitation (from weeks 5 to 8) is the transition from limited functional activity to aggressive functional activity. The actual exercise protocol is similar to any other type of patellofemoral rehabilitation. The only real difference with ORIF patella fracture is that a true fixation of the fracture has been obtained. Motion at the fracture site tends to activate secondary callus formation, especially with tension band wiring of a patella fracture. The danger in moving a nonfixated fracture (i.e., a fracture with no established callus formation) is that a nonunion may develop. A nonunion of bone is caused by excessive motion

TABLE 26-2 Patella Open Reduction and Internal Fixation

Rehabilitation Phase	Criteria to Progress to This Phase	Anticipated Impairments and Functional Limitations	Intervention	Goal	Rationale
Phase II Postoperative 5-8 wk	• No signs of infection • No significant increase in pain • No loss of range of motion	• Pain • Limited ROM • Limited strength • Limited gait	• Continuation and progression of interventions from phase I • Patellofemoral taping • Gait training; discontinue crutches when indicated • LE exercises continued from phase I • A/AROM—stationary bike used as a ROM assist for flexion • AROM—knee extension (when cleared by physician, usually between 6-8 wk)	• Self-manage pain • Decrease gait deviations • Increase LE strength • PROM of knee to 90% • Independent with home exercises	• Prepare patient for discharge • Assist patellofemoral mechanics • Promote return to unassisted gait in the community • Restore LE stability and strength • Promote restoration of normal joint mechanics • Initiate extensor mechanism strengthening and improve tolerance to patellofemoral compression with tracking

A/AROM, Active assistive range of motion; *AROM,* active range of motion; *LE,* lower extremity; *PROM,* passive range of motion.

directly at the fracture site, which keeps the callus from forming sufficiently. This underlines the importance of maintaining immobility in some patella fractures during the rehabilitative process.[49]

Another factor to consider is that patella fractures involve joint surfaces. Incongruency of the articular surfaces can lead to articular cartilage degeneration and possible early arthritis if not treated. Incongruity of the patellofemoral joint may alter the joint mechanics, producing areas of non-contact or excessive pressure over the patella.[50] Issues of patellofemoral contact area and joint reaction force must be evaluated during this phase of rehabilitation. The use of patellofemoral taping (see Figs. 20-1 to 20-3) can be useful in limiting imbalances over the fractured surface of the patella. By this phase, the patient is demonstrating increased competency in ambulating with the brace and decreased reliance (if any) on the crutches. Exercises are progressed as in phase I, and the patient is instructed to perform two sets per day (repetitions to fatigue). Closed-chain exercises are initiated on a progressive basis based on patient healing and quadriceps and LE control.

Modalities at this stage are primarily ice for pain control. ES of the quadriceps is continued as indicated to progress muscle recruitment. Moist heat can be used to prepare the knee for stretching after edema is controlled.

PROM stretches are progressed as indicated to obtain full flexion. The vigor of grades of mobilization is increased into resistance as indicated. AROM for the quadriceps is initiated between 6 to 8 weeks (or when the fracture is deemed stable enough to tolerate it). The stationary bike can be used as a ROM assistive device and progressed for strengthening and cardiovascular purposes after flexion allows full revolution without hip hiking. Surgeon approval is required before initiating resistance training on a bicycle.

The rehabilitation at this point begins to mimic that prescribed for the patient recovering from lateral release in terms of exercises and progressions. Taping can be initiated in this phase as deemed appropriate by the therapist.

Phase III (Advanced Phase)

TIME: 9 to 12 weeks after surgery

GOALS: Return to full function, develop endurance and coordination of the LE, continue to address limitations with steps and running (with physician clearance) (Table 26-3)

The advanced stage of rehabilitation (from weeks 9 to 12) focuses on functional, skill-specific activity. Most of the effort and work is spent on building back the patient's quadriceps, hamstring, and gastrocnemius-soleus muscle strength.

Depending on remaining deficits, exercises from the previous two phases are continued. The therapist should keep in mind that the time frame will vary depending on many factors, including type of fracture, fixation, and the patient's response to rehabilitation.

Furthermore, isokinetics should be avoided until the physician approves them. The need for taping should be minimal, but if continued taping is needed, patients are instructed in self-taping techniques. Monitoring for pain and joint effusion gives the therapist feedback on the way to progress activities aggressively. Long-term strengthening of the muscles surrounding the patellofemoral joint with the development of endurance and coordination over time are the goals of this phase.

By this stage, patients should be close to discharge because they are fairly functional with sitting, standing, and walking tolerances. Limitations with stairs and squatting activities

TABLE 26-3 Patella Open Reduction and Internal Fixation

Rehabilitation Phase	Criteria to Progress to This Phase	Anticipated Impairments and Functional Limitations	Intervention	Goal	Rationale
Phase III Postoperative 9-12 wk	• Pain free at rest • Range of motion 0°-90° • Good quadriceps control during gait • Minimal gait deviations	• Limited endurance with prolonged functional activities • Mild pain of patellofemoral joint during skill-specific exercises • Limited tolerance to stairs and single-limb squat and balance	• Closed-chain and stretching exercises as listed in phases I and II • Patella taping • Patella mobilization • PREs on leg press • Function-specific activity: bicycle, treadmill, isokinetic training (when cleared by physician) • Home exercises (see Suggested Home Maintenance section)	• Unlimited community ambulation • No gait deviations • Good sitting and standing tolerances • Good patella stability without taping • Patient self-management of symptoms	• Decrease pain with functional activities • Improve joint mechanics • Improve joint mobility and stability • Provide functional strengthening • Improve endurance of vastus medialis oblique • Increase reliance on patient self-management

PREs, Progressive resistance exercises.

continue to be present. Prolonged standing and walking should be continually improving, with the focus on a progressive increase in activities. Running and jumping should be initiated on an individual basis as determined by the surgeon (potentially after removal of hardware).

SUGGESTED HOME MAINTENANCE FOR THE POSTSURGICAL PATIENT

An exercise program has been outlined at the various phases. The home maintenance section outlines rehabilitation guidelines the patient may follow. The PT can use it in customizing a patient-specific program.

TROUBLESHOOTING

Issues that prevent a successful outcome are unstable fixation, incongruous reduction, poor patient compliance, and

delays in early PROM exercises. Patients with poor pain tolerance do not regain strength and ROM as easily and may be left with residual deficits. Return of maximal function after a patella fracture can take as long as 1 year.[10] Residual problems of anterior knee pain and stiffness are common complications.* An estimated 70% to 80% of patients recovering from patella ORIF have good to excellent results, although 20% to 30% have fair to poor results.[3] Residual loss of extensor strength has been recorded in the 20% to 49% range.

Prolonged immobilization is detrimental to the final result regardless of the treatment.[3] Although it produces a risk of wound infection, the benefits of ROM outweigh the risk of wound complications. However, this situation is especially tenuous in patients who suffer open patella fractures because they are at a higher risk for infection.

---

*References 24, 29, 34, 36, 43, 44..

 Suggested Home Maintenance for the Postsurgical Patient

Weeks 1 to 4
GOALS FOR THE PERIOD: Control pain, manage edema, gain 0° to 90° of PROM, improve quadriceps and hamstring contraction
1. Elevate and ice at home two to three times per day (preferably after exercises).
2. Perform ankle pumping and hamstring stretches with the extremity elevated and on ice (20 to 30 minutes).
3. Perform supine wall slides (when appropriate)—one set of five repetitions three to four times a day.

4. Perform active heel slides—one set of 10 repetitions performed three to four times per day.
5. Perform quadriceps sets (on clearance from the physician)—two sets of 10 repetitions performed three to four times per day. Even though general guidelines such as this may prescribe a number of sets and repetitions, if the patient fatigues and cannot continue to recruit a quality quadriceps contraction, then the exercise is over. *Patients are only to count repetitions with quality quadriceps contractions.* The heel should stay on the floor. Quadriceps sets also may be performed standing

if the patient finds it easier to activate the quadriceps in this position. The key to early strengthening is to find which position the patient is most successful in recruiting a quality quadriceps contraction.

Weeks 5 to 8
GOALS FOR THE PERIOD: Self-manage pain, increase strength, increase ROM to 90%, initiate quadriceps AROM (6 to 8 weeks), have minimal gait deviations on level surfaces
1. Perform the same exercises as in weeks 1 to 4, increasing the number of repetitions. Exercises should generally be performed in two sets of 10 to 20 repetitions per day (based on fatigue).
2. Initiate closed-chain exercises based on patient tolerance to resistance. Spider killers are initiated in pain-free ranges. In addition, simulated leg press exercises with elastic tubing can be performed. Patients begin with two sets of 10 repetitions and progress based on tolerance.

3. Perform self-taping as deemed appropriate by therapist.
4. Continue use of ice after exercises.

Weeks 9 to 12
GOALS FOR THE PERIOD: Return to full ADL function, develop endurance and coordination of the LE, continue to address limitations with steps and running (with physician clearance)
1. Depending on remaining deficits, continue exercises from the previous 8 weeks. The need for taping should be minimal; if continued taping is required, then patients are instructed in self-taping techniques.
2. Progress closed-chain exercises to include stepping exercises at home using threshold of doorway for balance.
3. Gradually return to functional activities while monitoring for pain and joint effusion.

CLINICAL CASE REVIEW

1 James is 45 years old and had patella ORIF 3 weeks ago. He arrives for his initial evaluation in an immobilizer with his incision well healed. He weighs 250 lb and is 5-feet 10-inches tall. What modality and procedures would be most appropriate to improve his gait pattern?

Given his size, pool therapy would be the most appropriate tool to improve his gait pattern and limit body weight stress on the patella. Warm water can help improve ROM and decrease pain, and stresses that land-based therapy place on the joint.

2 Meghan is 25 years old and had patella ORIF 6 weeks ago. She has only 60° of flexion and guards with any attempts at manual therapy (soft tissue mobilization, joint mobilization) to improve ROM. The "end feel" of her flexion is a soft end feel that does not provide much resistance (no catching or hard end feel). She also has been negligent in performing her home exercise program. What changes did the therapist suggest to improve Meghan's outcome?

Meghan was instructed to, when possible, take her pain medication before coming to therapy. The therapist also explained that 20% to 30% of patients have a "poor" outcome. If her case was to be successful (and the surgeon saw no reason why it should not be), then she

must gain flexion ROM. At some point she needs to take responsibility for her care. After this intervention, her ROM improved as did her tolerance to manual techniques.

3 Jessica is 40 years old. She fractured her patella when she fell off a footstool and onto her knees. She had a patella ORIF surgery 9 weeks ago. Her knee flexion ROM is limited, and peripatella pain is a factor when performing ROM stretches. ROM exercises for knee flexion have been emphasized during the past few treatments along with modalities for pain control. Little progress has been noted. What treatment techniques may be the most helpful?

The PT should assess the patellofemoral and the tibiofemoral joints for limited mobility. If mobility is limited, which is likely, then patella mobilizations using grades into resistance (grades 3 and 4) can be helpful. The therapist should receive clearance from the physician before initiating mobilization into resistance. If it is limited, then increasing inferior patella movement may particularly help knee flexion ROM. The patellofemoral contact area and reaction forces also must be evaluated. Patellofemoral taping can be useful in limiting imbalances over the fractured surfaces of the patella. Complaints of pain with flexion may decrease, particularly with closed-chain exercises. If restrictions are found in the tibiofemoral joint, mobilizations (grade 3 and 4) can be performed to increase flexion (posterior glides of the tibia on the femur).

4 Jessica's knee ROM is now full 12 weeks after surgery. She performs a series of exercises for leg strengthening. She begins by stretching her hamstrings and gastrocnemius-soleus muscles. She then performs the following:

- Standing minisquats against the wall
- Leg presses using 100 lb and keeping knee flexion less than 60°
- Lunges with 5-lb weights in a long-stride position
- Wall slides between 0° and 45° with a 1-minute hold
- Sit-stand
- Standing (four-wall) elastic tubing hip flexion, abduction, and adduction on the uninvolved side
- Step-downs on an 8-inch step, holding contraction until the heel of the opposite leg makes contact

Although she has minimal discomfort during the exercise regimen, she has increased complaints of pain for 2 days after the exercises. Which of these exercises is most likely to be an aggravating factor?

The 8-inch step-downs are the most aggressive exercises because they produce the highest patellofemoral compression forces. The knee is most likely flexed beyond 50° while performing an eccentric contraction during FWB on the affected extremity.

5 David is 3 weeks after surgery and just started therapy. He has been a patient in the past and his pain tolerance is not that good. He notes a constant 5/10 pain in his knee without evidence of infection or instability of the repair. What pain management techniques can be used?

ES for pain control is avoided because of the proximity of the screw and wires. However, ES can be used to assist in quadriceps contraction when appropriate. Gentle mobilization (grades 1 and 2 shy of resistance) of the patella also is used to control pain in addition to ice and elevation.

6 George is 7 weeks postoperation and has limited tolerance to weight bearing because it causes some increased pain around the patella. What procedures/techniques can be used to assist in managing his symptoms?

The use of patellofemoral taping can be useful in limiting imbalances over the fractured surface of the patella. By this phase, the patient is demonstrating increased competency in ambulating with the brace and decreased reliance (if any) on the crutches.

7 Lissette is 12 weeks postoperation and is frustrated that she is not able to return to running activities because of pain. What can be done to assist the patient with return to prior activities.

First and foremost the therapist should keep in mind, and educate the patient, that the time frame to return to prior activites will vary depending on many factors, including type of fracture, fixation, and the patient's response to rehabilitation. Accomplishing this early on and setting interim goals (i.e., partial weight bearing to FWB, double- to single-leg squat, single-leg squat with 50% body weight to 100% body weight) are helpful. Monitoring for pain and joint effusion gives the therapist feedback on the way to progress activities aggressively. Long-term strengthening of the muscles surrounding the patello-femoral joint with the development of endurance and coordination over time are the goals of this phase.

8 George is 12 weeks postoperation and has made slow progress (0° to 115°, fair quadriceps contraction, residual mild antalgia during gait/single-limb stance). What instructions can you give him to be successful over the next 6 months?

Patients with poor pain tolerance do not regain strength and ROM as easily and may be left with residual deficits. George was instructed to continue his home stretching/strengthening program with monthly reassessments. Return of maximal function after a patella fracture has been noted to take as long as 1 year.

REFERENCES

1. Böhler L: Technik der Knochenbruch Behandlung 12-13. Auflage. Wien: W. Maudrich, 1957.
2. McMaster PE: Fractures of the patella. Clin Orthop 4:24, 1954.
3. Nummi J: Fracture of the patella: A clinical study of 707 patellar fractures. Ann Chir Gynaecol Fenn 179(suppl):1-85, 1971.
4. Watson-Jones R: Fractures and other bone and joint injuries, Edinburgh, 1939, E&S Livingstone.
5. Piva SR, et al: Patella fracture during rehabilitation after bone-patellar tendon-bone anterior cruciate ligament reconstruction: 2 case reports. J Orthop Sports Phys Ther 39(4):278-286, 2009.
6. Keating EM, Haas G, Meding JB: Patella fracture after post total knee replacements. Clin Orthop Relat Res 416:93-97, 2003.
7. Miller MD, Nichols T, Butler CA: Patella fracture and proximal patellar tendon rupture following arthroscopic anterior cruciate ligament reconstruction. Arthroscopy 15(6):640-643, 1999.
8. Viola R, Vianello R: Three cases of patella fracture in 1,320 anterior cruciate ligament reconstructions with bone-patellar tendon-bone autograft. Arthroscopy 15(1):93-97, 1999.
9. Bostman O, et al: Fractures of the patella treated by operation. Arch Orthop Trauma Surg 102:78, 1983.

10. Hung LK, et al: Fractured patella: Operative treatment using tension band principle. Injury 16:343, 1985.
11. Lexack B, Flannagan JP, Hobbs S: Results of surgical treatment of patellar fractures. J Bone Joint Surg Br 67:416, 1985.
12. Weber MJ, et al: Efficacy of various forms of fixation of transverse fractures of the patella. J Bone Joint Surg Am 62:215, 1980.
13. Bostman O, et al: Comminuted displaced fractures of the patella. Injury 13:196, 1981.
14. Carpenter JE, et al: Biomechanical evaluation of current patella fracture fixation techniques. J Orthop Trauma 11(5):351-356, 1997.
15. Rabalais RD, et al: Comparison of two tension-band fixation materials and techniques in transverse patella fractures: A biomechanical study. Orthopedics 31(2):128, 2008.
16. Schnabel B, et al: Biomechanical comparison of a new staple technique with tension band wiring for transverse patella fractures. Clin Biomech (Bristol, Avon) 24(10):855-859, 2009.
17. Hughes SC, et al: A new and effective tension-band braided polyester suture technique for transverse patellar fracture fixation. Injury 38(2):212-222, 2007.
18. Sturdee SW, Templeton PA, Oxborrow NJ: Internal fixation of a patella fracture using an absorbable suture. J Orthop Trauma 16(4):272-273, 2002.
19. Patel VR, et al: Fixation of patella fractures with braided polyester suture: A biomechanical study. Injury 31(1):1-6, 2000.
20. Smith ST, et al: Early complications in the operative treatment of patella fractures. J Orthop Trauma 11(3):183, 1997.
21. DePalma AF: The management of fractures and dislocations, Philadelphia, 1959, Saunders.
22. Muller ME, Allgower M, Willinegger H: Manual of internal fixation: Technique recommended by the AO group, New York, 1979, Springer-Verlag.
23. Rorabeck CH, Bobechko WP: Acute dislocation of the patella with osteochondral fracture: A review of eighteen cases. J Bone Joint Surg 58A:237, 1976.
24. Andrews JR, Hughston JC: Treatment of patellar fractures by partial patellectomy. South Med J 70:809, 1977.
25. Anderson LD: In Crenshaw AH, editor: Campbell's operative orthopaedics, ed 5, St Louis, 1971, Mosby.
26. Brooke R: The treatment of fractured patella by excision: A study of morphology and function. Br J Surg 24:733, 1937.
27. Heineck AP: The modern operative treatment of fracture of the patella. I. Based on the study of other pathological states of bone. II. An analytical review of over 1,100 cases treated during the last ten years, by open operative method. Surg Gynecol Obstet 9:177, 1909.
28. Jakobsen J, Christensen KS, Rassmussen OS: Patellectomy—a 20-year follow-up. Acta Orthop Scand 56:430, 1985.
29. Peeples RE, Margo MK: Function after patellectomy. Clin Orthop 132:180, 1978.
30. Thompson JEM: Comminuted fractures of the patella: Treatment of cases presenting with one large fragment and several small fragments. J Bone Joint Surg 58A:537, 1976.
31. Watson-Jones R: Excision of the patella (letter). Br Med J 2:195, 1945.
32. West FE: End results of patellectomy. J Bone Joint Surg 62A:1089, 1962.
33. Burton VW: Results of excision of the patella. Surg Gynecol Obstet 135:753, 1972.
34. Duthie HL, Hutchinson JR: The results of partial and total excision of the patella. J Bone Joint Surg 40B:75, 1958.
35. Sanderson MC: The fractured patella: A long-term follow-up study. Aust N Z J Surg 45:49, 1974.
36. Sutton FS, et al: The effect of patellectomy on knee function. J Bone Joint Surg 58A:537, 1976.
37. Magnusen PB: Fractures, ed 2, Philadelphia, 1936, Lippincott.
38. Zionts LE: Fractures around the knee in children. J Am Acad Orthop Surg 10:345-355, 2002.
39. Makino A, et al: Arthroscopic-assisted surgical technique for treating patella fractures. Arthroscopy 18(6):671-675, 2002.
40. Johnson EE: Fractures of the patella. In Rockwood CA, Green DP, Bucholz RW, editors: Fractures in adults, ed 3, Philadelphia, 1991, Lippincott.
41. Bray TJ, Marder RA: Patellar fractures. In Chapman MD, Madison M, editors: Operative orthopaedics, ed 2, Philadelphia, 1993, JB Lippincott.
42. Crenshaw AH, Wilson FD: The surgical treatment of fractures of the patella. South Med J 47:716, 1954.
43. Einola S, Aho AJ, Kallio P: Patellectomy after fracture: Long-term follow-up results with special reference to functional disability. Acta Orthop Scand 47:441, 1976.
44. Wilkinson J: Fracture of the patella treated by total excision: A long-term follow-up. J Bone Joint Surg 59B:352, 1977.
45. MacAusland WR: Total excision of the patella for fracture: Report of fourteen cases. Am J Surg 72:510, 1946.
46. Lachiewicz PF: Treatment of a neglected displaced transverse patella fracture. J Knee Surg 21(1):58-61, 2008.
47. Lotke PA, Ecker ML: Transverse fractures of the patella. Clin Orthop 158:1880, 1981.
48. Benjamin J, et al: Biomechanical evaluation of various forms of fixation of transverse patella fractures. J Orthop Trauma 1:219, 1987.
49. Klassen JK, Trousdale RT: Treatment of delayed and non-union of the patella. J Orthop Trauma 11(3):188, 1997.
50. Sanders R: Patella fractures and extensor mechanism injuries. In Bronner BD, et al, editors: Skeletal trauma, Philadelphia, 1992, Saunders.

CHAPTER 27

Total Knee Arthroplasty

Julie Wong, Michael D. Ries

INTRODUCTION

Osteoarthritis (OA), also called osteoarthroses or degenerative joint disease, is the most common type of arthritis and one of the leading causes of disability worldwide. OA is a chronic condition characterized by the breakdown of the joint's cartilage. Cartilage is the part of the joint that cushions the ends of the bones and allows easy movement of joints. The breakdown of cartilage causes the bones to rub against each other, causing stiffness, pain, and loss of movement in the joint. In the United States, it is estimated that OA may affect 33 million adults.[1] When conservative management fails to decrease pain or restore mobility, surgical intervention becomes the treatment of choice. Arthroscopic surgeries may be beneficial in early stages with mechanical symptoms,[2] but when this also fails, a total knee arthroplasty (TKA) is usually recommended.

According to the American Academy of Orthopaedic Surgeons, approximately 581,000 knee replacements are performed each year. Most were performed on people aged 60 to 80,[3] reflecting the aging population of Baby Boomers. Understanding the surgical procedure of the TKA and designing appropriate programs for rehabilitation are essential to ensure successful and cost-effective outcomes in anticipation of this future growth. Self-report measures of perceived functional ability indicate that 1 year following TKA, individuals have regained 80% of normal functions. However, despite improvement compared with preoperative status, pain and stiffness can remain a problem for some of these people.[4]

The scope of this chapter focuses on primary TKA. It is referred to as TKA, rather than total knee replacement (TKR), to distinguish it from total knee revision (which is also referred to as TKR). In addition, minimally invasive surgery (MIS)-TKA is also described.

SURGICAL INDICATIONS AND CONSIDERATIONS

TKA is an effective treatment for symptomatic OA or inflammatory arthritis of the knee that is not responsive to conservative therapy. Earlier stages of arthritis may be treated with nonsteroidal antiinflammatory drugs, activity restrictions, exercise, bracing, orthotics, and weight loss. Other treatments include injections of hyaluronic acid or cortisone. However, when conservative measures fail and arthritic symptoms limit functional activity, surgery is a more appropriate treatment option. If symptoms are mechanical and associated with catching or locking more than weight-bearing pain, they may result from a torn or degenerative meniscus. Magnetic resonance imaging (MRI) is useful to delineate meniscal pathology from degeneration of the articular cartilage. Arthroscopic débridement may be beneficial for treatment of meniscal pathology but does not appear to be as helpful for management of articular cartilage degeneration.[5] If cartilage degeneration occurs primarily in the medial tibiofemoral (TF) compartment with varus deformity, then valgus osteotomy of the tibia can be effective in relieving medial-sided knee pain and delay the need for total joint replacement.[6] Osteotomy is most appropriate for treatment of unicompartmental OA in a young active patient, a knee with adequate range of motion (ROM), and limited varus deformity. Relative contraindications include obesity, flexion contracture, significant lateral compartment or patellofemoral arthritis, TF subluxation, and advanced age. For lateral compartment OA with valgus deformity, distal femoral rather than proximal tibial osteotomy is preferred. However, osteotomy generally requires a longer rehabilitation period, and outcomes are less predictable than for TKA.[7]

Prosthetic options include metallic interposition hemiarthroplasty, as well as unicompartmental, bicompartmental, and TKA. The McKeever and MacIntosh metallic interposition hemiarthroplasties were used before the development of TKA.[8,9] The implant is a metallic spacer placed between the femoral and tibial surfaces. Favorable results may be achieved most commonly in a patient with arthritic changes in one compartment who was not considered an appropriate candidate for osteotomy because of obesity, limited motion, or arthritic involvement of the opposite compartment.[10,11] However, pain may develop from articulation of the joint surface with the metallic implant. More recently a mobile metallic Uni spacer* has been used which is intended to distract the medial compartment and transfer loads to the lateral compartment.[12] However, results appear less predictable than unicompartmental or TKA.

Unicompartmental, bicompartmental, and TKA resurface both the femoral and tibial articular portions of the joint and are effective in relieving arthritic pain. Unicompartmental arthroplasty is indicated for degenerative arthritis limited to either the medial or lateral TF compartment with preservation of the opposite TF and patellofemoral (PF) compartments. Unicompartmental arthroplasty preserves both cruciate ligaments, the opposite TF compartment, and the PF joint, which is typically associated with more favorable knee kinematics, ROM, and overall joint function than TKA. However, failure of unicondylar arthroplasty may occur from the development of arthritic symptoms in the PF or opposite TF compartment, requiring conversion to TKA. Mechanical failure or polyethylene wear may also limit the longevity of unicondylar replacement. Although the indications for use of unicondylar replacement as an alternative to TKA are controversial, unicondylar replacement is generally considered less predictable in terms of longevity of the arthroplasty, particularly when used in situations in which some arthritic involvement of the opposite TF or PF compartment exists. Recent literature shows favorable functional results and patient satisfaction from unicompartmental knee arthroplasty (UKA), especially in the younger, high-demand, and active patients.[13] The advantages of UKA versus TKA include better ROM at discharge and a shorter hospital stay (77° versus 67° and 1.3 to 1.4 days versus 2.2 days). The average arc of motion at initial 6-week follow-up was 116° for the UKA patients and 110° for the TKA patients, with 56% of knees having greater than 120°. Early discharge for the patients appeared to be safe; in 97% of cases, patients were discharged directly to home, but 18% of the cases required home health physical therapy and 76% of the cases required outpatient physical therapy. Only 3% of the patients required a skilled nursing or postdischarge rehabilitation stay.[14]

Bicompartmental (combined medial and PF) arthroplasty is indicated for treatment of symptomatic medial compartment and PF OA.[15] Early results with bicompartmental arthroplasty indicate that satisfactory clinical results and restoration of normal kinematics can be achieved.[16] However,

since bicompartmental arthroplasty is a relatively new procedure, long-term results are not known.

TKA is an effective treatment for severe arthritic knee pain. Both the medial and lateral TF, and usually the PF compartments, are resurfaced in TKA. After TKA, reliable improvement in pain and function can be expected, and survivorship rates of 90% to 95% after 10 years have frequently been reported.[17-22] **Early failures may result from infection, instability, malalignment, stiffness, reflex sympathetic dystrophy, and patellar problems. Relative contraindications include active infection, extensor mechanism disruption, severe loss of bony or ligament support, and uncontrolled cardiac disease or medical comorbidities that substantially increase the risk of perioperative morbidity and mortality.** However, using proper surgical technique, implant selection, appropriate postoperative pain management, and rehabilitation can avoid these problems. Recent developments including computer-assisted surgery, more kinematic or high-flexion implant designs, use of MIS, and MRI-derived custom cutting blocks may further improve the results of TKA. TKA performed through a conventional skin incision centered over the rectus tendon proximally and extending distal to the tibial tubercle, with a medial parapatellar arthrotomy, is associated with reliable pain relief, improvement in function, and 90% to 95% 10-year survivorship.[17-22] However, many patients experience significant pain and inflammation, which typically occurs to some extent for 6 months after arthroplasty and may limit participation in rehabilitation exercises. Less invasive or MIS permits TKA to be performed with reduced soft tissue trauma, with average skin incision of 9.4 to 10.9 cm in the MIS group and 13.7 to 17.1 cm in the conventional group.[23] Reports indicate that MIS is associated with less blood loss, less pain, and earlier return of quadriceps function and ROM.[24-26]

Recent literature shows favorable results in the MIS surgery. In selected patients, the Berger and associates' study showed that outpatient MIS TKA was safe for discharge on the day of surgery with no short-term readmission or complications in 96% of the patients.[27] In Tanavalee's study, 82% of the MIS patients were able to do active knee extension on day 1 while none were able to do active knee extension in the conventional group. Additionally, patients who could walk on day 1 were 17 versus 2.[23] In another study, in the first 12 weeks after surgery, the MIS group had less flexion contracture and better flexion.[28] At 1 year postoperative, average passive range of motion was 131° in the MIS group and 121° in the conventional group; while active range of motion was 125° in the MIS group and 115° in the conventional group.[29]

However, a minimally invasive approach may compromise surgical exposure and result in increased complications. With use of small cutting blocks and avoiding dissection of the suprapatellar pouch, reliable results can be achieved with a complication rate that is not greater than conventional TKA.[24-26] Particularly, when combined with a preoperative patient education program and multimodal

---

*Centerpulse, Austin, Texas.

postoperative pain management, TKA performed through a minimally invasive approach appears to offer advantages compared with conventional TKA. However, more muscular patients, those with prior surgery, stiffness, poor skin vascularity, or significant deformity requiring soft tissue releases may not be appropriate candidates for a minimally invasive approach.

SURGICAL PROCEDURES—TRADITIONAL

Preoperative Evaluation

Preoperative evaluation always includes a thorough history and physical examination, determination of the type of arthritis, other joint involvement and functional status, walking distance, current and expected activity level, and sports involvement. Other significant concerns include history of deep venous thrombosis (DVT) or pulmonary embolus (PE) and previous surgery such as joint replacement, corrective osteotomy, and internal fixation of a hip, femur, or tibial fracture. Close attention is paid to joint alignment (varus or valgus), stability, ROM (especially the presence or absence of flexion contracture), muscle tone, and leg lengths.

Preoperative radiographs should include long weight-bearing films to demonstrate any femoral or tibial deformity and aid in determining overall lower extremity (LE) alignment. The angle between the mechanical and anatomic axis is measured on the femur to ensure that the distal femoral osteotomy will be perpendicular to the mechanical axis and parallel to the proximal tibial osteotomy (Fig. 27-1). Routine roentgenograms should also include anteroposterior (AP) standing films, as well as lateral and patellar views.

Procedure

Numerous implant and fixation choices are available for TKA:
1. Cemented, uncemented, or hybrid fixation
2. Metal-backed tibia or all-polyethylene tibia
3. Patella resurfacing or patella retaining
4. Posterior cruciate or bicruciate substituting, posterior cruciate-retaining, or mobile-bearing surfaces

The technique described here is the primary TKA using cemented fixation, a metal-backed tibia, an all-polyethylene patella, and posterior cruciate substitution (Fig. 27-2). Currently, this combination is the most commonly used with consistent long-term results published to date.[30-34]

Surgical Technique

An antithrombotic stocking or pump is placed on the uninvolved leg. The patient is questioned as to which knee is to be replaced as a final check to avoid the mistake of operating on the wrong knee. An intravenous antibiotic, usually first-generation cephalosporin, is given before the skin incision is made. The patient is placed supine on the operating room table with a tourniquet about the proximal thigh. A general endotracheal or regional anesthetic is required. However,

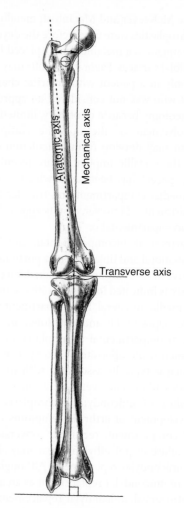

Fig. 27-1 The anatomic axis parallels the femoral shaft, whereas the mechanical axis is a straight line from the center of the femoral head to the center of the knee and the center of the ankle. (Courtesy Zimmer, Inc, Warsaw, Ind.)

peripheral nerve block of the femoral nerve has been shown to be effective in controlling pain whether through a local infusion (24 hours) or administered via percutaneous insertion of a catheter adjacent to the femoral nerve (a 2- to 3-day ambulatory continuous femoral nerve block).[35,36]

A sandbag is taped to the operating room table, or a commercial leg-holding device is often used to help stabilize the leg during the procedure. The entire LE is sterilely prepared and draped. The LE is exsanguinated with an Esmarch bandage, and a tourniquet is inflated to an appropriate pressure.

Exposure

A longitudinal midline skin incision is made extending from proximal to the patella to just distal to the tibial tuberosity. Full-thickness skin flaps, including the deep fascia, are developed medially and laterally (Fig. 27-3). A medial arthrotomy is made extending from the quadriceps tendon and ending medial to the tibial tuberosity. The patella is everted or subluxed laterally. After flexing the knee to 90°, the surgeon trims osteophytes from the femoral condyles, intercondylar notch, and tibial plateaus. The cruciate ligaments are excised.

Ligament Balancing

Ligamentous balance is addressed by inserting spreaders in the medial and lateral femoral tibial joints, both in flexion and extension. Equal spacing is then attained by excision of osteophytes and soft tissue releases. The three most common deformities encountered are varus, valgus, and flexion. Release of contracted soft tissues on the concave side of the deformity is achieved either by sequential subperiosteal longitudinal release of individual anatomic soft tissue constraints or use of multiple transverse stab wound incisions (pie crusting) into the contracted soft tissues.

Varus Deformity. Osteophytes protruding off the medial tibia are removed and the medial capsule is incised. If necessary, then the medial collateral ligament is subperiosteally stripped off the tibia. For deformities with combined varus and flexion contracture, release of the semimembranosus insertion is often necessary.

Valgus Deformity. A lateral retinacular release is commonly required. If the valgus deformity is more rigid in extension than in flexion, the iliotibial band is released. The popliteus tendon, lateral collateral ligament, and posterolateral capsule may also be released, depending on the severity of the deformity. Peroneal nerve neuropraxia can occasionally occur, especially with correction of flexion contracture in association with valgus deformity.

Flexion Deformity. Excising posterior femoral osteophytes and releasing posterior capsular adhesions usually address a minor contracture. Further correction requires resection of more bone from the distal femur and posterior capsular release.

Osseous Preparation. An intramedullary femoral guide is placed through a drill hole in the center of the trochlea (Fig. 27-4). The intramedullary rod must parallel the femoral shaft in both the AP and lateral planes, ensuring placement parallel to the anatomic axis of the femur. Cutting guides are attached to the intramedullary guide to allow precise osteotomies of the anterior and distal femur. The distal femoral osteotomy is usually made 6° to the anatomic axis to produce distal femoral alignment perpendicular to the mechanical axis (Fig. 27-5).

Either intramedullary or extramedullary tibial cutting guides are used. The proximal tibia is osteotomized with a sagittal saw perpendicular to its long axis, approximately 5 mm distal to its articular surface, and angled posteriorly approximately 3° to 5°. Small tibial defects are effectively addressed with cement. Larger defects require either bone grafting or metal augments.

An AP measuring guide is used to determine the appropriate size and position of the femoral component. An AP cutting block is placed to remove the anterior and posterior

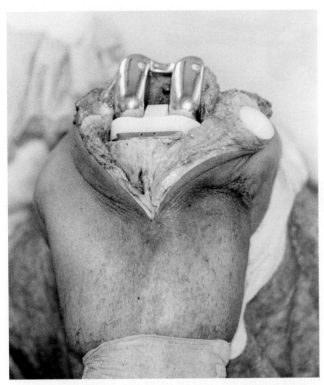

Fig. 27-2 Primary TKA using all polyethylene patella and posterior cruciate substitution. (Some physicians favor this approach; it is not the preference of Dr. Ries.)

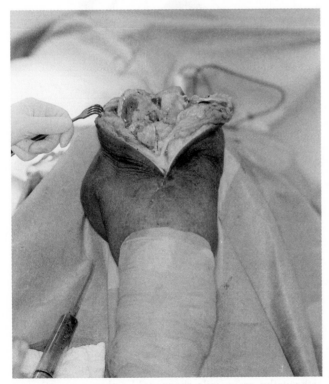

Fig. 27-3 Surgical exposure of the left knee. Note the full-thickness skin flaps, medial arthrotomy, and eversion of the patella. This varus knee demonstrates severe wear of the medial femoral condyle.

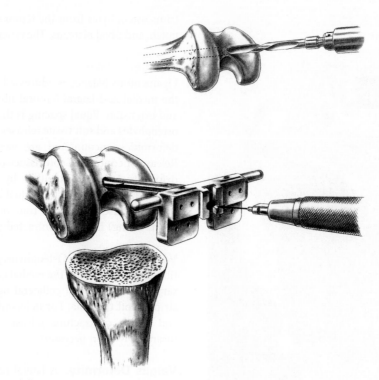

Fig. 27-4 The intramedullary femoral guide ensures placement parallel to the anatomic axis. (Courtesy Zimmer, Inc, Warsaw, Ind.)

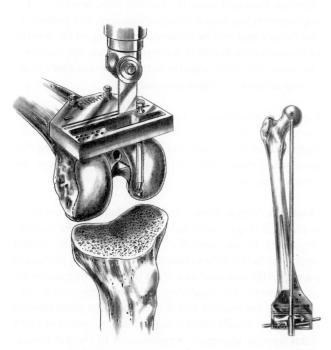

Fig. 27-5 The distal femoral guide attaches to the intramedullary guide with a proper amount of valgus (usually 6°) to ensure the osteotomy is made perpendicular to the mechanical axis. (Courtesy Zimmer, Inc, Warsaw, Ind.)

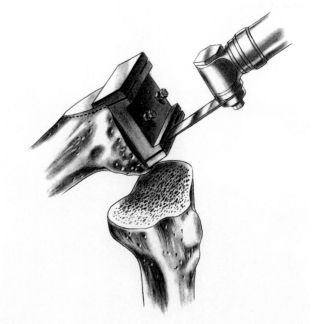

Fig. 27-6 Anterior and posterior femoral osteotomies. (Courtesy Zimmer, Inc, Warsaw, Ind.)

femoral condyles. This affords excellent visibility and access to remove any remaining meniscus, cruciate ligament, and osteophytes (Fig. 27-6).

The flexion and extension gaps are measured with standardized spacer blocks. Ideally, the same gap has been produced between the distal femur and tibia in extension and posterior femur and tibia in flexion. This ensures proper soft tissue tension and ligamentous balance. **If full extension is not attained, then further bone is removed from the distal femur.** For very severe flexion contractures, such as those encountered in some cases of hemophilic arthropathy or juvenile rheumatoid arthritis, resection of the distal femur to the level of the collateral ligament insertions may be required. Further bone resection is a relative

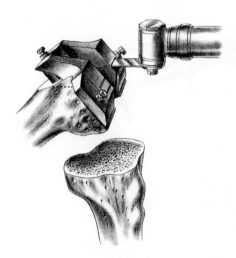

Fig. 27-7 Single guide used to perform anterior and posterior chamfers and to remove the intercondylar notch. (Courtesy Zimmer, Inc, Warsaw, Ind.)

contraindication to conventional TKA if the ligament insertions are compromised, and use of a more highly constrained or revision prosthesis is necessary. A guide is then used to chamfer the anterior and posterior femoral condyles and remove bone from the intercondylar notch (Fig. 27-7).

Sizing guides are used to determine the proper-sized tibial component.

After orienting the guide in the AP, medial, and lateral planes, the surgeon ensures proper rotation with the use of an alignment rod extending to the middle of the ankle joint. A bone punch is then used to compress the soft cancellous bone in the tibial metaphysis to accommodate the keel on the tibial component (Fig. 27-8). Trial tibial and femoral components are placed to ensure proper sizing, soft tissue tensioning, ligamentous balance, patellar tracking, and ROM.

Patellar thickness is measured with a caliper. The articular surface is removed with a power saw or reamer. A guide is used to drill one or more holes in the patella for additional peg fixation (Fig. 27-9). The component is usually placed slightly medial on the patella to assist in patella tracking. The thickness is again checked with the caliper; if the patella is thicker than before resection, then more patella is removed to restore normal patella thickness. Patella tracking is observed (Fig. 27-10) and if the patella tracks laterally, then a lateral retinacular release is performed. Efforts are made to preserve the superior lateral geniculate artery, thereby preserving the blood supply to the patella.

All trial components are removed, bony surfaces are cleansed with pulse lavage, and bone cement is mixed. All components may be cemented at one time, or a second batch of cement may be prepared to allow sequential implantation of the components. All excess cement is trimmed while soft. After the cement has hardened, the tibial spacer may be exchanged to allow final adjustments with regard to ROM and stability. The tourniquet is released and bleeding controlled.

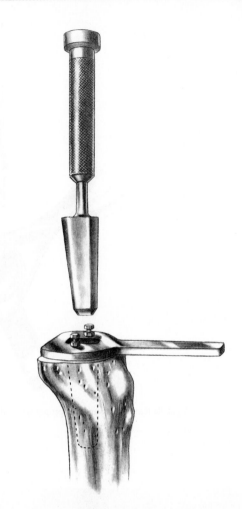

Fig. 27-8 A tibial template is rotationally aligned and sized appropriately to allow proper placement of the tibial stem punch. (Courtesy Zimmer, Inc, Warsaw, Ind.)

The wound is irrigated thoroughly and closed over a suction drain. A sterile dressing is applied. An antithrombotic stocking or compressive dressing is applied over the sterile dressing (Fig. 27-11).

MINIMALLY INVASIVE SURGERY

Surgical Technique

The minimally or less invasive skin incision extends from the superior pole of the patella to the tibial tubercle (Fig. 27-12). In most patients the length of the incision is approximately 10 to 12 cm, but it may be longer or shorter depending on the size of the patient. Full-thickness skin and subcutaneous tissue flaps are raised to mobilize the skin and subcutaneous layer and permit adequate deep exposure.

Either a medial parapatellar, midvastus, or quadriceps-sparing (subvastus) arthrotomy may be used to expose the knee. Excellent results have been reported using the minimidvastus approach, whereas the quadriceps-sparing approach is more restrictive and may only be appropriate for thin patients with mobile extensor mechanisms and no intraarticular deformity. Typically for muscular male

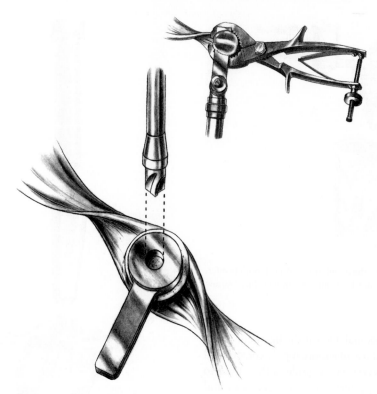

Fig. 27-9 A patella template ensures the proper size and placement of the patella component. (Courtesy Zimmer, Inc, Warsaw, Ind.)

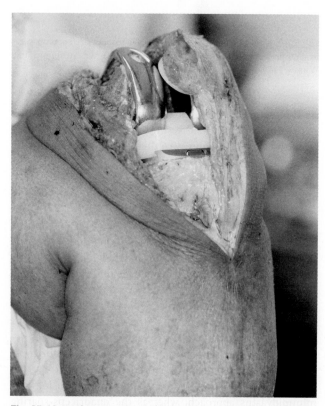

Fig. 27-10 Final component cemented in place. Central tracking of patella without finger pressure should be noted.

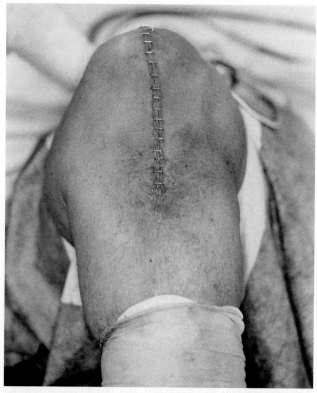

Fig. 27-11 The wound is closed in layers with nonabsorbable sutures in arthrotomy incisions, running absorbable sutures in subcutaneous layer incorporating the Scarpa fascia, and staples in the skin. Suction drainage is performed supralaterally to avoid quadriceps mechanism.

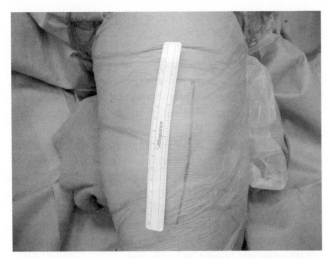

Fig. 27-12 Skin incision extends from the proximal pole of the patella to the tibial tubercle.

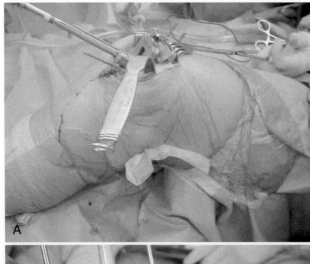

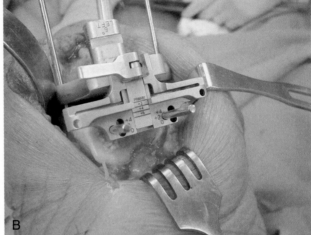

Fig. 27-14 **A,** To expose the distal femur, the knee is partially flexed to 45° to 60°, which moves the center of the skin incision more proximally. **B,** The distal femoral cutting block is positioned, and the distal femoral cut is made with the knee partially flexed.

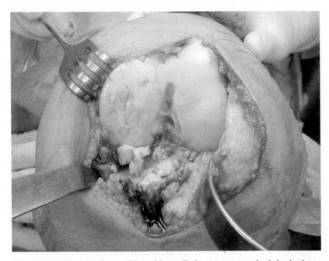

Fig. 27-13 The patella is subluxed laterally but not everted while the knee is flexed.

patients, either more proximal dissection of the vastus medialis (in a midvastus approach) or a medial parapatellar arthrotomy is necessary to displace the extensor mechanism laterally. A portion of the fat pad is excised to facilitate exposure. Lateral patellar subluxation is necessary, but eversion of the patella while the knee is flexed does not necessarily increase exposure and may contribute to quadriceps inhibition and postoperative knee pain (Fig. 27-13). The skin and subcutaneous tissue may be considered as a "mobile window." By extending the knee, the skin incision is moved more proximally and exposure is centered over the distal femur, whereas flexing the knee permits more distal exposure over the proximal tibia (Figs. 27-14 and 27-15). Cutting guides for MIS-TKA are smaller than conventional instruments but permit accurate bone cuts. Alternatively, custom disposable cutting guides can be used. These are derived from preoperative three-dimensional MRI images of the arthritic knee and

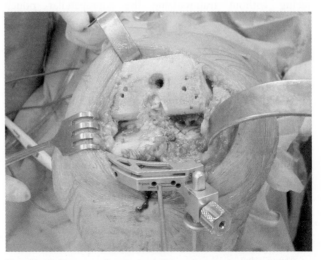

Fig. 27-15 To expose the proximal tibia and resect the tibial surface, the knee is fully flexed.

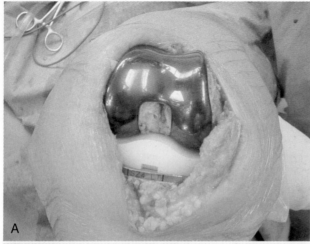

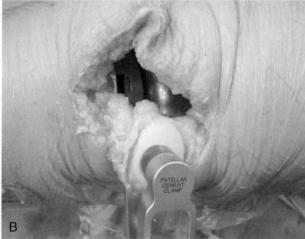

Fig. 27-16 A, The femoral and tibial components are implanted. **B,** With the knee fully extended, the patella is everted and resurfaced.

intended to provide precise orientation of the bone cuts. With the knee in extension, tension in the extensor mechanism is reduced and the patella may be everted for resurfacing without traumatizing the suprapatellar pouch (Fig. 27-16).

THERAPY GUIDELINES FOR REHABILITATION

Successful postoperative management of the patient ideally begins preoperatively. In many cases, the patient has already been seen by a physical therapist (PT) for a conservative course of treatment. Prescription of high- and low-resistance training exercises is an essential aspect of management for knee OA and both have significantly improved clinical effects.[37] Although the goal of rehabilitation at this time may be to avoid surgery, the PT must bear in mind that the treatment plan is similar to those for preoperative care:

1. Patient education regarding the disease process and prognosis
2. Behavioral and health modification for joint protection

3. Cardiovascular conditioning as an adjunct to weight loss
4. An individualized exercise program to address strength and flexibility issues
5. Functional training to maximize the patient's ability

Much can be done for these patients in this phase of the disease process. A successful outcome for postoperative TKA can be predicted by the patient's functional ability and status preoperatively.[38-40]

In the event that a TKA is the intervention of choice, then preoperative treatment is modified to include the assembly of a multidisciplinary team. This group includes the orthopedic surgeon, PT, nursing staff, occupational therapist, and social service worker. Although each team member is responsible for his or her area of expertise, all are committed to the common goal of providing the best possible care to get the maximal benefit and outcome.

During this phase the patient should be educated and familiarized with the surgical procedure and the phases of the rehabilitation process. This serves both to identify and anticipate any special problems or needs that the patient should incur. It will also reinforce the active role of the patient in his or her own long-term care. Recommendations may involve home planning, dental hygiene, and social planning.

In the era of managed care, many hospitals have formed preoperative educational classes for this purpose. In a group atmosphere, patients can begin to understand the rehabilitation process and formulate realistic goals and expectations. Informational pamphlets outlining all pertinent information are also helpful. Good preoperative care and communication between the team and the patient can guarantee a smooth transition through the postoperative process.

Phase I (Inpatient Acute Care)

TIME: 1 to 5 days after surgery
GOALS: Prevent complications, reduce pain and swelling, promote ROM, restore safety and independence (Table 27-1)

The goals for this initial period of rehabilitation are standard for any postoperative care. These pertain to the prevention of any possible complications. Medical considerations include (1) the prevention of infection, (2) the prevention of PE, (3) the prevention of DVT, and (4) the reduction of pain and swelling. Functional goals include (1) the promotion of ROM and (2) the restoration of safety and independence in activities of daily living (ADLs) and gait. The treatment plan is formulated with these specific considerations in mind.

Medical Considerations

Intravenous antibiotics are continued for 24 hours. DVT prophylaxis is initiated. This typically consists of antithrombotic pumps, Coumadin, low molecular weight heparin, or a combination of these treatments.

Monitoring the surgical incision for drainage, erythema, excessive pain, or swelling is continued throughout the

TABLE 27-1 Total Knee Arthroplasty

Rehabilitation Phase	Criteria to Progress to This Phase	Anticipated Impairments and Functional Limitations	Intervention	Goal	Rationale
Phase I Inpatient acute care 1-5 days	• Postoperative and cleared by physician to initiate therapy	• Edema • Pain • Limited ROM • Limited strength • Limited bed mobility and transfers • Limited gait	• CPM setup and patient instruction beginning with 0°-40° and progressing 5°-10° as tolerated 5-10 hr/day • Inspect wound for drainage, erythema, and excessive pain • Breathing exercises • Patient education to control edema (elevation and pumps) and positioning to prevent knee flexion contracture • PROM—knee extension and flexion, supine heel slides • Isometrics—quadriceps, hamstrings, and gluteal sets: 10 repetitions three times • AROM—ankle dorsiflexion, plantar flexion, and circumduction • Transfer and bed mobility training • Gait training with weight bearing as tolerated or as physician orders (using walker or crutches) in immobilizer until adequate quadriceps control is attained After second day, progress to: • Initiation of A/AROM exercises twice daily • AROM—heel slides (supine and seated) TKEs, SLRs	• Independent with the following: (1) Bed mobility; (2) don/doff clothing, and corset if indicated; (3) transfers; (4) gait using assistive device as appropriate • Demonstrate appropriate body mechanics with self-care and basic activities of daily living • Independent with gait for 100 ft on level surfaces using appropriate assistive device • Progress self-management of ROM exercises • Decrease pain and edema	• Restore ROM of knee • Improve wound healing, reduce adhesion formation, prevent complications • Wound and surgical site protection is important as patient begins to perform exercises and ambulation (Note: Infection and deep venous thrombosis are major postoperative complications of total knee arthroplasty.) • Use gravity feed and muscle pump to minimize edema and prevent deep venous thrombosis • Reduce reflex inhibition of quadriceps resulting from pain and edema • Prepare patient for independence with transfers • Begin to prepare extensor mechanism to accept loads • Restore independence with ambulation • Improve stability of involved lower extremity • Prevent disuse atrophy and reflex inhibition • Prepare for home disposition, facilitate independence

A/AROM, Active assistive range of motion; *AROM*, active range of motion; *CPM*, continuous passive motion; *PROM*, passive range of motion; *ROM*, range of motion; *SLR*, straight leg raises; *TKE*, terminal knee extension.

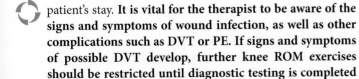

patient's stay. **It is vital for the therapist to be aware of the signs and symptoms of wound infection, as well as other complications such as DVT or PE. If signs and symptoms of possible DVT develop, further knee ROM exercises should be restricted until diagnostic testing is completed** **and DVT is ruled out or an appropriate level of anticoagulation therapy is achieved.** Specific signs, symptoms, and tests are discussed in the Troubleshooting section of this chapter. Any symptom must be brought to the immediate attention of the nursing staff and surgeon.

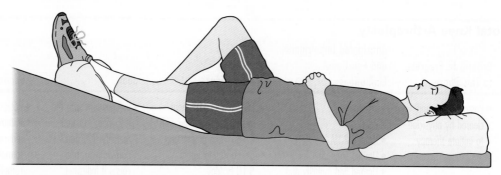

Fig. 27-17 With the leg straight, a pillow is positioned under the ankle to increase end-range extension and venous drainage and decrease compression of the posterior tibial vein.

Functional Considerations

Restoration of functional ROM is essential for the success of TKA. Continuous passive motion (CPM) has been used and shown to be beneficial in regaining early mobility, but may not necessarily affect the final ROM achieved. CPM can be initiated immediately after surgery in the recovery room.

In one study, CPM patients were able to achieve 90° of flexion in 9.1 days versus their non-CPM counterparts, who required 13.8 days to reach the same goal.[41,42] Unfortunately, CPM was found to be ineffective in the enhancement of knee extension.[41,43]

Many surgeons choose to begin immediate postoperative CPM.[44,45] Because of wound concerns, others choose to begin on postoperative day 2.[46] The beneficial effects of CPM include the improvement of wound healing,[47] accelerated clearance of hemarthrosis,[48] reduced muscle atrophy,[49,50] reduced adhesion formation,[51-54] reduction in the incident of DVT,[55] decreased hospital stay,[56] and decreased need for medication.[57,58] Although excellent function and ROM can be achieved without the use of CPM, many surgeons and patients find that CPM is useful in reducing the frequency of complications after TKA.[45,46,59]

The protocol of CPM application varies in the literature. In general, the initial settings range from 0° to 25° to 40° of flexion. The range is then either increased 5° to 10° per day or to patient tolerance. CPM can be used from 4 to 20 hours per day. Its use is discontinued at the end of the acute hospital stay or when maximum knee flexion of the CPM machine is attained.

Another modality that has been shown to be useful in improving ROM and quadriceps strength is neuromuscular electrical stimulation (NMES). **Mitigating quadriceps muscle weakness immediately after TKA using early NMES may improve functional outcomes, because quadriceps weakness has been associated with numerous functional limitations and an increased risk for falls.**[60] When NMES was added to a voluntary exercise program, deficits in quadriceps muscle strength and activation resolved quickly after TKA.[61] In conjunction with the CPM, the application of NMES was shown to reduce extensor lag and the length of stay in the acute care setting.[59]

Exercises are taught at bedside beginning on postoperative day 2 or 3.[44,62] Breathing exercises promote full excursion of the rib cage. Ankle ROM exercises (i.e., pumping, circumduction) along with instruction in proper elevation and positioning of the LE is encouraged (Fig. 27-17). The purpose of these exercises is to engage the muscle pump and passive gravity feed to decrease distal edema and avoid DVT.

Isometric gluteal sets, hamstring sets, and quadriceps sets are taught to prevent disuse atrophy and quadriceps reflex inhibition. Patients are encouraged to do these exercises independently, thereby increasing their active participation. It is recommended that this program be initially performed 10 repetitions every hour, and progressed to 20 repetitions, three times daily.[62]

This exercise program is advanced throughout the first week of rehabilitation. Active assistive range of motion (A/AROM) exercises, such as seated heel slides or therapist-assisted knee flexion and passive knee extension, are performed to improve mobility. Straight leg raises (SLRs) and terminal knee extensions (TKEs) further strengthen the quadriceps muscles, thus improving the dynamic stabilizers of the knee.[62,63] These exercises will become part of the home program once the patient is discharged.

The patient is also instructed in ADLs, such as dressing, bathing, transfers, reaching, and picking up items. Usually this comes under the supervision of the occupational therapist, although particularly in some smaller hospital settings, the PT may be responsible. The ADLs should be reviewed and performed until the patient can demonstrate safety and independence. The need for any special assistive devices is assessed and they are issued.

Progressive gait training begins with a walker or crutches on postoperative day 2 or 3,[62] proceeding throughout the acute care hospitalization. Safety, balance, and patient independence are the primary goals for this intervention. Negotiating level surfaces, ramps, curbs, stairs, or other activities relevant to the patient are practiced.

Current clinical care pathways recommend that the average length of stay in the acute hospital should be approximately 3 to 4 days,[62,64] with physical therapy sessions twice daily. The patient is discharged when deemed medically stable. Specifically, from a rehabilitation standpoint, the patient should be able to demonstrate 80° to 90° of motion, 30 transfer supine to sit and sit to stand independently, ambulate 15 to 100 feet, and ascend and descend three steps[65] or as the home situation dictates.[62] If unable to do these tasks or if any medical postoperative complications occur, then the patient may be transferred to an extended care unit (ECU) or skilled nursing facility for further care.

Phase IIa (Inpatient Extended-Care or Skilled Nursing Facility)

TIME: 6 to 14 days after surgery
GOALS: Prevent complications, reduce pain and swelling, promote ROM, restore safety and independence (Table 27-2)

The goals of this short-term rehabilitation phase are the same as for in the acute hospital. Treatment efforts continue, with physical therapy scheduled twice a day for a length of stay of approximately 3 to 7 days or until goals are met. Sometimes it becomes necessary to begin training family members or caregivers in assisting the patient during gait and transfers. Social services are often necessary to assist in planning home care needs or placement in long-term care facilities.

Phase IIb (Outpatient Home Health)

TIME: 2 to 3 weeks after discharge to home
GOALS: Become safe in home environment with transfers, gait, and most ADLs (Table 27-3)

Once discharged home, physical therapy treatments are reduced to three times weekly. During this phase of rehabilitation, the goals are expanded to facilitate functional ROM, endure safe and independent ADLs, transfers, and gait in the community. It is important for the therapist to assess the home for safety and make changes as appropriate.

TABLE 27-2 Total Knee Arthroplasty

Rehabilitation Phase	Criteria to Progress to This Phase	Anticipated Impairments and Functional Limitations	Intervention	Goal	Rationale
Phase IIa Extended care or skilled nursing (inpatient) 6-14 days	• No signs of infection • No significant increase in pain • No loss of ROM • Discharge from acute care • Progressive stiffness, wound drainage, other complications that may preclude home discharge • If patient is unsafe for home disposition, transfer to ECU • Discharge to home	• Edema and pain • Limited ROM • Limited strength • Limited gait tolerance	• Continuation and progression of interventions from phase I • Transfer training (car, sit-stand with varying seat heights) • Progressive gait training using appropriate assistive device • Aggressive knee extension and flexion exercises • PROM—flexion (prone and standing) • A/AROM—flexion (seated, on step, on bicycle) • AROM—SLR, heel raises, leg curls, step-ups, step-downs, one-fourth squats • Joint mobilization • Soft tissue and myofascial release (respecting incision) • Careful ongoing monitoring of edema	• Self-management of pain and edema • Independence with bed mobility and transfers • Independent gait in community distances (300-500 ft) • Knee PROM 0°-110° • Advance independence with home exercises • Improve functional lower extremity strength	• CPM may be discontinued if ROM is improving • Prepare for discharge from ECU (transition to home health or outpatient) • Promote return to unassisted gait in the community • Obtain close to if not functional ROM (110° necessary for stair climbing) • Maximize lower extremity strength and stability • Prevent disuse atrophy • Treat hip weaknesses resulting from altered weight-bearing and compensatory postural strategies (Note: Postoperative stiffness is a major complication of total knee arthroplasty. Manipulation criteria varies among surgeons—see text.)

A/AROM, Active assistive range of motion; *AROM*, active range of motion; *CPM*, continuous passive motion; *ECU*, extended care unit; *PROM*, passive range of motion; *ROM*, range of motion; *SLR*, straight leg raises.

TABLE 27-3 Total Knee Arthroplasty

Rehabilitation Phase	Criteria to Progress to This Phase	Anticipated Impairments and Functional Limitations	Intervention	Goal	Rationale
Phase IIb Home health 2-3 wk (depending on need for extended care unit or skilled nursing facility)	• No signs of infection • No significant increase in pain • No loss of ROM • If at home, good family support for assistance with ADLs and safety	• Limited ROM • Limited strength • Difficulty with gait on uneven surfaces and stairs • Unable to attend outpatient rehabilitation (homebound)	• Assess home safety and make changes as appropriate • Car transfers and gait training on uneven surfaces • Continuation of exercises as listed previously to increase knee ROM and strength • Progressive weight bearing per physician's orders and patient's ability	• Safe and independent in home setting • Independent ambulation using appropriate assistive device • Independent in community distances • ROM 0°-110°	• Prevent complications such as falling • Return to independent living • Prepare for discharge to outpatient rehabilitation facility • Strengthen lower kinetic chain • Prevent disuse atrophy • 110° of flexion required for stair climbing and use of stationary bicycle • Avoid postoperative contracture and need for manipulation

ADLs, Activities of daily living; *ROM,* range of motion.

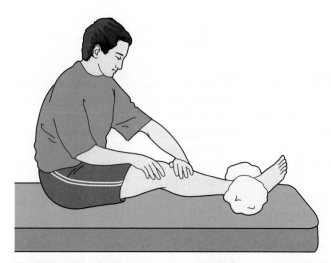

Fig. 27-18 TKE with passive overpressure. With the knee straight, a pillow is positioned under the ankle. Manual overpressure is applied above and below the patellofemoral joint to increase TKE passively.

Recommendations may include but are not limited to the installation of nonskid rugs, safety rails and ramps, and the elimination of potential obstacles around the house.

The home exercise program initiated in the inpatient setting is reviewed and refined. **If extension mobility is lacking, then more aggressive knee extension exercises are instructed** (Fig. 27-18). Postoperative pain may limit a patient's ability to perform knee ROM exercises. If postoperative pain is not adequately controlled, then more effective pain management strategies should be considered, including inpatient pain management for very severe cases. If knee flexion is limited, then more progressive active and active

assistive exercises are given (Fig. 27-19, *A* to *C*). Functional strengthening exercises are progressed in both the open- and closed-chain positions. Examples of closed-chain exercises are bilateral toe raises, sit-to-stand exercises (Fig. 27-20, *A* and *B*), one-quarter squats, and progressive step-ups and step-downs (Fig. 27-21, *A* and *B*). Closed-chain exercises have been shown to be highly effective in recruiting the vastus medialis oblique and vastus lateralis as compared with open-chain isometric exercises.[66-68] Specific transfers in the home and the car are practiced. Progression in gait includes advancing the patient to crutches or a cane as his or her balance dictates. Ambulation on uneven, ramped, and outdoor surfaces is also reviewed. Home physical therapy is discontinued when the patient is no longer home bound.

Phase III (Outpatient Care)

TIME: 3 to 12 weeks after surgery
GOALS: Normalize gait; reduce reliance on assistive devices; increase ROM; improve weight bearing, balance, strength, endurance, and proprioception (Table 27-4)

This phase of rehabilitation may begin on postoperative week 2 to 4 for the highly advanced and active patients or week 4 to 6 for those proceeding more routinely. The length of this stage is also dependent on factors such as the patient's goals and potential functional abilities. The therapist should review the insurance benefits and explain to the patient all options for rehabilitation if there are any insurance limitations.

Common difficulties encountered with TKAs include patellar instability and lack of motion. Routine functional

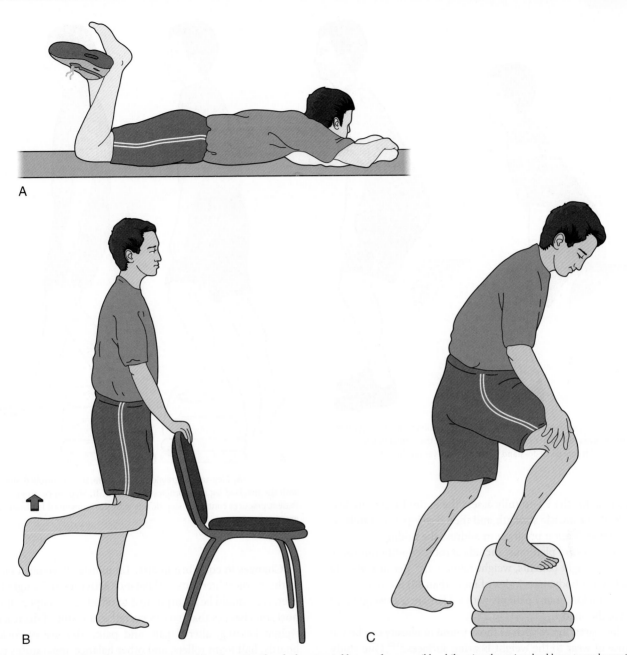

Fig. 27-19 **A,** Prone knee flexion. In a prone position the patient bends the operated knee as far as possible while using the uninvolved knee to apply passive overpressure to increase knee flexion. **B,** Standing open-chain knee flexion. In a standing position with upper extremity support, the patient actively bends the involved knee, bringing the heel to the buttocks while maintaining upright posture. **C,** Standing closed-chain knee flexion. In a standing position, the patient places the foot of the involved leg flat on a step; then the patient places the hands above the knee, slowly leans forward on the involved leg, and guides the knee into more flexion.

activities usually require ROM from 0° to 110°. **Full extension is necessary to normalize the gait cycle[69-71] and to facilitate quadriceps strength.**[64] Full normal ROM may not be a realistic goal for all patients. Postoperative ROM may be restricted, particularly if preoperative and intraoperative ROM is restricted. Stair climbing, sitting on a regular toilet seat or chair (17-inch height), and stationary bike riding requires 110° of knee flexion.[72] If motion is limited, then a manipulation under anesthesia (MUA) may be warranted.

General indications for a manipulation include less than 90° at postoperative week 6[73] or a progressive loss of

flexion.[73,74] **Manipulation carries a small risk of fracture or other complications that may further compromise the outcome of the TKA.**[73] Relative contraindications to manipulation include severe osteoporosis and markedly restricted intraoperative ROM.

Muscle strength and flexibility imbalances of the hip, knee, ankle, and foot can occur after knee injury or surgery.[75-78] Reflex inhibition, faulty joint mechanics, altered gait, presurgical disuse atrophy, immobilization, or nerve injury have been shown to cause altered function of the muscles in the lower kinetic chain.[79-82] Therefore it is

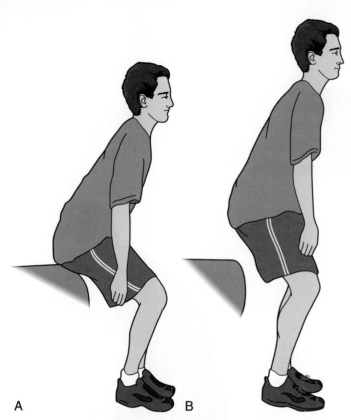

Fig. 27-20 Sit-to-stand exercise. **A,** Start position. **B,** End position. Without using the upper extremities for support, the patient practices controlled and balanced sit-to-stand transfers from various heights.

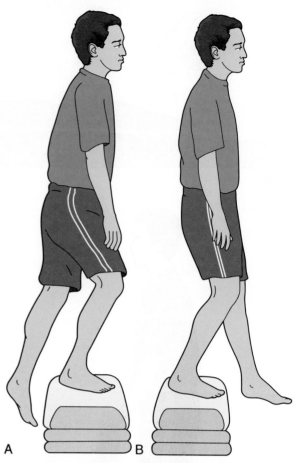

Fig. 27-21 **A,** Step-up progression. Patient practices controlled step-up with the involved leg from progressive heights. **B,** Step-down progression. Patient practices controlled step-downs with the uninvolved leg from progressive heights.

essential for the PT to fully assess the entire LE for any loss of ROM or muscle strength and then develop a comprehensive rehabilitation program to address the findings.

A successful plan must include aerobic conditioning and, for overweight patients, weight reduction.[83] Because obesity (defined as body mass index of more than 30) is often associated with OA, many patients with a TKA are overweight and deconditioned.

Increased forces such as those found in obesity can be the cause of wear to the weight-bearing surfaces.[84,85] One study found that subjects were 12 to 13 kg (25 to 30 lbs) heavier and had 4% to 6% more body fat 1 year after TKA.[120] On the other hand, after total joint replacement, many patients have been shown to resume routine walking and recreational activities that improved maximum oxygen consumption 1 year after the surgery.[86] Nonimpact activities such as stationary bicycling, distance walking, and swimming are suggested for cardiovascular conditioning.[85]

Aquatic therapy programs have proven to be effective in rehabilitation of total joint replacements.[87-89] The buoyant and warm environment can provide pain relief, increase circulation, and decrease weight bearing for the patient. Many can immediately start to work on ROM, strengthening, and normalizing gait without the assistance of a walker. The therapist can challenge the patient by progressing him or her from shoulder-deep water (approximately 24% weight bearing) to waist-deep water (50% weight bearing).

Changes in equilibrium after LE injuries have been cited in the medical literature.[90-94] Balance activities and single-leg exercises should be incorporated to offset any compensatory postural changes that have occurred as a result of decreased weight bearing, altered gait, and pain. The use of rocker boards, half foam rollers, and other balance apparatuses can be helpful to improve the patient's proprioception, balance, and postural control strategies.

With regard to long-term rehabilitation goals, the patient's primary concern should be to maintain a pain-free functional activity level for as long a period as possible. With a TKA, certain restrictions in activities are warranted. Generally those recreational activities and sports that involve high repetitive compression or impact loading are not encouraged because of the possibility of loosening or osteolysis of the joint implant.[76,95,96] Joint forces at the TF interface are 1.5 to 4.0 times body weight when walking,[38] 1.2 times body weight when cycling, and increase to 2.0 to 8.0 times body weight when running.[97] Patellofemoral joint forces also show comparable increases. During walking, these are 0.5 times body weight[98] and with running they increase to 3.0 to 4.0 times body weight.[99] Failures of TKAs may occur because of mechanical loosening or wear of the implant. Therefore

TABLE 27-4 Total Knee Arthroplasty

Rehabilitation Phase	Criteria to Progress to This Phase	Anticipated Impairments and Functional Limitations	Intervention	Goal	Rationale
Phase III Outpatient care 3-8 wk	• No longer homebound • Safe and independent with ambulation using assistive device • Safe and independent with care transfers • Patients may access outpatient care if caregiver or family member is assisting with transfers and gait	• Limited ROM • Limited community ambulation using assistive device • Limited lower extremity strength	• Initiate aquatic therapy if available with concurrent land-based treatment • Continuation of ROM stretches and soft tissue procedures • Progression of (repetitions or weight) intensity with previous exercises • Squats, leg press, and bridging • Bicycling, walking, or swimming for cardiovascular conditioning 20 minutes three to five times a week (as indicated per general health issues) • Hip external rotator exercises • BAPs (foam roller) • Return to previous activities (see text)	• Normalize gait pattern and reduce reliance on assistive device • Increase ROM to 110°-125° or as indicated by comparison with uninvolved knee • Single-leg half-squat to 65% body weight • Full weight bearing with single-leg stance • Improve balance, strength, endurance, and proprioception of lower extremity • Reduce stress on the compensatory muscle and joints to prevent chronic imbalance issues • Aquatic (buoyant) environments allow for increased ease of mobility and load-bearing stresses on joints • 0°-110° or 125° of flexion required to use bicycle and stairs • Improved extension and flexion reduces compensatory gait patterns such as "hip hiking"	• Decrease stress on the uninvolved leg with sit-stand transfers • Increase vastus medialis oblique and vastus lateralis in closed-chain exercises • Provide aerobic conditioning for weight control • Address hip weakness caused by altered weight-bearing and compensatory postural strategies • Improve tolerance to community ambulation and prevent falls • Resume previous activities to restore quality of life

BAPs, Balance and proprioception exercises; *ROM,* range of motion.

patients with joint replacement are encouraged to participate in those activities that maintain cardiovascular fitness while subjecting the implant to reduced impact-loading stresses.

In the gym, using a treadmill (walking only), ski machine, stair-climbing machine, elliptical machine, or stationary bicycle is acceptable. Outdoor sports that are allowable include golfing, hiking, cycling, cross-country skiing, swimming, fishing, hunting, scuba diving, sailing, and occasional light doubles tennis.[85] Baseball, basketball, football, martial arts, parachuting, singles tennis, racquetball, running, soccer, and volleyball are generally discouraged.

REHABILITATION FOR MINIMALLY OR LESS INVASIVE SURGERY TOTAL KNEE ARTHROPLASTY

Minimally invasive surgery is one of the most recent advancements in primary TKA. Because of the smaller incision, quadriceps muscle and tendon sparing, less intraoperative blood loss, deletion of patella eversion procedure, and reduction of pain, rehabilitation can occur on an accelerated timeline. Shorter hospital stays; less overall use of analgesics; and more rapid return of ROM, strength, and function are the benefits.[100-102]

In one observation, hospital length of stay was decreased from 7 days to 2 to 3 days.[89] Physical therapy can begin on postoperative day 1, with ROM, ADLs, and gait training. It has been shown that the average MIS-TKA patient regained 90° of flexion within 3.2 days after surgery.[101]

Depending on the patient's age, motivation, previous function, and fitness level, gait and ADL training is progressed immediately. Early studies after MIS-TKA show that patients used crutches or walkers for 1 to 2 weeks, then advanced to a cane for 1 to 2 weeks thereafter. Many ambulated without the use of an assistive device 4 weeks after surgery. Most were independent with bed and bath transfers and all other ADLs after 2 weeks. Many were climbing stairs at 1 month and descending stairs at 2 months. Driving is allowed at 3 to 6 weeks.

As with traditional TKAs, light-impact activities such as hiking, swimming, and cycling are permitted when comfortable. High-level activities such as running and singles tennis remain unadvisable in the long term.[100,103]

MIS-TKA outcomes show that a large percentage of patients were satisfied with the cosmetic benefit as well as the quicker recovery and excellent early function. Patients achieved discharge goals 18% faster than those who had traditional TKA. Good function and knee scores were achieved after 3 to 4 months as compared with the usual 1-year result.[100,101,103]

TROUBLESHOOTING

Although the treatment guidelines given here provide a framework for postoperative rehabilitation of TKA, they should not be used as strict protocols. In fact, modifications are expected because each patient has individual needs, abilities, and goals. Continual reassessment of the patient's status and subsequent alterations in the treatment plan are necessary to achieve optimal results. The therapist must have the necessary abilities and skills to anticipate any potential complications and implement appropriate changes in the treatment plan. The following section describes additional procedures and modalities that can be used to refine the therapy to meet the patient's individual needs.

Medical Complications

During the initial stage of postoperative care, the most serious complications are wound infection, PE, DVT, persistent joint effusion, and lymphedema. **As previously stated, the therapist must know all symptoms and signs that may indicate any of these medical problems. Any of these complications can severely deter rehabilitation progress in terms of time frame and overall prognosis.**

Wound Infection

Systemic signs of a potential wound infection include patient complaints of fever or chills. Knee pain can be severe and not relieved with rest. Knee flexion can increase skin tension. If skin necrosis develops, then ROM exercises should be limited until adequate soft tissue healing has occurred. Other symptoms of infection include increased warmth and erythema about the surgical site and wound drainage.[104] Wound dressings should be checked and changed daily until the staples are removed.[72] Although uncommon (less than 1%), infection remains a serious problem, usually requiring additional surgery and intravenous antibiotic therapy.

Methods to reduce the risk of infection include proper preoperative skin preparation; prophylactic antibiotics and local antibiotics in cement, particularly for immune-compromised patients (e.g., rheumatoid arthritis, diabetes mellitus, human immunodeficiency virus, cancer); and minimizing the length of surgery and tissue trauma.[105]

Pulmonary Embolus

PE is a potentially fatal, but rare, complication. PE can be life threatening and requires prompt diagnostic testing and treatment. Patients at risk for PE are those who may have proximal LE DVT. Proximal LE DVTs are located at or proximal to the trifurcation of the popliteal vein and considered the more dangerous form of LE DVT because the thrombi are larger than those associated with calf DVT and are more likely to embolize.[106]

Clinical signs of PE include tachycardia, distended cervical veins, hypotension, and chest pain. Pulmonary symptoms include tachypnea, rales, wheezing, and pleural effusion.[104] Sudden dyspnea is the most frequent symptom. Pleuritic pain is also common in patients with severe embolization. If any of these signs or symptoms occur, then the PT should immediately notify the nursing staff and physician.

Deep Venous Thrombosis

Because of decreasing lengths of hospitalization, patients are seen in outpatient settings with elevated risks of DVT. Significant signs and symptoms of DVT include complaints of pain and swelling in the involved extremity, calf tenderness, and a positive Homans sign. Specifically, the patient may report a dull ache, tight feeling, or frank pain in the calf or entire leg. The signs and symptoms include slight swelling in the involved calf; distention of the superficial venous collaterals; tenderness, induration, or spasm of the calf muscles, with or without pain, produced by dorsiflexion of the foot (Homans sign); warmth of the affected leg when both legs are exposed to room temperature; and a slight fever or tachycardia.[92] However, DVTs are also often asymptomatic. When signs and symptoms of possible DVT develop, further ROM exercises should be restricted until definitive diagnostic testing is performed.

Additionally, improved assessment of risk for DVT can be obtained by the use of a clinical decision rule (CDR). A series of studies found that patients could be categorized into low-, moderate-, and high-risk groups based on their CDR scores. The use of the CDR may aid in improving the accuracy of probability estimates of DVT and subsequent referral decisions.[106]

Persistent Joint Effusion

A patient sometimes complains of postoperative stiffness, pain, and swelling. The patient should be reassured that this usually decreases within the first few weeks after surgery. **Persistent joint effusion can forestall the rehabilitation process.** Knee ROM exercises can be continued if an effusion is present, but the effusion may limit motion and should be treated with ice before and after exercise. Soft tissue mobilization is an effective procedure that can enhance muscle recovery and reduce soreness after intense physical activity.[107,108] Increasing blood flow may increase oxygen delivery to the injured tissue, enhance healing, and restore homeostasis.[109] If edema, swelling, and inflammation are significant factors in muscle soreness sensation,[110,111] then massage may be able to reduce soreness in the involved muscles. Persistent effusion may be aspirated, not only to relieve pressure and stiffness but also to rule out an indolent infection.

Lymphedema and Total Knee Arthroplasty

Lymphedema is abnormal swelling caused by the presence of excess lymphatic fluid within the tissues. This swelling occurs when the lymphatic system malfunctions or is damaged from a decrease in developmental transport capacity of the lymph vessels, trauma, surgery, radiation, or infection. **Although lymphedema is a minor complication, persistent swelling can occur.**[112]

Lymphedema that is present before surgery should be minimized with use of support stockings and, if necessary, diuretic medications. If lymphedema develops after surgery, rehabilitation can be continued, but compressive stockings should be used to limit the amount of swelling. Because abundant lymph vessels are found at the medial aspect of the knee, trauma to this area or surgery can lead to lymphedema. Lymph flow swelling in this area of bottleneck occurs as a result of tissue trauma in this area. A patient who has venous insufficiency and undergoes TKA also has an increased risk of developing lymphedema after surgery.[112,113]

In treating lymphedema, therapy consists of manual lymph drainage, special compressive bandaging, exercise, and skin care. With proper treatment, edema can be reduced by as much as 60% and in some cases up to 74%. Once the limb is reduced, the patient graduates from the compressive bandages to a proper compression class stocking. Antiembolism stockings, such as TED hose stockings[114] (12 to 20 mm Hg), are worn postsurgery as DVT prophylaxis from bed rest, mild edema, or mild varicosities. Class I (20 to 30 mm Hg) are used for mild lymphedema, mild venous insufficiency, moderate varicose veins, or DVT prevention in individuals with clotting disorders. Higher grades of class II to IV (30 to ≥ 50 mm Hg) are available for individuals with moderate to severe lymphedema or cardiovascular insufficiency or for prevention of DVT in postthrombotic syndrome.[113,115]

Functional Complications

Peroneal Nerve Neuropraxia

Peroneal nerve neuropraxia may arise more frequently in patients with (1) flexion contractures associated with valgus deformity, (2) those who had epidural anesthesia for postoperative control of pain or previous laminectomy, and (3) those who had a previous proximal tibial osteotomy.[116]

In peroneal nerve neuropraxia, the common peroneal nerve and its branches are tethered at the fibular neck. Clinical findings of nerve entrapment or injury include local tenderness around the fibular neck with pain, diminished sensation, or paresthesia radiating over the lateral surface of the lower leg and the dorsum of the foot.[11,117] Nerve conduction velocity testing and electromyographic studies will be positive for neuropathic dysfunction in the motor distribution of the common peroneal nerve distal to the injury or entrapment site at the fibular neck. Clinically, the patient displays an inability to walk or stand on the heel because of the weakness of the ankle dorsiflexors. Additionally, instability when attempting toe walking results from the muscle imbalance and associated sensory abnormalities at the ankle joint. The muscles affected are those in the anterior and lateral compartments of the leg.

When the superficial peroneal nerve is compressed, a decrease in sensation is noted over the dorsum of the foot, with the exception of the first web space. The involvement of the deep peroneal nerve produces a diminution of sensation in the first web space of the foot and affects the muscles of the anterior compartment, including the extensor hallucis brevis and the extensor digitorum brevis.

Complete common peroneal nerve palsy results in a severely affected gait pattern. Without an ankle-foot orthosis, the patient suffers from a foot drop with associated steppage gait in profoundly affected cases or foot slapping in milder ones. The ankle is unstable and vulnerable to ankle inversion sprains. The functional result of partial peroneal nerve palsy depends on which nerve components are the most affected. Loss of the peroneal muscles in the lateral compartment results in a chronically inverted foot, with weight bearing occurring more laterally than normal and invariably affecting the position and stability of the foot and ankle throughout the stance phase of the gait cycle. Loss of the anterior compartment muscles, especially the tibialis anterior, affects the entire gait cycle. The loss of the dorsal intrinsic muscles of the foot has a relatively minor effect on basic weight-bearing functions.

Physical therapy interventions for nerve entrapment include examination of the joint mechanics of the proximal and distal tibiofibular joints and determination of the specific muscle weakness and sensory loss. Manual techniques include joint mobilization as appropriate, facilitation of the recruitment of the affected muscles, and dural nerve root stretches for the sciatic and peroneal nerves.

Muscle Imbalance

A detailed evaluation of the entire lower kinetic chain is necessary for the successful treatment of patients with TKA. Altered gait, faulty mechanics, and muscle imbalances have more than likely existed before the TKA. These factors contribute greatly to the eventual surgical outcome. Most of the present understanding regarding muscle imbalances and neuromotor retraining comes from the work of Janda,[118,119] Lewit,[120] and Sahrmann.[82] Muscle imbalance is a multifactorial problem and can be highly complex. In simplistic terms, the result of muscle imbalance is that the tight muscles become tighter, weak muscles become weaker, and motor control becomes asymmetric.[121]

According to Janda,[118,119] muscle balance is continually adapting the body's posture to gravity. When an injury occurs, faulty posture and weight bearing alter the body's center of gravity, which initiates mechanical responses requiring muscle adaptation. Change in the mechanical behavior of a joint causes neuroreflexive alteration of muscle function through aberrant afferent mechanoreceptor stimulation of articular reflexes.[122] Postural-tonic muscles respond to dysfunction with facilitation, hypertonicity, and shortening. Dynamic-phasic muscles respond with inhibition, hypotonicity, and weakness. In the lower quadrant, Janda[118,119] identified a common pattern of muscle imbalance. Hyperactive muscles include the iliopsoas, rectus femoris, tensor fascia latae, quadratus lumborum, the thigh adductors, piriformis, hamstrings, and the lumbar erector spinae musculature. Muscles that display inhibition or reflexive weakness include the gluteus maximus, medius, and minimus; quadriceps (vasti); rectus abdominis; and external and internal obliques. Sahrmann,[82] Dorman and associates,[123] and Bullock-Saxton, Janda, and Bullock,[79] similarly identified weakness in the entire LE in the presence of knee dysfunction.

Quadriceps weakness, especially in the early stages of TKA rehabilitation, must be addressed. Failure to adequately address the chronic muscle impairments has the potential to limit the long-term functional gains that may be possible following TKA. Postoperative rehabilitation addressing quadriceps strength should mitigate these impairments and ultimately result in improved functional outcomes.[124] These impairments with significant worsening of knee ROM, quadriceps strength, and performance on functional tests occurred 1 month after surgery. Quadriceps strength went through the greatest decline of all the physical measures assessed and never matched the strength of the uninvolved limb. The high correlation between quadriceps strength and functional performance suggests that improved postoperative quadriceps strengthening could be important to enhance the potential benefits of TKA.[125] A knee immobilizer may be needed for ambulation in the hospital setting if quadriceps strength is not great enough to stabilize the knee. Biofeedback or NMES can be beneficial in "jump starting" the

recruitment of the quadriceps. In cases of patella instability, quadriceps strength should be restored as soon as possible. Soft tissue work, friction massage, and assisted stretches to the iliotibial band may be beneficial.

Faulty joint mechanics at the hip, knee, and ankle affect the overall surgical result. A study by Dorman and associates[123] found that inhibition or facilitation of the gluteus medius is influenced by the position of the sacroiliac joint. An anterior rotation (an apparent long leg) manifested a significantly weaker muscle than one in posterior rotation (an apparent short leg). Exercises that address gluteus medius weakness include hip abduction and lateral hip rotation (Fig. 27-22).

Altered ankle movements and instability disturb the overall sense of balance and influence gait safety accordingly. Joint mobilization techniques to correct associated dysfunctions in the joints of the LE can be helpful. A stiff knee can be helped with contraction and relaxation techniques to the muscles that may be guarding or fatigued.[73,87]

Kneeling

Kneeling is an important functional activity frequently not performed after knee replacement, thus affecting a patient's ability to carry out basic daily tasks. Kneeling ability before surgery was poor in osteoarthritic patients but improves with knee arthroplasty surgery.[126] Despite no clinical reason preventing kneeling, many patients fail to resume this activity. Patients avoided kneeling because of uncertainties or recommendations from third parties (doctors, nursing staff, or friends). Inability to kneel may also be caused by scar position, skin hypoaesthesia, restricted range of flexion, involvement of other joints, or pain. The solution to this problem is to incorporate kneeling activity with PT intervention at 6 weeks after surgery because there was significant

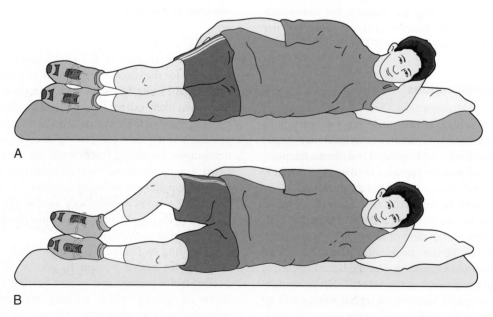

Fig. 27-22 Hip lateral rotation. **A,** Start position. The patient lies on the uninvolved side with the shoulders and hips perpendicular to the table and the knees flexed to 45°. **B,** End position. The patient then lifts the top knee toward the ceiling, keeping the feet in contact. The patient should emphasize movement from the hip and not allow the pelvis to roll backward.

improvement in patient reported kneeling 1 year after surgery in patients who received kneeling intervention.[125,127]

OUTCOMES

TKA is a method to improve "quality" of life. This is accomplished primarily through pain relief, resulting in increased functional mobility. Results are generally reported using the Hospital for Special Surgery[128] or the Knee Society[129] rating systems. Haas' patients[24] from the Hospital for Special Surgery who had MIS showed favorable outcomes (Table 27-5) compared with the traditional TKA. They were able to do an SLR on postoperative day 1, walk without a cane on postoperative day 8, alternate stair climbing by week 6, and perform full knee ROM by week 8.

It should be noted that despite extensive rehabilitation efforts, various studies have shown outcomes of diminished functional capacity. Self-report measures of perceived abilities indicate that at 1 year after TKA, most individuals have regained 80% of normal function. However, stiffness and pain occasionally still remained a problem.[93,130,131] Lingard's study[39,132] showed that the most improvement in pain reduction and functional improvement was made in the first 3 months after TKA, with little change after 12 months.[133,134] Walsh and associates[83] also showed that at 1 year after TKA, little pain was noted during activities of walking, stair climbing, and concentric muscle testing. However, after implantation of a total knee prosthesis, it only partly improved performance from sit to stand movement. After TKA, patients were able to fully load their operated leg, but they could not generate enough knee angular velocity during rising.[135] Additionally, the minimum 96° of hip and knee flexion is required at initial sit to stand movement. Without effective hip and knee joint extension post lift off from the chair, people were not able to do this task.[136] Sled and associates found in their study that following implementation of an 8-week home strengthening program for the hip abductor muscles, participants with knee OA had a decrease in knee pain and demonstrated a significant improvement in hip abductor strength and improved function in sit to stand.[137] Other functional deficits, including slower walking speeds for both males and females, were reported (62% and 25% decrease at normal pace and 31% and 6% decrease at fast pace, respectively). Clinical relevance points to the fact that 17% of these individuals were not able to cross safely at a typical city intersection. Other recent studies have shown slower sit-to-stand and up-and-go tests,[138] quadriceps weakness,[46,47] and smaller girth circumference[47] for individuals at greater than 1 year after surgery. Lastly, the first study that demonstrated patients with TKA had impaired balance and movement control because of lack of exercise interventions for this problem was done by Piva and associates. In this study, exercise programs that target balance and movement control improved functional performance, stiffness, and pain in patients after TKA.[139]

With these studies in mind, the development and implementation of a well-designed, comprehensive treatment plan is paramount. Addressing the entire lower quadrant with an appropriate exercise program will enhance the course of rehabilitation and ensure a more successful outcome.

TABLE 27-5 Functional Outcomes—Minimally Invasive Surgery Compared with Traditional Total Knee Arthroplasty

Functional Measure	Minimally Invasive Surgery	Traditional Total Knee Arthroplasty
• SLR	• Postoperative day 1	• Unable to do SLR
• Walk without a cane	• Postoperative day 8	• Days 6-14 with assistive device
• Knee flexion at 3 months after surgery	• 122° flexion	
• Knee flexion at 1 year after surgery	• 125° flexion	• 110° flexion
		• 116° flexion

SLR, Straight leg raises.

CLINICAL CASE REVIEW

1 John is 69 years old. He had a left TKR 8 days ago. He is now semireclined in his hospital bed. When the therapist helps him out of bed during transfer, John complains of feeling light-headed. He usually requires a few moments for his head to clear, but today he needs a little more time to adjust. Gait training is initiated, and suddenly John has difficulty breathing. What do these symptoms indicate?

Rapid heart rate, hypotension, and dyspnea are signs of a possible PE—a potentially fatal complication. Cardiovascular signs may include tachycardia, distended jugular veins, hypotension, and chest pain. Pulmonary symptoms include tachypnea, rales, wheezing, and pleural effusion. Sudden dyspnea is the most common symptom.

2 Randy is 52 and had a TKA 2 weeks ago. He presented for his initial evaluation with −30° extension and 75° flexion. What should be considered and addressed during his initial evaluation?

Prior functional level and preoperative ROM

Prior response to surgery and potential to develop adhesions

General health status (e.g., diabetes, PVD, CHF).

Current state of incision (infection potential) and edema (girth measurements)

Discussion with his home health PT will also give you an indication of his current response to treatment thus far.

All of the above are important to consider when evaluating and making a treatment plan.

3 What exercises should be emphasized with Randy?

Passive stretches (prone and supine hangs) should be performed regularly and, as appropriate and pain allows, weight should be added to the ankle and knee to provide increased compliance into extension. Passive flexion stretches should include supine heel slides with a towel or strap to allow the patient to provide overpressure as able. Also supine wall slides (with weight as appropriate). Duration of stretches should be progressed as able taking into account the response of the knee to stretches (minimal—no increase in residual pain, edema, or weight-bearing tolerance).

4 Sharon is a 60-year-old patient who had TKA 4 weeks ago. She complains that her operative leg is shorter than the other leg. No preoperative leg length difference was noted, and the physician noted that there were no relative changes made that would account for decreased leg length. What possible explanation could there be for this?

Upon further evaluation it was found that the patient had a posteriorly rotated ilium, creating an apparent leg length difference. Faulty joint mechanics at the hip, knee, and ankle affect the overall surgical result. Manual techniques and exercises were used to address the posterior rotation. Exercises that address gluteus medius weakness include hip abduction and lateral hip rotation (see Fig. 27-22).

5 Noreen is a 55-year-old patient who had TKR 7 weeks ago. Her pain levels have prevented ROM gains beyond −8° to 95°. Her preoperative ROM was −5° to 120°. Her ROM in the last week has plateaued and may have even decreased. What should be the therapist's next course of care be?

A phone call to the orthopedist is warranted to explore if she is appropriate for an MUA. After consultation with the physician, an MUA was scheduled and performed. The patient returned to therapy and gained full extension and 125° of flexion. The patient's post-MUA physical therapy should also include taking medication before her treatments to manage pain and maintain and improve the gains in ROM made from the MUA.

6 Gemma is 55 years old. She had severe degenerative joint disease in her right knee and underwent a TKR 8 weeks ago. She says the pain around the knee has considerably decreased. However, she complains of pain around the area of the fibular neck. The area also is sensitive to palpation. Gemma has intermittent pain radiating down the lateral surface of the lower leg. What is the probable cause of these symptoms?

The peroneal nerve travels around the fibular neck. The symptoms described indicate peroneal nerve irritation. On further investigation, the PT noted altered sensation over the dorsum of the foot, with the exception of the first web space. In addition, right dorsiflexion and eversion strength both equaled 4/5 to 5/5 (5/5 is "normal" strength on a manual muscle test [MMT]). Normal strength was demonstrated throughout the left LE. Dural nerve root stretches for the sciatic and peroneal nerve were initiated. After the first treatment using nerve tissue mobilization to target these nerves, strength returned to normal for dorsiflexion and eversion. After three treatments using dural mobilization, the pain was decreased by 90% and the sensation tested normal.

7 Ginny is 12 weeks postoperation, and while she demonstrates excellent ROM, she complains of medial knee pain with single-leg squat (SLS) exercises. What can be done to address this issue?

Up to this point in her rehabilitation she had not complained of any pain until SLS resistance increased. In observing her technique with SLS, it was noted that she began to allow her hip to internally rotate, causing a "valgus" collapse at the knee. With reinstruction in technique and hip abduction/external rotation strengthening, her symptoms subsided. It is important that strengthening exercises continue to progress inclusive of the entire LE.[140]

8 Nancy is 3 months postop and continues to complain of knee pain that has not improved and limits her weight bearing tolerance. What should be considered as a potential explanation of her symptoms?

Chronic knee pain is unfortunately a side effect for some patients. Differential diagnosis of continuing extra articular knee pain should consider:

Neurologic (lumbar origin, neuroma, complex regional pain syndrome)

Vascular claudication

Musculoskeletal (Hip arthritis, tendinitis, bursitis, stress fracture, and periprosthetic fracture)[141]

REFERENCES

1. Arthitistoday.org: What is osteoarthritis? Available at: http://www.arthritistoday.org/conditions/osteoarthritis/all-about-oa/what-is-oa.php accessed 6/11/10.

2. American Academy of Orthopaedic Surgeons: Osteoarthritis of the knee—a compendium of evidence-based information and resources, San Francisco, 2004, American Academy of Orthopaedic Surgeons.

3. American Academy of Orthopedic Surgeons: Total knee replacement. Available at: http://orthoinfo.aaos.org/topic.cfm?topic=A00389 (accessed 6/13/10).

4. Finch E, et al: Functional ability perceived by individuals following without total knee arthroplasty compared to age-matched individuals knee disability. J Orthop Sports Phys Ther 27(4):255, 1998.

5. Moseley JB, et al: A controlled trial of arthroscopic surgery for osteo-arthritis of the knee. N Engl J Med 347(11):81, 2002.

6. Koshino T, et al: Regeneration of degenerated articular cartilage after high tibial valgus osteotomy for medial compartmental osteoarthritis of the knee. Knee 10:229, 2003.

7. Stukenborg-Colsman C, et al: High tibial osteotomy versus unicompartmental joint replacement in unicompartmental knee joint osteoarthritis: 7-10-year follow-up prospective randomized study. Knee 8:187, 2001.

8. MacIntosh DL: Hemi-arthroplasty of the knee using a space occupying prosthesis for painful varus and valgus deformities. Proceedings of the joint meeting of the Orthopaedic Associations of the English Speaking World. J Bone Joint Surg 40A:1431, 1958.

9. McKeever DC: Tibial plateau prosthesis. Clin Orthop 18:86, 1960.

10. Emerson R, Potter T: The use of the McKeever metallic hemi-arthroplasty for unicompartmental arthritis. J Bone Joint Surg 67A:208, 1985.

11. Kopell HP, Thompson WAL: Peripheral entrapment neuropathies of the lower extremity. N Engl J Med 262(2):56, 1960.

12. Hallock RH, Fell BM: Unicompartmental tibial hemiarthroplasty: Early results of the UniSpacer knee. Clin Orthop Relat Res 416:154, 2003.

13. Saccomanni B: Unicompartmental knee arthroplasty: A review of literature. Clin Rheumatol 29(4):339-346, 2010.

14. Berend KR, Lombardi AV, Jr: Liberal indications for minimally invasive oxford unicondylar arthroplasty provide rapid functional recovery and pain relief. Surg Technol Int 16:193, 2007.

15. Argenson JA, et al: The new arthritic patient and arthroplasty treatment options. J Bone Joint Surg, 91:43, 2009.

16. Wang H, et al: Gait analysis after bi-compartmental knee replacement. Clin Biomech 24:751, 2009.

17. Berger RA, et al: Long-term follow-up of the Miller-Galante total knee replacement. Clin Orthop 388:58, 2001.

18. Buehler KO, et al: The press-fit condylar total knee system: 8- to 10-year results with a posterior cruciate-retaining design. J Arthroplasty 15:698, 2000.

19. Dixon MC, et al: Modular fixed-bearing total knee arthroplasty with retention of the posterior cruciate ligament: A study of patients followed for a minimum of fifteen years. J Bone Joint Surg 87A:598, 2005.

20. Laskin RS: The Genesis total knee prosthesis: A 10-year follow-up study. Clin Orthop 388:95, 2001.

21. Lyback CO, et al: Survivorship of AGC knee replacement in juvenile chronic arthritis: 13-year follow-up of 77 knees. J Arthroplasty 15:166, 2000.

22. Worland RL, et al: Ten to fourteen year survival and functional analysis of the AGC total knee replacement system. Knee 9:133, 2002.

23. Tanavalee A, Thiengwittayaporn S, Ngarmukos S: Rapid ambulation and range of motion after minimally invasive total knee arthroplasty. J Med Assoc Thai 87(Suppl 2):195, 2004.

24. Haas SB: Minimally invasive knee arthroplasty. Course notes, Western Orthopedic Association, Seascape, Calif, May 2005.

25. Laskin RS, et al: Minimally invasive total knee replacement through a mini-midvastus incision: An outcome study. Clin Orthop 428:74, 2004.

26. Tria AJ, Coon TM: Minimal incision total knee arthroplasty. Clin Orthop 416:185, 2003.

27. Berger RA, et al: Outpatient total knee arthroplasty with a minimally invasive technique. J Arthroplasty 20(7 Suppl 3):33, 2005.

28. McAllister CM, Stepanian JD: The impact of minimally invasive surgical techniques on early range of motion after primary total knee arthroplasty. J Arthroplasty 23(1):10, 2008.

29. Arnout N, et al: Avoidance of patellar eversion improves range of motion after total knee replacement: a prospective randomized study. Knee Surg Sports Traumatol Arthrosc 17(10):1206, 2009.

30. Colizza WA, Insall JN, Scuderi GR: The posterior stabilized total knee prosthesis: Assessment of polyethylene damage and osteolysis after a 10 year minimum follow up. J Bone Joint Surg 77A:1713, 1995.

31. Diduch DR, et al: Total knee replacement in young active patients: Long term follow up and functional outcome. J Bone Joint Surg 79A(4):575, 1997.

32. Ranawat CS, et al: Long-term results of the total condylar knee arthroplasty. Clin Orthop 286:94, 1993.

33. Rand JA, Illstrup DM: Survivorship analysis of total knee arthroplasty: Cumulative rates of survival of 9200 total knee arthroplasties. J Bone Joint Surg 73A:397, 1991.

34. Stearn SH, Insall JN: Posterior stabilized prosthesis: Results after follow up of 9 to 12 years. J Bone Joint Surg 74A:980, 1992.

35. Kardash K, et al: Obturator versus femoral nerve block for analgesia after total knee arthroplasty. Anesth Analg 105(3):853-858, 2007.

36. Ilfeld BM, et al: A multicenter, randomized, triple-masked, placebo-controlled trial of the effect of ambulatory continuous femoral nerve blocks on discharge-readiness following total knee arthroplasty in patients on general orthopaedic wards. Pain 150(3):477-484, 2010. Epub 2010 Jun 22.

37. Farr JN, et al: Activity levels in patients with early osteoarthritis of the knee: A randomized controlled trial. Phys Ther 90(3):356, 2010.

38. Kuster MS, et al: Joint load considerations in total knee replacement. J Bone Joint Surg 79B(1):109, 1997.

39. Lingard EA: Five-year patient reported outcomes of TKA. Poster presented at the 71st Annual Meeting of the American Academy of Orthopedic Surgeons, San Francisco, March 2004.

40. Ritter MA, et al: Predicting range of motion after TKA. J Bone Joint Surg Am 85-A(7):1278, 2003.

41. Chiarello CM, Gunderson L, O'Halloran T: The effect of continuous passive motion duration and increment on range of motion in total knee arthroplasty patients. J Orthop Sports Phys Ther 25(2):119, 1997.

42. Vince KG, et al: Continuous passive motion after total knee arthroplasty. J Arthroplasty 2(4):281, 1987.

43. Hassen CH, et al: Meta-analysis of continuous passive motion use in total knee arthroplasty: Research presented at the APTA Scientific Meeting, Orlando, Fla, 1998.

44. Munin MC, et al: Early in-patient rehabilitation after elective hip and knee arthroplasty. JAMA 279(11):880, 1998.

45. Yashar AA, et al: Continuous passive motion with accelerated flexion after total knee arthroplasty. Clin Orthop 345:38, 1997.

46. Maloney WJ, et al: The influence of continuous passive motion on outcome in total knee arthroplasty. Clin Orthop 256:162, 1990.

47. Ross MD, et al: A comparison of quadriceps strength and girth between involved and uninvolved limbs in individuals with total knee arthroplasty. Research presented at the APTA Scientific Meeting, Orlando, Fla, June 1998.

48. O'Driscoll SW, Kumar A, Salter RB: The effects of continuous passive motion in the clearance of hemarthrosis from synovial joint: An experimental investigation in the rabbit. Clin Orthop 176:305, 1983.

49. Anderson MA: Continuous passive motion. In Iglarsh ZA, Richardson JK, Timm KE, editors: Orthopaedic physical therapy clinics of North America, vol 1, Philadelphia, 1992, Saunders.

50. Dhert WJA, et al: Effects of immobilization and continuous passive motion of postoperative muscle atrophy in mature rabbits. Can J Surg 31:185, 1988.

51. Coutts RD: Continuous passive motion in the rehabilitation of the total knee patient, its role and effect. Orthop Rev 15(3):126, 1986.

52. Coutts RD, Toth C, Kaita JH: The role of continuous passive motion in the rehabilitations of the total knee patient. In Hungerford DS, Krackow DA, Kenna RV, editors: Total knee arthroplasty: A comprehensive approach, Baltimore, 1984, Williams & Wilkins.

53. Frank C, et al: Physiology and therapeutic value of passive joint motion. Clin Orthop 185:113, 1984.

54. Parisien JS: The role of arthroscopy in the treatment of postoperative fibroarthrosis of the knee joint. Clin Orthop 229:185, 1988.

55. Lynch JA, et al: Mechanical measures in the prophylaxis of postoperative thromboembolism in total knee arthroplasty. Clin Orthop 260:24, 1990.

56. Gosc JC: Continuous passive motion in the postoperative treatment of patients with total knee replacement: A retrospective study. Phys Ther 67(1):39, 1987.

57. Burks R, Daniel D, Losse G: The effect of continuous passive motion on anterior cruciate ligament reconstruction stability. Am J Sports Med 12:323, 1984.

58. Coutts RD, et al: The effect of continuous passive motion on total knee rehabilitation (abstract). Orthop Rev 7:535, 1983.

59. Goth RS, et al: Electrical stimulation effect on extensor lag and length of hospital stay after total knee arthroplasty. Arch Phys Med Rehabil 75(9):957, 1994.

60. Stevens JE, et al: Early neuromuscular electrical stimulation to optimize quadriceps muscle function following total knee arthroplasty: A case report. J Orthop Sports Phys Ther 37(7):364, 2007.

61. Petterson SC, Snyder-Mackler L: The use of neuromuscular electrical stimulation to improve activation deficits in a patient with chronic quadriceps strength impairments following total knee arthroplasty. J Orthop Sports Phys Ther 36(9):678, 2006.

62. Enloe LJ, et al: Total hip and knee replacement treatment programs: A report using consensus. J Orthop Sports Phys Ther 23(1):3, 1996.

63. Spencer JD, Hayes KC, Alexander IJ: Knee effusion and quadriceps reflex inhibition in man. Arch Phys Med Rehabil 65:171, 1984.

64. Mukand J, et al: Critical pathways for TKR—protocol saves time and money. Adv Phys Ther Rehab Med 6(8):31, 1997.

65. Shields RK, et al: Reliability, validity, and responsiveness of functional tests in patients with total joint replacement. Phys Ther 75(3):169, 1995.

66. Cuddeford T, Williams AK, Medeiros JM: Electromyographic activity of the vastus medialis oblique and vastus lateralis muscles during selected exercises. J Man Manip Ther 4(1):10, 1996.

67. Gryzlo SM, et al: Electromyographic analysis of knee rehabilitation exercises. J Orthop Sports Phys Ther 20(1):36, 1994.

68. Tippett SR: Closed chain exercise. Orthop Phys Ther Clin N Am 1:253, 1992.

69. Corcoran PJ, Peszczynski M: Gait and gait retraining. In Basmajian JV, editor: Therapeutic exercise, ed 2, Baltimore, 1978, Williams & Wilkins.

70. Hertling D, Kessler RM: Management of common musculoskeletal disorders, ed 2, Philadelphia, 1990, Lippincott.

71. Murray MP: Gait as a total pattern of movement. Am J Phys Med 46(1):290, 1967.

72. Aliga NA: New venues for joint replacement rehab. Adv Dir Rehab 17(4):43, 1998.

73. Lux PS, Hoernschemeyer DG, Whiteside LA: Manipulation and cortisone injection following total knee replacement (abstract). Paper presented at the 64th Annual Meeting of the American Academy of Orthopedic Surgeons, San Francisco, Feb 1997.

74. Esler CN, et al: Manipulation of TKR: Is the flexion gained retained? J Bone Joint Surg Br 81(1):27, 1999.

75. Elmqvist L, et al: Does a torn anterior cruciate ligament lead to change in the central nervous system drive of the knee extensors? Eur J Appl Physiol 58:203, 1988.

76. Herlant M, et al: The effect of anterior cruciate ligament surgery on the ankle plantar flexors. Isokinet Exerc Sci 2(3):140, 1992.

77. Jaramillo J, Worrell TW, Ingersoll CD: Hip isometric strength following knee surgery. J Orthop Sports Phys Ther 20(3):160, 1994.

78. Kisner C, Colby LA: Therapeutic exercise foundations and techniques, ed 2, Philadelphia, 1990, FA Davis.

79. Bullock-Saxton JE, Janda V, Bullock MI: Reflex activation of gluteal muscles in walking. Spine 18(6):704, 1993.

80. Patla-Paris C: Kinetic chain: Dysfunctional and compensatory effects within the lower extremity (manual). Orthop Phys Ther Home Study Course 91(1):1, 1992.

81. Ross M, Worrell TW: Thigh and calf girth following knee injury and surgery. J Orthop Sports Phys Ther 27(1):9, 1998.

82. Sahrmann SA: Diagnosis and treatment of movement impairment syndromes. Course notes, San Francisco, June 1997.

83. Walsh M, et al: Physical impairments and functional limitations: A comparison of individuals one year after total knee arthroplasty with control subjects. Phys Ther 78(3):248, 1998.

84. Foran JRH, et al: The outcome of total knee arthroplasty in obese patients. J Bone Joint Surg Am 86(8):1609, 2004.

85. Savory CG: Total joint replacement patients should stick to low-impact sports. Biomechanics 5(3):71, 1998.

86. Ries MD, et al: Improvement in cardiovascular fitness after total knee arthroplasty. J Bone Joint Surg 78:1696, 1996.

87. Cocchi R: No pain with gain—aquatic total knee replacement therapy. Adv Phys Ther Rehab Med 8(3):7, 1997.

88. Farina EJ: Aquatic vs. conventional land exercises for the rehabilitation of total knee replacement patients (abstract), VII World FINA Med & Sci Aspects of Aquatic Sports.

89. Toran MW: Pooling resources for sports medicine. Adv Dir Rehab 7(3):59, 1998.

90. Friden T, et al: Disability in anterior cruciate ligament insufficiency—an analysis of 19 untreated patients. J Orthop Res 6:833, 1988.

91. Gauffin H, et al: Function testing in patients with old rupture of the anterior cruciate ligament. Int J Sports Med 11:73, 1990.

92. Koralewicz LM, et al: Comparison of proprioception in arthritic and age-matched normal knees. J Bone Joint Surg Am 82:1592, 2000.

93. Swanik CB, et al: Stiffness after TKA. J Bone Joint Surg Am 86:328, 2004.

94. Tropp H, Odenrick P: Postural control in single-limb stance. J Orthop Res 6:833, 1988.

95. Amstutz HC, et al: Mechanism and clinical significance of wear debris-induced osteolysis. Clin Orthop 276:7, 1992.

96. Jasty M, Smith E: Wear particles of total joint replacements and their role in periprosthetic osteolysis. Curr Opin Rheumatol 4(2):204, 1992.

97. Ericson MO, Nisell R: Tibiofemoral joint forces during ergometer cycling. Am J Sports Med 14(4):285, 1986.

98. Ficat RD, Hungerford DS: Disorders of the patellofemoral joint, Baltimore, 1977, Williams & Wilkins.

99. Pitman MI, Frankel VH: Biomechanics of the knee in athletes. In Nicholas JA, Hershman EB, editors: The lower extremity and spine in sports medicine, St Louis, 1995, Mosby.

100. Bonutti P: Minimally invasive total knee arthroplasty—two year follow-up. Paper presented at the 71st Annual Meeting of the American Academy of Orthopedic Surgeons, San Francisco, March 2004.

101. Laskin RS: TKR through a mini midvastus MIS approach and comparison of standard approach TKR. Paper presented at the 71st Annual Meeting of the American Academy of Orthopedic Surgeons, San Francisco, March 2004.

102. Vaughan LM: Minimal incision TKA-5 year follow-up. Paper presented at the 71st Annual Meeting of the American Academy of Orthopedic Surgeons, Symposia AR Knee, San Francisco, March 10-14, 2004.

103. Nickenig T: Medical marvels. Adv Dir Rehab 13(10):40, 2004.

104. Krupp MA, Chatton MJ: Current medical diagnosis and treatment, Los Altos, Calif, 1979. Lange Medical.

105. Ranawat CS: Optimizing outcomes in orthopedic surgery. Course notes, 71st Annual Meeting of the American Academy of Orthopedic Surgeons, San Francisco, March 10-14, 2004.

106. Riddle DL, et al: Diagnosis of lower-extremity deep vein thrombosis in outpatients with musculoskeletal disorders: A national survey study of physical therapists. Phys Ther 84(8):717, 2004.

107. Cafarelli E, Flint F: The role of massage in preparation for and recovery from exercise. Sports Med 14:1, 1992.

108. Lehn C, Prentice WE: Massage. In Prentice WE, editor: Therapeutic modalities in sports medicine, St Louis, 1995, Mosby.

109. Hunt ME: Physiotherapy in sports medicine. In Torg JS, Welsh RP, Shephard RJ, editors: Current therapy in sports medicine, Toronto, 1990, Decker.

110. Smith LL: Acute inflammation: The underlying mechanism in delayed onset muscle soreness. Med Sci Sports Exerc 23:542, 1991.

111. Tidius PM: Exercise and muscle soreness. In Torg JS, Welsh RP, Shephard RJ, editors: Current therapy in sports medicine, Toronto, 1990, Decker.

112. Lymphnotes.com: Total knee replacement and lymphedema. Available at: http://www.lymphnotes.com/article.php/id/512/. Accessed 7/19/06.

113. Norton School of Lymphatic Therapy: The Basic MLD Certification Course. Course notes, Boston, August 2004.

114. Anti-embolism.com. Anti-embolism hosiery (TED). Available at: http://anti-embolism.com/. Accessed 8/28/06.

115. Weiss JM: Treatment of leg edema and wounds in a patient with severe musculoskeletal injuries. Phys Ther 78(10):1104, 1998.

116. Idusuyi OB, Morrey BF: Peroneal nerve palsy after total knee arthroplasty: Assessment of predisposing and prognostic factors. J Bone Joint Surg 78:177, 1996.

117. Piegorsch K: Peripheral nerve entrapment syndromes of the lower extremity (manual). Orthop Phys Ther Home Study Course 91(1):1, 1991.

118. Janda V: Muscles, central nervous motor regulation and back problems. In Korr I, editor: The neurobiologic mechanisms in manipulative therapy, New York, 1978, Plenum Press.

119. Janda V: Muscles as a pathogenic factor in low back pain in the treatment of patients. Proceedings of the IFOMT 4th Conference, Christchurch, NZ, 1980.

120. Lewit K: Manipulative therapy in rehabilitation of the motor system, London, 1975. Butterworth.

121. Greenman PE: Principles of manual medicine, ed 2, Baltimore, 1996, Williams & Wilkins.

122. Bookout MR, Geraci M, Greenman PE: Exercise prescription as an adjunct to manual medicine. Course notes, Tucson, March 1997.

123. Dorman TA, et al: Muscles and pelvic clutch. J Man Manip Ther 3(3):85, 1995.

124. Meier W, et al: Total knee arthroplasty: Muscle impairments, functional limitations, and recommended rehabilitation approaches. J Orthop Sports Phys Ther 38(5):246, 2008.

125. Jenkins C, et al: Kneeling ability after partial knee replacement. Phys Ther 88(9):1012, 2008.

126. Hassaballa MA, et al: Can knees kneel? Kneeling ability after total, unicompartmental and patellofemoral knee arthroplasty. Knee 10(2):155, 2003.

127. Palmer SH, et al: Ability to kneel after total knee replacement. J Bone Joint Surg Br 84(2):220, 2002.

128. Insall JN, et al: A comparison of four models of total knee-replacement prosthesis. J Bone Joint Surg 58A:754, 1976.

129. Insall JN, et al: Rationale of the Knee Society clinical rating system. Clin Orthop 248:13, 1989.

130. Finch E, et al: Functional ability perceived by individuals following total knee arthroplasty compared to age-matched individuals without knee disability. J Orthop Sports Phys Ther 27(4):255, 1998.

131. McAuley JP, et al: Outcome of knee arthroplasty in patients with poor preoperative ROM. Clin Orthop (404):203, 2002.

132. Lingard EA, et al: Predicting the outcome of total knee arthroplasty. J Bone Joint Surg Am 86:2179, 2004.

133. Dalury DF, et al: The long term outcome of TKA patients with moderate loss of motion. J Knee Surg 16 (4):215, 2003.

134. Jones CA, et al: Determinants of function after TKA. Phys Ther 83(8):696, 2003.

135. Boonstra MC, et al: Sit-to-stand movement as a performance-based measure for patients with total knee arthroplasty. Phys Ther 90(2):149, 2010.

136. Fotoohabadi MR, Tully EA, Galea MP: Kinematics of rising from a chair: Image-based analysis of the sagittal hip-spine movement pattern in elderly people who are healthy. Phys Ther 90(4):561, 2010.

137. Sled EA, et al: Effect of a home program of hip abductor exercises on knee joint loading, strength, function, and pain in people with knee osteoarthritis: A clinical trial. Phys Ther 90(6):895, 2010.

138. Hasson S, et al: An evaluation of mobility and self report on individuals with total knee arthroplasty. Research presented at the APTA Scientific Meeting, Orlando, Fla, June 1998.

139. Piva SR, et al: A balance exercise program appears to improve function for patients with total knee arthroplasty: A randomized clinical trial. Phys Ther 90(6):880, 2010.

140. Piva SR, et al: Contribution of hip abductor strength to physical function in patients with total knee arthroplasty. Phys Ther 91(2):225-233, 2011. Epub 2011 Jan 6.

141. Edward C, et al: The painful total knee arthroplasty: Diagnosis and management. Orthopedics 29(2):129, 2006.

CHAPTER 28

Lateral Ligament Repair of the Ankle

Robert Donatelli, Will Hall, Brian E. Prell, Graham Linck, Richard D. Ferkel

The ankle requires both static and dynamic stability. Mobility is crucial for normal ankle function in the midst of rapidly changing postures of the foot during sporting and everyday weight-bearing activities. Lateral ligament injuries of the ankle account for 13% to 56% of all injuries in sports requiring running or jumping such as soccer, basketball, and volleyball.[1,2] Ankle sprains also compromise 10% of the emergency room visits in the United States, with an incidence of 30,000 injuries per day.[3] The large majority of these injuries can be successfully treated conservatively with casting, bracing, nonsteroidal antiinflammatory drugs, and physical therapy. Approximately 85% of all ankle sprains involve the lateral structures of the ankle.[4,5] The majority of ankle sprains heal without any residual functional instability.[4] Despite adequate trials of conservative measures, however, approximately 10% to 30% of all acute ligamentous injuries have recurrent symptoms of chronic pain, swelling, and instability with activities.[4,6-9] Functional instability of the ankle is reported to be as high as 20% after ankle sprains.[10,11] Ligamentous instability has been thought to be related to the loss of mechanoreceptors[12] and can lead to the development of ankle joint degenerative changes.[13] When conservative measures fail to produce satisfactory proprioceptive performance and mechanical stability, surgical repair or reconstruction of the injured lateral ligament structures should be considered.

ANATOMY AND MECHANISM OF INJURY

The etiology of the unstable ankle is usually a forced plantar flexion inversion injury in which the body's center of gravity rolls over the ankle. This type of force results in injury to the anterior talofibular (ATF) ligament; and possibly the calcaneofibular (CF) ligament, the anterior inferior tibiofibular ligament, or the posterior talofibular (PTF) ligament.[3] The ATF ligament is the weakest of the lateral ligaments and blends with the ankle joint capsule. The CF ligament is the only extraarticular ligament among the complex and is larger and stronger than the ATF ligament[14]; it has been found able to withstand forces two to three-and-a-half times greater

than that of the ATF ligament.[15] The PTF ligament is the strongest of all the ligaments and is rarely injured with inversion sprains or associated with chronic ankle instability.[14] The unstable ankle is generally caused by a traumatic event such as an ankle sprain. It also can be associated with ankle fractures but virtually never develops insidiously.

SURGICAL INDICATIONS AND CONSIDERATIONS

A lateral ankle reconstruction is an elective surgery used to treat chronic instability that results from a continuum of ankle injuries. Ankle injuries can result in permanent damage to the ligaments that support the lateral ankle. Various studies have examined the benefits of surgical versus functional treatment in lateral ligament injuries of the ankle. These studies have shown that operative repair was associated with patients' delayed return to work, restricted range of motion (ROM), impaired ankle mobility, and increased complications after surgery, including undefined pain.[16-19] This is in contrast to conservative treatment, which includes functional bracing and early mobilization. Kannus and Renstrom reviewed 12 prospective studies and found that functionally or conservatively managed patients with grade III ankle sprains returned to work two to four times faster than those patients who underwent acute repair of the damaged ligaments.[20] Therefore, the surgical option is used when nonoperative treatments have failed, such as physical therapy, bracing, activity modification, and steroid injections. Postoperative physical therapy is a vital link in returning the patient to an active lifestyle.

Indications for reconstruction of the ankle's lateral ligaments include recurrent giving way with activities of daily living (ADLs) and sports that is refractory to conservative treatment, a positive physical examination, abnormal inversion, and/or positive anterior drawer stress x-rays (Fig. 28-1).

Patients of all ages and types are candidates for this type of surgery, but few patients older than 50 years undergo ankle reconstruction because of decreased activity levels and

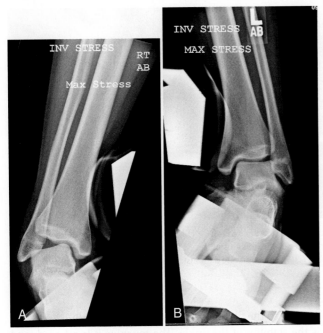

Fig. 28-1 Inversion stress testing on the Telos device. The right ankle (**A**) demonstrates increased talar tilt compared with the left ankle (**B**).

an increased ability to adjust functions and lifestyle to avoid recurrent buckling episodes. Surgeons should take care when considering this procedure for patients with generalized ligamentous laxity and collagen disorders that may result in failure. In addition, advanced degenerative joint disease or arthrofibrosis may be relative contraindications to this surgery.

SURGICAL PROCEDURES

More than 50 different surgical procedures for correction of lateral ankle instability have been described.[21] The majority of reconstructive procedures use part, or all, of the peroneal brevis tendon. Common procedures include the Watson-Jones, Evans, Chrisman-Snook, and Elmslie procedures and their modifications. Anatomic repair with direct suturing of the torn ligaments, imprecation, reinsertion to the bone, and in some instances augmentation with local tissue have increased recently in popularity.[10,22,23] Direct repair of the ATF and CF ligaments was described by Broström in 1966 and later modified by Gould in 1980.[22,24] Direct repair of torn lateral ligaments has the advantage of being simple and reliable, avoiding the use of normal tendons. It restores the original anatomy, requires less exposure, and maintains full ankle motion.

Procedure—Modified Broström

The modified Broström procedure, also termed the Broström-Gould procedure, is the method of choice for most patients with lateral ankle instability. The patient is taken to the operating room and examined under anesthesia. If the surgeon has any questions about the degree of ankle instability, stress x-ray films (stressing the ankle in both inversion and anterior drawer) are taken. The thigh is then secured on a well-padded thigh holder in preparation for ankle arthroscopy, as described in Chapter 30. The lower extremity is prepared and draped in standard fashion. Arthroscopy is performed first; the authors of this chapter have found that 93% of patients have additional intraarticular ankle pathology associated with lateral ankle instability in one study.[5] More recently, in another study, we found 95% of patients had associated intraarticular problems noted at arthroscopy before the Broström procedure.[25] In addition, a similar report by Taga showed 95% of patients have additional intraarticular pathology at the time of ankle reconstruction.[26] Hua and associates[27] found 91% of patients to have intraarticular lesions at the time of the modified Broström reconstruction.

The intraarticular pathology is identified and addressed through arthroscopic surgery. The scarred anterior talofibular (ATF) ligament is identified and assessed to make sure it is adequate for the modified Broström repair. After the arthroscopy is completed, the nurse removes the thigh support and places the leg flat on the surgical table. The ankle is reswabbed with a sterile antibacterial solution. An additional clean surgical drape is placed over the foot and ankle, and gloves are changed. New sterile instruments are used to perform the open portion of the procedure. Arthroscopic methods are now available for surgical reconstruction of the lateral ankle ligaments, but at this time open stabilization as described by Broström gives a better, more reproducible result. Recently, Corte-Real and Moreira,[11] Lui,[28] Nery and associates[29] reported on their arthroscopic method for chronic lateral ankle instability. The results had a high percentage of good-excellent results, but long-term studies are necessary to compare the arthroscopic with the open procedures before a recommendation can be made for switching to all-arthroscopic techniques.

After arthroscopy the ankle is prepared and the tourniquet inflated. An incision is made over the lateral aspect of the ankle. This incision may be obliquely shaped in the skin folds or more vertical from the fibula toward the sinus tarsi, depending on the surgeon's preference and the clinical situation. The senior author prefers the vertical incision because it allows better assessment of the peroneal tendons and can be extended distally and proximally if other procedures need to be done. Dissection is carried down through the subcutaneous tissues and the extensor retinaculum is carefully exposed because it is to be used for later reattachment. The surgeon must take care to avoid the intermediate dorsal cutaneous nerve, the lateral branch of the superficial peroneal nerve (which often lies near the end of the ATF ligament), and the sural nerve (which lies over the peroneal tendons). An oblique capsular incision is then made along the anterior border of the fibula from the AITF ligament to the CF ligament, leaving a small 3- or 4-mm cuff of tissue on the fibula for reattachment of the torn ligament complex (Fig. 28-2). The stretched ATF ligament is found as a thickening in the anterior capsule, and the CF ligament is found in the distal portion of the wound under the tip of the fibula, running

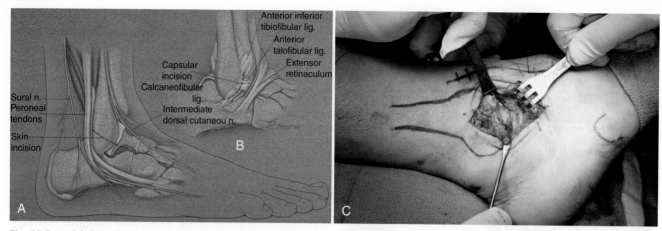

Fig. 28-2 Modified Broström reconstruction. **A,** An oblique incision is made over the fibula, in line with the ATFL and the extensor retinaculum and lateral ligaments are exposed. **B,** An oblique capsular incision is made along the anterior border of the fibula from the AITF ligament to the CF ligament, leaving a small 3- to 4-mm cuff of tissue on the fibula for reattachment of the ligament complex. **C,** Operative picture demonstrating opening the capsule with an oblique incision. (**A** and **B** copyright © Richard D. Ferkel, MD.)

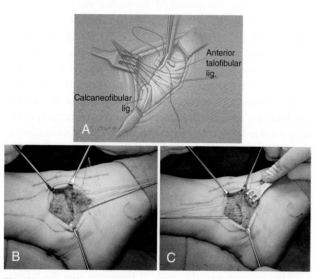

Fig. 28-3 Modified Broström procedure. **A,** The ATF and CF ligaments are reefed in a "pants-over-vest" fashion with nonabsorbable suture. **B** and **C,** Operative pictures showing the sutures in place before being tied. In **C,** the sutures are pulled proximally and a posterior drawer is applied on the ankle while the sutures are tied. (**A** copyright © Richard D. Ferkel, MD.)

deep to the peroneal tendons. The CF ligament often is attenuated or avulsed from the fibular tip.

A "pants-over-vest" overlapping suture technique is used to imprecate or shorten the torn ligaments and provide a double layer of reinforcement to the repair. Suturing is done starting from the ligament portion attached to the talus, so that the knots are tied distal and inferior to the fibula (Fig. 28-3). This helps prevent postoperative knot prominence and skin irritation with shoe wear. "O" nonabsorbable sutures are used in the majority of the repair, but one absorbable suture is used for the CF ligament near the peroneal tendon, to avoid irritation. The sutures are tied with the ankle in neutral position, and a posterior drawer is applied to reduce the talus. The ankle is checked to make sure full ROM has been maintained during the repair. The extensor retinaculum is then pulled proximal over the repair and

sutured to the fibular periosteum. ROM is again checked, as is the stability of the ankle. The tourniquet is released, and bleeding tissues are coagulated. The subcutaneous tissue and skin are then closed in the standard fashion. The patient is placed in a short-leg well-padded cast that is split in the recovery room to allow for swelling.

The patient's cast is changed at 1 and 2 weeks and the stitches are removed. Weight bearing is started at week 3 in a cast or cast boot, at the surgeon's discretion. Physical therapy with mobilization starts usually at week 6 or sometimes sooner.

Procedure—Anatomic Hamstring Reconstruction

Indications for an anatomic hamstring reconstruction include a high-stress, heavy athlete, generalized ligamentous laxity, deficient ATF ligament tissue for direct repair, talar tilt greater than 10° more than the opposite ankle, and a varus hindfoot. The incision used is the same as shown in Fig. 28-2, *A*. The lateral ligaments are released in the same oblique fashion for later reattachment over the hamstring repair. An autogenous or allograft semitendinosus graft is prepared with nonabsorbable sutures at both ends. A guidepin is inserted into the fibula to create two converging bony tunnels, beginning from insertion of the ATF ligament on the fibula, as well as the insertion of the CF ligament on the fibula. These tunnels are connected using a curved curette. Alternatively, as option B, the holes can be drilled out the posterior fibula to increase the bone bridge between the anterior talofibular ligament (ATFL) arm and the calcaneofibular ligament (CFL) arm. A reamer is then placed over the guidepin to create 5-mm tunnels. A guidepin is then inserted along the talar neck at the nonarticular portion and reamed to a predetermined size based on the diameter of the graft (Figs. 28-4 and 28-5). A passing device is placed from posterior to anterior through the fibula to facilitate graft passage (Fig. 28-6). The graft is then fixated on the talus with a special interference screw that helps push the tendon into

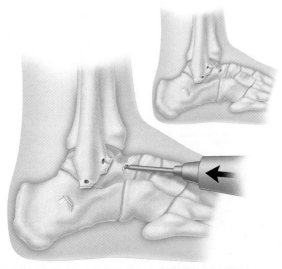

Fig. 28-4 The location of the tunnels on the talus and fibula are drawn in and the guidepin is inserted, aiming posteromedially on the talus.

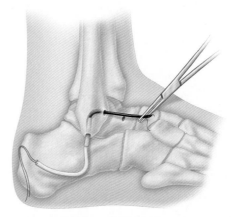

Fig. 28-6 The passing device is placed from posterior to anterior through the fibula to help make graft passage easier.

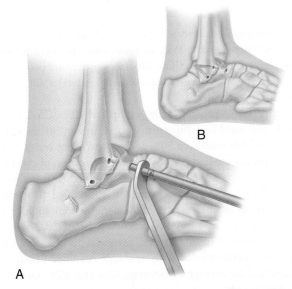

Fig. 28-5 Creating the tunnels. **A,** The tunnels created in a semicircular fashion in the fibula and the location and direction of the drill for the talar hole. **B,** An alternative placement of the drill holes coming out the posterior fibula.

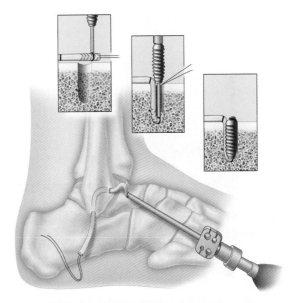

Fig. 28-7 The graft is fixated initially on the talus using an interference screw that helps push the graft into the talar tunnel.

the bone socket (Fig. 28-7). Alternatively, in option B, the graft can be passed from anterior to posterior and the ATF arm can be separately tensioned and fixed with an interference screw before tensioning the CFL arm (Fig. 28-8). This is usually done in slight plantar flexion because this is when the ATF ligament is the tightest. The tensioning on the CFL arm is done in slight dorsiflexion, and the tendon is passed underneath the peroneal tendons to exit into a drill hole made through the calcaneus. The CFL arm is cut so that 20 mm of the tendon will be in the calcaneus when it is secured with an interference screw (Fig. 28-9). This is done with the ankle in neutral position by bringing the sutures out through a poke hole on the medial heel and pulling tension on the sutures while the screw is inserted in the calcaneus

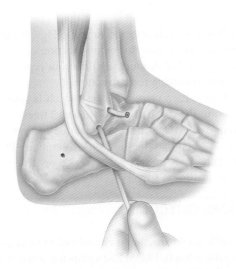

Fig. 28-8 Option B involves a fibular hole exiting the posterior fibula in a V fashion. This allows separate tensioning of each limb.

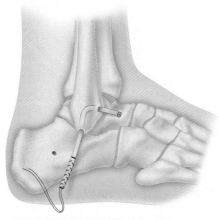

Fig. 28-9 The CFL is cut to the appropriate length so that at least 20 mm of tendon will end up in the calcaneus.

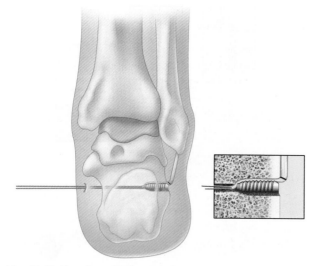

Fig. 28-10 The calcaneal hole is partially drilled, the guidepin creates a hole for the suture to exit medially. With the foot in appropriate position, tension is applied on the medial sutures through the calcaneus and an interference screw is inserted.

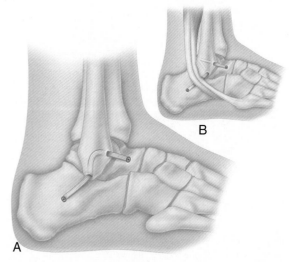

Fig. 28-11 Completed construct. **A,** The graft is fixated in the talus and calcaneus with a semicircular hole. **B,** A similar technique using the V-wedged holes.

(while pulling the graft into the tunnel) (Fig. 28-10). The final constructs gives anatomic reconstruction of the ATFL and CFL (Fig. 28-11). A modified Broström repair is then done over the hamstring reconstruction.

The patient is then placed in a cast which is split in the recovery room. The cast is changed at 1 and 2 weeks, and the stitches removed. Weight bearing is started at week 3 in a cast or a cast-boot at the surgeon's discretion. Physical therapy usually starts in the pool at week 6 or 8, depending on what else is done at surgery.

SURGICAL OUTCOMES

A lateral ankle reconstruction is considered to be successful when the patient has full ROM and a pain-free ankle and can return to all ADLs and sports without restriction. Liu and Baker[30] studied the static restraints of various surgical procedures in 40 cadaveric ankles. They found no significant difference between the Watson-Jones and Chrisman-Snook procedures, but the modified Broström procedure produced the least anteroposterior displacement and talar tilt at all different forces tested.

Hennrikus[31] prospectively compared the Chrisman-Snook and modified Broström procedures in 40 patients. Although both produced 80% good-to-excellent results, the former procedure had a much greater proportion of complications and the latter procedure had a higher functional score. Hamilton et al[34] performed the modified Broström procedure on 28 ankles; 54% of the patients were high-level ballet dancers. At 64 months' follow-up, he noted 27 of 28 good-to-excellent results. Peters[33] reviewed the literature and found 460 ankles treated with anatomic modified Broström repairs had an average of between 87% and 95% good-to-excellent results.

Ferkel and Chams[25] reviewed the results of 21 patients who underwent the modified Broström procedure. The average patient age was 27.5 years and the average follow-up occurred at 57 months. They found 95% good-to-excellent results with an American Orthopaedic Foot and Ankle Society's (AOFAS) ankle/hindfoot score of 97.1. When the ATF ligament is not adequate to use for a Broström repair, we use either an autogenous or allograft hamstring graft with biotenodesis screws through the talus and calcaneus to reconstruct the ATFL and CFL.[34-36]

Alternatively, the Broström-Evans procedure can be used in patients with the same indications as the hamstring reconstruction. In this procedure, the peroneal brevis is split using one third of it through a drill hole in the tip of the fibula, exiting the posterior fibula. The peroneal tendon is then secured with an interference screw and the Broström is placed over it. Results with the Broström-Evans procedure have also been good.[22]

CHALLENGES

Despite having a stable ankle postoperatively, some patients still complain of pain, aching, swelling, and crepitation.[26] Many of these complaints may be related to preexisting intraarticular pathology such as degenerative joint disease, osteochondral lesions of the talus, loose bodies, chronic synovitis, and chronic scarring. Occasionally the ankle can be made too tight at the time of reconstruction; this severely limits the patient's ability to invert. This is the single most serious complication after ankle reconstruction. If a patient does not have full motion after surgery, especially full inversion and eversion, rehabilitation is significantly compromised and the patient tends to develop a painful valgus hindfoot.

PRECAUTIONS AND CONTRAINDICATIONS

The physical therapist should increase the level of rehabilitation gradually for the patient after surgery. Too-vigorous exercise and the use of isokinetic machines can lead to increased pain, shear stress, and swelling that can last for weeks to months and stretch the reconstruction. If this occurs, the ultimate results can be compromised and the patient, physician, and physical therapist can all become quite frustrated. Every patient progresses at a different rate and the exercise program should be customized to the individual needs of each patient.

REHABILITATION CONCERNS

The therapist should contact the physician whenever pain appears to be out of proportion to expectations. In addition, any wound drainage, evidence of fever or infection, and increased laxity should alert the therapist to interact with the surgeon. If the patient has an acute episode of pain or feels a "pop" or significant change during rehabilitation or ADLs, the surgeon should be alerted immediately.

THERAPY GUIDELINES FOR REHABILITATION

The first 6 weeks after surgery are important for the succes of the surgery. Whether the reconstruction was done with primary ligamentous repair (as in the Broström procedure), with tendon augmentation (as in the Chrisman-Snook procedure), or with hamstring reconstruction, the initial tissue healing stage is important.[9,31] The surgical reconstruction to correct the ligamentous instability is only as good as the stability gained from soft tissue healing. Soft tissue healing is considered the maximal protection stage.

Evaluation

The initial postoperative evaluation gives the therapist a baseline from which to proceed in returning the patient to desired independent function. Initial ROM measurements are taken both for active range of motion (AROM) and passive range of motion (PROM). PROM is measured within a pain-free range, especially while measuring forefoot inversion.

The physical therapist has a responsibility to the surgeon and the patient to protect the lateral ligamentous reconstruction. Forefoot inversion stresses the reconstructed tissues and must be carefully engaged. Manual muscle testing to determine strength of the lower extremity can be part of the initial evaluation. However, muscle testing at the ankle is delayed until the patient has progressed and accommodated to resisted exercises at the ankle. **The therapist should avoid having the patient perform a single–leg heel raise, which is usually advocated to determine normal gastrocnemius-soleus strength, because of decreased proprioception and the significant muscle deficits resulting from the effects of immobilization.** The incision is assessed for mobility and hypersensitivity after complete healing has occurred. Operative damage to the sural nerve and the lateral branch of the superficial peroneal nerve has been reported as a cause of decreased sensation in the involved ankle.[10,37] Joint effusion and soft tissue edema can be factors in limited ROM, proprioception deficits, and the inability to strengthen the joint. Joint and soft tissue mobility also are assessed at the limits of ROM.

Phase I

TIME: Weeks 4 to 6 after surgery
GOALS: Decrease pain and swelling, restore joint and soft tissue mobility, increase strength in lower extremity and ankle, increase proprioception, normalize gait, maintain cardiovascular fitness, and provide patient education (Table 28-1)

During this maximal protection phase the patient is casted and allowed to progress from non–weight bearing to weight bearing. The patient remains non–weight bearing and the cast is removed at the first postoperative visit for wound inspection. A second cast is applied for an additional week and the stitches are removed. Weight bearing is initiated during the third week and the cast is removed at the sixth week. At this point the patient is placed in a controlled action motion (CAM) walker brace and compression stocking or in a small brace, depending on the individual patient. At 6 weeks the patient is started on ROM and strengthening exercises in physical therapy, as well as pool exercises. Some authors have advocated a limited ROM of 10° dorsiflexion and 10° of plantar flexion, with partial weight bearing from 2 to 6 weeks after surgery.[30] Formal physical therapy is usually initiated at 6 weeks when the cast is removed. At this time the tissues should be adequately healed and ready to tolerate stresses within a pain-free ROM. Studies have shown that motion is beneficial to nourish cartilage, prevent soft tissue contractures, and restore joint mobility.[37] After performing the initial evaluation, the physical therapist can implement appropriate treatment. Initially, the therapist performs grades I and II joint mobilization along with PROM, especially inversion, within pain-free ranges. At 6 weeks after

TABLE 28-1 Lateral Ligament Repair

Rehabilitation Phase	Criteria to Progress to This Phase	Anticipated Impairments and Functional Limitations	Intervention	Goal	Rationale
Phase I Postoperative 4-6 weeks	• Postoperative • Cleared by physician to begin rehabilitation	• Edema • Pain • Patient casted for 6 weeks • Limited weight bearing (non–weight bearing for 3 weeks, then progressive weight bearing per physician) • Limited ROM • Limited strength	• Patients usually begin therapy at about 6 weeks • Modalities as needed • PROM — (stretches within pain-free ranges) plantar flexion, dorsiflexion, and eversion; take care when gently stretching into inversion • Isometrics — submaximal multiangle exercises for all planes • AROM — ankle:supine and seated plantar flexion and dorsiflexion • Progressive resistance exercise — hip (all ranges) • Soft tissue mobilization • Joint mobilization as indicated • Gait training — progress to full weight bearing using appropriate assistive device • Patient education	• Manage edema • Decrease pain • Increase ROM • Increase tolerance of muscle contraction	• Provide maximal protection in this phase; patient is casted for 6 weeks; communication with physician is imperative regarding weight-bearing status • Begin restoring joint and soft tissue mobility • Initiate muscle contraction and prepare for strengthening exercises • Improve hip strength to prepare for normal gait • Provide gait training to improve tolerance to accepting weight on involved leg • Avoid overstressing healing tissues; adapt program as symptoms dictate

AROM, Active range of motion; *PROM,* passive range of motion; *ROM,* range of motion.

surgery the ligaments should have healed sufficiently to allow gentle active movement.[38]

However, at this stage the soft tissue is unable to withstand significant forces into inversion.[4] The patient is able to perform AROM for plantar flexion and dorsiflexion using pain as a guide; submaximal multiangle isometrics for all planes also are used at this stage of the rehabilitation. Soft tissue and joint mobilizations are started to reverse the effects of immobilization and surgical trauma. Effusion, pain, and soft tissue edema are treated with the appropriate modalities. Research has suggested that ice independently is not effective in reducing postoperative edema. Instead, studies have reported an increased effectiveness of reducing postoperative edema using cold compression therapy.[39-41] Efforts to normalize full weight-bearing gait without assistive devices should include gait training drills. Proper foot mechanics throughout the stance phase of gait can be emphasized if pain is minimal or absent. A home exercise program emphasizing increased frequency and decreased intensity of exercises should be initiated at this time. The therapist should clearly instruct the patient on precautions to protect healing tissues. The program may be altered as needed by the therapist.

Precautions

The therapist should take a few precautions during this phase.

Careful monitoring of exercise progression and intensity of the workout session is crucial to avoid overstressing healing tissues. The therapist must caution the patient to avoid aggressive stretching and strengthening of lateral ankle tissues early in the rehabilitation program; progress should be cautious and slow. Exercises that cause increased symptoms in the lateral ankle complex must be modified or avoided.

Phase II

TIME: Weeks 6 to 8 after surgery
GOALS: Return gait within normal range, maintain normal ROM, increase strength, control pain and swelling, increase proprioception (Table 28-2)

Phase II is overlapped with phase I as the patient's ROM begins to progress and therapeutic exercise options are expanded. At this stage rehabilitation is similar to that advocated in the literature for lateral ankle sprains.[11] Multiplane isometrics and AROM against gravity progress to exercises with appropriate grades of submaximal resistance using weights or rubber tubing. Peroneal strengthening is a major focus because repeated trauma resulting from the instability may lead to weakness of these muscles.[4] Activities to increase strength may occur on land or in a pool. On land, early proprioceptive activity is initiated with the use of a balance board as a means of increasing functional stability.[42,43] The

TABLE 28-2 Lateral Ligament Repair

Rehabilitation Phase	Criteria to Progress to This Phase	Anticipated Impairments and Functional Limitations	Intervention	Goal	Rationale

Phase II Postoperative 6-8 weeks	• No increase in pain
	• No loss of ROM
	• Improved tolerance to weight bearing
		• Mild edema
		• Mild pain
		• Limited strength
		• Limited ROM
		• Limited gait
			Continuation of phase I interventions as indicated
			• Isometrics—multiplane submaximal inversion and eversion (pain-free)
			• AROM—ankle (all ranges against gravity)
			  • Standing bilateral heel raises
			  • Squats and lunges
			• Treadmill
			• Stationary bicycle (using low resistance)
			• Elastic tubing (light resistance) exercises indicated late phase II; dorsiflexion, plantar flexion, inversion, and eversion
			• Balance board progressed from seated to standing with bilateral, then unilateral, support
			• Proprioceptive neuromuscular facilitation
			• Pool therapy—deep water running and light jumping
				• Control edema and pain
				• Increase strength
				• Promote equal weight bearing with sit-stand
				• Minimize gait deviations on level surfaces
				• Increase tolerance to single-limb stance
				• Improve proprioception and stability of ankle
				• Increase tolerance to advanced activities
					• Continue modalities to control edema and pain
					• Improve strength and stability of ankle joint in numerous directions
					• Improve strength with mild resistance initially
					• Progress exercises incorporating functional activities
					• Maintain consistent cadence and work on endurance
					• Later in phase II, ankle should be able to tolerate increased resistance with inversion and eversion motions
					• Proprioception exercises with varying degrees of weight bearing and manual resistance aids in return of proprioception
					• Buoyancy effect of water aids progression of more advanced activities

AROM, Active range of motion; *ROM,* range of motion.

patient progresses from sitting to standing, with bilateral and then unilateral support. One-leg standing also is initiated. Bilateral heel raises are started and progressed to unilateral as tolerated by the patient and according to the therapist's discretion. Proprioceptive neuromuscular facilitation (PNF) is an excellent strengthening tool for the lower kinetic chain. In the pool, activities may include light jogging and jumping exercises in shallow water. Lunges and squats also are effective. The patient should continue with deep water running exercises for increased cardiovascular fitness. Gait training is an important aspect of the rehabilitation program and should be given priority. An aberrant pattern reinforces itself and leads to continued limitations in ROM and strength. Walking on a treadmill at a moderate speed with a low-to-moderate grade as tolerated aids in gait training.

Phase III

TIME: Weeks 8 to 10 after surgery
GOALS: Focus on training to allow return to work and sports, continue ankle mobilization and passive stretching, prevent pain and swelling (Table 28-3)

When ROM and gait are within normal limits, isokinetic strengthening for inversion and eversion can be initiated. At this time the patient should be able to tolerate a submaximal strengthening program without exacerbation of symptoms. Resistive exercises for plantar flexion and dorsiflexion are initiated at 8 weeks. Inversion and eversion resistive exercises must be performed to the tolerance of the patient. Single-leg stance with opposite leg-resisted flexion, abduction, extension, and adduction can be performed with increasing resistive band tension. Patients may begin performing exercises on partial–weight bearing equipment such as the Shuttle MVP, including single/double leg press and toe raises. All resistive exercises should be performed without pain. Three-way lunge, single-leg stance with three-point reach and three-point step with the opposite leg can be initiated cautiously. The ability to perform pain-free weight training and isokinetic training is a good indication that soft tissue strength is progressing well.

The therapist must monitor the progression of resistive exercises to ensure that symptoms are not exacerbated. The patient may be ready for discharge after phase III or may progress to phase IV depending on the prior level of fitness or activity and goals.

TABLE 28-3 Lateral Ligament Repair

Rehabilitation Phase	Criteria to Progress to This Phase	Anticipated Impairments and Functional Limitations	Intervention	Goal	Rationale
Phase III Postoperative 8-10 weeks	• No loss of ROM • No increase in pain • Continued progress in therapy	• Limited gait on uneven surfaces • Limited ROM • Limited strength • Mild edema and pain associated with increased activity	Continue interventions as in phases I and II (joint and soft tissue mobilization performed as indicated) • Elastic tubing (mild to moderate resistance)—ankle (all ranges) • Isotonics—ankle (all ranges) • Isokinetics—Performed at pain-free intensities • Joint mobilization: grades III and IV to decrease stiffness and increase ROM • Single-leg stance with opposite leg-resisted flexion, abduction, extension, and adduction can be performed with increasing resistive band tension • Three-way lunge, single-leg stance with three-point reach, and three-point step with the opposite leg can be initiated cautiously	• Full AROM and PROM • 80% ankle strength • Self-management of edema and pain	• By the end of this phase, the patient should have full ROM and hands-on care can be eliminated • Exercises should use a combination of varying resistance in different positions to acquire proprioceptive strength and stability • Exercises are progressed to include activity-specific drills emphasizing specificity of training principles

AROM, Active range of motion; *PROM*, passive range of motion; *ROM*, range of motion.

TABLE 28-4 Lateral Ligament Repair

Rehabilitation Phase	Criteria to Progress to This Phase	Anticipated Impairments and Functional Limitations	Intervention	Goal	Rationale
Phase IV Postoperative 11-18 weeks	• Good progression through previous phases with the need to return to higher-level activities and sports • Normal ROM • Normal strength	• Limited strength and tolerance to higher-level activities	Continuation of exercises from phases I through III as indicated • Use ankle brace as appropriate • Plyometrics, trampoline activities, figure-8 drills, carioca, slide board, and lateral shuffle • Increase demand of pivoting and cutting exercises • Four-square hopping ankle rehabilitation (see Fig. 30-13) • Progress towards box drills	• Prevent reinjury with return to sport • Discharge to gym program • Return to sport	• Patient's opportunity for reinjury is highest with the addition of advanced exercises; clinicians should ensure proper performance of drills (plyometrics, pivoting, cutting) • Functional training for sports • After patients can perform drills safely and adequately, they are discharged with communication to coaches and trainer

ROM, Range of motion.

Phase IV

TIME: Weeks 11 to 18 after surgery
GOAL: Return to sporting activities (Table 28-4)

The goal of rehabilitation is, in general, for the patient to return to sporting activity 11 to 18 weeks after surgery; an ankle brace is used initially on return to sporting activities.[10,31] Exercise should continue with the therapist monitoring patient progress. Exercises in this phase are more advanced, and chances of reinjury are greater. In this final phase of rehabilitation the patient should be able to perform all exercises safely and correctly, with proper form and technique and with little verbal cueing from the therapist. After the AROM and PROM are within normal limits and strength has returned to normal, sport-specific and functional training can be implemented. Exercise options include plyometrics, trampoline activities, box drills, figure-8 drills, carioca, slide board, and lateral shuffles (Figs. 28-12 through 28-15). Many of the initial ankle injuries resulted from sporting activities such as cutting activities and movements requiring quick reflexes and balance. Although not in the scope of this chapter, retraining the vestibular system is also an important part of an athlete returning to their sport of choice. Incorporating vestibular exercises with sport-specific movements and exercises can help the athlete achieve his or her goals (Fig 28-16). These activities should be incorporated into the rehabilitation program.

SUGGESTED HOME MAINTENANCE FOR THE POSTSURGICAL PATIENT

An exercise program has been outlined at the various phases. The home maintenance box outlines rehabilitation suggestions the patient may follow. The physical therapist can use it in customizing a patient-specific program.

TROUBLESHOOTING

Limited dorsiflexion can be a problem with most patients because of limited talar tibia-fibula mobility as a result of joint restrictions and soft tissue tightness. If restrictions exist at the talocrural joint, long-axis distraction thrust techniques are useful. In addition, mobilization of the talus, tibia, and fibula can be useful. Anterior and posterior glides to these bones help restore dorsiflexion. The gastrocnemius and soleus muscle group can be the major limiting factor in dorsiflexion ROM. Low-load prolonged stretching techniques in combination with heat can be beneficial in increasing soft tissue extensibility.[44] The load of the stretch is to the patient's tolerance for 20 to 30 minutes, one or two times per day.

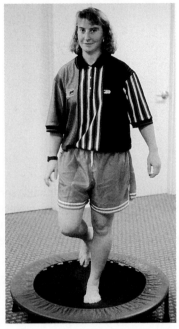

Fig. 28-13 Trampoline stork standing.

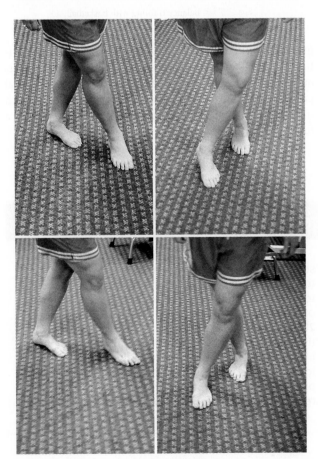

Fig. 28-12 Carioca.

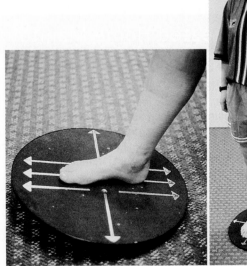
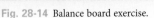

Fig. 28-14 Balance board exercise.

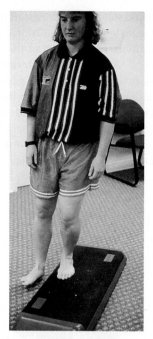

Fig. 28-15 Step-ups.

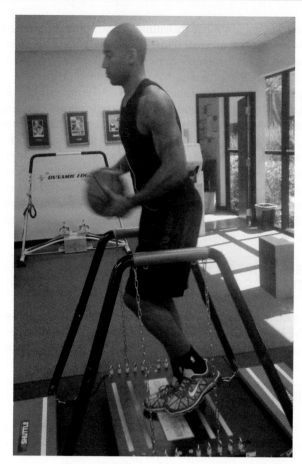

Fig. 28-16 Balance training with basketball.

Another method to prevent chronic ankle sprains is to use biomechanical foot orthotics. In theory, biomechanical foot orthotics are designed to enhance joint position, increasing the shock-absorbing capabilities of the lower limb and improving muscle function.

SUMMARY

A successful outcome for lateral ligamentous reconstruction includes no recurrent instability, normal ROM and strength, and no pain with weight-bearing activities. A successful functional outcome is achieved if the patient experiences no instability on returning to daily activities or sporting activities. The first step toward a good outcome is adequate postoperative stabilization. However, the success of the surgical procedure depends on postoperative rehabilitation in which the patient, surgeon, and therapist work closely to achieve a functional ankle.

 ## Suggested Home Maintenance for the Postsurgical Patient

Weeks 6 to 8

GOALS FOR THE PERIOD: Improve gait, increase ROM to normal, gradually increase strength, control pain and swelling, and increase proprioception
1. AROM in plantar flexion, dorsiflexion, and eversion
2. Isometrics for plantar flexion, dorsiflexion, and eversion
3. Towel calf non–weight bearing stretch for gastrocnemius-soleus muscle group
4. Towel-crunching exercise
5. Four-way hip non–weight bearing exercise to initiate total lower extremity strength
6. Seated heel and toe raises

Exercise Progression: Begin all exercises with two sets of 10 repetitions. If no adverse effects are noted to previous intensity level, progression can proceed to three sets of 10 repetitions, followed by 3 sets of 12 to 15 repetitions, and finally three sets of 20 repetitions. Once a patient is able to perform three sets of twenty repetitions of an exercise; the intensity of the exercise must be increased in some form (i.e., more resistance, longer duration) and the patient should start back with two sets of 10 repetitions and follow the same progression.

Weeks 8 to 10

GOALS FOR THE PERIOD: Maintain normal ROM, continue to increase strength and improve proprioception

1. Rubber tubing with appropriate resistance for dorsiflexion and plantar flexion
2. Submaximal isometric exercises of inversion and eversion (performed without pain)
3. Stationary bicycle
4. Heel raises (bilateral)
5. Step-ups, step-downs
6. Single-leg stance

Weeks 11 to 18

GOALS FOR THE PERIOD: Progress with strengthening, increase endurance, and return to previous level of function (sport activity)

1. Standing gastrocnemius-soleus stretch
2. Increased resistance of rubber tubing
3. Straight-ahead running if gait is normal
4. Heel raises progressing to single-leg raises
5. Sports-specific training
6. Functional training
7. Return to sport as cleared by the therapist and physician with ankle bracing

CLINICAL CASE REVIEW

1 Will, who is 18 years old, tore his ATF ligament while playing basketball. The tear occurred over a 1-year period after accumulating multiple ankle sprains. He had an ATF ligament repair 8 weeks ago. Since then his physical therapy has consisted of massage, ultrasound, AROM and PROM exercises, cryotherapy with compression, and a home exercise program. His main complaint is stiffness during gait, while ascending stairs, and during attempts to squat partially. Dorsiflexion is limited by 10° with moderate edema noted. What treatment is most likely to improve Will's dorsiflexion ROM and decrease edema?

The patient was reassessed for associated restrictions. A mobilization technique was performed at the proximal and distal fibula. An AP movement was applied to the proximal fibular head, and a posteroanterior (PA) movement was applied to the lateral malleolus to increase dorsiflexion. This was followed by stretching and ROM exercises to reinforce dorsiflexion. Will's dorsiflexion PROM increased to 18°. Pain with gait, stairs, and squatting was dramatically decreased after the first treatment.

2 Leigh is a 30-year-old woman who tore her left ATF ligament while performing step aerobics. She had an ATF ligament repair 10 weeks ago. She has complained of knee and back pain on the unilateral side. She has asymmetric pelvic imbalance, with left iliac crest higher than the right and the left anterosuperior iliac spine (ASIS)/posterior superior iliac spine (PSIS) higher than the right. Decreased knee extension left versus right. Progress with exercises has decreased because of pain during many of the closed-chain exercises such as single-leg stance, double-heel lifts, minisquats, and

walking more than 8 minutes on the treadmill. What types of activities can be performed for her unilateral imbalances while increasing core stability?

The therapist explained to Leigh that any activities causing her to substitute secondary to increased pain must be modified. The patient was reassessed, and associated restrictions at the pelvis were recorded. A long axis distraction was performed to correct pelvic asymmetry. Appropriate hamstring stretches were performed to increase muscle length. As exercises were modified and asymmetries were corrected, Leigh was able to perform the following closed-chain exercises: forward lunges, backward lunges, lateral lunges, heel raises with minisquat, and single-heel raises performed on a leg press machine using 70 lb. She was also able to perform backward walking, minimal walking on a treadmill, and jogging or running in the pool. As strength and tolerance to exercise increased, Leigh progressed to more challenging exercises, which included core stabilization activities.

3 Karen is 22 years old and plays basketball primarily on the weekends. She tore her ATF during a pick-up game when she stepped abnormally causing her ankle to turn into extreme inversion. She had an ATF ligament repair 11 weeks ago. Progress with exercise has decreased because of pain during many closed-chain activities. What factors could be involved that would cause pain during these activities?

During an additional assessment, it was found that Karen had restrictions with AP proximal fibular glides and PA distal fibular glides. Calcaneal eversion was also limited. Graded mobilizations were performed at the proximal and distal fibular heads, which released the calcaneal eversion and decreased the patient's pain during activity.

4 Jason is a 30-year-old man who suffered an ATF tear after slipping on wet grass while performing yard work. He had an ATF ligament repair 12 weeks ago. He reports that his ankle pain has started to decrease but that he is noticing progressively increased pain at the third through fifth distal metatarsal heads. The pain is progressing to affect gait. What should the therapist assess?

The therapist, when learning of this clinical change, assessed the foot position and compared findings bilaterally. The patient was found to have increased rear foot pronation and forefoot supination on the affected side as compared with the unaffected side. The therapist attempted a temporary orthotic trial and posted the patient using a 3° medial rear foot wedge and a 3° lateral forefoot wedge on the affected extremity. At the next session, the patient reported decreased ankle and distal metatarsal pain on the affected side. The patient would later be fitted for permanent orthotics.

5 Jim is 17 years old and tore his ATF while rounding second base during a high school baseball game. He had an ATF ligament repair 16 weeks ago. He has progressed well through rehabilitation but was having difficulty initiating higher-level activities. How did the therapist progress this athlete for him to return to baseball for the next season?

The therapist initiated activities that were sports specific to increase functional stability. The patient performed multidirectional single-leg hopping, including forward, backward, and side to side. The patient began box exercises, including shuffle sprint and box X with pivot. He was progressed in proprioceptive activities, including unilateral leg stand with opposite LE resistive-band flexion, extension, and abduction, and biomechanical ankle platform system (BAPS) board activities. The exercises were progressed, increasing the time from 1 to 2 minutes.

6 Steve is an 18-year-old senior track athlete being actively recruited by several Division I universities for pole vaulting. During a track meet, the patient performed his vault and, upon landing, severely inverted his right ankle. He entered the clinic with severe bruising around the ankle with +2 pitting edema. He was tender over the lateral malleoli and peroneals, as well as the lateral ligaments. He has no significant gait deviations and has reported that he has been jogging. What is the differential diagnosis and course of treatment?

The therapist first instructed Steve to cease jogging activities immediately and used the tuning fork and

tapping method to rule out possible fracture, which was negative. Radiographs later showed no fracture present. The patient was positive with talar tilt, anterior drawer, and high ankle sprain. The patient demonstrated MMT within normal limits for all ankle motions except ankle eversion, which showed pain and weakness at 3+/5. Grossly, the patient had full ROM with pain at end range. The course of treatment included initial edema reduction and pain management while maintaining full ROM. Because of peroneal involvement, the therapist was able to begin strengthening in all planes except eversion, which was limited to isometrics. The patient later performed proprioception and plyometric exercises and returned to pole-vaulting after 8 weeks, with an ankle-stabilizing orthosis (ASO) ankle brace.

7 Elizabeth is a 15-year-old competitive gymnast with a history of chronic ankle sprains to her right ankle during her gymnastics competitions. The most frequent occurrence of her injury involves the vault and tumbling with floor exercises. She has not undergone any surgical intervention but wishes to continue competing in her sport. What type of treatment plan should the therapist initiate to allow Elizabeth to return to her sport?

Upon evaluation, the therapist finds that she has the following objective findings: Restricted passive dorsiflexion/talar gliding, weakness with MMT to the peroneals, tenderness to palpation along the ATF ligament/sinus tarsi and also tenderness in her Achilles tendon, she was also noted to have significant propriocpetive deficits, and posterior hip strength deficits as well. Treatment began with modalities to decrease pain/inflammation and to help start scar tissue remodeling including: infrared light, ultrasound, crossfriction massage and soft tissue mobilization of the gastroc/soleus and Achilles tendon. The restricted dorsiflexion was addressed with long-axis distraction to the talocrural joint. She was put on a progressive strengthening program for her posterior hip muscle deficits, as well as an eccentric training regimen for her Achilles tendon. She was also performing progressive inversion/eversion strengthening with theraband and PNF diagonal strengthening with the therapist providing manual resistance. She then progressed to plyometric training first with partial–weight bearing equipment, such as the Shuttle MVP, and then to more aggressive plyometric training on devices such as the Vertimax with an emphasis on her landing mechanics. The patient was also placed on a progressive perturbation training program to address her proprioceptive deficits. Elizabeth was also advised to either tape her ankle or obtain a brace for her to use during competitions.

8 Elaine is 45-year-old female who injured her right ankle in an MVA while on vacation. Once she returned home, she was found to have torn her ATF ligament and underwent the Broström-Gould procedure to reconstruct the ligament. Upon coming to physical therapy 6 weeks following the procedure, Elaine is ambulating with crutches and a CAM boot. She reports pain over the lateral malleoli, ATFL, sinus tarsi, and lateral syndesmosis. She also has impaired sensation and increased scar tissue surrounding the incision. Atrophy and limited soft tissue mobility of the gastros/soleus comlex are noted as well. How would the therapist initiate treatment at her current level?

The patient was instructed in a HEP consisting of towel gastrocnemius/soleus stretching, desensitization and scar mobility exercises, submaximal and pain-free isometrics for inversion/eversion, and AROM exercise for plantar and dorsiflexion. While in the clinic; high-voltage electrical stimulation was used to address muscular atrophy of the gastrosnemius/soleus complex and cryotherapy with interferential electrical stimulation was used if there was pain following treatments. The patient began a progressive gait training program under the supervision of the therapist which began on two crutches, next to one crutch on the contralateral side, then a single-point cane and finally no assistive device. The final stage was allowed once the patient was able to ambulate with proper mechanics and a nonantalgic gait pattern.

9 Brandon is a 16-year-old male basketball player who has had recurrent ankle sprains. At the end of the season, he again sprained his ankle by landing on an opposing players' foot and severely inverting his foot while running. Brandon and his parents are concerned about the new injury/possible fracture and want to address the continued recurrent instability in his ankle that has occurred over the last year. What should the therapist do to address these issues?

To rule out the possible fracture the therapist can use the Ottawa ankle rules for fracture. The therapist can also use the tuning fork technique or attempt ultrasound over the painful area. If there is a fracture, ultrasound over the area will usually reproduce the patient's pain and indicate possible bony pathology. The therapist should arrange or contact the patient's orthopedic doctor and relay these concerns so that the surgeon can give the patient and family all of the possible treatment options and initiate diagnostic imaging if warranted. The therapist can also educate the patient and his family on the problems associated with recurrent ankle instability; such as early joint degeneration, impaired balance/proprioception, and decreased function with higher level activities (i.e., running, jumping, cutting sports).

10 Ryan is a 25-year-old who injured his ankle after falling off of his bicycle. He was taken to the emergency room and was stabilized. After the initial swelling had decreased Ryan underwent surgical reconstruction of his ATF ligament with arthroscopy to his talocrural joint. Ryan was a previous patient who the therapist had treated for other injuries over the past year. The day after the surgery, Ryan calls the therapist because he is concerned about his increase in pain/swelling following the procedure. He also reports numbness/tingling in his foot and tenderness in his calf. What should the therapist do?

Without the patient being seen in the clinic, assessment is limited. But the therapist should tell Ryan to follow-up with his surgeon immediately to rule out any possible compartment syndrome or deep vein thrombosis which may have occurred as a result of the procedure. If the therapist is familiar with the surgeon, he or she should then also call the surgeon to relay these symptoms and concerns to the physician so that he or she can appropriately address these issues.

11 Cliff is a 26-year-old Air Force officer who injured his ankle while doing his routine physical training regimen. While running he stepped off the side of the track and experienced a plantar flexion with inversion injury to his ankle. He then underwent surgical reconstruction and is currently 4 months postop and would like to begin running again. How should the therapist assist Cliff to return to running without exacerbating his pain?

Before beginning a running program, Cliff must demonstrate certain objective findings before attempting to begin the program. He should demonstrate no restrictions in ankle mobility specifically dorsiflexion, be able to perform three sets of 15 repetitions of single–leg calf raises without ankle pain, demonstrate near symmetric single-leg balance, and appropriate strength in the other lower extremity muscle groups (i.e., hip, quadriceps, and hamstring strength) involved with running. A nice precursor to running can be the elliptical machine, or running in deep water (no impact), or on an underwater treadmill at a certain percentage of his body weight. If Cliff has had no adverse reactions to the above precursors he can start with a progressive treadmill running program. He may begin with a light warm-up at a nice cadence for 3 to 5 minutes and then begin with an interval program at a pace that simulates a light jog for him. Intervals should start with 1 minute of jogging, followed by a minute of walking at a fast pace; then 2 minutes of jogging with 1 minute of walking and then 3 minutes of jogging; again followed by a walking/cool down period. He should remain with this intensity of training for at least a week to see how he is responding. If he is responding well he may begin to increase both the speed and duration of his jogging/running bouts over the ensuing weeks.

12 Ashley is a 17-year-old tennis player who has had recurrent ankle sprains to her left ankle over the past

2 years. She has increased inversion with the talar tilt test compared with her right ankle. She does not report any recurrent instability with normal daily activities, only with her athletic activities. She does not wish to undergo surgery and would like a conservative approach to address her ankle issues. What should the therapist do?

The therapist should do a full lower extremity evaluation examining lower extremity muscle strength, ROM, joint mobility/gliding, balance/vestibular testing, and foot/ankle mechanics for possible orthotic intervention. Deficits were found in Ashley's posterior hip musculature and ankle eversion strength. She was found to have proprioceptive deficits on the left with balance testing. Observation of her static and dynamic mechanics revealed increased femoral Q angle contributing to increased knee valgus with dynamic movements, she also demonstrated increased foot pronation with collapse of the midtarsals during the stance phase of gait. So to address these deficits, Ashley should be put on a progressive strengthening program for her posterior hip muscles and peroneals. She should also be fitted for orthotics to address her foot/ankle mechanics. A progressive balance and proprioceptive training program should also be initiated. While undergoing this treatment program, Ashley will need to reduce her tennis training, and it was recommended that she tape or brace her ankle in some fashion until her strength and mechanical issues were resolved.

13 Describe a progressive training program for the peroneals.

Initially after injury or surgery, the patient may begin with submaximal isometrics. Progression with isometrics can increase with the amount of force or with the duration of holding the isometric contraction. The next phase would be pain-free active range motions. The patient may begin first while sitting or lying and then to progress to a sidelying position so that the ankle is everting against gravity. Following this stage, he or she may progress to elastic tubing/Theraband exercises. Focus should also be placed on the eccentric component of these exercises which will assist with tendon strengthening. The therapist may also do PNF diagonals with manual resistance at this stage. Once he or she has completed these phases of the program, which were designed to isolate the peroneals, the focus of the program should shift to more whole body and sport-specifc movements, with emphasis on lateral and diagonal movement patterns.

REFERENCES

1. Ekstrand J, Trapp H: The incidence of ankle sprains in soccer. Foot Ankle 11:41-44, 1990.
2. Garrick JG: The frequency of injury, mechanism of injury and epidemiology of ankle sprains. Am J Sports 5(6):241-242, 1977.
3. Chan KW, Ding BC, Mroczek KJ: Acute and chronic lateral ankle instability in the athlete. Bull NYU Hosp Jt Dis 69(1):17-26, 2011.
4. DeMaio M, Paine R, Drez D: Chronic lateral ankle instability-inversion sprains: Part I & II. Orthopedics 15:87-96, 1992.
5. Komenda G, Ferkel RD: Arthroscopic findings associated with the unstable ankle. Foot Ankle Int 20(11):708-713, 1999.
6. Bahr R, Fetal P: Biomechanics of ankle ligament reconstruction: An in vitro comparison of the Broström repair, Watson-Jones reconstruction, and a new anatomic reconstruction technique. Am J Sports Med 25:424-432, 1997.
7. Balduini FC, et al: Management and rehabilitation of ligamentous injuries to the ankle. Sports Med 4:364-380, 1987.
8. Evans DL: Recurrent instability of the ankle: A method of surgical treatment. Proc R Soc Med 46:343-344, 1953.
9. Keller M, Grossman J: Lateral ankle instability and the Broström-Gould procedure. Foot Ankle 35:513-520, 1996.
10. Colville MR, Grondel RJ: Anatomic reconstruction of the lateral ankle ligaments using a split peroneus brevis tendon graft. Am J Sports Med 23:210-213, 1995.
11. Corte-Real NM, Moreira RM: Arthroscopic repair of chronic lateral ankle instability. Foot Ankle Int 30:213-217, 2009.
12. Colville MR: Surgical treatment of the unstable ankle. J Am Acad Orthop Surg 6(6):368-377, 1998.
13. Harrington KD: Degenerative arthritis of the ankle secondary to long-standing ligamentous instability. J Bone Joint Surg Am 61(3):354-361, 1979.
14. Taser F, Shafiq Q, Ebraheim NA: Anatomy of lateral ankle ligaments and their relationship to bony landmarks. Surg Radiol Anat 28(4):391-397, 2006.
15. Attarian DE, McCrackin HJ, DeVito DP: Biomechanical characteristics of human ankle ligaments. Foot Ankle 6(2):54-58, 1985.
16. Evans GA, Hardcastle P, Frenyo AD: Acute rupture of the lateral ligament of the ankle: To suture or not to suture? J Bone Joint Surg Br 66(2):209-212, 1984.
17. Kaikkonen A, Kannus P, Jarvinen M: Surgery versus functional treatment in ankle ligament tears: A prospective study. Clin Orthop Relat Res, May:(326):194-202, 1996.
18. Kerkoffs GM, et al: Surgical versus conservative treatment for acute injuries of the lateral ligament complex of the ankle in adults. Cochrane Rev 3, Apr 18(2):CD000380, 2007.
19. Specchiulli F, Cofano RE: A comparison of surgical and conservative treatment in ankle ligament tears. Orthopedics 24(7):686-688, 2001.
20. Kannus P, Renstrom P: Treatment for acute tears of the lateral ligaments of the ankle: Operation, cast, or early controlled mobilization. J Bone Joint Surg Am 73(2):305-312, 1991.
21. Berlet GC, Anderson RB, Davis WH: Chronic lateral ankle instability. Foot Ankle Clin 4:713, 1999.
22. Gould N, Seligson D, Gassman J: Early and late repair of lateral ligament of the ankle. Foot Ankle 1:84-89, 1980.
23. Karlsson J, et al: Reconstruction of the lateral ligaments of the ankle for chronic lateral instability. J Bone Joint Surg 70A:581-588, 1988.
24. Broström L: Sprained ankles VI. Surgical treatment of "chronic" ligament ruptures. Acta Chir Scand 132:551-565, 1966.
25. Ferkel RD, Chams RN: Chronic lateral instability: arthroscopic findings and long-term results. Foot Ankle Int 28:24-31, 2007.
26. Taga I, et al: Articular cartilage lesions in ankles with lateral ligament injury: An arthroscopic study. Am J Sports Med 21:120-126, 1993.

27. Hua Y, et al.: Combination of modified Broström procedure with ankle arthroscopy for chronic ankle instability accompanied by intraarticular symptoms. Arthroscopy 26:524-528, 2010.

28. Lui TH: Arthroscopic-assisted lateral ligamentous reconstruction in combined ankle and subtalar instability. Arthroscopy 23:554.e1-555.e5, 2007.

29. Nery C, et al: Arthroscopic-assisted Broström-Gould for chronic ankle instability: A long term follow-up. Am J Sports Med 39:2381-2388, 2011.

30. Liu SH, Baker CL: Comparison of lateral ankle ligamentous reconstruction procedures. Am J Sports Med 22:313-317, 1994.

31. Hennrikus WL, et al: Outcomes of the Chrisman-Snook and modified-Broström procedures for chronic lateral ankle instability: A prospective, randomized comparison. Am J Sports Med 24:400-404, 1996.

32. Hamilton WB, Thompson FM, Snow SW: The modified Broström procedure for lateral ankle instability. Foot Ankle 13:1-7, 1993.

33. Peters WJ, Trevino SG, Renstrom PA: Chronic lateral ankle instability. Foot Ankle 12:182-191, 1991.

34. Coughlin MJ, et al: Comprehensive reconstruction of the lateral ankle for chronic instability using a free gracilis graft. Foot Ankle Int 25:231-241, 2004.

35. O'Shea KJ: Technique for biotenodesis screw fixation in tendon-enhanced ankle ligament reconstruction. Tech Foot Ankle Surg 2:40-46, 2003.

36. Takao M, et al: Anatomical reconstruction of the lateral ligaments of the ankle with a gracilis autograft. Am J Sports Med 33:814-823, 2005.

37. Gebhard JS, et al: Passive motion: The dose effects on joint stiffness, muscle mass, bone density, and regional swelling. JBJS 75A:1636-1647, 1993.

38. Karlsson J, et al: Comparisons of two anatomic reconstructions for chronic lateral instability of the ankle joint. Am J Sports Med 25:48-53, 1997.

39. Sammarco GJ, Carrasquillo HA: Surgical revision after failed lateral ankle reconstruction. Foot Ankle Int 16:748, 1995.

40. Bleakley C, McDonough S, MacAuley D: The use of ice in the treatment of acute soft-tissue injury: A systematic review of randomized controlled trials. Am J Sports Med 32(1):251-261, 2004.

41. Scheffler NM, Sheitel PL, Lipton MN: Use of Cryo/Cuff for the control of postoperative pain and edema. J Foot Surg 31(2):141-148, 1992.

42. Wilke B, Weiner RD: Postoperative cryotherapy: Risks versus benefits of continuous-flow cryotherapy units. Clin Podiatr Med Surg 20(2):307-322, 2003.

43. Eils E, Rosenbaum D: A multi-station proprioceptive exercise program in patients with ankle instability. Med Sci Sports Exerc 33(12):1991-1998, 2001.

44. Lentell G, et al: The use of thermal agents to influence the effectiveness of a low-load prolonged stretch. J Orthop Sports Phys Ther 16(5):200-207, 1992.

ADDITIONAL READINGS

Chrisman OD, Snook GA: Reconstruction of lateral ligament tears of the ankle: An experimental study and clinical evaluation of seven patients treated by a new modification of the Elmslie procedure. J Bone Joint Surg 51A:904-912, 1969.

Ferkel RD, Chams RN: Chronic lateral instability: Arthroscopic and long term results. Foot Ankle Int 28(1):24-31, 2007.

Girard P, et al: Clinical evaluation of the modified Broström-Evans procedure to restore ankle stability. Foot Ankle Int 20:246-252, 1999.

Haraguchi N, Tokumo A, Okamura R, et al: Influence of activity level on the outcome of the treatment of lateral ankle ligament rupture. J Orthop Sci 14(4):391-396, 2009.

Shahrulazua A, et al: Early functional outcome of a modified Broström-Gould surgery using bioabsorable suture anchor for chronic lateral ankle instability. Singapore Med J 51(3):235-241, 2010.

Watson-Jones R: Fractures and other bone and joint injuries, Baltimore, 1940, Williams & Wilkins.

CHAPTER 29

Open Reduction and Internal Fixation of the Ankle

Graham Linck, Danny Arora, Robert Donatelli, Will Hall, Brian E. Prell, Richard D. Ferkel

INTRODUCTION

The treatment of ankle fractures dates back to antiquity. Evidence of healed ankle fractures has been noted in the remains of mummies from ancient Egypt.[1] Hippocrates recommended that closed fractures be reduced by traction of the foot, but few other advances in the understanding and treatment of ankle fractures were made until the middle of the eighteenth century.[2-4] Operative treatment of ankle fractures was popularized by Lambotte[5] and Danis[6]; the AO group began a systematic study of fracture treatment in 1958.[7-9] Since these original investigators, significant progress has been made in the treatment of ankle fractures.

Much of the current understanding of the mechanism of ankle fractures has developed from the work of Lauge-Hansen.[4] In his system, the position of the foot (pronation or supination) at the time of the injury is described first and the direction of the deforming force is described second. Ankle fractures currently are classified most commonly by two systems: Lauge-Hansen[4] and Danis-Weber[10,11] (Fig. 29-1). The latter system is based on the location of the fracture of the fibula: infrasyndesmotic, transsyndesmotic, and suprasyndesmotic. Fractures also are classified by the number of bones that are affected—that is, a bimalleolar fracture involves injury to both medial and lateral malleoli, whereas a trimalleolar fracture indicates that the medial, lateral, and posterior malleoli have all been fractured.

An ankle fracture is a debilitating injury, especially if the fracture is unstable. The treatment of choice for an unstable ankle fracture is open reduction and internal fixation (ORIF). Surgical treatment of a displaced, unstable ankle fracture centers on anatomic restoration of the bony and ligamentous structures that surround the joint. As technology and surgical techniques have advanced, so have the outcomes for ORIF.[12-14]

SURGICAL INDICATIONS AND CONSIDERATIONS

Ankle fractures can be treated conservatively if the ankle mortise remains stable. The medial clear space (space between medial malleolus and talus) or lateral clear space (space between lateral malleolus and talus) must measure less than 3 mm on a mortise radiographic view, or less than 5 mm on a stress radiographic view. It is important to ensure that the talus is well reduced beneath the tibia plafond and not subluxated forward or backward. The following specific injuries are indications for conservative treatment: isolated non-displaced medial malleolar fracture or tip avulsion fracture, isolated lateral malleolar fracture with less than 3 mm displacement and no talar shift, and a posterior malleolar fracture with less than 25% joint involvement or less than 2-mm stepoff. Conservative management usually entails immobilization in a short-leg cast or boot, which extends to the tips of the toes with the foot in an appropriate position for the type of fracture deformity. Any fracture of the ankle with a residual talar tilt or subluxation, in which the ankle mortise is not anatomically reduced, warrants surgical fixation.

In general, ORIF should be performed on all patients, regardless of age, gender, activity level, or vocation, as long as they are healthy enough to undergo the procedure. However, exceptions do exist, including paraplegics and quadriplegics, and patients who are nonambulatory and lack sensation to the lower extremities.

Preoperative variables that predict a successful outcome include an otherwise healthy patient who is well motivated to recover after surgery. Systemic diseases such as osteoporosis, diabetes, peripheral vascular disease, alcoholism, and tobacco abuse can all affect the ultimate outcome of surgery. These variables affect wound healing, as well as the healing of the fracture itself.

DANIS-WEBER

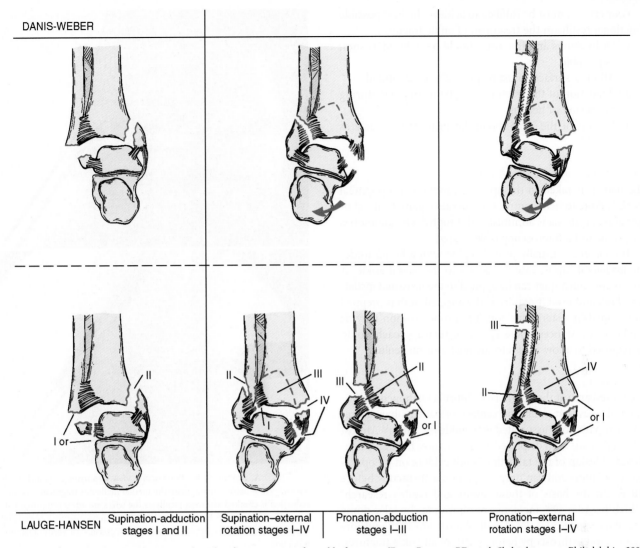

| LAUGE-HANSEN | Supination-adduction stages I and II | Supination–external rotation stages I–IV | Pronation-abduction stages I–III | Pronation–external rotation stages I–IV |

Fig. 29-1 The Lauge-Hansen and Danis-Weber classification systems for ankle fractures. (From Browner BD, et al: Skeletal trauma, Philadelphia, 2009, Saunders.)

SURGICAL PROCEDURES

Patient Evaluation

It is important to get a history on the mechanism of injury, and if possible, the position of the ankle, as well as the direction of force. This will not always be possible, because most patients will only be able to describe a twisting or rolling type of injury. Completing your history with current medical comorbidities and social habits is necessary for patient outcomes. Physical examination includes inspection, palpation, and neurovascular examination. It is crucial to note any gross deformity, which may indicate possible dislocation, and would necessitate early closed reduction and splinting, as well as any wounds around the ankle, which may indicate an open fracture, and would require emergent surgical irrigation and débridement.

A careful preoperative assessment of not only the patient's health, but also the fracture and the patient's swelling and skin tension, is important to a successful outcome. In some cases surgery may have to be delayed for as long as 14 days to allow swelling to resolve so the skin can be closed at the end of surgery without a wound slough. Recently, a foot and ankle pump device has been used to reduce swelling rapidly to permit earlier surgery and fewer complications.

Initially, patients may be too swollen to wear a cast. In this instance a bulky dressing with cast padding and bias type of compression wrap is applied with a posterior splint. The patient remains non–weight bearing with crutches and elevates the injured ankle above the heart to promote reduction of swelling.

Surgical Technique

The currently accepted method for fracture ORIF is the AO (Arbeitsgemeinschaft für Osteosynthesefragen, or Association for the Study of Internal Fixation) technique developed in Switzerland. This technique emphasizes the use of plates, screws, and wires as needed to achieve rigid fixation.

Four criteria must be fulfilled to achieve the best possible functional results in the treatment of ankle fractures:

1. Dislocations and fractures should be reduced as soon as possible.
2. All joint surfaces must be precisely reconstituted.
3. Reduction of the fracture must be maintained during the period of healing.
4. Motion of the joint should be instituted as early as possible.

Anesthesia and Positioning

The patient is taken to the operating room and a popliteal block is done to help control postoperative pain. General or epidural anesthesia is administered. Prophylactic antibiotics are given, and a fluoroscopy table is used.

The patient is usually placed supine with a bump under the ipsilateral hip to ease the access to the lateral ankle. A pneumatic tourniquet can be applied to the proximal ipsilateral thigh and used if required. The affected limb is prepped and draped in a sterile fashion. The prone position may be used in rare instances where a posterolateral approach would be required to allow access to the posterior malleolus.

Procedure

Recent research at the Southern California Orthopedic Institute indicates that a high percentage of patients have intraarticular pathology associated with ankle fractures.[13] Almost 75% of patients with displaced ankle fractures have an osteochondral lesion of the talus that is not evident on preoperative x-ray films and can only be seen on arthroscopy before ORIF. On the basis of these results and Lantz's research[8] (which found a 49% incidence of injuries to the talar dome articular cartilage in isolated malleolar fractures), the authors recommend arthroscopy before ORIF of all ankle fractures. This approach is also supported by Hintermann's study[15] that showed a 79% incidence of osteochondral lesions of the talus with an ankle fracture.

The arthroscopic evaluation is done as described in Chapter 30. All intraarticular pathology is documented and appropriately treated. The surgeon must examine carefully for osteochondral lesions of the talus, tears of the deltoid, anterior talofibular and syndesmotic ligaments, and dislocations of the posterior tibial tendon, which may impede fracture reduction. Some fractures can be reduced and internally fixated by arthroscopic means alone.[16] A typical example is a patient with a fracture of the medial malleolus that was débrided arthroscopically and fixated percutaneously with two cannulated screws (Fig. 29-2). We have also had good long-term results treating Tillaux fractures in an arthroscopic manner. After the arthroscopic portion of the procedure is completed, if the fracture is not amenable to all-arthroscopic reduction, the ankle is prepared and draped again, gloves are changed, and new sterile instruments are used.

Incisions are made over the lateral, medial, or posterior malleolus, depending on the nature of the fractures. When a fracture apparently involves only the medial malleolus, the surgeon should search for an injury to the syndesmosis with

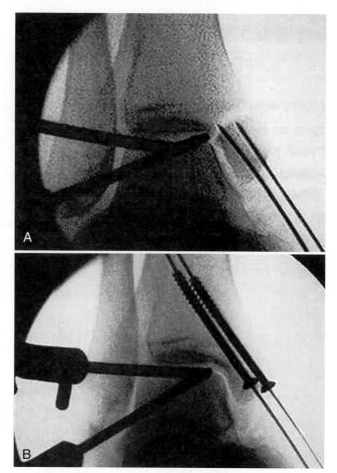

Fig. 29-2 A, Intraoperative fluoroscopy view confirming parallel guide wire insertion used to manipulate the medial malleolus fragment. Fracture reduction is checked arthroscopically as the wires are advanced proximally across the fracture site. **B,** Cannulated screws are subsequently inserted and checked under fluoroscopy and also arthroscopically to verify anatomic reduction.

subsequent tearing of the interosseous membrane, which may result in a high fibular fracture. This type of fracture, which also is known as a Maisonneuve type of fracture, could even occur at the fibular head and may be missed if the surgeon is not diligent. In this instance, the medial malleolar fracture is reduced anatomically, usually with two screws inserted proximally through a small incision from the tip of the medial malleolus. The deltoid ligament is split in line with its fibers, and the two screws are inserted parallel to each other under fluoroscopic control. If the syndesmosis and interosseous membrane have been torn and are unstable, one or two syndesmotic screw(s) are inserted through the fibula and tibia, exiting the medial border of the tibia with the foot in dorsiflexion. The screw(s) are not placed with compression because compressing the syndesmosis restricts motion postoperatively.

When a Weber B fracture occurs with disruption of the deltoid, syndesmosis, and interosseous membrane, anatomic reduction of the medial and lateral clear spaces is critical (Fig. 29-3). After arthroscopically débriding the ankle and cleaning out the torn ligaments, ORIF is performed.

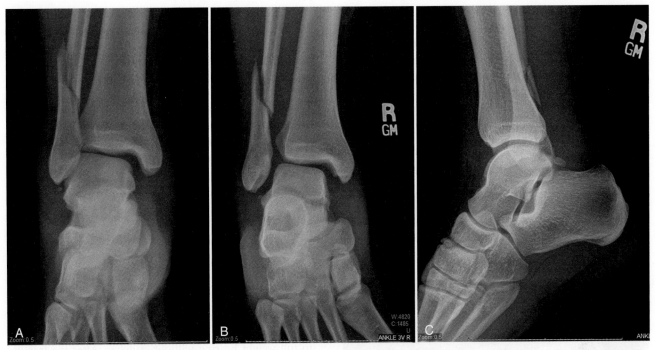

Fig. 29-3 Weber C fracture-dislocation. Anteroposterior (AP) **(A)**, mortise **(B)**, and lateral **(C)** radiographs showing a high fracture of the fibula with disruption of the syndesmosis and deltoid ligaments.

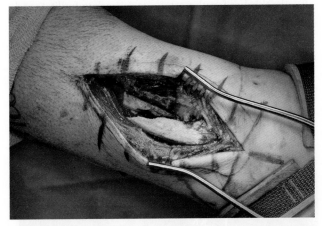

Fig. 29-4 The lateral malleolus fracture of the right ankle is exposed and the periosteum is elevated with sharp dissection to reveal the fracture site.

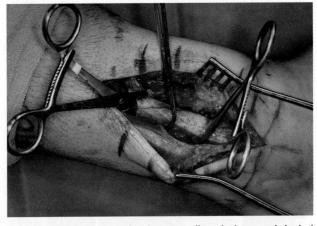

Fig. 29-5 The fracture is reduced anatomically with clamps and checked under fluoroscopy.

The surgeon makes an incision over the fracture site and extends it proximally and distally on the fibula. Dissection is carried down to the periosteum and the fracture site. Care is taken to identify the superficial peroneal nerve, which crosses the field approximately 7 cm proximal to the distal tip of the fibula. The fracture is exposed and the periosteum is elevated with sharp dissection (Fig. 29-4). The surgeon uses a curette to remove the hematoma and applies reduction clamps to assist in reducing the fracture. Reduction of the fracture usually also requires traction and rotation of the foot and ankle (Fig. 29-5). When anatomic reduction has been achieved, frequently one or two lag screws are used to provide interfragmentary compression across the fracture site. After this is accomplished, an appropriately sized plate is centered over the fracture site and stabilized with screws.

One or two syndesmosis screws or a screw and tightrope are then inserted to reduce the ankle, and the reduction is checked under fluoroscopy (Fig. 29-6). Postoperative radiographs are taken to verify anatomic reduction of the fractures and syndesmosis, and appropriate positioning of the screws and plate (Fig. 29-7).

When both the medial and lateral malleoli have been fractured, the lateral malleolus is approached first (Fig. 29-8). An incision is then made over the medial malleolus as previously described, the fracture site is exposed, the hematoma is removed, and the fracture is reduced. The surgeon inserts one or two screws. Postoperative x-ray films demonstrate anatomic reduction of the fractures with good position of the plate and screws (Fig. 29-9).

In ORIF of a trimalleolar fracture, the lateral and medial malleoli are addressed as previously mentioned. Using the fluoroscope, the surgeon then reduces the posterior malleolar fracture by manipulating the fragment into place and making a small incision along the anterolateral aspect of the distal tibia. Two guide pins are inserted to reduce the fragment and one or two cannulated screws are inserted from anterior to posterior to hold the posterior malleolar

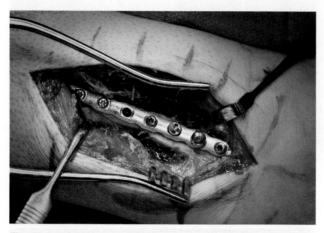

Fig. 29-6 A lag screw is used to provide interfragmentary compression across the fracture site. An appropriately sized plate is then centered over the fracture site, and the fracture is stabilized with screws. A syndesmosis screw and tightrope are then inserted to reduce the mortise.

fragment in place. In general, posterior malleolar fracture fragments do not require internal fixation if they involve less than 25% of the articular surface. If the posterior malleolus needs to be addressed directly, a posterolateral approach can be used.

Postoperative Plan

After surgery the patient is splinted in a well-padded short-leg cast in the neutral position; the cast is split in the recovery room to allow for swelling. Patients are asked to keep the limb elevated as much as possible for the first postoperative week. The procedure can be done on an outpatient basis if the pain level is not too severe, but in some instances the patient may be required to stay 1 or 2 days in the hospital. After discharge the patient is non–weight bearing on crutches for at least 4 weeks. The cast is changed at 1 week after surgery, the wound is inspected, and all new dressings are applied. At 2 weeks after surgery, the stitches are removed and a new short-leg cast is applied for 2 additional weeks. At 4 weeks after surgery, another short-leg cast is applied and the patient starts partial weight bearing, gradually increasing to full weight bearing without crutches. After the fracture has healed, the patient can wear a supportive brace and start pool and then land physical therapy. In patients with stable, reliable fixation, early motion can sometimes be initiated after the third or fourth postoperative week to facilitate early return of motion and strength.[17] Patients are restricted from operating an automobile for 9 weeks following right-sided ankle fractures.

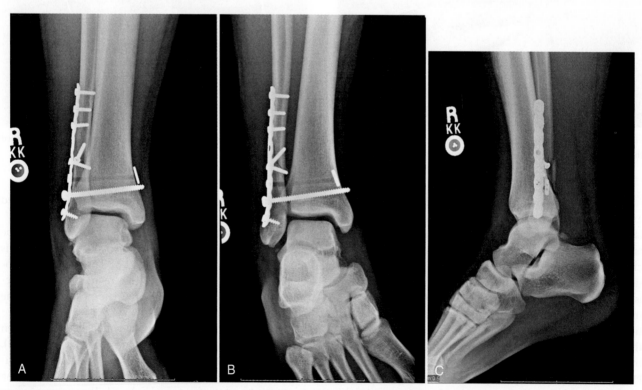

Fig. 29-7 Postoperative radiographs. AP (**A**), mortise (**B**), and lateral (**C**) radiographs demonstrate anatomic reduction of the mortise with normal measurements of the medial and lateral clear spaces with hardware in place.

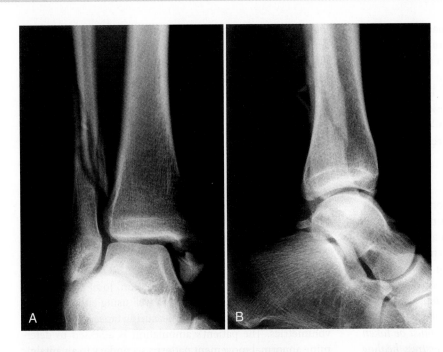

Fig. 29-8 Bimalleolar ankle fracture. AP (**A**) and lateral (**B**) radiographs demonstrating fractures of the medial and lateral malleoli.

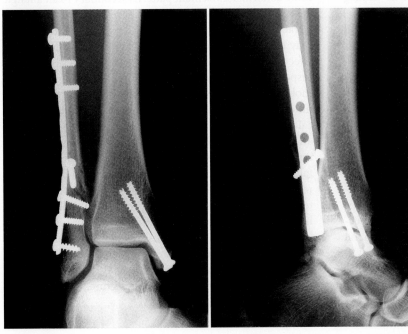

Fig. 29-9 Postoperative radiographs. AP (**A**) and lateral (**B**) radiographs demonstrating anatomic reduction of the fractures with appropriate position of the screws and plate.

If a syndesmosis screw or screws were inserted during fixation, the patient must be non–weight bearing for 6 to 8 weeks. The screw(s) is removed at 12 to 16 weeks postoperatively, since it can break with weight bearing if left in place. Physical therapy is started 6 to 8 weeks after surgery. After the screw(s) is removed, the patient can be more aggressive with physical therapy and weight-bearing activities.

Surgical Outcomes

A successful outcome is defined as a fully healed fracture, with the patient achieving near full or complete range of motion (ROM) with normal strength and function.[9] Function is defined differently for each patient—an athlete's function is different from that of a sedentary, elderly patient.

Several different grading systems, including subjective, objective, and functional data, are used to evaluate ankle fracture results. However, ankle fracture results are difficult to compare because of the multitude of fracture patterns and different circumstances of treatment. Results can be affected by many things, including severity and type of injury, associated intraarticular problems, preexisting arthritis,[3] age and reliability of the patient, quality of the bone, and other site injuries. Finally, it should be noted that there is a potential for superficial nerve injury after surgical repair, as well as syndesmosis instability.[18]

Younger age, male sex, absence of diabetes, and a lower American Society of Anesthesia class are predictive of a good functional recovery at 1 year following ankle fracture surgery.[11] Anand and Klenarman[19] report that, in a sample of 80 patients older than 60 years, 88.5% were satisfied with their postoperative outcome. Ankle fractures are the fourth most common fracture in those older than 65 years and usually are the result of significant trauma.[12] Recent studies have not demonstrated any age-related risks to surgery beyond those posed by other comorbidities.[14,20] Therefore, the criteria for surgery should not be different for elderly patients than for younger individuals.

Postoperative Considerations

In patients with stable, reliable fixation, sometimes early motion can be initiated after the third or fourth postoperative week to facilitate early return of motion and strength.[17] Early motion and exercise have been found to have beneficial effects following ankle ORIF. *Patients have demonstrated decreased activity/functional restrictions, decreased pain, and improved ankle range of motion with early mobility. However, a higher rate of adverse events following ankle ORIF was associated with early exercise/mobility so care must be taken by both the therapist and patient to not overstress healing tissues.*[21]

When a syndesmosis screw has been inserted, the patient must be non–weight bearing for 6 to 8 weeks; the screw is removed at 10 to 12 weeks postoperatively. The screw will break with weight bearing if it is left in place. Physical therapy is started 6 to 8 weeks after surgery. After the screw is removed, the patient can be full weight bearing and initiate physical therapy.

Complications

Minor complications include incidence of 4% to 5% wound problems (epidermolysis and superficial infection) and peroneal tendinitis with painful hardware. Major problems include nonunion, hardware failure, 1% to 2% deep infections (up to 20% in diabetic patients with peripheral neuropathy), posttraumatic arthritis, and compartment syndrome. *Patients who have any condition (i.e., diabetes, peripheral artery disease) that might compromise circulation in the distal extremities are at an increased risk for complications relating to wound healing and closure.*[22]

THERAPY GUIDELINES FOR REHABILITATION

The physical therapist normally evaluates the patient approximately 6 weeks after surgery. In most cases, the patient has been in a cast for those 6 weeks and has had partial weight-bearing status between 2 and 4 weeks. Studies have reported that clinical outcomes may be improved in patients with trimalleolar fractures who have full weight-bearing status in an ankle orthosis between 2 to 4 weeks after surgery.[23] *A recent systematic review article evaluated nine randomized control studies that compared early motion of the ankle with 6 weeks of cast immobilization and found that early mobility is associated with quicker return to work and improved ankle range of motion after 12 weeks. However, other article's authors found that early motion was associated with increased risk of wound infection.*[23,24] Some authors also suggest early active range of motion (AROM) for plantar flexion and dorsiflexion as soon as the surgical incision has healed.[24,25] *For those patients who are having issues with wound healing, a number of new technologies have been developed to try to accelerate wound healing, such as hyperbaric oxygen therapy, low level laser therapy, nano/microcurrent technology, and infrared light.*[22,26-28]

EVALUATION

The initial evaluation establishes the baseline deficits from which further goals and treatment are formulated (Box 29-1). AROM and passive range of motion (PROM) are assessed within the patient's tolerance. ROM is a primary limitation noted at the initial evaluation. Joint effusion and soft tissue edema are evaluated as well using either a "figure 8" technique, with a standard measuring tape, or by applying volumetrics. The patient's ambulation is assessed to determine abnormal movement patterns secondary to an antalgic gait. At this stage the patient may have acute pain and be in a fracture boot or other type of orthosis. Often, the patient may experience hardware-related pain, which may have an affect on functional outcomes.[29] The physical therapist inspects and evaluates scar mobility. Joint and soft tissue mobility is assessed with an emphasis on the way restrictions limit ROM and function. After enough mineralization and calcium formation have occurred according to the physician, an assessment of the arthrokinematic movements of the ankle joint can be done. For example, posterior glide of the talus is often markedly restricted and has been correlated to restrictions in dorsiflexion and normal gait. In addition, posterior and anterior glide of the proximal and distal fibular heads have been shown to increase AROM and PROM.

After evaluation and discussion, the physical therapist and patient formulate a treatment plan and goals. Belcher et al[30] reported impaired function as long as 24 months after an ORIF surgery for a trimalleolar fracture.

PHASE I

TIME: Weeks 6 to 8 after surgery
GOALS: Minimize pain and swelling, normalize ROM, initiate AROM and therapeutic exercises, normalize

---

BOX 29-1   Evaluation Goals

Assess PROM within pain tolerance.
Assess AROM within pain tolerance.
Assess joint effusion and soft tissue edema.
Assess ambulation secondary to antalgic gait.
Assess scar mobility.
Assess soft tissue mobility (including muscle tightness).
Assess joint mobility after 8 to 10 weeks (after enough mineralization and calcium formation has occurred per physician).

gait, increase joint and soft tissue mobility, maintain cardiovascular fitness, and provide patient education (Table 29-1). Treatment goals initially are to decrease pain and swelling, increase ROM and strength, and normalize gait. AROM and PROM are initiated immediately for all planes of movement under the supervision of the physical therapist. AROM can progress from movement with lessened gravity (e.g., in a pool) to movement using gravity as resistance. Soft tissue mobilization of restricted structures is particularly useful in decreasing pain and increasing ROM. Around 8 weeks, with physician approval, joint mobilization of the ankle is implemented using distraction and glide maneuvers.[31]

Ankle joint mobilizations into resistance are deferred until enough mineralization and calcium formation have occurred (usually 8 weeks). The rehabilitation program also includes gait training and lower extremity strengthening in shallow and deep water in addition to land therapy. Recently, some harness treadmill systems have been developed that can unload the patient's body weight and decrease his or her fear of falling, allowing the patient to focus more on his or her gait mechanics. Ankle AROM exercises also are initiated in the pool.

The patient should avoid jumping and running exercises in shallow water at this time. However, if lack of ROM and gait are significant problems at the time of the patient's initial physical therapy evaluation, the therapist may decide to begin land therapy in combination with pool therapy to address specific problems and monitor the patient more closely.

A compressive stocking is useful to help control soft tissue edema and joint effusion, especially during initial weight-bearing activities. The patient is instructed in a home exercise program incorporating ice, elevation, compression, and light active exercises, such as stationary bicycling or AROM

TABLE 29-1 Ankle Open Reduction and Internal Fixation

Rehabilitation Phase	Criteria to Progress to this Phase	Anticipated Impairments and Functional Limitations	Intervention	Goal	Rationale
Phase I Postoperative 6-8 wk	• Cleared by physician to begin rehabilitation postoperation	• Limited weight-bearing per physician • Pain • Edema • Limited ROM • Limited strength	• Encourage use of compression stocking • Cryotherapy with compression • ES (with pads carefully placed) • Elevation • PROM (pain free) for ankle dorsiflexion, plantar flexion, inversion, and eversion • Joint mobilization grades II and III (at 8 wk with physician approval) • Isometrics (submaximal) for ankle dorsiflexion, plantar flexion, inversion, and eversion • AROM (pain free) for ankle dorsiflexion, plantar flexion, inversion, and eversion • PNF patterns • Weight-shifting exercises • Stationary bicycle • Seated balance board activities • Soft tissue mobilization • Gait training as indicated by weight-bearing status • Instruction for locating neutral pelvic position • Initial core stabilization exercises • Home exercise program	• Manage edema • Decrease pain • Increase PROM • Increase strength • Decrease gait deviations, improve tolerance to weight bearing • Improve soft tissue mobility • Improve joint mobility	• Control edema and decrease pain using ES, rest, ice with compression, and elevation • Improve ROM in pain-free ranges to avoid increase in edema and pain • Movement nourishes the articular cartilage and improves tolerance to exercise • Physician must give weight-bearing status to progress gait; weight-shifting exercises and intermittent loading (bicycle) can be useful in progressing tolerance of the ankle and foot to compression • Soft tissue and joint mobilization is useful in restoring ROM and gating pain • Core stabilization to maintain neutral pelvic position and improve gait biomechanics • Self-manage exercises

AROM, Active range of motion; *ES,* electrical stimulation; *PNF,* proprioceptive neuromuscular facilitation; *PROM,* passive range of motion; *ROM,* range of motion.

exercises, to reduce soft edema and joint effusion. Pain and swelling are managed with appropriate modalities, such as pulsed ultrasound or electrical stimulation. However, these modalities should not be performed over the metal implants. *Just as with quadriceps stimulation following knee surgery, high voltage electrical stimulation may be beneficial in the early phase of recovery to retard any further muscle atrophy of the gastroc/soleus complex that may have resulted secondary to immobilization or weight-bearing restriction.*[32]

PHASE II

TIME: Weeks 9 to 12 after surgery
GOALS: Minimize pain and swelling, normalize ROM, normalize gait, decrease soft tissue restrictions, increase strength of intrinsic and extrinsic foot and ankle muscles (Table 29-2)

The second phase is initiated after pain and swelling have subsided, usually 9 to 12 weeks after surgery. The second phase of treatment blends with the first as ROM and gait progress to normal. Progressive resistive exercises are used to strengthen the anterior and posterior tibialis, peroneals, and gastrocnemius and soleus muscle groups. A home program, using elastic tubing for resistance, is helpful to augment supervised physical therapy in the office. Treatment options for strengthening exercises include the stationary bicycle, stair-climbing machine, step-ups, step-downs, calf raises, and isokinetic exercises. Specific muscle strengthening for the gastrocnemius and soleus muscles is important to examine because of the likelihood of muscle atrophy. A total lower extremity strengthening program is indicated, as well as a program to maintain cardiovascular fitness. Joint and soft tissue mobilization is continued as indicated. Submaximal isokinetics can be implemented using high speeds such as 120° to 180° per second. The higher velocities prevent excessive resistance that could exacerbate the patient's symptoms. Proprioceptive activities are increased as the patient begins to demonstrate increased balance; use of a balance board is helpful in developing proprioception. The patient progresses heel raises from sitting to standing to single-leg

TABLE 29-2   Ankle Open Reduction and Internal Fixation

Rehabilitation Phase	Criteria to Progress to This Phase	Anticipated Impairments and Functional Limitations	Intervention	Goal	Rationale
Phase II Postoperative 9-12 wk	• No signs of infection • No loss of ROM • No significant increase in pain	• Edema and pain present but under control • Limited ROM • Limited strength • Gait deviations	• Continue interventions, as in phase I, as indicated • Modalities as needed • PROM (stretches) — Gastrocnemius/soleus, tibialis posterior and anterior • AROM — Sitting heel raises (bilateral and progressed to single leg and from sitting to standing). • Isotonic or elastic tubing exercises — dorsiflexion, plantar flexion, inversion, eversion • Passive resistance exercises • Treadmill • Stationary bicycle • Stair-climbing machine • Multihip exercises • Knee flexion/extension • Closed-chain exercises • Leg press machine • Bilateral heel raises • Step-ups and step-downs • Lateral step ups and step-downs • Minisquats • Partial lunges • Isokinetics (submaximal) — 120°-180° per second • Balance exercises	• Self-manage edema • Decrease pain • Increase ROM • Increase strength • Decrease gait deviations • Improve functional strength of gait • Increase endurance • Increase proprioception and prevent reinjury	• Progress home exercises and use modalities as indicated • Provide specific LE stretches • Improve tolerance to body weight as resistance for exercises • Use varying resistance to progress strength • Use gym equipment to progress functional strength and endurance; progress to cardiovascular levels when able • Use closed-chain and balance exercises to strengthen foot intrinsic and ankle muscles in a weight-bearing position

AROM, Active range of motion; *LE,* lower extremity; *PROM,* passive range of motion; *ROM,* range of motion.

standing. Modalities such as compression wraps and ice packs are used as indicated for postexercise pain and swelling. Electrical stimulation may be used if the pads are appropriately placed away from plates and pins. The intensity of the rehabilitation should be altered if pain or swelling limit the rehabilitation progression. **Weight-bearing exercises and resisted exercises done too aggressively will exacerbate the symptoms and could delay the rehabilitation process for several weeks.**

PHASE III

TIME: Weeks 13 to 18
GOALS: Maintain normal limits of ROM, joint and soft tissue mobility, gait, and muscle strength; increase coordination for higher level activities; improve balance and proprioception (Table 29-3)

The third phase of rehabilitation begins approximately 13 to 18 weeks from the time of surgery. The fracture is usually healed by this phase of rehabilitation.[25] The patient has progressed to normal ROM and demonstrates a normal gait and increased strength with manual muscle testing. Before progressing to a more aggressive program the patient should be cleared by the surgeon. Therapeutic exercises should progress to include strengthening exercises that are 60% to 70% of maximal effort. This submaximal effort is best determined by the patient's ability to lift a specific amount of weight 10

times. The ninth and tenth repetitions should be difficult for the patient. Isokinetic strengthening programs can be initiated. The use of various speeds during the workout session is referred to as velocity spectrum. We have found velocity spectrum training useful in promoting strength and power of the extrinsic muscles of the foot and ankle.

Functional training should be initiated for the patient wishing to return to sporting activities or vigorous work. Treadmill walking on an incline or retrograde can be an excellent method of training for the endurance athlete. Pool activities can be used initially for running and jumping.

PHASE IV

TIME: Week 19 and beyond
GOALS: Return to sporting activities or daily activities without restrictions (Table 29-4)

Phase IV is the last phase, starting at 19 weeks after surgery. This phase is used to condition the patient for a return to sports, work, or any activity requiring vigorous movement. Sport-specific activities are carefully implemented with the use of an ankle brace.

Plyometric exercises simulate many sporting activities because of the prestretch to the muscle before contraction. Some examples of plyometric exercises include depth jumping, trampoline, hopping, and jumping over obstacles. However, plyometric exercises are stressful to joints and soft

TABLE 29-3 Ankle Open Reduction and Internal Fixation

Rehabilitation Phase	Criteria to Progress to This Phase	Anticipated Impairments and Functional Limitations	Intervention	Goal	Rationale
Phase III Postoperative 13-18 wk	• Continued progression with phase II activities • No loss of ROM • No increase in pain	• Limited strength • Limited gait • Limited progression with jumping and running*	• Continuation of phase I and II interventions as indicated • Treadmill using incline and retrograde • Isokinetic velocity spectrum • Agility drills—Lateral shuffles, carioca, and initiate low-level plyometrics • Pool therapy—Running and jumping in chest- to waist-deep water as indicated	• Full ROM • No gait deviations • Ankle muscle strength 80%-90% • Increase coordination, balance, and proprioception • Prepare for return to sport	• Progress phases from I and II as indicated; discontinue reliance on modalities to control pain. • Use uneven surface ambulation and agility drills to improve tolerance of the ankle and foot to the community environment, and return to sport • Progress isokinetics to train ankle for endurance activities • Use water to aid in progression of tolerance to advance activities while unweighted • Use FCE to determine work tolerances if activity is in question

FCE, Functional capacity evaluation; *ROM*, range of motion.
*The patient should begin on progressive run and jump training programs during this phase. However, care needs to be taken to ensure that the patient does not experience exacerbations. Adequate rest and recovery time between bouts of activities is essential. If a patient experiences a problem (e.g., increased pain or swelling), the therapist should treat it as an acute injury and should reduce the symptoms before progressing to the next phase.

TABLE 29-4 Ankle Open Reduction and Internal Fixation

Rehabilitation Phase	Criteria to Progress to This Phase	Anticipated Impairments and Functional Limitations	Intervention	Goal	Rationale
Phase IV Postoperative 19+ wk	• Continued progress in phases I to III	• Limited with higher level activities	• Continuation of exercises from phases I to III as indicated • Plyometrics • Work- and sport-simulated exercises • FCE	• Return to work and sport activities	• Use specificity of training principles to return to previous activities • Use FCE to determine work tolerances if activity is in question

FCE, Functional capacity evaluation.

tissue structures and should be initiated after normal muscle strength is obtained throughout the lower limb.

PRECAUTIONS

A trimalleolar fracture is a serious injury. Secondary problems and complications can occur during postoperative rehabilitation. Occasionally low back or sacroiliac pain develops as a result of the antalgic gait with the cast or fracture boot. This is treated symptomatically with emphasis on the need to normalize gait as soon as possible or restrict ambulation activities.

Overuse injuries such as plantar fasciitis secondary to a preexisting overpronation may be treated with modalities and foot orthosis. Because limited dorsiflexion is sometimes an issue, a low-load prolonged stretch for dorsiflexion over 2 to 30 minutes is effective. This can be done in conjunction with moist heat or ultrasound to the gastrocnemius and soleus muscle group.

SUGGESTED HOME MAINTENANCE FOR THE POSTSURGICAL PATIENT

An exercise program has been outlined at the various phases. The home maintenance box outlines rehabilitation suggestions the patient may follow. The physical therapist can use it in customizing a patient-specific program.

TROUBLESHOOTING

Residual problems after surgical anatomic restoration of the ankle joint include chronic pain, loss of motion, recurrent swelling, and perceived instability. The cause of such poor outcomes is often unclear, but it may be related to missed occult intraarticular injury.[10,33-35] Other postoperative problems that can develop include malunion or nonunion, loosening or fracture of the internal fixation devices, infection, and wound problems. These complications are rare. Unless contraindicated, the physical therapist must work on mobilization of the scar or scars, as well as general stretching and mobilization of the joint. Care should be taken to increase soft tissue and ankle flexibility gradually and not to stretch or stress the joint excessively to gain more rapid and improved ROM. Pool therapy should be used initially, with some land therapy; as the patient progresses, land therapy increases and pool therapy diminishes. The physical therapist also must take care to avoid pushing the ankle too hard, resulting in increased swelling, pain, and subsequent loss of motion.

The physician should be notified immediately if the patient develops significantly increased pain, swelling, loss of motion, or wound healing problems. In addition, if signs of infection or loosening of the internal fixation develop, the physician should be notified immediately.

SUMMARY

In the next century, continued advances in surgical techniques and rehabilitation will allow patients to return earlier to their work and sports activities. As additional physicians and physical therapists specialize in foot and ankle problems, more basic and clinical research will be carried out to "push the envelope" of progress to improve foot and ankle care.

Suggested Home Maintenance for the Postsurgical Patient

Weeks 6 to 8
GOALS FOR THE PERIOD: Minimize pain and swelling, improve ROM, initiate AROM and therapeutic exercises, improve gait, and maintain cardiovascular fitness
1. AROM of the ankle (plantar flexion, dorsiflexion, inversion, and eversion)
2. Stretching exercises for the gastrocnemius and soleus muscle groups in a non–weight-bearing position (use of a towel or strap to stretch these muscles is recommended)
3. Seated heel and toe raises
4. Ice, elevation, and compression
5. Lower extremity conditioning using the stationary bicycle and/or pool
   Exercise progression: Begin all exercises with 2 sets of 10 repetitions. If no adverse effects are noted to previous intensity level, progression can proceed to 3 sets of 10 repetitions, followed by 3 sets of 12 to 15 repetitions, and finally 3 sets of 20 repetitions. Once a patient is able to perform 3 sets of 20 repetitions of an exercise, the intensity of the exercise must be increased in some form (i.e., more resistance, longer duration, etc.) and the patient should start back with 2 sets of 10 repetitions and follow the same progression.

Weeks 9 to 12
GOALS FOR THE PERIOD: Normalize ROM and gait, increase strength of the intrinsic and extrinsic foot and ankle musculature, and improve cardiovascular condition
1. Standing heel raises
2. Resistive exercises using elastic bands or tubing for all ankle movements

3. Step-ups and step-downs
4. Single-leg standing progressed to standing on a pillow with eyes open and then with eyes closed (for balance and proprioception)
5. Walking program, including hills as appropriate
6. Lower extremity conditioning using a stationary bicycle, stair-climbing machine, treadmill, pool, leg press, and toe raises
7. Weight-bearing stretching exercises to the posterior calf muscles

Weeks 13 to 18
GOALS FOR THE PERIOD: Maintain normal ROM, gait, and strength; increase coordination for higher level activities; improve balance and proprioception; and transition to sporting activities
1. Strengthening exercises with increasing resistance
2. Pool activities such as jumping, running, and cutting drills
3. Agility drills such as side shuffles, backward walking, and carioca
4. Lower extremity conditioning continued from phase II

Week 19 and Beyond
GOALS FOR THE PERIOD: Return to previous level of function (sport- and activity-specific exercises) without restrictions
1. Maximal strengthening of lower extremity muscles
2. Land-based functional activities, such as running, jumping, and cutting
3. Sports simulated activities

CLINICAL CASE REVIEW

1 Amy is a 30-year-old female who suffered a bimalleolar fracture while playing soccer. She underwent an ORIF procedure on her ankle 15 weeks ago. Amy complains of tightness, which progressively increases throughout the day as she performs her functional daily activities. How did the therapist address this issue in her treatment plan?

When a patient complains of stiffness, it is always necessary to determine if the problem is joint or soft tissue in nature. The therapist assessed the patient and found significant restrictions with proximal fibular anteroposterior (AP) glides and distal fibular posteroanterior (PA)

glides. These were treated appropriately, and the patient immediately noticed a decrease in her "stiffness."

2 Lauren is a 23-year-old female who suffered a bimalleolar fracture secondary to a motor vehicle accident. Lauren has progressed well; however, she has noticed increased purulent discharge from her incision at an area that is having difficulty closing. Upon assessment, increased skin temperature and redness around the incision was also noted. What was done?

The physician was notified, and the patient was sent for a follow-up visit. Tests showed the patient had developed an infection at the incision site, and she was placed on a broad-spectrum antibiotic. Whirlpool treatment was initiated, maintaining the water at 98° F to 100° F for 20 minutes, three times per week. General wound care was provided, and her rehabilitation schedule continued in a modified fashion.

3 Brittany is a 30-year-old female who suffered a bimalleolar fracture and had ORIF 16 weeks ago. Brittany has returned to her position as an art teacher, which requires her to stand frequently throughout the day. Since returning, Brittany reports she has had increased lateral ankle pain, which is greater in the afternoon and evening. How did the therapist treat this patient?

Brittany was assessed and it was found that her AROM and strength were within normal limits. She had the option of having the hardware removed once healing occurred; however, Brittany refused to have additional surgery. Brittany was issued a home TENS unit and was instructed in its use, as well as precautions and contraindications. She was also issued an ankle-stabilizing orthosis (ASO) brace to wear during work and with activities requiring prolonged walking and running. Finally, the therapist discussed various options for allowing changes in the length of time she stands during the day (the therapist recommended she use a stool while lecturing).

4 Sarah is a 23-year-old college senior who suffered a right ankle bimalleolar fracture and had ORIF 6 weeks ago. On arriving to the clinic for a treatment session, she complained of experiencing increased right calf pain exacerbated with weight bearing. Sarah also reported that she noticed her right calf felt "hot" to touch as compared with the left. She has not slept well the last two nights secondary to the previously mentioned symptoms. How did the therapist proceed?

Further assessment by the therapist revealed a positive Homans sign at the right calf. The physician was notified, and the patient was sent immediately to the hospital for an ultrasound, which showed the patient had developed a deep vein thrombosis (DVT). The patient was admitted to the hospital where anticoagulant therapy was initiated.

5 Braeden is a 19-year-old male who suffered a bimalleolar fracture 20 weeks ago with corresponding ORIF. He received physical therapy at another facility after his surgery for 10 weeks. Braeden has been referred to the therapist's facility with a chief complaint of pain inferior to the lateral malleolus and at the Achilles tendon insertion. Pain is minimal in the morning and progressively worsens throughout the day. The patient was noted to have decreased calcaneal abduction and demonstrated increased pronation on the affected side. The patient was

also noted to have 5° of dorsiflexion. How did the therapist proceed?

Grades III and IV joint mobilization was performed for AP talar glides and grades III and IV physiologic calcaneal abduction. A contract-relax technique was initiated to increase dorsiflexion. The patient was then taught how to perform the contract-relax technique as a home exercise. Exercises to increase strength in the peroneals and the gastrocnemius and soleus complex were also performed. Additionally, a 3° wedge was inserted into the right shoe medially to decrease the angle of pronation. The patient was later casted for custom orthotics.

6 Eric is a 26-year-old football player who injured his ankle when his foot got caught under another player. His injury resulted in a compound fracture to both his right tibia and fibula. His injury was treated with ORIF, and he is presenting to the therapist for his initial evaluation 8 weeks following the surgery. He was non–weight-bearing for the entire period before beginning therapy. How should the therapist begin treatment of Eric at this time?

The initial assessment should include examination of the ankle's active and passive range of motion within limits of his pain tolerance. The therapist should inspect the surgical sites for signs of possible infection. Strength testing should be deferred at this stage. Treatment may begin with modalities to promote healing and reduce excessive scar tissue formation, such as infrared light, ultrasound, and scar massage if warranted. If visible atrophy of the gastroc/soleus complex is noted, the therapist can take circumferential or volumetric measurements and initiate high-voltage electrical stimulation. The patient should be given a home program, including active and active assistive range of motion exercises, for plantar flexion, dorsiflexion, inversion, and eversion, which should not induce pain. Eric then should be educated on how to progress with his gait training. For example, he should start with bilateral axillary crutches and WBAT. Once he has proper mechanics and is able to ambulate without pain he can be weaned to one axillary crutch on the contralateral side, then to a single point cane, and finally no assistive device.

7 Lorraine is 30-year-old female who injured her ankle in a rollover all terrain vehicle (ATV) accident. She was found to have fractured her left distal tibia, along with a Lis Franc fracture in her left foot. Both injuries were addressed with ORIF. After undergoing rehabilitation for the first 4 months, she has now begun to return to work at a retail sales position. She reports increased lateral foot pain, lateral swelling, and pain along the distal medial tibia extending into her arch. How would the therapist address her complaints?

Upon evaluation of Lorraine's gait mechanics, a collapse of the midtarsal joints was found during the stance phase of gait. To address this and her medial distal tibia tenderness, custom orthotics were fabricated to help support the midtarsal area during ambulation. Lorraine also was noted to have restricted dorsiflexion of the talocrural joint, restricted cuboid mobility, and limited first metatarsophalangeal joint mobility. The following manual therapy techniques were used to improve her joint mobility: talocrural distraction; anterior and posterior glides of the talus; anterior/posterior glides of the cuboid; and traction with anterior/posterior glides of the first metatarsophalangeal joint. Lorraine was educated on trying to take more frequent breaks while working, so that her ankle does not become as swollen following her work activities.

8 Kate is a 21-year-old who fractured both of her ankles in a fall. She required both external fixation and ORIF procedures to restore proper alignment and to allow for proper bone healing. Kate was non–weight-bearing for 4 months after the injury. She now presents to PT approximately 1 year after the injury. She has recently began to return to running and is complaining of bilateral Achilles tendinitis. What type of exercise program should Kate be placed on to address her problem?

Eccentric exercise programs have been shown to have beneficial results in tendon strengthening. However, initially the patient must be started at an exercise intensity that does not exacerbate the tissue while it is still inflamed. The initial treatments may consist of modalities to reduce pain, swelling, or tenderness in the area and begin a gentle gastroc/soleus towel stretching program. The exercise progression may begin starting with double leg calf raises, three sets of 15 repetitions, adding one to two sets every week of treatment, depending on the patient's response to the exercise program. After 4 to 6 weeks of double leg calf raises, the patient may progress to single leg calf raises and start the program over along the same progression as before. Kate will start the exercise by standing on the edge of a step and raising up on her toes as high as she can. After pausing at the apex, she should then start slowly lowering herself back to the ground, if possible, at a 5- to 7-second descent is ideal.

9 Sally is a 45-year-old female who fractured her left ankle when she fell off of her horse. She was treated with ORIF in the days following the injury and has progressed through rehabilitation after initially being non–weight-bearing for 8 weeks. She is now approximately 4 months out from surgery and is ambulating without any assistive device. Sally has been complaining of left medial knee pain and swelling with prolonged weight-bearing activities. Upon further evaluation the therapist is concerned of possible cartilage/meniscal pathology, how should the therapist proceed?

After a severe traumatic injury, such as an ankle fracture that requires ORIF, the immediate concern is to stabilize the injury and prevent any secondary injury; for example, compartment syndrome or infection. Sometimes in these types of injuries, other pathology further up the kinetic chain may not be recognized until later in the treatment process once the patient begins to perform more aggressive weight-bearing activities. The patient should be referred back to her orthopedist, and the therapist should contact the orthopedist and relay his or her concerns and objective findings. In Sally's case, she had medial joint line tenderness, occasional crepitus, and pain with stair climbing, as well as positive Apley compression and Thessaly meniscal special tests. The patient underwent imaging after seeing the orthopedist and was found to have a medial meniscus tear, which was addressed with arthroscopy.

10 Allan is a 25-year-old basketball player who fractured his right ankle while landing on an opponents foot during a game. His fracture was stabilized with ORIF, and he was placed in a controlled ankle movement (CAM) boot approximately 4 weeks after the procedure. He has been progressing with his rehabilitation and is now 6 months after his surgery. He has recently begun sport-specific activities, such as running, jumping, and cutting. Describe a proper exercise progression for Allan at this stage of his rehabilitation.

Before beginning higher impact activities, including running, jumping, and cutting required for sports like basketball, the patient must demonstrate necessary lower extremity strength and sufficient soft tissue and joint mobility before attempting more vigorous activities. Also, the patient should have been placed on a neuromuscular and perturbation training program with an emphasis on landing mechanics and proprioception before beginning the more advanced weight-bearing activities. To begin, Allan may begin jumping either in a pool or on devices (i.e., Shuttle MVP) that allow for partial weight-bearing—first beginning with bilateral lower extremity exercises and then progressing to unilateral. Once he has progressed through this phase, Allan may begin more full weight-bearing exercises, such as jump squats, single leg hops over obstacles, and multidirectional lunges. The last phase should incorporate sport-specific agility drills while maintaining focus on proper mechanics and joint protection. For example, Allan may perform a shuttle drill with a different basketball skill or maneuver required at each station of the drill.

11 Angela is a 55-year-old female who experienced an open fracture of her left ankle when she fell off of a step. She underwent surgical repair of the injury, but had issues with wound closure following the procedure and required a skin graft. Angela is a diabetic and has issues with circulation to her distal extremities secondary to her diabetes. She presents to physical therapy 8 weeks after the injury. Her wound has still not fully healed but does not demonstrate signs of infection (i.e., warmth, redness, tenderness, or drainage surrounding the wound). What should the therapist do to assist with wound healing at this stage in her recovery.

The therapist should contact the referring doctor to relay concerns regarding the patient's slow wound healing. Recently, newer technologies have been developed to assist those who may have issues with wound healing. Treatment options that may be considered by the surgeon and therapist include hyperbaric oxygen treatments, infrared light therapy, microcurrent/nanocurrent electrical stimulation devices, and traditional wound care (using a variety of topical creams and/or dressings). Angela should be educated on not trying to stress the healing area excessively while the tissue is still fragile; for example, being on her feet for a number of hours continuously leading to increased swelling, which may further delay healing. Also, the patient needs to be educated on reducing other lifestyle factors, which might impede healing, such as smoking or illicit drug use, nutritional status, proper rest and recovery, or any medications that may delay healing. Wound healing needs to be obtained first before the patient may progress to the next phase of the rehabilitation process.

REFERENCES

1. Elliot S, Wood J: The archeological survey of Nubia: Report for 1907-1908, vol 2, Cairo, 1910 Ministry of Finance, Egypt, National Printing Department.
2. Adams F: The genuine works of Hippocrates, London, 1849, C and J Adlard.
3. Jarde O, et al: Malleolar fractures: Predictive factors for secondary osteoarthritis. Retrospective study of 32 cases. Acta Orthop Belg 16(4):382-388, 2000.
4. Lauge-Hansen N: "Ligamentous" ankle fractures: Diagnosis and treatment. Acta Chir Scand 97:544-550, 1949.
5. Lambotte A: Chirurgie operatoire des fractures, Paris, 1913, Masson & Cie.
6. Danis R: Le vrai but et les dangers de l'ostesynthese. Lyon Chirugie 51:740-743, 1956.
7. Allgower M, Muller ME, Willenegger H: Techniques of internal fixation of fractures, Berlin, 1965, Springer-Verlag.
8. Lantz BA, et al: The effect of concomitant chondral injuries accompanying operatively reduced malleolar fractures. Int Orthop Trauma 5(2):125-128, 1991.
9. Wiss DA, editor: Masters techniques in orthopaedics: Fractures, ed 3, Philadelphia, 2012, Lippincott Williams & Wilkins.
10. Michelson JD: Ankle fractures resulting from rotational injuries. J Am Acad Orthop Surg 11:403-412, 2003.
11. Wiesel SW, editor: Operative techniques in orthopaedic surgery, Philadelphia, 2011, Lippincott Williams & Wilkins.
12. Jensen SL, et al: Epidemiology of ankle fractures: A prospective population-based study of 212 cases in Aalborg, Denmark. Acta Orthop Scand 69:48-50, 1998.
13. Loren GJ, Ferkel RD: Arthroscopic assessment of occult intraarticular injury in acute ankle fractures. Arthroscopy 18(4):412-421, 2002.
14. Pagliaro AJ, Michelson JD, Mizel MS: Results of operative fixation of unstable ankle fractures in geriatric patients. Foot Ankle Int 22:399-402, 2001.
15. Hintermann B, et al: Arthroscopic findings in acute fractures of the ankle. J Bone Joint Surg 82B:345-351, 2000.
16. Loren GJ, Ferkel RD: Arthroscopic strategies in fracture management of the ankle. In Chow JCY, editor: Advanced Arthroscopy, New York, 2001, Springer.
17. Godsiff SP, et al: A comparative study of early motion and immediate plaster splintage after internal fixation of unstable fractures of the ankle. Injury 24(8):529-530, 1993.
18. Redfern DJ, Sauvé PS, Sakellariou A: Investigation of incidence of superficial peroneal nerve injury following ankle fracture. Foot Ankle Int 24(10):771-774, 2003.
19. Anand N, Klenarman L: Ankle fractures in the elderly: MVA versus ORIF. Injury 24:116-120, 1993.
20. Chaudhary SB, et al: Complications of ankle fracture in patients with diabetes. J Am Acad Orthop Surg 16:159-170, 2008.
21. Lin CWC, Moseley AM, Refshauge KM: Rehabilitation for ankle fractures in adults (review). Cochrane Collaboration 3, 2008.
22. Kleinman Y, Cahn A: Conservative management of Achilles tendon wounds: Results of a retrospective study. Ostomy Wound Manage 57(4):32-40, 2011.
23. Thomas G, Whalley H, Modi C: Early mobilization of operatively fixed ankle fractures: a systematic review. Foot Ankle Int 30(7):624-666, 2009.
24. Ahl T, et al: Early mobilization of operated on ankle fractures. Acta Orthop Scand 64:95-99, 1993.
25. Hovis WD, Bucholtz RW: Polyglycolide bioabsorbable screws in the treatment of ankle fractures. Foot Ankle Int 18(3):128-131, 1997.
26. Eskes A, et al: Hyperbaric oxygen therapy: solution for difficult to heal acute wounds? Systematic review. World J Surg 35(3):535-542, 2010.
27. Landau Z, Migdal M, Lipovsky A, et al: Visible light-induced healing of diabetic or venous foot ulcers: a placebo-controlled double blind study, Photomed Laser Surg. World J Surg 29(6):399-404, 2011.
28. Lee B, et al: Ultra-low microcurrent in the management of diabetes mellitus, hypertension and chronic wounds: Report of twelve cases and discussion of mechanism of action. Int J Med Sci 7:1, 2010.
29. Brown OL, Dirschl DR, Obremskey WT: Incidence of hardware-related pain and its affect on functional outcomes after open reduction and internal fixation of ankle fractures. J Orthop Trauma 15(4):271-274, 2001.
30. Belcher GL, et al: Functional outcome analysis of operatively treated malleolar fractures. J Orthop Trauma 11:106-109, 1997.
31. Donatelli R: Biomechanics of the foot and ankle, Philadelphia, 1996, FA Davis.
32. Hasegawa S, et al: Effect of early implementation of electrical stimulation to prevent muscle atrophy and weakness in patients after anterior cruciate ligament reconstruction. J Electromyogr Kinesiol 21(4):622-630, 2011.
33. Anderson IF, et al: Osteochondral fractures of the dome of the talus. J Bone Joint Surg 71A:1143-1152, 1989.
34. Rozzi SL, et al: Balance training for persons with functionally unstable ankles. J Orthop Sports Phys Ther 8:478-486, 1999.
35. Schmidt R, et al: The potential for training of proprioceptive and coordinative parameters in patients with chronic ankle instability. Z Orthop Ihre Grenzgeb 143(2):227-232, 2005.

ADDITIONAL READINGS

Eilis E, Rosenbaum D: A multi-station proprioceptive exercise program in patients with ankle instability. Med Sci Sports Exerc 33(12):1991-1998, 2001.

Hommen JP, Ferkel RD: Arthroscopic treatment of the juvenile Tillaux ankle fracture, submitted for publication.

Hughes SPF: A historical view of fractures involving the ankle joint. Mayo Clin Proc 50:611, 1975.

Lauge N: Fractures of the ankle. Analytic historic survey as the basis of new, experimental, retrogenologic and clinical investigations. Arch Surg 56:259, 1948.

Leeds HC, Ehrlich MG: Instability of the distal tibiofibular syndesmosis after bimalleolar and trimalleolar ankle fractures. J Bone Joint Surg Am 66(4):490, 1984.

Michelson J, Curtis M, Magid D: Controversies in ankle fractures. Foot Ankle 14:170-174, 1993.

Renström PA: Persistently painful sprained ankle. J Am Acad Orthop Surg 2:270-280, 1994.

Simanski CJ, et al: Functional treatment and early weightbearing after an ankle fracture: A prospective study. J Orthop Trauma 20(2):108-114, 2006.

Stone JW: Osteochondral lesions of the talar dome. J Am Acad Orthop Surg 4:63, 1996.

Taga I, et al: Articular cartilage lesions in ankles with lateral ligament injury. An orthoscopic study. Am J Sports Med 21:120, 1993.

Weber BG: De verletzungen des oberon Sprunggellenkes, Aktuelle Probleme in der Chirurgie, Bern, 1966, Verlag Hans Huber.

CHAPTER 30

Ankle Arthroscopy

Tom Burton, Danny Arora, Benjamin Cornell, Lisa Maxey, Richard D. Ferkel

The first arthroscopic inspection of a cadaveric joint was performed by Takagi in Japan in 1918.[1] In 1939 he reported on the arthroscopic examination of an ankle joint in a human patient.[1] With the advent of fiberoptic light transmission, video cameras, instruments for small joints, and distraction devices, arthroscopy has become an important diagnostic and therapeutic modality for disorders of the ankle. Arthroscopic examination of the ankle joint allows direct visualization during stress testing of intraarticular structures and ligaments about the ankle joint. Various arthroscopic procedures have been developed with less attendant morbidity and mortality to patients.[2-6] With the advent of better, smaller joint arthroscopes and instrumentation, and the introduction of more efficient noninvasive distraction devices, ankle arthroscopy is now state of the art. It has become a standard procedure in many institutions as a diagnostic and therapeutic tool for the practicing surgeon.

SURGICAL INDICATIONS AND CONTRAINDICATIONS

Foot and ankle arthroscopy has become a valuable adjuvant to the diagnosis and treatment of an increasing amount of disorders. Diagnostic indications (Box 30-1) for ankle arthroscopy include unexplained pain, swelling, stiffness, instability, hemarthrosis, locking, and abnormal snapping or popping.

Operative indications for ankle arthroscopy include loose body removal, excision of anterior tibiotalar osteophytes, débridement of soft tissue impingement and arthrofibrosis, and treatment of osteochondral lesions and ankle instability. Other indications include arthrodesis for posttraumatic degenerative arthritis and treatment for ankle fractures and postfracture defects.

Absolute contraindications for ankle arthroscopy include localized soft tissue or systemic infection, and severe degenerative joint disease (DJD). With end-stage DJD, occasionally successful distraction may not be possible, precluding visualization of the ankle joint. Relative contraindications include complex regional pain syndrome (CRPS), moderate DJD with restricted range of motion (ROM), severe edema, and tenuous vascular supply.

PATIENT EVALUATION

Successful outcomes following ankle arthroscopy depend on accurate diagnosis and concise preoperative planning. It is important to understand the nature of the patient's complaint and gather the following information: date of injury, duration and severity of symptoms, provocative events, previous injuries and presence of any redness, swelling, instability, stiffness, locking, or popping.

A general medical examination should be obtained, with special attention to rheumatologic disorders. The physical examination should include: inspection, palpation, ROM, and special tests. The contralateral side should always be inspected for comparison. Stability of the ankle and the subtalar joint should be evaluated. Often, a local anesthetic agent can be injected into a specific joint to aid in diagnosis.

Routine blood tests should be performed to check for systemic and rheumatologic conditions and infection. Aspiration of the ankle joint and analysis of the joint fluid can be helpful in distinguishing inflammatory from septic conditions of the ankle joint.

Routine radiographs (anteroposterior [AP], lateral, and mortise view) should be obtained for all patients. Stress radiographs can provide useful information when instability is suspected. Computed tomography (CT) and/or magnetic resonance imaging (MRI) are often helpful in evaluating soft tissue and bony disorders about the foot and ankle. Three-phase bone scans can also aid in distinguishing soft tissue from bony pathology.

SURGICAL TECHNIQUE

Ankle arthroscopy is usually performed in one of four ways: (1) in the supine position, (2) with the knee bent 90° over the end of the table, (3) in the decubitus position, or (4) in

BOX 30-1 Surgical Indications and Contraindications

Indications

Loose bodies
Anterior tibiotalar osteophytes
Soft tissue impingement
Osteochondral lesions
Synovectomy
Lateral instability
Arthrodesis
Ankle fractures

Contraindications

Infection*
Severe degenerative joint disease*
Complex regional pain syndrome[†]
Moderate degenerative joint disease[†]
Severe edema[†]
Tenuous vascular supply[†]

*Absolute contraindications.
[†]Relative contraindications.

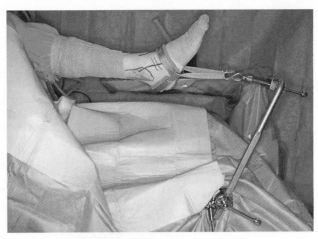

Fig. 30-1 Setup for ankle and foot arthroscopy with the patient's thigh secured on a support and soft tissue distraction applied across the ankle.

the prone position for posterior ankle arthroscopy. The method of choice is a surgeon's preference, while taking into account specific surgical circumstances. Different types and sizes of arthroscopic equipment can be used depending on surgeon's preference and availability of equipment. The procedure described is that used most commonly by the senior author of this chapter; a more detailed description of ankle arthroscopy can be found in his textbook.[2]

Positioning

The patient is taken to the operating room and placed in the supine position. The hip is flexed to 45°, and the thigh is placed onto a well-padded support placed proximal to the popliteal fossa and distal to the tourniquet. The lower extremity (LE) is then prepared and draped so that good access is available posteriorly. A tourniquet is applied as needed. A noninvasive distraction strap is placed over the foot and ankle. Distraction is used to separate the distal tibia from the talus so that at least 4 mm of joint space opening is obtained (Fig. 30-1). Without distraction, the surgeon has difficulty positioning the arthroscopic instruments in the ankle without scuffing the articular cartilage; visualizing the central and posterior portions of the ankle also is difficult without adequate joint separation. The distraction device is carefully positioned so as not to injure the neurovascular structures, and approximately 30 to 40 lb of force is placed across the ankle for no more than 60 to 90 minutes. Before applying the distraction strap, the surgeon should identify and outline the dorsalis pedis artery, the deep peroneal nerve, saphenous vein, tibialis anterior tendon, peroneus tertius tendon, and superficial peroneal nerve and its

branches on the skin with a marker. Identification of the superficial peroneal nerve and its branches is facilitated by inverting and plantar flexing the foot and flexing the toes.

Arthroscopic Portal Placement

The surgeon uses three primary portals or access areas to insert the arthroscope and instrumentation (Fig. 30-2). These include the anteromedial, anterolateral, and posterolateral portals. Accessory portals can be used as needed but are rarely required. Portals are made by nicking the skin only, then with the use of a clamp spreading through the subcutaneous tissue and into the ankle joint. The surgeon must take great care to avoid injuring the neurovascular and tendinous structures.

The anteromedial portal is established first and a 2.7-mm, 30° oblique small joint videoscope is inserted. The surgeon establishes the anterolateral portal under direct vision, using extreme care to avoid injuring the superficial peroneal nerve branches. The arthroscope is then positioned in the posterior portion of the ankle so the posterolateral portal can be made just lateral to the Achilles tendon, entering the ankle beneath the posterior ankle ligaments.

In recent years, techniques have been developed for arthroscopy in the prone position, using the posterolateral and posteromedial portals. This allows access for treatment of a variety of problems, including osteochondral lesions of the talus (OLT), os trigonum, and flexor hallucis longus tendinitis or tears.[7-10] The senior author of this chapter occasionally uses this position.

Arthroscopic Examination

A 21-point arthroscopic examination of the ankle is performed to ensure a systematic evaluation.[2] After completing the arthroscopic evaluation, the surgeon identifies the pathology and treats it accordingly, using small joint instrumentation ranging in size from 2.0 to 3.5 mm. These instruments include baskets, knives, intraarticular shavers, and burrs. Scar tissue is removed using baskets and an

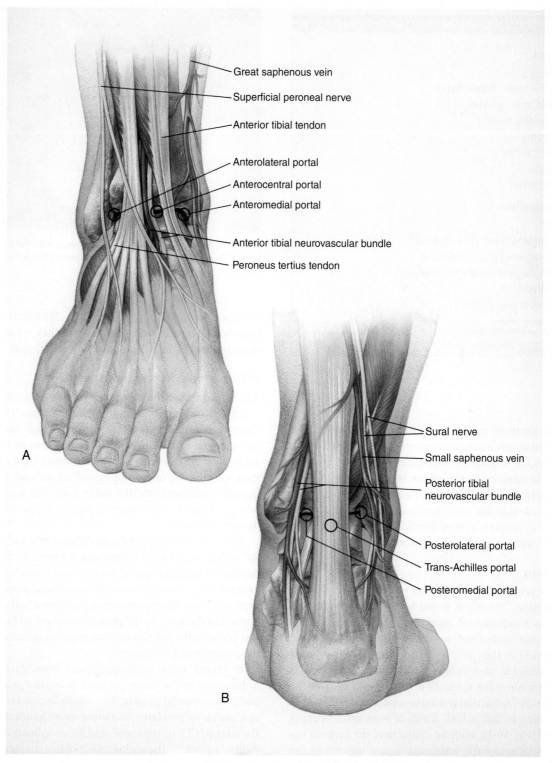

Great saphenous vein

Superficial peroneal nerve

Anterior tibial tendon

Anterolateral portal

Anterocentral portal

Anteromedial portal

Anterior tibial neurovascular bundle

Peroneus tertius tendon

A

Sural nerve

Small saphenous vein

Posterior tibial
neurovascular bundle

Posterolateral portal

Trans-Achilles portal

Posteromedial portal

B

Fig. 30-2 A, Anterior arthroscopic ankle portals. The anterocentral portal is usually not used. **B,** Posterior arthroscopic ankle portals. The Achilles portal is not normally used. (From Ferkel RD: An illustrated guide to small joint arthroscopy, Andover, MA, 1989, Smith & Nephew Endoscopy.)

intraarticular shaver. Synovectomy is performed with an intraarticular shaver (Fig. 30-3). OLT are carefully evaluated and, if they are found to be loose, excised with a ring curette and banana knife. The surgeon can use transmalleolar or transtalar drilling, and/or microfracture techniques, to promote fibrocartilage formation and new circulation in the avascular area (Fig. 30-4). Acute ankle fractures can be evaluated arthroscopically; the surgeon can perform percutaneous screw insertion while monitoring fracture reduction arthroscopically (see Chapter 29).

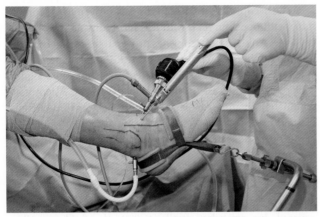

Fig. 30-3 Arthroscopic surgery of the right ankle. Notice the small joint arthroscope is in the anteromedial portal, the intraarticular shaver is in the anterolateral portal, and inflow is coming in through the posterolateral portal.

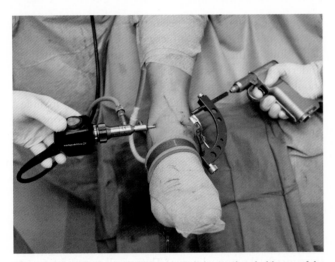

Fig. 30-4 Transmalleolar drilling of a medial osteochondral lesion of the talus in a right ankle. Notice the arthroscope is visualizing through the anterolateral portal.

After the procedure is performed, the wounds are closed with a nonabsorbable suture, and a compression dressing and posterior splint are applied.

Postoperative Plan

The patient remains non–weight bearing on crutches for 1 week. The splint and the stitches are then removed. If an osteochondral lesion has been treated with one of the previously mentioned methods, the patient may be required to be non-weight bearing for 4 to 6 weeks. During this time, the patient is initially in a removable splint and is allowed to exercise the ankle actively to promote new fibrocartilage formation. The type of arthroscopic procedure performed and individual patient goals determine weight-bearing status and rehabilitation.

SOFT TISSUE IMPINGEMENT

Ankle sprains are one of the most common injuries in sports. One inversion sprain occurs per 10,000 persons per day. It

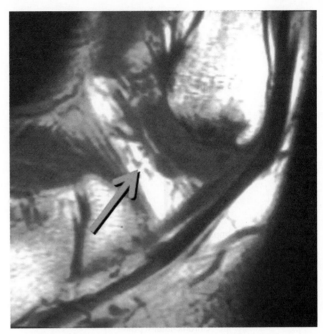

Fig. 30-5 Sagittal T-1 weighted MRI showing low-signal intensity, consistent with anterolateral soft tissue impingement of the ankle.

has been estimated that 10% to 50% of patients will have some degree of chronic ankle pain.

The primary cause of chronic ankle pain after an ankle sprain is soft tissue impingement. This can occur along the syndesmosis, the syndesmotic interval between the tibia and fibula, or the medial, lateral, and/or posterior gutters. Most commonly it is located anterolaterally given the common occurrence of a common inversion ankle sprain.[11] Diagnosis is done by careful history, physical examination, and selective injections. MRI can also be very helpful in assessing the problem (Fig. 30-5).[12]

The sequence of lateral ankle pain after a sprain can be explained as shown in Fig. 30-6.

A distraction device may be necessary to identify some of the synovial pathology involving the posterolateral corner of the ankle, because such identification can be sometimes difficult. The inflamed synovium, thickened adhesive bands, osteophytes, and loose bodies are débrided arthroscopically using motorized shavers and burrs, graspers, and baskets (Fig. 30-7).

Postoperatively, patients are splinted for 1 week, and then put into a CAM (controlled angle motion) walker for 2 to 3 weeks. Subsequently, they wear a soft ankle brace and begin formal physiotherapy. Return to activity or sport is allowed only after all rehabilitation goals are achieved.

Arthroscopic treatment of anterolateral soft tissue impingement of the ankle has been proven successful at alleviating chronic ankle pain after an inversion sprain. Numerous authors have reported a good to excellent outcome in approximately 80% to 85% of patients.[11,13,14]

OSTEOCHONDRAL LESIONS

Controversy persists regarding the cause, treatment, and prognosis of osteochondral and chondral lesions of the

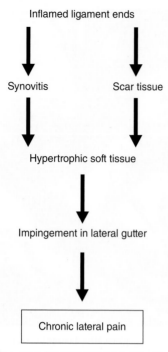

Fig. 30-6 Sequence of lateral ankle pain.

ankle. OLT comprise 4% of all osteochondral defects. Males are slightly more predominant than females between the ages of 20 to 30 years. Medial talar dome lesions are more common than lateral.

There are many possible causes for OLT. Trauma is believed to play a major role, but there are also instances where atraumatic presentations are possible, secondary to idiopathic avascular necrosis. The diagnosis of OLT requires a high index of suspicion because symptoms may be mild and imaging is not readily available. Patients may present in an acute traumatic setting, complaining of persistent ankle pain (i.e., inversion ankle sprain), or may have a chronic complaint of ongoing ankle pain. The literature has shown that the location of pain is not correlative with the location of the lesion, therefore adding to the vague nature of the condition. Other common symptoms include stiffness, deep aching pain, swelling, clicking, locking, or even instability.

OLT that do not respond to conservative treatment are treated arthroscopically. Most chronic OLT in adults are loose and have to be excised. The osteochondral lesion bed is then microfractured and/or drilled. Occasional they can be pinned back (Fig. 30-8).

Postoperatively, patients are splinted for 1 week in neutral position. Once the portal incisions have healed (approximately 1 to 2 weeks), ROM exercises are begun, since early motion appears to facilitate cartilage healing. Patients remain non–weight bearing for 6 to 8 weeks, depending on the size of the lesion. Usually by 4 to 6 weeks, patients start physical therapy in the pool and then progress to land exercises. Cutting, shear stress, or impact activities are avoided for 6 months.

Arthroscopic treatment of OLT has proven to be comparable with open surgery, with less morbidity and less recovery time. Ankle arthroscopy has proven to be one of the most reliable methods in classifying OLT. Recently, clinical management of articular cartilage defects has generated significant research interest in the orthopedic world. Attempts to stimulate a hyaline cartilage response have included transplantation of various cells, including periosteal and perichondral tissues, woven carbon-fiber pads, and osteochondral autografts/ allografts.

In addition, chondrocyte transplantation has been studied extensively now in the United States. With further research, it is hoped that osteochondral defects can be successfully covered by articular cartilage instead of fibrocartilage replacement.[9]

OVERALL SURGICAL OUTCOMES

Numerous papers have been published regarding the outcome of arthroscopic surgery of the ankle. Results vary depending on the type of procedure and the study that was undertaken.[15-23] In general, a large percentage of patients should achieve a successful outcome depending on the nature of the pathology. Expectations after surgery include a full ROM, strength, and full function. The preoperative ROM, strength, and severity of the pathologic condition heavily influence the results.

COMPLICATIONS

All arthroscopic procedures have potential complications.[24] The most common complications in foot and ankle arthroscopy are injuries to the neurovascular structures, especially the superficial peroneal nerve.[8] The overall complication rate has varied with the transition from invasive to noninvasive distraction. Current complication rates are between 6.8% and 9%.[25,26] The physical therapist should report to the physician any problems they note after surgery. Sometimes, excessive massage over the portals can even irritate the nerves and cause tingling and numbness. In general, we wait 2 to 3 weeks to initiate physical therapy after ankle and foot arthroscopy to avoid wound problems and increased pain while the soft tissues are healing.

THERAPY GUIDELINES FOR REHABILITATION

Several factors must be considered in planning a successful rehabilitation program for the postoperative ankle arthroscopy patient. Rehabilitation guidelines can vary greatly for the same injury depending on the patient's age, severity/chronicity of injury, healing rate of tissue, general medical health, and previous level of activity. The physician, physical therapist, and patient must work together as a team to create an appropriate, effective, and efficient treatment plan that will allow the patient to optimize his or her recovery. The phases in each of the following rehabilitation protocols may

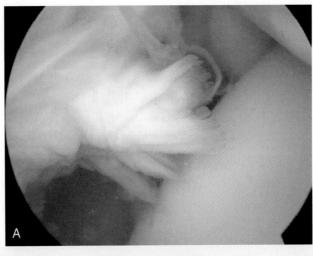

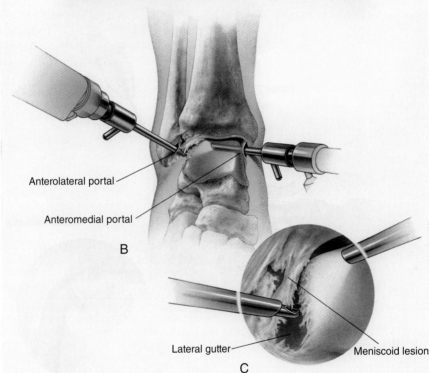

Anterolateral portal

Anteromedial portal

B

Lateral gutter

Meniscoid lesion

C

Fig. 30-7 Soft tissue impingement of the ankle. **A,** Arthroscopic picture in a right ankle of synovitis and scarring of the anterolateral talar dome. **B,** Débridement of anterolateral soft tissue impingement with synovitis and fibrosis at the anterolateral gutter in a right ankle. **C,** Arthroscopic drawing showing the scar bands and inflammation as a portion of the anterior inferior talofibular ligament fascicle abrading the lateral talar dome in a right ankle. (*B and C from Ferkel RD: An illustrated guide to small joint arthroscopy, Andover, MA, 1989, Smith & Nephew Endoscopy.*)

overlap 1 to 3 weeks depending on the factors mentioned previously and individual progress.

The physical therapist should consider the following 6 basic principles when planning an ankle rehabilitation protocol:

1. Protect the healing tissue. What tissues were directly and indirectly affected during the procedure? Was the tissue healthy or frayed?

2. It is not just about strengthening. Control of acute symptoms and restoration of normalized mobility need to be addressed before embarking on an ankle strengthening regimen. Incorporation of propriocep-

tive training in conjunction with the patient's strengthening program will improve overall outcomes.

3. Minimize the effects of immobilization.

4. Encourage a neutral subtalar position during exercise to optimize functionally efficient training. This may require orthotics.

5. The ultimate goal of rehabilitation is to optimize the patient's function, minimize pain, and restore the patient to a reasonable and acceptable quality of life.

6. Take into account the whole patient. The ankle is just one part of the patient's kinetic chain. It is this kinetic chain that needs to be addressed in optimizing

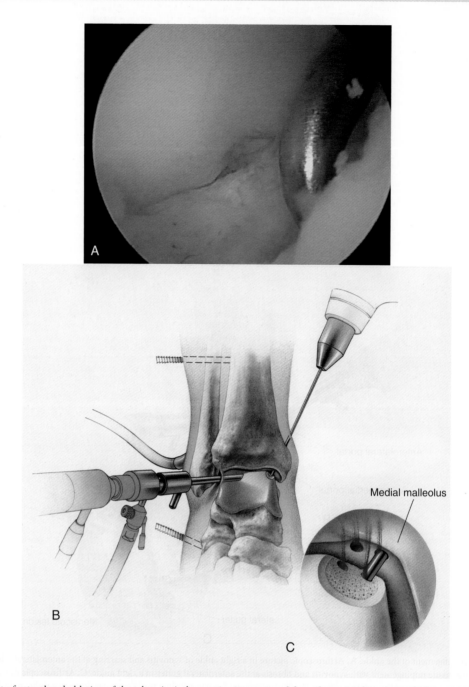

Medial malleolus

Fig. 30-8 Treatment of osteochondral lesion of the talus. **A,** Arthroscopic picture viewed from the posterolateral portal of an osteochondral lesion of the medial talar dome with microfracture holes being placed through the anteromedial portal in a right ankle. **B,** Transmalleolar drilling of the osteochondral lesion through the medial malleolus into the talus, while viewing from the anterolateral portal. **C,** Arthroscopic drawing showing how the K-wire goes through the medial malleolus into the talus to create bleeding channels. (*B* and *C* from Ferkel RD: *An illustrated guide to small joint arthroscopy,* Andover, MA, 1989, Smith & Nephew Endoscopy.)

outcomes. Putting a plan of care that includes the patient's UEs, trunk, core, and LEs will improve successful return to function. Recognizing and addressing any dysfunctions within the kinetic chain will improve functional outcomes and lessen future problems.

The following rehabilitation program was designed for a patient who has chronic pain because of a recurring inversion sprain suffered during the basketball season. The patient underwent an arthroscopic procedure to débride the anterolateral soft tissue because of impingement.

Preoperative Phase

GOALS: Restore functional ROM; normalize gait; apply corrective orthoses to improve mechanical neutrality; gait train with the appropriate assistive device(s), taking into consideration postoperative weight-bearing status; create patient's initial

TABLE 30-1 Ankle Arthroscopy

Phase	Criteria to Progress to This Phase	Anticipated Impairments and Functional Limitations	Intervention	Goal	Rationale
Preoperation	• Physician determines patient is a surgical candidate	• Limited ROM • Poor gait quality • No formal exercise program • Patient uncertainty as to what to expect	• ROM, mobilization, HEP to improve ROM • Gait training specific to assistive device needed and weight-bearing restrictions considering community barriers • Educate patient on an HEP for preoperative and postoperative wk 1 with hand out • Educate patient on surgery and usual postoperative care and timelines	• Restore functional ROM • Normalize gait pattern using the necessary assistive devices following the normal postoperative weight-bearing statuses • Independent HEP to include postoperative HEP • Patient well informed as to upcoming events	• Patient's return of ROM postoperation improves if ROM preoperation is improved • Patient safety is important during early preoperative phase. Poor gait or poor weight-bearing status follow-through could limit overall outcomes • Patient's ability to practice HEP before surgery will improve likelihood of correct HEP technique after and patient compliance • Patients will do better if they have a better understanding of what to expect and what is expected of them

HEP, Home exercise program; *ROM,* range of motion.

postoperative home exercise program (HEP) to bridge the gap from surgery to initiation of formal postoperative rehabilitation with surgeon's input; educate patient as to what the next few months will entail and answer any questions the patient may have (Table 30-1)

Phase I: Acute Phase

Initial Postoperative Examination

Palpation
- Incision site
- Local muscles and tendons (gastrocnemius, soleus, Achilles tendon)
- Check for pitting edema
- Dorsalis pedis pulse

Active range of motion (AROM)/passive range of motion (PROM) measurements
- Dorsiflexion, plantar flexion, inversion, eversion
- Hallux dorsiflexion
- Knee and hip joints

Girth measurements
- Figure 8 or volumetric measure

Strength of uninvolved LE muscles
- Quadriceps
- Hamstrings
- Hip flexors
- Hip extensors
- Hip abductors
- Hip adductors
- Hip internal rotators
- Hip external rotators
- Abdominals

Functional disability measure
- Lower extremity functional scale
- Foot and ankle disability index

Tests requiring caution
- Weight-bearing tests if non–weight bearing
- Strength testing if patient's irritability is high

TIME: Week 1 Postoperative

GOALS: Protect the healing tissue; control postoperative pain and swelling; initiate HEP; maintain patients overall level of fitness (Table 30-2)

Postoperatively, the patient will be in a splint and have weight-bearing restrictions. The patient should follow all postoperative instructions unless told otherwise by the surgeon. Elevation and intermittent icing (including cryopneumatic device) will help control postoperative swelling and pain. The patient's HEP can be initiated based on the program designed preoperatively. This may include upper extremity (UE) AROM/resistive exercises, trunk and core training, isometric strengthening of the glutes, and quads and hamstrings bilaterally with AROM exercises for the uninvolved side.

Phase II: Early Rehabilitation

TIME: Weeks 2 to 5 Postoperative

GOAL: Decrease inflammation and pain; increase ankle ROM; restore soft tissue flexibility/mobility; restore normal gait; progress weight-bearing and non–weight bearing exercises; maintain patient's general cardiovascular fitness (Table 30-3)

The splint can be removed under the surgeon's directive. Patient can progress to weight bearing as tolerated (WBAT)

TABLE 30-2 Ankle Arthroscopy

Phase	Criteria to Progress to This Phase	Anticipated Impairments and Functional Limitations	Intervention	Goal	Rationale
Phase I Postoperative wk 1	• Patient is postoperation and cleared to initiate therapy by the surgeon • Specific precautions, if any, are communicated by the surgeon to the therapist	• Protect healing tissue • Pain and swelling • Patient's overall fitness	• Follow surgeon-directed weight-bearing restrictions • Elevate, frequent ice applications (cryopneumatic device or cold packs) • Patient to begin exercise for noninvolved leg, trunk, and upper extremities • Initiate surgeon-approved home exercise program	• Protect healing tissue • Control pain and swelling • Initiate home exercise program • Maintain overall physical fitness	• Quickly progressing to weight bearing could lead to worsening of symptoms and delay of therapy • Control of pain and swelling will improve patient tolerance to slow, steady progressions • Patient will need to maintain fitness when it is time to safely return to activity

TABLE 30-3 Ankle Arthroscopy

Phase	Criteria to Progress to This Phase	Anticipated Impairments and Functional Limitations	Intervention	Goal	Rationale
Phase II postoperative wk 2-5	• Surgeon has cleared patient for weight bearing as tolerated • Surgeon-approved removal of splint	• Pain and swelling • Immobility • Difficulty walking • Decreased strength • Potential for decreased general fitness	• Ice, electrical stimulation, manual therapy (soft tissue and grade I-II joint mobilizations) • ROM exercises and progress on home exercise program • Gait training • Pool therapy (where available) • Beginning proprioception • General fitness program keeping any operative side restrictions in mind	• Reduced pain and swelling • Improved ROM • Restore soft tissue flexibility • Restore gait with good compliance to weight-bearing restrictions. • Maintain/progress LE, UE, and trunk exercises program.	• Status postsurgery + pain + swelling + immobilization is a common formula for restriction of normal joint and tissue function • Pool therapy offers a very functional means of training a patient while controlling weight bearing

LE, Lower extremity; *ROM,* range of motion; *UE,* upper extremity.

and eventually full weight bearing (FWB) as long as there is no evidence of compensation. If the surgical sites are closed/dry/healed *and* the surgeon has approved, initiate pool therapy when available. Pool therapy should include normalized gait, weight-bearing exercises, balance, and deep water cardiovascular exercises. Land therapy may also begin progressing through AROM exercises, exercise bike, beginning weight-bearing exercises, and passive resistance exercises. Care needs to be taken to not progress the patient too quickly, which could lead to an unwanted inflammatory response and probable setback. General physical fitness should continue to be addressed. PROM, A/AROM, AROM, and joint mobilization can be initiated to address the patient's restricted ROM at the ankle and the surrounding joints. The soft tissue will need to be addressed as well, since it is an integral component of normal joint function Balance activities can also be progressed as the patient is able to tolerate when on land.

Start with static positioned exercises such as single-limb stance (SLS) and progress by varying the standing surfaces (pads/towels/trampoline) and adding dynamic activities such as the PlyoBack.

The following are some ideas to address the goals for phase 2.

Decrease Inflammation and Pain

- Ice and elevate. The incorporation of compression is also very helpful. This can be found in devices like the "Game Ready" and "CryoCuff".
- Electrical stimulation.
- Kinesio tape.
- Soft tissue mobilization. This can help with concomitant spasms that are not uncommon after surgery or injury. Lymphedema techniques can also assist with inflammation.

- Phonophoresis/iontophoresis. The use of ultrasound or electricity to drive medication into the affected area. Oftentimes this can be a steroid. This will need to be cleared by the surgeon. Introduction of medications into an area too soon in the postoperative phase can slow/deter healing.
- Active ankle pumps and circles.
- Grade I to II forefoot, midfoot, and hindfoot joint mobilization. Sustained stretching techniques after ankle and foot mobilization can be used as a beginning technique to stretch the joint capsule. The gentle oscillations involved with grade I and II mobilizations can assist in decreasing swelling and pain. Grade III and IV mobilizations can be used to improve limited joint ROM once pain and swelling have been reduced. The following are a few recommendations for accessory joint mobilizations:
  - Forefoot and metatarsal anterior and posterior glides
  - Talar rock (for calcaneal movement)
  - Anterior glide of the talocrural joint (to increase plantar flexion)
  - Posterior glide of the talocrural joint (to increase dorsiflexion) (see Fig. 29-8)
  - Distraction of the talocrural joint (increase joint play in the mortise) (see Fig. 29-6) and subtalar joint (see Fig. 29-8)
  - Medial and lateral subtalar glides (to increase eversion and inversion) (Fig. 30-9)

Restore Normal Gait

As the patient transitions to partial weight bearing (PWB), WBAT, and FWB, emphasis on proper heel to toe patterning should be made. This will limit compensatory patterning as the patient transitions off of assistive devices. This should carry over into the pool with his or her aquatic program and on land. It needs to be noted that normalizing ROM and strength not only in the involved foot and ankle, but in the proximal lower quarter of the surgical side as well as the nonsurgical side will lessen the possibility of a compensated patterning. Use of orthotics can be considered to assist in supporting the foot in a mechanically correct position.

Increase Ankle Joint ROM and Restore Soft Tissue Flexibility

The use of joint mobilization and soft tissue mobilization combined with exercise is an effective way to improve ROM and soft tissue function. As would be expected, a patient who has had an injury or surgery and is splinted or immobilized can quickly develop restrictions in the soft tissues and joints at and around the affected area. The following techniques should be considered if deemed safe to the surgical area:

- Joint Mobilizations. Progressing to grade II to III joint mobilizations will help restore normalized joint function and decrease capsular restriction.
- Soft tissue mobilization to reduce any soft tissue restrictions including adhesions, spasm, edema.
- Gastroc/soleus, FHL, anterior tib, hamstring, quads, glutes, and hip flexor stretching in weight bearing and non–weight bearing.
- AROM exercises in all planes.

Increase Strength

It is important to progress slowly in a well-paced manner to avoid aggravating the ankle. Aggravation of symptoms could require a 1 to 2 week delay. This can be avoided by making the patient aware that over activity with exercises and or functional weight bearing could lead to irritation and overstressing the healing tissues. Adding a few exercises at a time, working at minimal resistances, and progressing with each success by either adding new exercises or progressing the resistance/repetitions of their present exercises is one method of lessening the risk of any exacerbations. The following are a few examples:

- Manual resistance exercises in all planes. Resistance is mild progressing to moderate.
- Intrinsic muscle strengthening (towel curls, marble pick up) to stabilize the metatarsophalangeal joints during propulsion.
- "Windshield wipers".
- Active resistive exercises using elastic bands (progress from lightest to heavier) (Fig. 30-10).

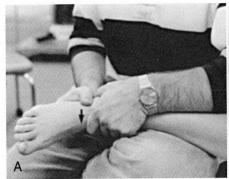
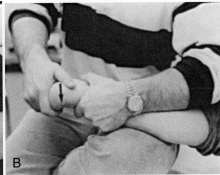

Fig. 30-9 **A,** Medial glide of the calcaneus on the talus to increase calcaneal eversion (pronation). **B,** Lateral glide of the calcaneus on the talus to increase calcaneal inversion (supination). (From Andrews JR, Harrelson GL, Wilk KE: *Physical rehabilitation of the injured athlete,* ed 3, Philadelphia, 2004, Saunders.)

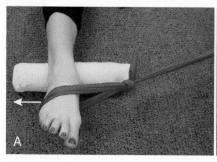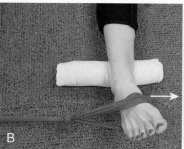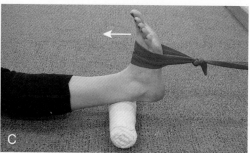

Fig. 30-10 Elastic bands or surgical tubing can be used for resisted exercises. **A,** Eversion; **B,** Inversion; **C,** Dorsiflexion. (From Andrews JR, Harrelson GL, Wilk KE: Physical rehabilitation of the injured athlete, ed 4, Philadelphia, 2012, Saunders.)

- Very low resistance leg presses and total gym within pain-minimized ranges.
- Incorporate weight bearing toe ups/heel ups.
- Continue UE, trunk, and proximal lower quarter exercises.
- Incorporate beginning cardiovascular exercises with the exercise bike at low resistance.

Increase Proprioception

Strengthening the stabilizing muscle groups will offer improved support through movement and increased safety on surfaces that are less stable. It will also offer improved reaction when loss of balance occurs. The following are some examples to help improve this:

- SLS exercises (see Fig. 28-5). Beginning with static flat surface SLS progressing to the use of variable firmness balance pads. With success, progression to dynamic SLS activities such as using the rebounder and Thera-Band. The BAPS (Biomechanical Ankle Platform System) Board can be used in sitting as a mild weight-bearing AROM exercise program and progressed to FWB in stance (see Fig. 28-6).

Maintain Cardiovascular Fitness

It is important to support and progress the overall fitness of the patient while in rehab. A patient's general fitness level is important to his or her ability to sustain activity in a safe, mechanically correct manner. If a body part fatigues but the activity continues, other areas of the body must work harder to sustain that activity. This can lead to overuse issues and potentially to injury. The following are ideas to help sustain fitness:

- Stationary (exercise) bike. There are standard and recumbent options.
- Upper body ergometer.
- Deep water pool running/bicycling.
- High repetition, lower resistance exercises progressed in a manner of a "push" followed by a "pull" exercise without a break between the alternating sets.
- The elliptical is an excellent piece of equipment (once the patient is allowed FWB) that trains a patient in a more functional way with minimal impact.

- There is a variety of unweighting equipment that can be used in conjunction with a treadmill.

Increase Patient Knowledge and Awareness

By educating the patient, the physical therapist is involving the patient as an active participant in his or her own care. The therapist can empower the patient by having a dramatic effect on his or her response to therapy, including how to avoid exacerbations and how to progress with each success. The following are ways to increase a patient's knowledge and awareness:

- Allow the patient a safe enough environment to ask questions. Encourage an open line of communication.
- Give specific instructions concerning the pathology of an injury, how healing occurs, precautions and limitations with activities to avoid flare ups, what to do for themselves in the case of a flare up, keys to progression, expectations/goals with treatment, why each component of the treatment is chosen, and the importance of consistency in treatment.

Phase III: Advanced Rehabilitation

TIME: Weeks 6 to 8 Postoperative
GOALS: Alleviate pain and swelling; normalize functional ROM; normalize functional strength; normalize functional proprioception (Table 30-4)

At this point, the patient should be progressing well with therapy. ROM and strength should be to a point that the patient is able to walk with a near normal gait pattern and progressing with the exercise program that should consist of a variety of weight-bearing and non–weight-bearing exercises.

Alleviate Pain and Swelling

Modalities specific to the issue(s) being treated should continue. Work with the patient to help problem solve if there are mechanical dysfunctions or behaviors that may be precipitating the patient's symptoms. The patient is far enough into the healing phases to consider iontophoresis or phonophoresis (it should still be cleared by the surgeon as to not interrupt any anticipated healing). Encourage the patient to

TABLE 30-4 Ankle Arthroscopy

Phase	Criteria to Progress to This Phase	Anticipated Impairments and Functional Limitations	Intervention	Goal	Rationale
Phase III postoperative wk 6-8	• Able to walk with a normal or near-normal gait pattern • ROM progressing • Strengthening progressing • Pain and swelling reduced • Tolerating a variety of weight-bearing and proprioceptive exercises	• Residual pain and swelling • Residual joint and soft tissue restrictions inhibiting full functional ROM • Strength not full • Potential for decreased general fitness	• Modalities, electrical stimulation as needed • Continued soft tissue and joint mobilizations (progressed to grade III-IV) • Progressed therapeutic exercises, proprioceptive exercises, cardiovascular exercises	• Alleviate pain and swelling • Normalize functional ROM • Normalize functional strength • Normalize functional proprioception • Progressed HEP • Maintain/progress cardiovascular and muscular fitness	• Soft tissue healing timeframes normally indicate 6 wk as a time that soft tissue is healed

HEP, Home exercise program; *ROM,* range of motion.

continue using home applied modalities such as ice. Modification of activities may need to continue with some refining.

Restore Normalized ROM

The patient should be near normal ROM at this point with the goal to achieve normalized ROM during this phase. Mobilizations should continue combined with a strong soft tissue mobilization program and stretching program. ROM during this phase can be made more aggressive with the use of body weight for stretching. Muscle energy can be an effective technique to improve ROM. Continue with general LE ROM as well. Stretching before and after a workout can be very effective. Help the patient in realizing that the efforts made outside of therapy (under the therapist's guidance) will not only bridge the gap between treatments, but continue his or her progress.

Improve Strength

As the patient is able to tolerate, progress the resistances in the therapeutic exercise program:

- Proprioceptive neuromuscular facilitation (PNF) for the ankle and the lower quarter to progress to moderate and maximal resistances.
- Increase elastic band resistance.
- Add resistance to Windshield wipers and towel curls.
- Concentric and eccentric gastrocnemius/soleus training in weight bearing. Increase resistance by either holding onto weights, resistance bands, or weight vests. If using a leg press machine, increase weight.
- Step up/downs. Add resistance and increase heights of steps (see Fig. 28-15).
- Increase resistance and time on exercise bike, elliptical, treadmill. Okay to incorporate elevation.
- Closed kinetic chain exercises using elastic bands, sports cord (start with light resistance and progress) (Fig. 30-11).
- Front and side LE lunges (add weight as tolerated).

- Lateral steps, lateral shuffles, lateral sidestep with elastic band.
- Slide board.
- Continued ongoing UE and trunk strengthening and conditioning.

Improve Proprioception and Balance

Balance and proprioception become more important in this phase because the patient is getting nearer to returning to sport. With that in mind, modifications in the stability of the base of support should be added (i.e., wobble boards, Dyna-Disc, etc.). Additionally, perturbations to balance using manual contact or external loads such as weight or bands will challenge the patient's balance strategies.

- SLS varied surface static and dynamic including uninvolved side resistive exercises
- BAPS board
- Wobble boards
- DynaDisc
- Trampoline for balance weight shifting
- Varied position on incline board (Fig. 30-12)

Continue with precautions and limitations with activities, rate of progression, and specific goals.

Phase IV: Specificity of Sport

TIME: Weeks 9 to 12 Postoperative

GOALS: Provide sport-specific training to allow return to the required physical demands of the sport and the athlete's specific position; independent home and gym exercise program (HEP, GEP) (Table 30-5)

This final phase of rehab is critical to the success of the athlete's return and is oftentimes an area not included in his or her rehabilitation. It is often heard that an athlete can return to play when he or she has full strength and ROM. The problem is full strength and full ROM does not imply

TABLE 30-5 Ankle Arthroscopy

Phase	Criteria to Progress to This Phase	Anticipated Impairments and Functional Limitations	Intervention	Goal	Rationale
Phase IV postoperative wk 9-12	• Surgeon approval • Normal ROM and strength • Pain free • Good proprioception	• Inability to perform sport- and position-specific physical skills at appropriate speeds and efforts	• Sport-and position-specific training progressing to expected full speeds and efforts	• Successful return to full functional activity	• Full ROM and strength do not indicate that an athlete or patient will be able to safely and successfully perform at the speeds and efforts necessary to their sport or position

ROM, Range of motion.

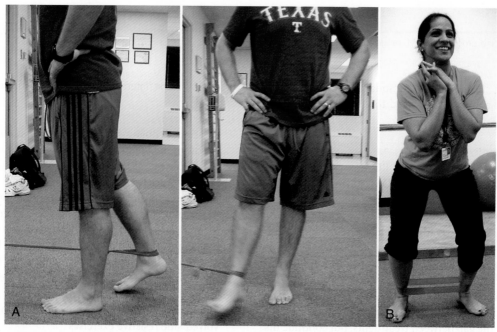

Fig. 30-11 **A,** Contralateral kicks to simulate closed chain pronation and supination. The elastic band goes around the unaffected LE. **B,** Tubing-resisted side steps. (From Andrews JR, Harrelson GL, Wilk KE: *Physical rehabilitation of the injured athlete,* ed 4, Philadelphia, 2012, Saunders.)

readiness to return to a sport safely and successfully. This safety and readiness comes with sport- or position-specific training. As the athlete prepares to return to sports, he or she will need to be progressed through a grouping of higher-level activities to recreate the expected stresses, forces, and movements for his or her sport and position.

It is important to note that an athlete before starting this phase of their rehabilitation should be:

Pain free

Without swelling

Full ROM

Full strength

Good proprioception

During this phase, the athlete will be working on advanced strengthening/proprioceptive/conditioning training. The exercises need to be tailored not only for the physical requirements of the sport, but also the physical requirements of the

position. A football kicker would require a much different training regimen than a football offensive lineman. That said, the following exercises and progressions are useful for rehabilitating a basketball player:

- Running on a treadmill
  - Vary the speeds from jogging to sprint (if available).
  - Vary the elevations.
  - Consider lateral shuffle and carioca.
- Jogging to sprint on flat hard surface
- Resisted running (chute, sport cord)
- Bilateral jumping
- Agility drills (progressing to sport-specific surface and to competition speeds) (see Fig. 28-12)
  - "A" skip (high knees skip)
  - "B" skip (high knees skip with knee extension)
  - Carioca

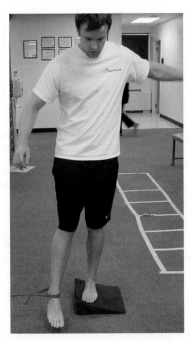

Fig. 30-12 Proprioceptive training on inclined surfaces. The elastic band goes around the unaffected LE. (From Andrews JR, Harrelson GL, Wilk KE: *Physical rehabilitation of the injured athlete*, ed 4, Philadelphia, 2012, Saunders.)

- Back pedaling
- Figure 8 drills
- Cutting drills
- Plyometrics all directions
- Trampoline work
- Four-square hopping (single limb) (Fig. 30-13)
- Sports drills
  - Dribbling
  - Lay ups
  - Shooting
  - Boxing out
  - Pick and rolls
- Videotaping the athlete playing and reviewing the tape with him or her to discuss any noted areas of weakness or biomechanic issues that could predispose him or her to further reinjury or new injury (Correct these areas to remove weakness and mechanical issues).

In review, the athlete can be guided in returning to sports activities with some basic progressions:
- Non–weight-bearing exercises
- PWB exercises
- Full weight-bearing exercises
- Stable surface balance training
- Walking
- Weight-bearing balance board training (start with bilateral and go to unilateral)
- Stepping in all planes
- Cariocas
- Rebounder jogging
- Jogging

- Running
- Bilateral jumping and hopping
- Backpedaling
- Figure 8 running
- Cutting and twisting
- Plyometrics
- Single-leg hopping and jumping

The program should be challenging for the athlete while keeping in mind where that patient is in the healing cycle. Stresses should be progressed when the physiology will allow for it and as the patient is able to demonstrate success. Continue to train the athlete into the physical requirements of his or her sport and position. Safe and successful return is the ultimate goal.

Before ending the formal rehabilitation program, the physical therapist should review proper training technique as it applies to the athlete's HEP. The athlete needs to be independent in his or her program.

If the athlete is part of a team that has training staff, with the athlete's approval, discuss the ongoing training program with the team trainer for consistency during this transition. Speed and duration of these exercises should meet what is expected for the sport or activity to ensure a safe return. If the patient has increased swelling or pain that lasts more than a day or two with these activities, then the patient is not ready to return to that particular level of play. Be sure to communicate with the surgeon the athlete's status in the discharge note. Be sure to comment on the HEP and that the training staff has been contacted.

TROUBLESHOOTING

It is not uncommon after ankle surgery to have soreness, numbness, and tingling over the portal sites. There may also be residual swelling and discoloration. Physical therapy can begin within 1 to 3 weeks postoperatively. If the therapy is too aggressive too soon, significant swelling and pain may develop and lead to loss of motion, loss of strength, decreased functional ability, and diminished confidence. It will take time to reverse this and it can delay therapy for 2 to 3 weeks or more. Although it is desirable to achieve weight bearing early in the rehabilitation process, caution should be taken in removing assistive devices if the patient is continuing to walk with an antalgic gait. Some patients may require special precautions depending on the surgery performed, the tissues involved, and the normal physiologic healing that is expected. The physical therapist should review the operative notes and discuss any precautions with the surgeon.

Complications can occur in ankle arthroscopy as with any surgery. It was previously discussed that a 6.8% to 9% complication rate exists. The most common of these complications is injury to the surrounding nerves, with injury to the superficial peroneal nerve accounting for the most frequent complication seen with ankle arthroscopy. There would be transient or permanent numbness on the dorsum of the foot extending into the toes. The therapist should notify the surgeon immediately if:

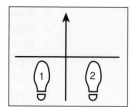

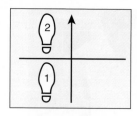

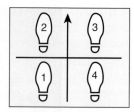

Side to side: Hop laterally between two quadrants.

Front to back: Hop forward and backward between two quadrants.

Four square: Hop from square to square in a circular pattern. Sets are performed clockwise and counterclockwise.

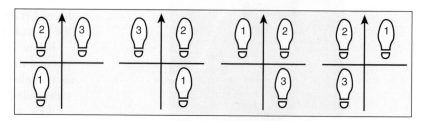

Triangles: Hop within three different quadrants. There are four triangles, each requiring a different diagonal hop.

Fig. 30-13 Four-square hopping ankle rehabilitation. The eight basic hopping patterns in the four-square ankle rehabilitation program are arranged in order of increasing difficulty. The arrows denote the direction the athlete is facing. No. 1 is the starting point. (From Toomey SJ: Four-square ankle rehabilitation exercises. Phys Sports Med 14:281, 1986.)

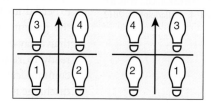

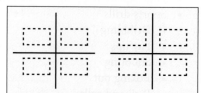

Crisscross: Hop in an X pattern.

Straight-line hop: Hop forward and then backward along a 15- to 20-ft. line.

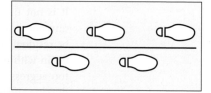

Line zigzag: Hop from side to side across a 15- to 20-ft. line while moving forward and then backward.

Disconnected squares: While performing the first five patterns, hop into squares marked in the quadrants.

- Drainage, redness, swelling, increased pain is evident at any of the surgical sites.
- Patient develops a fever.
- Abnormal redness, swelling of the lower leg is seen.
- Lack or loss of sensation develops.
- Sudden inability to tolerate therapy, HEP, function is evident.
- Patient stops attending therapy.
- Patient is noncompliant to any part of or all of rehabilitation.

Be sure that the athlete/patient always has a progress note when returning to the physician. This will allow the surgeon to know where the patient is in rehabilitation, any gains made, any issues that exist, and any recommendations to consider with his or her ongoing care. Keep the lines of communication open always.

CONCLUSION

Therapy for the postoperative ankle should follow an agreed upon plan set up by the surgeon. Sticking to a program that allows for progression of a patient taking into account the physiologic healing that is occurring will allow for a well-progressed rehabilitation with a minimal amount off exacerbations. Progressing the patient with success and making sure the patient has met all goals before progressing to the next phase of rehabilitation will continue steady, forward progress. Only when the athlete/patient has successfully returned to full functional ROM/strength/proprioception in a pain minimized/alleviated state *and* is able to meet the necessary physical requirements of normal activities should he or she be allowed to return to normal activities (whether it be professional sports or gardening at home). Do not forget the other three-fourths of the patient when rehabilitating the surgical ankle. Remember, the patient will need to be able to perform *all* required functions of his or her normal activities, which means the need to be fully functional and strong. The patient must also exhibit sustained endurance. Lastly, and perhaps most importantly, if there are any questions or issues that come up, talk with the surgeon. This open line of communication is paramount to the patient's/athlete's ultimate outcome.

CLINICAL CASE REVIEW

1 Paul had arthroscopic ankle surgery for an excision of an anterior tibiotalar osteophyte. He had surgery 7 weeks ago and has returned to working as a store manager. He is on his feet most of the day. He is anxious about recovering quickly and doing his usual routine. During his last visit he complained of increased soreness at times. The pain has not been decreasing, and swelling persists. During his home exercises, Paul works hard on the resisted exercises. How can the therapist help Paul to progress?

Paul was told that progressing his function or exercising too aggressively could lead to increased symptoms and potential delays in his progress. Paul's physician was able to write a prescription for compression stockings to help with the swelling and Paul was advised to sit and elevate his leg whenever possible. Paul was put on an icing regimen to elevate and ice three times a day as well. Paul's HEP was reviewed, with adjustments to resistances and repetitions to lessen the likelihood of irritation. Steady progress staying below the threshold of symptoms and exacerbations will keep Paul progressing with his therapy/function with minimal delays and setbacks.

2 Christine is a 32-year-old woman who underwent an ankle arthroscopy procedure for débridement of soft tissue impingement 5 weeks ago. Since then her physical therapy has consisted of massage, ultrasound, AROM and PROM exercises, resisted exercises, cryotherapy, and a HEP. Her main complaint is pain during gait, while descending stairs, and during attempts to squat partially. Dorsiflexion is limited, and minimal swelling persists. What treatment may be particularly helpful to Christine?

Mobilization of the talocrural joint was performed with an AP movement applied to the talus while stabilizing the distal tibia. Distal fibular mobilizations were performed as well to assist with the talus' ability to move into the ankle mortise. This was followed by stretching and ROM exercises to reinforce dorsiflexion. The increase in ROM to 15° with this treatment addition reduced her pain dramatically with gait, stairs, and squatting.

3 Jessica is a 40-year-old woman who had an ankle arthroscopy done with the removal of a loose body from an osteochondral lesion 9 weeks ago. She was non–weight bearing for 5 weeks and has been in therapy; progress with exercise has decreased because of pain during many of the closed chain exercises, such as SLS, double heel lifts, minisquats, and walking more than 8 minutes on the treadmill. What type of closed chain exercises can Jessica do to progress with her strengthening?

The therapist explained that any activities that cause prolonged pain and swelling need to be put on hold and techniques reviewed with the physical therapist. Any changes and modifications can be made so the exercise is successful. If success is not able to be achieved, the exercises that are symptomatic should be stopped until such time that the patient is able to perform without symptoms. Jessica was able to perform the following exercises without issue: forward lunges, backward lunges, lateral lunges, and single heel raises performed on a leg press machine set at 75 lb. She could backward walk and lessen the time on the treadmill. Use of a pool for gravity-minimized exercises is ideal in this situation as well. As her tolerance improved, she was able to progress her therapeutic exercises successfully and without exacerbation.

4 Rebecca is a 45-year-old mother of young children. She underwent ankle arthroscopy surgery for a synovectomy 5 weeks ago. When she is on her feet for more than a couple of hours, she has prolonged soreness. Yesterday, she was on her feet for several hours in the afternoon and intermittently for the rest of the day. Today, she is in for treatment. She has minimal to moderate swelling and complains of minimum to moderate levels of pain with weight-bearing activities. What type of treatment should Rebecca receive today?

When pain and/or swelling limits the progress of rehabilitation, the intensity of rehabilitation needs to be modified. The therapist, in this case, focused on controlling pain and decreasing swelling. Joint mobilizations using glides and distraction maneuvers were performed on the talocrural joints. Gentle PROM was performed. AROM and resisted exercises were placed on hold because of the pain and swelling. Soft tissue mobilization was performed to assist with swelling and to address any soft tissue/fascial restrictions. Ice packs with compression was performed as well. The patient was encouraged to avoid any known aggravating factors. The patient's swelling and pain lessened and the patient was able to get back on track.

5 Jennifer is a 22-year-old ballet dancer. She underwent arthroscopic ankle surgery 10 weeks ago for posterior soft-tissue impingement. She has begun to resume dance practice but still feels some pinching discomfort in her posterior ankle when in an en pointe (on toes) position. What treatment may be particularly helpful to Jennifer at this stage of her rehabilitation?

A mobilization technique was performed at the talocrural joint. A posterior to anterior (PA) glide was applied to the talus, while stabilizing the distal tibia, to increase plantarflexion. To address the end range position needed for ballet, the mobilization was performed in an end range plantarflexion position with a grade IV technique to improve capsular stretching. Following treatment, Jennifer was able to go en pointe with significantly less pinching in her posterior ankle.

6 James is a 30-year-old recreational soccer player. Because of multiple ankle sprains over many years of playing, he suffered an osteochondral lesion of his medial talus. He underwent arthroscopic loose body débridement 9 weeks ago. He has been jogging without symptoms for up to 15 minutes on a treadmill or a track. Over the weekend, he went out to run on the soccer field and began to feel soreness. He states he did no cutting, only running straight up and down the field. What can be done to help James achieve his goal of returning to soccer when he is unable to run on grass pain free?

Despite James' pain-free running on flat surfaces, the grass poses a new challenge because of its inherent instability. James may need to spend more time working on his ankle proprioception during dynamic activities before running on grass. Running on level ground with small changes in direction will provide his ankle the stimulus to control the lateral movements of the subtalar joint. He may also be able to achieve his goal by breaking down the task and doing shorter jogs on the grass with rest before discomfort to allow his body to adjust to the new situation.

7 You have been seeing Sharon in physical therapy for 1 week following her surgery for ankle arthroscopy 2 weeks ago. Today she is complaining of worsening pain and redness along her surgical portals. Upon inspection you notice localized edema, erythema, and warmth along the surgical portal. In addition, there is a small amount of yellow exudate from the wound. How should your physical therapy plan change based on today's findings?

You should immediately contact the surgeon as there is a chance that the wound has become infected.

8 For 2 weeks following arthroscopic surgery for synovitis of his ankle, Bill complains of numbness and tingling along his lateral foot. He noticed it to be more pronounced after splint removal and the onset of weight bearing 1 week ago. He often feels it when pointing his toes during his active ROM exercises. What other objective testing should you perform at this time to help in your treatment of Bill?

Decreased neural mobility in the foot and ankle can occur following any immobilization. Straight leg raise or slump testing should be completed to determine if this might be causing Bill's symptoms.

REFERENCES

1. Takagi K: The arthroscope. J Jpn Orthop Assoc 14:359, 1939.
2. Ferkel RD: Arthroscopic surgery: The foot and ankle, Philadelphia, 1996, Lippincott-Raven.
3. Ferkel RD, Hommen JP: Arthroscopy of the ankle and foot. In Mann RA, Coughlin M, Saltzman C, editors: Surgery of the foot and ankle, ed 7, St Louis, 2006, Mosby.
4. Ferkel RD, Scranton PE, Jr: Arthroscopy of the ankle and foot. J Bone Joint Surg Am 75(8):1233-1242, 1993.
5. Jackson J, Ferkel RD, Nam EK: Ankle and subtalar arthroscopy. In Thordarson DB, editor: Foot and ankle: Orthopaedic surgery essentials, ed 2, Philadelphia, 2012, Lippincott Williams & Wilkins.
6. Stetson WB, Ferkel RD: Ankle arthroscopy. Part I: Technique and complications. Part II: Indications and results. J Am Acad Orthop Surg 4(1):17-34, 1996.
7. Acevedo JI, et al: Coaxial portals for posterior ankle arthroscopy: An anatomic study with clinical correlation on 29 patients. Arthroscopy 16:836-842, 2000.
8. Sitler DF, et al: Posterior ankle arthroscopy. J Bone Joint Surg 84A:763-769, 2002.
9. van Dijk CN, de Leeuw PAJ, Scholten PE: Hindfoot endoscopy for posterior ankle impingement: surgical technique. J Bone Joint Surg Am 91(Suppl 2):287-298, 2009.

10. van Dijk CN, Scholten PE, Krips R: A 2-portal endoscopic approach for diagnosis and treatment of posterior ankle pathology. Arthroscopy 16:871-876, 2000.

11. Ferkel RD, et al: Arthroscopic treatment of anterolateral impingement of the ankle. Am J Sports Med 19:440-446, 1991.

12. Ferkel RD, et al: MRI evaluation of anterolateral soft tissue impingement of the ankle. Foot Ankle Int 31(8):655-661, 2010.

13. Bassett FH, et al: Talar impingement by the anteroinferior tibiofibular ligament: A cause of chronic pain in the ankle after inversion sprain. J Bone Joint Surg 72A:55-59, 1990.

14. Liu SH, et al: Arthroscopic treatment of anterolateral ankle impingement. Arthroscopy 10:215-218, 1994.

15. Bazaz R, Ferkel RD: Results of endoscopic plantar fascia release. Foot Ankle Int 28(5):549-556, 2007.

16. Ferkel RD, Chams RN: Chronic lateral instability: Arthroscopic findings and long-term results. Foot Ankle Int 28(1):24-31, 2007.

17. Ferkel RD, Hewitt M: Long-term results of arthroscopic ankle arthrodesis. Foot Ankle Int 26(4):275-280, 2005.

18. Ferkel RD, et al: Surgical treatment of osteochondral lesions of the talus. Instr Course Lect 59:387-404, 2010.

19. Ferkel RD, et al: Arthroscopic treatment of osteochondral lesions of the talus: Long-term results, submitted for publication Am J Sports Med 36:1750-1762, 2008.

20. Gregush RV, Ferkel RD: Treatment of the unstable ankle with an osteochondral lesion: Results and long-term follow-up. Am J Sports Med 38:782-790, 2010.

21. Loren GJ, Ferkel RD: Arthroscopic assessment of occult intra-articular injury in acute ankle fractures. Arthroscopy 18:412-421, 2002.

22. Williams MM, Ferkel RD: Subtalar arthroscopy: Indications, techniques, and results. Arthroscopy 14:373-381, 1998.

23. Zengerink M, et al: Current concepts: treatment of osteochondral ankle defects. Foot Ankle Clin 11:331-359, 2006.

24. Ferkel RD: Complications in ankle and foot arthroscopy. In Ferkel RD, editor: Arthroscopic surgery: The foot and ankle, Philadelphia, 1996, Lippincott-Raven.

25. Nickisch F, et al: Postoperative complications in patients after posterior ankle and hindfoot arthroscopy. J Bone Joint Surg Am 94:439-446, 2012.

26. Young BH, Flanigan RM, Digiovanni BF: Complications of ankle arthroscopy utilizing a contemporary noninvasive distraction technique. J Bone Joint Surg Am 93(10):963-968, 2011.

CHAPTER 31

Achilles Tendon Repair and Rehabilitation

Jane Gruber, Eric Giza, James Zachazewski, Bert R. Mandelbaum

Achilles tendon injuries, whether acute or chronic, occur in many individuals. The severity of these injuries varies from mild, overuse-related inflammatory responses to acute, traumatic tendon rupture. Nonoperative treatment options are immobilization with a cast or functional bracing, while surgical options are operative repair with open or percutaneous procedures. Postoperative management varies with the length of immobilization and timing of early motion. This chapter describes current trends in surgical intervention, outlines rehabilitative guidelines and techniques, and details the rationales associated with treating Achilles tendon ruptures.

SURGICAL INDICATIONS AND CONSIDERATIONS

Anatomy

The Achilles tendon complex is composed of contributions from the gastrocnemius, soleus, and plantaris (collectively known as the triceps surae) and inserts directly into the central third of the posterior calcaneal surface. The tendon is round in cross section to a level 4 cm proximal to calcaneus, where it flattens and rotates 90° so that its medial fibers insert posteriorly. This biomechanical "winding" of the fibers increases stored energy for higher shortening velocity and muscle power.[1]

During dorsiflexion, the tendon articulates with the superior third of the calcaneus. This articulation is cushioned by the retrocalcaneal bursa, which lies between the tendon and the superior third of the calcaneus.

The Achilles tendon does not possess a true synovial sheath. The peritendinous structures of the Achilles are composed of a triple-layered tissue.[2] The superficial layer of tissue is the most durable and is analogous to the deep fascia. This layer comprises the posterior boundary of the superficial posterior compartment. The middle layer, the mesotendon, provides the major blood supply for the central portion of the Achilles tendon. The deepest layer of tissue is quite delicate and thin; however, it can always be isolated from the most superficial layer of the tendon, the epitenon.

The Achilles tendon is supplied with blood and nutrients by three different sources.[2] The most abundant supply is at the proximal and distal portions of the tendon, and the poorest is in the central portion of the tendon. As originally demonstrated by Lagerrgren and Lindholm[3] and corroborated by others,[4,5] a gradual decrease occurs in the number of blood vessels in the central part of the tendon 2 to 6 cm proximal to the calcaneal insertion (Fig. 31-1).

Nutrient branches emanate directly from the muscle to nourish the distal gastrocnemius aponeurosis and proximal portion of the tendon.[6] The insertion of the Achilles tendon is supplied by anastomotic branches between the periosteal vessels and the tendon vessels. As already noted, the major blood supply comes from the mesotendon. Vessels enter the tendon itself via a network of fine connections with the deepest peritendinous layer. These vessels come off the deepest layer radially and enter the tendon perpendicular to its long axis. They then course proximally and distally. Because of the external forces that may be encountered by the posterior aspect of the tendon as a result of friction supplied by the skin, most of these fine vessels are found along the anterior aspect of the tendon, where they are afforded more protection (Fig. 31-2).

Pathogenesis

The theoretic explanation for tendon injuries suggests a continuum of events, including hypovascularity and repetitive microtrauma, that results in localized tendon degeneration and weakness and ultimately rupture with the application of an otherwise normal load that exceeds the tendon's physiologic capacity. Based on clinical and histologic findings, the traditional description of Achilles tendonitis is not preferred,[7] and Achilles tendon pathology is classified into three different categories: (1) paratendinitis, (2) paratendinitis with tendinosis, and (3) pure tendinosis.[8-10]

Paratendinitis involves inflammation only in the paratenon, regardless of whether it is lined by synovium. The paratenon thickens, and adhesions may form between the paratenon and the tendon.[11] However, patients will rarely have isolated

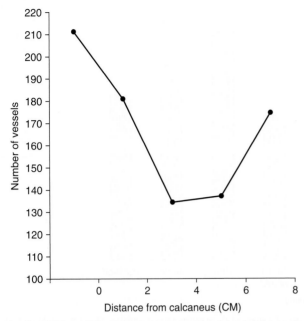

Fig. 31-1 The number of intratendinous vessels of the Achilles tendon varies depending on the distance from the calcaneus. (From Carr AJ, Norris SH: The blood supply of the calcaneal tendon. J Bone Joint Surg Br 71B:100, 1989.)

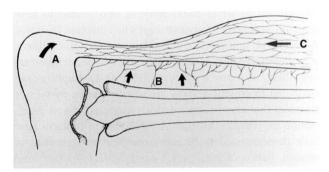

Fig. 31-2 Diagram of the blood vessels of the Achilles paratenon, showing supply for the osseous junction (A), the mesotendon (B), and the musculotendinous junction (C). (From Carr AJ, Norris SH: The blood supply of the calcaneal tendon. J Bone Joint Surg Br 71B:100, 1989.)

paratendinitis, and some authors believe that this process is the predecessor to tendinosis.[7]

Paratendinitis with tendinosis involves not only inflammation of the paratenon but also a degenerative change within the substance of the tendon. Paddu, Ippolito, and Postacchini[10] and Kvist and Kvist[11] have noted thickening, softening, and yellowing of the tendon, as well as cleavage planes and vascular budding during surgery for this condition. As in tendinitis, pain also is commonly noted because of the inflammatory process.

Pure tendinosis often appears as a nodule that is mobile with plantar flexion.[7] It can present as a chronic nodule in the sedentary middle-aged person or as a contribution to the pathology of rupture in the tendons of persons older than 35 years who have suffered spontaneous rupture.[12] Histopathologic changes such as hypoxic and mucoid

degeneration, lipomatous infiltration, and calcifying tendinopathy have been noted at the time of surgical repair of acute ruptures.[10,12]

Hippocrates was the first to record an injury to the Achilles tendon, while Ambrose Pare was the first to describe Achilles tendon ruptures in 1575, and Gustave Paoaillon was the first to report operative repair of the tendon.[1,2,13] Theories implicating the degenerative changes that take place in the Achilles tendon with the increased mechanical loads associated with various activities are the most common explanations of the pathogenesis of these ruptures.[13,14] A combination of hypovascularity and repetitive microtrauma results in degenerative changes and inflammation, putting the tendon at risk for rupture. Healing and regeneration are hindered or halted because of poor blood supply to the tendon and recurrent microtrauma. Alfredson, Thorsen, and Lorentzon[15] have shown that microtears in the tendon lead to areas of chronic damage that lack normal levels of prostaglandin E2, which are needed for healing. The combination of these factors may account for the fact that most ruptures occur 2 to 6 cm proximal to the tendon's insertion into the calcaneus. Associated intrinsic factors include age (which leads to decreased vascularity and decreased deoxyribonucleic acid [DNA] synthesis),[16-18] endocrine function, and nutrition.[19] Extrinsic factors of compression and friction on the posterior aspect of the tendon (from the skin and inappropriately compressive footwear) further hinder vascularity, healing, and regeneration. Fluoroquinolone antibiotics are also associated with Achilles tendon rupture. Their use inhibits transcription of decorin, a protein important in collagen architecture, and the odds ratio for tendon rupture in patients taking the medication is 4.2.[20] Acute Achilles ruptures are also often the result of corticosteroid injection for chronic inflammation of the tendon.[7]

Normally, tendons are able to tolerate high forces associated with daily activities and athletics. However, if degenerative changes take place, then the mechanical load usually tolerated may exceed the tendon's physiologic capacity. Mechanically, a tendon may be damaged or ruptured by a sudden application of force. This often involves a forceful lengthening or eccentric muscle contraction. Sudden maximal muscle activation results in a larger than normal force that is applied rapidly to the tendon, causing the rupture. The high load forces that cause such rupture are usually associated with vigorous activities such as sports. The forces to which the Achilles tendon is exposed during activities such as running and jumping have been calculated to be between 4000 and 5500 N[21-23]; they are summarized in Fig. 31-3.[19] Arner and Lindholm[24] describe three activities that can rupture a tendon:

1. Pushing off with weight bearing on the forefoot while extending the knee (e.g., running, sprinting, jumping)
2. Sudden dorsiflexion with full weight bearing as might occur with a slip, fall, or sudden deceleration
3. Violent dorsiflexion when jumping from a height and landing on a plantar-flexed foot

Curwin[19] best summarized the possible progression of tendon injury (Fig. 31-4).

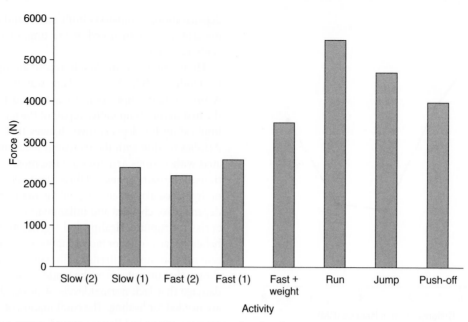

Fig. 31-3 Increasing Achilles tendon forces during toe-raising exercises over the edge of a step and three sports-related activities. Slow (2), weight on both feet, slow speed; Slow (1), weight on one foot, slow speed; Fast (2), weight on both feet, fast speed; Fast (1), weight on one foot, fast speed; Fast + weight, extra weight added to body; Run, spring running; Jump, landing from 50 cm; Push-off, change in direction from backward to forward running. The slow and fast movements represent progressive steps in the clinical exercise program to treat Achilles tendinitis. (From Curwin SL: Tendon injuries: pathophysiology and treatment. In Zachazewski JE, Magee DG, Quillen WS, editors: Athletic injuries and rehabilitation, Philadelphia, 1996, Saunders.)

Epidemiology

Reports regarding the incidence, cause, and conservative, surgical, and postoperative management of Achilles tendon ruptures have increased during the past 50 to 60 years. The number of cases reported may be attributed not only to the observation and diligence of the health care community in publishing their research and thus improving patient care but also to the fact that the general population has increased its level of participation in recreational activity.

Although spontaneous tendon ruptures are rare, the Achilles tendon appears to be the one that is most frequently ruptured. Kannus and Jozsa[12] report that 44.6% (397 out of 891) of tendon ruptures treated surgically between 1968 and 1989 involved the Achilles tendon, whereas the biceps brachii accounted for 33.9%. Achilles tendon ruptures are usually traumatic and occur between the ages of 30 and 40 years,[25-27] which is younger than for other tendon ruptures (Fig. 31-5).

Most ruptures are suffered by recreational athletes rather than highly competitive, very active athletes. Of the 105 patients with Achilles ruptures described by Nistor,[28] only 9 participated in competitive sports. Of the remaining patients, 35 exercised twice a week, 41 once a week, 20 took walks and occasionally exercised, and two were physically inactive. Of the 111 patients who ruptured their Achilles tendon while participating in a sports activity in Cetti and colleagues' report,[26] 92 (83%) averaged only 3.6 hours of athletic activity per week. Of the 292 Achilles tendon ruptures documented by Jozsa and associates,[27] 59% occurred during recreational athletic activity—141 of these (83.2%) in men and 29 (16.8%) in women. No patients in this study by Jozsa and colleagues participated in competitive athletics. In their study, more than 625 of the Achilles tendon ruptures occurred in

professional or white collar workers who tended to have generally sedentary lifestyles except when involved in sports. A review of numerous studies demonstrates that athletic activities that require sudden acceleration or deceleration are most likely to cause a rupture (Table 31-1). Ruptures not attributed to athletic activity are usually caused by falls or stumbles that also produce sudden acceleration and deceleration movements. Overall, Achilles tendon ruptures have been demonstrated to be more common in men than in women. Ratios of 2:1,[29] 4:1,[30] 1.6:1,[31] 8.7:1,[28] 10:1,[25] and 12:1[10] have been reported.

Diagnosis of Acute Achilles Tendon Rupture

In most situations the history is diagnostic. Patients describe hearing a pop as though someone had shot them in the back of the ankle. Prodromal symptoms of Achilles aching have been reported in 5% to 30% of cases.[12,32] The rupture commonly occurs in the "watershed area," between 2 and 6 cm proximal to the calcaneus.[3] Avulsion fractures of the calcaneus are relatively uncommon.[4] A careful history and physical examination are important because it has been shown that 22% of primary care physicians miss the diagnosis of acute Achilles rupture.[26] The physical examination is characterized by palpation of the defect and documentation by Thompson test,[33] which indicates discontinuity and loss of plantar flexion when the calf is squeezed. The Thompson test is performed by asking the patient to kneel on a chair with the feet hanging over the edge and the calf muscles relaxed. In this prone position, the examiner can usually denote a difference in resting angle from the contralateral side. Radiographic evaluation rules out the presence of a bony injury. Magnetic resonance imaging (MRI) can be helpful in

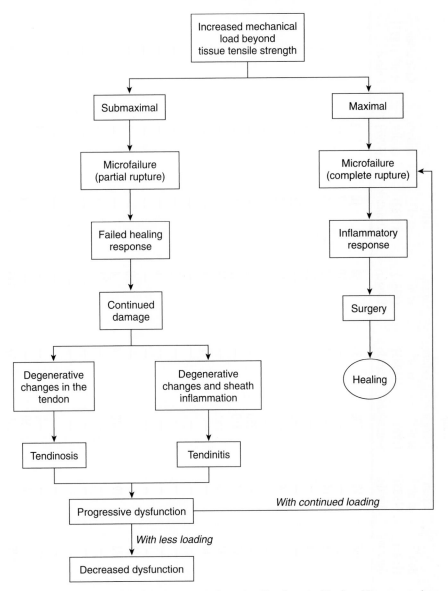

Fig. 31-4 Progression of tendon injury. The inflammatory response may be limited and barely noticed by the athlete, even as degenerative changes continue. As the remaining collagen fibers are overloaded and more are damaged, the inflammatory response recurs, possibly weeks or months after the initial injury. After the tendon is in the inflammatory stage, it can be treated as an acute injury and should heal normally. In rare cases the tendon may rupture because applied forces exceed the tensile strength of the now-weakened tendon. (Adapted from Curwin SL: Tendon injuries: Pathophysiology and treatment. In Zachazewski JE, Magee DG, Quillen WS, editors: Athletic injuries and rehabilitation, Philadelphia, 1996, Saunders.)

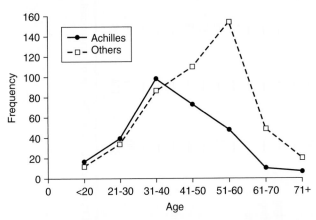

Fig. 31-5 Age distribution of patients with Achilles tendon ruptures. (From Josza L, et al: The role of recreational sport activity in Achilles tendon rupture. Am J Sports Med 17:338, 1989.)

demonstrating the presence, location, and severity of tears of the Achilles tendon. MRI also is helpful in assessing the status of an Achilles tendon repair.[34] Ultrasonography has been used to define Achilles tendon discontinuity[35] in countries where MRI is not routinely used. No one clinical test has been shown to be superior; however, a combination of a complete history and physical examination along with radiographic studies (if necessary) will lead to an accurate diagnosis.[36]

After an accurate diagnosis is made, a definitive physical therapy and rehabilitation program can be implemented by establishing the objectives for management. If any questions remain regarding the diagnosis or severity of the tear, then MRI and ultrasonography can be used to enhance diagnostic accuracy. The physical therapist (PT) should define the

TABLE 31-1 Distribution of Achilles Tendon Ruptures According to Sport

Sport	Frings[129] (1969) Germany	Nillius et al[130] (1976) Sweden	Inglis et al[31] (1976) USA	Cetti and Christenson[131] (1983) Denmark	Holz[132] (1983) Germany	Schedl et al[133] (1983) Austria	Zolinger et al[134] (1983) Switzerland	Kellam et al[99] (1985) Canada	Jozsa et al[135] (1987) Hungary	Cetti et al[126] (1983) Denmark	Soldatis et al[100] (1997) USA	Karjalainen et al[90] (1997) Finland
Soccer	102	35	18	7	168	13	300	33	58	10	3	2
Handball	32	9	4	19	57	—	—	—	10	7	—	1
Volleyball	—	—	4	—	6	14	—	5	3	3	4	2
Basketball	—	—	29	—	6	—	—	—	23	—	10	1
Badminton	4	38	—	20	—	—	—	—	—	58	—	7
Tennis	5	15	20	—	23	4	—	—	12	3	3	3
Table tennis	4	5	20	—	—	—	—	—	2	—	—	—
Other ball games	9	—	—	5	—	—	230	—	5	—	—	—
Gymnastics	43	19	—	—	47	7	110	—	12	10	—	1
Running	46	6	5	—	42	5	—	17	14	—	—	—
Jumping	31	—	—	—	18	—	—	—	14	—	—	—
Climbing	—	—	—	1	—	—	—	—	—	—	—	—
Rock climbing	—	—	—	—	—	—	—	—	3	—	—	—
Weight lifting	—	—	—	—	—	—	—	—	6	—	—	—
Trampoline	—	—	1	1	—	—	—	—	—	1	—	—
Bicycling	—	—	12	—	39	—	—	—	3	—	—	—
Skiing	6	—	10	—	73	19	570	4	4	—	—	1
Dancing	—	—	9	—	—	—	—	—	7	1	—	—
Jogging	—	—	—	—	—	—	—	—	—	—	—	—
Racquetball	—	—	—	—	—	—	—	—	—	—	2	—
Aerobics	—	—	—	—	—	—	—	—	—	—	4	—
Baseball	—	—	—	—	—	—	—	—	—	—	4	1
Others	30	7	—	—	—	6	30	—	—	19	4	1
Total	317	134	131	53	479	68	1240	59	173	111	30	20

Study

Adapted from Jozsa L, et al: The role of recreational sport activity in Achilles tendon rupture: A clinical, pathoanatomical, and sociological study of 292 cases. Am J Sports Med 17(3):338, 1989.

patient's functional and athletic goals, personal needs, and temporal priorities before making therapeutic judgments.

Nonoperative Versus Operative Management

Treatment for Achilles tendon ruptures was nonoperative until the twentieth century. It included immobilization with strapping, wrapping, and braces for varying periods of time.[37] In 1929 Quenu and Stoianovitch[38] stated that a rupture of the Achilles tendon should be operated on without delay. Christensen[30] (1953) and Arner, Lindholm, and Orell[4] (1958) compared patients treated surgically and those managed nonoperatively; the surgical group had better results. As the field of sports medicine progressed with new surgical techniques, including rigid internal fixation combined with rehabilitation, the optimal treatment for Achilles tendon rupture became controversial. Some studies supported nonoperative management of Achilles ruptures,[28,39] as shown in the following editorial statement made in 1973: "In view of the excellent results obtainable by conservative treatment, it is doubtful whether surgical repair in closed rupture of the Achilles tendon can be justified.[40]" In an updated meta-analysis of reports on Achilles tendon injury, Khan and associates[41] found that open operative treatment of acute Achilles tendon ruptures significantly reduces the risk of rerupture compared with nonoperative treatment, but it produces a significantly higher risk of other complications, including wound infection. Significance varied among studies included. In total, reruptures in the operative groups were 3.5% versus 12.5% in the nonoperative groups. Rates for other complications (infection, adhesions, disruptions in sensation) in the operative groups were 34% versus 2.7% in the nonoperative groups.

In 2003, Weber and colleagues[42] compared the results of acute ruptures in 23 patients treated nonoperatively to 24 patients treated operatively. Patients in the nonoperative group were allowed full weight bearing in 20° patellofemoral casts for 6 weeks and were verified with weekly ultrasonography and cast changes. Patients in the operative group were placed in casts and were non–weight bearing for 6 weeks with variable rehabilitation protocols. The results showed a decreased return to work and crutch time for nonoperative cases, with 4 of 23 reruptures at 7 to 12 weeks. Patients in the operative group had only 1 of 24 reruptures at 3 years. This study demonstrates that nonoperative treatment may be acceptable for some patient populations, but that operative treatment, even with traditional postoperative immobilization, yields a lower rerupture rate. The surgeon must explore the goals and expectations of the patient and decide which treatment is most appropriate. Indications for nonoperative treatment include concomitant illness in the patient, a sedentary lifestyle, or lower functional and athletic goals.

Early nonoperative options were well accepted and tolerated. But in the past 20 years, patient expectations and functional goals have increased so that surgical options have gained acceptance and preference.

Less invasive surgical procedures were first noted in the literature by Ma and Griffith.[43] A lower overall rate of complications (particularly infection) in the percutaneously treated group has been noted.[41,44,45] Studies comparing open versus percutaneous techniques have a relatively small number of subjects, limiting their reliability.

The patient selected for operative repair should be an individual who is extremely interested in optimal functional restoration.

In 2010 the American Academy of Orthopaedic Surgeons published guidelines on the treatment of acute Achilles tendon ruptures. A meta-analysis of all existing literature showed similar outcomes in operative and nonoperative treatment. The study demonstrated two moderate-strength recommendations that included suggestions for early postoperative protective weight bearing and for the use of protective devices that allow for postoperative mobilization in those patients who have surgical treatment.[36]

Functional postoperative treatment programs, regardless of surgical technique, avoid cast immobilization and are well tolerated, safe, and effective with well-motivated athletes and patients who especially desire the highest functional outcome.[13,46-50]

Acute Care of the Achilles Tendon Rupture

In the last century, the literature has proposed numerous approaches to the management of acute Achilles tendon ruptures. The most important design principles of the option selected should include the following:

1. The option and procedure are safe and effective.
2. The method allows the patient to accomplish realistic goals.
3. The surgeon can execute the method successfully.
4. The risks of the method are acceptable to the patient and surgeon.

The categorical options for the surgical treatment of acute Achilles tendon rupture include repair, repair with augmentation, and reconstruction.

SURGICAL PROCEDURE

Repair

The rationale for any repair method is to restore continuity of the ruptured tendon end, facilitate healing, and restore muscle function. The technical difficulty is taking relative "mop ends" and opposing them in a stable fashion. Bunnell[51] and Kessler[52] were the first to popularize the end-to-end suture technique for ruptured tendons. Ma and Griffith[43] described a percutaneous repair in 1977; however, a higher rerupture rate also occurred in their series. Beskin[25] introduced the three-bundle suture, and Cetti[46] demonstrated the suture weave in 1988, which was further modified by Mortensen and Saether[53] in 1991 as a six-strand suture technique. Nada[54] described the use of external fixation for Achilles tendon ruptures in 1985. Richardson, Reitman, and Wilson[55] described good results using a pull-out wire, which has the advantage of minimal suture reaction but requires a second procedure for suture removal. More recently, a commercial device has become available that allows for the percutaneous passing of a suture to repair a rupture through a minimally invasive incision. Jung and colleagues evaluated 30 patients with limited open repair for Achilles tendon rupture using a commercial device with an average 18 months follow-up and found that 16 patients were very satisfied, 11 were satisfied, and 3 were dissatisfied.[56]

Each of these techniques has advantages and disadvantages, hence the wide spectrum of options. The surgeon's selection of a method should be based on technical training, an accurate pathoanatomic diagnosis, and the patient's goals and desires.

Repair With Augmentation

Historically, augmentation procedures evolved to supplement the repair construct of mop ends plus suture. Most augmentation procedures involved the local use of gastrocnemius fascia flaps or the plantaris tendon if available. Christensen[30] described the use of the gastrocnemius aponeurosis flap to augment Achilles tendon repair in 1981. Silfverskiold[57] described a central rotation gastrocnemius flap, and Lindholm[58] devised a method of two turndown flaps. Lynn[59] used the plantaris tendon, fanning it out to use the membrane to reinforce the repair. Kirschembaum and Kellman[60] modified the technique in 1980 by placing the fascial flaps centrally rather than separating them. Chen and Wertheimer[61] demonstrated the use of suture anchors distally at the calcaneus to repair the gastrocnemius turndown flap with semirigid fixation. Overall, these methods can facilitate the continuity and strength of the repair construct when doubt persists concerning the repair's integrity. In practice these techniques are applied only in limited situations, but they should still be in the surgeon's armamentarium.

Reconstruction

Acute ruptures are usually managed with the repair techniques already described with or without augmentation. Usually these are appropriate to promote continuity and healing of acute ruptures. Neglected, chronic ruptures, however, require reconstruction with endogenous or exogenous materials. Endogenous materials include fascia lata,[62] peroneus brevis transfer,[63] flexor digitorum longus,[64] and flexor hallucis longus.[65] Exogenous materials include carbon fiber,[66] Marlex mesh,[67] Dacron vascular grafts,[49] polylactic acid implant, and a polypropylene braid.[68] Once again, the surgeon must be familiar with these procedures and understand their advantages and disadvantages before applying them in appropriate scenarios.

Concepts of Achilles Tendon Repair

Prolonged cast immobilization has been used with both operative and nonoperative treatment of Achilles tendon ruptures. Although cast immobilization may promote healing, it also promotes one or more of the following manifestations of "cast disease"[69,70]:

- Muscle atrophy
- Joint stiffness
- Cartilage atrophy
- Degenerative arthritis
- Adhesion formation
- Deep venous thrombosis

Immobilization after tendon surgery was considered the single factor most responsible for postsurgical complications as long ago as 1954.[24,30,43] Various clinical studies in the literature document residual isokinetic strength deficits between 10% and 16% after cast immobilization of Achilles tendon injuries, regardless of whether they were managed operatively or nonoperatively.[9,28,71-73]

The AO Group of Switzerland found that stable and rigid internal fixation of bone fractures allows early range of motion (ROM) and maximal rehabilitation, thus minimizing atrophy and the manifestations of cast disease. This principle indicates that early mobilization of tendon ruptures should be promoted as long as stable fixation is ensured. In support of this concept, it has been demonstrated that early motion limits atrophy,[74] promotes fiber polymerization to collagen,[75] and increases the organization of collagen at the repair site, leading to increased strength.[76-79] Krackow, Thomas, and Jones[80] initially described a suture technique that allows "rigid" internal fixation without tendon necrosis. This technique, coupled with complete repair of the peritenon, should result in progressive and successful healing of the Achilles tendon rupture without postoperative cast immobilization.

Mandelbaum, Myerson, and Forster[13] reported on the successful use of the Krackow modified suture technique in a series of 29 athletes with acute Achilles tendon rupture. Postoperatively the patients were not rigidly immobilized and were started on early ROM and conditioning programs. No patients in this series experienced rerupture, persistent pain, frank infection, or skin necrosis as a complication. By 6 weeks after surgery, 90% of patients had full ROM. By 6 months, 92% had returned to sports participation; strength deficits were less than 3% on isokinetic testing. Rigid internal fixation of Achilles tendon tears allowed a more functional rehabilitation process in this series, including early motion and weight bearing. Maffulli and colleagues,[32] who reported on the operative results of 42 patients who were randomized to a traditional protocol of postoperative immobilization or a full weight bearing protocol, strengthened these results. In the full weight-bearing group, patients were placed in a full weight-bearing cast for 2 weeks, then a full weight-bearing dorsiflexion splint for 4 weeks. In the traditional protocol, the patients were immobilized in a cast for 4 weeks, then a full weight bearing cast for 2 more weeks. They found that the full weight-bearing group had no crutch use at 1.5 weeks, a quicker return to work, less calf atrophy, greater patient satisfaction, less patient visits, and isometric strength equal to the traditional group.[32] This method of accelerated but controlled postoperative management has proven to be safe and highly effective at returning the athlete and patient to activities of daily living (ADLs) and sports with the highest level of function.[13,14,81]

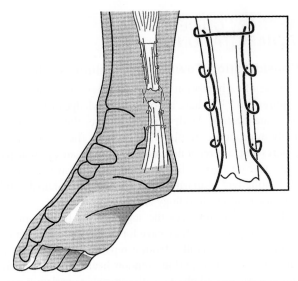

Fig. 31-6 Krackow suture technique. (Courtesy Santa Monica Orthopaedic and Sports Medicine Group, Santa Monica, Calif.)

Preoperative Treatment

After the diagnosis is made, the patient should be placed in a compressive elastic or cohesive tape wrap to minimize swelling. They should be encouraged to use ice and elevate the extremity. If possible, the patient should be allowed to ambulate in a cam walker boot or with a cane to promote circulation and prevent venous thrombosis. Surgery should be performed in an outpatient setting 7 to 10 days after the injury. This delay allows consolidation of the tendon ends, making repair technically easier.

Surgical Technique

Surgery is performed with the patient in the prone position under general, regional, or local anesthesia. Care should be taken to note the resting tension of the opposite foot. To be most accurate, both feet can be prepped to allow accurate side-to-side comparison of tendon length. Either a straight midline or an anteromedial incision is made just medial to the gastrocnemius. A direct incision is made through the peritenon, which is split and tagged. Before repair of the tendon, any adhesions between the anterior surface of the muscle and tendon unit and the paratenon are removed. A relaxing incision in the anterior surface of the paratenon is made down to the muscle of the flexor hallucis longus, which will facilitate closure of the paratenon. Each end of the tear is sewn with a No. 2 nonabsorbable suture using the Krackow suture technique (Fig. 31-6). The recently introduced synthetic, polyethylene sutures such as Fiberwire* or Orthocord† are now commonly used for the repair and have been shown to have superior strength to traditional braided sutures.[82] The sutures are tensioned appropriately to achieve the same resting angle as the contralateral extremity. If any doubt exists regarding the amount of tension, then the

contralateral side may be used for comparison. The suture knots are passed to the anterior aspect of the tendon and secured. The peritenon is then closed anatomically with 4-0 absorbable suture. The ankle is taken through a ROM to evaluate the stability of the repair construct. The wound is closed with dermal mattress sutures, with the knots based on the medial side to protect the tendon; a posterior splint is applied. On the second day after surgery, the splint is removed and the ankle is taken gently through active range of motion (AROM). Gentle ROM exercises are begun. The sutures are removed by about day 14, and a progressive weight-bearing program is initiated using a walker boot.

Percutaneous Repair

Percutaneous repair of the Achilles tendon has become an acceptable alternative method to open repair. Proponents of the technique have cited a lower wound complication rate and similar rerupture rates.[83-87] Halasi, Tallay, and Berkes[46] performed an endoscopically assisted repair on 123 patients and had no wound problems, a return to sport in 4 to 6 months, and no wound complications. Although sural nerve irritation can be a complication of the technique, it has been postulated that endoscopic assistance of the procedure lowered the sural nerve complication rate.

Percutaneous Repair Technique

Buchgraber and Pässler[83] described the following surgical technique. Patients are placed in a prone position and given a short-acting general anesthetic. The tendon defect is identified by palpation, and a transverse or longitudinal incision is made along the skin folds across its center. The associated hematoma is deliberately left in place. Using a 15.3-mm blade, stab incisions are made at the medial and lateral aspects of the tendon approximately 10 to 12 cm above the site of the tear. Another two stab incisions of the same length are made above the calcaneus, medial and lateral to the insertion of the Achilles tendon. To prevent sural nerve injury, a mosquito clamp is placed in the proximal lateral stab incision to retract the skin and the underlying fascia. With the help of a cutting needle,* a 1.2-mm polydioxanone suture (PDS) cord is pulled through proximally from the medial to the lateral stab incision. Then the cutting needle is introduced through the incision overlying the tear, passed through the tendon proximally, and advanced toward the lateral proximal stab incision. Using the cutting needle, the end of the PDS cord at this site is passed out through the central incision. Next the cutting needle is pushed into the tendon tissue from the lateral distal stab incision, brought out centrally to load it with the lateral end of the PDS cord, and pulled out distally. This end of the cord is grasped with the needle and introduced through the medial distal stab incision, brought out through the lateral distal stab incision, and pulled through medially. In the final step, the needle is passed through the proximal tendon end from the central

*Arthrex, Naples, Fla.
†DePuy Mitek, Norwood, Mass.

*Aesculap, Tuttlingen, Germany

incision and brought out at the medial proximal stab incision. The foot is put repeatedly through the full ROM to ensure that the cord will dig into the tendon tissue. The ends of the cord are tied with the foot in slight plantar flexion. Once the first knot is tied, the foot is dorsiflexed several times to check the tension on the cord. The procedure is concluded with another two knots added in a crisscross pattern.[83]

Potential Complications

The major complication with nonoperative treatment is a higher rerupture rate and an incomplete return of function and performance. Complications associated with the surgical technique include infection, anesthetic problems, rerupture, deep vein thrombosis, and an incomplete return of function. Infection can be a disastrous complication because soft tissue coverage is a major problem and can only be resolved with vascularized flaps and a reconstructive tendon procedure.[88]

THERAPY GUIDELINES FOR REHABILITATION

Consideration Toward the Healing Tendon

The use of early motion during postoperative rehabilitation requires the PT to have a working knowledge of the process of tissue healing. With this knowledge, the therapist can apply appropriate amounts of stress at the correct times, progressing the rehabilitation program at an optimal pace and ensuring a good clinical outcome. Extensive summaries by Leadbetter,[89] Curwin,[19] and Curwin and Stanish[22] fully describe tendon physiology and healing.

Fig. 31-7 summarizes the stages of the healing process and the implications they have for traditional postoperative management of Achilles tendon repairs and motion in the early postoperative period. Tendon healing occurs in four consecutive, related phases, with somewhat overlapping time frames.

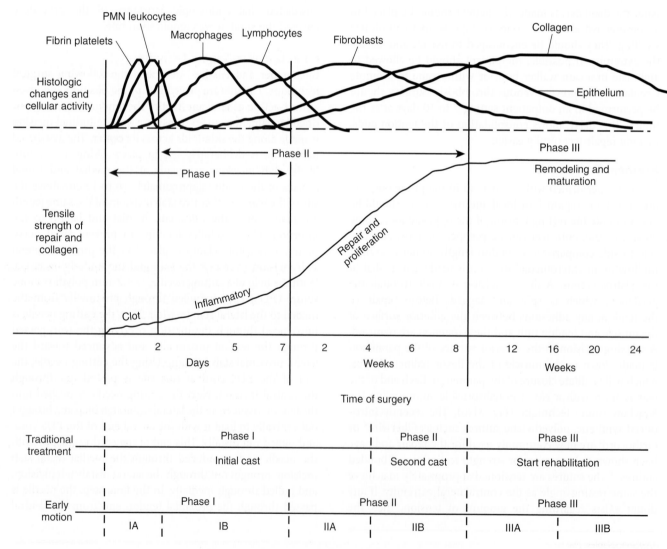

Fig. 31-7 Phases of tissue healing and rehabilitation timelines.

Stages of Healing

Inflammatory Response

Minutes after injury, laceration, or the initiation of surgical repair, a coagulation response occurs, triggering the formation of a fibrin clot. This clot contains fibronectin, which is essential to reparative cell activity. Fibronectin eventually creates a scaffold for cell migration and supports fibroblastic activity. Soon after this clot forms, polymorphonuclear leukocytes and macrophages invade the area to clear cellular and tissue debris. The resulting arachidonic acid cascade is the primary chemical event during this stage. This stage is usually complete in less than 6 days unless infection and wound disturbance occur.

Repair and Proliferation

The repair and proliferation stage may begin as early as 48 hours after injury and may last for 6 to 8 weeks. Tissue macrophages are the key factors early in this stage. The macrophage is mobile and capable of releasing various growth factors, chemotactants, and proteolytic enzymes when necessary or appropriate for the activation of fibroblasts and tendon repair.[89] Fibroblastic proliferation continues and produces increasing amounts of collagen. Type III collagen, which has poor cross-link definition, small fibril size, and poor strength, is initially deposited rapidly. As the repair process continues, collagen deposition shifts to type I collagen, which has greater cross-link definition, fibril size, and strength. The deposition of type I collagen accelerates and continues throughout this stage and well into the remodeling and maturation stage.

Changes in the postoperative internal structure of 21 surgically repaired Achilles tendons have been documented by Karjalainen and colleagues[90] during the healing process using MRI. After surgery, patients were placed in casts in equinus position for 3 weeks without weight bearing and for another 3 weeks in a short walking cast in neutral position, with weight bearing as tolerated. After cast removal, patients began AROM and walking exercises. MRI was repeated at 3 weeks, 6 weeks, 3 months, and 6 months after repair to document changes (Fig. 31-8). During this stage the postoperative cross-sectional repaired area Achilles tendon increased dramatically, measuring 2.9 and 3.4 times the size of the uninjured contralateral tendon at 3 and 6 weeks, respectively. A diffuse, high-intensity heterogeneous signal was present at the repair site for all 21 tendons at 3 weeks and in 13 of 21 tendons at 6 weeks. In the other eight tendons, early formation of high-intensity intratendinous signal was present in the center of the tendon at the level of repair.

Remodeling and Maturation

Remodeling and maturation of collagen fibrils and crosslinks characterize the third healing stage. Overall a trend toward decreased cellularity and synthetic activity, increased organization of the extracellular matrix, and a more normal biochemical profile is evident.[91] Functional linear alignment

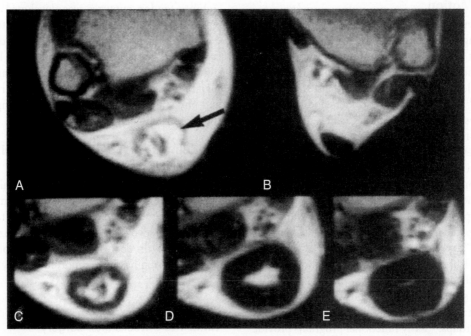

Fig. 31-8 T_2 weighted MRI (TR, 2000 msec; TE, 80 msec) of the normal reunion process of ruptured and surgically repaired Achilles tendon. **A,** The affected tendon shows a high-intensity signal *(arrow)* with a peripheral thin rim of low-intensity signal area and also low-intensity elements centrally. **B,** The unaffected side. **C,** At 6 weeks the intratendinous lesion and the margin of the Achilles tendon are better visualized. **D,** At 3 months the periphery of the healing tendon has returned to its normal low-intensity signal level. The intratendinous lesion inside the tendon is rather small. The cross-sectional area is seven times as large as the unaffected side (**B**). **E,** At 6 months the scar is barely visible and the edema around the tendon has decreased compared with previous images. (From Karjalainen PT, et al: Magnetic resonance imaging during healing of surgically repaired Achilles tendon ruptures. Am J Sports Med 25[2]:164, 1997.)

of the collagen fibrils is usually present by 2 months.[89] Although maturation appears to be complete a number of months after the injury, biochemical differences in collagen type and arrangement, water content, DNA content, and glycosaminoglycan content persist indefinitely. The material properties of these scars never become identical to those of intact tendon.[8] Biomechanical properties can be reduced by as much as 30% despite the completion of all stages of healing and maturation.[8,22,92,93] Karjalainen and associates[61] found that the cross-sectional area of the tendon continues to increase. The area is 6.1 times the size of the unaffected tendon at 3 months and 5.6 times the size at 6 months. A variably sized, high-intensity signal demonstrating a central intratendinous lesion was detected in 19 of 21 repaired tendons at 3 months. The development of an intratendinous lesion appears to be a normal part of the healing process after surgical repair and casting.

Future Directions

Gene therapy and growth factors have an emerging role in the treatment of bone, cartilage, and tendon healing.[94,95] Tendon callus can be influenced by cartilage derived morphogenic protein-2 (CDMP-2).[95] Using an animal model of rabbit Achilles tendon tears, Forslund and Aspenberg[96] showed that failure load and stiffness in a CDMP-2 group were greater at 14 days compared with controls. Future treatments may include addition of growth factors to the repair site.

Postoperative Management: Traditional Immobilization and Remobilization Versus Early Motion

Since surgical repair of Achilles tendon ruptures began almost 50 years ago,[37] the traditional method of postoperative management has been to immobilize the repair in a plaster cast or other type of restrictive device until healing is considered complete, and then begin ROM and strengthening exercises.[12,26,31,32,97-102] Based on an understanding of connective tissue physiology and the success achieved with other types of surgical repairs, such as anterior cruciate ligament reconstruction, several authors have begun using early postoperative motion to minimize the deleterious effects of immobilization on joints (e.g., stiffness and loss of muscle strength, endurance, and flexibility)[74,93,103,104] and facilitate an earlier return to preoperative functional levels.* Numerous studies have compared immobilization to early postoperative motion[12,32,101,108-110] and early weight bearing.[12,32,101,102,109-111] In a meta-analysis, Khan found that functional bracing and early motion resulted in fewer adhesions, disturbed sensitivity, hypertrophic scarring, and infection with no difference in the rerupture rates between early motion and traditional immobilization groups.[41] Early functional programs provide better patient satisfaction without an increase in rerupture rates compared with cast immobilization.[109] However, no

studies have compared different early motion rehabilitation regimens. Varying protocols make comparison between studies difficult. The guidelines presented are a compilation of various approaches considering appropriate tendon healing.

Outcomes Measurements

Several outcomes measurement instruments have been used in Achilles tendon rupture research. In addition to objective clinical measures such as ROM, calf circumference, and muscle testing, instruments for function and patient satisfaction help the clinician to set goals and determine success of treatment. Early research used nonvalidated scoring methods for pain, stiffness, activity limitations, footwear restrictions, patient satisfaction, strength, and ROM.[111-114] The Victorian Institute of Sport Assessment was validated as an index of severity for patients with Achilles tendinopathy and has been used in Achilles tendon rupture research.[32,115] Although found to be reliable and valid, the degree of responsiveness has not been established. Patients use a visual analogue scale to score eight items for morning stiffness, pain with walking, descending stairs, heel raises, single-leg hops, and ability to participate in sports and physical activities.[116]

The foot and ankle ability measure (FAAM) assesses activity limitations and vocational and avocational restrictions for individuals with general musculoskeletal foot and ankle disorders. The FAAM uses a Likert scale for a 21-item ADL/activities subscale and an 8-item sport subscale for a perfect score of 100 with a minimal clinically important difference (MCID) of 8 points for ADL and 9 points for sports.[117,118] In 2007 an outcomes measurement specific to Achilles tendon ruptures was developed and found to be valid and reliable but has not been reported in a randomly controlled trial.[110,119,120] The Achilles tendon total rupture score (ATRS) uses 10 items rated on a 10-point scale for difficulty with strength, fatigue, stiffness, pain, ADLs, walking on level surfaces, ascending stairs or hills, running, jumping, and physical labor. We suggest that a change of 10 points in the score is clinically relevant.[119]

Guidelines for Traditional Immobilization and Remobilization

Immobilization might be in a conventional cast[12,32,45,101,102] or a fixed-angle ankle foot orthosis.[109] The time of immobilization has been reported from 4 weeks[102,109] to 8 weeks.[101] Cast changes can occur during the immobilization period for wound care or decreasing the degree of plantar flexion. Weight bearing has been reported as early as 2 weeks.[102]

Phases I and II

TIME: 1 to 8 weeks after surgery
GOALS: Minimize deconditioning, control edema and pain, encourage independent gait (*non–weight bearing until cleared by the physician to progressive weight bearing, usually at 4 weeks*) with assistive device as appropriate

---

*References 12-14, 32, 49, 101, 102, 105-108.

During traditional postoperative rehabilitation of surgically repaired Achilles tendon ruptures, a cast is usually in place throughout phases I and II of the healing process (Table 31-2). The PT can do little to influence healing and affect the outcome of the surgical repair. Casting incorporates varying degrees of plantar flexion to protect the repair from stress. Casts that were initially applied with the foot in plantar flexion are usually changed to neutral (0° dorsiflexion) for the final 3 to 4 weeks of immobilization. During this period, a conditioning program is designed to maintain the patient's general strength and cardiovascular conditioning. After the cast is removed, the PT can further protect the tendon from full stress by using a heel lift of varying heights for as long as 8 weeks, if needed. Crutches with progressive weight bearing also may be used to control mechanical stress.

Phase III

TIME: 9 to 16 weeks after surgery
GOALS: Normalize gait, increase ROM and strength, improve scar mobility

With the traditional approach, the rehabilitation program does not truly begin until phase III. The scar and tissue have begun to mature and therefore ROM, joint mobilization, stretching, strengthening, gait training, and return to function may progress as tolerated (Table 31-3). The sequence of treatment depends more on resolving the patient's physical impairments and functional limitations than on the timeline of healing. Impairments are resolved to reestablish function, develop skills, and return the patient to full activity and sports participation.

The initial goal is to restore ROM. Restoration of mobility must occur before the patient can begin to work on strength. Active exercises in the sagittal (dorsiflexion and plantar flexion) and transverse (inversion and eversion) planes are initiated and progressed with the knee flexed and extended. The therapist should use joint mobilization techniques to assist in gaining joint ROM and stretching exercises to gain muscle flexibility and improve joint ROM (see figures in the Chapter 29 describing mobilization of the ankle).

Any symptoms of pain and swelling that occur must be controlled during this phase through the use of appropriate modalities and adjustments in the intensity of the

TABLE 31-2 Achilles Tendon Repair (Traditional Rehabilitation)

Rehabilitation Phase	Criteria to Progress to This Phase	Anticipated Impairments and Functional Limitations	Intervention	Goal	Rationale
Phase I Postoperative 1-4 wk	• Postoperative	• Edema • Pain • Non–weight bearing • Cardiovascular and muscular deconditioning	• Immobilize in equinus • Provide elevation and ice • Instruct and monitor progressive weight-bearing crutch gait on all surfaces • Design and implement cardiovascular- and muscular-conditioning program	• Control edema and pain • Protect repair • Minimize deconditioning	• Immobilization in equinus minimizes stress on surgical repair during healing process • Elevation and ice assist in minimizing pain and swelling • Non–weight bearing status protects repair • Maintenance of cardiovascular and muscular conditioning crucial to general health and return to preoperative level of function when out of cast
Phase II Postoperative 5-8 wk	• Stable edema and pain • Well-healed incision present at cast change	• Abolished or diminishing postoperative pain and swelling • Atrophy of lower leg and foot muscles • Progressive weight-bearing status allowed • Cardiovascular and muscular deconditioning	• Recasted in neutral dorsiflexion • Elevation and ice as needed • Instruct in progressive weight bearing to full weight bearing using appropriate assistive devices • Modify cardiovascular and muscular conditioning program as appropriate	• Control symptoms of edema and pain if they occur • Continue to protect repair • Encourage full weight bearing during gait cycle • Minimize deconditioning	• Decreased rate of atrophy occurs when muscles are immobilized in a lengthened position[93] • Progressive weight bearing to full weight bearing allows loading and proprioceptive input • Conditioning program should be progressed as the patient's condition allows

TABLE 31-3 Achilles Tendon Repair (Traditional Rehabilitation)

Rehabilitation Phase	Criteria to Progress to This Phase	Anticipated Impairments and Functional Limitations	Intervention	Goal	Rationale
Phase III Postoperative 9-16 wk	• Out of cast • No increase in pain • No increased loss of ROM • Incision healed	• Altered gait cycle (preswing phase of gait) • Limited joint ROM and muscle flexibility • Atrophy and limited strength • Soft tissue edema and joint swelling • Tendon hypertrophy • Scar tissue adhesion • Limited cardiovascular fitness	• Ice, elevation, and nonsteroidal antiinflammatory drugs • Therapeutic ultrasound and/or whirlpool • PROM (stretches)—gastrocnemius-soleus, peroneals, tibialis anterior, tibialis posterior • Exercises, pool therapy, and joint mobilization as listed under the early motion program • AROM and isometrics in all directions, progressing to resisted exercises using tubing or manual resistance (proprioceptive neuromuscular facilitation) • Gait training—heel lift if required; return to progressive weight bearing with appropriate assistive devices (crutches or cane) to obtain normal gait cycle if necessary to avoid secondary overuse/tendonitis syndrome; progress as indicated based on symptoms of gait cycle	• Control edema and pain if occur • Initiate normalization of gait cycle • Obtain full ROM • Improve strength of all foot and ankle musculature • Reduce scar tissue adhesion • Promote cardiovascular and muscular conditioning	• Modalities have been demonstrated to improve ease of tissue deformation when used in conjunction with mobilization and stretching • Restore normal ROM • Initiate strength through ROM to improve overall function • Increase strength and endurance • Gait deficits in the preswing phase may result from limited dorsiflexion and decreased plantar flexion strength—heel lifts assist in reducing stress on musculotendinous structures in foot and ankle during the early gait cycle out of cast; heel lift can be decreased or eliminated as indicated • Overuse symptoms should be addressed as appropriate to minimize their severity and longevity
Phase IV Postoperative 17-20 wk	• No symptoms from ROM, flexibility, and strengthening exercises initiated during wk 9-16 • Able to sustain isometric single-leg toe raise and lower body weight eccentrically under control • AROM dorsiflexion 5° • PROM dorsiflexion 10° • Symmetric plantar flexion, inversion, and eversion • No assistive devices required for ambulation	• Mild or minimal alteration in gait cycle without assistive devices • Restricted joint ROM and muscle flexibility • Unable to do repeated single-leg heel raise • Limited strength • Limited proprioception • Soft tissue edema • Tendon hypertrophy • Minimal scar tissue adhesion • Cardiovascular and muscular deconditioning	• Continue intervention from phase III as indicated • Continue joint mobilization techniques as appropriate • Continue stretching exercises; initiate body weight stretching over edge of step • Continue strength program for foot and ankle musculature as listed in early motion program • Modify cardiovascular and muscular conditioning program as needed • Isokinetics and body weight resistance exercises such as heel raises (if no increase in symptoms occurs with previous exercises) • Balance and proprioceptive activities (e.g., Biomechanical Ankle Platform System board, single-leg balance activities) • Near the end of the phase, begin running progression and sport-specific skill development	• Normal gait cycle on level surfaces; initiate running program when normal gait cycle is evident • Full symmetric ankle joint ROM and muscle flexibility • Continue to improve foot and ankle strength; repeated single-leg heel raise • Symmetric single-limb balance • Reduce scar tissue adhesion • Promote cardiovascular and muscular conditioning	• Progress intensity of rehabilitation program as indicated • Restore arthrokinematics • Promote patient self-management and stretching program • Prepare for discharge • Promote symmetric strength of foot and ankle via single-limb balance, isokinetic testing, and progressive plyometric program initiated in water and progressed to land • Continue and progress based on each patient's response to intervention • Provide a good cardiovascular maintenance program based on patient's needs • Increase strength and improve function • Improve balance and coordination on uneven surfaces • Transition into high-level occupational activities or sports

AROM, Active range of motion; *PROM*, passive range of motion; *ROM*, range of motion.

treatment plan and home program. For return to progressive weight bearing use appropriate assistive devices (crutches or cane) to obtain normal gait cycle if necessary to avoid secondary overuse/tendonitis syndrome. Progress as able based on symptoms of gait cycle. Soft tissue mobilization can be used to reduce scar adhesion. These adjuncts for restoring ROM, muscle and tendon flexibility, and strength are continued throughout the program as appropriate (see Table 31-3).

Phase IV

TIME: 17 to 20 weeks after surgery
GOALS: Demonstrate normal gait on level surfaces, initiate running program, have full ROM, increase strength, improve balance and coordination

The therapist can initiate strengthening as ROM progresses. Initially, isometric techniques are used for all motions. Strength training then progresses to the use of elastic tubing and manual resistive techniques, such as proprioceptive neuromuscular facilitation. Isokinetic exercise and body weight resistance can be added if symptoms do not arise from the other techniques. The patient should begin double-heel raises before single-heel raises to reduce tensile stress and the potential for symptoms such as pain and swelling. The heel raises should initially be performed on a level, flat surface, after which the patient can progress to doing them over the edge of a stair to use the full ROM available. Proprioceptive and balance activities should be initiated concurrently with strengthening. The PT can begin a running progression, sport-specific skill development, and functional activities after the patient has a normal gait and full ROM and can rapidly perform heel raises. Isokinetic measurement of strength, power, and endurance at 4 to 6 months may assist in the determination of return to sport activity, but it is not the sole determining factor.

The success of Achilles tendon repair using traditional immobilization and rehabilitation has been favorably measured, primarily by rerupture rates, strength, calf circumference, tendon width, and return to previous activity levels. In a meta-analysis comparing cast immobilization and functional bracing, Khan reported a pooled rerupture rate for traditional immobilization of 5% and other complications (adhesions, infection, and disturbed sensibility) at 35.7%.[41] Early weight bearing in a cast was found to have no adverse effect as compared with the non–weight bearing group.[102] The weight-bearing group discarded crutches approximately 3 weeks earlier than the non–weight bearing group, with no differences noted in tendon size measured by ultrasound and in isometric strength. Strength measurements include the ability to perform single-toe raises, manual muscle tests, and isokinetic strength measurements. Authors using peak torque measurements of isokinetic plantar flexion strength have reported that the gastrocnemius and soleus strength of the repaired Achilles tendon ranges from 83% to 101% of the uninvolved extremity.[37] Some authors use combined

isokinetic deficits at several speeds, ranking results poor to excellent, with good to excellent results in 71% to 79% of the subjects.[112,114] Outcome measures in studies that have been reported in the literature are difficult to use in comparing various studies.[37] These studies used different operational definitions, set forth different methodologies, and collected data at different times, making meaningful comparison difficult.

Guidelines for Early Motion

As early as 1984, in an effort to reduce the effects of immobilization, various authors began to present methods of repair that would allow early motion and rehabilitation.[13,49,86,106,120-123] Orthoses or specialized splinting were developed to protect the repair after surgery.* Only one report, a case series, described an early motion protocol, no postoperative fixation, and no postoperative complications within 24 weeks. Protected AROM begins as early as day 1.[120] In some cases AROM begins at 2 weeks.[32,109,123] The functional orthosis is removed most frequently at 6 weeks, sometimes with use of a heel lift for several weeks. Weight bearing begins immediately[32,101,110] or up to 2 weeks after surgery[109] and is generally progressed as tolerated. **Regardless of the type of repair, rehabilitation programs that emphasize early motion must consider the strength and integrity of the repaired Achilles tendon as it changes during the various stages of healing.**

Phase Ia

TIME: 1 to 2 days after surgery
GOALS: Prevent infection, control edema and pain, increase AROM, prevent complications, promote independent gait using assistive device as appropriate

Phase Ib

TIME: 3 to 7 days after surgery
GOALS: Demonstrate AROM dorsiflexion to 5° and plantar flexion 50% of uninvolved side, control edema and pain

When using an early motion program for postoperative **rehabilitation, the therapist must keep in mind the phases of tissue healing and the degree to which tissues can tolerate tensile stress.** During phases Ia and Ib of the early motion program, the primary concerns are evaluating wound status, decreasing swelling, and initiating ROM exercises (Table 31-4). *However, ROM should not be pushed aggressively. The patient should work through PROM within the limits of pain and swelling intermittently throughout the day.* The PT may prescribe ice, compression, and elevation to decrease swelling.

---

*References 12, 32, 101, 105, 107, 109, 123.

TABLE 31-4 Achilles Tendon Repair (Early Motion)

Rehabilitation Phase	Criteria to Progress to This Phase	Anticipated Impairments and Functional Limitations	Intervention	Goal	Rationale
Phase Ia Postoperative 1-2 days	• Postoperative	• Pain • Soft tissue and joint edema • Altered weight bearing, non–weight bearing with crutches	• Instruct in surgical site protection • Provide ice, compression, and elevation • Teach toe curls and pumps • AROM (out of splint) — ankle dorsiflexion, plantar flexion within pain limits two times a day • Patient education • Instruction and monitoring of non–weight bearing crutch gait	• Monitor wound status for drainage • Prevent wound infection • Control pain and swelling • Increase AROM • Prevent complications	• Surgical site inspection and cleanliness is crucial when patient is out of splint for ROM • Ice, compression, and elevation with an ice cuff over a sterile wound dressing minimizes swelling • Toe curls and AROM dorsiflexion and plantar flexion provide muscle pump to minimize edema
Phase Ib Postoperative 3-7 days	• No signs of infection	• Pain • Soft tissue and joint edema • Altered weight bearing, non–weight bearing with crutches until day 14	• Monitor wound for infection • Provide ice, compression, and elevation • AROM — increase frequency to three times a day for dorsiflexion and plantar flexion • Therapeutic ultrasound • Instruction and monitoring of progressive crutch gait	• Minimize joint stiffness • Facilitate healing • Reduce soft tissue and joint swelling • Active dorsiflexion to −5° • 50% active plantar flexion ROM compared with opposite side	• As in phase Ia • Therapeutic ultrasound has been demonstrated to assist in fibroblastic proliferation and facilitate collagen development along lines of stress.[124,125,127]

AROM, Active range of motion; *ROM*, range of motion.

Phase IIa

TIME: 2 to 4 weeks after surgery
GOALS: Increase AROM and PROM, strength, and weight-bearing tolerance

During phase IIa (Table 31-5) of the early motion program, emphasis is placed on gaining active dorsiflexion past neutral, following a full weight-bearing program in a protective splint or boot with a fixed hinge (Fig. 31-9), and **initiating a gentle strength-training program of all the muscle groups in a range that minimizes tensile stress on the repair.**

During phases Ia and IIa, therapeutic ultrasound can be used to assist in the healing response. In some instances therapeutic ultrasound has been shown to increase collagen synthesis and tensile strength in experimentally repaired rabbit Achilles tendon.[79,124-126] Enwemeka[125] and Enwemeka, Rodriguez, and Mendosa[124] reported favorable results that enhanced the healing response using 1 MHz at doses of 0.5 W/cm² and 1 W/cm² for 5 minutes during nine consecutive treatments. Jackson, Schwane, and Starcher[126] noted changes in collagen synthesis and breaking strength as early as 5 days after injury when giving continuous therapeutic ultrasound at 1.5 W/cm² for 4 minutes over 8 consecutive days and then every other day for up to 21 days. Freider and associates[127] reported similar results in partially ruptured, nonsurgically repaired Achilles tendons of Marland rats that received continuous therapeutic ultrasound at 1.5 W/cm² three times a week for either a 2- or a 3-week period. Ng reported no significant difference among treatment groups in the collagen fibril size in severed rat Achilles tendons after treatment with 1 Mhz continuous therapeutic ultrasound at 0.5, 1.2, and 2 W/cm². There was a significant difference comparing treatment groups to control of sham ultrasound.[128]

Although the results of studies using animal models may not be directly applicable to the human response, the therapeutic use of therapeutic ultrasound in the inflammatory and proliferative stages could prove beneficial. Using therapeutic ultrasound during these stages is a common clinical intervention.

TABLE 31-5 Achilles Tendon Repair (Early Motion)

Rehabilitation Phase	Criteria to Progress to This Phase	Anticipated Impairments and Functional Limitations	Intervention	Goal	Rationale
Phase IIa Postoperative 2-4 wk	• Absence of wound drainage and infection • Stable edema and pain levels • Diminishing postoperative pain • No increase in pain with touchdown weight bearing using crutches • A well-healed incision should be present by wk 3 to progress to the more active interventions (pool therapy) outlined in this phase	• Diminishing postoperative pain • Diminishing soft tissue and joint swelling • Scar adhesion • Touchdown and progressive weight-bearing status • Restricted ROM • Decreased strength • Altered cardiovascular endurance and conditioning	• Continue interventions as noted in phase I • Joint mobilization progress techniques for distraction—anteroposterior and medial-lateral glides • Progressive soft tissue mobilization and scar massage • Progressive weight-bearing exercises and gait training in walking splint • Start touchdown weight bearing on day 8; progress from partial to full weight bearing as pain and symptoms allow beginning on day 14 • Isometrics—out of splint • Ankle in neutral—inversion and eversion • Start plantar flexion isometrics in late phase IIa • Pool therapy—walk or run under full buoyancy conditions (non–weight bearing only) • AROM (out of splint)—ankle (early phase IIa, all directions, knee flexed and extended; late phase IIa, gentle dorsiflexion stretching with towel or strap, knee flexed and extended towel curls with toes) • Gait training wearing protective splint, with weight bearing to tolerance • Elastic tubing or band exercises—inversion, eversion, and plantar flexion and dorsiflexion; progress as tolerated if pain and symptoms allow • Isotonics—weight training program for all unaffected muscle groups • Cardiovascular exercise using stationary bicycle to tolerance in walking splint	• Minimize joint stiffness • Facilitate healing • Decrease edema • Minimize scar adhesion • Increase weight bearing tolerance to full weight bearing, beginning on day 14 • Initiate isometric strength program • Improve general muscular strength and endurance • Early phase IIa: active dorsiflexion to 0° with knee extended, 5° with knee flexed • Late phase IIa: active dorsiflexion to 0°-5° with knee extended, 5°-10° with knee flexed • Minimize cardiovascular deconditioning	• Therapeutic ultrasound is most effective in first 3 wk and less effective thereafter; discontinued by late phase IIa • Repair is strong enough and symptoms are stable enough to initiate full weight bearing in protective brace; reduce weight-bearing status as necessary based on symptom fluctuation and patient activity pattern • Isometrics to facilitate strengthening and to diminish edema and atrophy are performed in neutral position to reduce stress on repair • Pool exercises facilitate ROM and strength in non–weight-bearing environment • Ice, compression, and elevation with a Cryo Cuff over sterile wound dressing minimizes swelling • Toe curls and AROM dorsiflexion and plantar flexion provide muscle pump to minimize edema • Sufficient strength present at repair site based on healing and surgical technique to allow AROM to 0° dorsiflexion and all other motions to symptom tolerance with knee flexed and extended • Towel curls facilitate muscle pump action to diminish edema and atrophy • By 4 wk, sufficient strength to allow start of plantar flexion isometrics and isotonics within symptom limits, using light resistance; performed in non–weight bearing • Maintenance of general muscular strength and cardiovascular endurance necessary to resume full activities of daily living and recreational activities when feasible; walking splint protects repair during activity

AROM, Active range of motion; *ROM,* range of motion.

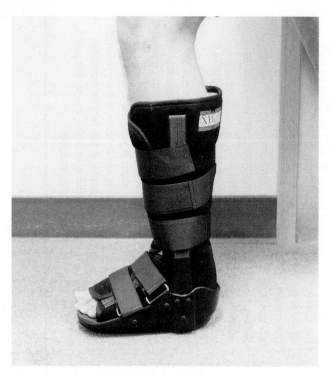

Fig. 31-9 Protective splint and boot for initiating progressive and full weight bearing. A fixed hinge should be used.

Phase IIb

TIME: 5 to 8 weeks after surgery
GOALS: Demonstrate normal gait on level surfaces, encourage full ROM (symmetric), increase strength and proprioception

During phase IIb (Table 31-6), the patient should strive to obtain full symmetric ROM, achieve a normal gait cycle on level surfaces and in controlled environments without the protective boot, progress the strength program, and initiate proprioceptive training.

Phase IIIa

TIME: 9 to 16 weeks after surgery
GOALS: Demonstrate normal gait for all activities, have full weight bearing, increase strength and endurance; initiate walking with progression toward a jogging program (as appropriate), isokinetics, and pool therapy plyometrics as appropriate (toward end of phase)

TABLE 31-6 Achilles Tendon Repair (Early Motion)

Rehabilitation Phase	Criteria to Progress to This Phase	Anticipated Impairments and Functional Limitations	Intervention	Goal	Rationale
Phase IIb Postoperative 5-8 wk	• No loss of ROM • No increase in symptoms • Full weight bearing in walking splint • Incision healed • Mild edema • Pain controlled • AROM • Dorsiflexion to neutral or better • Plantar flexion, inversion/eversion symmetric	• Minimal postoperative pain • Limited ROM • Limited strength • Tendon hypertrophy and continued soft tissue swelling • Altered gait cycle out of walking splint • Unable to do a single-leg heel raise • Altered proprioception and joint reaction time	• Continue interventions as noted in phases I and II • PROM—initiate weight-bearing dorsiflexion stretch with knee extended and flexed • AROM (out of splint) • Gait training out of walking splint to tolerance • Strength training—initiate double-leg heel raises • Isokinetics—submaximal velocity spectrum • Plantar flexion and dorsiflexion, emphasizing endurance • Weight training program for all unaffected muscle groups • Stationary bicycle to tolerance without walking splint • Pool therapy for ROM (walking or running under total buoyant conditions); heel raises in waist- to chest-deep water	• Full symmetric ROM in all motions • Normal gait cycle on level surfaces and controlled environments out of walking splint • Initiate isokinetic and isotonic strength-training program for gastrocnemius-soleus complex • Improve cardiovascular conditioning • Improve muscular strength and endurance • Improve proprioception and joint reaction time	• Continue mobilizations to increase soft tissue strength and mobility and restore joint ROM sufficient to initiate gait training out of splint; gait should be practiced in controlled environment out of splint for safety as appropriate; discontinue use of splint at physician's and therapist's discretion • Weight-bearing dorsiflexion required for normal ADLs; repair should be sufficiently strong; discontinue if symptoms occur • Gastrocnemius-soleus/repair initially conditioned with isometrics; repair now strong enough to tolerate increased strength training on a progressive weight and force basis

ADLs, Activities of daily living; *AROM,* active range of motion; *PROM,* passive range of motion; *ROM,* range of motion.

Phase IIIb

TIME: 17 to 20 weeks after surgery
GOALS: Return to preoperative level of activity or sport

During phase IIIa (Table 31-7), emphasis is on increasing the velocity of activity, increasing the patient's strength to perform a repeated single-leg heel raise, and improving the endurance of the gastrocnemius and soleus group to tolerate a functional progression. During phase IIIb (Table 31-8), a full functional progression is initiated to return the patient to the desired level of function.

All authors using an early functional program, regardless of the type of augmentation used during surgery, have reported excellent results. Success was measured by the same methods as for traditional rehabilitation. Limitation of ROM for dorsiflexion and plantar flexion are rare; patients are able to walk heel-toe and do single-leg raises at the time of

TABLE 31-7 Achilles Tendon Repair (Early Motion)

Rehabilitation Phase	Criteria to Progress to This Phase	Anticipated Impairments and Functional Limitations	Intervention	Goal	Rationale
Phase IIIa Postoperative 9-16 wk	• No longer requires walking splint for ADLs; may require use of splint for extended ambulatory periods in early parts of phase • Pain-free gait during ADLs walking out of splint • Minimal difference in dorsiflexion range of motion versus uninvolved side • Full plantar flexion, inversion, and eversion	• Gait deviations in preswing phase of gait resulting from limited plantar flexion, strength, and endurance, not insufficient dorsiflexion • Unable to perform single-leg heel raise • Unable to jump and run • Mild pain and muscle and tendon fatigue at end of day if walking for a significant period • Limited tolerance to tendon-loading activities (concentric and eccentric)	• Continue interventions from phases I and II as indicated, especially weight-bearing dorsiflexion stretch • AROM—progress toward single-leg heel raises, add resistance up to 1.5 times body weight as symptoms dictate • Gait training—treadmill walking on level surfaces and slight incline, uneven surface walking, stair climbing; progress to jogging toward end of phase if symptom free (no sprinting, cutting, or jumping activities); jogging on minitrampoline • Isokinetics—submaximal effort velocity spectrum plantar flexion and dorsiflexion • Pool therapy (waist-deep)—plyometrics (hopping, bounding, and jumping in waist-deep water) • Cardiovascular exercises	• Discontinue use of walking splint • Repeated single-leg heel raise from level surface • Normal gait cycle for all ADLs • Full symmetric weight-bearing dorsiflexion • Initiate fast-walking or jogging program • Decrease complaints of mild pain or muscle and tendon fatigue at end of day with walking activities • Increase plantar flexion strength and endurance • Improve plantar flexion strength and endurance at maximal velocities • Prepare for land-based agility drills • Improve cardiovascular fitness level	• Plantar flexion weakness will compromise gait; emphasis is placed on improving functional plantar flexion strength and endurance (single-leg heel raise); higher gait velocities affected until late in this phase or into phase IIIb • Incline treadmill use will develop strength and endurance of gastrocnemius-soleus muscles • Uneven surface and stair training improves proprioception and community ambulation • Jogging and running must be initiated only if patient is symptom free, has a normal gait, and is able to perform multiple single-leg heel raises at moderate to high velocities to avoid overloading tendon and initiating an inflammatory cycle • Use of minitrampoline will facilitate achievement of dorsiflexion at varying velocities, simulate higher level function, and develop higher velocity eccentric load tolerance • Continued development of strength and endurance required throughout this phase to achieve full ADLs and recreational function • Plyometric activities in the pool facilitate functional use without full weight-bearing stress • Use gait training activities and stair machine to provide aerobic training

ADLs, Activities of daily living; *AROM,* active range of motion.

TABLE 31-8 Achilles Tendon Repair (Early Motion)

Rehabilitation Phase	Criteria to Progress to This Phase	Anticipated Impairments and Functional Limitations	Intervention	Goal	Rationale
Phase IIIb Postoperative 17-20 wk	• Normal gait on all surfaces and inclines • Able to fast walk or jog without gait deficits • Able to do repeated single-leg heel raises with moderate to high velocities • Asymptomatic with all activities of daily living, treadmill walking, and jogging	• Unable to hop or jump on single leg without performance deficit or compensatory movement • Difficulty with sprinting or cutting during higher level recreational activities	• Review of past rehabilitation program to address areas that may not have been appropriately addressed • Development of individualized strength, flexibility, ROM, and functional progression program to alleviate impairments and functional limitations	• Resolve all impairments and functional limitations that limit full return to preoperative level of function	• Most patients and athletes have only minor performance deficits by this time; deficits (which may continue to exist) require individualized attention based on their presentation and the way they affect the athlete or patient in question; these areas may not have been appropriately addressed earlier or the patient might have tried to progress too fast; any impairments or functional limitations are usually resolved within this phase and time period

ROM, Range of motion.

follow-up examination. In addition, isokinetic peak torque levels are within 5% of the uninvolved side.[13,105]

Reruptures are rare and are usually attributed to lack of retraining before a return to sports[123] or return to vigorous activity against advice.[101] However, these outcomes are also difficult to compare for the same reasons as cited for traditional rehabilitation programs.

SUMMARY

The superiority of early motion for Achilles tendon repairs compared with traditional postoperative casting cannot yet be fully determined. Although studies reported to date state that the results are excellent, the different rehabilitation philosophies cannot be compared critically because of differences in operational definitions, criteria monitored, postoperative time when the data are collected, and surgical technique. Although the ultimate level of function achieved appears to be the same regardless of the rehabilitative program, the authors of this chapter believe that using early motion after Achilles tendon repair enables the patient to obtain a more independent and active quality of life sooner than that seen with traditional postoperative casting. However, patient compliance and ongoing oversight of the rehabilitation program are crucial factors that must always be considered.

Suggested Home Maintenance for the Postsurgical Patient

Adherence to a home exercise program is crucial for a successful return to full ADLs and recreational function after Achilles tendon repair. The suggestions provided in this chapter do not constitute a fixed protocol. The home program for any patient must be individually determined based on the patient's postoperative condition, anticipated follow-through, and individual needs. Frequency, sets, and repetitions are determined similarly based on the therapist's professional opinion of what is needed in a particular situation.

Suggested Home Maintenance for the Postsurgical Patient: Traditional Rehabilitation Program

Weeks 1 To 4
GOALS FOR THE PERIOD: Manage symptoms (edema and pain), improve function, minimize deconditioning
1. For edema and pain: Use ice and elevation; perform toe curls and pumps.
2. For function: Use non–weight bearing crutch gait, progress depending on surgeon preference, type of immobilization, and as tolerated.
3. For deconditioning: Modify cardiovascular and muscle conditioning as tolerated. (Continue progressive program throughout rehabilitation.)

Weeks 5 To 8
GOALS FOR THE PERIOD: Manage symptoms, improve function
1. For symptoms: Use ice, compression, and elevation as needed; perform toe curls and pumps as needed.
2. For function: Progress to full weight bearing to tolerance with appropriate assistive devices if needed.

Weeks 9 To 16
GOALS FOR THE PERIOD: Improve ROM, continue strength training, and achieve functional improvement
1. For ROM:
   a. Initiate non–weight bearing stretching exercises for all ankle motions (dorsiflexion, plantar flexion, inversion, and eversion).
   b. Initiate weight-bearing dorsiflexion stretch with knee flexed and extended.
2. For strength training:
   a. Initiate isometric and elastic band strengthening exercises for all muscle groups.
   b. Progress to double-leg heel raises as tolerated.

3. For function:
   a. Begin ambulation out of cast to symptom tolerance.
   b. Use heel lift and cane or crutches as appropriate to limit symptoms.

Weeks 17 To 20
GOALS FOR THE PERIOD: Improve ROM, continue strength training, achieve functional improvement
1. For ROM: Continue all stretching exercises.
2. For strength training:
   a. Initiate single-leg heel raises.
   b. Progress to additional weight heel raises with up to 1.5 times body weight provided no symptoms of pain, swelling, or inflammation develop.
3. For function:
   a. Initiate walking on all types of surfaces and inclines and declines.
   b. Progress to fast walking and jogging toward the end of this phase if no symptoms have occurred and patient is able to do single-leg toe raises repeatedly.
   c. **No sprinting, cutting, or jumping allowed.**

Week 20 And Beyond
GOALS FOR THE PERIOD: Continue strength training, achieve functional improvement
1. For strength training:
   a. Do single-leg heel raises over the edge of a step.
   b. Do weight lifting to tolerance.
2. For function:
   a. Initiate jogging when able.
   b. Initiate hopping, skipping, and jumping activities.
   c. Return to all recreational and sports activities.

Suggested Home Maintenance for the Postsurgical Patient: Early Motion Program

Week 1
GOALS FOR THE WEEK: Manage symptoms (edema, pain), improve ROM, begin work on function, minimize deconditioning
1. For symptoms: Use ice, compression, and elevation; perform toe curls and pumps.
2. For ROM: Perform active range of motion (AROM) three times daily; perform plantar flexion and dorsiflexion out of the splint within pain limits with the knee flexed and extended.
3. For function: Use non–weight bearing crutch gait; progress depending on surgeon preference, type of immobilization, and as tolerated.
4. For deconditioning: Modify cardiovascular and muscle conditioning as tolerated. (Continue progressive program throughout rehabilitation.)

Weeks 2 To 4
GOALS FOR THE PERIOD: Manage edema, improve ROM, continue strength training, work on function
1. For edema: Use ice, compression, and elevation as needed; perform toe curls and pumps as needed.
2. For ROM in early phase IIa (days 7 to 21): Perform AROM three times daily in all directions out of the splint (plantar flexion, dorsiflexion, inversion, and eversion) with the knee flexed and extended.
3. For ROM in late phase IIa (days 21 to 28): Perform gentle dorsiflexion stretching with a towel or strap with the knee flexed and extended three times daily.
4. For strength training in early phase IIa (days 7 to 21): Perform isometric inversion and eversion in neutral dorsiflexion.
5. For strength training in late phase IIa (days 21 to 28): Perform isometric plantar flexion and dorsiflexion; progress to light elastic band exercises if free of pain and swelling.
6. For function (note: use walking boot at all times): Start touchdown weight bearing on day 8; perform progressive weight bearing at day 14 if no increase in pain and symptoms is noted.

Weeks 5 To 8
GOALS FOR THE PERIOD: Improve ROM, continue strength training, improve function
1. For ROM:
   a. Continue phase IIa activities as appropriate.
   b. Initiate weight-bearing dorsiflexion stretch with knee flexed and extended.
2. For strength training:
   a. Continue phase IIa activities as appropriate.
   b. Initiate double-leg heel raises.
3. For function:
   a. Begin ambulation out of the walking splint to symptom tolerance.
   b. Use heel lift and cane as appropriate to limit symptoms.

Weeks 9 To 16
GOALS FOR THE PERIOD: Improve ROM, continue strength training, improve function
1. For ROM: Continue phase IIb activities as appropriate to gain full ROM.
2. For strength training:
   a. Progress towards single-leg heel raises.
   b. Progress to additional weight heel raises with up to 1.5 times body weight if no symptoms of pain, swelling, or inflammation occur.
3. For function:
   a. Initiate walking on all types of surfaces and inclines and declines.
   b. Progress to jogging toward end of phase if no symptoms have occurred.
   c. **No sprinting, cutting, or jumping allowed.**

Weeks 17 To 20
GOALS FOR THE PERIOD: Continue strength training, achieve functional improvement
1. For strength training:
   a. Do single-leg heel raises over the edge of a step.
   b. Perform weight lifting to tolerance.
2. For function:
   a. Initiate hopping, skipping, and jumping activities.
   b. Return to all recreational and sports activities.

CLINICAL CASE REVIEW

1 What are the three stages of healing?

(a) Inflammatory response—Minutes after injury, laceration, or the initiation of surgical repair. (b) Repair and proliferation—The repair and proliferation stage may begin as early as 48 hours after injury and may last for 6 to 8 weeks. (c) Remodeling and maturation—can last months.

2 Scott is 35 years old and is undergoing his initial evaluation 7 days after surgery. What part of his history will help the therapist avoid being too aggressive and putting the repair at risk?

His general health, family, and past medical history are keys to determining if any factors may delay the healing process. Diabetes, peripheral vascular disease, medications (corticosteroids/NSAIDs), anticoagulants, smoking, past responses to healing (surgical, nonsurgical, or both), pain tolerance, nutrition, and high body mass index all influence soft tissue healing response.

3 Nancy is following an early motion program and began therapy at 1 week postoperation with an ATRS score of 10. At 6 weeks, she has made clinically significant progress as demonstrated by an ATRS score of 44. How do you use this data to plan her continued therapy?

Review the detailed scores to find that Nancy is limited more so in her activity scores than in pain, stiffness, and strength which correlates with your objective findings. Evaluate Nancy's ADLs, vocational, and recreational activity goals to begin activity-specific training.

4 Kerry had an Achilles tendon repair 7 weeks ago. She is partial weight bearing and uses a fixed protective splint. At 9 weeks she will initiate non–weight bearing stretching exercises for all ankle motions. During phases I and II (weeks 1 through 8) of the healing process, fibroblastic proliferation continues, producing a rapid increase in the amount of collagen. Even though collagen amounts are increased, the repaired tissue is weak and requires protection (e.g., restricted weight bearing and nonaggressive ROM stretches). Why do the healing tissues remain weak despite the increase in collagen fibers?

Type III collagen is deposited; it has poor cross-link definition, small fibril size, and poor strength. As the repair process continues, the collagen deposition shifts to type I collagen, which has better cross-link definition, fibril size, and strength.

5 Kim is 40 years old and ruptured her Achilles tendon playing tennis. She had surgery 7 weeks ago and is eager to resume her prior activity level. What exercises can she safely perform, laying the foundation for her return to the court?

At this stage of Kim's rehabilitation, she can safely perform deep-water running (in a floatation vest without her feet touching the bottom), core training exercises that avoid straining the repair (sitting or supine using a medicine ball), and upper extremity exercises (scapula stabilization and rotator cuff program).

6 Doug is 43 years old and underwent an Achilles tendon repair 9 weeks ago. The physician has chosen the traditional immobilization approach for rehabilitation. He presented today 1 week after cast removal and is still quite painful with ambulation (stance phase). What can the therapist do to help control his symptoms?

The PT can assist in protecting the tendon from full stress by using a heel lift of varying heights, and wean the height as able. In addition, by using crutches, progressive weight bearing may be used to control mechanical stress. Modalities can also be used to help manage any residual pain and inflammation.

7 Brian is 3 months postoperation and is concerned that his repaired Achilles tendon looks much larger than his unaffected side. Is this normal?

The area of repair can be 6.1 times the size of the unaffected tendon at 3 months and 5.6 times the size at 6 months. A variably sized, high-intensity signal demonstrating a central intratendinous lesion was detected in 19 of 21 repaired tendons at 3 months. The development of an intratendinous lesion appears to be a normal part of the healing process after surgical repair and casting.

8 Tom is 3 weeks postoperation in the early motion guidelines. What can be done to assist his healing response.

Once the incision is healed and dry, therapeutic ultrasound can be used to help assist in the healing response. In some instances therapeutic ultrasound has been shown to increase collagen synthesis and tensile strength.

9 Dan is 22 weeks postoperation and demonstrates good ROM and strength. He has a normal gait on level surfaces, and he initiated the Return to Running program. He appears to be holding back his effort on some agility drills and he mentions that he "just doesn't feel that he can trust it." What can you do as a clinician to alleviate his concerns?

Reruptures are rare and are usually attributed to lack of retraining before a return to sports. The demands of his sport should be broken down into phases and accomplished one phase at a time. This will allow him to be successful in smaller demand activities and gain confidence that he can "trust" his repair. Refer to the chapters on Return to Running and Return to Jumping for a complete program.

REFERENCES

1. Romanelli D, Almekinders L, Mandelbaum B: Achilles rupture in the athlete: Current science and treatment. Sports Med Arthrosc Rev 8:377, 2000.
2. Schuberth JM: Achilles tendon trauma. In Scurran BL, editor: Foot and ankle trauma, ed 2, New York, 1996, Churchill Livingstone.
3. Lagerrgren C, Lindholm A: Vascular distribution in the Achilles tendon: An arteriographic and microangiographic study. Acta Chir Scand 116:491, 1959.
4. Arner O, Lindholm A, Orell SR: Histologic changes in subcutaneous rupture of the Achilles tendon. Acta Chir Scand 116:484, 1959.
5. Carr AJ, Norris SH: The blood supply of the calcaneal tendon. J Bone Joint Surg 71B(1):100, 1989.
6. Schatzker J, Branemark PI: Intravital observation of the microvascular anatomy and microcirculation of tendon. Acta Orthop Scand Suppl 126:3, 1969.
7. Alfredson H, Lorentzon R: Chronic Achilles tendinosis: Recommendations for treatment and prevention. Sports Med 29:135, 2000.
8. Amadio PC: Tendon and ligament. In Cohen IK, Diegelmann RF, Lindblad WJ, editors: Wound healing: Biochemical and clinical aspects, Philadelphia, 1992, Saunders.
9. Bradley JP, Tibone JE: Percutaneous and open surgical repairs of Achilles tendon ruptures. Am J Sports Med 18:188, 1990.
10. Paddu G, Ippolito E, Postacchini F: A classification of Achilles tendon disease. Am J Sports Med 4(4):145, 1976.
11. Kvist H, Kvist M: The operative treatment of chronic calcaneal paratendonitis. J Bone Joint Surg 62B(3):353, 1980.
12. Kannus P, Jozsa L: Histopathological changes preceding spontaneous rupture of a Achilles tendon. J Bone Joint Surg 73A(10):1507, 1991.
13. Mandelbaum BR, Myerson MS, Forster R: Achilles tendon ruptures: A new method of repair, early range of motion, and functional rehabilitation. Am J Sports Med 23(4):392, 1995.
14. Mandelbaum BR, Hayes WM, Knapp TP: Management of Achilles tendon ruptures. Foot Ankle 2(3):1, 1997.
15. Alfredson H, Thorsen K, Lorentzon R: In situ microdialysis in tendon tissue: High levels of glutamate, but not prostaglandin E2 in chronic Achilles tendon pain [see comment]. Knee Surg Sports Traumatol Arthrosc 7:378, 1999.
16. Almekinders LC, Deol G: The effects of aging, antiinflammatory drugs, and ultrasound on the in vitro response of tendon tissue. Am J Sports Med 27:417, 1999.
17. Hastad K, Larsson HG, Lindholm A: Clearance of radiosodium after local deposit in the Achilles tendon. Acta Chir Scand 116:251, 1959.
18. Strocchi R, et al: Human Achilles tendon: Morphological and morphometric variations as a function of age. Foot Ankle 12:100, 1991.
19. Curwin S: Tendon injuries: Pathology and treatment. In Zachazewski JE, Magee DJ, Quillen WS, editors: Athletic injuries and rehabilitation, Philadelphia, 1996, Saunders.
20. van der Linden PD, et al: Increased risk of Achilles tendon rupture with quinolone antibacterial use, especially in elderly patients taking oral corticosteroids [see comment]. Arch Int Med 163:1801, 2003.
21. Curwin SL: Force and length changes of the gastrocnemius and soleus muscle-tendon units during a therapeutic exercise program and three selected activities, master's thesis, Halifax, Nova Scotia, Canada, 1984, Dalhousie University.
22. Curwin S, Stanish W: Tendinitis: Its etiology and treatment, Lexington, Mass, 1984. Collamore Press.
23. Gregor RV, Komi PV, Jarvinen M: Achilles tendon forces during cycling. Int J Sports Med 8(suppl):9, 1987.
24. Arner O, Lindholm A: Avulsion fracture of the os calcaneus. Acta Chir Scand 117:258, 1959.
25. Beskin JL, et al: Surgical repair of Achilles tendon ruptures. Am J Sports Med 15:1, 1987.
26. Cetti R, et al: Operative versus nonoperative treatment of Achilles tendon rupture: A prospective randomized study and review of the literature. Am J Sports Med 21(6):791, 1993.
27. Jozsa L, et al: The role of recreational sport activity in Achilles tendon rupture: A clinical, pathoanatomical, and sociological study of 292 cases. Am J Sports Med 17(3):338, 1989.
28. Nistor L: Surgical and non-surgical treatment of Achilles tendon rupture. J Bone Joint Surg 63A(3):395, 1981.
29. Carden DG, et al: Rupture of the calcaneal tendon: The early and late management. J Bone Joint Surg 69B:416, 1987.
30. Christensen IB: Rupture of the Achilles tendon: Analysis of 57 cases. Acta Chir Scand 106:50, 1953.
31. Inglis AE, et al: Ruptures of the tendo Achilles. J Bone Joint Surg 58A:990, 1976.
32. Maffulli N, et al: Early weightbearing and ankle mobilization after open repair of acute midsubstance tears of the Achilles tendon. Am J Sports Med 31:692, 2003.
33. Thompson TC, Doherty JH: Spontaneous rupture of tendon of Achilles: a new clinical diagnostic test. J Trauma 2:126, 1962.
34. Mink JH, Deutsch AL, Kerr R: Tendon injuries of the lower extremity: magnetic resonance assessment. Top Magn Reson Imaging 3:23, 1991.
35. Harcke H, Grisson LE, Finkelstein MS: Evaluation of the musculoskeletal system with sonography. AJR Am J Roentgenol 150:1253, 1988.
36. Chiodo CP, et al: The diagnosis and treatment of acute Achilles tendon rupture. J Am Acad Orthop Surg 18(8) 503, 2010.
37. Wills CA, et al: Achilles tendon rupture: A review of the literature comparing surgical versus non-surgical treatment. Clin Orthop 207:156, 1986.
38. Quenu J, Stoianovitch I: Les ruptures du tendon d'Achilles. J Chir (Paris) 67:647, 1929.
39. Laseter JT, Russell JA: Anabolic steroid-induced tendon pathology: A review of the literature. Med Sci Sports Exerc 23:1, 1991.
40. Achilles tendon rupture (editorial). Lancet 1:189, 1973.
41. Khan RJ, et al: Treatment of acute Achilles tendon ruptures: A meta-analysis of randomized, controlled trials. J Bone Joint Surg Am 87:2202-2210, 2005.
42. Weber M, et al: Nonoperative treatment of acute rupture of the Achilles tendon: results of a new protocol and comparison with operative treatment. Am J Sports Med 31:685, 2003.

43. Ma GW, Griffith TG: Percutaneous repair of acute closed ruptured Achilles tendon: A new technique. Clin Orthop 128:247, 1977.

44. Wong J, Varrass V, Maffulli N: Quantitative review of operative and non-operative management of Achilles tendon ruptures. Am J Sports Med 30(4) 565, 2002.

45. Tang KL, et al: Arthroscopically assisted percutaneous repair of fresh closed Achilles tendon rupture by Kessler's suture. Am J Sports Med 35(4):589, 2007.

46. Cetti R: Ruptured Achilles tendon: Preliminary results of a new treatment. Br J Sports Med 22:6, 1988.

47. Cetti R, Henriksen LO, Jacobsen KS: A new treatment of ruptured Achilles tendons. Clin Orthop 308:155, 1994.

48. Crolla RMPH, et al: Acute rupture of the tendo calcaneus. Acta Orthop Belg 53:492, 1987.

49. Levy M, et al: A method of repair for Achilles tendon ruptures without cast immobilization. Clin Orthop 187:199, 1983.

50. Rippstein P, Jung M, Assal M: Surgical repair of acute Achilles tendon rupture using "mini-open" technique. Foot Ankle Clin 7(3):611, 2002.

51. Bunnell S: Primary repair of severe tendons. Am J Surg 47:502, 1940.

52. Kessler I: The grasping technique for tendon repair. Hand 5:253, 1973.

53. Mortensen NHM, Saether J: Achilles tendon repair: A new method of Achilles tendon repair tested on cadaverous materials. J Trauma 31:381, 1991.

54. Nada A: Rupture of the calcaneal tendon. J Bone Joint Surg 67B(3):449, 1985.

55. Richardson LC, Reitman R, Wilson M: Achilles tendon ruptures: Functional outcome of surgical repair with a "pull-out" wire. Foot Ankle Int 24:439, 2003.

56. Jung HG, et al: Outcome of Achilles tendon ruptures treated by a limited open technique. Foot Ankle Int 29(8):803-837, 2008.

57. Silfverskiold N: Uber die subkutane totale Achillessehn-enruptur und deren Behandlung. Acta Chir Scand 84:393, 1941.

58. Lindholm A: A new method of operation in subcutaneous rupture of the Achilles tendon. Acta Chir Scand 117:261, 1959.

59. Lynn TA: Repair of the torn Achilles tendon, using the plantaris tendon as a reinforcing membrane. J Bone Joint Surg 48A:268, 1966.

60. Kirschembaum SE, Kellman C: Modification of the Lindholm procedure for plastic repair of ruptured Achilles tendon: A case report. J Foot Surg 19:4, 1980.

61. Chen DS, Wertheimer SJ: A new method of repair for rupture of the Achilles tendon. J Foot Surg 31:440, 1992.

62. Bugg EI, Jr, Boyd BM: Repair of neglected rupture or laceration of the Achilles tendon. Clin Orthop 56:73, 1968.

63. Teuffeur AP: Traumatic rupture of the Achilles tendon: Reconstruction by transplant and graft using the lateral peroneus brevis. Orthop Clin North Am 5:89, 1974.

64. Mann RA, et al: Chronic rupture of the Achilles tendon: A new technique of repair. J Bone Joint Surg 73A:214, 1991.

65. Wapner KL, Hecht PJ, Mills RH, Jr: Reconstruction of neglected Achilles tendon injury. Orthop Clin North Am 26:249, 1995.

66. Jenkins DHR, et al: Induction of tendon and ligament formation by carbon implants. J Bone Joint Surg 59B:53, 1977.

67. Hosey G, et al: Comparison of the mechanical and histologic properties of Achilles tendons in New Zealand white rabbits secondarily repaired with Marlex mesh. J Foot Surg 30:214, 1991.

68. Giannini S, et al: Surgical repair of Achilles tendon ruptures using polypropylene braid augmentation. Foot Ankle 15:372, 1994.

69. Haggmark T, et al: Calf muscle atrophy and muscle function after non-operative vs. operative treatment of Achilles tendon ruptures. Orthopaedics 9(2):160, 1986.

70. Muller ME, et al: General considerations. In Muller ME, et al, editors: Manual of internal fixation: Techniques recommended by the AO-Group, Berlin, 1979, Springer-Verlag.

71. Inglis AE, Sculco TP: Surgical repair of ruptures of the tendo Achilles. Clin Orthop 156:160, 1981.

72. Leppilahti J, et al: Isokinetic evaluation of calf muscle performance after Achilles rupture repair. Int J Sports Med 17:619, 1996.

73. Shields CL, et al: The Cybex II evaluation of surgically repaired Achilles tendon ruptures. Am J Sports Med 6:369, 1978.

74. Booth FW: Physiologic and biochemical effects of immobilization on muscle. Clin Orthop 219:15, 1987.

75. Pepels WRJ, Plasmans CMT, Sloof TJH: The course of healing of tendons and ligaments (abstract). Acta Orthop Scand 54:952, 1983.

76. Enwemeka CS: Inflammation, cellularity, and fibrillogenesis in regenerating tendon: Implications for tendon rehabilitation. Phys Ther 69:816, 1989.

77. Enwemeka CS: Connective tissue plasticity: ultrastructural, biomechanical, and morphometric effects of physical factors on intact and regenerating tendons. J Orthop Sports Phys Ther 14(5):198, 1991.

78. Enwemeka CS, Spielholz NI, Nelson AJ: The effect of early functional activities on experimentally tenotomized Achilles tendon in rats. Am J Phys Med Rehabil 67:264, 1988.

79. Gelberman RH, et al: Flexor tendon repair in vitro: A comparative histologic study of the rabbit, chicken, dog, and monkey. J Orthop Res 2:39, 1984.

80. Krackow KA, Thomas SC, Jones LC: A new stitch for ligament-tendon fixation: Brief note. J Bone Joint Surg 68A:764, 1986.

81. Soma CA, Mandelbaum BR: Repair of acute Achilles tendon ruptures. Orthop Clin North Am 26(2):239, 1995.

82. De Carli A, et al: Effect of cyclic loading on new polyblend suture coupled with different anchors. Am J Sports Med 33:214, 2005.

83. Buchgraber A, Pässler HH: Percutaneous repair of Achilles tendon rupture: Immobilization versus functional postoperative treatment. Clin Orthop Relat Res 341:113, 1997.

84. Haji A, et al: Percutaneous versus open tendo Achilles repair. Foot Ankle Int 25:215, 2004.

85. Halasi T, Tallay A, Berkes I: Percutaneous Achilles tendon repair with and without endoscopic control. Knee Surg Sports Traumatol Arthrosc 11:409, 2003.

86. Lim J, Dalal R, Wasseem M: Percutaneous vs open repair of the ruptured Achilles tendon—a prospective randomized controlled study. Foot Ankle Int 22(7):559, 2001.

87. Tomak SL, Fleming LL: Achilles tendon rupture: An alternative treatment. Am J Orthop 33:9, 2004.

88. Leppilahti J, et al: Free tissue coverage of wound complications following Achilles tendon rupture surgery. Clin Orthop 328:171, 1996.

89. Leadbetter WB: Cell matrix response in tendon injury. Clin Sports Med 11(3):533, 1992.

90. Karjalainen PT, et al: Magnetic resonance imaging during healing of surgically repaired Achilles tendon ruptures. Am J Sports Med 25(2):164, 1997.

91. Laurant TC: Structure, function and turnover of the extracellular matrix. Adv Microcirc 13:15, 1987.

92. Gamble JG: The musculoskeletal system: Pathological basics, New York, 1988, Raven Press.

93. Gelberman RH, et al: Effects of early intermittent passive mobilization on healing canine flexor tendons, J Hand Surg 7(2):170, 1982.

94. Hannallah D, et al: Gene therapy in orthopaedic surgery. J Bone Joint Surg Am 84:1046, 2002.

95. Rodeo SA: What's new in orthopaedic research. J Bone Joint Surg Am 85:2054, 2003.

96. Forslund C, Aspenberg P: Improved healing of transected rabbit Achilles tendon after a single injection of cartilage-derived morphogenetic protein-2. Am J Sports Med 31:555, 2003.

97. Fitzgibbons RE, Hefferon J, Hill J: Percutaneous Achilles tendon repair. Am J Sports Med 21(5):724, 1993.

98. Gerdes MH, et al: A flap augmentation technique for Achilles tendon repair, postoperative strength and functional outcome. Clin Orthop 280:241, 1992.

99. Kellam JF, Hunter GA, McElwain JP: Review of the operative treatment of Achilles tendon rupture. Clin Orthop 201:80, 1985.

100. Soldatis JJ, Goodfellows DB, Wilber JH: End to end operative repair of Achilles tendon rupture. Am J Sports Med 25(1):90, 1997.

101. Costa ML, et al: Immediate full weight bearing mobilization for repaired Achilles tendon ruptures: A pilot study. Injury 34:874-876, 2003.

102. Maffulli N, et al: No adverse effect of early weight bearing following open repair of acute tears of the Achilles tendon. J Sports Med Phys Fitness 43:367-379, 2003.

103. Malone TR, Garrett WE, Zachazewski JE: Muscle: deformation, injury, repair. In Zachazewski JE, Magee DJ, Quillen WS, editors: Athletic injuries and rehabilitation, Philadelphia, 1996, Saunders.

104. Zachazewski JE: Muscle flexibility. In Scully R, Barnes ML, editors: Physical therapy, Philadelphia, 1989, Lippincott.

105. Carter TR, Fowler PJ, Blokker C: Functional postoperative treatment of Achilles tendon repair. Am J Sports Med 20:459, 1992.

106. Fernandez-Fairen M, Gimeno C: Augmented repair of Achilles tendon ruptures. Am J Sports Med 25(2):177, 1997.

107. Solveborn SA, Moberg A: Immediate free ankle motion after surgical repair of acute Achilles tendon ruptures. Am J Sports Med 22(5):607, 1994.

108. Sorrenti SJ: Achilles tendon rupture: Effect of early mobilization in rehabilitation after surgical repair. Foot Ankle Int 27:407-410, 2006.

109. Suchak AA, et al: The influence of early weight bearing compared with non–weight bearing after surgical repair of the Achilles tendon. J Bone Joint Surg Am 90:1876-1883, 2008.

110. Yotsumoto T, Miyamoto W, Uchio Y: Novel approach to repair of acute Achilles tendon rupture early recovery without postoperative fixation or orthosis. Am J Sports Med 2(38):287, 2009.

111. Metz R, et al: Acute Achilles tendon rupture: Minimally invasive surgery versus nonoperative treatment with immediate full weight bearing—A randomized controlled trial. Am J Sports Med 36:1688, 2008.

112. Kangas J, et al: Early functional treatment vs early immobilization in tension of the musculotendinous unit after Achilles rupture repair: A prospective, randomized, clinical study. J Trauma 54(6):1171, 2003.

113. Boyden EM, et al: Late versus early repair of Achilles tendon rupture clinical and biomechanical evaluation. Clin Orthop Relat Res 317:150-158, 1995.

114. Leppilahti J, et al: Outcome and prognostic factors of Achilles rupture repair using a new scoring method. Clin Orthop Relat Res 346:152-161, 1998.

115. Don R, et al: Relationship between recovery of calf muscle biomechanical properties and gait pattern following surgery for Achilles tendon rupture. Clin Biomech 22:211-220, 2007.

116. Robinson JM, et al: The VISA-A questionnaire: A valid and reliable index of the clinical severity of Achilles tendinopathy. Br J Sports Med 35:335-341, 2001.

117. Martin RL, et al: Evidence of the validity for the Foot and Ankle Ability Measure (FAAM). Foot Ankle Int 26(1):968-983, 2005.

118. Carcia CR, et al: Achilles pain, stiffness, and muscle power deficits: Achilles tendinitis clinical practice guidelines linked to the International Classification of Functioning, Disability, and Health from the Orthopaedic Section of the American Physical Therapy Association. J Orthop Sports Phys Ther 40(9):A1, 2010.

119. Nilsson-Helander K, et al: The Achilles Tendon Total Rupture Score (ATRS): Development and validation. Am J Sports Med 35(3):421-426, 2007.

120. Maffulli N, et al: Favorable outcome of percutaneous repair of Achilles tendon ruptures in the elderly. Clin Orthop Relat Res 468:1039-1046, 2010.

121. Kerkoffs GM, et al: Functional treatment after surgical repair of acute Achilles tendon rupture: Wrap vs walking cast. Arch Orthop Trauma Surg 122(2):102, 2002.

122. Mortenson NH, Skov O, Jenson PE: Early motion of the ankle after operative treatment of a rupture of the Achilles tendon: A prospective, randomized clinical and radiographic study. J Bone Joint Surg Am 81(7):983, 1999.

123. Motta P, Errichiello C, Pontini I: Achilles tendon rupture: A new technique for easy surgical repair and immediate movement of the ankle and foot. Am J Sports Med 25(2):172, 1997.

124. Enwemeka CS, Rodriguez O, Mendosa S: The biomechanical effects of low intensity ultrasound on healing tendons. Ultrasound Med Biol 16:801, 1990.

125. Enwemeka CS: The effect of therapeutic ultrasound on tendon healing: A biomechanical study. Am J Phys Med Rehabil 67:264, 1988.

126. Jackson BA, Schwane JA, Starcher BC: Effect of ultrasound on the repair of Achilles tendon injuries in rats. Med Sci Sports Exerc 23(2):171, 1991.

127. Freider S, et al: A pilot study: The therapeutic effect of ultrasound following partial rupture of Achilles tendons in male rats. J Orthop Sports Phys Ther 10(2):39, 1988.

128. Ng GY, Fung DT: The effect of therapeutic ultrasound intensity on the ultrastructural morphology of tendon repair. Ultrasound Med Biol 33(11):1750-1754, 2007.

129. Frings H: Uber 317 falle von operrierten subkutanen Achil-lesrupturen be sportiern und sportlerinnen. Arch Orthop Unfallchir 67:64, 1969.

130. Nillius SA, Nilsson BE, Westin WE: The incidence of Achilles tendon rupture. Acta Orthop Scand 47(1):118, 1976.

131. Cetti R, Christenson SE: Surgical treatment under local anesthesia of Achilles rupture. Clin Orthop 173:204, 1983.

132. Holz U: Die Achilles shenen ruptur–klinische und ultratrukturelle aspekte. In Chapchal G, editor: Sportverletzungen und Sportschagen, Stuttgart, 1983, Georg Tieme.

133. Schedl R, Fasol P, Spangler H: Die Achillessehnen-ruptur als sportverletzung. In Chapchal G, editor: Sportverletzungen und Sportschagen, Stuttgart, 1983, Georg Tieme.

134. Zolinger H, Rodriquez M, Genoni M: Zur atiopathogeneseund diagnostik der Achillesehnenrupturen im sport. In Chapchal G, editor: Sportverletzungen und Sportschagen, Stuttgart, 1983, Georg Tieme.

135. Jozsa L, et al: Pathological alterations of human tendons. Morphol Igazsagugy Orr Sz 27(2):106, 1987.

CHAPTER 32

Bunionectomies

Joshua Gerbert, Neil McKenna

DEFINITIONS

The term "bunion" refers to the any enlargement around the first metatarsal phalangeal joint (MTPJ). The term "hallux valgus" has been used as a catch-all phrase to include all types of bunions without being specific. The actual definition of "hallux valgus" is a frontal plane deformity of the great toe in which the plantar aspect of the toe is beginning to face the second toe. "Hallux abductus" is a transverse plane deformity of the great toe in which it is moving toward, abutting, overriding, or underriding the second toe. In most cases the surgeon will make a diagnosis of "hallux abductus with bunion deformity" (Fig. 32-1) or "hallux abducto-valgus with bunion deformity" depending upon the preoperative position of the great toe. A "dorsal bunion" is an enlargement over the dorsal aspect of the first MTPJ and in most situations is indicative of limited first MTPJ motion known as "hallux limitus."

ETIOLOGIES

Bunion deformities are complex problems and dynamic, meaning that over time the deformity will most likely progress regardless of the conservative measures employed. This is especially true if there is any structural malalignment of the bones that comprise the first ray. Once a "bunion" deformity has developed there are no conservative measures that will reverse the situation. Conservative measures may halt the progression of the deformity and/or reduce the symptoms associated with it. The etiologies are varied and at times are the result of several different causes. The following are the more common causes of bunion deformities:
- Structural malalignment of one or more of the bones that make up the first ray
- Biomechanical imbalance in the lower extremity (LE) in which the patient functions with abnormal pronation during gait
- Metabolic (arthritides creating degenerative joint disease of the first MTPJ and bone spur proliferation)

It should be noted that once the intrinsic and extrinsic muscles of the LE abnormally function during gait and the patient significantly pronates, the hallux begins to deviate toward the second toe and retrograde forces on the first metatarsal begin to move this bone more medially. The more transverse plane mobility that exists at the first metatarsal cuneiform joint (MCJ), the more the first metatarsal may splay from the second metatarsal. The more sagittal plane mobility that exists at the first MCJ, the more the first metatarsal will migrate dorsally and produce limited first MTPJ motion (hallux limitus rather than a medial bunion deformity with a hallux abductus).

INDICATIONS AND CONSIDERATIONS FOR SURGICAL CORRECTION

A very detailed clinical examination of the foot and LE is required both non–weight bearing and weight bearing to determine areas of pathology contributing to the "bunion" deformity. Objective measurements of the first MTPJ range of motion (ROM) (dorsiflexion and plantarflexion) are obtained non–weight bearing (Fig. 32-2). The amount of dorsiflexion deemed necessary for a normal propulsive gait is approximately 65° (Fig. 32-3). Since plantarflexion of the first MTPJ is not a motion required for gait, there are really no normal values usually considered other than knowing that the first MTPJ can plantarflex to some degree without discomfort. Evaluation of mobility at the first MCJ on both the transverse and sagittal planes is important to detect any hypermobility. If sagittal plane hypermobility of the first ray appears to exist, then one should dorsiflex the hallux at the first MTPJ and evaluate the motion again. By dorsiflexing the hallux, one is engaging the plantar fascia (windlass mechanism). If the abnormal sagittal plane motion is no longer present, then the use of an orthotic device will most likely halt any deforming forces caused by hypermobility of the first ray, which are usually jamming of the first MTPJ in gait, limited first MTPJ motion, and transfer metatarsalgia. However, if by engaging the windlass mechanism by

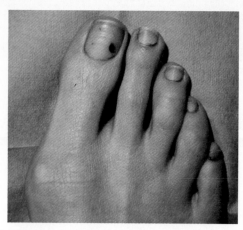

Fig. 32-1 Photograph showing a patient with a hallux abductus with bunion deformity.

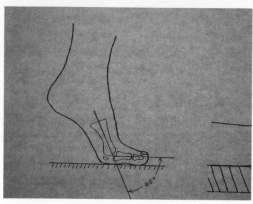

Fig. 32-3 The 65° of dorsiflexion that is needed for a propulsive gait. Some patients may not need this amount of dorsiflexion to achieve a normal propulsive gait.

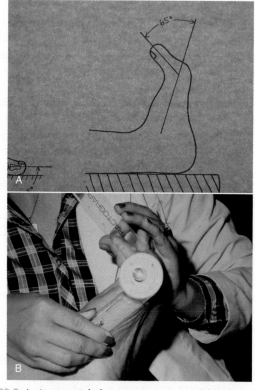

Fig. 32-2 **A,** A non–weight bearing measurement of dorsiflexion of the first metatarsal phalangeal joint. A line is drawn along the declination angle of the first metatarsal and extended straight out. Any movement in a dorsal direction from that line is measured as dorsiflexion. **B,** The actual measurement of first dorsiflexion with a tractograph.

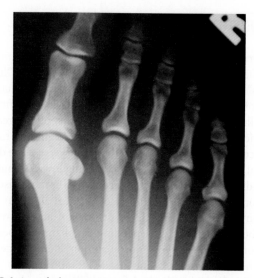

Fig. 32-4 A weight-bearing anteroposterior radiograph showing the deformity demonstrated in Fig. 32-1. The hallux is deviated toward the second digit and the intermetatarsal angle between the first and second is increased. In this case there is a soft tissue imbalance at the first metatarsal phalangeal joint and a structural malalignment of the first metatarsal.

dorsiflexing the hallux and the hypermobility appears to remain, then a surgical procedure aimed at stopping this motion is usually needed, such as a fusion of the first MCJ known as a Lapidus procedure. Symptoms may not always be the indication for pursuing a surgical correction of the "bunion." A patient who has a progressive hallux abductus and a bunion deformity in which the hallux is significantly abutting the second toe but is asymptomatic may require a surgical correction of the deformity to prevent deformity of the second toe and dislocation of the second MTPJ.

Weight-bearing radiographic evaluation of the foot is extremely important in the evaluation of the "bunion" deformity to determine any structural malalignment of the first ray and at which level or levels the pathology exists (Fig. 32-4). A unique aspect of the first MTPJ is the presence of two sesamoid bones on the plantar aspect of the metatarsal head (Fig. 32-5), which serve as a fulcrum for the tendons of the flexor hallucis brevis muscle that attaches to the plantar aspect of the base of the proximal phalanx. At times the fibular sesamoid bone may become a very powerful deforming force and the surgeon may need to release its soft tissue attachments or excise it (Fig. 32-6). This maneuver can create scar formation to such an extent as to limit first MTPJ dorsiflexion postoperatively.

Various angular measurements are taken and correlated with the clinical examination.

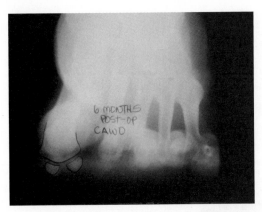

Fig. 32-5 A weight-bearing plantar axial radiograph showing the two sesamoid bones plantar to the first metatarsal head that make up part of this joint complex. They serve to provide a better mechanical advantage for the flexor hallucis brevis muscle in maintaining good hallux toe purchase.

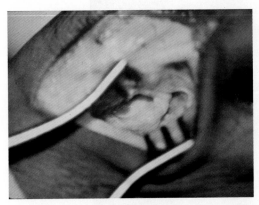

Fig. 32-6 An intraoperative photograph showing a release of the fibular sesamoid apparatus in the first interspace through the dorsal incision used to correct the bunion deformity. At times the dissection to perform this maneuver or excise the sesamoid can produce excessive scar formation and/or a hematoma in the interspace, creating postoperative problems for the patient.

The surgeon must also take into consideration the patient's overall medical health, body type, age, occupation, and home environment before deciding which surgical procedure or procedures would best correct that patient's "bunion" deformity. While the clinical and radiographic evaluation data may indicate an "ideal" surgical correction, the specific medical and/or social data on that specific patient may dictate a lesser surgical correction.

SURGICAL PROCEDURES

Since there are a wide variety of surgical procedures used to correct a "bunion" deformity, and in many cases the surgeon may perform more than one procedure to correct the deformity, I thought it would be beneficial to the physical therapist to put the procedures in categories as they relate to postoperative management and to briefly describe the major aspect of the procedure. This chapter does not allow me to cover every type of procedure used to correct

"bunion" deformities. However, the following are the more common ones.

Category 1

Category 1 procedures are those in which the patient can begin immediate propulsive ambulation following surgery and return to high impact activities within 2 to 3 weeks.
1. Soft tissue rebalancing of the first MTPJ—McBride type (rarely performed as an isolated procedure) (Fig. 32-7)
2. First MTPJ prosthesis—total or hemi (Fig. 32-8)
3. Cheilectomy—removal of bone spurs from the dorsal aspect of the first MTPJ in hallux limitus (dorsal bunion deformity) (Fig. 32-9)
4. Resectional arthroplasty of the first MTPJ—Keller type (usually performed in a very elderly patient with a non-salvageable first MTPJ) (Fig. 32-10)

Category 2

Category 2 procedures are those in which the patient can bear weight immediately; however, the propulsive phase of gait must be eliminated for 2 to 3 weeks following surgery and the patient cannot resume high impact activities for 8 weeks.
1. Metatarsal head procedures to create a relative reduction of the intermetatarsal angle (Fig. 32-11)
2. Decompressional metatarsal head procedure to shorten the metatarsal and open the first MTPJ space to allow for more joint motion (Fig. 32-12)
3. SCARF metatarsal shaft procedure (Fig. 32-13)

Category 3

Category 3 procedures are those in which the patient can bear weight immediately; however, the propulsive phase of gait must be eliminated for 4 to 6 weeks following surgery and the patient cannot resume high impact activities for 12 weeks.
1. Hallux osteotomies—Akin type (Fig. 32-14)
2. Fusion of the first MTPJ (Fig. 32-15)

Category 4

Category 4 procedures are those in which the patient must remain non–weight bearing for 6 to 7 weeks following surgery and the patient cannot resume high impact activities for 12 to 16 weeks.
1. Metatarsal base osteotomies (Fig. 32-16)
2. Fusion of the first MCJ (Fig. 32-17)

Category 5

Category 5 procedures are those in which a bone graft was used at the osteotomy site or fusion site and the patient must remain non–weight bearing until the bone graft has become incorporated, which depending upon the size of the graft may take 3 months.
1. Metatarsal base osteotomy with bone graft (Fig. 32-18)
2. Fusion of the first MTPJ or first MCJ with bone graft (Fig. 32-19)

Text continued on page 589

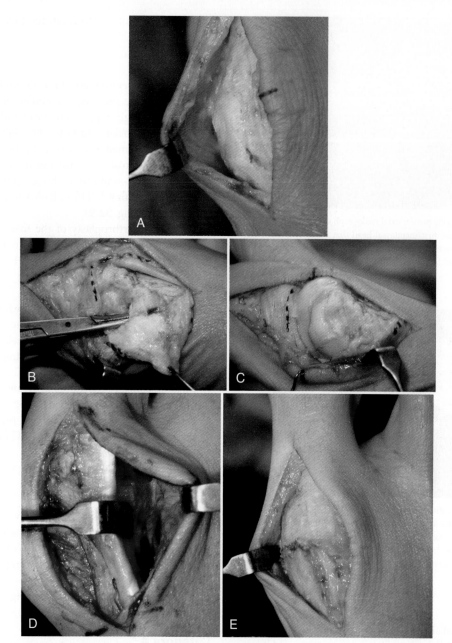

Fig. 32-7 **A,** An intraoperative photograph showing a dorsal incision with exposure of the dorsal and medial aspect of the first metatarsal phalangeal joint in the initial stages of performing a soft tissue type bunionectomy to rebalance the tissues around the joint. **B,** An intraoperative photograph showing the medial aspect of the joint capsule being dissected and cutting the collateral ligament to expose the bunion site. **C,** The medial aspect of the first metatarsal head exposed to remove a portion of the medial aspect of the metatarsal head that is enlarged. **D,** The dissection that is now performed into the first interspace to release abnormally tight lateral structures and release of the fibular sesamoid if necessary. **E,** The closure of the medial and dorsal aspects of the first metatarsal phalangeal joint capsule in which redundant tissue was removed to realign the hallux into a better transverse plane position.

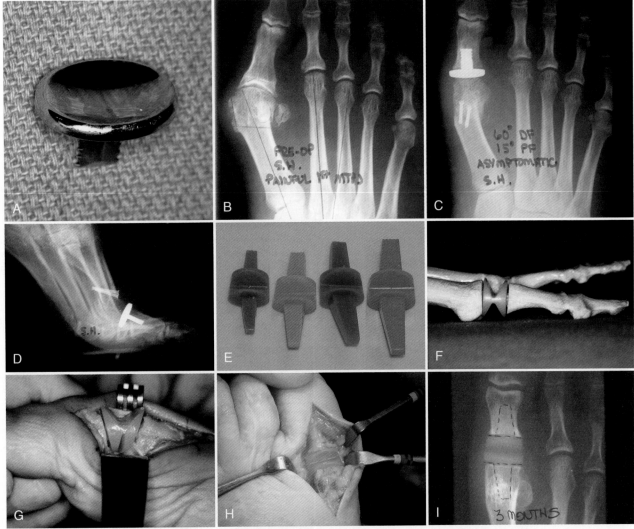

Fig. 32-8 A, A "hemi" type metallic joint prosthesis that replaces the base of the proximal phalanx. **B,** An anteroposterior weight-bearing preoperative radiograph showing a degenerative first metatarsal phalangeal joint that was painful with motion, an abnormal increase in the intermetatarsal angle with a bunion deformity, and a hallux abductus deformity. The treatment for this condition was a combination of a metatarsal head osteotomy to reduce the distance between the first and second metatarsals, realign the soft tissue structures around the first metatarsal phalangeal joint, and to replace the base of the proximal phalanx with a hemiimplant. **C,** A postoperative radiograph following the metatarsal osteotomy with two screws for fixation, soft tissue rebalancing around the joint, and insertion of a hemiimplant with resultant adequate first metatarsal phalangeal joint dorsiflexion and elimination of pain. **D,** A lateral radiograph of this patient simulating propulsion to demonstrate the movement of the implant gliding over the metatarsal head. **E,** Implant sizers for a total silicone hinge joint prosthesis. **F,** An implant inserted into a "sawbone" model to demonstrate its position and the amount of bone that is needed to be removed both from the metatarsal head and base of the proximal phalanx. Minimal bone is normally removed from the metatarsal head and the majority of bone is removed from the base of the proximal phalanx to preserve some weight bearing under the first metatarsal head. Because of the amount of bone needed to be removed from the base of the proximal phalanx, the insertion of the flexor hallucis brevis muscle is eliminated. **G,** An intraoperative photograph from a medial view showing the total hinge implant. **H,** The total hinge implant from a dorsal view. **I,** A postoperative anteroposterior weight-bearing radiograph showing the total hinge implant.

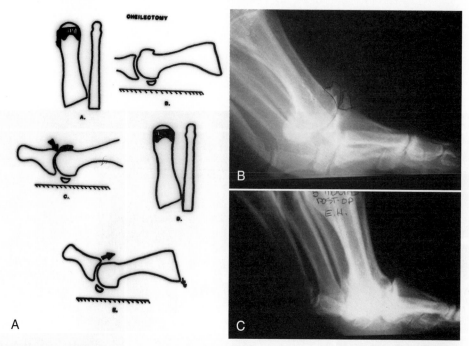

Fig. 32-9 **A,** A cheilectomy procedure in which the dorsal, medial, and lateral bone spurs are removed from the metatarsal head and base of the proximal phalanx. **B,** A lateral preoperative radiograph simulating propulsion showing the significant bone spurs at the dorsal aspect of the first metatarsal phalangeal joint that were the cause of the pain and limitation of motion. **C,** A postoperative lateral photograph stimulating propulsion with normal motion once the bone spurs had been removed.

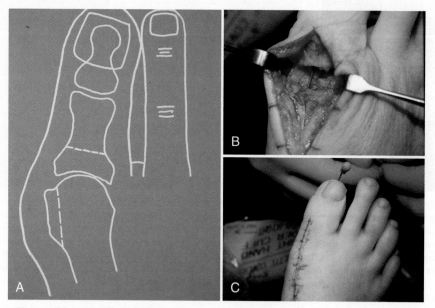

Fig. 32-10 **A,** The amount of bone to be removed from the base of the proximal phalanx in performing a resectional arthroplasty (Keller) bunionectomy. **B,** A dorsal view intraoperatively following this procedure in which a k-wire has been inserted through the hallux and into the metatarsal head to hold the hallux in a corrected position on the transverse and sagittal planes until scarring can occur within the void that was created by removing the base of the phalanx. **C,** A postoperative view following the surgery with the k-wire inserted through the hallux and metatarsal. Note that the hallux does shorten as a result of this procedure, which will result in transfer metatarsalgia in many patients.

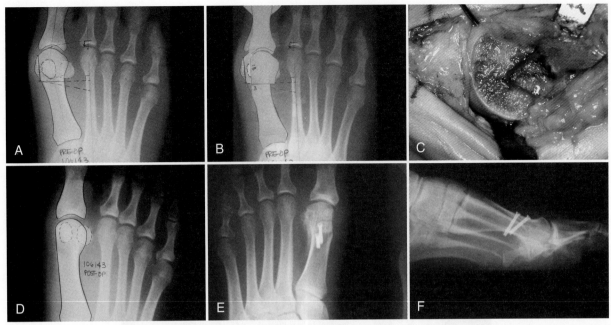

Fig. 32-11 **A,** A preoperative anteroposterior weight-bearing radiograph showing a hallux abductus with bunion deformity in which the underlying patholo-gies are soft tissue imbalance around the first metatarsal phalangeal joint and an increase in the intermetatarsal angle creating the bunion. **B,** A paper template constructed to demonstrate the metatarsal osteotomy to be performed in which the metatarsal head is transposed laterally to achieve a relative reduction of the intermetatarsal angle and eliminate the bunion. A soft tissue procedure (McBride) will need to be performed to rebalance the soft tissue structures around the joint. **C,** A medial view intraoperatively following a "chevron" (Austin) osteotomy through the metatarsal neck. **D,** A postoperative weight-bearing radio-graph following the Austin/McBride bunionectomy. Fixation was accomplished with absorbable rods. **E,** An anteroposterior radiograph showing the same type of procedure in which the osteotomy was fixated with two screws. **F,** A lateral radiograph showing the procedure fixated with two screws.

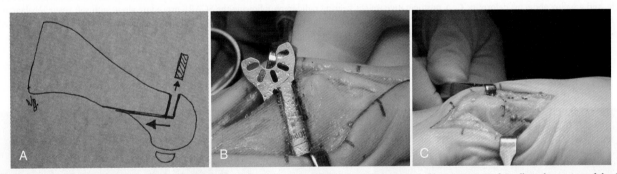

Fig. 32-12 **A,** A decompressional osteotomy performed at the metatarsal head level in which a section of bone is removed to allow shortening of the first metatarsal, which relaxes the soft tissue structures around the first metatarsal phalangeal joint permitting increased range of motion. **B,** A dorsal view during surgery of the first metatarsal head following removal of a section of bone to allow shortening of the first metatarsal. **C,** A medial view following fixation of the decompressional osteotomy using two screws from dorsal to plantar.

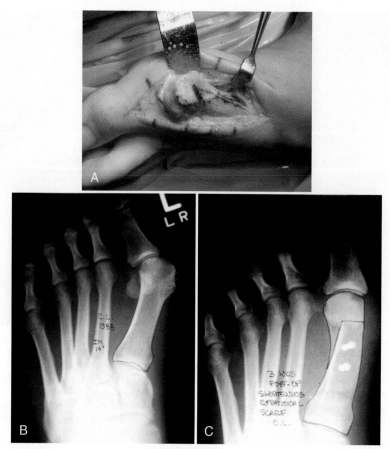

Fig. 32-13 **A,** An intraoperative photograph showing the medial aspect of the first metatarsal in which a long "Z" type osteotomy is performed in the shaft of the metatarsal known as a SCARF procedure. **B,** A preoperative weight-bearing radiograph showing a long first metatarsal, an increase in the intermetatarsal angle, and a hallux abductus deformity. **C,** A postoperative weight-bearing radiograph following the SCARF procedure along with soft tissue rebalancing of the first metatarsal phalangeal joint fixated by several screws. Note that the intermetatarsal angle has been reduced, the metatarsal length has been reduced to a more normal parabola, and the first metatarsal phalangeal joint has been realigned.

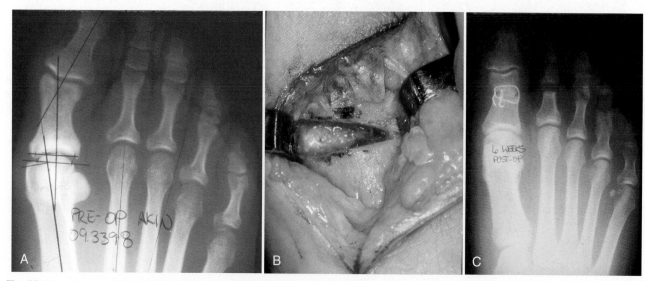

Fig. 32-14 **A,** A preoperative weight-bearing radiograph showing an abnormal abductus at the level of the interphalangeal joint of the hallux. The patient does not have a bunion. **B,** A dorsal intraoperative photograph showing a medial wedge of bone having been removed from the distal aspect of the proximal phalanx. When this osteotomy is closed it will reduce the abnormal abductus deformity and straighten the toe. **C,** A weight-bearing postoperative anteroposterior radiograph showing the reduction of the deformity using a distal Akin osteotomy with stainless steel wire fixation. No soft tissue rebalancing was performed in this procedure.

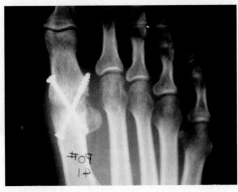

Fig. 32-15 A postoperative weight-bearing radiograph showing a primary fusion of the first metatarsal phalangeal joint using two crossed screws. Once the fixation is secured, the position of the hallux on the frontal plane, sagittal plane, and transverse plane cannot be altered.

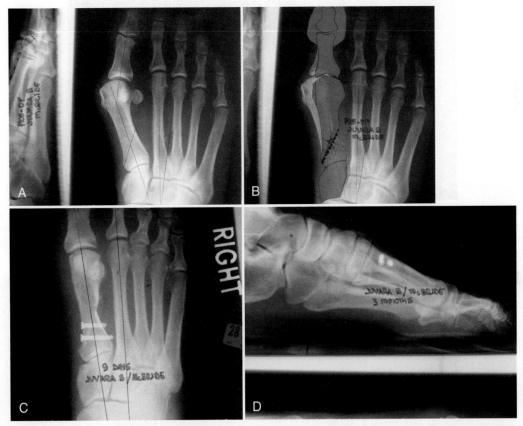

Fig. 32-16 **A,** A preoperative anteroposterior weight-bearing radiograph showing a hallux abductus with bunion deformity in which there is a significant increase in the intermetatarsal angle and a deviated first metatarsal phalangeal joint. The intermetatarsal angle is too large to be corrected with a metatarsal head osteotomy. **B,** The same radiograph with a paper template demonstrating the proposed metatarsal base osteotomy to be used to reduce the large intermetatarsal angle. It shows the removal of a lateral wedge of bone with the apex medially. **C,** A postoperative radiograph showing the reduction of the intermetatarsal angle following the base osteotomy in which two screws were used for fixation and a McBride soft tissue rebalancing was performed at the first metatarsal phalangeal joint. **D,** A lateral radiograph of that patient showing the normal sagittal plane alignment of the first metatarsal following the procedure. Note that the dorsal cortex of the first metatarsal is parallel to that of the second metatarsal, thus ensuring a normal weight-bearing position of the first.

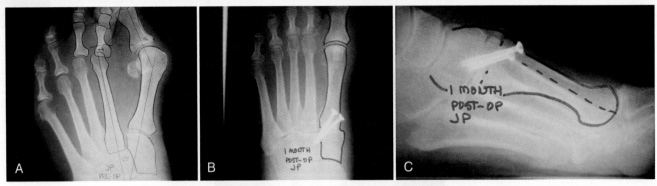

Fig. 32-17 **A,** A preoperative anteroposterior weight-bearing radiograph showing a hallux abductus with bunion deformity in which there is a significant increase in the intermetatarsal angle. Clinically the first metatarsal was shown to be hypermobile with abnormal sagittal plane motion at the first metatarsal cuneiform joint. The second metatarsal phalangeal joint has dorsal dislocated and the second toe has migrated over the dorsal aspect of the hallux because of the long-standing bunion deformity. **B,** A postoperative anteroposterior radiograph following a fusion of the first metatarsal cuneiform joint (Lapidus procedure) along with a McBride soft tissue rebalancing of the first metatarsal phalangeal joint. Two screws were used to fixate the fusion site. Several procedures were performed to relocate the second metatarsal phalangeal joint and realign the second digit. **C,** A lateral radiograph following the metatarsal cuneiform joint fusion showing that the first metatarsal is in normal sagittal plane alignment relative to the lesser metatarsals. The dorsal cortex of the first metatarsal is parallel to the dorsal cortex (dotted lines) of the second metatarsal.

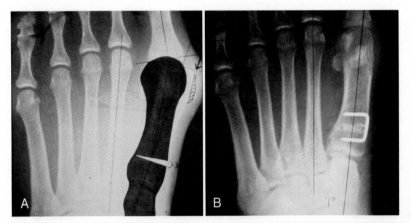

Fig. 32-18 **A,** A preoperative anteroposterior weight-bearing radiograph in which a paper template has been constructed to demonstrate a medial opening wedge osteotomy at the metatarsal base to reduce a significantly high intermetatarsal angle. A bone graft will need to be inserted into the opening osteotomy site. **B,** An anteroposterior radiograph following the opening wedge osteotomy with bone graft in which a staple was used for fixation. A McBride soft tissue rebalancing was performed at the first metatarsal phalangeal joint.

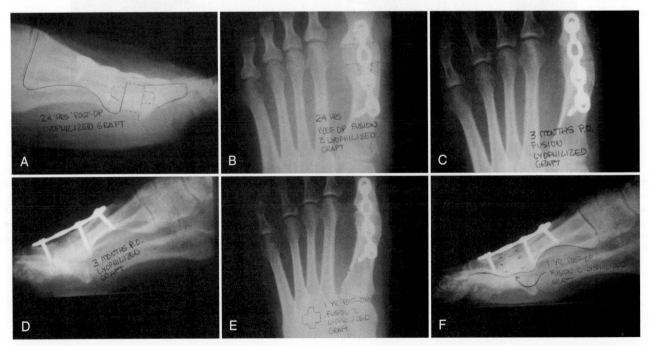

Fig. 32-19 **A,** A postoperative lateral radiograph following a first metatarsal phalangeal joint fusion in which a bone graft was used. This was necessary because a total implant failed, and once removed the graft was needed to preserve length of the hallux. A low profile bone plate was used dorsally to fixate the site. **B,** An anteroposterior postoperative radiograph at 24 hours following the procedure with the graft. **C,** An anteroposterior radiograph at 3 months following the graft arthrodesis procedure. **D,** A lateral radiograph at 3 months following this procedure. **E,** An anteroposterior radiograph of that patient at 1 year with complete reconstitution of the bone and solid first metatarsal phalangeal joint fusion. **F,** A lateral view of that patient at 1 year postoperative.

Underlying Pathology

In the majority of "bunion" deformities, the underlying pathology is a combination of both a soft tissue imbalance at the first MTPJ and a structural malalignment involving one or more of the bones comprising the first ray. Therefore the surgeon may need to perform combinations of procedures, such as an Akin osteotomy of the hallux, a McBride soft tissue rebalancing around the first MTPJ, and a metatarsal base osteotomy. The postoperative management would be dictated by the procedure that requires the most protection. So in the example given, the patient would need to remain non–weight bearing for 6 to 7 weeks because of the metatarsal base osteotomy. If the surgeon used rigid internal fixation and believed the patient to be compliant, then the patient may be allowed to begin early first MTPJ ROM and not be placed in a below the knee cast. This would of course allow for faster rehabilitation once the patient could resume weight bearing and return to normal activities.

SURGICAL PROCEDURE FOR A METATARSAL HEAD OSTEOTOMY (CATEGORY 2) AND SOFT TISSUE REBALANCING OF THE FIRST MTPJ (CATEGORY 1)

One of the more common bunionectomy procedures involves a first metatarsal osteotomy (Austin or Chevron procedure) and a soft tissue rebalancing (McBride procedure) to correct both a positional and a structural malalignment (see Fig. 32-11, A). A pneumatic ankle cuff is used to stop all blood flow into the foot and allow for a dry field during the procedure, which usually requires 45 to 60 minutes to complete. After a sterile preparation of the foot, a dorsal medial incision is made over the first MTPJ and by using blunt and sharp dissection the subcutaneous tissues and neurovascular elements are separated from the dorsal and medial aspect of the first MTPJ capsule (see Fig. 32-7, A). The surgeon then uses one of many capsulotomies to enter and expose the first MTPJ.

Fig. 32-7, B shows an inverted "L" capsulotomy having been performed and the incision through the medial suspensory and collateral ligaments. Following this maneuver, the surgeon then is able to expose the medial and dorsal aspects of the first metatarsal head as shown in Fig. 32-7, C. Based on the preoperative x-ray and a preoperative template, if constructed, the surgeon is able to determine how much of the medial eminence of the metatarsal head needs to be removed as seen in Fig. 32-11, B. Once the medial eminence has been removed, the surgeon can use a sterile marker and create the proposed osteotomy site. At this time and before performing the osteotomy, the surgeon decides whether to perform a lateral release of the first MTPJ or remove the fibular sesamoid bone; then further dissection is performed in the first interspace as shown in Fig. 32-7, D. Some surgeons elect to perform this maneuver through a second incision over the dorsal aspect of the first interspace. This portion of the procedure is performed to release any abnormally tight soft tissue structures that are holding the hallux in the abductus position. Using some type of power instrumentation, the bone is cut completely through from medial to lateral, severing all cortical surfaces as shown in Fig. 32-11, C. Then based upon the surgeon's evaluation of the preoperative x-ray and/or preoperative template, the metatarsal head is transposed laterally toward the second metatarsal by a certain number of millimeters. Once the metatarsal head has been transposed to the desired amount, the osteotomy site is fixated based upon the surgeon's preference and the medial overhang of bone on the metatarsal shaft is removed flush. Fig. 32-11, D is a postoperative radiograph in which the osteotomy site was fixated with absorbable rods, which are radiolucent. Fig. 32-11, E and F, are postoperative radiographs in which the osteotomy site for this type of procedure was fixated with two cannulated screws.

Once fixation is completed, the structural component now has been corrected. The next portion of the procedure is the completion of the soft tissue rebalancing. In this specific example an inverted "L" capsulotomy was performed medially. The surgeon's assistant holds the hallux into a corrected position on the transverse plane, and the surgeon can then appreciate how much redundant medial capsular tissue is present. This medial redundant tissue is excised and the medial capsule closed using suture material of the surgeon's preference (see Fig. 32-7, E). The dorsal portion of the capsule is then closed again using suture material of the surgeon's preference. Some surgeons will elect to close the subcutaneous tissues and others will insert several buried knot sutures in the dermal layer to take the tension off the skin before skin closure. Skin closure is accomplished usually with a nonabsorbable material, again based on the surgeon's preference.

Bandages are applied in such a manner as to control postoperative edema and reinforce the soft tissue realignment of the first MTPJ. The patient is placed either in a surgical postoperative shoe or a removable walking boot. Both devices allow for the patient to begin immediate ambulation with elimination of the propulsive phase of gait, which is needed because of the osteotomy procedure.

POTENTIAL COMPLICATIONS

For the physical therapist to better develop an effective rehabilitation program for a specific patient following a bunionectomy, the therapist needs to appreciate certain inherent anatomic changes associated with the procedures being performed. Furthermore, there are certain complications created intraoperatively by the surgeon that no amount of physical therapy will resolve. If possible the physical therapist should attempt to at least see a preoperative x-ray of the deformity because there are patients who have unrealistic cosmetic expectations of the end result.

The following are some of the more common complications associated with a bunionectomy procedure and possible causes:

1. Chronic edema at the surgical site
   a. Surgical correction involving multiple osteotomy procedures that resulted in increased surgical dissection
   b. Noncompliant patient who kept the foot in a dependent position for prolonged periods immediately following the surgery
   c. Development of a hematoma, especially in the first interspace
   d. Prolonged cast immobilization
2. Delayed bone healing following a procedure involving an osteotomy
   a. Noncompliant patient who ambulated too soon following the procedure
   b. Poor internal fixation of the osteotomy site
   c. Medical factors (smoker, systemic steroid usage, osteoporosis, etc.)
   d. Traumatic event involving the surgical foot following surgery
3. Limited first MTPJ ROM
   a. Overtightening of soft tissue structures around first MTPJ
   b. Dorsiflexion of the first metatarsal following an osteotomy of the metatarsal
   c. Prolonged immobilization
   d. Capsulodesis following removal of significant bone from the dorsal surface of the first metatarsal head
   e. Failure of surgeon to create a congruous first MTPJ
   f. Soft tissue fibrosis and/or damage of the hallucal sesamoids at the plantar aspect of the first MTPJ
   g. Noncompliant patient who will not exercise first MTPJ or ambulate with a propulsive gait
   h. Weakness of the peroneus longus muscle or overpowering of the anterior tibial muscle
4. Lack of hallux toe purchase when the patient is standing
   a. Shortening osteotomy of the first metatarsal, which creates loss of tension of the flexor tendons and plantar fascial slip to the hallux (decompressional procedures)
   b. Loss of insertion of the flexor hallucis brevis tendons into the base of the hallux (joint prosthesis, resectional arthroplasty procedures)
   c. Capsulodesis of the first MTPJ following remodeling of the dorsal aspect of the first metatarsal head (cheilectomy, joint prosthesis procedures)
   d. Overtightening dorsally of soft tissue structures at first MTPJ
   e. Chronic edema at plantar aspect of the first MTPJ (metatarsal head osteotomy procedures)
5. Hallux separation from the lesser toes (Hallux varus)
   a. Overtightening of soft tissue structures at medial aspect of first MTPJ
   b. Overcorrection of the intermetatarsal angle
   c. Overcorrection of an osteotomy procedure of the hallux

PHYSICAL THERAPY CONSIDERATIONS BEFORE DEVELOPMENT OF A TREATMENT PLAN

The following are some facts that the physical therapist should attempt to know before establishing a treatment plan for a specific patient following a bunionectomy.

1. **Was an osteotomy performed and, if so, where was it performed and what type of fixation was used?** Bone normally requires 6 weeks to heal in the best circumstances. An osteotomy performed in the diaphyseal section of the proximal phalanx or first metatarsal will usually take 7 weeks to adequately heal. Bone healing is prolonged in a patient who is a smoker. Two points of fixation, especially screws, will allow for a more aggressive approach to establishing good first MTPJ ROM.
2. **Was a bone graft used and if so how large and where was it inserted?** Bone grafts take longer to heal than an osteotomy since they need to be revascularized and new bone produced to take the place of the graft material. The larger the graft the longer the healing. A bunionectomy that at times requires bone grafting is the Lapidus procedure (first metatarsal-cuneiform fusion). For these patients the need to remain non–weight bearing may be 3 months, again depending upon the size of the graft. Further, unless a plate was used across the dorsal aspect of the MCJ, attempts to reestablish first MTPJ ROM must be limited since any aggressive dorsiflexion movements will create plantarflexion forces on the first metatarsal and could disrupt the fusion site.
3. **What type of fixation was used and how much?** Large metallic fixation devices, especially if located at the dorsal aspect of the first MCJ, may be a contraindication to the use of ultrasound because of the build up of heat in the devices.
4. **How long was the patient kept either non–weight bearing or in a nonpropulsive type gait and was the patient immobilized in a cast?** The longer the period of time that the first MTPJ motion was eliminated or limited, the greater incidence of restricted motion once the patient is seen by the physical therapist. If the therapist determines that there is significant fibrosis of the first MTPJ and/or the patient is not performing adequate exercises to increase ROM, the patient should be referred back to the surgeon as soon as possible for reevaluation to make certain that the lack of motion is not due to some abnormal malalignment of the joint. If the joint and associated structures are in good alignment, then the surgeon should anesthetize the first MTPJ and forcibly manipulate the joint and record the amount of dorsiflexion and plantarflexion obtained at that visit. The patient should be referred back to the therapist along with this information so that further joint manipulation can be performed.
5. **Is the patient compliant?** Most surgeons have an appreciation of whether or not the patient is compliant and this

information should be related to the physical therapist. Unfortunately, most physical therapy prescription forms do not ask for this information and surgeons are reluctant to state this information on the form. Perhaps a box should be added on the physical prescription form that the surgeon can check requesting the therapist to contact the surgeon for additional information regarding that specific patient.

EXPECTED OVERALL OUTCOME FOLLOWING A BUNIONECTOMY

For the majority of bunionectomies the following signs and/ or symptoms to some extent may be present for 5 to 6 months postoperatively, even if the surgery was performed correctly and the patient had an uneventful postoperative recovery.

1. Residual edema at surgical site after prolonged ambulation or after exercise that resolves upon rest and elevation of the foot
2. Dermatologic color changes over the dorsum of the foot at the end of the day or after having the foot immersed in warm water for a prolonged period of time
3. Mild transient neuritis of some superficial nerves at the surgical site
4. Increased sensitivity at the surgical scar
5. Some limited first MTPJ ROM, especially in plantarflexion as compared with the preoperative measurements
6. Induration with palpation of the first interspace

THERAPY GUIDELINES FOR REHABILITATION

Preoperative Considerations

A biomechanical imbalance of the LE that results in excessive foot pronation is a common cause for bunion deformities. Physical therapists have a role in evaluating this inefficient motor plan. They can get the rehabilitative process started before surgery since this will ultimately need to be addressed. Plantar pressure of the medial foot during normal gait should be included in the preoperative evaluation if the therapist has the means to assess it. First metatarsal phalangeal (MTP) joint dorsiflexion and plantar flexion ROM measurements should be ascertained for baseline purposes. Strength testing of the LE musculature, in particular the peroneals and flexor hallucis longus/brevis, should be performed. Schuh and associates[1] recommend using the metatarsophalangeal-interphalangeal score of the American Orthopedic Foot and Ankle Society as a functional survey.

Initial Postoperative Examination

Patients should be both cognizant and compliant with their weight-bearing precautions, depending on the procedure(s) performed, to decrease their risk for complications. Therefore, it is imperative that the physical therapist is aware of the type of surgery that was performed and discusses it with the patient. It is also helpful to view the imaging studies to understand the full extent of the patient's preoperative deformity. Refer to Box 32-1 for objective measures that should be included in the evaluation.

Please remember that patients who have undergone **procedures in categories 4 and 5 (metatarsal base osteotomies with or without a bone graft, fusion of the first MCJ, and fusion of the first MCJ or MTPJ with bone graft) require additional time for healing. Passive range of motion of these joints would be contraindicated if healing is not sufficient at this point. Therefore, it is imperative to consult with the surgeon regarding the integrity of the region before applying any therapist- or patient-generated forces across these joints.**

THERAPY GUIDELINES

There are no specific time parameters associated with these phases because of the variations in the types of procedures used. Procedures that include a metatarsal base osteotomy require 6 to 7 weeks of non–weight bearing. In comparison, the SCARF procedure allows for immediate weight bearing; however, the propulsive phase of gait cannot begin until the third to fourth week postoperatively.

The use of a bone graft in category 5 of the surgical procedures will preclude a patient from beginning therapy until the fusion site has adequately healed. The surgeon will ascertain this on subsequent postoperative follow-up visits. This may occur as early as 8 weeks, but can take up to 3 months. When this patient can begin physical therapy, you will place him or her in the appropriate treatment category depending on the weight-bearing status and specific postsurgical precautions.

Those patients that receive a procedure in category 4 (metatarsal base osteotomies and fusion of the first MCJ) may begin therapy earlier than those in category 5. The surgeon will refer the patient to physical therapy once the area is adequately healed; however, the patient may still be non–weight bearing.

In summary, selection of the appropriate rehabilitation phase depends on the patient's weight-bearing status and associated stage of healing. Please refer to the tables for the guidelines related to each specific treatment category.

Phase I (Non–Weight Bearing) (Table 32-1)

It is common for the patient to demonstrate edema in the foot after a bunionectomy. It is imperative to control this via modalities, manual treatment, graded exercise, and patient compliancy with limited dependent positioning. Since the patient is non–weight bearing, he or she should be independent in the use of the assistive device. This will help avoid falls and compensatory pain patterns from occurring.

The ROM limitations that likely result from immobilization of the foot and ankle need to be addressed to avoid contractures that can lead to gait compensations and functional limitations. In the case in which the patient received a bone graft or fusion of a joint, it is imperative to protect

---

BOX 32-1 Initial Postoperative Examination

- Measurement of edema: volume change is preferred method, less reliable are girth measurements
- Range of motion (ROM): first joint metatarsal phalangeal (MTP) dorsiflexion and plantarflexion; non–weight bearing, and weight bearing only if not contraindicated (as described by Shamus et al[3]) (Fig. 32-20)
  - Talocrural joint dorsiflexion
  - Subtalar joint eversion and inversion
- Joint arthrokinematics: all joints of the foot, including the talocrural joint and distal/proximal tibiofemoral joints. Please be aware of the type of procedure, since a fusion may have been performed. Some procedures also remove or reposition the sesamoids.
- Assessment of the surgical site:
  - Look for possible signs of infection
  - Assess for tethering of the scar to underlying structures without directly pulling on the incision itself
  - Note the boundaries of edema
  - Note any vasomotor dysfunction (pale and cyanotic compared with red and warm)
  - Look for trophic changes (coarse hair, brittle nails, and change in skin texture)
- Movement assessment (if not contraindicated):
  - If patient is non–weight bearing, make sure that he or she is completely independent in the use of the selected assistive device with ambulation. You should reassess the assistive device to make sure that it fits him or her properly.
  - For the full weight-bearing patient, plantar pressure assessment during gait is a valuable tool to help identify decreased medial toe loading. This can be achieved with the use of a Harris Mat, force plate, or other device. Step-downs and squats should also be included to assess lower extremity

- kinematics and its relationship to foot pronation for the full weight-bearing patient.
- Muscle strength:
  - First MTP joint plantarflexion for the full weight-bearing patient: Shamus et al[3] recommend using a pinch gauge dynamometer for assessing this
  - MMT of the peroneal muscle complex, since midfoot pronation is required for optimal loading of the medial forefoot
  - MMT of hip and knee musculature, especially if the patient was initially non–weight bearing after the procedure
- Soft tissue mobility:
  - Pay particular attention to the peroneal tendon tract. There needs to be optimal gliding to appropriately strengthen this muscle complex
  - Techniques to the anterior tibialis are helpful to decrease muscle tone and allow improved function of the peroneals
  - Assessment of the abductor hallucis, adductor hallucis, and flexor hallucis longus because of chronic length changes
- Lower extremity peripheral nerve mobility:
  - As long as ROM of the ankle is allowed, gliding dynamics of the sural, tibial, and peroneal nerves should be assessed in either the slump position or straight leg raise position
- Proprioception for the full weight-bearing patient:
  - Single-limb stance assessment with eyes open and closed
  - Pay particular attention to the willingness of the patient to allow for midfoot pronation. If you observe relatively decreased ipsilateral midfoot pronation, you may need to encourage this motion during subsequent treatment sessions to restore proper plantar loading of the medial foot.

---

the region as mobility is gained elsewhere. **The physical therapist should consult with the surgeon before applying any manual forces across a surgically fixated joint.** All of the structures that cross the ankle have the potential of demonstrating tightness; therefore the treatment needs to address myofascial and neural mobility as well.

The surgical site needs to be monitored for excessive scar formation and possible tethering because of the decrease in overall functional movement. If this area requires treatment, avoid tensioning the healing skin directly because this may adversely affect wound healing.

Disuse atrophy and weakness is another potential complication resulting from this non–weight bearing status. The physical therapist needs to take into consideration the prior functional level of the patient when creating this portion of the program. For example, if the patient is a tennis player,

his program should include core and upper extremity strengthening exercises because of the relative disuse of these systems during this period.

Phase IIa (Partial Weight Bearing) (Table 32-2)

The patient in this category will likely have a walking boot or supportive shoe. Edema control remains imperative at this stage. This is an opportune time to educate the patient on the relationship of swelling and initial weight bearing. It is not uncommon to experience increased swelling as the patient transitions into partial weight bearing. The patient should understand that a large increase in swelling that does not subside with rest may indicate periods of prolonged and/or excessive weight bearing. The patient will therefore need to modify her activity level to help minimize this inflammatory response. Mobility of the foot and ankle complex should

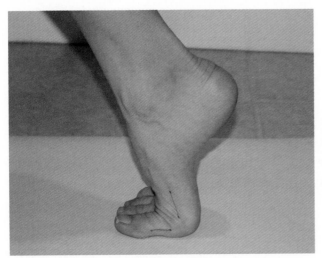

Fig. 32-20 As described by Shamus and associates,[3] first draw a line bisecting the first metatarsal and a line bisecting the first phalanx. Place a dot on the center of the metatarsal phalangeal joint. Then place table paper on the floor. Have the patient take eight steps on this paper, thereby creating a footprint template. Then guide the patient back to the footprints and have them place their feet in the respective footprints. You will be assessing the trail limb in this instance. Ask the patient to raise his or her heel as high as he or she can while maintaining both the step length and the hallux contact on the ground. You will measure with a goniometer using the landmarks you have already marked. Take three measurements, and record the highest measurement you get.

be progressed as well. Remember to consider the various tissues that cross the ankle in addition to the arthrokinematics of the foot and ankle. Since the patient is beginning to ambulate, normal talocrural dorsiflexion should be achieved in this stage. Scar tissue monitoring and treatment of the surgical area needs to be included in this stage as well. **Direct scar tissue massage on the affected skin should be avoided for the first 4 weeks postoperatively.**

Strengthening of the LE and other functionally dependent regions should be initiated or maintained. Unloaded exercise is a valuable adjunct to this treatment as it helps to restore neuromuscular coordination associated with functional movement. Since the patient has begun to bear weight, proprioception of the LE becomes very important. Sitting on an exercise ball with unilateral leg support is an effective means for both assessment and treatment. He or she should demonstrate symmetry between both sides by the end of this phase.

Phase IIb (Initial Full Weight Bearing)
(Table 32-3)

The patient in this category may have a walking boot or supportive shoe. The patient will likely demonstrate increased swelling with the onset of full weight bearing. He or she needs to be educated on the direct relationship of excessive and/or prolonged loading and the inflammatory response. This will help to gradually return the patient to pain-free, full weight-bearing status.

The patient should have symmetric ankle dorsiflexion during this stage, and demonstrate at least 55° of first MTP

joint dorsiflexion by the end of this stage. There should be enough first MTP joint plantarflexion so that the metatarsal head can rest normally on the ground. **Regarding joint mobilizations, manual distraction of the first MTP joint should not occur until the sixth week postoperatively if absorbable rods were used.** Symmetric soft tissue integrity of the foot/ankle complex and neural mobility should be accomplished as well. There should be no signs of scar tissue hypomobility by the end of this phase.

The strengthening program should be progressed to allow for functional weight-bearing exercises, such as squatting, stepping, heel raising, and lunging. Prescription of these exercises depends on the type of procedure. Category 2 procedures do not allow for forward propulsion during the first 2 to 3 weeks postoperatively. Therefore, this patient cannot step down with the nonsurgical foot first, as this will create the dorsiflexion at the affected first MTP joint that occurs during propulsion (Fig. 32-21). This is the same for category 3 patients; however, they need to avoid propulsion for the first 4 to 6 weeks. As a safety precaution, step-downs should begin from a step 7 inches or less in height. Forward lunges are appropriate; however, extension of the affected first MTP joint should again be avoided. This is accomplished by lunging forward in place and avoiding heel-off of the trail leg (Fig. 32-22).

As the patient performs these exercises, the physical therapist needs to monitor the quality and quantity of medial foot loading. **Excessive medial loading needs to be immediately controlled.** Limited medial loading may result from a combination of several factors: weakness or poor control of the peroneals and/or flexor hallucis brevis/longus, tightness of the medial foot (in the absence of an arthrodesis), limited subtalar joint eversion and/or talocrural joint dorsiflexion, restricted first metatarsal plantarflexion, or limited hip internal rotation. Pain and/or apprehension are another possibility. Once identified, the therapist should include treatment of the impairment(s) in the plan of care. Kernozek and associates[2] demonstrated that although patients who received a distal metatarsal osteotomy 12 months prior had favorable outcomes (appropriate joint motion of both the ankle and first MTP joint and decreased pain with ambulation), they did not increase the loading of their medial foot compared with their presurgery data. These patients performed ROM exercises given by the surgeon and did not receive physical therapy. Shamus and associates[3] found that increasing the ROM of the first MTP joint, improving the strength of the flexor hallucis, and gait training achieved a decrease in pain that was statistically significant from the control group in those diagnosed with hallux limitus. These studies illustrate the need for gait training and functional exercises that encourage appropriate LE mechanics, especially during this phase of the rehabilitative process.

Proprioception training should progress to standing activities. These should be tailored to the individual's current impairment level and progressed in a fashion that best replicates the patient's prior functional level.

TABLE 32-1 Bunionectomy Rehabilitation

Rehabilitation Phase	Criteria to Progress to This Phase	Anticipated Impairments and Functional Limitations	Intervention	Goal	Rationale
Phase I	• Postoperative • Non–weight bearing	• Edema and pain • Non–weight bearing • Decreased mobility • Postoperative and disuse weakness	• Effleurage techniques • Patient education on elevation and icing • Use of cryotherapy • Intermittent compression (avoid constant compression) • Gait training • Graded mobilizations of the first MTP, sesamoids, talocrural, subtalar, Lisfranc, transverse tarsal, and tibiofibular joints. Because of the nature of the procedure, grade IV mobilizations should not be attempted until patient response has been thoroughly ascertained via implementation of grade II then III mobilizations. *Distraction of the first MTP joint is contraindicated during the early stages of rehabilitation, especially if absorbable rods were used for osteotomies of the hallux head.* • STM of skin adjacent to surgical incision. Make sure to avoid tensioning the incision itself. • STM of peroneals, anterior tibialis, abductor hallucis, adductor hallucis, and flexor hallucis longus • Gliding techniques of the lower extremity neural system in slump sitting or straight leg raise positions if restrictions are noted • Non–weight bearing gluteals strengthening: clam shells, side-lying hip abduction, prone hip extension • Quadriceps and hamstring strengthening: SLR, SAQ, prone knee flexion, bridging with heels on exercise ball • Peroneals: begin with manually resisted, than progress to Thera-Band once movement pattern is correct • AROM great toe: AROM flexion, extension, abduction; progress to manually resistive as tolerated. Marble pickups, towel curls, and isometric contractions of the flexor hallucis should be included.	• Control edema and pain • Make sure that patient is independent with the assistive device they are using • Maintain or progress the arthrokinematic motion of the various joints • Normalize tissue mobility • Normalize muscle play and tendon sliding • Improve the sliding mechanism of the lower extremity neural system • Increase strength	• Assist in lymphatic and venous circulation • To control the amount of edema • Constant compression may facilitate avascular necrosis of the distal segment • To avoid a fall that can ultimately compound the recovery process • To allow for improved foot and ankle mechanics upon return to full weight bearing • To help prevent tethering and excessive scar formation • To allow for optimal contractile functioning during strengthening activities • To help prevent excessive tensioning of the nerves once higher level functional activities are initiated • To minimize gait impairments when weight bearing is allowed • To eventually allow for the forefoot pronation that is required for optimal plantar loading during gait • To improve great toe function • Strengthening of first MTP joint plantarflexion will help with plantar loading when ambulation begins

AROM, Active range of motion; *MTP*, metatarsal phalangeal; *SAQ*, short arc quadriceps; *SLR*, straight leg raise; *STJ*, subtalar joint; *STM*, soft tissue mobilization; *TCJ*, talocrural joint.

TABLE 32-2 Bunionectomy Rehabilitation

Rehabilitation Phase	Criteria to Progress to This Phase	Anticipated Impairments and Functional Limitations	Intervention	Goal	Rationale
Phase IIa	• Partial weight bearing • May be in a walking boot or supportive shoe	• Edema and pain • Decreased mobility • Postoperative impairments in muscle function • Gait impairments • Impaired proprioception	• Continue interventions from phase I as needed • Talk with surgeon regarding the use of Coban or other compression garment if the edema has been present for at least 4 wk • Continue interventions from phase I as needed. Avoid grade IV mobilizations for the first 3 wk of the first MTPJ, unless your patient progressed to this phase from phase I • *Distraction of the first MTPJ should be avoided during the first 6 wk from surgery if absorbable rods were used during an osteotomy of the hallux head* • Continuation of previous phase exercises • Unloaded squatting (total gym), seated heel raises; the resistance will need to be less than body weight • Unloaded walking (body weight supported system or pool ambulation) • This needs to be pain-free • Seated on exercise ball with affected lower extremity as support lower extremity	• Control edema and pain • Maintain or progress the quality of motion of the various joints and soft tissues • Increase strength and motor control • Pain-free partial weight-bearing ambulation • Symmetrical control of bilateral lower extremity	• Assist in lymphatic and venous circulation • To control the amount of edema • To allow for improved foot and ankle mechanics upon return to full weight bearing • To minimize gait impairments when weight bearing is allowed • To eventually allow for the forefoot pronation that is required for optimal plantar loading during gait • To improve great toe function • To help minimize the potential for compensatory gait pattern upon return to full weight bearing • To allow for improved foot and ankle mechanics upon return to full weight bearing

MTPJ, Metatarsal phalangeal joint.

TABLE 32-3 **Bunionectomy Rehabilitation**

Rehabilitation Phase	Criteria to Progress to This Phase	Anticipated Impairments and Functional Limitations	Intervention	Goal	Rationale
Phase IIb	• Full weight bearing with ground reaction forces not to exceed those of normal ambulation • May be in a supportive shoe	• Decreased mobility • Postoperative impairments in muscle function • Gait impairments • Impaired proprioception	• Continue interventions from phase IIa as needed. Grade IV mobilizations are appropriate for this stage. Use of ROM splinting is appropriate at this stage if ROM gains are slow; however, in many cases this treatment option may not be covered by insurance. • Continuation of previous phase exercises • Standing squats • Forward lunge avoiding trail limb forefoot rocker (heel stays on ground) (see Fig. 32-22) • Steps (however, the affected foot needs to lead the step-down motion) (see Fig. 32-21, A) • Unloaded heel raises on Total Gym (performed with resistance less than body weight) • Monitor for appropriate plantar loading of first MTPJ and the compensation of excessive adduction of the ipsilateral hip (see Fig. 32-25, B) • Manual cueing for medial foot loading during midstance and terminal stance • This needs to be pain-free • Single-limb stance, perturbations	• By the end of this phase, patient should have 55° of first MTPJ PROM dorsiflexion and enough plantarflexion so that the first metatarsal head can rest on the ground • Any soft tissue dysfunctions should be improved as well by the end of this phase • The peroneals and intrinsics should be adequately strong by this point • Pain-free ambulation • Symmetric control of bilateral lower extremity	• To allow for optimal foot and ankle mechanics • To minimize gait impairments as weight bearing is progressed • To eventually allow for the forefoot pronation that is required for optimal plantar loading during gait • To improve great toe function • To allow for return to higher level activities • To allow for optimal proprioceptive control required for higher level activities

MTPJ, Metatarsal phalangeal joint; *PROM,* passive range of motion; *ROM,* range of motion.

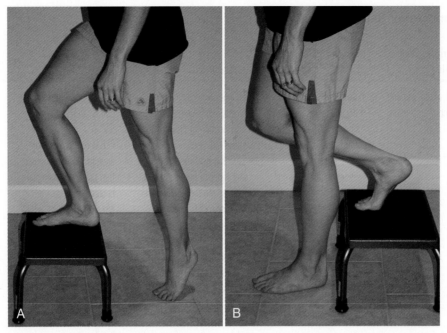

Fig. 32-21 **A,** Starting position for the step up for the affected right lower extremity. Notice the amount of first metatarsal phalangeal joint dorsiflexion in the trail limb at the onset of this exercise. For this reason, the patient needs to have no propulsive precautions in the event that she was to alternate the legs. **B,** End position for an unaffected left lower extremity step down. Notice the amount of first metatarsal phalangeal joint dorsiflexion in the right foot as it maintains contact on the step. For this reason, the patient needs to have no propulsive precautions to perform this portion of the exercise.

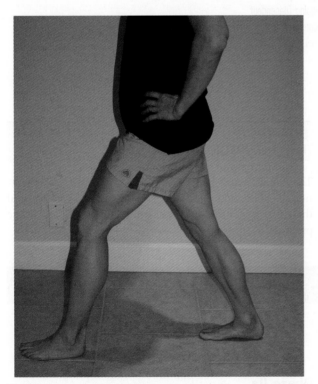

Fig. 32-22 Lunge stretch with heel maintained on the ground. This is the end position for the affected right lower extremity. Avoiding the forefoot rocker will restrict the first metatarsal phalangeal joint from dorsiflexing.

Phase III (Full Weight Bearing Without Precaution) (Table 32-4)

The patient in this category has no restrictions. They may have continued edema because of the progressed functional level. The patient should have symmetric bilateral ankle dorsiflexion, at least 55° to 65° of first MTP joint dorsiflexion, and the first metatarsal head should be resting on the ground naturally during stance.

The main emphasis during this phase is to achieve the above stated goals and to begin with progressive loading beyond the normal gait pattern. This program should be highly individualized and based primarily on the prior functional level of the patient. The exercises should not produce pain, rather they should gradually progress pain-free loading.

By the end of this phase, the patient should have no gait deviations (especially limited medial foot loading). He or she should be able to perform a bilateral heel raise with full body weight with little to no pain. In terms of higher functioning patients, running and jumping will depend on the precautions associated with the type of procedure they received.

TROUBLESHOOTING

The physical therapist may encounter a patient who complains of hyperesthesia near the surgical region toward the onset of therapy. Desensitization techniques are extremely valuable at the onset of care to help manage complex regional pain dysfunctions. The patient should also be educated on the importance of self-desensitization techniques, as well as graded exposure to weight bearing and self-ROM methods to help reduce the patient's anxiety over great toe function. This patient will require extra helpings of positive feedback regarding their progress throughout therapy.

Nerve entrapment of the superficial nerves surrounding the first MTP joint is another potential problem. As a precaution, activities that encourage toe flexion with concomitant ankle plantarflexion will help to mobilize this region. An

TABLE 32-4 Bunionectomy Rehabilitation

Rehabilitation Phase	Criteria to Progress to This Phase	Anticipated Impairments and Functional Limitations	Intervention	Goal	Rationale
Phase III	• Full weight bearing without precaution	• Decreased mobility • Postoperative impairments in muscle function • Anxiety and/or impaired motor control during impact activities	• Continue with aggressive mobilizations and stretching • Continuation of previous phase exercises • Standing heel raises with ball squeeze between heels, lunges with promotion of forefoot rocker, and step training (see Fig. 31-28) • Monitor for appropriate plantar loading of first MTPJ and the compensation of excessive adduction of the ipsilateral hip • Jump: stops on minitrampoline or foam pad, unloaded jogging (body weight support system or pool) progressed to full impact jogging (dependent on procedure and surgical precautions)	• By the time of discharge, patient should have 55°-65° of first MTPJ PROM dorsiflexion and enough plantarflexion so that the first metatarsal head can rest on the ground • The patient does not require cueing for appropriate loading of the medial foot during all exercises • Patient is pain-free with all exercises • Pain-free jumping and running (dependent on procedure and surgical precautions)	• To allow for optimal foot and ankle mechanics upon return to high-level activities • To normalize motor control of the lower extremity for return to high level activities

MTPJ, Metatarsal phalangeal joint; *PROM,* passive range of motion.

example of this would be the use of marble pickups with the patient's calcaneus hovering above the ground. Soft tissue techniques during the onset of therapy should help to mitigate this problem as well.

In the case that you suspect nerve compression (burning symptoms, cramping of the dorsal region, and/or unrelenting pain), confer with the surgeon regarding the use of iontophoresis.

SUGGESTED HOME MAINTENANCE FOR THE POSTSURGICAL PATIENT

The home maintenance section outlines the postoperation rehabilitation the patient is to follow. The physical therapist can use it in customizing a patient-specific program.

 Suggested Home Maintenance for the Postsurgical Patient

Phase I
1. Edema control
   • Recommend icing and elevation
2. Soft tissue mobilization of scar
3. Gentle self-mobilizations/stretching of first MTPJ
4. Strengthening of peroneals and foot intrinsics
   • Windshield wipers, towel curls, marble pick-ups
5. Strengthening of gluteals and knee musculature as appropriate
6. Gym equipment
   • Avoid: any standing exercises and those that put pressure through the foot (e.g., leg presses)

   • Approved: seated hip abduction machine, seated or prone hamstring curls, and leg extensions as approved by therapist

Phase IIa
1. Edema control as needed
2. Soft tissue mobilization of scar as needed
3. Self mobilizations in non–weight bearing positions
4. Strengthening
   • Seated heel raises
   • Continue with phase I exercises as appropriate
5. Proprioception training
   • UE supported (elbows on table) weight shifting

6. Gym Equipment
   • Avoid: any standing exercises
   • Approved: leg presses with sub-body weight load, as long as it is pain-free

Phase IIb

1. Edema control as needed
2. Soft tissue mobilization of scar as needed
3. Self-mobilizations
   • These have progressed to weight-bearing stretches to allow for more ROM gains
4. Wedge first MTP joint extension (Fig. 32-23)
5. Calf stretching against wall
6. Lunge stretch with first MTP dorsiflexion (Fig. 32-24)
7. Strengthening
   • Resisted lateral walking
   • Bilateral heel raises with elbows on table top through pain-free ROM
8. Proprioception training
   • Single-limb stance progressed to perturbations and eyes closed
9. Gym Equipment
   • Avoid: any activities that load the foot beyond typical gait, such as plyometric and jumping exercises
   • Approved: weighted sitting heel raises, leg presses, and squatting

Phase III

1. Continue with self-mobilizations if range is not acceptable at this point
2. Continue with strengthening exercises from phase II if strength is not acceptable
   • Include lunges with trailing leg forefoot rocker
3. Monitor for excessive knee valgus of the trailing limb during the lunge
4. Try to encourage plantar loading the medial forefoot (Fig. 32-25)
   • Bilateral heel raises with ball squeeze (Fig. 32-26)
5. The following exercise will help to keep the patient's weight from shifting to the lateral borders of the feet as the patient rises onto his or her toes
   • Unilateral squatting with multiplanar LE reaches
6. Proprioception training
   • Unilateral stance with triplanar perturbations progressed to labile surface

After Discharge

1. Any underlying impairments that may have been identified throughout the course of therapy that contributed to the deformity should be addressed as the patient returns to their prior functional level:
   • Restricted ankle dorsiflexion
   • Limited hip extension
   • Lunges and heel raises to help maintain first MTP joint dorsiflexion

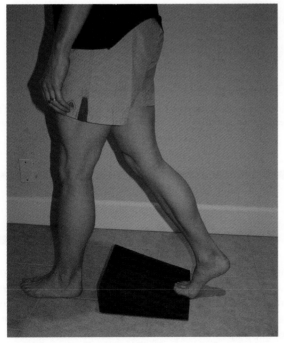

Fig. 32-23 Wedge self first metatarsal phalangeal joint dorsiflexion stretch. This is the end position for the right lower extremity. The patient should not push through the restriction during this stretch; rather, he or she should bring it up to the level of tightness and hold for 5 to 10 seconds. After a few repetitions, the range of motion should improve and the patient should be able to dorsiflex further.

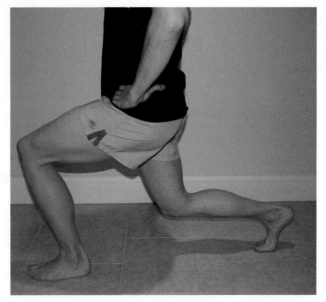

Fig. 32-24 Lunge stretch for the affected right lower extremity, allowing first metatarsal phalangeal joint dorsiflexion. The end position is gauged by how much the patient can dorsiflex their metatarsal phalangeal joint. The patient should not push through the restriction during this stretch but should bring it up to the level of tightness and hold for 5 to 10 seconds.

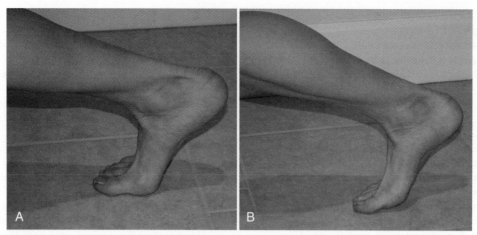

Fig. 32-25 **A,** An example of appropriate medial forefoot plantar loading during the lunge exercise. **B,** An example of insufficient medial forefoot plantar loading. Notice how the weight is shifted toward the center and lateral aspects of the foot. This should be improved throughout therapy to allow for eventual effective propulsion and to decrease the risk of compensatory pain patterns from the beginning.

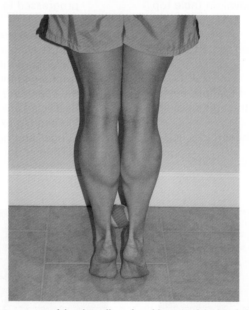

Fig. 32-26 The use of a ball between the posterior aspects of the tibias allows for adduction of the hip, helping to shift weight to the medial aspects of the feet during a heel rise. This will allow for use of first metatarsal phalangeal joint dorsiflexion. Placing the ball at the calcanei tends to create hindfoot inversion, possibly shifting the weight to the lateral borders of the feet.

CLINICAL CASE REVIEW

1 What information can the physical therapist give regarding postdischarge shoe fitting for the patient who received a bunionectomy?

Recommendations from the American Academy of Orthopaedic Surgeons[4]: have the feet measured regularly as this can change with aging; measure both feet and fit to the largest foot; perform the fitting at the end of the day when the feet are the largest; stand during the fitting; make sure there is ⅜ to ½ inch from the longest toe to the end of the shoe; the ball of the foot should fit well into the widest portion of the shoe; do not purchase shoes that feel tight in hopes of stretching them to fit; and there should be a minimum amount of heel slippage.

2 Katrina comes to the physical therapy department for her initial evaluation. She brings her intake information and her prescription. The prescription states, "s/p bunionectomy, PT evaluation and treat." Is this enough

information for the therapist before he or she manually assesses the foot?

The physical therapist needs to know the type of procedure(s) that were performed for the bunionectomy. Each procedure has its own set of precautions in terms of weight-bearing status, when propulsion during gait can be initiated, and whether or not the therapist can apply manual forces across the joints of the medial forefoot.

3 What other areas should be included in a physical therapy evaluation besides assessment of the local region following a bunionectomy?

Because of the functional significance of regional interdependence, the therapist should identify the quality and quantity of motion at the individual "links" of the kinetic chain. This should be conducted with the patient's surgical precautions in mind. Of particular importance are the hip and ankle joints. To minimize the transverse stress on the first MTP joint, one needs to have appropriate hip extension and ankle dorsiflexion ROM. Weakness of the gluteus medius and/or posterior tibialis may also contribute to poor control of pronation, leading to an increase in stress. There are many other possibilities that may contribute to the hallux valgus deformity. Therefore, the physical therapist should have a thorough understanding of each patient's functional movement and address what can be improved upon throughout the rehabilitative process.

4 Keri received a cheilectomy and McBride soft tissue rebalancing 1 week ago and has come for her physical therapy initial evaluation. Why should the physical therapist assess the integrity of the first medial MTP joint soft tissue during this visit?

A portion of Keri's medial MTP joint capsule may have been excised during this procedure. There may have been a surgical release of the lateral sesamoid as well. Therefore, it is imperative for the physical therapist to help prevent excessive scarring on the medial and medial-plantar aspects of this joint. This will help to minimize the likelihood of resultant limited hallux adduction, and possibly a hallux valgus deformity.

5 What peripheral nerve may be affected in patients who receive a bunionectomy? How would it present if it were affected?

Because of the location of the incision either dorsomedially or medially, the dorsal digital branches of the superficial peroneal nerve may become entrapped if there is excessive scar formation. Paresthesia of the medial great toe, and possibly second and third toes, may be reported. A slump test and/or straight leg raise with superficial peroneal nerve bias would be helpful in identifying altered neurodynamics when compared with the uninvolved side.

6 Simone underwent a SCARF procedure 3 weeks ago. During her treatment session, the therapist prescribes marble pickups and great toe flexion isometrics. Why?

Having the appropriate ROM and strength of first MTP joint flexion will facilitate medial foot loading. This motion is important for propulsion during activities such as running and jumping. Decreased medial foot loading may also place increased stress to the lateral foot, lateral knee, hip joint, and lumbar spine.

7 Brian underwent a bunionectomy, is currently in stage 3, and has no weight-bearing precautions. He has been performing heel rises at home; however, he has begun to complain of ipsilateral fifth metatarsal pain. What should the physical therapist inspect in relation to this exercise?

Brian may be excessively loading the lateral aspect of his foot upon the heel rise motion. This could be due to many variables, including decreased strength of the flexor hallucis, limited first MTP joint dorsiflexion, pain, apprehension, peroneal weakness, and/or poor movement strategies. If the impairment were apprehension and/or poor movement strategy, placing a ball between both posterior tibias would help to facilitate the plantar loading of the medial foot. Otherwise, the physical therapist would need to treat the impairment and then reassess the response subsequently.

8 Bernice received a fusion of the first MCJ with a bone graft 8 weeks ago. She has begun to bear weight, but reports a significant increase in swelling. Should the physical therapist be concerned? Why?

It is common to report an increase in swelling upon an increase in functional demand. However, the therapist needs to always consider the integrity of the graft, especially at transitional times of function. The duration and frequency of weight bearing needs to be gradually progressed within patient tolerance. The presence of ipsilateral pitting edema in the absence of vascular disease may indicate potential strain to the graft and should be communicated to the surgeon.

9 When trying to increase dorsiflexion at the first MTP joint, how should the physical therapist mobilize the joint?

Since the head of the metatarsal is convex and the proximal end of the phalanx is concave, the proximal phalanx should be dorsally mobilized to improve dorsiflexion.

10 Casey is currently full weight bearing without precaution following her bunionectomy 8 weeks ago. Casey demonstrates minimal loading of the medial aspect of her foot during the stance phase of gait when compared with the nonoperative side. Her ambulation is currently pain-free. The physical therapist has noted that her first MTP joint passive range of motion and active range of motion dorsiflexion and plantarflexion are within normal limits. The manual muscle testing of the flexor hallucis was a 5/5 bilaterally. What could this scenario indicate?

There are many possibilities that can explain this gait pattern. The therapist needs to ascertain if only one factor is responsible, or if there is an interaction of several impairments. Pain and/or apprehension are likely. If Casey demonstrates normal and pain-free squatting and stepping mechanics, then apprehension is the likely culprit. Restrictions in subtalar joint eversion, hip adduction, and hip internal rotation are likely explanations as well. In this case, the therapist would likely observe the same dysfunction upon squatting and stepping motions.

REFERENCES

1. Schuh R, et al: Rehabilitation after hallux valgus surgery: importance of physical therapy to restore weight bearing of the first ray during the stance phase. Phys Ther 89(9):934-945, 2009.
2. Kernozek TW, Sterriker SA: Chevron (Austin) distal metatarsal osteotomy for hallux valgus: Comparison of pre- and post-surgical characteristics. Foot Ankle Int 23(6):503-507, 2002.
3. Shamus J et al: The effect of sesamoid mobilization, flexor hallucis strengthening, and gait training on reducing pain and restoring function in individuals with hallux limitis: A clinial trial. JOSPT 34(7):368-376, 2004.
4. American Academy of Orthopaedic Surgeons: Bunion surgery. Retrieved August 11, 2010, from http://orthoinfo.aaos.org/topic.cfm?topic=a00140, 2001.

ADDITIONAL READING

Burns AE: Surgical Procedures of the Hallux. In Banks AS, et al, editor: McGlamry's comprehensive textbook of foot and ankle surgery, Philadelphia, 2001, Lippincott Williams and Wilkins.

Chang TJ: Distal metaphyseal osteotomies in hallux abducto valgus surgery. In Banks AS, et al, editor: McGlamry's comprehensive textbook of foot and ankle surgery, Philadelphia, 2001, Lippincott Williams and Wilkins.

Chang TJ, Camasta CA: Hallux limitus and hallux rigidus. In Banks AS, et al, editor: McGlamry's comprehensive textbook of foot and ankle surgery, Philadelphia, 2001, Lippincott Williams and Wilkins.

Coughlin MJ, Mann RA: Surgery of the foot and ankle, ed 8, Philadelphia, 2007, Mosby.

Gerbert J: Textbook of bunion surgery, ed 3, Philadelphia, 2001, Saunders.

Gudas CJ: scarf Z-osteotomy. In Banks AS, et al, editor: McGlamry's comprehensive textbook of foot and ankle surgery, Philadelphia, 2001, Lippincott Williams and Wilkins.

Mothershed RA: Osteotomies of the first metatarsal base. In Banks AS, et al, editor: McGlamry's comprehensive textbook of foot and ankle surgery, Philadelphia, 2001, Lippincott Williams and Wilkins.

Yu GV, Shook JE: Arthrodesis of the First metatarsophalangeal joint. In Banks AS, et al, editor: McGlamry's comprehensive textbook of foot and ankle surgery, Philadelphia, 2001, Lippincott Williams and Wilkins.

CHAPTER 33

Transitioning the Jumping Athlete Back to the Court

Christine Prelaz

Lower extremity injuries are prevalent in athletics. These injuries can range from minor sprains or strains to those that result in significant functional limitation and loss of time from work and/or sport.[1] An estimated 3 to 5 million injuries occur each year among recreational and competitive athletes in the United States[1] with the worldwide annual cost being estimated at $1 billion.[2] The National Collegiate Athletic Association (NCAA) reported that more than 50% of injuries occurred in the lower extremity with the most common sites being the ankle and knee over a 16-year period.[3] These data come from the NCAA Injury Surveillance System, which summarized surveillance data for 15 NCAA sports over a 16-year period.[3] Research studies indicate that both intrinsic and extrinsic factors play a role in sustaining lower extremity injuries.[2,4] Recent attention in the literature has focused on identifying modifiable and nonmodifiable associated risks with the overall goal of reducing such injuries. Given the frequency and cost of these injuries, the clinician is challenged not only with restoring function of the injured athlete but also with implementing interventions to prevent future injury. In today's competitive environment, the health care team is faced with higher levels of pressure from the athlete, coaches, and parents to return the athlete back to sport as expediently and as safely as possible. Ongoing assessment and proper program design based on current evidence-based research can provide the clinician with the best information possible and guide him or her to determine an athlete's readiness to return to sport.

PROGRAM DESIGN

Numerous lower extremity rehabilitation protocols exist for both conservative management and surgical procedures. Each clinician has his or her unique approach to the rehabilitation of a specific athletic injury. For example, a survey of practices in ACL reconstruction by the American Orthopedic Society for Sports Medicine showed that rehabilitation protocols were *the* most variable factor among other practice factors that were surveyed.[5] Other factors included in the survey were weight bearing, immobilization, bracing, length of physical therapy, and when to return to a sport. Such variability in protocols can lead to confusion as to what is appropriate and/or foster the practice of a "one size fits all" rehabilitation approach. Whatever the injury, a team approach consisting of close communication between the physician, physical therapist, athletic trainer, and other medical specialists should provide the best environment for returning the athlete to the sport. The clinician must have a comprehensive understanding of the structures involved, the surgical procedures, surgeon preferences, and tissue healing constraints. Because it is beyond the scope of this chapter to outline a program for each specific sport or injury, the goal of this chapter is to provide general rehabilitation guidelines, ideas, and resources for returning jumping athletes back to their respective sports successfully and safely.

Readiness to Prepare for Return

Regardless of the injury or surgical procedure, it is the clinician's responsibility to determine the athlete's level of readiness to progress to each phase of rehabilitation.

Continual monitoring of tissue tolerance by the clinician as the athlete progresses through each rehabilitation phase is critical. Knowledge of the type and extent of injury, surgical procedure, pain levels, swelling, ROM, strength, endurance, flexibility, patient's goals, and psychologic readiness are all factors that should assist in the clinical decision process.

Individual goals must be set for each athlete dependent upon his or her current functional level, the level of competition to which they are to return, and the specific sport of the athlete. In general, the goals of the training program are to restore and/or improve flexibility, endurance, strength, balance, and agility. Once the athlete has completed his or her acute phase rehabilitation, the concept of a needs analysis may assist in establishing more sports-specific goals. The needs analysis takes into account the fitness needs of both the activity/sport and the individual athlete, thus designing a more customized versus a "cook book" program. To develop a needs analysis, both a physiologic and biomechanical analysis must be completed. When considering a specific event, one must look at the muscles involved, the energy system needs, speed/strength/power/endurance requirements, and any other specific needs of the event itself.[6] Next, the current status and prior history of the athlete is determined and a program is then designed to progress him or her toward those specific goals. Sport-specific training is fundamental in returning the athlete back to his or her respective sport. The rehabilitation program should incorporate a whole body approach including core strengthening and exercises for the noninjured extremity.

Flexibility

Controversy exists in the literature regarding static stretching.[7] Several studies have shown that there is little evidence to support its role in injury prevention and determined that preexercise static stretching may actually negatively affect performance.[8] Some researchers found decreases in muscle strength[9] and decreases in jumping ability[10] after passive stretching. The concept of using a dynamic warm-up instead of static stretching has gained popularity in both the literature and on the field. Some of the proposed benefits of a dynamic warm-up versus static stretching are that the muscles are in more continuous movement, thus increasing the overall temperature and achieving a more "true warm-up." Dynamic stretching can also use more sports-specific movements to incorporate balance and motor control and mental preparation for the athlete, which may help to prime the neuromuscular system for the upcoming event.[11] A few examples of dynamic warm-up exercises are heel/toe walking, marching, skipping, long leg kicks, gluteal kicks, lunge walking, carioca, and lateral slides. This does not mean that static stretching should be abandoned, however. Shrier[8] contends that regular stretching as part of a comprehensive program and not before exercise can increase force, jump height, and speed.[8] Athletes who need greater range of motion or need to increase overall flexibility may still benefit from static stretching (Box 33-1). Stretching after activity may also tend to relax the tissues and prevent general postactivity stiffness.

Strength

Before starting any training program, it is important to have a full understanding of the demands of the sport and the individual athlete. The needs analysis will enable the clinician to design a comprehensive specific program to develop strength, endurance, power, speed, agility, and balance.

Special considerations must be given to injured athletes with regard to strengthening. Rehabilitation of knee injuries in particular has presented the clinician with a challenge. For example, the main goal of rehabilitation following ACL reconstruction is to restore lower extremity strength while protecting the reconstructed graft and the patellofemoral joint from excessive stresses. Selective quadriceps muscle atrophy occurs following injury and/or immobilization. Strength deficits in the quadriceps of up to 10% have been

---

> ### BOX 33-1 Flexibility
>
> **General Guidelines for Static Stretching**
> - Initial warm-up
> - Stretch slowly, no bouncing
> - Stretch until mild tension is felt, not painful
> - Hold each stretch 20 to 30 seconds
> - Repeat 2 to 3 repetitions for each muscle group
>
> **Major Muscle Groups to Stretch**
> - Hamstrings
> - IT band
> - Gastrocnemius-soleus complex
> - Quadriceps
> - Low back
> - Hip flexors
> - Pectorals/biceps
> - Latissimi/triceps

reported by Shelbourne and associates[12] at an average follow-up of 4 years following ACL surgery. Debate exists between the uses of open kinetic chain (OKC) versus closed kinetic chain (CKC) exercises to build quadriceps strength (Fig. 33-1). Several authors have advocated the use of both after ACL reconstruction.[13,14] A literature review by Ross and associates[15] on OKC versus CKC exercises following ACL reconstruction indicates that the greatest amount of ACL strain and patellofemoral joint stress occurs at approximately 40° of knee flexion to full extension.[16,17] It was therefore recommended that OKC exercises for quadriceps strengthening be performed with knee angles greater that 40° to avoid excessive stress on these structures. Closed chain activities beyond 60° were to be avoided since maximum stress on the patellofemoral joint occurs between 60° and 90° of flexion.[17]

Because of the predominant atrophy of type I (slow twitch) muscle fibers following injury or immobilization, high repetitions (6 to 10 sets, 12 to 15 repetitions) with low resistance is recommended early in the rehabilitation program.[15] Establishing normal muscle balance for both involved and uninvolved limbs is one of the primary goals. A comprehensive strength training program should address core, hip, calf, and ankle musculature, as well as establish appropriate quadriceps/hamstring ratios. Strengthening of the hamstrings using both closed and open chain methods is important because of their role in assisting in the control of anterior tibial translation. Traditional and functional techniques can be incorporated for both variety and effectiveness (Box 33-2).

There has been an increasing amount of literature in recent years regarding the relationship of hip and core strength as factors in lower extremity injuries. Unfortunately, this relationship is not quite clear. For example, weakness of the hip abductors and external rotators has been shown to contribute to increased hip adduction and internal rotation motion observed in female runners with patellofemoral

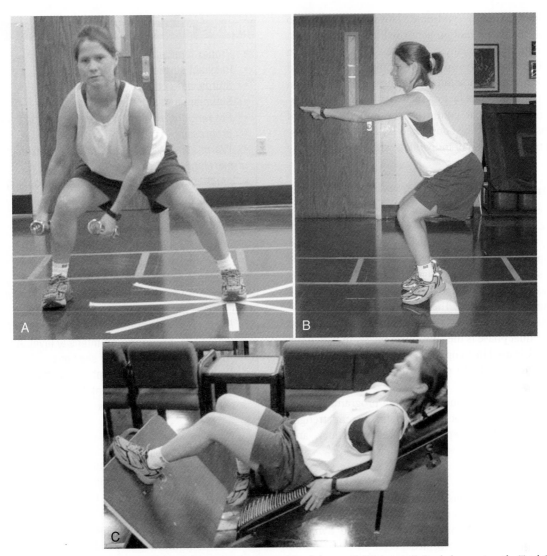

Fig. 33-1 CKC exercises. **A,** Example of closed chain strengthening: multiangle lunges. **B,** Minisquat. **C,** Single-leg squat on the Total Gym.

BOX 33-2 Strengthening

Guidelines: high repetitions, low resistance—4 to 6 sets of 12 to 15 repetitions for lower extremity exercises in early rehabilitation phases. Upper extremity and core strengthening can follow standard strengthening guidelines. Use combinations of traditional and functional training techniques.

- Open kinetic chain knee extension 90° to 45° (as per physician and clinician philosophy)
- Closed kinetic chain exercises 0° to 60°
  - Total Gym squats (double leg, single leg)
  - Leg press (double leg, single leg)
  - Minisquats (double leg, single leg) with proper form and control
  - Lunges—multidirectional (weights, sport cord, cable column resistance)
  - Forward/backward/lateral step

- Hamstrings
- Hip abductors/adductors
- Calf raises—bent and straight knee
- Core strengthening—abdominals, hip musculature, low back
- Upper body:
  - Chest
  - Deltoids
  - Latissimus/posterior shoulder
  - Bicep
  - Triceps

pain or iliotibial band syndrome. However, it has also been shown that these motion abnormalities can exist even though no strength deficits are present. This indicates an apparent disconnect between muscle strength and observed abnormal kinematics in some cases. Therefore, it has been suggested that additional factors such as altered proprioception and neuromuscular control of the lumbo-pelvic and hip regions should also be considered in the clinical assessment and treatment plan of individuals with lower extremity injuries.[18]

Plyometrics

General Principles

Plyometric exercises use the stretch-shortening cycle to store potential energy. The stretch-shortening cycle consists of the eccentric phase where preloading occurs as the muscle is placed on stretch, thus storing potential energy. The amortization phase refers to the time period between the eccentric and concentric contraction. The amortization phase must be kept short; the longer it is, the greater the loss of stored energy. The final phase is the concentric phase, in which the stored energy is used in an opposite reaction (i.e., the muscle contracts concentrically to provide the force necessary for the required movement).[19]

When designing a plyometric training program, consideration must be given to age, body weight, current strength and conditioning level, experience, previous injury, and demands of the sport (Boxes 33-3 through 33-5).[19,20]

Warm Up/Cool Down

Warm-up exercises can consist of a combination of general and specific skill enhancement drills such as marching, skipping, shuffling, and footwork drills.[20] Static and dynamic stretching should also be performed.

Proper Technique

Proper instruction and monitoring of technique is critical not only for proper neuromuscular retraining but also to avoid injury. Verbal, visual, and manual cues may be used to teach the athlete proper control. If the athlete fails to demonstrate proper control during any part of the exercise, he or she should be stopped and given a brief rest period before continuing. If improper technique is still present, the exercise should be discontinued for that session. Explaining and reinforcing the importance of proper technique to the athlete will help to prevent overuse and injury during the training program.

Frequency

Perform one to three sessions per week. Two sessions is the norm for most off-season sports programs.[21] Frequency should be determined by the intensity of the sessions and the phase of rehabilitation or cycle in the sport season.

Volume

Volume is expressed in number of foot contacts per workout. Volume should be 60 to 100 foot contacts for beginners; 100

BOX 33-3 Plyometrics Guidelines

- Proper footwear
- Resilient surface
- Sturdy, safe equipment
- Sufficient and safe training area
- *Proper control and technique for all drills before progressing*
- *Warm-up:* static/dynamic stretching; skipping, marching, bounding, etc.
- *Frequency:* 2 to 3 times per week depending on intensity and other program components
- *Volume:*
  - Beginner—60 to 100 foot contacts
  - Intermediate—100 to 150 foot contacts
  - Advanced—120 to 200 foot contacts
  - Elite—200 to 400 foot contacts
- *Intensity:* Low, medium, high. Decrease volume as intensity increases.
- *Recovery:* 30 seconds to 3 minutes between repetitions, depending on intensity level. Allow 48 to 72 hours between training sessions.
- *Direction:* choose drills that are sport specific for enhancing vertical, horizontal, lateral, or combinations or directions

Progression

Basic Guidelines

- Start simple, progress to complex
- Low volume to higher volume
- General drills progressing to sport-specific exercises
- Bilateral to unilateral exercises
- Stable to unstable surfaces
- Slow speed to faster speeds

Level of Difficulty Progression

- Jumps in place
- Standing jumps
- Multiple hops/jumps
- Bounding/cone drills
- Box/depth jumps

Data from Nutting M: Practical progressions for upper body plyometric training. NSCA Performan Train J 3(2):14-19, 2004.

---

to 150 for intermediate level and 120 to 200 for advanced off-season workouts.[20] If intensity is high, volume should be low to medium. Volume may also be expressed as a specific distance.[21] Adjust the number of contacts down for younger, inexperienced or postinjury individuals. Elite athletes may perform 200 to 400 foot contacts.[19]

Intensity

Intensity refers to the amount of stress on the tissues during the plyometric activity. It can be classified as low (Fig. 33-2), medium, or high (Fig. 33-3). **In general, as intensity increases, volume should decrease. Athletes weighing**

BOX 33-4 Plyometric Exercise Examples

Low Intensity
- Prancing, galloping, skipping, marching
- Skipping rope
- Wall jumps
- Squat jumps
- Two feet ankle hops
- Side, forward/backward hops
- Dot drill—double leg
- Broad jumps

Medium Intensity
- Tuck jumps
- Split squat jumps
- Scissor jumps
- Barrier jumps (forward/backward, lateral)
- Single-leg hops
- Dot drill—single leg
- Bounding
- Double-leg diagonal barrier jumps
- Single-leg dot drills
- Hip-twist ankle hops
- 180° twist

High Intensity
- Single-leg triple jump and sticks
- Single-leg diagonal jumps
- Single-leg vertical power jumps
- Single-leg tuck jumps

Shock
- Depth jumps
- Box jumps

BOX 33-5 Plyometric Guidelines

General Principles
Frequency:
- One to three sessions per week
- Two sessions is the norm for off-season

Intensity:
- Low, medium, high
- As intensity increases, volume should decrease
  Recovery:
- 30 seconds to 3 minutes between sets
- Allow 48 to 72 hours between sessions

Volume
- Expressed as number of foot contacts per session
- Beginners: 60 to 100 contacts
- Intermediate: 100 to 150
- Advanced: 120 to 200
- If intensity is high, volume should be medium to low
- Adjust down for younger, inexperienced, or postinjury individuals
- Elite athletes may perform 200 to 400 contacts per session

Progression
- Adequate strength and conditioning levels should be present before beginning a plyometric program
- Start with simple, progress to more complex drills
- Start with low volume and intensity, progressing to high
- Start with general drills, progressing to sport specific
- Start with bilateral, progressing to single leg
- Stable surfaces before unstable
- Slow speed to faster speeds
- Low height to higher heights

---

more than 220 lb should not perform depth jumps from heights greater than 18 inches.[19]

Progression

Adequate strength and conditioning levels should be present before the athlete can progress. It is recommended that the athlete be able to squat 1.5 times body weight before starting shock types of plyometric training such as depth jumps.[22] Progression should be based on a current evaluation of the athlete, the establishment of sport-specific goals, attainment of proper technique and control, and the absence of any signs or symptoms of overuse. In general, the following progression guidelines are suggested to avoid overtraining and to prevent injury during the plyometric program[23]:

- Start with simple drills and progress to complex
- Low volume progressing to high volume
- General to specific drills/exercises
- Bilateral to unilateral exercises
- Use stable before unstable surfaces
- Slow speed to faster speeds
- Low height to higher height

Recovery

Adequate recovery time must be given between repetitions and sets, as well between workout sessions. Plyometrics are not intended to be an aerobic conditioning workout. Rest time between repetitions and sets is dependent upon the intensity of the exercise and the individual. Allow 30 seconds up to 3 minutes for recovery.[19] Plyometric sessions should not be performed on consecutive days. In general, plyometric workouts should allow 48 to 72 hours between sessions.[24]

Direction of Motion

A needs analysis should determine if the sport requires speed and power in a vertical plane, horizontal plane, lateral or diagonal directions, or a combination. Most sports require a combination of directions. Drills that specifically enhance the required components of the sport should be chosen for the program.

Proper technique and control is crucial before progressing to the next level.

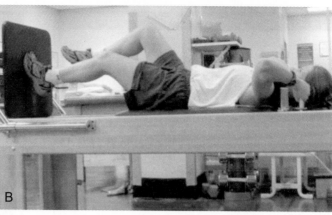

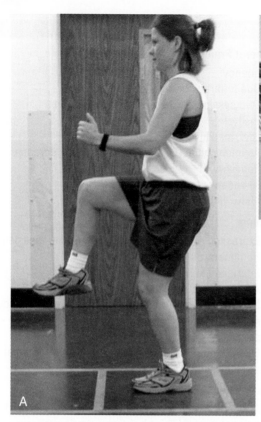

Fig. 33-2 Low-intensity plyometric exercises. **A,** Marching. **B,** Simulated jumping on the Pilates Reformer.

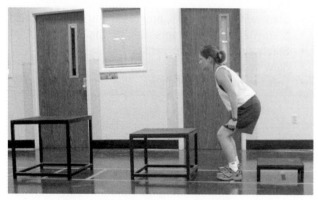

Fig. 33-3 High-intensity plyometric drill: box jumps.

Speed and Agility

Agility is the ability to rapidly change body direction, accelerate, or decelerate. It is influenced by balance, strength, coordination, and skill level. Agility can be improved by first developing an adequate base of strength and conditioning that is appropriate for the difficulty level of the athlete. After this is achieved, drills designed to enhance reactive and explosive motor skills can be progressively incorporated (Fig. 33-4).

Guidelines for speed and agility training are as follows:
- Allow adequate warm-up
- The athlete should have an appropriate strength/conditioning base for the selected drills

- Speed and agility should be performed early in the training session or preferably on separate days to maximize training effect, avoid fatigue, and prevent overuse
- Allow adequate rest between sets and repetitions. Heart rate and respiration should return to almost normal levels after the drill. A 1:4-6 work-to-rest ratio is recommended.[22]
- Number of sessions per week may vary depending on the sport, the individual's current level, history of injury, intensity of the drill, and/or period of the mesocycle. Two times per week can be used as a general rule.
- Volume: two to five sets of each exercise
- Quality not quantity

Box 33-6 lists various speed and agility drills. This list provides examples only; the reader may wish to refer to specific resources on speed, agility, and plyometric training for a more comprehensive list and description of drills.[20,22,25,26]

Neuromuscular Training

Neuromuscular control is the ability to produce controlled movement through coordinated muscle activity.[27] It is the efferent motor response to sensory input from the somatosensory (proprioceptive and kinesthetic) system, the visual system, and the vestibular system. Stability is achieved by continuous feedback to the central nervous system from the integration of input from these three systems. The somatosensory system uses several different types of sensory input from proprioceptors and the sensory nerve terminals found

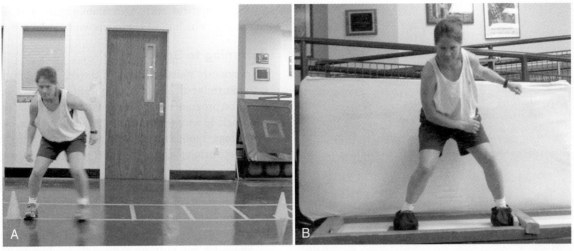

Fig. 33-4 Agility drills. **A**, Lateral shuffles. **B**, Slide board.

BOX 33-6 Speed/Agility

Speed and Agility Guidelines

- Adequate strength/conditioning base
- Warm-up
- Perform early in the training session, preferably on separate days
- Allow adequate rest between sets and repetitions. A 1:4-6 work-to-rest ratio is recommended
- Number of sessions per week may vary; two times per week can be used as a general rule
- Volume: two to five sets of three to five exercises; 15 seconds progressing to 30 seconds or measured in distance
- Emphasize quality not quantity

Speed and Agility Exercise Examples

- High knees
- Gluteal kickers
- Resisted running drills
- Step hurdles
- Foot-tapping
- Shuttle runs
- Ladder drills
- Cariocas
- Lateral shuffles
- Side to side box shuffles
- Directional mirror drills
- T drills
- 5 dot drills—double leg, single leg
- Figure eights with cones

---

in muscles, tendons, and joint capsules. Proprioceptors relay information relating to movement and position sense.

Visual input received in the cortex and vestibular nuclei provides information for the vestibular and somatosensory systems to make adjustments to maintain stability and balance. Dynamic joint stability is the ability of the joint to remain stable under the rapidly changing loads during activity.[27]

Following an injury, deafferentation to ligament and capsular mechanoreceptors may occur. The presence of tissue swelling and pain can also compound sensory damage by disrupting sensory feedback that can alter reflexive joint stabilization and neuromuscular coordination.

Neuromuscular training programs aimed at enhancing or restoring neuromuscular control following injury have been developed and have been shown to reduce the incidence of injury.[28-32] A comprehensive neuromuscular program would integrate exercises that challenge all three regulatory systems: the somatosensory, visual, and vestibular systems. The neuromuscular program should incorporate a multilevel approach, which includes combinations of strength training, flexibility, balance, agility, and plyometric exercises. Activities that induce adaptations to the system may include open and/or closed chain exercise, eccentric training, balance activities, reflex facilitation, stretch-shortening, biofeedback training, and controlled position training. Balance training might include stationary and dynamic surfaces, such as wobble boards, balance beams, and foam pads, to enhance both static and dynamic balance. Functional training, such as jumping and landing, agility, and perturbation training, should also be included depending on sport demands. Fig. 33-5 illustrates several examples of neuromuscular training exercises.

As mentioned previously, the clinician must continually monitor the athlete for tissue tolerance and to determine readiness to proceed to the next phase in the rehabilitation process. Myer and associates have proposed a progressive end-stage return to sport protocol following ACL reconstruction that is based on the athlete meeting specific criteria before being able to progress to the next phase.[33] The protocol consists of four stages: dynamic stabilization, functional strengthening, power development, and sports performance symmetry. One significant limitation of this protocol is that some of the criteria were based on the use of specialized

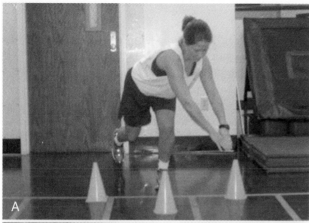

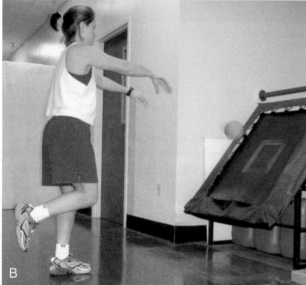

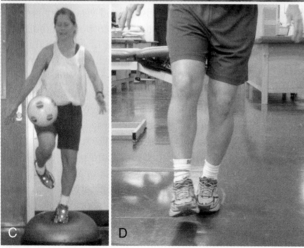

Fig. 33-5 Neuromuscular training exercises. **A,** Cone reaches–balance exercise. **B,** Plyotoss—proprioception drill/neuromuscular control. **C,** Functional activity incorporated with balance (on BOSU). **D,** Four way leg kicks—balance/proprioception.

testing equipment such as a stabilometer and isokinetic equipment, which most clinicians would not have available.

Returning to Sport

As previously stated, the goal of the rehabilitation program is to return the athlete to the highest functional level. Rehabilitation programs are based on current scientific principles that include knowledge of the healing process, anatomy/physiology, biomechanics, and kinematics. Keep in mind that these principles and concepts are ever-changing as new research becomes available.

Typically, return to sport is based on various subjective and objective criteria. Many clinicians have either developed their own compilation of tests or have adopted those used by others to determine when an athlete is ready to return to sport.

Single-leg hop tests are commonly used to determine an athlete's progress in his/her rehabilitation program and to determine the readiness to return to sport. Various single-leg hop tests either used alone or in combination have been described in the literature.[34-38] These tests include single-leg hop and stop tests,[36] single-leg hop for distance and time, triple hop, and the triple crossover hop.[34-39] Several studies have shown these tests to be reliable with intraclass coefficients between 0.66 to 0.97.[40-42] Barber and associates recommended using at least two hop tests and achieving a limb symmetry score of 85%.[34]

Other test measures have been used to determine return to sport as well. Vertical jump height (Fig. 33-6) and

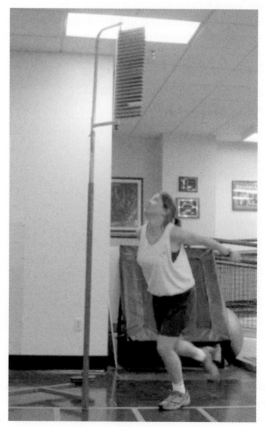

Fig. 33-6 Vertical jump test.

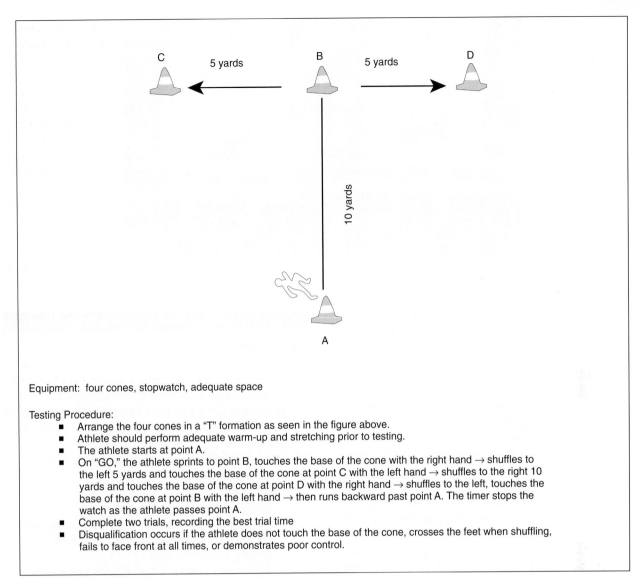

Equipment: four cones, stopwatch, adequate space

Testing Procedure:
- Arrange the four cones in a "T" formation as seen in the figure above.
- Athlete should perform adequate warm-up and stretching prior to testing.
- The athlete starts at point A.
- On "GO," the athlete sprints to point B, touches the base of the cone with the right hand → shuffles to the left 5 yards and touches the base of the cone at point C with the left hand → shuffles to the right 10 yards and touches the base of the cone at point D with the right hand → shuffles to the left, touches the base of the cone at point B with the left hand → then runs backward past point A. The timer stops the watch as the athlete passes point A.
- Complete two trials, recording the best trial time
- Disqualification occurs if the athlete does not touch the base of the cone, crosses the feet when shuffling, fails to face front at all times, or demonstrates poor control.

Fig. 33-7 T test. (Adapted from Semenick DM: Testing protocols and procedures. In Baechle TR, editor: The essentials of strength training and conditioning, Champaign, Ill, 1994, Human Kinetics.)

isokinetic testing have been used to assess function and strength.[43,44] A 1 repetition maximum (RM) leg press test or squat can also be used to assess strength. The shuttle run and figure eight run have been used to test the ability to run, cut, and pivot.[34,45,46] The T-test (Fig. 33-7) and the Edgren side step test are two tests that can be used to assess agility and body control.[47] These tests can also be used in the rehabilitation program as functional drills.

Speed tests measure the body's displacement per unit of time. Testing speed for clinical purposes is usually limited because of lack of appropriate space. The majority of the research on these tests has been with ACL deficient or ACL reconstruction individuals; however, the tests may be used in other lower extremity patient populations as well. Standard health and fitness tests for flexibility, local endurance, aerobic power, and agility/speed such as those described in *The Essentials of Strength and Conditioning*[47] may also be incorporated into the testing protocol and compared with available normative data.

Davies[48] has developed a functional testing algorithm that uses a systematic functional progression of testing and exercise. It is designed to progressively increase stresses on the athlete while gradually lessening clinical control. The algorithm includes the following: subjective information, basic measurements, KT 1000 test, balance testing, closed and open chain strength testing, two-leg jump test, unilateral hop test, lower extremity functional test, and sports-specific testing.[48] Very specific criterion must be met before the athlete is allowed to progress to the next level. Frequent testing and monitoring of the patient allows the clinician to always know the status of that patient. A specific rehabilitation program can then be designed to address individual deficits instead of following a preset clinical protocol.

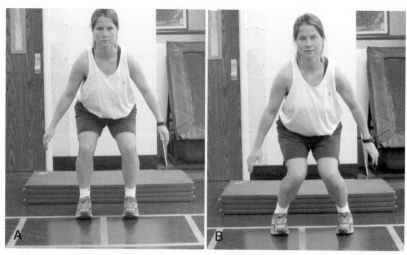

Fig. 33-8 **A,** Proper landing form with good lower extremity alignment. **B,** Improper landing form with increased lower extremity valgus.

Recent research by Hewett and associates[49] has focused on biomechanical loading measurements in female athletes in an attempt to predict those who are at risk for ACL injury. They concluded that increased valgus motion and valgus moments at the knee were key predictors for potential ACL injury (Fig. 33-8). If predictive factors associated with lower extremity injuries can be identified, specific screening programs and training programs could potentially be designed to reduce the risk for injury.

In general, there is currently no standard accepted series of tests to determine when an athlete is ready to return safely to sport. The decision should be based on ROM, strength, symptomatology, and functional testing. Box 33-7 provides a list of tests that the clinician may select to assist in the decision. It is recommended that a minimum of two hop tests,[34] a strength assessment, and an agility/body control test be used. The athlete must demonstrate proper form and technique throughout the test procedures. A deficit of 10% or less with good control is currently used in many facilities to allow return to sport. There are obvious limitations to the tests; however, they appear to be the most commonly used in various combinations. Further research is needed not only to determine risk factors, but also to determine what testing procedures would be best to predict safe return to sport.

SUMMARY

Returning the jumping athlete back to sport as safely and efficiently as possible is the primary goal of the rehabilitation program. The length of time to return depends on many factors. It is the clinician's responsibility to have the scientific knowledge base and clinical skills to determine when and how the athlete is to progress through the program. Current testing procedures have their limitations; however, they provide some objective data to assist the clinician in deciding when the athlete may resume sport activities. It is impossible to design one rehabilitation protocol for all athletes lest it be

---

BOX 33-7 Example of Criteria Return to Sport Criteria

Assessment
- Range of motion
- Self-report scores (optional): Lysholm, Knee Outcome Survey, International Knee Documentation Committee, Cincinnati Knee Rating Scale, foot/ankle outcomes, or other functional outcome assessment self-reports
- Strength: 1 RM leg press, squat test, isokinetics
- *Stability:* Manual tests, KT-1000
- *Functional Tests:*
  - Vertical jump
  - Hop tests (single-leg hop for distance, triple hop for distance, single-leg hop for time over 6 meters, cross-over hop)
  - Agility/body control: T-test, Edgren side step test, shuttle run
  - Lower extremity functional test
  - Balance testing

Criterion for Return to Sport
- No complaints of pain
- No giving way/sensation of instability
- No effusion
- Full and pain-free range of motion
- Strength deficit 10% or less compared with uninvolved side
- Establish proper muscle balance ratios
- Functional test score 10% or less deficit compared with uninvolved side. Must demonstrate good technique and control.

---

a cookbook approach. Table 33-1 provides only one example of how the various training components can be combined. It was the goal of this chapter to provide the clinician with guidelines, ideas, and resources for returning the jumping athlete back to sport; hopefully, it accomplished its goals.

TABLE 33-1 Example Program

Day	Weeks 1-3	Weeks 4-6	Weeks 5-8
Monday	• Strengthening • Upper body plyometrics • Core strength • Cardio	• Strengthening • Upper body plyometrics • Core strength • Cardio	• Strengthening • Upper body plyometrics • Core strength • Cardio
Tuesday	• Low-intensity plyometrics — 4 drills • Agility • Cardio	• 2 low-intensity, 2 medium-intensity plyometric drills • Progress to 4 medium-intensity plyometric drills • Agility • Sport-specific drills • Cardio	• 2 medium-intensity plyometric drills, 2 high-intensity plyometric drills • Progress to 4 high-intensity drills • Agility • Sport-specific drills • Cardio
Wednesday	• Strength training • Upper body plyometrics • Core strength	• Strength training • Upper body plyometrics • Core strength	• Strength training • Upper body plyometrics • Core strength
Thursday	• Low-intensity plyometrics — 4 drills • Agility • Cardio	• 2 low-intensity, 2 medium-intensity plyometric drills • Progress to 4 medium-intensity plyometric drills • Agility • Sport-specific drills	• 2 medium-intensity plyometric drills, 2 high-intensity plyometric drills • Progress to 4 high-intensity drills • Agility • Sport-specific drills • Cardio
Friday	• Strength training • Core strength • Cardio	• Strength training • Core strength • Cardio	• Strength training • Core strength • Cardio

CLINICAL CASE REVIEW

1 Matt is a 42-year-old male who has had an ACL reconstruction. He has completed his early postoperative rehabilitation and is in phase I (dynamic stabilization and strengthening) of his return to a sport program. What criteria might you use to assess whether Matt is ready to progress to functional strengthening exercises (stage II)?

• No pain
• No swelling
• Full ROM
• Single-limb squat and hold symmetry (60° knee flexion, 5-second hold)
• Audibly rhythmic foot strike patterns with treadmill running
• Acceptable single-leg balance measures

These criteria are based on the Return to Sport algorithm developed by Myer and associates.[33] Matt should have been allowed to progress from stage I into stage II by having a minimum International Knee Documentation Committee score of 70 and baseline strength scores. This algorithm is somewhat limiting because much of the testing uses equipment that is not available to most clinicians. However, the clinician may still incorporate this criterion-based approach by using other "low technology" tests and measures: a 1 RM test, the lateral step test, and the Star Excursion Balance test are a few examples.

2 Matt is now 6 months after surgery for an ACL/meniscal repair. He had been going to the gym to work on his strengthening and cardiovascular training while attending rehabilitation sessions once per week to progress and focus on his functional training. He had been progressing extremely well—good control with landings and agility exercises, etc. He is very motivated and eager to return to basketball. At 6 months after surgery, he performed a functional assessment that included four single-leg hop tests. Although he had no pain or symptoms during the test, the following day Matt experienced significant swelling and discomfort in the knee. How would you modify his program at this point?

• Reexamine the knee for signs of instability or possible meniscal pathology
• Apply modalities to reduce effusion and pain

- Notify physician and/or refer to physician if any suspicion of reinjury
- ROM and light strengthening as indicated if no signs of significant reinjury to prevent loss of ROM and strength
- As symptoms subside, gradually progress him back to the appropriate rehabilitation stage based on the Return to Sport algorithm

3 Julie is a 36-year-old woman with a grade II ankle sprain who plays recreational volleyball. She has had several sprains in the past, but this was her worst. Her walking boot was discontinued several weeks ago and she is progressing well with her rehabilitation. Although Julie's physician released her to return to volleyball, she still has mild swelling and slight pain with some of the light plyometric exercises. Should she be allowed to return to play?

Julie did not return to play at that time for the following reasons:
- She had pain with even light plyometric and agility drills
- She demonstrated 4/5 ankle evertor strength
- She had balance deficits on the Star Excursion Balance test
- Julie is a recreational player and not under any pressure to return

4 Andy has completed a rehabilitation program following a grade II hamstring strain. He returned to tennis but reinjured the hamstring after only 3 weeks. He had no complaints of pain with jogging, cutting, or jumping. He demonstrated 5/5 strength with manual muscle testing. What factors could have lead to his reinjury?

It has been reported that nearly one third of hamstring strain injuries will recur within the first year after return to sport. This high recurrence rate suggests inadequate rehabilitation, premature return to sport, or a combination of both. Heiderscheit and associates[50] proposed

recommendations for diagnosis, rehabilitation progression, and injury prevention. Factors that may contribute to reinjury may include persistent weakness, decreased extensibility of the musculotendinous unit, and/or compensatory changes in biomechanics and motor patterns following injury. Proper diagnosis through examination, appropriate phase progression, and use of the best available evidence to determine return to sport may be beneficial in reducing recurrence rates. Therapeutic exercises that strengthen and promote neuromuscular control of the lower extremity and lumbo-pelvic musculature should be key components of the program. Manual therapy techniques to restore mobility should be included as indicated.[50]

Strength testing to assist with determining return to play should be performed prone with the knee at both 90° and 15° of flexion. The athlete should be able to perform four pain-free maximal effort contractions. Isokinetic testing would be more optimal if available and should demonstrate a less than 5% deficit in the ratio of eccentric hamstring to concentric quadriceps strength.[50]

5 Matt is now 7-months postoperation for an ACL/meniscal repair. What testing criteria might you use to determine if he is ready to return to basketball?

The choice of testing depends on the physician and/or clinician's preference, as well as the specific sport demands of the patient. The following are examples of commonly used criteria:
- No complaints of pain
- No giving way/sensation of instability
- No effusion
- Full and pain-free ROM
- Strength deficit of 10% or less compared with uninvolved side
- Establish proper muscle balance ratios
- Functional test score of 10% or less deficit compared with uninvolved side. Must demonstrate good technique and control (see Box 33-7).

REFERENCES

1. Kraus JF, Conroy C: Mortality and morbidity from injuries in sport and recreation. Annu Rev Public Health 5:163-192, 1984.
2. Murphy DF, Connolly DA, Beynnon BD: Risk factors for lower extremity injury: A review of the literature. Br J Sports Med 37:13-29, 2003.
3. Hootman JM, Dick MA, Angel J: Epidemiology of collegiate injuries for 15 sports: Summary and recommendations for injury prevention and initiatives. J Athl Train 42(2):311-319, 2007
4. Bahr R, Holme I: Risk factors for sports injuries: A methodological approach. Br J Sports Med 37(5):384-392, 2003.
5. Delay BS, Smolinski RJ, Wind WM, et al: Current practices and opinions in ACL reconstruction and rehabilitation: Results of a survey of the American Orthopedic Society for Sports Medicine. Am J Knee Surg 14(2):85-91, 2001.
6. Cissick J: You need a needs analysis, http://www.coachr.org, accessed July 8, 2010.
7. Croner C: Stretching out. J Biomech 10:1-8, 2004.
8. Shrier I: Stretching out before exercise does not reduce the risk of local muscle injury: A critical review of the clinical and basic science literature. Clin J Sports Med 9:221-227, 1999.
9. Fowles JR, Sale DG, MacDougall JD: Reduced strength after passive stretch of the human plantar flexors. J Appl Physiol 89:1179-1188, 2000.
10. Cornwell AG, et al: Acute effects of passive muscle stretching on vertical jump performance. J Hum Mov Stud 40:307-324, 2000
11. Stein A: Warming up: The dynamic alternative to static stretching, http://www.pponline.co.uk/encyc/warming-up-the-dynamic-alternative-to-static-stretching-1051, accessed July 8, 2010.

12. Shelbourne KD, Whitaker HJ, McCarroll JR: Anterior cruciate ligament injury: Evaluation intraarticular reconstruction of acute tears without repair—Two to seven year follow-up of one hundred and fifty five athletes. Am J Sports Med 18:484-493, 1990.

13. DeCarlo M, Klootwyk TE, Shelbourne KD: ACL surgery and accelerated rehabilitation: Revisited. J Sport Rehabil 6:144-156, 1997.

14. Mangine RE, Kremchek TE: Evaluation-based protocol of the anterior cruciate ligament. J Sport Rehabil 6:157-181, 1997.

15. Ross MD, Denegar CR, Winzenried JA: Implementation of open and closed kinetic chain quadriceps strengthening exercises after anterior cruciate ligament reconstruction. J Strength Cond Res 15(4):466-473, 2001.

16. Beynnon BD, et al: The strain of the anterior cruciate ligament squatting and active flexion-extension: A comparison of an open and closed kinetic chain exercise. Am J Sports Med 25:823-829, 1997.

17. Steinkamp LA, et al: Biomechanical considerations patellofemoral joint rehabilitation. Am J Sports Med 21:438-444, 1993.

18. Heiderscheidt B: Lower extremity injuries: Is it just about hip strength? J Orthop Sports Phys Ther 40(3):39-41, 2010

19. Kutz MR: Theoretical and practical issues for plyometric training. NSCA Perform Train J 2(2):10-12, 2002.

20. Chu DA: Jumping in to plyometrics. Champaign, Ill, 1998, Human Kinetics.

21. Allerheiligen WB: Speed development and plyometric training. In Baechle TR, editor: The essentials of strength training and conditioning, Champaign, Ill, 1994, Human Kinetics.

22. Brown LE, Ferrigno VA, Santana JC: Training for speed, agility, and quickness. Champaign, Ill, 2000, Human Kinetics.

23. Nutting M: Practical progressions for upper body plyometric training. NSCA Perform Train J 3(2):14-19, 2004.

24. Cissik JM: Plyometric fundamentals. NSCA Perform Train J 3(2):9-13, 2004.

25. Boyle M: Functional training for sports. Champaign, Ill, 2004, Human Kinetics.

26. Radcliffe JC, Farentinos RC: High-powered plyometrics, Champaign, Ill, 1999, Human Kinetics.

27. Williams GN, et al: Dynamic knee stability: Current theory and implications for clinicians and scientists. J Orthop Sports Phys Ther 31(10):546-566, 2001.

28. Caraffa A, et al: Prevention of anterior cruciate ligament injuries in soccer: A prospective controlled study of proprioceptive training. Knee Surg Sports Traumatol Arthrosc 4:19-21, 1996.

29. Hewett TE, et al: The effect of neuromuscular training on the incidence of knee injury in female athletes: A prospective study. Am J Sports Med 27:699-706, 1999.

30. Hewett TE, et al: Plyometric training in female athletes: Decreased impact forces and increased hamstring torques. Am J Sports Med 24:765-773, 1996.

31. Risberg MA, et al: Design and implementation of a neuromuscular training program following anterior cruciate ligament reconstruction. J Orthop Phys Ther 31(11):620-631, 2001.

32. Fitzgerald GK, Axe MJ, Snyder-Mackler L: The efficacy of perturbation training in nonoperative anterior cruciate ligament rehabilitation programs for physically active individuals, Phys Ther 80:128-140, 2000.

33. Myer GD, et al: Neuromuscular training techniques to target deficits before return to sport after anterior cruciate ligament reconstruction, J Strength Conditioning Res 22(3):987-1014, 2008

34. Barber SD, et al: Quantitative assessment of functional limitations in normal and anterior cruciate ligament-deficient knees, Clin Orthop 255:204-214, 1990.

35. Fitzgerald GK, et al: A decision-making scheme for returning patients to high-level activity with nonoperative treatment after anterior cruciate ligament rupture. Knee Surg Sports Traumatol Arthrosc 8:76-82, 2000.

36. Juris PM, et al: A dynamic test of lower extremity function following anterior cruciate ligament reconstruction and rehabilitation. J Orthop Sports Phys Ther 26:184-191, 1997.

37. Noyes FR, et al: Abnormal lower limb symmetry determined by function hop tests after anterior cruciate ligament rupture. Am J Sports Med 19:513-518, 1991.

38. Wilk, KE, et al: The relationship between subjective knee scores, isokinetic testing, and functional testing in the ACL-reconstructed knee. J Orthop Sports Phys Ther 20:60-73, 1994.

39. Fitzgerald, GK, et al: Hop test as predictors of dynamic knee, stability. J Orthop Sports Phys Ther 31(10):588-597, 2001.

40. Bandy WD, Rusche KR, Tekulve FY: Reliability and symmetry for five unilateral functional tests of the lower extremity. Isokinet Exerc Sci 4:108-111, 1994.

41. Bolgla LA, Keskula DR: Reliability of lower extremity functional performance tests. J Orthop Sports Phys Ther 26:138-142, 1997.

42. Brosky JA, et al: Intrarater reliability of selected clinical outcome measures following anterior cruciate ligament reconstruction. J Orthop Sports Phys Ther 29:39-48, 1999.

43. Blackburn JR, Morrissey MC: The relationship between open and closed chain strength of the lower limb and jumping performance. J Orthop Sports Phys Ther 27:430-435, 1998.

44. Petschnig R, Baron R, Albrecht M: The relationship between isokinetic quadriceps strength and hop tests for distance and one-legged vertical jump test following anterior cruciate ligament reconstruction. J Orthop Sports Phys Ther 28:23-31, 1998.

45. Tegner Y, Lysholm J: Derotation brace and knee function in patients with anterior cruciate ligament tears. Arthroscopy 4:264-267, 1985.

46. Tegner Y, et al: A performance test to monitor rehabilitation and for evaluation of anterior cruciate ligament injuries. Am J Sports Med 14:156-159, 1986.

47. Semenick DM: Testing protocols and procedures. In Baechle TR, editor: The essentials of strength training and conditioning, Champaign, Ill, 1994, Human Kinetics.

48. Davies GJ, Zillmer DA: Functional progression of exercise during rehabilitation. In Ellenbecker TS, editor: Knee ligament rehabilitation, New York, 2000, Churchill Livingstone.

49. Hewett TE, et al: Biomechanical measures of neuromuscular control and valgus loading of the knee predict anterior cruciate ligament injury risk in female athletes. Am J Sports Med 33:492-501, 2005.

50. Heiderscheit BC, et al: Hamstring strain injuries: Recommendations for diagnosis, rehabilitation, and injury prevention. J Orthop Sports Phys Ther 40(2):67-81, 2010.

CHAPTER 34

Transitioning the Patient Back to Running

*Steven L. Cole**

For many patients a return to prior activity is a measure of the success of their rehabilitation. Usually an athlete's first question is "When can I start running?" As clinicians our responsibility is to make sure that patients can return to some form of physical activity that stresses their cardiovascular system. For the purposes of this chapter, that form of exercise is running. Dr. Fries of Stanford University[1] completed a 21-year longitudinal study comparing runners against a control group, and although the study had some limitations, it found that runners tended to have decreased disability and a better survival rate than the control group.

Regardless of the injury or the surgical procedure, it is the clinician's responsibility to determine the patient's level of readiness to progress to each stage of rehabilitation. Many programs exist on how to progress patients back to running and it the goal of this chapter to provide the clinician a framework from which to develop a comprehensive program while keeping in mind the factors that led to the initiation of a return to run program. The factors to consider are age, type and extent of injury, current and prior surgical procedures, pain levels, swelling, range of motion (ROM), strength, endurance, flexibility, patient goals, and psychological readiness.[2]

Most clinicians who will be initiating a return to run program are the same ones who have been treating patients through their postoperative rehabilitation. However, it is imperative in cases in which the patient is seen for the first time to initiate a running program and to communicate with the sports medicine team physician (surgeon, team: physician), physical therapist, certified athletic trainer, and so forth.

ASSESSMENT

Knowledge of the patient's prior physical status and progression through his or her postoperative rehabilitation course is important in setting achievable goals. The patient's overall physical condition level must be assessed: aerobic capacity (usually submaximal on bike), flexibility (ROM), strength (of the whole body not just the injured body part), balance, and coordination. A thorough gait analysis is also performed to assess any biomechanical deficiencies. Shoe wear should be assessed by a qualified professional and the patient's shoes should be properly fit before this program is initiated.

FLEXIBILITY, STRENGTH, AND BALANCE/COORDINATION

In the running motion the clinician must consider all the joints that are directly involved once the foot hits the ground and transitions that force up the kinetic chain. While acknowledging that the upper quarter (cervical spine, thoracic spine, and upper extremities) also play an important role in the running motion, for the purposes of this chapter we will focus on the lumbar spine down to the foot. After a period of immobilization from surgery, the patient needs to reestablish normal ROM and efficient flexibility in the hip, knee, and ankle regions. The following major muscle groups should be assessed: lumbar paraspinals, latissimus dorsi, multifidus, gluteals, piriformis, hip flexors/adductors, hamstrings, iliotibial band, hip rotators, quadriceps (especially rectus femoris), gastrocnemius, and soles complex.

AMBULATION

The patient needs to reestablish a normal gait pattern before starting an aggressive closed-chain exercise program. In most cases, gait training should have been completed during the patient's postoperative rehabilitation. As a rule, if the patient cannot walk without a limp, he or she should be using crutches and/or a shortened stride length. If ambulation results in increased swelling, the patient should be using crutches and is not ready to progress until he or she can ambulate without deviations.

The tests in the following paragraphs are used to assess the ability of the lower extremity to provide a stable base during static and dynamic postures. The patient must successfully complete these tests before progressing.

*Special Acknowledgement: Assistance with the Core Stability section provided by Kristina Carter, DPT, Advanced Specialty Center, Williamsburg Physical Therapy, Williamsburg, Va.

Baseline Balance Test

Have patient can stand on both feet with equal distribution, free standing, with his or her eyes closed, and maintain balance for 20 seconds.

Tandem Stance

Have patient stand heel to toe with his or her nondominant foot in back, weight evenly distributed on both feet, with his or her hands on the hips and eyes closed. Count the number of times he or she moves out of that position in a 20-second period. To progress, the patient should have no more than 4 errors (such as lifting the hands off the hips, opening eyes, lifting the forefoot or heel, step, stumbling, or falling).

Balance Progression

- Have the patient stand on both feet with equal weight distribution. Start with assisted balance with hands on the edge of a table, eyes open, and progress to free standing away from table and then with eyes closed.
- Have the patient stand on both feet, dominant foot in front of the other, heel to toes, with equal weight distribution. Start with assisted balance with hands on the edge of a table, eyes open, and progress to free standing away from table and then with eyes closed.
- Have the patient stand on the involved leg. Start with assisted balance with hands on the edge of a table, eyes open, and progress to free standing away from table and then with eyes closed.
- Have the patient stand on the involved leg approximately 24 inches from a wall, throw a tennis ball against the wall, and catch it. Progress to place four marks on the wall—two at a level approximately 12 inches above head level and 12 inches beyond shoulder width; the other two should be at waist level and 12 inches beyond hip width. Throughout the exercise, alternate the mark at which to throw the ball.

Time each attempt at each level; as balance improves and the patient is able to maintain a stable position, progress to the next level.

STRENGTH/ENDURANCE

Strength of the trunk/core and the entire lower extremity should be assessed. The assessment should encompass not only isometric testing but also concentric and eccentric, since all are important to the acceleration and deceleration involved in the running motion. The patient must have the ability to maintain active control of spinal and pelvic posture during dynamic loading and movement. During running, good core strength will allow the patient to appropriately distribute force, allow for efficient and controlled movement, absorb ground impact forces, and decrease compression forces. The patient will need good core strength and balance before progressing into an aggressive return to running program.

Core Stability

Testing core stability forces the patient to move and control motion in multiple planes: sagittal, frontal, transverse, and multiplanar. It is essential to stabilize the proximal segment (in this case, trunk and pelvis) to allow efficient distal mobility.[3-5] The following are simple tests for core stability that are easy to administer and can be measured both qualitatively and quantitatively.

Sagittal plane tests motion in a forward/backward or anteroposterior direction—stability here helps the runner move the body forward or slow down when stopping or descending a hill.

Bridge—Sagittal Plane:

Instructions:

- Lie on your back with knees bent
- Tighten abdominal and gluteal muscles
- Slowly raise buttock from the table
- Attempt to hold for 30 seconds

Bridge with Good Stability (Fig. 34-1):

- Hips remain level (Fig. 34-1, *A*)
- Lower extremities remain in proper alignment (Fig. 34-1, *A*)

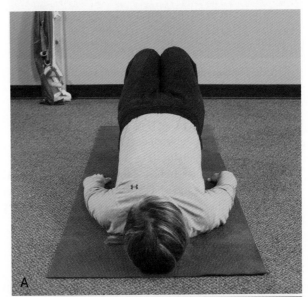

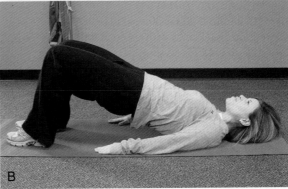

Fig. 34-1 Bridge with good stability. **A,** Hips remain level, and lower extremities remain in proper alignment. **B,** Back does not arch or sag.

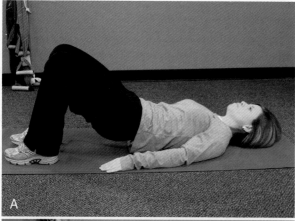

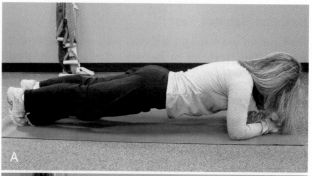

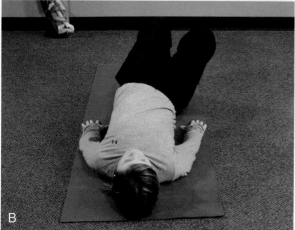

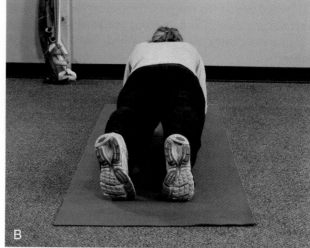

Fig. 34-2 Bridge with poor stability. **A,** Side view. **B,** Top view.

Fig. 34-3 Prone bridge with good stability. **A,** Back does not arch or sag. **B,** Hips are level.

- Back does not arch/sag (Fig. 34-1, *B*)
- Able to hold for 30 seconds

Bridge with Poor Stability (Fig. 34-2):
- Back sags, and she wobbles with wobbling (Fig. 34-2, *A*)
- Hips not level (and she's cheating by squeezing her knees together to use her adductors as a compensatory movement) (Fig. 34-2, *B*)

Prone Bridge—Sagittal Plane:
Instructions:
- Begin lying on stomach
- Tighten abdominals and gluteals while propped on forearms and balls of feet
- Attempt to hold for 30 seconds

Prone Bridge (Plank) with Good Stability (Fig. 34-3):
- Able to hold for 30 seconds
- Back does not arch/sag (Fig. 34-3, *A*)
- Hip level (Fig. 34-3, *B*)

Prone Bridge with Poor Stability (Fig. 34-4):
- Back sags (Fig. 34-4, *A*)
- Hips not level (Fig. 34-4, *B*)

Frontal plan stability and transverse plane stability help to keep the runner moving forward—weakness here makes the movement inefficient; there is wasted energy with side to side or rotational motion.

Side Bridge (Plank)—Frontal Plane:
Instructions:
- Begin on one side (test both sides)
- Prop on forearm and the foot that is in contact with the table
- Tighten abdominals
- Attempt to hold for 30 seconds

Side Bridge with Good Stability (Fig. 34-5):
- Able to hold for 30 seconds
- Hip that is facing downward does not sag (Fig. 34-5, *A*)
- Shoulders and feet remain in alignment (Fig. 34-5, *B*)

Side Bridge with Poor Stability (Fig. 34-6):
- Cannot keep shoulders and feet alignment or maintain balance (Fig. 34-6, *A*)
- Hips sag (Fig. 34-6, *B*)

Bridge with Knee Extension—Transverse Plane (Fig. 34-7):
Instructions:
- Lie on back with both knees bent
- Contract abdominal and gluteal muscles
- Slowly raise bottom from the table
- Extend one knee while remaining in the bridge position
- Attempt to hold for 10 seconds on each side

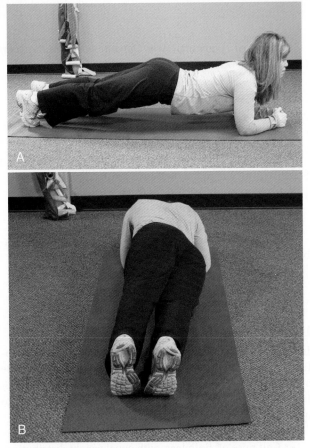

Fig. 34-4 Prone bridge with poor stability. **A,** Back sags. **B,** Hips are not level.

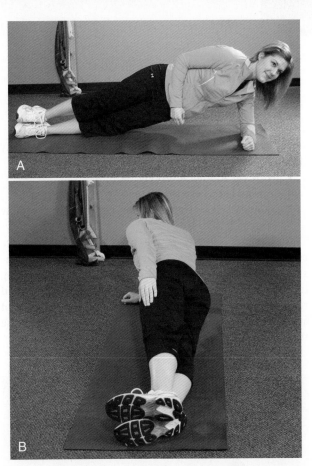

Fig. 34-6 Side bridge with poor stability. **A,** Shoulders and feet are not aligned, and balance is not maintained. **B,** Hips sag.

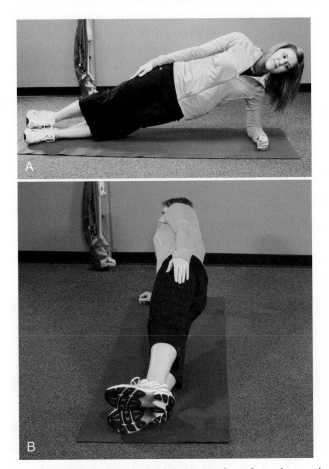

Fig. 34-5 Side bridge with good stability. **A,** Hip that is facing downward does not sag. **B,** Shoulders and feet remain in alignment.

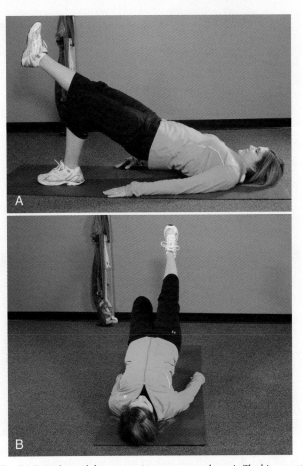

Fig. 34-7 Bridge with knee extension: transverse plane. **A,** The hips are at a high level, and there his no movement or hip sag. The extended leg is parallel with the opposite leg. **B,** The hips are level.

Bridge with Knee Extension with Good Stability:
- Able to hold for 10 seconds on each side
- Hips remain level
- Knee remains straight
- Back remains flat against the table

Bridge with Knee Extension with Poor Stability (Fig. 34-8):
- Hips sag and not level (Fig. 34-8, *A*)
- Cannot keep knee straight
- Shoulders and back are not flat against the table (Fig. 34-8, *B*)

Multiplanar stability is the most functional, because running is a dynamic movement of the body in three dimensions simultaneously with one side of the body working independently of the other, all the while controlling ground reaction forces and delivering propulsion forces. Lack of adequate multiplanar stability has been shown to increase the risk of lower extremity injuries.[6]

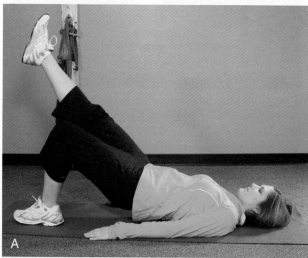

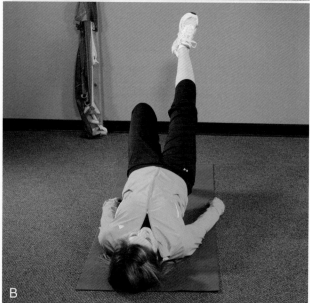

Fig. 34-8 Bridge with knee extension with poor stability. **A,** Hips sag and are not level. **B,** Shoulders and back are not flat against the floor.

Quadruped Opposite Arm/Opposite Leg—Multiplanar (Fig. 34-9):

Instructions:
- Begin on hands and knees
- Tighten abdominals
- Slowly extend one arm and the opposite leg
- Attempt to hold for 10 seconds

Quadruped Opposite Arm/Opposite Leg with Good Stability:
- Able to hold for 10 seconds on each side
- Back does not arch/sag
- Arm and leg do not drop downward

Quadruped Opposite Arm/Opposite Leg with Poor Stability (Fig. 34-10):
- Hips sag and not level (Figure 34-10, *A*)
- Arm and leg drop (Fig. 34-10, *B* and *C*)
- Cannot maintain balance

Lower Extremity Stability

In preparation to return to running, it is important to establish a strong initial contact base (gastroc-soleus). This can be accomplished progressively through closed-chain exercises focusing on technique and quality with progression into quantity.

Calf Raise Progression into Single-Leg Hop:
- Calf raise off both legs, with equal weight distribution; start with assistance with hands on the edge of a table; progress to free standing away from table.
- Calf raise on the uninvolved leg, maintaining a balanced, stable position (10 to 25 reps). This will serve as the "norm" for the involved side.
- Calf raise on the involved leg; start with assisted with hands on the edge of a table, progress to free standing away from table. The movement should be of the same quality (height, speed, and control of movement) as that of the uninvolved leg.
- Hop off both legs, with equal weight distribution.
- Hop off the uninvolved leg multiple times (10 to 25 reps). This will serve as the "norm" for the involved side.
- Hop off the involved leg. The movement should be of the same quality (height, speed, and control of movement) as that of the uninvolved leg.

The emphasis should be on the quality of the movement and high repetition. Points of emphasis on quality are the

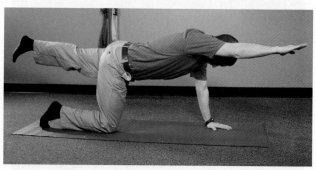

Fig. 34-9 Quadruped opposite arm/opposite leg: multiplanar.

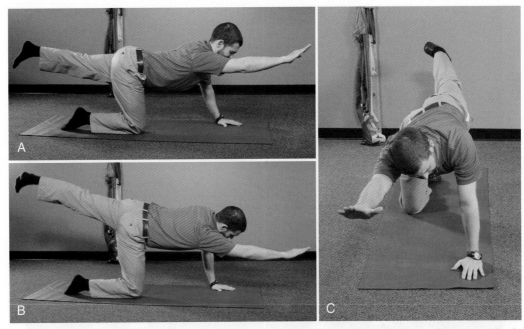

Fig. 34-10 Quadruped opposite arm/opposite leg with poor stability. **A,** Hips sag and are not level. **B** and **C,** Arm and leg drop.

height of the movement, rapid raise, slow controlled descent and landing, and maintaining balance. Repetitions should start with 5 and progress to 25.

Single-Leg Squat Test—Multiplanar (Fig. 34-11):

Instructions:

- Stand with one foot on a stool, keep foot flat on stool during descent
- Keep lower leg perpendicular to the floor and knee behind and within toes
- Slowly lower the other foot toward the ground
- Perform this five times on each side

Single-Leg Squat Test with Good Stability:

- Able to complete five repetitions with good form
- Knee remains in line with the second toe
- Hip does not internally rotate
- Patient does not lose balance

Single-Leg Squat Test with Poor Stability (Fig. 34-12):

- Top left—too much adduction—weak glutes (Fig. 34-12, *A*)
- Top right—knee wobble—weak quads or weak glutes
- Bottom—hip drop (Fig. 34-12, *C*)

Useful objective measurement tools for assessing a patient's ability for force absorption and force production with a lower extremity injury are the leap test and the hop and stop test (Fig. 34-13).[7] Before attempting either test, the patient must have established normal ambulation, progressed through the calf raise progression, and phase I (walking program) and progressed through phase II (plyometric program) of the return to running progression.

PAIN MANAGEMENT

It is important to have a consistent, objective way of grading the patient's pain level. Try grading the level of pain the patient has over a period of several days to weeks. Is the pain

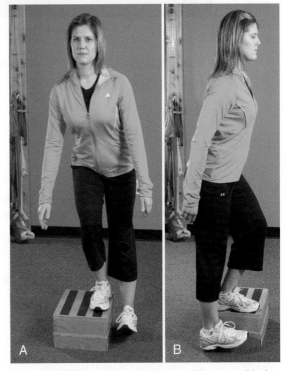

Fig. 34-11 Single-leg squat test: multiplanar. **A,** There is good body stabilization. The knee is over the toes on descent. The foot on the step is pointed straight ahead. The shoulders are level. **B,** The back is straight, and the knee does not extend past the toes.

getting worse, staying the same, or gradually dissipating? Use a pain scale of 0 to 10, in which 0 is normal and 10 is the worst.[8]

- Getting worse: need total rest; decrease to previous activity level and decrease intensity of exercise.
- Staying the same: decrease activity level to previous level and maintain until pain decreases.

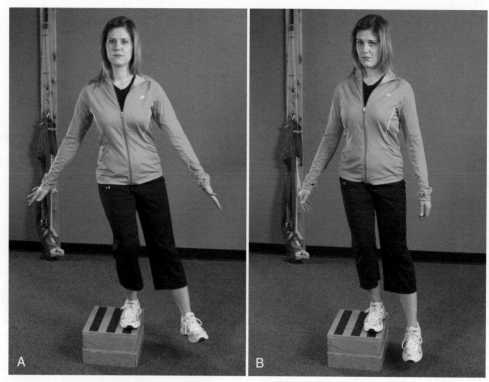

Fig. 34-12 Single-leg squat test with poor stability. **A,** Top left. **B,** Bottom.

Leap Test (Takeoff on uninvolved leg and land on the involved leg; stick the landing)

Leap Test:

1: _____ Inches

2: _____ Inches

3: _____ Inches

Divide distance of involved leap test by distance of involved hop test for percentage: _____%

Goal: Distance of involved leap test should be less than 109% of the involved hop test; less than 109% indicates that the patient needs to work on force absorption for the involved leg.

Developed by: Paul Juris, PhD

A

Hop and Stop Test (Takeoff and land on same leg, stick the landing)

Hop Test:	Uninvolved	Involved
1:	_____ Inches	_____ Inches
2:	_____ Inches	_____ Inches
3:	_____ Inches	_____ Inches

Patient's Height: _____ (inches)

Divide distance of uninvolved hop by patient's height for percentage: _____%

Divide distance of involved hop by distance of uninvolved hop for percentage: _____%

Divide distance of involved hop by patient's height for percentage: _____%

Goal: Distance of uninvolved hop test should equal the patient's height; a score of less than 89% indicates that the patient needs to work on force production for the uninvolved leg. A score of less than 89% indicates that the patient needs to work on force production for the involved leg.

Developed by: Paul Juris, PhD

B

Fig. 34-13 **A,** Leap test. **B,** Hop and stop test.

For the successful progression of the return to running program, it is critical to understand the level, location, and nature of discomfort that may develop as the patient increases the activity level. In general the patient should apply moist heat before the activity and stretch thoroughly, then ice immediately after the activity for 15 to 20 minutes. **If the patient develops swelling in a joint or muscular pain that lasts longer than 72 hours, he or she has done too much and needs to decrease activity (duration and/or intensity) and increase rest between workouts.** Consultation with the physician should occur immediately if there is pain with weight bearing or antalgic persists.

Here are some useful tips: If the patient develops tightness during activity, he or she should stop and perform a static stretch (at least 3 repetitions, hold each for a 30 count each) of the affected area, then resume activity. If tightness returns, the patient should stop and stretch the affected area again. If pain develops or after three stretching sessions and the tightness remains, the patient needs to stop the activity and apply ice to the involved area for 20 minutes.

It is important for the patient to identify the exact location of the pain and to differentiate if the pain is in a constant location or if it "moves around" in a general area.

- Constant location: **be very cautious, incorporate more rest between exercise sessions, and keep the intensity low and exercise on level, soft surfaces**.
- "Moves around": **continue with progression but do not increase the intensity.**

It is important for patients to identify when they have pain:

- **Type I:** After activity. Plan: stretch affected area well (at least 3 to 5 repetitions, hold each for at least a 30 count); do long, slow, gentle stretches, then ice for 20 minutes. Continue to progress program if discomfort appears to be muscle soreness. **If any joint pain and/or swelling develops, increase rest between exercise sessions and decrease activity level to previous level. Consult physician.**
- **Type II:** During activity (muscular), or at beginning then dissipates. Plan: maintain same activity level and low intensity until symptoms dissipate.
- **Type III:** During activity (muscular), gradually developing and intensifying with activity. Plan: decrease intensity of activity, stop and stretch to relieve symptoms; stop activity if these steps do not relieve symptoms. Maintain same activity level; if symptoms continue, decrease activity to previous level.
- **Type IVa:** Upon waking in the morning then dissipat, which is usually a sign of more to come. Plan: decrease activity to previous level and keep intensity low.
- **Type IVb:** At night, keeps patient up or wakes patient. **This is a warning sign that the patient is doing too much or that the muscle/joint is not tolerating the amount of work.** Plan: total rest until symptom free; decrease activity to previous level and keep intensity low.

RETURN TO RUNNING PROGRAM

Phase I: Walking Program

To progress to phase II (plyometric routine), the patient must be able to walk pain-free, aggressively (roughly 4.2 to 5.2 miles per hour), and preferably on a level treadmill, for 30 minutes before beginning the plyometric and walk/jog program. The patient must be pain-free, without residual swelling or loss of strength/ROM on the following day, especially upon waking.

Start each session with an easy warm up for at least 5 minutes. During the warm up, the patient should be able to maintain normal, comfortable stride mechanics and maintain a conversation. After the initial 2 minutes, the patient should increase the speed by 0.5 mph every 30 seconds for the remaining 3 minutes of the warm up.

End each session with an easy cool down for at least 5 minutes. During cool down, the patient should be able to maintain normal, comfortable stride mechanics and maintain a conversation. Decrease the speed by 0.5 mph every 30 seconds for the 5 minutes of the cool down period.

If the patient experiences pain or is unable to complete an exercise, stop, stretch, and apply ice to the involved area. If the patient is pain-free the next day, attempt to restart the routine.

Progression

Complete a walking session (5 minute warm up, 30 minutes of aggressive walking, 5 minute cool down) for 2 consecutive days; take a day off, complete 2 more consecutive days. If pain-free, without residual swelling or loss of strength/ROM, progress to phase II after a day off.

Goal

The patient should be able to walk, pain-free, aggressively (roughly 4.2 to 5.2 mph), preferably on a level treadmill, for 30 minutes. He or she should be able to aggressively walk at a pace and stride mechanics just below the threshold where he or she would be jogging. During an aggressive walk, the patient maintains a heel/toe gait pattern without a flight segment (maintains contact with the surface with both feet).

Phase II: Plyometric Routine

Plyometric exercises are essential to include in a return to a running program. Plyometrics works on the stretch-shortening cycle of the running motion to improve running efficiency and performance.[9] To progress to the phase III walk/jog progression, the patient should complete the entire cycle within the time intervals without residual swelling, loss of strength or ROM, and pain. The patient must be pain-free the following day, especially on waking.

Rationalization

A mile run generally consists of 1500 foot contacts, 750 per foot. The program integrates 470 foot contacts per leg, which would be equivalent to two thirds the foot contacts of a mile.

TABLE 34-1 Closed-Chain Progression

Exercise	Sets	Foot Contacts/Set	Total Foot Contact
Step 1: Two-leg ankle hops: in place	3	30	90
Step 2: Two-leg ankle hops: forward/backward	3	30	90
Step 3: Two-leg ankle hops: side to side	3	30	90
Step 4: One-leg ankle hops: in place	3	20	60
Step 5: One-leg ankle hops: forward/backward	3	20	60
Step 6: One-leg ankle hops: side to side	3	20	60
Step 7: One-leg broad hop	4	5	20

22 sets for a total of 470 total foot contacts.
Note: The "one-leg" activities are performed on the involved extremity.
Rest intervals: Between sets, 90 seconds; between exercises, 3 minutes.

Successfully completing the routine (Table 34-1) is a good indicator of a patient returning to running a half to three quarters of a mile distance.

I prefer that the exercises be performed on a "forgiving" surface, such as a rubber mat. Gastrocnemius-soleus, quadriceps, and hamstrings should be stretched between exercises. Clinicians should stress quality of the movement, emphasizing toe-heel landing, triple flexion (hip and knee flexion, ankle dorsiflexion), triple extension (hip and knee extension, plantar flexion), and soft landing. Patients recovering from a knee, thigh, or hip injury should incorporate a greater degree of knee and hip flexion.

If the patient develops persistent tightness or increased discomfort during the exercise session, he or she should stop and note the foot count for the activity upon the onset of symptoms, such as if pain developed on repetition 21 of the third set in step 3, which is foot contact no. 261. This will provide a measurement of progress for future attempts.

If the patient experiences pain or is unable to complete an exercise, he or she should stop, stretch, and apply ice to the involved area. If pain free the next day, he or she should attempt to restart the routine.

Phase III: Walk/Jog Progression (Table 34-2)

The patient may begin this program on level ground if he or she:

1. The patient completed phases I and II
2. The patient has no pain or swelling with normal daily activities (on a pain scale of 0 to 10, in which 0 is normal and 10 is the worst, he or she must be at 0)
3. The injured area no longer hurts when pressed on

Program Progression

- If jogging hurts, the patient should stop, apply ice, and return to the previous stage the next day if there is no

TABLE 34-2 Walk/Jog Progression

Stage	Walk	Jog	Repetitions	Total Time
Stage I	5 minutes	1 minute	5 times	30 minutes
Stage II	4 minutes	2 minutes	5 times	30 minutes
Stage III	3 minutes	3 minutes	5 times	30 minutes
Stage IV	2 minutes	4 minutes	5 times	30 minutes
Stage V	1 minute	5 minutes	5 times	30 minutes
Stage VI	Jog every other day with a goal of reaching 30 consecutive minutes. Begin with 5 minutes of walking, gradually increasing the pace. End with 5 minutes of walking, gradually decreasing the pace to a comfortable walk.			

residual swelling, or loss of strength or ROM, and pain, especially on waking. If pain/discomfort remains or increases, the patient should continue to return to a previous level until discomfort stabilizes or decreases.

- If there is no pain when doing this activity level or afterward and there is no discomfort or tightness that limits normal movements the next morning, the patient should proceed to the next stage.
- The patient should not attempt more than two stages on consecutive days; he or she should take a day off before progressing to next the stage.

Phase IV: Timed Running Schedule

During this phase, the duration of the running program progresses. The patient should try to jog/run on a flat, forgiving surface (i.e., golf course, athletic field) before hilly courses or even surfaces and follow the Ten Percent Rule[10]: only increase the weekly mileage by 10% of the previous week. If no pain is experienced when doing an activity level or afterward and there is no discomfort or tightness that limits normal movements the next morning, he or she can proceed to the next stage.

The intensity (how hard/fast) of the jog/run is increased before the duration (how long). When the patient increases the frequency (how many days per week) of the jog/run workouts, the clinician should also have them decrease the duration of the workout. When the patient begins running multiple days in a row, increases (duration or intensity) are made on the first day of activity after a day of rest, the duration of activity is decreased to the previous level.

If the patient develops persistent tightness or increased discomfort to a point of dysfunction (develops a limp or altered gait pattern) during the activity, he or she should stop and note the time of onset of symptoms (during a 30-minute planned exercise session, symptoms develop after 21 minutes). Consider splitting the duration of activity between two workouts, with each exercise session shorter than the time of the onset of symptoms during the previous attempt. For example, if during a 30-minute planned exercise session, symptoms develop after 24 minutes, each of the two exercise sessions would be 20 minutes long. The exercise sessions should be separated by 6 to 8 hours. The clinician should refer to the section on Pain Management in this chapter if the patient begins to develop pain/swelling and remember: **If pain/discomfort remains or increases, continue to return to a previous level until discomfort stabilizes or decreases.**

Phase IV: Timed Running Schedule—Intermediate (Table 34-3)

The patient may begin this program on level ground if they have completed phases I, II, and III.

The intermediate schedule is designed for the patient restarting running training or recovering from an injury, such as a stress fracture or significant illness that has kept them "off their feet" or on non–weight bearing activities for 4 weeks or longer. To allow for soft tissue adaptation, the patient should run every other day for 8 weeks. He or she should cross-train or be on active or total rest on days off. The patient's pace should be 8 to 9 minutes per mile.

Phase IV: Timed Running Schedule—Advanced (Table 34-4)

The advanced schedule is designed for the patient/runner who is recovering from a soft tissue injury, such as a strained muscle, which has forced him or her to cross-train for less than 4 weeks. The patient may begin this program on level ground if he or she has completed phases I, II, and III. To allow for soft tissue adaptation, the patient runs every other day for 8 weeks. He or she should cross-train or be on active or total rest on days off. The patient's pace should be 7.5 to 8 minutes per mile.

Mileage Schedule

To allow for soft tissue adaptation. The patient should run every other day for 2 weeks, then a maximum of 5 days a week for the next 4 weeks. If the patient/runner's previous level of training was less than 4 miles per session, the patient should follow the mileage schedule indicated in Tables 34-5 through 34-7.

TABLE 34-3 Timed Running Schedule—Intermediate

| | Day | | | | | | | |
	1	2	3	4	5	6	7	Week
Minutes	30	—	30	—	30	—	35	1
	—	30	—	30	—	35	—	2
	35	—	30	—	35	—	35	3
	—	35	—	40	—	35	—	4
	35	—	40	—	40	—	35	5
	—	40	—	40	—	40	—	6
	45	—	40	—	40	—	45	7
	—	45	—	40	—	45	30	8*
	—	45	35	—	45	40	—	9
	45	45	—	45	45	30	—	10
	45	45	35	—	45	45	40	11
	—	45	45	45	—	45	45	12

*Run multiple days in a row after 8 weeks.

FUTURE CONSIDERATIONS

Currently there is a lot of interest in the mechanics of running and the use (or nonuse) of running shoes. Of consideration is foot contact while running. Some authors have found a reduced rate of injury in barefoot runners whose initial

TABLE 34-4 Timed Running Schedule—Advanced

| | Day | | | | | | | |
	1	2	3	4	5	6	7	Week
Minutes	30	—	30	30	—	35	30	1
	—	35	35	—	40	35	—	2
	40	40	—	45	40	—	45	3
	45	—	45	40	30	—	45	4
	40	35	—	45	40	40	—	5
	45	45	40	—	45	45	45	6*
	45	—	50	50	45	—	50	8
	50	50	—	55	50	50	—	9
	55	55	50	—	55	55	55	10
	—	60	55	55	—	60	60	11
	55	—	60	60	60	—	65	12

*This activity level at 6 weeks is the same as the activity level at 12 weeks with the intermediate program and uses a higher intensity (faster running pace).

TABLE 34-5 Mileage Table for Runners Below 4 Miles Per Session

| | Day | | | | | | | |
	1	2	3	4	5	6	7	Week
Miles	½	—	½	—	½	—	1	1
	—	1	—	1	—	2	—	2
	2	1	—	2	2	—	3	3
	2	—	3	3	—	4	3	4
	—	4	4	—	4	4	—	5

TABLE 34-6 Mileage Table for Runners Between 4 and 6 Miles Per Session

| | Day | | | | | | | |
	1	2	3	4	5	6	7	Week
Miles	1	—	1	—	1	—	2	1
	—	2	—	2	—	3	—	2
	3	2	—	3	3	—	4	3
	3	—	4	4	—	5	4	4
	—	5	5	—	6	5	—	5

Note: Return to previous preinjury mileage level in 4-6 weeks.

TABLE 34-7 Mileage Table for Runners Between 40 and 60 Miles Per Week

				Day				
	1	2	3	4	5	6	7	Week
Miles	2	—	2	—	2	—	3	1
	—	3	—	3	—	4	—	2
	4	3	—	4	4	—	5	3
	4	—	5	5	—	6	5	4
	—	6	6	—	7	6	6	5

Note: Return to preinjury mileage level in 4-6 weeks.

contact is on the forefoot instead of the heel. Mechanically, this make sense from a force distribution standpoint because the ground forces acting on the lower extremity are decelerated via eccentric dorsiflexion (using forefoot-gastrocnemius-soleus) versus heel strike, which absorbs and distributes the forces through the calcaneus-tibia and deceleration happening at the knee. There is, however, a learning curve to adapt to this type of training, which stresses the soft tissues (foot and ankle plantarflexor soreness). Although there is controversy surrounding these mechanics, it is an interesting approach and may allow patients to run with less compressive force on the skeletal system. Running shoes provide an important barrier to environmental hazards (surface irregularities, sharp objects, extreme hot/cold) and foot mechanic deviations (e.g., over pronation). Further research is needed to quantify the benefit to foot contact and the need for "running" shoes.[11,12]

SUMMARY

Many programs are available to clinicians to return their patients to running. The progression and tables in this chapter have been effective for me in successfully returning patients to running. The clinician should continually evaluate the patients' mechanics and ensure that they are performing their strength, flexibility, and balance program regularly and cross-training as appropriate. Mileage progression may vary depending on a number of factors (e.g., muscle soreness, level of fitness). Shoe wear is another factor to consider when returning to running. Assessments of show wear should be performed by qualified professional, with foot mechanics thoroughly evaluated and taken into account.

CLINICAL CASE REVIEW

1 The patient has been progressing through the return to running program and is pain free with activity. However, the morning after completing phase II (plyometric routine), the patient has tightness and pain in the Achilles tendon with the first several steps of the day. After walking around the house for a short period, the pain and tightness dissipates. What should the patient do for activity that day?

Take the day off, do gentle stretching, and ice the involved area. The following day, the patient should repeat the activity level from the previous attempt.

2 The patient presents 3 months after partial hip labrum resection and wishes to return to running activity. What factors should be considered before he or she returns to running?

He or she should be fully evaluated for adequate ROM/flexibility, strength, and balance, making sure to focus on the whole body, not just the surgical site.

3 The patient is progressing through the timed running schedule (phase IV) and is ready to start running multiple days in a row. Describe for the patient how increasing timed running periods should be approached.

Increase the timed session by 5 minutes after a day off, then decrease the timed session by 5 minutes the next day, then take a day off. When running 3 days in a row, the timed sessions are built on the front end of the sequence.

4 The patient has passed the balance baseline test. What functional activities should be considered before the patient begins a running progression?

The patient must have normal ambulation and core stability.

5 What is the importance of good core strength for a runner?

It allows for the appropriate distribution of forces, leads to the control and efficiency of movements, helps with the absorption of ground impact forces, and decreases compression forces.

6 Paul had a meniscus repair and was cleared to begin a return to running program. He has made good progress through phase I and initiated phase II, but after the second week he has delayed onset of pain and swelling in his knee. What should be considered?

On reexamination it was found that his symptoms were aggravated by tibial compression and rotation (suspicious of a tear of the repair). Edema management techniques were initiated, and he was referred back to his surgeon.

REFERENCES

1. Chakravarty EF, et al: Reduced disability and mortality among aging runners: A 21-year longitudinal study. Arch Intern Med 168(15):1638-1646, 2008.

2. Kulund DN: The injured athlete, Philadelphia, 1988, Lippincott, Williams, and Wilkins.

3. Kibler WB, Press J, Sciascia A: The role of core stability in athletic function. Sports Med 36(3):189-198, 2006.

4. Willson JD, et al: Core stability and its relationship to lower extremity function and injury. J Am Acad Orthop Surg 13(5):316-325, 2005.

5. Bliss LS, Teeple P. Core stability: The centerpiece of any training program. Curr Sports Med Rep 4(3):179-183, 2005.

6. Zazulak BT, et al. Deficits in neuromuscular control of the trunk predict knee injury risk: A prospective biomechanical-epidemiologic study. Am J Sports Med 35(7):1123-1130, 2007.

7. Munro AG, Herrington LC: Between-session reliability of four hop tests and the agility T-test. J Strength Cond Res 25(5):1470-1477, 2011.

8. 50mg of Benadryl and some morphine. Feb. 8, 2010. http://firefighter-paramedicstories.blogspot.com/2010/02/50mg-of-benadryl-and-some-morphine.html.

9. Kawamoto J-E: Go ahead and jump: Using plyometric training to improve running performance. June 25, 2010. http://running magazine.ca/2010/06/sections/health-nutrition/body-work/go-ahead-and-jump-using-plyometric-training-to-improve-running-performance/.

10. Buist I, et al: The GRONORUN study: Is a graded training program for novice runners effective in preventing running related injuries? Design of a randomized controlled trial. BMC Musculoskelet Disord 8:24, 2007.

11. Warburton M: Barefoot running. Sportscience 5(3), 2001. sportsci.org/jour/0103/mw.htm.

12. Lieberman DE, et al: Foot strike patterns and collision forces in habitually barefoot versus shod runners. Nature 463(7280):531-535, 2010.

INDEX

Page numbers followed by "f" indicate figures, "t" indicate tables, and "b" indicate boxes.

628